Cancer Prevention, Detection, and Control:

A Nursing Perspective

Editors

Kathleen Jennings-Dozier, PhD, MPH, RN, CS, and
Suzanne M. Mahon, RN, DNSc, AOCN®, APNG(c)

Oncology Nursing Society
Pittsburgh, PA

ONS Publishing Division
Publisher: Leonard Mafrica, MBA, CAE
Director, Commercial Publishing, Barbara Sigler, RN, MNEd
Technical Publications Editor: Dorothy Mayernik, RN, MSN
Senior Staff Editor: Lisa M. George
Copy Editors: Toni Murray, Lori Wilson
Creative Services Assistant: Dany Sjoen
Secretary: Amy Zahn

Cancer Prevention, Detection, and Control: A Nursing Perspective

Library of Congress Control Number: 2002106898

ISBN 1-890504-27-0

Publisher's Note

This book is published by the Oncology Nursing Society (ONS). ONS neither represents nor guarantees that the practices described herein will, if followed, ensure safe and
effective patient care. The recommendations contained in this book reflect ONS's judgment regarding the state of general knowledge and practice in the field as of the date of
publication. The recommendations may not be appropriate for use in all circumstances.
Those who use this book should make their own determinations regarding specific safe and
appropriate patient-care practices, taking into account the personnel, equipment, and
practices available at the hospital or other facility at which they are located. The editors
and publisher cannot be held responsible for any liability incurred as a consequence from
the use or application of any of the contents of this book. Figures and tables are used as
examples only. They are not meant to be all-inclusive, nor do they represent endorsement of any particular institution by ONS. Mention of specific products and opinions
related to those products do not indicate or imply endorsement by ONS.

ONS publications are originally published in English. Permission has been granted by
the ONS Board of Directors for foreign translation. (Individual tables and figures that are
reprinted or adapted require additional permission from the original source.) However,
because translations from English may not always be accurate and precise, ONS disclaims
any responsibility for inaccurate translations. Readers relying on precise information should
check the original English version.

Printed in the United States of America

Oncology Nursing Society
Integrity • Innovation • Stewardship • Advocacy • Excellence • Inclusiveness

To my husband, Darryl, and daughter, Taylor. Thank you for your unconditional love. And to Sue Holman-Audi, BSN, RN, who challenged me to be a better nurse, and who showed me how to fight cancer gracefully.

Kathleen Jennings-Dozier

To my parents, Ted and Jackie Dubuque, who encouraged me from a young age to pursue my interests.

To my husband, Jerry, who has supported me throughout my professional career.

To my three beautiful daughters, Emily, Maureen, and Elaine, who are a constant source of joy and a sign of hope for the future.

Suzanne M. Mahon

This book is dedicated to the memory of co-editor Kathleen Jennings-Dozier, who died shortly before its publication. It was her dream that this textbook be available as a reference for all of those with an interest in and need for information on issues related to cancer control.

She continued to work on the project during her difficult illness; through this book, she will continue to contribute to the advancement of nursing education on cancer prevention and detection.

"Not unto us, Oh Lord, not unto us, but unto thy name give glory, for thy mercy, and for thy truth's sake."

Psalm 115:1

Contributors

Co-Editors

Kathleen Jennings-Dozier, PhD, MPH, RN, CS
Associate Professor
College of Nursing and Health Professions
MCP Hahnemann University
Philadelphia, PA
Chapter 2 – An Epidemiological Approach to Cancer Prevention and Control

Suzanne M. Mahon, RN, DNSc, AOCN®, APNG(c)
Assistant Clinical Professor
Division of Hematology and Oncology
Saint Louis University
St. Louis, MO
Overview Section I, Overview Section II, Overview Section III, Overview Section IV, Overview Section V, Chapter 17 – Tertiary Prevention: Improving the Care of Long-Term Survivors of Cancer, Chapter 20 Vignette – Tertiary Prevention in Long-Term Survivors of Breast Cancer

Authors

Terri B. Ades, MS, APRN-BC, AOCN®
Director, Quality of Life/Health Promotion Strategies
American Cancer Society, Inc.
Atlanta, GA
Chapter 25 – Information Resources for Patients and Families

Jennifer Aikin, RN, MSN, AOCN®
Former Director, Clinical Coordinating Section
NSABP Foundation, Inc.
Pittsburgh, PA
Chapter 8 – Chemoprevention

Corlis L. Archer, MD
Clinical Instructor, Urology Department
University of Connecticut Health Center
John Dempsey Hospital
Farmington, CT
Chapter 14 – Urologic and Male Genital Cancers

Carol Reed Ash, EdD, RN, FAAN
Eminent Scholar/Professor
Kirbo Endowed Chair, Oncology Nursing
University of Florida College of Nursing
Professor, Cancer Nursing
American Cancer Society, Inc.
Gainesville, FL
Chapter 20 Vignette – GatorSHADE™ Sun Protection Program at the University of Florida College of Nursing

Laural A. Aubry, RN, BSN, OCN®
Patient Care Coordinator
Community Cancer Care Specialists
Shelby Township, MI
Chapter 24 – Health-Education Issues for Patients in Cancer Prevention and Early Detection

Sandy Balentine, RN, BBA, OCN®
Manager of Clinical Oncology
Valley Hospital
Paramus, NJ
Chapter 20 Vignette – The Breast and Cervical Cancer Early Detection Project, Chapter 20 Vignette – The Regional Hereditary Cancer Evaluation Program

James K. Bennett, MD
Clinical Associate Professor of Urology
Emory University School of Medicine
Midtown Urology
Atlanta, GA
Chapter 14 – Urologic and Male Genital Cancers

Deb Bisel, RN, MSN, OCN®
Oncology Coordinator
Spectrum Health
Grand Rapids, MI
Chapter 20 Vignette – Colon Cancer Screening Program

Carol S. Blecher, RN, MS, AOCN®, CNS, C
Oncology Clinical Nurse Specialist
Valley Health System
Elizabeth, NJ
Chapter 24 – Health-Education Issues for Patients in Cancer Prevention and Early Detection

Janice V. Bowie, PhD, MPH
Assistant Professor
Department of Health Policy and Management
Bloomberg School of Public Health
Faculty of Social Services and Behavioral Sciences
Johns Hopkins University
Baltimore, MD
Chapter 3 – Human Behavior and Health Education

Catherine C. Burke, APRN, BC
Nurse Practitioner
Professional Education for Prevention and Early Detection
University of Texas M.D. Anderson Cancer Center
Houston, TX
Chapter 15 – Skin Cancer Prevention and Early Detection, Chapter 20 Vignette – Professional Education for Prevention and Early Detection

Faith Callif-Daley, MS, CGC
Genetic Counselor
The Children's Medical Center
Dayton, OH
Chapter 20 Vignette – The Regional Hereditary Cancer Evaluation Program

Marianne E. Casale, RN, MSN, CS, AOCN®
Oncology Clinical Nurse Specialist
Amgen Inc.
Maple Shade, NJ
Chapter 20 Vignette – Skin Cancer Awareness at the Races

Janine K. Cataldo, PhD, RN, CS
Lecturer, Psychiatric-Medical Health Nursing Specialty
Yale University School of Nursing
New Haven, CT
Chapter 9 – Smoking and Cancer

Dianne D. Chapman, RN, MS
Nurse Coordinator, Comprehensive Breast Center
Rush Cancer Institute
Rush-Presbyterian-St. Luke's Medical Center
Chicago, IL
Chapter 20 Vignette – Comprehensive Breast Center

Carol Cherry, RNC, BSN, OCN®
Project Manager, Family Risk Assessment Program
Fox Chase Cancer Center
Philadelphia, PA
Chapter 20 – Evolution of a Community-Based Family Risk Assessment Program: An Oncology Nursing Perspective

Mary E. Cooley, PhD, CRNP, AOCN®
Research Associate/Adult Nurse Practitioner
Smoking Cessation Research Program
Harvard Medical School/Harvard School of Dental Medicine
Boston, MA
Chapter 9 – Smoking and Cancer

Cathy A. Coyne, PhD
Assistant Professor
Department of Community Medicine
West Virginia University
Morgantown, WV
  *Chapter 3 – Human Behavior and Health
  Education*

Robin L. Coyne, MS, RN, CS-FNP
Nurse Practitioner
University of Texas M.D. Anderson Cancer Center
Cancer Prevention Center
Houston, TX
  *Chapter 16 – Prevention and Detection of
  Head and Neck Cancers*

Regina S. Cunningham, MA, RN, AOCN®
Chief Nursing Officer
Director of Ambulatory Services
Cancer Institute of New Jersey
Clinical Assistant Professor
University of Medicine and Dentistry of
New Jersey
New Brunswick, NJ
  *Chapter 22 – Advancing the Cancer Control
  Agenda: The Role of Advanced Practice Nurses*

Margaret M. Doyle, RN, BSN
Per-Diem Nurse
Hunterdon Regional Cancer Center
Flemington, NJ
  Chapter 20 Vignette–Development of a Comprehensive Cancer Program

Janie Eddleman, RN, OCN®
Cancer Care Coordinator
ValleyCare Health System
Pleasanton, CA
  Chapter 24 – Health-Education Issues for Patients in Cancer Prevention and Early Detection

Nancy Eisemon, RN, MPH, CGRN, APN/
CNS
Nurse Endoscopist
Central DuPage Hospital
Winfield, IL
  Chapter 20 Vignette – Colon Cancer Screening Program Preventive Healthcare Program Using Nurse Endoscopists

Jennifer Flach, BS
Clinical Research Program Specialist
National Cancer Institute
Division of Cancer Prevention
Bethesda, MD
  *Chapter 6 – An Overview of Bioethical Issues
  and Approaches in Cancer Prevention, Detection, and Control*

Ann Foltz, DNSc, RN
Adjunct Faculty
University of Central Florida
Orlando, FL
  *Chapter 2 – An Epidemiological Approach to
  Cancer Prevention and Control*

Bertie Ford, RN, MSN, AOCN®
Oncology Clinical Specialist
Amgen Inc.
Columbus, OH
  *Chapter 20 Vignette – Men Against Cancer
  Program*

Marilyn Frank-Stromborg, EdD, JD, FAAN
Chair and Presidential Research Professor
Northern Illinois University School of Nursing
DeKalb, IL
  *Chapter 1 – The Evolution of Nursing's Role
  in the Prevention and Early Detection of Cancer*

Donna Garrett, RN, MSN, CCRN
Cardiovascular Clinical Nurse Specialist
Spectrum Health
Grand Rapids, MI
  *Chapter 20 Vignette – Tobacco Free for Good
  Tobacco Cessation Program*

Ellen Giarelli, EdD, RN, CS, CRNP
Postdoctoral Research Fellow in Psychological Oncology and HIV/AIDS
Funded by the National Institute of Nursing Research, NIH (5-T32-NR-07036)
University of Pennsylvania School of Nursing
Philadelphia, PA
  *Chapter 4 – Cancer Prevention, Screening,
  and Early Detection: Human Genetics, Chapter 9 – Smoking and Cancer*

Cathleen M. Goetsch, MSN, ARNP, AOCN®
Hereditary Cancer Risk Consultant
Cancer Prevention Clinical Trials Coordinator
Virginia Mason Medical Center
Seattle, WA
  Chapter 20 Vignette – Enacting Cancer Prevention Clinical Trials in a Community Setting, Chapter 20 Vignette – Assessing Hereditary Cancer Risk

Karen E. Greco, RN, MN, ANP
Full-time Doctoral Student; Minor, Genetics
School of Nursing
Oregon Health & Science University
Portland, OR
  Chapter 18 – Genetic Counseling and Screening

Carol Grimm, MD, MPH
Medical Director, Cancer Risk Assessment Program
Roger Maris Cancer Center
Fargo, ND
  Chapter 20 Vignette – Family Cancer Risk Assessment Program

Mary Magee Gullatte, RN, MN, ANP, AOCN®, FAAMA
Director of Nursing
Winship Cancer Institute, Emory University Hospital, and Crawford Long Hospital
Adjunct Clinical Faculty
Nell Hodgson Woodruff School of Nursing
Emory University
Atlanta, GA
Adult Nurse Practitioner, Primary Care
Marietta, GA
  Chapter 14 – Urologic and Male Genital Cancers

Jacquelin Holland, RNC, CRNP
Screening Services Director
Columbus Cancer Clinic
Columbus, OH
  Chapter 20 Vignette – Men Against Cancer Program

Deborah M. Hudson, BS, RRT
Program Coordinator

Indiana University Cancer Center, Nicotine Dependence Program
Indianapolis, IN
  Chapter 20 Vignette – Indiana University Nicotine Dependence Program

Linda A. Jacobs, PhD, CRNP, AOCN®, BC
Clinical Assistant Professor
Coordinator, Living Well After Cancer Program
University of Pennsylvania Cancer Center
Philadelphia, PA
  Chapter 4 – Cancer Prevention, Screening, and Early Detection: Human Genetics

Jean Jenkins, PhD, RN, FAAN
Clinical Nurse Specialist Consultant
National Cancer Institute
Bethesda, MD
  Chapter 4 – Cancer Prevention, Screening, and Early Detection: Human Genetics

Linda U. Krebs, RN, PhD, AOCN®
Assistant Professor
University of Colorado Health Sciences Center School of Nursing
Aurora, CO
  Chapter 20 Vignette – University of Colorado Comprehensive Cancer Center Screening Clinic

Jane A. Lipscomb, RN, PhD, FAAN
Associate Professor
University of Maryland School of Nursing
Baltimore, MD
  Chapter 10 – Environmental Health and Cancer Control

Agnes Masny, RN, MPH, MSN, CRNP
Nurse Practitioner
Fox Chase Cancer Center
Philadelphia, PA
  Chapter 20 Vignette – Establishment of a Breast Cancer High-Risk Registry at Community-Based Institutions

Noella Devolder McCray, RN, MN
Nurse Manager
University of Kansas Hospital
Kansas City, KS
  Chapter 24 – Health-Education Issues for Patients in Cancer Prevention and Early Detection

Diane McElwain, RN, OCN®, MEd
Oncology Coordinator
York Cancer Center
York, PA
Chapter 20 Vignette – Breast Health Outreach

Shirley Frederick McKenzie, RN, BSN, OCN®
Former Manager, Breast Program
Breast Health Access for Women With Disabilities Program
Consultant
Alta Bates Comprehensive Cancer Center
Berkeley, CA
Chapter 20 Vignette – Breast Health Access for Women With Disabilities

Cindy H. Melancon, RN, MN
President, Editor, Creator
CONVERSATIONS! The International Ovarian Cancer Connection
Amarillo, TX
Chapter 20 Vignette – CONVERSATIONS! The International Ovarian Cancer Connection

Patti Moser, RN, BSN, OCN®
Outreach Coordinator
Via Christi Cancer Center
Wichita, KS
Chapter 20 Vignette – Buddy Check™ 10: A Breast Cancer Awareness Program, Chapter 20 Vignette – Development of an Oncology Public Education Plan, Chapter 20 Vignette – Health Education Kits: Safe Sun and Don't Get Hooked on Smoking

Linda C. Nebeling, PhD, MPH, RD, FADA
Chief
Health Promotion Research Branch, Behavioral Research Program/DCCPS
National Cancer Institute
Bethesda, MD
Chapter 7 – Diet and Cancer Prevention: Why Fruits and Vegetables Are Essential Players

Bridget E. O'Brien, ND, RN, CS-FNP, OCN®
Nurse Practicioner
Robert H. Lurie Comprehensive Cancer Center of Northwestern University

Chicago, IL
Chapter 12 – Gastrointestinal Malignancies

Kathleen Farley Omerod, RN, MS, AOCN®
Education Consultant
NM Academy, Northwestern Memorial Hospital
Chicago, IL
Chapter 13 – Gynecologic Cancers

Marcia L. Patterson, MSN, RN, CS, ANP, GNP
Nurse Practitioner
Genitourinary Medical Oncology
University of Texas M.D. Anderson Cancer Center
Houston, TX
Chapter 20 Vignette – Professional Education for Prevention and Early Detection

Jennifer Douglas Pearce, RN, MSN, CNS
Associate Professor of Nursing
University of Cincinnati Raymond Walters College
Blue Ash, OH
Chapter 21 – Preparation of Nurse Generalists for Cancer Prevention and Detection Practice: Experiences of Associate-Degree Nursing Programs

Janice Mitchell Phillips, PhD, RN, FAAN
Program Director
National Institute of Nursing Research
Bethesda, MD
Chapter 11 – Breast Cancer Prevention and Detection: Past Progress and Future Directions

Marva Mizell Price, DrPH, MPH, RN, CS
Assistant Professor of Nursing
Family Nurse Practitioner Program
Duke University School of Nursing
Durham, NC
Chapter 11 – Breast Cancer Prevention and Detection: Past Progress and Future Directions

Ann Reiner, RN, MSN, OCN®
Director of Education and Outreach

Oregon Health & Science University Cancer Institute
Portland, OR
Chapter 20 Vignette – Skin Cancer Screening in the Metropolitan Area of Portland, OR

Kimberly Rohan, MS, RN, AOCN®
Manager/Clinical Nurse Specialist
Edward Cancer Center
Naperville, IL
Chapter 1 – The Evolution of Nursing's Role in the Prevention and Early Detection of Cancer

Barbara Sattler, RN, DrPH
Associate Professor and Director of Environmental Health Education Center
University of Maryland School of Nursing
Baltimore, MD
Chapter 10 – Environmental Health and Cancer Control

Anne Marie Shaftic, RN, C, BSN, OCN®
Oncology Nurse Educator for Inpatient, Outpatient, Radiation Oncology and Professionals
Holy Name Hospital
Teaneck, NJ
Chapter 24 – Health-Education Issues for Patients in Cancer Prevention and Early Detection

Lisa Stucky-Marshall, RN, MS, AOCN®
Gastrointestinal Oncology Advanced Practice Nurse
Northwestern Memorial Hospital
Robert H. Lurie Comprehensive Cancer Center of Northwestern University
Chicago, IL
Chapter 12 – Gastrointestinal Malignancies

Carol Stoner, MS, RN
Clinical Nurse Specialist in Oncology Nursing
Valparaiso, IN
Overview Section IV

Linda Sveningson, MS, RN, AOCN®
Nurse Coordinator, Cancer Risk Assessment Program

Roger Maris Cancer Center
Fargo, ND
Chapter 20 Vignette – Family Cancer Risk Assessment Program

Linda J. Trapkin, DO
Clinical Assistant Professor
Upstate Medical Center, State University of New York
Attending Pathologist
St. Joseph's Hospital Health Center
Syracuse, NY
Chapter 5 – Pathology and the Clinical Laboratory in Cancer Control

Mary Ann S. Van Duyn, PhD, MPH, RD
Chief
Health Promotion Branch, Outreach and Partnerships
Office of Communications
National Cancer Institute
Bethesda, MD
Chapter 7 – Diet and Cancer Prevention: Why Fruits and Vegetables are Essential Players

Jill W. Varnes, EdD, CHES
Professor in Health Science Education
College of Health and Human Performance
University of Florida
Gainesville, FL
Chapter 20 Vignette – GatorSHADE™ Sun Protection Program at the University of Florida College of Nursing

Claudette G. Varricchio, DSN, RN, FAAN
Chief, Office of Extramural Programs
National Institute of Nursing Research
Bethesda, MD
Chapter 19 – The Role of the Nurse in Cancer Control

Jane Williams, MSN, APRN, BC, FNP
Nurse Practitioner
Genitourinary Medical Oncology
University of Texas M.D. Anderson Cancer Center
Houston, TX
Chapter 20 Vignette – Professional Education for Prevention and Early Detection

Melanie Williams, RN, BSN
Health Science Associate
Merck & Co., Inc.
Ballwin, MO
Chapter 17 – Tertiary Prevention: Improving the Care of Long-Term Survivors of Cancer

Bessie Woo, RN, MSN, OCN®
Clinical Education Coordinator
Chinese Hospital
San Francisco, CA

Chapter 24 – Health-Education Issues for Patients in Cancer Prevention and Early Detection

Annette B. Wysocki, PhD, RN, C
Director, Wound Healing Program
National Institute of Dental and Craniofacial Research
Bethesda, MD
Chapter 23 – Research Training Opportunities

Contents

Foreword

The National Cancer Institute projects that one of every two men and one of every three women in the United States will develop some type of cancer over the course of their lives. There is no question that cancer is prevalent and that everyone knows someone whose life has been directly affected by its threat or diagnosis. The editors of this text have taken an important step in giving educators, students, and clinicians a comprehensive guide of what is known and what can be done about preventing and detecting cancer early. They have enlisted the help of authors who are experts on understanding cancer, its consequences, and how it affects human behavior. Some of the contributors are my former pre- and postdoctoral graduates who have committed their professional careers to ensuring positive outcomes for people who face the threat of cancer or experience it firsthand. The authors are themselves either seasoned researchers or experienced clinicians who are sensitive to the hard realities of trying to translate knowledge into clinical practice.

The virtual explosion of new research in cancer prevention, detection, and control in recent years warrants the evolution of this text. This book does a great service by positioning cancer prevention and control in its most meaningful place within the broad scope of quality cancer care. Achieving the best outcomes for people at risk for developing cancer or who develop it requires widespread application of the state-of-art cancer management strategies. This book includes successful efforts targeted at underserved populations and underrepresented minority groups. We need to continue to strive to improve programs to help to prevent, detect, and control cancer in all segments of the populations.

The Oncology Nursing Society's support of this book symbolizes their continued commitment to the rapid transfer of knowledge from its discovery to widespread clinical use. I believe this is an outstanding book that will find its place on most educators' and expert clinicians' bookshelves. It will be used repeatedly as a reference book to validate facts and provide answers to those searching for solutions. The book should be required reading for all students in nursing and medical oncology programs. Consumers need to hold their providers accountable for the content associated with the recommended guidelines for prevention, screening, early detection, and treatment of site-specific cancers. The book provides critical linkages to bring advancement in these areas to patients, families, and the public.

Perhaps the most important accomplishment of this text is its insistence of incorporation of all the elements of cancer care into one informative and coherent book. As a cancer survivor of 12 years, I learned firsthand that knowledge alone is not enough to win the fight against the threat of cancer. We also must have timely access to diagnostic tests, competent professionals to communicate the results, and clear and understandable options for treatment even when controversy surrounds the outcomes. Nurses often are with patients during times when they are contemplating available options and a course of action. At these times, it is not only our knowledge but also our presence that helps to relieve the situational distress that accompanies times of crisis. As outlined in the Institute of Medicine's report *Ensuring Quality Cancer Care*, the authority to organize, coordinate, and improve cancer care services rests largely with service providers and insurers. The challenge for us as professionals and members of the interdisciplinary team of cancer experts is to create systems that will facilitate our abilities to work together. *Interdisciplinary care* refers to the reliance on healthcare and other providers with a range of backgrounds and expertise. Comprehensive, coordinated care is the ability to fully access necessary services and have components of care efficiently planned and integrated. Clear and ongoing communication among care providers and among patients and family members is a prerequisite to coordinated care. Too often, adults who are suspected of having cancer or who are newly diagnosed see several doctors sequentially, without having an overall plan of care devised at the outset by, or in consultation with, an interdisciplinary team (Hewitt & Simone, 1999).

Many gaps remain between knowledge gained through science and the translation of that information to the actual experience of people at risk for, diagnosed with, or surviving cancer. This book helps us to look back with pride to all that has been accomplished and forward to the many important next steps needed to continue. I congratulate Kathleen Jennings-Dozier and Suzanne Mahon on giving us this up-to-date and comprehensive text that will guide us on our journey to ensure that all Americans have access to quality cancer care when they need it.

Hewitt, M., & Simone, J. (Eds.). (1999). *Ensuring quality cancer care.* Washington, DC: National Academy Press.

Ruth McCorkle, PhD, FAAN
The Florence S. Wald Professor of Nursing
Yale University School of Nursing
New Haven, CT

Preface

Cancer control is an ever-growing and ever-changing field. The public and healthcare professionals scrutinize issues related to cancer control, including cancer prevention and early detection, because it serves as the best hope of decreasing the morbidity and mortality associated with cancer.

Many issues in cancer control are controversial. Every development in cancer control leads to different questions. For example, statistics demonstrate that cancer incidence and mortality rates have dropped for some malignancies in the last decade. Mammography has led to more breast cancers being detected early, when the hope of long-term survival is best and less radical surgery may be indicated. If mammography is effective, why does a disparity exist with its use in some populations? Every woman who is 40 years of age and older should have a mammogram. When should mammograms stop being performed? Should they be discontinued when a woman is 70, 80, 90, or 100 years old? Is the disparity in mammography use because of cost, accessibility, cultural differences, or educational barriers? The answers to these and many other questions are not readily evident. These questions point to the progress that has been made in some areas of cancer control and identify the challenges that remain.

The Oncology Nursing Society Position on Prevention and Early Detection of Cancer (see page xix) addresses why cancer control is important and why it is becoming a priority area in oncology nursing practice and research. Cancer control is a field in which oncology nurses really can make a difference. Principles of cancer risk assessment, issues relating to genetic testing, applying primary cancer prevention practices, selecting appropriate cancer screening tests, and educating patients about symptoms to report and how to conduct self-examinations are only a few examples of the roles oncology nurses can assume in cancer control. Oncology nurses must deliver these services in an environment that respects the culture and personal beliefs of those served and also consider the ethical issues that surround cancer screening.

A decade ago, oncology nurses rarely worked in cancer control. This implies that many nurses, including those with graduate degrees, may not have had the opportunity to study about cancer control issues or be mentored by someone with expertise in cancer control. This book examines many of the developments in the field of cancer control and can serve as a reference for nurses who work in cancer control, students trying to learn more about cancer control, and oncology nurses who take care of patients and families in active treatment who want to better understand principles of cancer control.

Section I provides an overview of the theoretical constructs that guide cancer control. Although this literature may be unfamiliar to some, the reader is encouraged to consider these principles that guide primary, secondary, and tertiary prevention. Section II describes issues and progress in cancer prevention. Primary cancer prevention often is overlooked. Primary cancer prevention, however, holds promise for patients who want to try to control their cancer risks. Secondary cancer prevention or cancer screening for major tumor sites is discussed in Section III, as well as issues related to cancer genetics risk assessment and management and tertiary cancer prevention in long-term survivors of cancer. Section IV translates the information from the first three sections into examples of how nurses from diverse geographic regions, practice settings, and academic backgrounds implement principles of cancer control into their daily practice. The creativity of these programs truly is remarkable and offers hope that nurses can implement cancer control into their practice settings. Section V addresses issues related to education for the oncology nurse as a professional and considerations for educating patients and the public about cancer control.

On a more personal note, every oncology nurse needs to consider his or her own personal risk for developing cancer. We hope the information in this book will challenge each oncology nurse to carefully assess his or her own personal risk for developing cancer, consider the means to reduce this risk through primary prevention, and engage in appropriate and regular cancer screening. Oncology nurses who engage in these practices will serve as role models to the patients and families they serve.

This book is an attempt to address issues related to cancer control, describe the current progress in cancer prevention and early detection, highlight controversial issues, and demonstrate the important and real role that oncology nurses play in cancer control. Every effort has been made to identify the ramifications of each issue for clinical practice, public and professional education, and future nursing research. We sincerely hope that every oncology nurse will make cancer control a priority in his or her personal and professional life.

Oncology Nursing Society Position on Prevention and Early Detection of Cancer in the United States

In the United States, more than 1,200,000 new cancers are diagnosed in individuals across the lifespan each year. The lifetime risk of developing cancer in the United States is one in two for men and one in three for women. Cancer is the second leading cause of death in the United States, with one in every four deaths caused by cancer. Cancer is the leading cause of death in individuals 40–79 years of age (American Cancer Society [ACS], 2001). Consequently, cancer is a major public health problem in the United States. Adopting healthier lifestyles and avoiding carcinogen exposure could prevent many cancers. According to ACS, institution of prevention measures and early detection of cancer are two of the most important and effective strategies for reaching important public health goals of saving lives lost from cancer, diminishing suffering from cancer, and eliminating cancer as a major health problem.

It Is the Position of the Oncology Nursing Society (ONS) That

Professional Education
- Oncology nurses, at both the generalist and advanced practice levels, must have educational preparation in the behavioral, biologic, educational, and economic principles of cancer prevention and early detection.
- Continuing education and specialized educational programs must be developed and provided to practicing nurses to facilitate integration of cancer prevention and early detection into clinical practice.
- Oncology specialty certification examinations and nursing licensure examinations should include evaluation of knowledge related to cancer prevention and detection practices in the general population.

Public Education
- All oncology nurses are well suited to provide education to the general public about prevention measures and general population screening guidelines for the early detection of cancer.
- Oncology nurses also are well suited to provide the necessary information and education to facilitate client decision making about participation in cancer prevention and control clinical trials.

- Oncology nurses must strive to provide comprehensive cancer prevention education and early detection services in a manner consistent with the cultural background and healthcare beliefs of individuals and families. Educational materials should be used that are in the appropriate language and are targeted to the appropriate level of literacy.
- Oncology nurses must be involved in the development of educational resources that have a focus on wellness, including the prevention and early detection of cancer in at-risk populations.
- Education programs must be developed and provided on the primary prevention of cancer (e.g., smoking cessation programs, nutritional counseling, avoidance of exposure to ultraviolet light) beginning in childhood and throughout the lifespan to encourage people to adopt healthy lifestyles.

Cancer Prevention and Detection Services

- Oncology nurses need to develop, implement, and evaluate measures to ensure that individuals and families have access to education about cancer prevention and appropriate cancer screening.
- Advanced practice oncology nurses can obtain, document, and interpret cancer risk assessments; recommend appropriate cancer early detection and prevention strategies to individuals and families; and arrange or provide comprehensive cancer screening examinations based on the individual's level of risk. These practices must be consistent with guidelines defined by the appropriate state's nurse practice act, educational preparation, and role scope, along with standards of oncology nursing practice.
- As genetic technology evolves and knowledge of cancer genetics expands, healthcare providers must respond by informing patients, families, and the public about the implications of these developments for cancer prevention, early detection, and treatment. Nurses providing comprehensive cancer genetic counseling must be advanced practice oncology nurses with specialized education in hereditary cancer genetics.
- Individuals who have survived a cancer diagnosis also should receive age-appropriate cancer screening for other cancers.
- Programs that are focused on delivering services for the early detection of individual cancers (e.g., breast, prostate) also should ensure that patients receive education and are referred for screening for other common cancers. An immediate opportunity exists to implement this approach in men and women who are covered by Medicare and already eligible for reimbursement of the respective screening tests for breast, cervical, colorectal, and prostate cancers.
- Individuals should be assessed for eligibility for chemoprevention trials based on personal level of risk and referred for consideration at the appropriate clinical site.
- Individuals should be fully informed of their options for managing their personal risks for developing cancer and should understand the limitations, benefits, and risks of each strategy.

Research

- Oncology nurses need to conduct research to further assess the efficacy of cancer prevention and early detection programs, the psychological impact of cancer prevention and detection strategies, and promotion of participation in prevention and early detection activities.
- Research related to cancer prevention and detection strategies must be integrated into practice.

Health Policy

- The development and evaluation of cancer prevention and detection health policy should be based on current cancer control research and involve multidisciplinary academicians and clinicians (including oncology nurses) and the public.
- Payors must be encouraged to provide coverage for prevention measures, counseling on prevention strategies, nutrition, and smoking cessation and for early detection and screening services based on individual risk levels.
- The ability to identify individuals who are at increased risk for developing cancer because of inherited altered (mutated) cancer predisposition genes is possible through cancer predisposition genetic testing. Risk assessment counseling and cancer predisposition genetic testing are components of comprehensive cancer care, and payors should cover them.
- Payors should cover clinical trials evaluating cancer prevention and detection strategies and chemoprevention.

Background

Primary cancer prevention refers to the prevention of cancer through health promotion and risk reduction. This includes carcinogen avoidance and, more recently, the use of chemoprevention agents and consideration of prophylactic surgeries in individuals at high risk for developing cancer, such as those with genetic predispositions. Secondary cancer prevention refers to the early detection and treatment of subclinical disease or early disease in people without signs or symptoms of cancer. Early detection is defined as the application of a test to detect a potential cancer in individuals who have no signs or symptoms of the cancer. Cancer screening refers to looking for cancer in a population at risk for a particular cancer. Cancer screening and early detection are forms of secondary cancer prevention aimed at detecting cancer early, when it is most treatable in asymptomatic people. Tertiary cancer prevention refers to the prevention and early detection of second primary cancers in individuals who have been diagnosed with cancer. This includes the application of specific tests to detect cancer and the use of chemoprevention agents to prevent the development of additional cancers.

Cancer continues to be a significant health problem in the United States. Everyone is at risk for developing cancer. Many cancers could be prevented by avoidance of carcinogens and mutagens. ACS (2001) estimated that 171,000 cancer deaths result annually from tobacco use and 19,000 deaths are related to excessive alcohol use. An additional 185,000 cancer deaths are attributed to diet, nutrition, and other lifestyle factors and are probably preventable. Many of the 1.3 million skin cancers diagnosed annually could be prevented or controlled if people decreased their exposure to ultraviolet light. These facts underscore the importance of educating the public about the importance of a healthy lifestyle and strategies that can be instituted for the prevention of cancer. Public policy should support programs that provide education to the public about cancer prevention measures. Public education about the importance of cancer prevention measures and recommended cancer screening guidelines is an important component of oncology nursing practice and should occur both across the lifespan and the continuum of cancer care.

Cancer morbidity and mortality could be reduced further by the early detection of cancer in asymptomatic individuals. Cancers of the breast, colon, rectum, cervix, prostate, testis, oral cavity, and skin can be detected early, when treatment is more likely to be effective. These cancers alone account for about one-half of all cancer cases diagnosed annually in the United States. The ACS (2001) estimated that the current five-year relative survival rate for these cancers is about 80%. If all Americans participated in regular cancer screening, this rate could increase to 95%. Payors must include coverage of cancer screening services to achieve this goal.

Approved by the ONS Board of Directors, April 2001.

The Board of Directors acknowledges the collective wisdom, contributions, and recommendations of these ONS members with recognized experience in the prevention and detection of cancer: Suzanne M. Mahon, RN, DNSc, AOCN®, assistant clinical professor in the Division of Hematology and Oncology at Saint Louis University in Missouri; Lois J. Loescher, PhD, RN, cancer prevention fellow at Arizona Cancer Center at the University of Arizona in Tucson; and Kathleen Jennings-Dozier, PhD, MPH, RN, CS, associate professor at MCP Hahnemann University College of Nursing and Health Professions in Philadelphia, PA.

Reference

American Cancer Society. (2001). *Cancer facts and figures, 2001.* Atlanta: Author.

Additional Resources

- Carroll-Johnson, R.M. (Ed.). (2000). Cancer prevention and early detection: Oncology nursing's next frontier. *Oncology Nursing Forum, 27*(Suppl. 9), 1–61.
- National Cancer Institute, www.nci.nih.gov

Acknowledgments

Dr. Suzanne Mahon supported and believed in my vision for this book, sight unseen, and no questions asked—thanks. To Barbara Sigler, RN, MNEd, and her staff at the Oncology Nursing Society, you have the patience of Job. A special thank-you to Drs. Gloria F. Donnelly and Patricia Gerrity for their support and encouragement. Finally, to Drs. Douglas Weed and Ronald E. Myers, who taught me the fundamentals of cancer prevention and control, and to Drs. Sandra Millon Underwood and Ruth McCorkle who convinced me that, in order to make a real difference, nurses must have their say.

—Kathleen Jennings-Dozier

I would like to acknowledge those people who were particularly helpful to me during the preparation of this book. It would not have been possible without the continual assistance and encouragement from the ONS Publishing Division. In a special way I would like to thank Barbara Sigler and Lisa George for their support and insight at every step of publication. It has been a pleasure to work with Kathleen Jennings-Dozier on this project, as well.

The willingness and dedication of each author also should be noted. Each author generously shared her expertise. These authors met deadlines and complied with requests when needed.

Special thanks to my past and present employers, who have challenged me to find new and creative means to implement cancer control programs in the clinical setting. Without their support and willingness to allow a nurse to assume responsibility for such programs, I would not have been able to have the opportunity to practice in this dynamic area of oncology nursing. I also want to thank those patients who continually remind me each and every day of why cancer control is so important.

Finally, I extend sincere thanks to my family, who stood by me during the publication process and helped out whenever they could. Their encouragement and assistance did not go unnoticed.

—Suzanne M. Mahon

SECTION I

Fundamentals of Cancer Prevention, Detection, and Control

Chapter 1.

The Evolution of Nursing's Role in the
Prevention and Early Detection of Cancer

Chapter 2.

An Epidemiological Approach to Cancer Prevention and Control

Chapter 3.

Human Behavior and Health Education

Chapter 4.

Cancer Prevention, Screening, and Early Detection: Human Genetics

Chapter 5.

Pathology and the Clinical Laboratory in Cancer Control

Chapter 6.

An Overview of Bioethical Issues and Approaches in
Cancer Prevention, Detection, and Control

OVERVIEW

Section I

Suzanne M. Mahon, RN, DNSc, AOCN®, APNG(c)

Cancer control is defined as the efforts to prevent, detect, and manage the disease of cancer. To ultimately decrease the morbidity and mortality associated with malignancy, effective means to prevent and detect cancer early must be developed and implemented. Section I provides a detailed examination of the conceptual considerations related to cancer control.

Documentation of efforts to treat cancer can be traced back to 5 B.C. In Chapter 1, Rohan and Frank-Stromborg provide a comprehensive history of cancer-control efforts. This chapter highlights the major roles nurses have played in the development of effective means to educate, prevent, and detect cancers early. An understanding of this historical perspective provides insight into the dramatic advances that have been made in the effort to prevent and detect cancer when it is most easily treated. This information can serve as hope to patients and families that cancer control truly can become a reality. Nurses need to share this hope and historical legacy as they provide patient and public education about cancer control.

Much of the progress that has been made in cancer control stems from epidemiologic research that aims to understand environmental, genetic, and population risks for developing specific cancer(s). In Chapter 2, Jennings-Dozier and Foltz provide a detailed discussion and definition of epidemiologic principles and the application of the principles to cancer control. This discussion includes definitions and clinical examples of statistical measures commonly used in epidemiologic studies and reports. The clinical applications of this technical information are enormous. Nurses constantly are challenged to construct and interpret cancer risk assessments to patients and their families. This demands that nurses be able to accurately interpret epidemiologic studies of cancer risk. The information in Chapter 2 provides the framework for understanding epidemiologic reports and the implications of these reports for clinical practice.

Lifestyle factors are also a major risk factor for many cancers. Although many of these risk factors are within an individual's control, getting individuals to change behaviors is a major challenge for nurses who work in the cancer-control arena. All cancers caused by heavy tobacco or alcohol use could be prevented. The American Cancer Society (ACS, 2001) estimated that in 2001, 172,000 cancer deaths were related to tobacco use, and an additional 19,000 deaths were caused by excessive alcohol use. Further, ACS estimated that at least one-third of the 535,400 deaths from cancer this year would be related to nutrition, physical activity, and other lifestyle factors that could be prevented. These figures do not consider the nonmelanoma skin cancers that are a direct result of ultraviolet light exposure.

ACS (2001) also estimated that cancers of the breast, colon, gynecologic organs, prostate, testicles, oral cavity, and skin account for half of all of the new cancer cases that are diagnosed annually. Currently, the relative five-year survival rates for these cancers are 81% (ACS). If regular screenings were implemented, this rate probably would increase to 95%.

Improving lifestyle practices and engaging in cancer-screening activities could significantly decrease the morbidity and mortality associated with cancer. Although the adoption of positive health behaviors and participation in a regular screening program seem very simple and relatively cost effective to implement, getting people to change health-related behaviors is extremely challenging. In Chapter 3, Coyne and Bowie examine the complex issues that surround human behavior and health education, especially as it relates to wellness. Before implementing any program for cancer prevention or early detection, nurses need to consider the health and human behaviors and beliefs of the target audience. After assessing these factors, nurses can choose appropriate and effective means to communicate information about cancer prevention and early detection that hopefully will lead to a decrease in the morbidity and mortality associated with cancer.

Recently, the science and developments in cancer genetics have dramatically affected cancer-control efforts. The ability to identify individuals and families who are at a significantly higher risk for developing cancer because of their genetic backgrounds offers the hope of targeting aggressive screening and prevention to those who stand to reap the most benefit. Many undergraduate and graduate programs provide limited instruction on genetics and human disease. The importance of understanding these complex scientific principles cannot be underestimated, especially in relation to cancer control. These principles lay the foundation for cancer risk assessments. Genetic testing rapidly is becoming an important tool in cancer control. In Chapter 4, Giarelli, Jacobs, and Jenkins review human physiology and genetic concepts in relation to cancer control. These authors address historical landmarks in genetics research, the basic scientific concepts of genetics and inheritance, and the mechanisms of mutation and carcinogenesis of some common cancers, as well as implications for nurses. Nurses need to consider these concepts when interpreting risk assessments to patients and making recommendations for cancer prevention and early detection.

Laboratory science also is playing an ever-increasing important role in cancer control. In Chapter 5, Trapkin discusses how nurses must consider clinical and laboratory findings in relation to cancer control. Nurses should look at the sensitivity, specificity, and predictive value of various laboratory tests used in cancer detection (e.g., Pap smear) or diagnosis (e.g., pathology of a colorectal polyp). An understanding of these concepts is necessary to recommend the appropriate screening or diagnostic testing and assist in the interpretation of the findings. Both patients and the public must receive education about the inherent strengths and limitations of various laboratory and radiological procedures used in cancer control for true informed consent. Nurses have a responsibility to communicate this information to patients in understandable terms. By understanding the limitations of laboratory testing, the nurse is in a better position to correlate the clinical expectations with the laboratory result and educate the patient regarding appropriate follow-up.

Ethical considerations and dilemmas can arise in the area of cancer control. In particular, issues with managed care, allocation of cancer research costs, population diversity and serving at-risk populations, genetic testing, and issues related to confidentiality can be particularly challenging in cancer prevention and early detection. In Chapter 6, Flach provides a detailed examination of these issues and suggests a framework for bioethical decision making. Nurses are challenged to consider these bioethical issues and dilemmas when implementing cancer-control education, prevention, and detection programs.

For nurses to provide effective cancer-control services to the patients and families they serve, they must be knowledgeable about the science and principles that guide the current understanding of cancer control. These principles must be applied to clinical practice consistently and interpreted to patients and families in understandable terms so they can make the best and most-informed choices possible about how to prevent and detect cancer early. For oncology nurses conducting and interpreting research about cancer-control issues, these conceptual considerations provide the framework for future oncology nursing research. Without a background and knowledge about these conceptual considerations and scientific principles, oncology nurses cannot develop effective programs for cancer control. Section I provides a framework to help meet these challenges.

Reference

American Cancer Society. (2001). *Cancer facts and figures, 2001*. Atlanta: Author.

CHAPTER 1

The Evolution of Nursing's Role in the Prevention and Early Detection of Cancer

Kimberly Rohan, MS, RN, AOCN®, and
Marilyn Frank-Stromborg, EdD, JD, FAAN

Introduction

According to current estimates, 1,220,100 new cases of invasive cancer and an additional 1,371,200 noninvasive cancers will have been diagnosed in the United States in 2000 (Greenlee, Murray, Bolden, & Wingo, 2000). Fortunately, the age-adjusted incidence rates for all cancer sites combined continues to decrease, with the incidence rates for the leading cancers diagnosed either declining or slowing down (Woolam, 2000). Unfortunately, African Americans continue to exhibit the highest cancer incidence rates and are 33% more likely to die of their cancer (Woolam). These statistics point to the need for aggressive prevention and early detection strategies to minimize the morbidity and mortality from cancer.

Nurses play a pivotal role in cancer prevention and early detection. Nurses, the largest healthcare group in this country, practice in more diverse settings and work with more people than any other group of healthcare professionals. The focus of this chapter is the incidence, prevention, and early detection of cancer in the major sites with an emphasis on the related nursing role that has emerged for each. The American Cancer Society (ACS) has established the goal of a 25% reduction in the overall age-adjusted cancer incidence rate and a 50% reduction in the overall age-adjusted cancer mortality rate by 2015 (Seffrin, 2000). These goals are aggressive but attainable. Nurses will be paramount in the effort by providing creative approaches to cancer prevention and early detection.

History of Prevention and Early Detection

A glimpse at the evolution of cancer nursing reveals a stark contrast from the past to the present. In the 17th century B.C., the perception of cancer as untreatable pervaded the attitudes of even the patients' physicians. For example, the oldest written description of a patient with cancer appeared in the Edwin Smith Papyrus from Egypt: "Thou should say concerning him . . . 'There is no treatment.'" (Yarbro, 2000). While such an assertion is now known to be false, a number of efforts were fundamental in the expansion of the cancer field over the years. As advances were made in technology and research, the role of the oncology nurse became more significant in the battle against cancer. Additionally, the efforts of numerous cancer-focused organizations helped to promote research and to educate medical professionals and the public. Consequently, the role of the modern oncology nurse expanded beyond its traditional roles as the need for nurses in specialized areas of cancer prevention and treatment increased (Yarbro, 1996).

The Early Years

Historical efforts in the field of oncology laid the foundation upon which advances have been made over time. Documentation of cancer treatment exists from the fifth century B.C., in which the common philosophy on cancer treatment was to *not* treat the patient at all (Yarbro, 2000). While this notion, formulated by Hippocrates, persisted for a number of years, medical progress became apparent in Europe in the 18th century when those in the medical field began to investigate this disease (Yarbro, 2000). In 1740, the first facility for patients with cancer opened in Rheims, France, but was later moved because of residents' fears that cancer was contagious (Yarbro, 1996). In 1761, Giovanni Morgagni laid the groundwork for scientific oncology when he correlated the clinical course of cancer to the pathological findings at autopsy (Yarbro, 2000). Furthermore, at the beginning of the 19th century, a committee of English physicians and surgeons gathered to formulate investigatory questions regarding cancer, such as, "Are there any proofs of cancer being a hereditary disease?" (Yarbro, 1996). Interestingly, this is a question those in the field of oncology would find themselves asking almost two centuries later. Many in the medical field touched on the first notions of prevention when they speculated that there were associations between human action and cancer—such as using snuff and sweeping chimneys (Yarbro, 1996). However, the concern surrounding cancer was primarily focused on treatment rather than on prevention and detection. Further advances in science and technology facilitated doctors' and nurses' efforts to address the needs of patients with cancer. For instance, the emergence of anesthesia and the first successful "painless" surgery performed by surgeon John C. Warren in 1846 induced more patients to undergo surgery at that time (Yarbro, 1996). The introduction of the radical mastectomy for breast cancer and the discovery of x-rays and radium followed soon thereafter in 1894, 1895, and 1898, respectively (Yarbro, 1996). The next century built on these breakthrough accomplishments.

The Changing Roles of Nurses

As surgery was the primary form of cancer treatment in the mid-1800s and the early 20th century, nursing was primarily concerned with the bedside care of those patients who had undergone surgery (Yarbro, 1996). However, at least one nurse helped to expand the role of nurses in the mid-1800s. The legendary Florence Nightingale obtained a job in 1851 at Kaiserswerth Hospital in Germany (Underwood, 1999). Three years later, the British Secretary of War asked her to organize a group of nurses to accompany her to Turkey to assess and possibly change the poor conditions causing numerous deaths of the British soldiers in the Crimean War (Underwood). Subsequently, Nightingale's success on the battle-field resulted in not only a large grant of money to open an education facility for nurses but also the recognition of the expanding role of nurses.

While Nightingale certainly was not the first nurse in history, she played a key role in professionalizing the nursing occupation. More specifically, she promoted preventive medicine policies long before they became reality. She said she wanted to "inoculate the country with the view of preventing instead of cure" (Yarbro, 2000, p. 6). Nurses continued to gain more recognition in the medical field as the demand for them increased before the turn of the century. Specifically, a need for trained nurses became apparent during the Civil War; subsequently, the first school of nursing opened in Boston in 1872, the New England Hospital School of Nursing (Yarbro, 1996).

The 20th Century

Long after the Crimean War ended, the battle against cancer raged on into the 20th century. More time and resources were expended on research, technology, and education as time progressed. In 1915, laboratory animals were induced with cancer for the first time when coal-tar was applied to a rabbit's skin (Yarbro, 2000). Moreover, the use of ionizing radiation in the diagnosis of, treatment of, and surgical procedures for cancer was extensive (Yarbro, 1996). As surgery was the principal form of cancer treatment, cancer nurses' primary role was to comfort patients with cancer. Although much knowledge was attained pertaining to cancer in the 18th century, the death rate from cancer still was at 99% in the early 1900s (Yarbro, 1996). A contributing factor to this high mortality rate may have been the persistent focus on cancer treatment rather than preventing the onset of cancer or detecting it in its initial stages. Data indicate that the early detection of cancer greatly improves the prognosis (Greenwald, 1995). Cancer rarely was discussed openly, and many still believed cancer to be contagious and without a cure (Yarbro, 1996). The need for more education of the public, as well as those in the medical profession, was apparent.

Although governmental intervention in the fight against cancer was not immediate, private cancer-focused organizations began to emerge in the early 1900s. The government addressed the need for improvements in the health field by passing the Sheppard-Towner Act in 1921 (McCabe & Piemme, 1996). The Act provided for governmental funding to the state for programs through the Public Health Service. A few years later, the Randall Act authorized the National Institutes of Health and governmental funding for research (McCabe & Piemme). In 1913, at the private level, prominent business leaders from New York City and a group of American Gynecological Society surgeons formed two organizations that emphasized cancer control: the American Society for the Control of Cancer and the American Association for Cancer Research (ACS, 2000; Greenwald, 1995). In 1927, the American Society for the Control of Cancer developed the slogan "Fight Cancer with Knowledge," emphasizing the movement to educate physicians (Yarbro, 1996). Both organizations offered a great deal of valuable services.

The next decade saw the development of a number of cancer organizations that continued to address the need for more cancer prevention-related research and education of the public, physicians, and nurses. For example, the American College of Surgeons established standards for doctors and nurses to use in their evaluations of patients with cancer (Yarbro, 1996). Furthermore, the American Society for the Control of Cancer developed the Women's Field Army (ACS, 2000; Yarbro, 1996). As a result of the Women's Field Army's efforts to educate the public about cancer and to raise money, volunteers active in cancer control increased tenfold from 1935 to 1938 (ACS; Yarbro, 1996).

The government began to propel the issue of cancer control into the public eye. Specifically, Congress passed an act in 1937 establishing the National Cancer Institute (NCI), the first of the National Institutes of Health (Marino, 1981; Yarbro, 1996). The objective of the organization was to "provide for, foster, and aid in coordination research relating to cancer" (Marino, p. 36). Funds for NCI increased dramatically over the next few years, allowing for the formation of clinical research programs and the Cancer Chemotherapy National Service Center. The chemotherapy center was particularly significant to the progress made by NCI because many universities' research centers participated collectively in cancer research clinical trials for patients with advanced stages of cancer. Moreover, during the next several years, NCI helped to shift the emphasis of cancer from treatment to prevention by promoting, for example, demographic research on the cause and natural history of cancer (Marino). Over time, NCI has been instrumental in providing funding for research, educational programs, and access to reliable information through the Cancer Information Service (Greenwald, 1995).

From the reorganization of the American Society for the Control of Cancer in 1945 emerged another significant cancer control organization—ACS (2000). The objective of ACS, carried over from the American Society for the Control of Cancer, was to "disseminate knowledge concerning the symptoms, treatment, and prevention of cancer; to investigate conditions under which cancer is found; and to compile statistics in regard thereto" (Marino, 1981, p. 38). While this 1913 objective targeted cancer prevention, ACS truly advocated prevention in 1947 when it began its public education campaign about the signs and symptoms of cancer (ACS). As ACS grew over the years, it offered more services, such as self-help organizations, research grants, public awareness campaigns, and financial support (ACS; Marino). ACS today prides itself as being a nationwide, community-based, voluntary health agency dedicated to eliminating cancer as a health problem by preventing cancer, saving lives, and diminishing suffering through research, education, advocacy, and service (ACS).

Knowledge surrounding cancer continued to expand as medical professionals utilized cancer organizations' financial support and services. The antitumor activity of nitrogen mustard, an agent of the chemical warfare program, was discovered at Yale (Yarbro, 1996). Another advance in chemotherapy occurred in 1947, when Sidney Farber, MD, of Children's Hospital in Boston achieved the first leukemia remission in a 10-year-old boy using the antineoplastic agent aminopterin (Yarbro, 1996). As the focus of cancer control shifted to cancer prevention, early detection was promoted through breast self-examination and the development of the Papanicolaou test to detect cervical cancer (Yarbro, 1996). Additionally, in 1955, NCI developed a national chemotherapy program to test chemicals that might be effective against cancer (Yarbro, 1996).

Just as knowledge about cancer increased, so did the educational opportunities for medical professionals in the field of oncology—particularly for nurses. The first university course in oncology nursing was offered at Teachers' College, Columbia University, in New York City in 1947 (Galassi, 2000). NCI also was instrumental in increasing educational opportunities for nurses. For instance, the organization instituted a three-week educational program on cancer nursing in 1950 (Yarbro, 1996). Congress demonstrated its support for nursing education when it passed the Health Amendment Act of 1956. The Act provided financial support for nurses pursuing leadership careers in teaching, administration, clinical practice, and public health (McCabe & Piemme, 1996). Additionally, ACS continued to support oncology nursing. In 1957, ACS addressed the lack of cancer nursing literature by publishing *A Cancer Source Book for Nurses* (ACS, 1957). While educational opportunities for nurses multiplied during the 1950s, the need for more opportunities was apparent. Specifically, a 1958 ACS survey of graduate nursing programs showed that only 2 of the 22 schools that responded offered programs with cancer content (Hilkemeyer, 1985). As nursing roles in oncology became more clearly defined in the 1960s, oncology nursing evolved into a specialty area (Yarbro, 1996). As a result, hospitals began to establish specific positions for oncology nurses (Yarbro, 1996). One of the first hospitals to establish such a position was St. Jude Children's Research Hospital in Memphis, which did so in 1969 (Yarbro, 1996).

The U.S. government officially placed cancer in the limelight in 1971 when President Nixon passed the National Cancer Act. The Act not only prioritized the defeat of cancer but also provided for expansion of NCI's programs and services (Marino, 1981). Additionally, the Act authorized an annual needs budget for the National Cancer Advisory Board, in which fund requests were sent directly to the president without undergoing scrutiny from any other areas of the administration (McCabe & Piemme, 1996). This legislation also allowed for the development of numerous services, including cancer centers, community oncology programs, and nurse's training (McCabe & Piemme, 1996). National funding for cancer also increased to $379 million in 1972 from $255 million in 1971 (Yarbro, 1996).

Nurses continued to solidify their role in the fight against cancer. In 1972, the University of Texas System Cancer Center opened the first curriculum for rehabilitation of patients with cancer; here, oncology nurses were responsible for teaching patients about rehabilitative procedures (Hilkemeyer, 1985). Likewise, ACS sponsored the First National Cancer Nursing Conference in Chicago in 1973 (Hilkemeyer). In 1975, the Oncology Nursing Society (ONS) was founded (Nielsen et al., 1996). ONS rapidly established itself in the cancer community in the early 1980s and initiated the certification process for the advancement and recognition of those in the field of oncology nursing (Nielsen et al.). The Oncology Nursing Certification Corporation (ONCC), formed by ONS, was responsible for overseeing the certification process; in 1986, 1,607 registered nurses took the first Oncology Nursing Certification Exam (Nielsen et al.). As more nurses took the exam each year, ONCC continued to evaluate and revise the exam and to study nurses' decision-making and critical thinking processes as related to nursing certification exams (Nielsen et al.).

Cancer prevention and treatment methods implemented over the years began to be reflected in the statistics. In the 1980s, half of all patients with cancer were considered to be cured of their disease (Yarbro, 1996). In addition, more cancer care shifted from the academic setting to the community setting, and approximately 80% of patients with cancer were treated by oncologists in the community setting (Yarbro, 1996). The available education for cancer nursing also made great strides, as 13 graduate cancer nursing programs existed in 1981 and more than 44 such programs were in place at the end of the 1980s (Yarbro, 1996). Furthermore, cancer control efforts stretched around the world, as cancer nurse experts continued to gain recognition on an international level in 1980, at the Second International Cancer Nursing Conference in London (Yarbro, 1996).

Finally, more than 16,000 nurses were oncology certified during the past two decades as oncology nursing became more established and branched into numerous areas of specialty (Nielsen et al., 1996). Additionally, in response to a 1983 Institute of Medicine study regarding medical research, the Health Research Extension Act authorized the National Center for Nursing Research (NCNR) in 1985 to support and maintain a program of grants and awards to promote nursing research (McCabe & Piemme, 1996). Finding strength in numbers, many nursing organizations undertook effective measures to influence more legislation. For example, in 1993, the American Nurses Association initiated the Nurses Strategic Action Team, a grass roots effort to influence healthcare legislation (McCabe & Piemme). As cancer is a political as well as a medical, social, and economic issue, oncology nurses need to progressively integrate their practice into each of these areas to effectively continue the emphasis on cancer prevention and detection at various sites, which will be detailed in the following sections (ACS, 2000).

Nurses' Involvement in Cancer Prevention and Control

Skin Cancer

A review of the literature indicated that nurses are actively involved in educating the public about skin cancer and the risks of ultraviolet (UV) exposure. Nurses have (a) planned, implemented, participated in, and evaluated skin cancer screening programs in the employment and community settings; (b) coordinated clinics for pigmented lesions and individuals who are at risk for skin cancer, (c) published articles on the prevention of skin cancer for the public; and (d) conducted research designed to determine approaches to effective primary prevention (Anderson & Munson, 1990; Bargoil, 1991; Coody, 1987; Fraser, 1981, 1982; Kelly, 1991; Koh,

Lew, & Prout, 1989; Larson, 1986; Lawler, 1990; Lawler & Schreiber, 1989; Loescher & Hazelkorn, 1983; Madsen, 1988; McGuire, 1979, 1985; Roberts, 1997; Schleper, 1991; Stewart, 1990).

The nurse's role in melanoma screening, which has been detailed by multiple nurse authors (Buckley & Cody, 1990; Larson, 1986; Madsen, 1988; Roberts, 1997; Schleper, 1991), was described as educational in terms of teaching patients to recognize their own skin changes, modify their sun exposure, and participate in surveillance and early detection programs. Nurses also were urged to include in their assessment questions about first-degree relatives having either melanoma or large, unusual-looking moles (Larson). Coody (1987), of the M.D. Anderson Hospital and Tumor Institute (now the University of Texas M.D. Anderson Cancer Center), also discussed the role of the special risk nurse in a Special Risk Clinic. The special risk nurse is responsible for "obtaining risk assessment information, providing genetic and behavioral modification and surveillance counseling, instructing patients in cancer screening techniques, and coordinating clinical and basic science cancer control research" (Coody, p. 90). The high-risk clinic at M.D. Anderson Hospital was designed for families with familial cancer syndromes (e.g., polyposis coli, dysplastic nevi, cancer of the colon). Fraser (1981, 1982) at the Cancer Nursing Service, National Institutes of Health, also detailed the role of a nurse working with high-risk individuals for malignant melanoma, stressing the educational role of the nurse, which includes providing high-risk individuals "with the knowledge, skills, support, and motivation needed to prevent and control melanoma" (Fraser, 1981, p. 92). McGuire (1979, 1985), in her discussion of the educational and psychosocial needs of families with hereditary cutaneous malignant melanoma, supported the educational role of the nurse that Fraser advocated when working with high-risk groups. She stated that nurses must continue to act as role models, practice "sun sensibility," and educate patients, colleagues, friends, families, and the community at large.

Misconceptions abound about the safety of indoor tanning because tanning booths have been incorrectly advertised as "safe" and capable of protecting the skin from further ultraviolet B (UVB) damage. Stewart (1990), therefore, advocated that nurses take an active role in educating the public about the implications of indoor tanning and preventing skin damage. Such education should include the information that tanning represents the body's response to injury, causes premature aging, and may cause increased damage to an area of the body not normally exposed to the sun.

An innovative approach to educating the general public and promoting screening for early skin cancer was discussed by Anderson and Munson (1990). The oncology nursing staff at North Memorial Medical Center in Minnesota designed and implemented a day-long skin cancer fair. Titled "Be Smart in the Sun: Slip, Slop, Slap," the fair provided an on-site educational program covering information on the incidence, risk factors, early detection, and prevention of skin cancer. The fair included displays, music, refreshments, minilectures, consultation sessions with on-staff dermatologists, and give-aways of sun protection materials, colorful posters, and handouts. Organizers used a quiz to measure participants' knowledge of sun protection to evaluate the effectiveness of the fair.

Kelly (1991) discussed another innovative approach to educating the public about skin cancer. Occupational health nurses throughout Texas were involved in the state skin cancer/melanoma awareness project, instructing employees at a multiplicity of worksites during the campaign. The nurses enlisted the cooperation of the Texas Cosmetology Commission to do a mass mailing. The letter from the commission urged the cosmetologists to examine the scalp, head, and neck areas of their clients for signs of skin cancer. One occupational nurse who was employed by a large outdoor amusement park convinced management to sponsor a skin cancer awareness day at the park, which included the distribution of educational materials, hats, and sunscreen samples. The success of the campaign was confirmed by the scores on post-tests given by an independent survey agency, showing a significant increase in skin cancer awareness and knowledge.

The healthcare professional's important role in changing behavior was documented by Buller, Callister, and Reichert (1995). They found the parents who more frequently received information from healthcare providers practiced more prevention strategies. Buller et al. (1995) noted that "nurses and other healthcare providers are influential sources of skin cancer prevention information . . . healthcare providers must be a main source of skin cancer prevention messages" (p. 1565).

The "Slip! Slop! Slap!" message originally was developed in 1981 in Australia by the Anti-Cancer Council of Victoria. It stands for *slip* on a shirt, *slop* on some sunscreen, and *slap* on a hat ("Education," 1988) A Slip! Slop! Slap! kit was made available to Australian primary schools, t-shirts with this message were worn by life guards, and TV messages were designed for the Australian population.

Nurses have been involved in research to determine the most effective methods of educating individuals at risk for skin cancer. Kersey and Kroll (1985) conducted a Sunscreen Consulting Project with 31 people with malignant melanoma and/or dysplastic nevus syndrome. In this project, the physician or nurse counseled these high-risk patients in measures to prevent a second primary skin cancer. A pretest/post-test research design demonstrated that this multidisciplinary approach to cancer prevention increased the awareness of the danger of UV exposure and the need to use sunscreens. Marlenga (1995) surveyed 202 Wisconsin farmers and found that, although they were knowledgeable about skin cancer and acknowledged their own high risk, they did not practice sun protection. The author suggested that nurses help to develop skin cancer prevention education that addresses the barriers to the use of sunscreen and protective clothing. These strategies include working with sunscreen manufacturers to develop and market products that farmers could apply easily while doing farm work. Developing magnets or bumper stickers would help to create awareness among farmers to protect their skin with sunscreen, as would writing articles for magazines, newspapers, radio, and television targeted to agricultural workers on skin cancer prevention.

Owen (1989) also studied the psychosocial effects of having a history of melanoma. Her research findings pointed out that intervention strategies to promote melanoma-preventive health practices must stress the benefits of performing skin self-examination and minimize the perceived barriers to observing this primary prevention practice.

The nurse's role in helping to lower the incidence of skin cancer involves urging people to modify sun-seeking behavior (i.e., indoor and outdoor tanning). Trying to change the popular mind-set about having that "healthy glow" is not easy. Tan, weathered skin used to be identified with the working class, but now it indicates a person has the time and money to enjoy outdoor leisure. The nursing assessment should speak to the individual's attitude about tanning, identify those who use tanning booths, document the history of sun exposure and family history of skin diseases (especially genetically related diseases, such as dysplastic nevus syndrome), and assess the skin for suspicious lesions and moles that warrant a physician referral. Routine skin self-examination should be taught to all individuals who are frequent users of indoor tanning booths.

Oral Cancer

A review of 20 years of the abstracts submitted to ONS for presentation at annual ONS Congresses showed very few abstracts related to the prevention and early detection of oral cancer. The following submitted abstracts are two examples of the many areas available for nurses to conduct research and teach about prevention at the same time.

Klatt-Ellis (1988) surveyed high school students in grades 9–12 to determine their usage of and knowledge of the health implications of smokeless tobacco. Her findings showed a heavy usage of smokeless tobacco among boys (37%) and the need for more surveys of this type in high schools in different geographic areas. "Information gleaned from an assessment study such as this can guide educational programming in the high-school setting" (p. 126).

A similar research approach was taken by Schulmeister (1986). In collaboration with a dentist, Schulmeister surveyed 200 adults from the dental practice about the symptoms of oral cancer and related risk factors. Data showed widespread misconceptions about the early symptoms of oral cancer and total lack of knowledge about conducting oral self-assessments. When given a pamphlet explaining how to conduct oral self-assessment, the majority of these adults indicated that they probably would not do it because "sores are so common." These findings led Schulmeister to advocate that "teaching, screening, and detecting oral cancer by oncology nurses is critically needed" (p. 63).

White (1983, 1986) and Frank-Stromborg (1986, 1989; Frank-Stromborg & Cohen, 1997; Frank-Stromborg, Johnson, & McCorkle, 1987; Frank-Stromborg, Heusinkveld, & Rohan, 1996), two nurses who have published extensively on the nurse's role in primary and secondary prevention of cancer, proposed numerous responsibilities related to oral cancer for nurses. Nurses should (a) routinely obtain information from patients regarding their risk factors for oral cancer; (b) when appropriate, conduct an oral assessment using the physical assessment techniques of inspection and palpation; (c) teach all high-risk individuals oral self-assessment and emphasize the importance of this self-examination technique; (d) stress the relationship of tobacco and alcohol to the development of oral cancer; and (e) make community referrals to assist high-risk individuals who are interested in stopping use of tobacco and/or decreasing alcohol intake.

The literature review documented that nurses who were involved in the prevention and early detection of oral cancer tended to function in ambulatory settings exclusively devoted to cancer screening (O'Rourke, Gypson, & Weitberg, 1986; Nelson-Marten & Krebs, 1991; Warren & Pohl, 1990). Nurses in traditional settings (e.g., staff nursing, public health nursing, occupational nursing) do not appear to be using available opportunities to conduct risk assessments and oral examinations or to provide information on performing oral self-assessment and the relationship between risk factors and the development of oral cancer. Exceptions to this statement are the recent articles by Aubertin (1997), Shugars and Patton (1997), and Bonner (1998), which may herald a change in approach to oral cancer. Aubertin detailed all the ways home healthcare nurses could be involved in performing oral cancer screening examinations on the elderly. Shugars and Patton provided an educational article for nurse practitioners engaged in primary care on conducting screening examinations for the early detection of oral cancer. Bonner wrote about the national Oral Cancer Awareness Program developed by the Oral Health Education Foundation. This multidisciplinary program is designed to facilitate cooperation among the various healthcare disciplines, including nursing.

The importance of having nurses in all settings involved in conducting oral examinations is underscored by the Healthy People 2010 goal to increase to at least 40% the proportion of people age 50 years or older who have received an oral examination while visiting a healthcare provider during the preceding year ("Examinations," 1994). In 1992, the Centers for Disease Control and Prevention (CDC) analyzed data from the National Health Interview Survey—Cancer Control supplement to determine the frequency of oral cancer examinations among the public. Overall, only 14.3% of the survey respondents reported that they had been examined for oral cancer. What is even more disturbing is that current smokers, a high-risk group, were less likely to report an examination than were former smokers. As a result of the survey, the CDC convened a national conference in 1997 on the early detection of oral cancer and established priority strategies that included the promotion of a multidisciplinary approach to the early detection of oral cancer ("Preventing and Controlling Oral and Pharyngeal Cancer," 1998). If the Healthy People 2010 goal related to oral cancer is to be achieved, nurses are going to have to be actively involved regardless of specialty or practice setting.

Gastric Cancer

Nurses can take several specific actions toward the primary prevention of gastric cancer. These include being knowledgeable about the risk factors for this type of cancer, the research-based recommended dietary changes, and the screening procedures that can decrease one's risk. Because the risk of developing gastric cancer is believed to be determined by exposures occurring in the first two decades of life, educational programs should be aggressively targeted to parents of young children (Frank-Stromborg, 1989). These educational programs should detail the specific dietary changes that will lower an individual's risk and should be incorporated into the family's dietary lifestyle. When dietary changes are recommended, it is best to keep any suggestions simple, practical, and cost-effective.

A review of abstracts submitted to ONS for presentation at the annual ONS Congresses during the past decade, as well as the abstract books and proceedings of the second through sixth International Conference on Cancer Nursing, uncovered no abstracts related to the primary and secondary prevention of gastric cancer. Sawyers and Eaton (1992) published an article on gastric cancer in Korean Americans that details the cultural practices of Korean Americans that may increase their risk for gastric cancer and influence response to treatment. Although gastric cancer is one of the leading causes of cancer-related deaths in many countries of the world, there does not appear to be much energy directed to prevention by nurses outside of the United States. The incidence of gastric cancer has dramatically decreased in the United States, but this picture may change with the aging of the American population. More people are living longer, and increased age is a significant risk factor for this type of cancer.

Esophageal Cancer

Mackel and Greski (1990) examined the nurse's role related to the early detection of esophageal cancer. The Tucson Veteran's Medical Center set up a nursing clinic to follow patients with Barrett's esophagus. Barrett's esophagus, a complication of chronic gastroesophageal reflux, is an acquired premalignant condition of the esophagus. Many of the patients seen in this clinic are smokers and/or heavy alcohol drinkers. The nursing role in this clinic includes early cancer detection, patient education, lifestyle and risk-factor modification, symptom control, and assistance with chemoprevention trials being conducted with this high-risk population.

Pervan (1988), a nurse in the Republic of South Africa, wrote about the high incidence of esophageal cancer in this region as well as the enormous difficulties associated with instituting early detection measures with rural Africans. Rural Africans are at high risk for this cancer because of their diet of maize, which is low in vitamin B content and tends to be infected with aflatoxin, and their high incidence of smoking. The author cited the need for oncology nurse involvement in community education at the grass roots level, which incorporates the tribal healer as well as the health beliefs of the African culture. This example of culturally sensitive intervention can be generalized to all ethnic or racial groups.

In general, the role of the nurse in the primary prevention of esophageal cancer involves taking an active part in patient counseling and programs geared toward prevention and cessation of all forms of smoking and alcohol abuse. Another preventive aspect involves education of high-risk individuals about the dangers of routinely eating and drinking excessively hot foods or beverages. Although it is recommended that nurses provide prevention-oriented education at the individual level, it is recognized that the prevention of cancer of the esophagus necessitates a broader, more comprehensive approach (Frank-Stromborg, 1989). Nurses can assume an active role in working with the government in establishing primary prevention programs at the local and national levels.

Colorectal Cancer

Colorectal screening has been found to be beneficial in detecting colorectal cancers in their earliest stages, which improves the likelihood of survival. Nurses play a key role in educating the public on these prevention and screening strategies. Occupational health nurses and cancer education nurses have been successful in providing worksite programs to employees on the early warning signs of colorectal cancer and recommended screening protocols. Messner and Gardner (1985) realized an 80% compliance rate in serial guaiac stool screening in the work setting. The authors attribute their success to the relationships that they had already developed with employees and their families.

One goal of *Healthy People 2010* is to reduce the number of colorectal cancer deaths in the United States to no more than 13.2 per 100,000 people from the age-adjusted baseline of 14.4 per 100,000 in 1987 (U.S. Department of Health and Human Services, 1990). Burris and McGovern (1993) recommended that occupational health nurses make educating employees about colorectal cancer screening a priority. These recommendations take into account the company's need to be fiscally sound and provide the greatest benefit to all employees. Minimizing the number of sick days taken and the amount of monetary reimbursement is an advantage to both. The recommendations include educating employees on the known risk factors and disease signs and symptoms; in an environment where the prevalence warrants a mass screening, to identify the high-risk individuals for the appropriate screening method; and to support follow-up and referral procedures (Burris & McGovern).

Colorectal cancer incidence and mortality rates are higher and survival rates lower for African Americans than for Whites. Frank-Stromborg, Johnson, and McCorkle (1987) developed workshops specifically for African American nurses that included information about cancer epidemiology in African Americans, cultural attitudes toward cancer, and early detection procedures for this population. Continuation of these workshops throughout the United States and related research by Olsen and Frank-Stromborg (1991) documented the positive impact of the educational intervention on the African American community. These programs assist in reaching the populations at high risk and ultimately have an impact on overall cancer mortality by increasing survival rates for colorectal cancer. Mitchell-Beren, Dodds, Choi, and Waskerwitz (1989) reached out to the African American population by educating African American nurses and helping them to set up programs in their churches. The authors found this approach to be effective in getting the information to the parishioners and in gaining compliance with screening strategies.

ACS, in conjunction with school health-education teachers, developed interactive programs to teach children the dietary recommendations for cancer prevention. However, Krohner, McBurney, and Wadelin (1988) found few studies or programs that focused on the prevention of colon cancer by educating children about diet during their formative years. They recommended more programs like ACS's "Great American Pigout" to aid in educating school-age children on proper nutrition in the prevention of colon and other cancers.

High-risk individuals have special needs and require specific surveillance measures. Nurses working with high-risk families are in a "pivotal role by teaching surveillance and early detection measures, assisting in role-playing, explaining hereditary cancer risk factors, supporting families through the ambivalence of a diagnosis of a hereditary disease, and fostering positive coping behaviors in general" (Fitzsimmons, Conway, Madsen, Lappe, & Coody, 1989, p. 93). Nurses are involved in multiple areas of primary and secondary prevention of colorectal cancer. They are educating patients in the dietary modifications necessary to decrease the incidence of this cancer. Nurses also are encouraging individuals to follow the guidelines established by ACS through community-based, creative, nontraditional educational offerings. Furthermore, they are educating individuals about serial guaiac testing, sigmoidoscopy, and the rationale for radiographic testing (Post-White, Herzan, & Drew, 1988; Wilkes & Bersani, 1983). In selected institutions in the United States, nurses and nurse practitioners are performing fiber-optic sigmoidoscopies. Research conducted by Spencer and Ready (1977) demonstrated that having specially trained nurses perform sigmoidoscopies significantly increased the number of elderly people who could be screened. The literature documents that nurses are involved with individuals from families at increased risk for the development of colorectal cancer through specialized clinics and programs. Nursing research conducted with high-risk populations found that the needs of these individuals are diverse and the psychosocial implications are far-reaching (Coody, 1987).

If the Healthy People 2010 goal is to be reached, all nurses must make a concerted effort to educate individuals on risk factors and screening modalities. Nurses must be actively involved in screening activities and support the guidelines established.

Testicular Cancer

The major role nurses play in the prevention and early detection of testicular cancer is to educate young men on the importance of practicing regular testicular self-examination (TSE). The best defense against testicular cancer is a well-educated male population that practices TSE and understands the importance of seeking medical attention when a lump is discovered. This point is key for school and pediatric nurses, who have the most contact with young men. Authorities advocate that education about TSE begin in the grammar schools as part of health education classes (Carlin, 1986; Marty & McDermott, 1983; Williams, 1981). Nursing research has demonstrated that college-age men were lacking in knowledge regarding testicular cancer and self-examination and benefited from nursing efforts aimed at educating them on testicular cancer and self-examination (Rudolf & Quinn, 1988). Stack (1979) developed a plan and teaching tool for high-school students regarding testicular cancer that provided a standard and an organized method to follow.

The lack of knowledge regarding testicular cancer and TSE is not limited to men. Stanford (1987) conducted a research study in England and found that 64.5% of the nurses surveyed did not remember being taught TSE in their nursing programs. Additionally, although two-thirds of the nurses felt it was their role to teach TSE, very few had actually taught anyone the technique. Similar findings were demonstrated in studies conducted by Warren and Pohl (1990) and Conroy (1986).

The majority of research has demonstrated a lack of knowledge regarding testicular cancer risk factors and screening. Studies have shown the effectiveness of nursing education in increasing the number of men performing self-examination (Rudolf & Quinn, 1988). Nurses, therefore, need to focus on educating men and their significant others on testicular examination to increase the number of men performing monthly TSE. The key to long-term survival and a decrease in morbidity requires early detection through the simple self-examination. Nurses need to continue to find strategies for getting this information to men in a way that will be heard, considered, and acted upon. Instilling in very young men the importance of this screening and developing the habit at a young age will lead to a lifelong commitment.

Prostate Cancer

In an article written in 1991 on the nurse's role in cancer prevention and early detection, Frank-Stromborg and Rohan (1992) noted that they could not locate any reports devoted solely to the nurse's role in preventing or detecting prostate cancer. Rather, they found several reports about nurse-run screening/prevention clinics that included prostate cancer screening. Stoltzfus and Ashby (1990) reported a mobile screening program that was a joint venture between the City of Hope National Medical Center in Duarte, CA, and ACS. This mobile screening program was designed to educate and screen individuals within the workplace, senior citizen centers, and community ethnic groups. A nurse practitioner conducted the examination, which included screening for testicular, prostate, and rectal cancer. In 34 months of operation, 10,500 people were educated and nearly 7,700 individuals were screened, with a 25.9% referral rate for suspicious findings. Nelson-Marten and Krebs (1991) reported a nurse-managed cancer prevention/screening clinic that evaluated the cancer risk and concerns of healthy, asymptomatic adults. The nursing role in this clinic included performing a cancer risk assessment and physical examination and teaching risk reduction. In eight months of operation, 100 healthy adults were seen, and about one-third were referred to a specific physician or to another clinic for follow-up.

A more recent review of the literature revealed a plethora of articles and abstracts detailing numerous roles nurses have assumed in the early detection of this cancer (Casale, 1999; Collins, 1997; Greco & Kulawiak, 1994; Lazzaro & Thompson, 1997; Mahon, 1995; McKee, 1994; Peate, 1998; Plowden, 1998; Tingen, Weinrich, Heydt, Boyd, & Weinrich, 1998; Weinrich, Weinrich, Boyd, & Atkinson, 1998; Zimmerman, 1997). Many of the articles detailed nursing research designed to determine the factors that influence men to attend a prostate screening program; typical of this line of research is the work of Tingen et al. Weinrich et al. investigated if perceived benefit was a predictor of participation in free prostate cancer screening. They found that predictors of participation in free screening programs were perceived benefit, being White, having at least a high school education, being married, and the type of educational intervention delivered. When all demographic variables and educational interventions were controlled, perceived benefit was significant as a predictor for men participating in the prostate screening program.

Weinrich et al. (1998) also documented that men who had more knowledge of prostate cancer were more likely to participate in a free prostate cancer screening. This finding was the result of a year-long series of community-based educational programs conducted throughout a southern state by a team of nurse researchers. The educational offerings were presented in churches, barber shops, senior citizen mealsites, housing projects, and National Association for the Advancement of Colored People (NAACP) headquarters. The educational programs were race-specific to appeal to both White and African American male audiences. The researchers determined that nurses should target African American and socioeconomically disadvantaged men for prostate cancer screening and educational programs to increase early detection of the disease. Collins' (1997) research supports the concept of providing educational programs to African American men to increase their participation in screening programs. The importance of educating men about this specific cancer is underscored by the work of Zimmerman (1997) and Peate (1998). Peate conducted her research in England, were she found that only 3 of 40 men asked to identify the prostate gland were able to do so. "These results indicate that men's perceptions of their bodies may be incorrect. It is evident that more work is needed to inform men of their bodies and promote their health" (p. 199). Zimmerman's research documented that promoting awareness of this cancer is one of the most effective strategies for increasing prostate screening participation among Hispanics.

Because prostate cancer is the primary cancer in men, nurses play an essential role in prevention and early detection of this cancer (Plowden, 1998). A recent literature review clearly demonstrated the involvement of nurses in the education, counseling, and screening of men for this cancer. Nurses must find ways to disseminate information on prostate cancer to the African American male population and encourage their participation in early detection programs. The best way to reduce prostate cancer mortality is by diagnosing men when they are asymptomatic, and nursing research can determine the best means of attaining this goal.

Gynecological Cancers
Cervical Cancer

Nurses have played various roles in the prevention and early detection of cervical cancer, including role modeling, educating, and performing gynecologic examinations. Role modeling involves practicing the prevention strategies recommended and following the screening guidelines. McMillan (1990) surveyed RNs in southwest Florida and found that the majority (57%) of nurses who responded to her survey reported having had a Pap test within the past three years; an additional 22% had undergone a hysterectomy and, thus, were not eligible for cervical smears.

Nurses have taken a very active role in educating women who are at increased risk for the development of cervical cancer. Schulmeister and Lifsey (1999) assessed Vietnamese women's knowledge, behaviors, and beliefs regarding cervical cancer screening and found that this high-risk group does not adhere to the screening guidelines; interventions need to focus on this group, taking into account their cultural beliefs. Kim et al. (1999) conducted a similar study in the Korean American population and found that only 34% of respondents reported having had a Pap smear. Both of these studies point toward the need to develop strategies for educating these two high-risk groups on the importance of screening and then making the screening available. Mahon (1996) developed a brochure on Pap testing and found it to be effective in educating a large number of women about gynecologic cancers.

Cava, Greenberg, Fitch, Spaner, and Taylor (1997) developed a community coalition in two low-income communities in North York. The goal of the coalition was to reduce mortality and morbidity related to cervical cancer by developing a program to reduce barriers to Pap screening among young low-income women. They accomplished this goal through involving the community, educating the women, providing a supportive environment, educating healthcare professionals, and providing advocacy. The authors found that a multiple-strategy approach with a team of individuals dedicated to the ultimate goal was needed. A similar approach was taken by nurses in an inner-city clinic in Chicago to reach the high-risk women they serve (Ansell, Lacey, Whitman, Chen, & Phillips, 1994). These types of programs should be set up in all areas where the need is the greatest.

Nurses' involvement in the early detection of cervical cancer also is important in developing countries. In Ireland and Finland, public health nurses are trained in performing cervical smears and educate women on the need for screening (Gillat, 1984; Massingberd, 1988). Nurses have set up mobile health vans to deliver education and screening to elderly women who may not be able to get to a clinic or hospital (Melillo, 1985).

Nurses have taken an active role in the prevention and early detection of cervical cancer by seeking innovative ways to reach the public, but the need continues for further development of programs to help the women at greatest risk. Complacency would be easy because cervical cancer incidence is decreasing, but in certain cultures and low-income areas, the number of invasive cancers continues to rise. They are the ones for which strategies need to be developed and priorities set.

Endometrial Cancer

Nurses' role in prevention and early detection of endometrial cancer focuses on education. Nurses must make women aware of the importance of undergoing an annual pelvic examination—especially the elderly. Smith (1995) developed a Women's Health Promotion project in a nurse-managed center to promote annual cancer screening for breast, cervical, and endometrial cancer in the elderly. More programs such as this need to be developed to reduce the mortality and morbidity of these cancers in the elderly, who are at the greatest risk. Nurses will need to assist patients in determining their risk for endometrial cancer and weighing that risk with their risk for heart disease, osteoporosis, and breast cancer in helping them to determine whether to take hormone replacement and/or tamoxifen.

Ovarian Cancer

Nurses need to teach women the risk factors for ovarian cancer and instruct them on the benefits of a low-fat, high-vitamin-A diet. Nurses should provide education on personal hygiene with emphasis on minimizing perineal exposure to chemicals. Nurses play a key role in clinics that provide screening for women at increased risk for the development of ovarian cancer. They make significant contributions to genetic counseling and maximizing screening strategies (Farley, 1999). If the incidence of gynecologic cancer is to be decreased, more nurses will need to be educated in and become active in the primary and early detection of ovarian cancer. More nursing research is indicated to investigate effective strategies in the dissemination of information regarding gynecologic cancers, especially in high-risk populations.

Lung Cancer

Nurses have been instrumental in the implementation of legislation to create smoke-free settings, smoking cessation counseling, antismoking education, and structured smoking cessation programs. Most importantly, nurses must act as role models by not smoking and by enforcing no-smoking policies. Because research has clearly documented that attitudes of healthcare professionals may influence patients to start or stop smoking, extensive writing and research had been conducted about the smoking habits and smoking-related attitudes of nurses (Casey, Haughey, Dittmar, O'Shea, & Brasure, 1989; DeMello, Hoffman, Wesmiller, & Zullo, 1989; Feldman & Richard, 1986; Gritz & Kanim, 1986). It is encouraging that research has shown a decline in nurse smokers. In a comparison study of critical-care nurses and medical-surgical nurses, DeMello et al. found that oncology clinical nurse specialists had the lowest prevalence of cigarette smoking among the nursing groups. Nurses must stand strong against the tobacco industry, play a role in antismoking campaigns, and work diligently to encourage adolescents to never start to smoke.

Breast Cancer

Tamoxifen has been shown in clinical trials to prevent the occurrence of cancer in the opposite breast of women who have been diagnosed with breast cancer. The Study of Tamoxifen and Raloxifene (STAR) trial is under way to compare tamoxifen to raloxifene in postmenopausal women who are at increased risk for the development of breast cancer. This trial may lead to the use of these drugs as a cancer prevention strategy for all women. Nurses play an integral role in data management and educating women about participation in the trial.

A review of the literature documented nursing involvement in many aspects of early detection of breast cancer. Nurses have been more involved in breast cancer prevention and early detection than in any other cancer site. Nurses teach breast self-examination (BSE) and have conducted research into the factors that encourage or impede women from doing BSE (Champion, 1987; Fletcher et al., 1990; Hallal, 1982; Houfek, Waltman, & Kile, 1997; Massey, 1986; Olson & Mitchell, 1989; Rutledge & Davis, 1988). Nurses have investigated the use of BSE in women in rural areas (Gray, 1990); in women with learning disabilities (Fletcher, 1998); in African American women (Brown & Williams, 1994; Nemcek, 1989; Willis, Davis, Cairns, & Janiszewski, 1989; Wilson, 1989); Mexican American women (Gonzalez, 1990; Longman, Modiano-Revah, & Saint-Germain, 1990); Chinese American women with a history of breast cancer (Doyle & Simonich, 1991; Facciponti & Cartwright, 1988); and adolescents (Kitson, 1989; Sheehan, Michalek, & Cassidy, 1981). Nurses have conducted research on their peers' attitudes about and ability to perform BSE (Cole & Gorman, 1984; Lillington, Padilla, Sayre, & Chlebowski, 1993). Nurses have investigated performance issues related to teaching BSE

(Ford & Martin, 1995; Leslie & Roche, 1997; Marty, McDermott, & Gold, 1983; Smith, 1991). Several nurses have established programs to reach the elderly in long-term facilities (Kenny & Keenan, 1991) and in home care (Williams, 1989). Caplan & Coughlin (1998) conducted a review of worksite breast cancer screening programs and found this to be an effective strategy for reaching women, but there is a need to establish more of these programs and monitor their impact on early detection.

Future Roles for Nursing in Cancer Prevention and Early Detection

Nursing interventions have focused primarily on the prevention and early detection of cancer in a few selected anatomic sites (e.g., breast, prostate); our control efforts in other cancer sites have been limited. In a previous report on the roles of nursing in cancer prevention and control (Frank-Stromborg & Rohan, 1992), the authors concluded that nurses need to broaden their primary prevention activities to include more anatomical sites. They argued that nurses had expended tremendous time and energy on the primary prevention of breast cancer and little time on other cancers. Today, much more information is available on nurses' primary prevention activities for oral, gastric, liver, and testicular cancers. Still, there is much room for improvement.

The "graying of America" underscores the need to expand the number of cancer sites included in primary prevention activities. By 2004, it is estimated that more than 25% of the population will be over age 65, with the fastest-growing segment being those over age 75. Many cancers become more prevalent with aging, such as gastric cancer, with the peak age of occurrence after age 75. Nurses should prepare to provide prevention and screening care for the cancers that will occur concomitantly with the aging of the American population.

Another strong recommendation is that nurses should have a more prominent role in primary prevention clinical trials. Nurses are essential in the development and management of clinical trial research. Unfortunately, the public view of clinical trial nurses appears to be limited to collecting data or other fairly restrictive roles. Nursing needs to take leadership roles in primary prevention clinical trials and ultimately serve in the principal investigator role. Nursing must take a stronger stance in the emerging areas of chemoprevention, genetic research, and genetic counseling. If nursing does not become actively involved in genetic counseling related to cancer prevention/early detection, other disciplines will step in and claim this territory. Nurses in doctoral programs need to be actively encouraged to do their dissertations and to focus their long-term research efforts in the area of primary prevention. This would put nurse PhDs in position to take leadership roles in related clinical trials.

Many of the primary prevention programs discussed by Frank-Stromborg and Rohan (1992) took place in traditional settings within hospitals or hospital systems. More programs need to be offered in community and workplace settings.

The workplace programs that nurses have conducted owe their success to three main factors: they were convenient, had the approval and support of management, and required little effort to attend. Nurses need to conduct prevention and early detection programs throughout every community in culture-specific settings. Bringing programs to churches, ethnic social organizations, fraternal societies, sisterhoods, religious communities, and self-help groups are just a few ways nurses can reach people.

The need exists for more creative, community-based prevention/early detection programs that address all age groups rather than continuing to concentrate efforts primarily on adults. The ideal educational approach is to begin primary prevention programs in preschool settings, build on these themes throughout the entire educational experience, and carry them over into the workplace, military, and religious settings. Presently, primary prevention programs are offered sporadically and based on the availability of funds, personnel, and national trends.

A primary prevention educational approach that permeates all aspects of our society requires a national commitment to this idea. Nurses need to become politically active and work for legislation to meet this goal. Increasing the visibility of nursing's agenda to lawmakers would be the first step toward increased Medicare coverage for cancer screening and funds for teaching school children about primary prevention. Oncology nurses need to be involved in setting the national agenda for cancer primary prevention and work to bring the different health interest groups together to deliver one unified message. The national organizations devoted to preventing heart disease, respiratory disease, and cancer could join together to deliver a strong message about lifestyle changes that would lower the risk for all three. A hospital in Illinois offers both a mammogram and an ultra-fast heart scan at the same screening program.

Wonderful strides have been made in bringing cancer prevention/early detection activities to minority and rural communities by educating minority nurses in the principles of primary prevention. In the 1980s, ONS, with funding from the NCI, offered a series of national workshops specifically designed for African American, Hispanic, Native American, and Asian /Pacific Islander nurses. These workshops were designed to provide minority nurses with the knowledge and skills to design and implement prevention and screening programs in their communities. Much more is needed to ensure that economically disadvantaged and remote rural residents have access to cancer prevention/early detection services. National statistics continue to reflect that minority populations (e.g., African Americans, Hispanics) have their cancers diagnosed at later stages and have lower survival rates than other groups. Nurses need to work with other disciplines in offering community-based programs to minorities and underserved communities. Nursing tends to engage in cancer prevention/early detection activities within the profession rather than working to establish and coordinate a multidisciplinary team approach. Involving other health professions would enable nurses to offer more creative and broader-based primary prevention programs.

The last recommendation is for nursing to continue to be involved in the design and implementation of antismoking programs. In the 1970s and 1980s, there was an antitobacco movement in the United States, and nurses were actively involved in its promotion. In the 1990s, society's focus changed to anti-drug efforts, and the antitobacco movement took a back seat. As a result, increasing numbers of teenagers are smoking cigarettes and cigars. Tobacco use in developing countries is epidemic. Even in the wake of the tobacco settlement, regulations against tobacco product advertising, and the increase in the number of smoke-free settings, one cannot assume that there is no longer a need to continue antitobacco efforts. Each new year brings a cohort of children who need to be educated about the dangers of smoking and use of other tobacco products.

While great strides have been made by oncology nursing in many areas, the war remains and the goals remain unmet. The accomplishments that can be attributed to nursing during the last 150 years are no less than awesome. Nurses' contributions to oncology have helped to make it what it is today—a place where people are cured of what was once incurable. Nurses have taken what Florence Nightingale taught them about preventing illness and applied it to preventing cancer. Nursing research has made a difference in the quality of life for so many people. The innovative ideas of nurse researchers inspire others to find better ways of solving health problems. A high point in the history of the nursing profession is the effort directed toward the prevention, detection, and control of cancer. It is the authors' hope that the chapters that follow will help in this effort.

References

American Cancer Society. (1957). *A cancer source book for nurses.* New York: Author.

American Cancer Society. (2000). *ACS history and mission.* Retrieved August 25, 2000 from the World Wide Web: http://www2.cancer.org/about_acs/index.cfm?sc=1

Anderson, S., & Munson, N. (1990). Skin cancer fair in the hospital setting [Abstract 268]. *Oncology Nursing Forum, 17,* 204.

Ansell, D., Lacey, L., Whitman, S., Chen, E., & Phillips, C. (1994). A nurse-delivered intervention to reduce barriers to breast and cervical cancer screening in Chicago inner city clinics. *Public Health Reports, 109,* 104–111.

Aubertin, M. (1997). Oral cancer screening in the elderly: The home healthcare nurse's role. *Home Health Nurse, 15,* 594–602.

Bargoil, S. (1991). Skin cancer prevention: "Do you know which sunscreen to use?" [Abstract 135]. *Oncology Nursing Forum, 18,* 383.

Bonner, P. (1998). The National Oral Cancer Awareness Program. *ORL-Head and Neck Nursing, 16*(2), 15–19.

Brown, L.W., & Williams, R.D. (1994). Culturally sensitive breast cancer screening programs for older black women. *Nurse Practitioner, 19*(3), 21–31.

Buckley, M., & Cody, B. (1990). Prevention and early detection of skin cancer: A comprehensive overview [Abstract 225]. *Oncology Nursing Forum, 17,* 194.

Buller, D., Callister, M., & Reichert, T. (1995). Skin cancer prevention by parents of young children: Health information sources, skin cancer knowledge, and sun-practices. *Oncology Nursing Forum, 17,* 204.

Burris, J., & McGovern, P. (1993). Mass colorectal cancer screening: Choosing an effective strategy. *American Association of Occupational Health Nurses Journal, 41*(4), 186–191.

Caplan, L.S., & Coughlin, S.S. (1998). Worksite breast cancer screening programs: A review. *AAOHN Journal, 46,* 443–453.

Carlin, P.J. (1986). Testicular self-examination: A public awareness program. *Public Health Reports, 101,* 98–102.

Casale, M. (1999). Using focus groups to assess participation in a prostate cancer screening program: A qualitative perspective [Abstract 118]. *Oncology Nursing Forum, 26,* 383.

Casey, F., Haughey, B., Dittmar, S., O'Shea, R., & Brasure, J. (1989). Smoking practices among nursing students: A comparison of two studies. *Journal of Nursing Education, 28,* 397–401.

Cava, M., Greenberg, M., Fitch, M., Spaner, D., & Taylor, K. (1997). Towards an inclusive cervical cancer screening strategy: Approaches for reaching socioeconomically disadvantaged women. *Canadian Oncology Nursing Journal, 7*(1), 14–18.

Champion, V. (1987). The relationship of breast self-examination to health belief model variables. *Advances in Nursing Research, 10,* 375–382.

Cole, C.F., & Gorman, L.M. (1984). Breast self-examination: Practices and attitudes of registered nurses. *Oncology Nursing Forum, 11*(5), 37–41.

Collins, M. (1997). Increasing prostate cancer awareness in African American men. *Oncology Nursing Forum, 24,* 91–95.

Conroy, C. (1986). A pilot project implementing breast self-exam (BSE) and testicular self-exam (TSE) teaching on one hospital unit [Abstract 52]. *Oncology Nursing Forum, 13*(2), 68.

Coody, D. (1987). Special risk clinic [Abstract 35A]. *Oncology Nursing Forum, 14*(2), 90.

DeMello, D.J., Hoffman, L.A., Wesmiller, S.W., & Zullo, T.G. (1989). Smoking and attitudes toward smoking among clinical nurse specialists, critical care nurses, and medical-surgical nurses. *Oncology Nursing Forum, 16,* 795–799.

Doyle, M.A., & Simonich, W. (1991). Comparison of breast self-examination (BSE) practices in women with breast cancer versus women with a non-breast primary [Abstract 193]. *Oncology Nursing Forum, 18,* 392.

Education about skin cancer. (1988). *Cancer News, 11,* 9–12.

Examinations for oral cancer—United States, 1992. (1994). *Morbidity and Mortality Weekly Report, 43,* 198–200.

Facciponti, C.A., & Cartwright, F. (1988). Identifying barriers to breast self examination practice in post mastectomy patients [Abstract 235]. *Oncology Nursing Forum, 15,* 160.

Farley, K. (1999). Ovarian cancer early detection program. *Oncology Nursing Forum, 26,* 833.

Feldman, B., & Richard, E. (1986). Prevalence of nurse smokers and variables identified with successful and unsuccessful smoking cessation. *Research in Nursing and Health, 9,* 131–138.

Fitzsimmons, M., Conway, T., Madsen, N., Lappe, J., & Coody, D. (1989). Hereditary cancer syndromes: Nursing's role in identification and education. *Oncology Nursing Forum, 16,* 87–94.

Fletcher, M.C. (1998). Breast awareness project for women with a learning disability. *British Journal of Nursing, 7,* 774–778.

Fletcher, S.W., O'Malley, M.S., Earp, J.L., Morgan, T.M., Lin, S., & Degnan, D. (1990). How best to teach women breast self-examination: A randomized controlled trial. *Annals of Internal Medicine, 112,* 772–779.

Ford, M.B., & Martin, R.D. (1995). Longitudinal evaluation of a breast cancer training module: Preliminary results. *Cancer, 76 (Suppl.* 10), 2125–2132.

Frank-Stromborg, M. (1986). The role of the nurse in early detection of cancer: Population sixty-six years of age and older. *Oncology Nursing Forum, 13*(3), 66–74.

Frank-Stromborg, M. (1989). The epidemiology and primary prevention of gastric and esophageal cancer. A worldwide perspective. *Cancer Nursing, 12*(2), 53–64.

Frank-Stromborg, M., & Cohen, K. (1997). Cancer risk and assessment. In S.L. Groenwald, M.H. Frogge, M. Goodman, & C.H. Yarbro (Eds.), *Cancer nursing: Principles and practice* (4th ed.) (pp. 108–132). Boston: Jones and Bartlett.

Frank-Stromborg, M., Heusinkveld, K., & Rohan, K. (1996). Evaluating cancer risk and preventive oncology. In R. McCorkle, K. Grant, M. Frank-Stromborg, & S.B. Baird (Eds.), *Cancer nursing: A comprehensive textbook* (2nd ed.) (pp.155–189). Philadelphia: W.B. Saunders.

Frank-Stromborg, M., Johnson, J., & McCorkle, R. (1987). A program model for nurses involved with cancer education of black Americans. *Journal of Cancer Education, 2*(3), 145–151.

Frank-Stromborg, M., & Rohan, K. (1992). Nursing's involvement in the primary and secondary prevention of cancer. Nationally and internationally. *Cancer Nursing, 15*(2), 79–108.

Fraser, M. (1981). Self-care: A plan for melanoma-prone families [Abstract 193]. *Oncology Nursing Forum, 8*(2), 92.

Fraser, M. (1982). The role of the nurse in the prevention and early detection of malignant melanoma. *Cancer Nursing, 5,* 351–360.

Galassi, A. (2000). Role of the oncology advanced practice nurse. In C.H. Yarbro, M.H. Frogge, M. Goodman, & S.L. Groenwald (Eds.), *Cancer nursing: Principles and practice* (5th ed.) (pp. 1712–1725). Boston: Jones and Bartlett.

Gillatt, A. (1984). Aspects of oncology nursing in the community of Ireland. In *Cancer Nursing in the 80s: Proceedings of the 3rd International Conference on Cancer Nursing* (pp. 173–177). Melbourne, Australia: Organizing Committee, 3rd International Conference on Cancer Nursing.

Gonzalez, J. (1990). Factors related to practice of breast self-examination among low-income Mexican American women. *Cancer Nursing, 13*(2),134–142.

Gray, M. (1990). Factors related to practice of breast self-examination in rural women. *Cancer Nursing, 13*(2), 100–107.

Greco, K., & Kulawiak, L. (1994). Prostate cancer prevention: Risk reduction through lifestyle, diet, and chemoprevention. *Oncology Nursing Forum, 21,* 1504–1511.

Greenlee, R.T., Murray, T., Bolden, S., & Wingo, P.A. (2000). Cancer statistics, 2000. *CA: A Cancer Journal for Clinicians, 50,* 7–33.

Greenwald, P. (1995). Introduction: History of cancer prevention and control. In P. Greenwald, B.S. Kramer, & D.L. Weed (Eds.), *Cancer prevention and control* (pp. 1–7). New York: Marcel Dekker.

Gritz, E., & Kanim, L. (1986). Do fewer oncology nurses smoke? *Oncology Nursing Forum, 13*(3), 61–64.

Hallal, J.C. (1982). The relationship of health beliefs, health locus of control, and self-concept to the practice of breast self-examination in adult women. *Nursing Research, 31,* 137–142.

Hilkemeyer, R. (1985). A historical perspective in cancer nursing. *Oncology Nursing Forum, 12*(Suppl.1), 6–15.

Houfek, J.F., Waltman, N.L., & Kile, M.A. (1997). The nurse's role in promoting breast cancer screening. *Nebraska Nurse, 30*(3), 4–9.

Kelly, P. (1991). Skin cancer and melanoma awareness campaign. *Oncology Nursing Forum, 18*, 927–931.

Kenny, J.C., & Keenan, P.W. (1991). A survey of breast cancer detection methods in long-term care facilities. *Journal of Gerontological Nursing, 17*(4), 20–22.

Kersey, P., & Kroll, B. (1985). Be sunsible! [Abstract 17P]. *Oncology Nursing Forum, 12*(Suppl. 2), 44.

Kim, K., Yu, E.S.H., Chen, E.H., Kim, J., Kaufman, M., & Purkiss, J. (1999). Cervical cancer screening knowledge and practice among Korean-American women. *Cancer Nursing, 22*(4), 297–302.

Kitson, J.K. (1989). Breast self-exam and the high-risk adolescent [Abstract 280]. *Oncology Nursing Forum, 16*(Suppl. 2), 198.

Klatt-Ellis, T. (1988). Adolescent use and knowledge of smokeless tobacco: Implications for school programming [Abstract 100]. *Oncology Nursing Forum, 15*, 126.

Koh, H.K., Lew, R.A., & Prout, M.N. (1989). Screening for melanoma/skin cancer: Theoretic and practical considerations. *Journal of the Academy of Dermatology, 20*, 159–172.

Krohner, K.M., McBurney, B.H., & Wadelin, J.W. (1988). Assessing cancer prevention learning needs of parents and their 6th, 7th, and 8th grade children. *Oncology Nursing Forum, 15*, 59–64.

Larson, R. (1986). The role of the nurse in the melanoma screening process [Abstract 91]. *Oncology Nursing Forum, 13*, 78.

Lawler, P.E. (1990). The prevention of skin cancer: A nursing challenge. *Cancer Nursing News, 8*, 1–2.

Lawler, P.E., & Schreiber, S. (1989). Cutaneous malignant melanoma: Nursing's role in prevention and early detection. *Oncology Nursing Forum, 16*, 345–352.

Lazzaro, M., & Thompson, M. (1997). Update on prostate cancer screening. *Primary Care Practitioner, 1*, 408–418.

Leslie, N.S., & Roche, B.G. (1997). The effectiveness of the breast self-examination facilitation shield. *Oncology Nursing Forum, 24*, 1759–1765.

Lillington, L.B., Padilla, G.V., Sayre, J.W., & Chlebowski, R.T. (1993). Factors influencing nurses' breast cancer control activity. *Cancer Practice, 1*, 307–314.

Loescher, L., & Hazelkorn, K. (1983). Development of a skin cancer early detection and prevention program [Abstract 75]. *Oncology Nursing Forum, 10*(2), 65.

Longman, A.J., Modiano-Revah, M., & Saint-Germain, M. (1990). Breast cancer prevention for older Hispanic women [Abstract 80]. *Oncology Nursing Forum, 17*, 157.

Mackel, C., & Greski, P. (1990). Barrett's esophagus: A model for monitoring and intervening in preneoplasia [Abstract 105]. *Oncology Nursing Forum, 17*, 164.

Madsen, N. (1988). Cutaneous malignant melanoma, dysplastic nevi, and heredity [Abstract 111]. *Oncology Nursing Forum, 15*, 129.

Mahon, S.M. (1995). Using brochures to educate the public about the early detection of prostate and colorectal cancer. *Oncology Nursing Forum, 22*, 1413–1415.

Mahon, S.M. (1996). Educating women about early detection of gynecologic cancers using a brochure. *Oncology Nursing Forum, 23*, 529–531.

Marino, L.B. (1981). The organizational structure of cancer health care. In L.B. Marino (Ed.), *Cancer nursing* (pp. 35–49). St. Louis, MO: Mosby.

Marlenga, B. (1995). The health beliefs and skin cancer prevention practices of Wisconsin dairy farmers. *Oncology Nursing Forum, 22,* 681–686.

Marty, P.J., & McDermott, R.J. (1983). Teaching about testicular cancer and testicular self-examination. *Journal of School Health, 101,* 98–102.

Marty, P.J., McDermott, R.J., & Gold, R.S. (1983). An assessment of three alternative formats for promoting breast self-examination. *Cancer Nursing, 6,* 207–211.

Massey, V. (1986). Perceived susceptibility to breast cancer and practice of breast self-examination. *Nursing Research, 35,* 183–185.

Massingberd, K. (1988). The role of nurses in comprehensive cancer screening programme for women in Finland. In A.P. Pritchard (Ed.), *Cancer nursing: A revolution in care. Proceedings of the Fifth International Conference on Cancer Nursing* (pp. 135–137). New York : Springer.

McCabe, M.S., & Piemme, J.A. (1996). Cancer legislation. In R. McCorkle, M. Grant, M. Frank-Stromborg, & S.B. Baird (Eds.), *Cancer nursing: A comprehensive textbook* (2nd ed.) (pp. 1409–1423). Philadelphia: W.B. Saunders.

McGuire, D.B. (1979). Familial cancer and the role of the nurse. *Cancer Nursing, 2,* 443–452.

McGuire, D.B. (1985). Preventive health practices and educational needs in families with hereditary melanoma. *Cancer Nursing, 8,* 29–36.

McKee, J. (1994). Cues to action in prostate cancer screening. *Oncology Nursing Forum, 21,* 1171–1176.

McMillan, S. (1990). Nurses' compliance with American Cancer Society guidelines for cancer prevention and detection. *Oncology Nursing Forum, 17,* 21–27.

Melillo, K.D. (1985). Who needs health maintenance? *Journal of Gerontological Nursing, 11,* 18–21.

Messner, R.L., & Gardner, S.S. (1985). Colorectal cancer screening in the workplace. *Occupational Health Nursing, 33,* 561–565.

Mitchell-Beren, B.E., Dodds, M.E., Choi, K.L., & Waskerwitz, M. (1989). A colorectal cancer prevention, screening, and evaluation program in community black churches. *CA: A Cancer Journal for Clinicians, 39,* 115–118.

Nelson-Marten, P., & Krebs, L. (1991). Designing and implementing a nurse-run cancer screening/prevention clinic [Abstract 270A]. *Oncology Nursing Forum, 18,* 357.

Nemcek, N. (1989). Factors influencing black women's breast self-examination practice. *Cancer Nursing, 12,* 339–343.

Nielsen, B.B., Scofield, R.S., Mueller, S., Tranin, A.S., Moore, P., & Murphy, C.M. (1996). Certification of oncology nurses: A history. *Oncology Nursing Forum, 23,* 701–708.

Olsen, S., & Frank-Stromborg, M. (1991). Practical application for improving the quality of life of African-Americans [Abstract 137A]. *Oncology Nursing Forum, 18,* 343.

Olsen, S., & Frank-Stromborg, M. (1996). Cancer screening and early detection. In R. McCorkle, M. Grant, M. Frank-Stromborg, & S.B. Baird (Eds.), *Cancer nursing: A comprehensive textbook* (2nd ed.) (pp. 265–297). Philadelphia: W.B. Saunders.

Olson, R.L., & Mitchell, E.S. (1989). Self-confidence as a critical factor in breast self-examination. *Journal of Obstetric, Gynecologic, and Neonatal Nursing, 18,* 476–481.

O'Rourke, A., Gypson, B., & Weitberg, A. (1986). Developing a cancer screening center [Abstract 163]. *Oncology Nursing Forum, 13*(2), 95.

Owen, P. (1989). Health beliefs and preventive practices among adults with a history of melanoma [Abstract 68A]. *Oncology Nursing Forum, 16*(Suppl. 2), 145.

Peate, I. (1998). Cancer of the prostate. 2: The nursing role in health promotion. *British Journal of Nursing, 7*(4), 196–200.

Pervan V. (1988). Cultural aspects of oesophageal cancer. In A.P. Pritchard (Ed.), *Cancer nursing: A revolution in care. Proceedings of the Fifth International Conference on Cancer Nursing* (pp. 125–126). New York: Springer.

Plowden, K. (1998). Using the health belief model in understanding prostate cancer in African American men. *Association of Black Nursing Faculty Journal, 10*(1), 4–8.

Post-White, J.L., Herzan, D., & Drew, D. (1988). Prevention of dietary associated cancer [Abstract 21]. *Oncology Nursing Forum, 15*, 107.

Preventing and controlling oral and pharyngeal cancer. Recommendations from a national strategic planning conference. (1998). *Morbidity and Mortality Weekly Report, 47*, 1–12.

Roberts, T. (1997). Skin cancer prevention. *Nursing Standard, 11*, 42–45.

Rudolf, V.M., & Quinn, K.M. (1988). The practice of TSE among college men: Effectiveness of an educational program. *Oncology Nursing Forum, 15*, 45–48.

Rutledge, D., & Davis, G. (1988). Breast self-examination compliance and the Health Belief Model. *Oncology Nursing Forum, 15*, 175–179.

Sawyers, J., & Eaton, L. (1992). Gastric cancer in the Korean-American: Cultural implications. *Oncology Nursing Forum, 19*, 619–623.

Schleper, J. (1991). Teaching skin self-examination. *Dermatology Nursing, 3*, 174–176.

Schulmeister, L. (1986). Screening for oral cancer: Collaborating with dentistry [Abstract 32A]. *Oncology Nursing Forum, 13*(2), 63.

Schulmeister, L., & Lifsey, D.S. (1999). Cervical cancer screening knowledge, behaviors, and beliefs of Vietnamese women. *Oncology Nursing Forum, 26*, 879–887.

Seffrin, J.R. (2000). An endgame for cancer. *CA: A Cancer Journal for Clinicians, 50*, 4–5.

Sheehan, A.P., Michalek, A.M., & Cassidy, M.H. (1981). Outcomes of a BSE program for adolescents [Abstract 191]. *Oncology Nursing Forum, 8*(2), 92.

Shugars, D., & Patton L. (1997). Detecting, diagnosing, and preventing oral cancer. *Nurse Practitioner, 22*, 105, 109–110, 113–115.

Smith, M. (1995). Implementing annual cancer screenings for elderly women. *Journal of Gerontological Nursing, 21*, 12–17.

Smith, P.E. (1991). A comparison of two educational methods for teaching women about breast cancer and early detection and their effects on knowledge, attitudes, and behavior [Abstract 205]. *Oncology Nursing Forum, 18*, 394.

Spencer, R., & Ready, R. (1977). Looking ahead: Utilization of nurse endoscopists for sigmoidoscopic examination. *Diseases of the Colon and Rectum, 20*, 94–96.

Stack, T.D. (1979). Testicular cancer—The need for education and early detection [Abstract 84]. *Oncology Nursing Forum, 6*(2), 45.

Stanford, J. (1987). Testicular self-examination: Teaching, learning, and practice by nurses. *Journal of Advanced Nursing, 12*, 13–19.

Stewart, D.S. (1990). Indoor tanning: The nurses role in preventing skin damage. In C. Reed-Ash & J. Jenkins (Eds.), *Enhancing the role of cancer nursing* (pp. 79–94). New York: Raven.

Stoltzfus, T., & Ashby, A. (1990). Bringing cancer prevention and detection to the workplace utilizing a mobile screening unit [Abstract 199P]. *Oncology Nursing Forum, 17,* 187.

Tingen, M., Weinrich, S., Heydt, D., Boyd, M., & Weinrich M. (1998). Perceived benefits: A predictor of participation in prostate cancer screening. *Cancer Nursing, 21,* 349–357.

Underwood, A. (1999). *Nightingale, Florence.* Retrieved December 18, 2000 from the World Wide Web: http://www.britannica.com/bcom/eb/article

U.S. Department of Health and Human Services. (1990). *Healthy people 2000: National health promotion and disease prevention objectives* (DHHS Publication No. PHS 91-50213). Washington, DC: U.S. Government Printing Office.

Warren, B., & Pohl, J. (1990). Cancer screening practices of nurse practitioners. *Cancer Nursing, 13,* 143–151.

Weinrich, S., Weinrich, M., Boyd, M., & Atkinson, C. (1998). The impact of prostate cancer knowledge on cancer screening. *Oncology Nursing Forum, 25,* 527–534.

White, L. (1983). The nurse's role in cancer prevention. In O.R. Newell (Ed.), *Cancer prevention in clinical medicine* (pp. 91–111). New York: Raven.

White, L. (1986). Cancer prevention and detection: From twenty to sixty-five years of age. *Oncology Nursing Forum, 13*(2), 59–64.

White, L., Cornelius, J., Judkins, A., & Patterson, J. (1978). Screening of cancer by nurses. *Cancer Nursing, 1*(1), 15–20.

White, L., & Faulkenberry, J. (1985). Screening by nurse clinicians in cancer prevention and detection. *Current Problems in Cancer, 9,* 1–42.

Wilkes, B., & Bersani, G. (1983). Development of a community colorectal cancer program [Abstract 79]. *Oncology Nursing Forum, 10*(2), 66.

Williams, H.A. (1981). Screening for testicular cancer. *Pediatric Nursing, 7*(5), 38–40.

Williams, R.D. (1989). Breast cancer detection in home health care of the older woman. *Home Healthcare Nurse, 8*(4), 25–29.

Willis, M.A., Davis, M., Cairns, N.U., & Janiszewski, R. (1989). Interagency collaboration: Teaching breast self-examination to black women. *Oncology Nursing Forum, 16,* 171–180.

Wilson, P. (1989). Breast self examination. *Journal of the Royal College of General Practice, 39,* 35.

Woolam, G.L. (2000). Cancer statistics, 2000: A benchmark for the new century. *CA: A Cancer Journal for Clinicians, 50,* 6.

Yarbro, C.H. (1996). The history of cancer nursing. In R. McCorkle, M. Grant, M. Frank-Stromborg, & S.B. Baird (Eds.), *Cancer nursing: A comprehensive textbook* (2nd ed.) (pp. 12–23). Philadelphia: W.B. Saunders.

Yarbro, J. (2000). Milestones in our understanding of cancer. In C.H. Yarbro, M.H. Frogge, S. Goodman, & S.L. Groenwald (Eds.), *Cancer nursing: Principles and practice* (5th ed.) (pp. 3–15). Boston: Jones and Bartlett.

Zimmerman, S. (1997). Factors influencing Hispanic participation in prostate cancer screening. *Oncology Nursing Forum, 24,* 499–504.

CHAPTER 2

An Epidemiological Approach to Cancer Prevention and Control

Kathleen Jennings-Dozier, PhD, MPH, RN, CS, and
Ann Foltz, DNSc, RN

Introduction

Epidemiology is the study of how disease is distributed in a population (Cookfair & Cookfair, 1996). Epidemiologists believe that disease, illness, and poor health are not randomly distributed (Gordis, 2000) and that individuals have certain characteristics, exposures, or behaviors that increase their risk of developing disease or that may protect them from specific diseases. The goal of epidemiology is to determine the origins of specific diseases by examining factors that influence their frequency of occurrence and distribution in a population (Friis & Sellers, 1999). According to Gordis, epidemiology is used to

1. Identify the etiology of a disease and its risk factors.
2. Determine the extent of disease found in a community.
3. Study the natural history and prognosis of a disease.
4. Evaluate both existing and new prevention and treatment measures and methods of healthcare delivery.
5. Provide the basis for public health policy and regulatory decisions regarding environmental issues.

Epidemiology originated as a result of the need to identify risk factors and strategies for controlling infectious diseases, which were once the major cause of death worldwide (Nelson, 2001). Improved sanitation and the development of vaccines have reduced mortality from infectious disease and substantially lengthened the life spans of many people in the United States and other developed countries. Subsequently, epidemiology has evolved into a discipline that now includes specialists in chronic diseases such as cancer and heart disease, which have surpassed infectious diseases as the major causes of death in the United States (Centers for Disease Control and Prevention [CDC], 2000). Epidemiologists specialize in genetics, molecular biology, and environmental health, among other disciplines.

How Does Epidemiology Relate to Nursing?

Epidemiology and nursing both evolved from "problem-solving processes" (Harkness, 1995). The problem-solving process provides a framework for investigating health-related problems, gathering new knowledge, and implementing interventions. The "nursing process" is an extension of the problem-solving process and is defined as a critical thinking competency that allows nurses to make judgments and take reasoned actions (Potter & Perry, 1998). The nursing process contains five steps (assessment, nursing diagnosis, planning, implementation, and evaluation) and is used to diagnose and treat human responses to health and illness. Epidemiology also employs a multi-step reasoning process (Gordis, 2000). First, epidemiology seeks to determine whether an association exists between individuals having certain characteristics and the development of a specific disease or condition. Second, epidemiology seeks to develop accurate inferences regarding a potential causal relationship from the observed patterns of association.

Epidemiology and nursing also are interdependent. Nurses use findings from epidemiological research to guide clinical decision making, to identify people or populations at increased risk for disease, and in the planning, implementation, and evaluation of health programs and services (Arthur & McGarry, 1999; Cookfair & Cookfair, 1996; Harkness, 1995; Mulhull, 2000; Pedersoli, Antonialli, & Vila, 1998). Further, nursing-based interventions have been used for implementing public health initiatives based on the findings from epidemiological studies (Pedersoli et al.; Shortridge & Valanis, 1992).

Nursing, Epidemiology, and Cancer Control

According to Jennings-Dozier and Mahon (2000), nurses are in a unique position to address the statistics that continue to challenge our nation's cancer control agenda. Nurses link patients, families, and communities to cancer-care services. To effect change, nurses also must become better informed about the scientific principles that guide the current understanding of cancer prevention and detection, which includes the study of epidemiology. In addition, nurses must be competent in the application of epidemiology to clinical practice (Harkness, 1995). The marriage of nursing, epidemiology, and cancer control has resulted in nurses becoming greater participants in cancer prevention and control practice, education, and research. Principles of cancer risk assessment, genetic testing, primary and secondary prevention, and the ethical issues surrounding cancer screening are just a few examples of the outcome of nursing, epidemiology, and cancer control working together. Yet, with the need for more nurses in the battlefield fighting the war against cancer, competency in epidemiology, cancer prevention, detection, and control is essential.

Understanding Cancer Risk

Nurses need to be aware of factors that influence the risk of developing cancer; this knowledge will allow them to answer patients' questions about their personal risk of developing cancer and suggest ways that this risk can be reduced. The existence of a "causal relationship" between a suspected risk factor and a particular disease can be determined by examining the

- **Strength of association**—the incidence of the disease is significantly higher among individuals who have been exposed to the factor than those who have not.
- **Specificity of association**—the stronger the association, the more likely the factor is to be a cause of the disease or conditions.
- **Temporal sequence**—"cause (i.e. factor/exposure)" precedes the effect
- **Coherence/biological plausibility**—the association makes sense biologically.
- **Consistency of findings**—the effect produces the same disease across time, person, and place.
- **Dose response relationship**—increasing amounts of the cause increases the effects.

Because of the multifactorial environment in which cancer occurs and the stringent causality criterion, establishing a single agent as the "cause" of a cancer often is difficult. As a consequence, epidemiologists generally refer to factors believed to be associated with the development of cancer as a risk factor rather than a "cause" (CDC, 2000).

This chapter provides a nursing perspective on the use of epidemiological methods in cancer prevention and control. The chapter is divided into four major sections and will discuss the role of descriptive epidemiology in the measurement of cancer occurrence, analytical epidemiologic study designs, cancer screening and surveillance, and expressing cancer prognosis and outcomes. These sections also will summarize important information for the nurse involved in cancer prevention and control and will provide a nursing perspective on how epidemiology may be useful in the efforts to reduce the burden of cancer in the population.

Descriptive Epidemiology: Measuring the Occurrence of Cancer

Figure 2-1 shows the natural history of disease and lists types of data that are generated at various points in the disease trajectory (Gordis, 2000). Data that can be used for research are generated from patients' family histories, medical records, treatment records, health insurance records, pathology reports, and death certificates at several points in the disease trajectory. When aggregated, these data provide information or *describe* the frequency of the occurrence, natural history, current treatment patterns, length of survival, rate of recurrence, and mortality from specific diseases in a population during a specific period of time. This section introduces a brief overview of the basics of descriptive epidemiology and defines basic statistical concepts useful in explaining the cancer morbidity and mortality noted in the epide-

Figure 2-1. Natural History of Disease and Sources of Data Relating to Each Interval

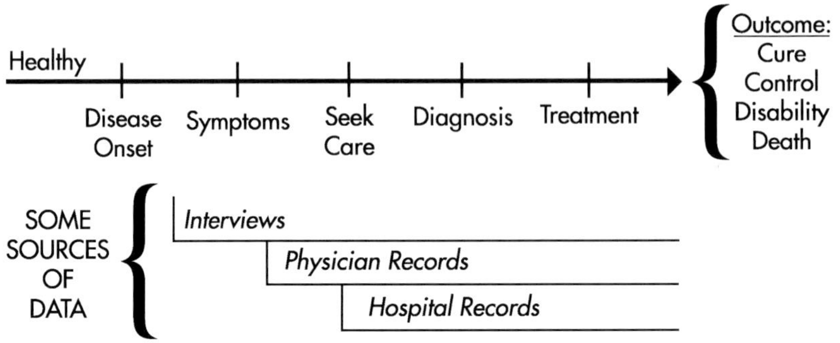

Note. From *Epidemiology* (2nd ed.) (p. 31), by L. Gordis, 2000, Philadelphia: W.B. Saunders. Copyright 2000 by W.B. Saunders. Reprinted with permission.

miological and nursing literature. Included are explanations of how hypothesis testing, measures of association, and descriptive studies are helpful aspects of descriptive epidemiology in understanding the burden of cancer in a population.

Using Descriptive Statistics

Table 2-1 defines some basic concepts used when measuring the occurrence of cancer. Descriptive statistics allow researchers and clinicians to summarize data into more meaningful forms that provide information about population characteristics. These include the mean, median, variance, standard deviation, and rates and proportions. (For more details, see Jung, 2001; Pagano & Gauvreau, 2000.)

Mean and Median

The *mean* and *median* measure the central or middle value of a distribution. The mean is the average value and the median is the middle value. Because the mean represents the average value, a few outlying or extremely high or low values that are not characteristic of the data set can have a substantial impact on the mean. In contrast, the median represents the value that is in the middle of the distribution and is not affected by the magnitude of outlying values. The median is the preferred measure of central tendency in cases where the data set contains extreme values.

Variance and Standard Deviation

The variance describes the amount of variability in a sample. Specifically, the variance provides information about how close, on average, individual values are to the mean value. The greater the variance, the more scattered the individual values (i.e., the greater the amount of difference in individual values). The standard deviation is the square root of the variance and provides a measure of the standard distance from the mean and describes the amount of variability among members of the population (Glantz, 1997). A small standard deviation indicates that the values typically are close to the mean, and a large standard deviation indicates that values generally are far from the mean.

Table 2-1. Basic Statistical Concepts

Concept	Description
Mean	The mean is the sum of all the values divided by the total number of values (members of the population). The mean is very sensitive to extreme values and may not represent the majority of the points.
Median	The median is the middle value in terms of magnitude. Sorting the observations from smallest to largest, the median has half of the data below and half of the data above. It is insensitive to extreme values.
Range	The difference between the largest and smallest observations in the sample.
Standard deviation	The square root of the variance. It is a measure of variation to show how far observations tend to vary from the mean.

Note. Based on information from Glantz, 1997; NCI, 1994; Rosner, 1995.

Rates, Ratios, and Proportions

A rate is a summarization of the frequency of an event or attribute in a population (Abramson, 2001). The rate actually is a ratio in which the numerator is the number of events (e.g., new cases of disease, deaths, recurrences, other event), and the denominator is the number of individuals in the population or the number of individuals at risk of having the event.

To control for the effect of the population size on the frequency of the event and to allow for comparison of rates between populations, the rate usually is presented per a specified population size (Abramson, 2001). Rates are most commonly expressed per 100,000; however, other population sizes can be used. Rates also can be calculated for specific groups such as race or ethnic group, marital status, cancer site or any other subgroup of the population where the appropriate numerator and denominator data are available. A rate may be reported as crude rate (unadjusted), age-specific, or adjusted by age, gender, or some other factor.

Crude Rates

Crude (unadjusted) rates provide an estimate of the absolute risk of cancer in the total population, whereas age-specific rates provide information on how disease risks vary between age groups and populations. A limitation of using crude rates to compare populations is that populations differ in distributions of characteristics such as age, race, or ethnicity, which may have an independent influence on the rate (Abramson, 2001; Gordis, 2000).

Standardized Rates

Standardized rates or adjusted rates frequently are used to report cancer data (CDC, 2001). Age is the most frequent variable that is controlled or adjusted in cancer rates. This is because of age differences in the risk of developing cancer and differences in the age distributions of specific populations. In general, because cancer incidence increases with age, it would be expected that older populations would have a higher incidence of cancer than younger ones. A comparison of crude (unadjusted) rates of two populations with substantially different age distributions is more likely to reflect differences in the proportion of older individuals (who are at a higher risk of developing cancer) than actual risk of developing a specific cancer (Gordis, 2000). An age-standardized (or age-adjusted) rate provides information on what the cancer rate would be if the age distribution of the populations being compared was similar. Many of the rates reported in cancer prevention and control literature are age-adjusted rates.

Age-Specific Rates

Age-specific rates provide valuable information about how disease risks vary between age groups and populations (Abramson, 2001). For example, data from the Surveillance Epidemiology and End Results Registry (SEER) show that overall age-adjusted breast cancer incidence is higher among White women than African-American women (see Table 2-2). However, additional calculations reveal that the age-specific breast cancer incident rates for White women who are younger than 35 years of age is 32.9/100,000 and is 46.7/100,000 for African American women (Ries et al., 2000). The overall age-adjusted rate is 13.8% higher among White women than African American women; however, the age-specific rates for women who are younger than 35 show that rates for African Americans are more than 40% higher than those for Whites.

Table 2-2. Age-Specific and Age-Adjusted Incidence Rates for Female Patients With Breast Cancer (1993–1997)*

Age	African American	White
0–4	0.0	0.0
5–9	0.0	0.0
10–14	0.0	0.0
15–19	0.5	0.0
20–24	2.9	1.1
25–29	11.3	7.8
30–34	32.0	24.0
35–39	64.4	57.4
40–44	116.5	117.1
45–49	199.3	201.9

*The incidence rates are per 100,000 and are age adjusted to the 1970 U.S. standard population.

Note. Based on information from Ries et al., 2000.

Incidence

Incidence refers to the number of *new* cases of a disease that occur during a specified period of time in a population at risk for developing the disease (Carmel & Reid, 1997; Gordis, 2000). Incidence rates can be used to evaluate the changing patterns of cancer frequency within a population. In addition, trends in incidence rates, stratified by stage of disease, can lend quantitative information on the effectiveness of cancer screening programs (Carmel & Reid; Pastides, 2001). Because incidence is a measure of the frequency of new events (cases of disease) that occur, incidence rates also provide information about the risk of developing a disease or condition. An incidence rate can be calculated using the following formula:

$$\text{Incidence rate} = \frac{\begin{array}{c}\text{Number of new cases of cancer that occur} \\ \text{during a specific time period}\end{array}}{\begin{array}{c}\text{Number of people at risk for developing} \\ \text{cancer during a specific time period}\end{array}} \times 100{,}000$$

Prevalence

The prevalence of a disease or condition is the proportion of individuals in a specific population who have the disease or condition at a specific point or during a specified period in time. The prevalence rate includes both newly diagnosed and existing (previously diagnosed or ongoing) cases of a given disease or condition (Carmel & Reid, 1997; Friis & Sellers, 1999). Cancer prevalence data provide information on the current impact that a specific cancer has on a population and, thus, may have implications for the scope of cancer health services needed in a given community.

Mortality

Cancer mortality rates measure the number of cancer deaths occurring in a defined population during a given period of time (Shambaugh et al., 1994), usually one year. Cancer mortality data are widely available and can come from a variety of sources, including death certificates, hospital records, and national databases. The National Center for Health Statistics (NCHS) collects data on all deaths occurring within the United States. These deaths can be classified by sex, age, race, and cancer site so that cancer mortality for a given period can be determined for the entire United States or for selected areas (Shambaugh et al.) or groups. Annual mortality rates can be calculated using the following formula:

$$\begin{array}{c}\text{Annual mortality rate for all cancer} \\ \text{cases (per 100,000 population)}\end{array} = \frac{\begin{array}{c}\text{Total number of cancer} \\ \text{deaths in one year}\end{array}}{\begin{array}{c}\text{Number of people in the} \\ \text{population (at risk of dying} \\ \text{in that one year)}\end{array}} \times 100{,}000$$

Like morbidity rates, mortality can be reported as rates or illustrated in the form of graphs and diagrams. Figure 2-2 illustrates an estimate of the gender-specific cancer deaths in the United States for 2001. These data show estimate trends in mortality rates for six specific cancer sites and suggest an excess number of deaths caused by lung cancer for both men and women.

Case-Fatality Rates

Cancer case-fatality rates provide information about the likelihood of dying from cancer among those suffering from the disease. Case fatality also can provide information about the impact of a specific cancer on a population and the efficacy of new cancer therapies. Case-fatality rates differ from mortality rates in that the

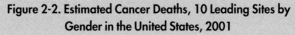

Figure 2-2. Estimated Cancer Deaths, 10 Leading Sites by Gender in the United States, 2001

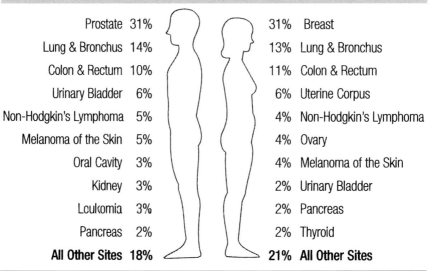

Prostate	31%		31%	Breast
Lung & Bronchus	14%		13%	Lung & Bronchus
Colon & Rectum	10%		11%	Colon & Rectum
Urinary Bladder	6%		6%	Uterine Corpus
Non-Hodgkin's Lymphoma	5%		4%	Non-Hodgkin's Lymphoma
Melanoma of the Skin	5%		4%	Ovary
Oral Cavity	3%		4%	Melanoma of the Skin
Kidney	3%		2%	Urinary Bladder
Leukemia	3%		2%	Pancreas
Pancreas	2%		2%	Thyroid
All Other Sites	**18%**		**21%**	**All Other Sites**

*Excludes in situ carcinomas except urinary bladder.
Percentages may not total 100% due to rounding.

Note. From "Cancer Statistics, 2001," by R.T. Greenlee, M.B. Hill-Harmon, T. Murray, and M. Thun, 2001, *CA: A Cancer Journal for Clinicians, 51*, p. 18. Copyright 2001 by the American Cancer Society. Reprinted with permission.

denominator in a mortality rate represents an *entire* population at risk of dying from cancer and includes those who do and do not have cancer. In contrast, cancer case-fatality rates use denominators that include only *those who have* the disease. Case fatality provides information about the severity of a certain cancer compared to other diseases or cancer sites.

$$\text{Case-fatality rate} = \frac{\text{Number of people dying from a specific cancer}}{\text{Number of people with a specific cancer}} \times 100$$

Using Hypothesis Testing

Once the occurrence of cancer has been measured in a population, tentative hypotheses or explanations that fit the descriptive data and identify the most common cancer type (e.g., breast, colorectal) or a population involved (e.g., women younger than 50, industry employees) are developed (Harkness, 1995). A hypothesis is an educated guess about an association that is testable in a scientific investigation (Morton, Hebel, & McCarter, 2000). It is a statement about the association between a variable and an outcome. Two hypotheses are set up in opposition to each other: the *null hypothesis*, against which the healthcare professional hopes to gather information, and the *alternative hypothesis*, the hypothesis for which the professional wishes to gather supporting evidence.

After establishing the null and the alternative hypothesis, the nurse must decide what test and significance level are to be used to determine whether to reject the null hypotheses. Several statistical tests are used in epidemiology for testing research hypotheses. The test that is used depends on the type of data that are used for hypothesis testing. For example, chi-square tests can compare proportions or risk ratios calculated from categorical data, which are arranged in categories, whereas T-tests compare means from continuous or count data (e.g., age, number of cigarettes smoked per day).

p value

The significance level or *p* value is the probability of detecting an association between two variables when one does not exist (Glantz, 1997). Most researchers use a significance level of 5% (*p* value = 0.05 or more) as the level below that the null hypothesis (of no association) is rejected. If the null hypothesis (no association) is rejected, the researcher concludes that a statistically significant association exists between the variable (risk factor) and the outcome. If the *p* value is greater than or equal to 0.05, then the null hypothesis is not rejected, and the researcher concludes that no statistically significant association exists between a particular variable and the outcome.

Confidence Interval

Confidence intervals (CI) provide information about the reliability of the risk estimate or statistic. A 95% CI usually is reported, although a 90% or 99% CI is sometimes used. A statistically significant association between a variable and an outcome is said to be present if the CI around the risk estimate does not include 1. If the confidence contains 1, the value of no effect or no difference, the observed relationship between the study variable and the outcome variable may be caused by sampling variation or chance (Glantz, 1997).

Using Measures of Association

Once a hypothesis has been developed, measures of association are special statistics used to indicate the strength of the association between two variables, or, in this case, the development of cancer and exposure to a risk factor. The most commonly used measures of association are the *relative risk* and *odds ratio*.

Relative Risk

Relative risk or rate ratio (RR) is the likelihood of a person developing a disease among those exposed to a risk factor relative to those who are not exposed (Gordis, 2000; Morton et al., 2000). The relative risk can be obtained from cohort studies (see pages 47–49 for definitions of cohort studies).

$$\text{Relative risk} = \frac{\text{Risk in exposed}}{\text{Risk in nonexposed}}$$

Interpreting Relative Risk

Values of relative risk range from zero to infinity. If relative risk is greater than 1, then its numerator is greater than its denominator, which means the risk for exposed people is greater than the risk for nonexposed people. For example, a study on the effects of second-hand cigarette smoke in relation to lung cancer reported that the relative risk for women whose husbands smoke cigarettes was 1.2 (Cardenas et al., 1997). This means that the sample of women in the study who were married to smokers (exposed) had a 20% greater risk for dying from lung cancer in comparison to women whose husbands were nonsmokers (nonexposed).

If the relative risk is less than 1, the risk in exposed people is less than the risk in nonexposed people. A relative risk less than 1 is evidence of a negative association and may be an indication of a "protective effect"(Gordis, 2000). Speizer, Colditz, Hunter, Rosner, and Hennekens (1999) reported that the RR of developing lung cancer among women who consume five or more carrots per week was 0.4 (95% CI = 0.2– 0.8) compared to women who consumed fewer or no carrots. This means that women who ate five or more carrots per week were 60% less likely to develop lung cancer in comparison to women who ate fewer or no carrots per week. These results also suggest that eating carrots may have provided some protection against developing lung cancer in female smokers. If the RR is equal to 1, then the risk in the exposed is equal to the risk in the unexposed. Thus, the risk factor is not associated with the outcome.

Odds Ratio

The *odds ratio* (OR) is a measure of association that provides similar information to the RR. ORs measure the odds of having the exposure among those with the disease compared to the odds of having the exposure among those who do not have the disease. Because relative risk cannot be directly calculated in case-control studies, ORs are used. Because of the selection process of case-control studies, the incidence of cancer in the exposed population (cases) or the nonexposed population (noncases) is not known; therefore, ORs must serve as an estimate of relative risk. (Note: many epidemiology and nursing pieces of literature report ORs as an approximation of cancer relative risk. See Gordis, 2000, p. 165, for conditions of use). In case-control studies, the odds of an event can be defined as the ratio of the number of ways the event can occur to the number of ways the event cannot occur (Gordis). Therefore, one should consider the OR of a cancer event as a measure of association of exposure and disease in a case-control study.

	Cases (with cancer)	Noncases (without cancer)
Exposed cancer cases	A	B
Not exposed cancer cases	C	D
Total	A+C	B+D
Proportions exposed to cancer	$\dfrac{A}{A+C}$	$\dfrac{B}{B+D}$

The illustration above denotes the odds of a case having been exposed to cancer (see A/C). The figure also shows the odds of a noncase being exposed (see B/D). To consider the OR of both the cases and noncases that were exposed to cancer, calculate the information from the figure.

$$\frac{(A/D)}{(B/D)} = \frac{AD}{BC}$$

Therefore, AD/BC represents the OR for a case-control study.

In cohort studies, odds ratios also are used to answer the question of whether an association exists between the exposure and the disease. ORs are defined as the odds of developing a disease in an exposed person to the odds of developing a disease in a nonexposed person (Gordis, 2000).

Interpreting Odds Ratio

ORs are interpreted in a manner similar to the RR. For example, an OR equal to 1 means no association exists; an OR different from 1 means the presence of an association—positive if greater than 1 and negative if less than 1. An OR of 1 suggests that the odds of exposure to a disease are equivalent among the cases and controls and that a particular exposure is not a risk factor. An OR of 2 suggests that the cases were twice as likely as the controls to be exposed to the risk factor for the disease in question. Interestingly, ORs are used as an estimate of relative risk in case-control studies; the discussion of how to calculate and interpret such an association is beyond the scope of this chapter.

Descriptive Studies

Descriptive studies describe patterns of disease occurrence within a population (Kelsey, Whittemore, Evans, & Thompson, 1996). These studies are helpful in understanding how disease patterns differ by racial or ethnic group, gender, geographic area, socioeconomic status, and other important characteristics. Information obtained from descriptive studies can be useful in forming hypotheses to be examined in analytical studies. Because descriptive studies often are based on the analysis of routinely collected data, they are sometimes less expensive and require less time to complete than analytical studies (Gordis, 2000). The three major types of descriptive studies are case reports and case series, correlational studies, and cross-sectional surveys. A summary of study designs and their strengths and limitations is provided in Table 2-3.

Case Reports and Case Series

Case reports and case series are used to report unusual manifestations of disease or patient history. Case reports describe the experience of one patient whereas case series describe the experiences of several patients (Gordis, 2000). Case reports and case series are important in epidemiology as they often provide the first evidence of an epidemic, a new disease, or a new risk factor for disease. Case reports and case series, however, cannot be used to establish a statistical association between an exposure and a disease.

Correlational and Ecologic Studies

Correlational studies use aggregate measures, such as geographic region, as the unit of analysis rather than individuals. Correlational studies are used to determine if disease rates are higher among aggregate units (e.g., regions, census tracts, states) with higher average levels of exposure. For example, Schwartz, Skinner, and Duncan (1998) used data from the Florida Cancer Data System, a population-based cancer registry, to compare county-specific pancreatic cancer incidence rates to county cigarette smoking prevalence and the amount of municipal solid waste collected.

Table 2-3. The Strengths and Limitations of Selected Epidemiological Study Designs

Design	Strengths	Limitations	Estimates and Statistics	Strength of the Evidence for a Causal Relationship
Clinical trial	Best design for controlling the influence of confounding variables Good for testing the efficacy of treatment regimens Can provide a sounder rationale for intervention than other study designs	Findings may not be generalizable to the population. Can be costly and time intensive Can present ethical dilemmas	Survival Incidence Relative risk Attributable risk	Strong
Cohort	Good for the study of rare exposures Multiple effects of a single exposure can be studied. Can establish a temporal relationship between the exposure and disease Incidence can be measured directly.	Generally requires a large number of subjects Not an efficient design for the study of rare diseases unless attributable risk is high Prospective studies often are expensive and time consuming. Retrospective study requires the availability of adequate records. Loss to follow-up can have a substantial impact on the validity of study results.	Survival Incidence Relative risk Attributable risk	
Case-control	Optimal for the study of rare diseases Multiple etiologic factors for the same disease can be studied. Smaller sample sizes are required.	Unless the study is population based, incidence rates cannot be computed directly. May be difficult to establish the temporal relationship between the exposure and the disease	Odds ratio	

(Continued on next page)

Table 2-3. The Strengths and Limitations of Selected Epidemiological Study Designs (Continued)

Design	Strengths	Limitations	Estimates and Statistics	Strength of the Evidence for a Causal Relationship
Case-control (cont.)	Good for the study of disease with long latent periods	In general, more susceptible to recall and selection bias than other study designs		
		Not an efficient design for the study of rare exposures		
Cross-sectional	Usually population based	Difficult to establish causal relationships	Prevalence rates	
	Can be completed in a relatively short time, thus minimizing loss to follow-up	Not practical for the study of rare diseases		
Correlational/ ecological	Can be completed in a relatively small amount of time with little expense	Cannot link exposure with disease in specific individuals	Correlation coefficient	
	Uses routinely collected data	Cannot control for potential confounding factors		
Case series	Useful in identifying the beginning or presence of a epidemic	Cannot be used to test for a statistical association between an exposure and a disease	None	
Case reports	Can be the first clues to new diseases or the adverse effects of exposures	Based on the experience of one individual	None	Weak

Note. Based on information from Hennekens & Buring, 1987.

Correlational studies generally require less time to complete because they use routinely collected data. Because individual exposure levels are not directly measured, it is not possible to determine if individuals who develop disease have higher exposure levels than others. Results from the Schwarz et al. (1998) study revealed a significant correlation between county-specific pancreatic cancer incidence and county-specific levels of cigarette smoking, income, and yard trash. One cannot conclude from these findings that an association exists between individual smoking, income, or amount of yard trash and the incidence of pancreatic cancer. Inappropriate conclusions about the association between exposure and disease at the individual level, based on findings from aggregate level exposure and disease data, can result in ecologic fallacies (Kelsey et al., 1996). Findings of correlational studies should be confirmed with analytical studies based on the individual level of data.

Cross-Sectional Studies

Cross sectional studies or prevalence studies examine the exposure or disease status of individuals in a population at a specific point in time or over a short period of time (Kelsey et al., 1996). At the onset of a cross-sectional study, both the exposure and disease have occurred. Data from study participants then are analyzed by exposure and disease status. Cross-sectional studies are useful for describing the distribution of risk factors and diseases in a population. Cross-sectional studies can be used to gather information on the prevalence of behavioral or lifestyle risks, such as cigarette smoking, or of certain diseases or conditions, such as hypertension or diabetes, within a specified population. Cross-sectional surveys are relatively quick to perform, are not expensive, and also can provide information on the possible association of a risk factor with a disease. Because cross-sectional studies collect exposure and disease data at the same time, it is difficult to establish causal relationships (Newman, Browner, Cummings, & Hulley, 2000).

Althuis et al. (2000) conducted a cross-sectional community-based survey in 1994 of women who were diagnosed with nonmetastatic primary breast cancer and also used tamoxifen. The survey examined time since last mammogram, time since last clinical breast examination, frequency of breast self-examination, self-rated health status, smoking status, participation in regular exercise, family history of cancer, and the development of a breast cancer recurrence (e.g., contralateral breast cancer, endometrial cancer). Data on the frequency of surveillance for uterine abnormalities among women previously treated for breast cancer are presented in Table 2-4.

These data show that a statistically significant association exists between tamoxifen use status and the prevalence of regular surveillance for uterine abnormalities among patients with breast cancer (p < 0.01). The prevalence of regular surveillance is highest among current tamoxifen users followed by former users and never users, respectively.

Table 2-4. Frequency of Surveillance for Uterine Abnormalities Among Patients With Breast Cancer Who Use Tamoxifen

| Tamoxifen Use | Frequency of Surveillance | | | |
| | Never | Irregularly | Regularly | |
	% (n)	% (n)	% (n)	p Value
Current user	38 (66)	19 (34)	43 (76)	< 0.01
Former user	38 (17)	27 (12)	35 (16)	
Never used	68 (112)	17 (27)	15 (25)	

Note. From "Surveillance for Uterine Abnormalities in Tamoxifen Treated Breast Carcinoma Survivors," by M.D. Althuis, M. Sexton, P. Langenberg, T.L. Bush, K. Tkaczuk, J. Magaziner, and L. Khoo, 2000, *Cancer, 89,* p. 806. Copyright 2000 by the American Cancer Society. Adapted with permission.

Analytical Epidemiology: Types of Study Designs

The previous section on descriptive epidemiology provided a helpful way to identify variations in the distribution of cancer occurrence in a population. When analyzed, descriptive epidemiology provides information to formulate hypotheses about the health status of a population. Analytical epidemiology differs from descriptive epidemiology in that it focuses on identifying the determinants of health as they relate to cancer prevention and control. According to Harkness (1995), analytical epidemiology provides strategies to test previously developed hypotheses in an attempt to find the reasons or determinants that are associated with variations noted in descriptive epidemiology. In general, the goal of analytical cancer studies is to determine whether an association exists between a particular exposure and disease status (e.g., cancer occurrence, recurrence, progression). Analytical studies are classified as observational or intervention. In observational studies, the researcher observes participant exposure and disease status. Observational study designs include cohort, case control, and cross-sectional studies (Correa, 1995). In contrast, researchers assign participants in intervention studies to receive or not receive a specific exposure (e.g., drug, treatment regimen, lifestyle change—exercise, diet) and then compare changes in disease status. Intervention studies are broadly referred to as clinical trials.

Cohort Studies

Cohort studies follow a group of people during a time period (Correa, 1995). The studies may involve more than two groups and may follow participants for several weeks, months, or years. A cohort study can be retrospective or prospective (also known as concurrent) (see Figure 2-3).

Retrospective Cohort Studies

In a retrospective cohort study, also called a historical or nonconcurrent cohort study, participants are identified by some past characteristic or exposure (e.g., asbestos). Existing records then are reviewed to determine changes in the participant's disease status that occurred after the exposure. At the time the researcher begins a retrospective cohort study, both the exposure and outcome of interest already have occurred (see Figure 2-3) (Gordis, 2000).

Retrospective cohort studies frequently use data (e.g., medical records, hospital discharge records, other administrative records) that are not specifically collected for the research study. A limitation of retrospective cohort studies is that existing data sets may not contain all of the data required to address the research question, such as smoking status, physical activity level, or dietary intake (Friis & Sellers, 1999). Retrospective cohort studies are relatively inexpensive compared to other designs and require less time to complete than prospective cohort studies. Retrospective studies are useful for studying diseases that have long latency periods, such as cancer.

Ellison (2000) retrospectively examined data on male participants of the 1970–1972 Nutrition Canada Survey to assess the relationship between tea, coffee, cola, and alcohol and the risk of developing prostate cancer. The Canadian Cancer Registry was used to obtain data on cancer cases diagnosed among male participants of the nutrition survey during 1969–1993. Patients diagnosed with cancer prior to 1970 or who had missing information on tea consumption were excluded from the

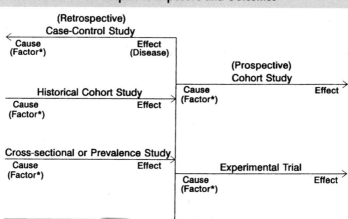

Figure 2-3. Timing of Analytic Epidemiological Studies With Respect to Exposure and Outcomes

*Hypothesized etiologic (causative) characteristic under study

Note. From *SEER Program Self-Instructional Manual for Cancer Registrars, Book 7: Statistics and Epidemiology for Cancer Registries* (NIH Publication No. 94-3766) (p.162), by E.M. Shambaugh, J.L. Young, C. Sippin, D. Lum, C. Akers, and M.A. Weiss, 1994, Bethesda, MD: National Cancer Institute, National Institutes of Health.

retrospective study. Thus, of the 3,584 males who participated in the original nutrition survey, only 3,400 were included in the retrospective study. One hundred and forty-five of the males in the retrospective study developed prostate cancer. Data on the levels of tea consumption and the risk of developing prostate cancer are provided in Table 2-5. Results indicated that no relationship existed between tea consumption and the risk of developing prostate cancer (all CIs contain 1).

Prospective Cohort Studies

At the beginning of a prospective cohort study, the *exposure* has occurred but the *outcome* of interest has not (see Figure 2-3). The exposure is measured at the onset of the study, and the cohort then is followed into the future and monitored to see if and when participants develop cancer or other outcomes of interest (Gordis, 2000). Prospective cohort studies also are called longitudinal studies. An advantage of prospective cohort studies is that they can be used to examine several exposures or diseases simultaneously. Data obtained from the Nurses Health Study, a prospective cohort study that began in 1976, have provided information regarding the risk of developing breast and ovarian cancers associated with the use of exogenous estrogens (Bain et al., 1981; Hennekens et al., 1979; Willett, Bain, Hennekens, Rosner, & Speizer, 1981), the use of permanent hair dyes and the risk of skin cancer (Hennekens et al.), and oral contraceptive use and myocardial infarction (Bain et al.). Prospective cohort studies are expensive, are time intensive, and generally require large sample sizes (Friis & Sellers, 1999). Because participants often are followed for long peri-

Table 2-5. Prostate Cancer Risk* and Tea Consumption (Nutrition Cancer Survey Cohort, 1970–1993)

Tea Intake (ml/day)	Males Who Developed Prostate Cancer	Person-Years	Relative Risk	95% Confidence Interval
0	23	7,325	1.00	Referent group
> 0–250	33	9,029	1.22	0.72–2.08
> 250–500	34	7,534	1.27	0.75–2.16
> 500–750	30	8,299	1.00	0.58–1.73
> 750	25	7,113	1.03	0.58–1.82
Any tea intake	122	31,975	1.13	0.72–1.76

*Data were adjusted for five-year age group.

Note. From "Tea and Other Beverage Consumption and Prostate Cancer Risk: A Canadian Retrospective Study," by L.F. Ellison, 2000, European Journal of Cancer Prevention, 9, p. 128. Copyright 2000 by Lippincott, Williams, & Wilkins. Adapted with permission.

ods of time, loss to follow-up also can be a substantial problem. The reliability of data derived from a prospective cohort study can be diminished by high attrition rates. Therefore, establishing several means of maintaining contact or gathering follow-up data on study participants is critical (Friis & Sellers).

Data from the Nurses Health Study also were used to examine aspirin use and the risk of developing colorectal cancer (Colditz, Hoaglin, & Berkey, 1997). The study originally included 121,701 female registered nurses who were between the ages of 30 and 55 in 1976. Follow-up questionnaires were mailed biennially to update risk factor data and document major medical events. In 1980, participants were asked to complete a supplementary questionnaire that collected data on medication use and diet. Only participants who completed the 1980 questionnaire, who had no previous diagnosis of cancer, except for skin cancer, and had not been diagnosed with familial polyposis syndrome or ulcerative colitis were included in the study of aspirin use and the risk for colorectal cancer (see Table 2-6).

Data show a slightly lower nonsignificant risk of developing colorectal, colon, and rectal cancer among participants who regularly used aspirin for five or more years. Participants who regularly used aspirin for 20 years or more had a statistically significant reduction in the risk of developing colorectal cancer and a nearly significant reduction in the risk of developing colon cancer. The regular use of aspirin for 20 years or more did not significantly reduce the risk of developing rectal cancer. Results from this study indicate that the regular use of aspirin for 20 years or more is associated with a statistically significant reduction in the risk of developing colorectal cancer.

Currently, several national cancer-control cohort studies are under way (see Figure 2-4). These studies are providing information on the development of cancer in humans and will yield important data that will be useful in the prevention and control of cancer.

Table 2-6. Relative Risk of Colorectal Cancer by Number of Consecutive Years of Regular Aspirin Use (Nurses Health Study, 1984–1992)

Years of Aspirin Use	Person-Years	Site	Total Cases	Relative Risk	95% Confidence Interval
0	357,905	Colorectal cancer	226	1.0	–
		Colon cancer	159	1.0	–
		Rectal cancer	43	1.0	–
1–4	70,820	Colorectal cancer	48	1.06	0.78–1.45
		Colon cancer	29	0.91	0.61–1.35
		Rectal cancer	12	1.39	0.74–2.63
5–9	42,306	Colorectal cancer	24	0.84	0.55–1.28
		Colon cancer	17	0.85	0.51–1.40
		Rectal cancer	7	1.29	0.58–2.88
10–19	28,709	Colorectal cancer	14	0.70	0.41–1.20
		Colon cancer	9	0.64	0.33–1.25
		Rectal cancer	3	0.81	0.26–2.56
> 20	52,259	Colorectal cancer	19	0.56	0.36–0.90
		Colon cancer	14	0.59	0.34–1.01
		Rectal cancer	4	0.63	0.23–1.74

Note. From "Aspirin and the Risk of Colorectal Cancer in Women," by E. Giovannuci, K.M. Egan, D.J. Hunter, M.J. Stampfer, G.A. Colditz, W.C. Willett, and F.E. Speizer, 1995, *New England Journal of Medicine, 333,* p. 612. Copyright 1995 by Massachusetts Medical Society. Adapted with permission.

Figure 2-4. Examples of Cancer Cohort Studies

• American Cancer Society Hammond-Horn Study: Cigarette smoking on death rates from cancer and other diseases
• Benzene Study Group: Benzene exposure in Chinese factory workers
• Breast Cancer Prevention Trial
• Framingham Heart Study: Nutritional factors and cancer
• Framingham Offspring Study: Nutritional factors and cancer
• Long Island Study: Environmental exposure and breast cancer risk
• National Cancer Institute–American Association of Retired Persons Study: Dietary exposure and risk for major cancers, especially those of the breast, large bowel, and prostate
• Nurses Health Study: Environmental exposure and breast cancer risk, dietary exposure and colorectal cancer risk
• Study of Tamoxifen and Raloxifene (STAR) Trial: Evaluation of tamoxifen and raloxifene for breast cancer prevention

Case-Control Studies

A case-control study is a retrospective study in which the exposures or past attributes of individuals with a particular condition or disease (cases) are compared with individuals who do not have the disease (controls) (CDC, 2001; Gordis, 2000). Case-control studies require smaller sample sizes than cohort studies, are optimal for the study of rare diseases, and are good for the study of diseases with long latency periods, such as cancer. Another advantage of case-control studies is that multiple risk factors for the same disease can be studied simultaneously. A disadvantage of case-control studies is that incidence rates cannot be calculated directly unless the study is population based. Differential recall of the exposure between cases and controls also can be problematic (Carmel & Reid, 1997). Because patients often are searching for an explanation for their disease, they may more accurately recall certain exposures. At the onset of a case-control study, both the disease and the exposure already have occurred. Participants in case-control studies are recruited on the basis of their disease status (Carmel & Reid). Cases can be selected from a variety of sources, including tumor registries, hospital medical records, physician practices, and clinics. Selecting cases from population-based registries, such as the SEER registry, improves the ability to generalize results to the general population. Controls often are selected from population-based databases, such as state driver license lists or the Centers for Medicare and Medicaid Services, or from population-based sampling methods such as random digit dialing.

Cohen, Kristal, and Stanford (2000) examined the association of fruit and vegetable intake (exposure) with prostate cancer risk (disease) in a population-based case-control study of men ages 40–64. The Seattle-Puget Sound SEER registry was used to identify 628 African American and White men from King County, WA, who were newly diagnosed with prostate cancer—January 1993–December 1996. Random-digit dialing was used to recruit 602 male controls from King County that were frequency matched to cases. Patients were ineligible for study participation if they did not have a residential telephone. Data were collected by personal interview and from a self-administered food frequency questionnaire, which assessed dietary intake during the three- to five-year period prior to diagnosis (cases) or study recruitment (controls). ORs for prostate cancer risk associated with fruit and cruciferous vegetable intake are provided in Table 2-7.

Table 2-7. Consumption of Fruits and Cruciferous Vegetables and Prostate Cancer Risk

Servings Per Week	Number of Cases	Number of Controls	Odds Ratio	95% Confidence Interval
Total fruit, five-a-day method				
Less than 3.5	120	109	1.0*	–
3.5–6.9	167	167	0.94	0.64–1.37
7–13.9	212	182	0.96	0.66–1.39
≥ 14	129	144	0.80	0.53–1.23
Cruciferous vegetables				
≤ 1	209	172	1.0*	–
1–2.9	269	245	0.90	0.69–1.18
≥ +3	150	185	0.67	0.50–0.90

*Referent group

Note. From "Fruit and Vegetable Intakes and Prostate Cancer Risk," by J.H. Cohen, A.R. Kristal, and J.L. Stanford, 2000, Journal of the National Cancer Institute, 92, p. 62. Copyright 2000 by Oxford University Press. Adapted with permission.

The results of the study revealed no statistically significant association between fruit intake and prostate cancer risk. The consumption of cruciferous vegetables 1–2.9 times per week was not associated with reduced prostate cancer risk; however, there was a statistically significant lower risk of prostate cancer associated with the consumption of three or more cruciferous vegetables per week.

Clinical Trials

Clinical trials are an important and specialized category of cohort studies. A clinical trial is defined as a prospective study that is designed to compare the effect and value of an intervention against a control in human subjects (Friedman, Furberg, & DeMets, 1998). That is, the outcomes from an intervention in one group are compared to the outcomes of a control group, which does not receive the intervention. The intervention could be a behavioral change, a new drug, or a new surgical method and may be intended to be prophylactic, diagnostic, or therapeutic. The major advantage of the clinical trial design lies within the strength of evidence for a causal relationship. Further, the clinical trial is the best design for controlling other factors that can influence outcomes (Friedman et al.). Several basic clinical trial study designs are available: historical control trial, nonrandomized control trial, and the randomized control trial.

Historical Control Trials

In the historical control trial, participants are given a new intervention, and their outcomes are compared to patients from a prior trial or series. These trials are not randomized and are subject to bias as a result of potential problems with the comparability of study participants. Historical control trials, however, can be useful for evaluating the effect of vaccines.

Nonrandomized Control Trials

As the name implies, participants in nonrandomized control trials are not randomized to the intervention or control group (Correa, 1955). Frequently, whether a participant receives the intervention is dependent upon specific clinical criteria. Because participants are not randomized to the intervention, these trials require larger sample sizes than randomized clinical trials. The major disadvantages of this study design are the potential for lack of comparability between participants and bias introduced by the somewhat subjective allocation of study participants (Correa).

Randomized Control Trials

Probably the best-known clinical trial design is the randomized control trial. Friedman et al. (1998) stated that the randomized control study is the standard against which all other study designs must be compared. In a randomized control trial, study participants are assigned to the intervention or control group by chance. Randomizing study participants can help to reduce the potential for biased allocation of participants to the intervention or control group. In addition, randomizing can provide intervention and control groups with similar distributions of baseline characteristics and aid in the production of data with greater comparability and generalizability.

Blinding in Clinical Trials

There are several examples of blinding that can occur in clinical trials. A trial is said to be unblinded when both the participants and the investigator know whether the participant was assigned to receive the intervention or to the control group. Unblinded trials are useful for interventions involving surgical procedures or lifestyle changes (Friedman et al., 1998) but are less useful for studies of new drugs. The major disadvantage of the unblinded trial is bias attributed to the influence of knowing whether a participant is receiving the intervention and the investigator's and participant's perception of outcomes. Further, patients who know that they are not receiving the intervention may lose interest in the trial and withdraw, leading to differential rates of attrition between the intervention and control groups, which biases study results. Blinding the participants or both the investigator and the participants to the assignment of the intervention or control group adds complexity to the study while alleviating many of the problems associated with unblinded studies.

In the single-blinded study, only the participants are blinded as to their assignment to the intervention or control group. In a double-blinded study, neither the participant nor the investigator involved with the conduct of the study knows whether a specific participant has been randomized to the study intervention or control group. Because of the necessity of keeping the intervention/control status of participants blinded from the participant and the investigator, double-blinded studies can be complex and difficult to carry out. For example, it can be difficult to maintain blinding if substantial characteristic side effects are associated with an interventional drug (Friedman et al., 1998).

Drug Trials

Clinical trials that involve the testing of a new drug or intervention proceed in an orderly series of steps called phases (NCI, 2001b). This allows researchers to ask and answer questions in a way that results in reliable information about the drug or intervention and protects the patients.

Phase I clinical trials are usually the first study of a drug or intervention on human subjects. (Studies performed prior to phase I trials are "pre-clinical trials" using mice or other animal models.) The main goal of a phase I drug trial is to establish the maximum tolerated dose of the intervention agent. A phase I trial usually enrolls only a small number of patients, sometimes as few as a dozen (NCI, 2001a). Phase I trials are not randomized, and every participant receives the intervention.

A phase II trial continues to test the safety of the drug or intervention and begins to evaluate how well the new intervention works (Greenwald, 1995). The goal of the phase II trial is to evaluate safety and efficacy trends and side effects and to define the appropriate dose. Phase II trials also provide information with regard to the metabolism of the drug, drug interactions, and its pharmacologic properties. Unlike phase I trials, participants in phase II trials are randomized to the intervention or control group.

The focus of phase III trials is to determine efficacy but only after a treatment seems to work in phase I and II trials. Phase III trials compare the results of participants who are receiving the investigational/new treatment with the results of people taking the standard treatment (i.e., which group has fewer recurrences, better survival rates, or fewer side effects). Typically, the sample sizes of phase III trials are considerably larger than those of phase I and II studies and frequently involve the collaborative effort of several institutions (NCI, 2001).

After a treatment has been approved and is being marketed, it is studied in a phase IV trial (postmarketing surveillance studies) to evaluate side effects that may not have been apparent in the phase III trial. Phase IV studies evaluate the long-term effects of the drug and its safety and efficacy among individuals in the general population. Thousands of people often are involved in a phase IV trial (NCI, 2001).

Cancer Treatment Trials

In cancer treatment trials, the control group receives the standard medication or treatment, or usual care, and the experimental (or intervention) group receives the new, untested treatment. Although these studies seek to improve methods of preventing or treating cancer, cancer clinical trials ultimately involve the withholding of a potentially beneficial treatment from the control group or the administration of a potentially risky new treatment to the experimental group (Polit & Hungler, 1999). As with all clinical trials, this type of research requires the careful consideration of ethical perspectives (see Chapter 6). A clinical trial should be scientifically, ethically, and methodologically justified. Investigators should carefully consider the amount of risk to participants, the necessity for a placebo, inclusion/exclusion criteria, and whether alternative ways are available of obtaining the same information prior to the onset of a clinical trial.

Findings From a Recent Breast Cancer Clinical Trial

Recent clinical trials have demonstrated the effectiveness of tamoxifen in reducing the risk of breast cancer among women at increased risk of developing the disease (Smigel, 1998), the lack of benefit of preoperative chemotherapy in the treatment of surgically resectable carcinoma of the thoracic esophagus (Malthaner & Fenlon, 2001), and the equivalence of outcomes from breast-conserving surgery with radiation compared to mastectomy among patients with early-stage breast cancer. These findings are used as a basis for treatment recommendations. NCI's Physician Data Query currently recommends breast-conserving surgery as an acceptable alternative to mastectomy for early-stage breast cancer (NCI, 2001c), and tamoxifen has been approved for use in the chemoprevention of breast cancer (U.S. Department of Health and Human Services, 1998). Clinical trials also have provided valuable information about risk factors for cancer (Greenwald, 1996). Clinical trials that evaluated the effect of alcohol consumption and tobacco use demonstrated the usefulness of reducing exposure to these substances and are examples of major research studies that have had a positive impact on the health behavior of many Americans (Buring & Hennekens, 1996; NCI, 2001a).

Supportive Care Trials

Supportive care trials are special studies that examine ways to improve the quality of life for patients with cancer and cancer survivors (NCI, 2001d). Supportive care trials may study drugs to reduce side effects from chemotherapy and other primary treatments and focus on problems (e.g., fatigue, nausea, pain, weight loss, a risk for second cancers, depression) encountered by patients with cancer. Other supportive care studies look for beneficial effects of nutrition, group therapy, and other approaches. Nurses serve as investigators and research team members on supportive care trials.

Challenges of Clinical Trials

Conducting clinical trials requires the consideration of many scientific and social issues (Friedman et al., 1998; Gordis, 2000). One major challenge facing clinical trials is minimizing or avoiding bias. Bias is defined as a systematic error in design, conduct, or analysis of a study that may result in a mistake estimate of an exposure's effect on the risk of disease (Friedman et al.; Gordis). Bias can be introduced into a study in several ways: faulty participant enrollment (selection bias), unstructured methods that result in differences between the groups within a study (observational bias), or study participants who may inaccurately remember different study events (recall bias). Nursing interventions should focus on reducing or avoiding bias in clinical trials. Such efforts should involve reducing error in the design and conduct of a study, reporting an actual or perceived bias, and taking such findings into consideration when interpreting the results of the study.

Another challenge facing the clinical trial results is its generalizability. According to Gordis (2000), the ultimate objective of conducting a clinical trial is to generalize its results beyond the study population. A study that readily allows its findings to generalize to the population at large is said to have high external validity (Pagano & Gauvreau, 2000). The degree of successfulness in eliminating confounding variables within the study itself is referred to as internal validity. The use of randomization or assigning study participants to a control group or to an experimental group ensures internal validity. External and internal validity are not all-or-none, present-or-absent dimensions of a clinical trial but rather vary along a continuum from low to high (Pagano & Gauvreau).

Finally, ethical patient care of the clinical trial participant involves putting the health interests of the patient first. The involvement of nurses helps to facilitate the rapid reporting of adverse events that occur as a result of clinical trial participation and respecting of patients' decisions about continued trial participation (Aikin, 2000). Ethical patient care is not contingent upon clinical trial participation; therefore, of patients should receive optimal care irrespective of their decision regarding participation in a clinical research study protocol. Clinical guidelines regarding the implementation of informed consent (Klimaszewski, Anderson, & Good, 2000), management of conflicts of interest (Cabriales, 2000a), and nursing guidelines for the ethical conduct of the clinical trials nurse are available (Cabriales, 2000b) and should be considered when developing nursing interventions related to the ethical conduct of clinical trials.

The Role of Nursing in Cancer Clinical Trials

Nurses are involved in almost every aspect of clinical trials, either as research nurses, data managers, protocol treatment nurses, advanced practice nurses, or nurse researchers (Aikin, 2000). According to Aikin, when nurses are actively involved in clinical trials, patients may be followed more closely and receive a greater standard of care when compared to patients who are not participating in clinical trials. Nurses also provide needed patient and family support, make referrals, and provide important information on the availability of clinical trials. Nurses who care for patients who participate in a cancer-control trial also collect objective and subjective data (DiGiulio et al., 1996; Edens & Safcsak, 1998; Sadler, Lantz, Fullerton, & Dault, 1999). Such data provide important feedback on the efficacy of the trial. Table 2-8 lists the types of cancer clinical trials, with examples of selected ongoing trials. Table 2-9 describes the role of nursing in cancer clinical trials.

Cancer Screening and Surveillance

Cancer screening, or secondary prevention, is used in the hope of improving a patient's prognosis. In Section III of this book, for the major cancer types, screen-

Table 2-8. Types of Cancer Clinical Trials With Selected Examples of Ongoing Trials

Type of Trial	Purpose of Trial	Example of Ongoing Trials
Treatment trials	To test new treatments such as a new cancer drug, new approaches to surgery or radiation therapy, new combinations of treatments, or new methods such as gene therapy	Phase I study of estramustine, docetaxel, and carboplatin in patients with hormone refractory prostate cancer
Prevention trials	To test new approaches to reduce or prevent the development of cancer or cancer recurrence. These can include lifestyle changes such as diet and physical activity, chemopreventive agents such as tamoxifen, and dietary supplements such as vitamins and minerals.	Study of Tamoxifen and Raloxifene (STAR) for the prevention of breast cancer
Screening trials	To test the effectiveness and feasibility of methods designed to screen for cancer in the general population	Diagnostic study of computed tomography and magnetic resonance imaging in the pretreatment evaluation of patients with invasive cervical cancer
Quality-of-life (supportive care) trials	To explore ways to improve comfort and quality of life for patients with cancer.	Randomized study of the quality of life in patients who have previously or currently received treatment for childhood cancers

Note. Based on information from NCI, 2001d.

Table 2-9. Nursing Characteristics and Roles in Cancer Clinical Trials

Title	Preparation and Characteristics	Responsibility	Potential Impact on Patient Care Outcome
Research nurse, clinical trials nurse, clinical research coordinator, protocol nurse	Registered nurse degree to advanced degrees. Ideally have experience in oncology nursing, familiar with administering protocol agents and symptom management strategies.	Administrative and clinical responsibilities, patient recruitment and eligibility, screening, medical management, patient and staff education, protocol compliance	Monitor patient's response to reduce toxicities and negative outcome to protocol; facilitate communication among patient, family, and research team; contribute to continuity of care by providing updates to team members.
Data managers clinical research associate (The roles of a nurse and data manager are sometimes combined or work in complimentary roles.)	Registered nurse or medical records professional. Have knowledge of oncology and medical terminology, anatomy, cancer staging, and data abstraction and clinical methodology.	Organize and collect data in a clinical trial. Design forms, enter data into computer, monitor patient accrual, provide periodic reports, and conduct audits.	Accurate data on patient enrollment, treatment responses, and outcome provide important feedback on the progress of the trial. More data are needed to accurately measure the effects of the role of the data manager.
Protocol treatment nurse	None provided; possible registered nurse	Administer treatments according to protocol guidelines; communicate with physicians and the research nurse; educate patients and family regarding side effects.	Patient benefits from close and careful monitoring when communication is available from health providers.
Advanced practice nurse, oncology clinical nurse specialist, nurse practitioner	Registered nurse degree with an advanced degree (e.g., MSN). Qualities of the research coordinator—expert symptom and clinical judgment and expanded scope of practice.	Administrative roles; develop new protocols and nursing care guidelines. Serve as resource for research nurses and data managers. Assist with adverse reporting.	Provide direct clinical care of patients, and participate in day-to-day activities of cooperative clinical trials group.
Nurse researcher	Doctorally prepared or master's degree in nursing	Often involved in conducting companion studies in association with existing medical studies	The outcomes of companion studies often provide data on basic, clinical, or behavioral outcomes. More nurse researcher–driven data are needed.

Note. Based on information from Aikin, 2000.

ing, and early-detection methods that currently are available will be reviewed. In the following section, the validity and reliability of cancer screening tests will be discussed, and some of the methodological considerations will be reviewed concerning inferences about the benefits of undergoing screening with such tests. Clinical Example 1 illustrates how the recognition of the differences in disease incidence in a population of interest can assist in choosing a guideline.

Clinical Example 1

Because incidence and prevalence vary significantly within a population, screening test choice and intervals may be different in institutions that serve different populations. For example, the most common cancers in the general United States population are lung, breast, prostate, and colon. In an Asian community, breast cancer incidence is quite low and gastric cancer incidence is high. These differences carry over even when people immigrate. Thus, an institution serving a largely first- or second-generation Asian American community may choose to use U.S. Protective Services Task Force recommendations to begin mammography at age 50 and then repeat every one to two years. In addition, such an institution may want to participate in gastric cancer screening trials. Another institution, serving largely Caucasian or African American populations, may choose guidelines and offer screening mammography to women beginning at age 40. This second institution also may consider offering in-depth risk assessment, counseling, and genetic testing for high-risk women and involvement with chemopreventive trials.

Note. From "Issues in Determining Cancer Screening Recommendations: Who, What, and When," by A. Foltz, 2000, *Oncology Nursing Forum, 27*(Suppl. 9), p. 14. Copyright 2000 by the Oncology Nursing Press, Inc. Reprinted with permission.

Validity of Screening Tests

How do nurses determine the quality of cancer screening and diagnostic tests for their patients? One way is to evaluate the validity of a screening test. The validity of a test can be defined as the ability of the test to distinguish people who have cancer. Validity has two dimensions: sensitivity and specificity (see Table 2-10). The sensitivity of a screening test is its ability to correctly identify patients who have cancer (Harkness, 1995). Accordingly, sensitivity reports the probability of testing positive if a cancer diagnosis truly is present. The specificity of a screening test is its ability to correctly identify patients who do not have cancer (Harkness). The specificity of a cancer-screening test explains the probability of a person testing negative if a cancer diagnosis truly does not exist.

As the sensitivity of a screening tests increases, its specificity decreases, and vice versa. Unfortunately, these differences may leave cases of cancer undetected (or classified as false negatives) or cases diagnosed with cancer that do not have it (false positives). When screening cases for cancer, the issue of false positives is important because these cases are brought back into the healthcare system for more sophisticated testing (Harkness, 1995). The resource needs and emotional burden placed on patients labeled as having cancer when they do not can be problematic. The problem of false negatives is also important. Failure to detect curable, early-stage cancers because of a false-negative result could represent long-term disability or even mortality.

Nurses can help to minimize the existence of some false-negative and false-positive cases by recommending the use of a screening test that is considered the "gold standard." A gold standard is a method, procedure, or measurement that is widely accepted as being the best available to detect the existence or nonexistence of a disease (Evidence Based Medicine Working Group, 2001b). For example, in comparison to digital or computer-enhanced screening, ultrasound, and magnetic resonance imaging, the mammogram is considered the gold standard test for the early detection of breast cancer and is the only current technology shown to lower breast cancer death rates (Institute of Medicine, 2001). Table 2-11 illustrates other important measures to improve sensitivity and specificity of cancer screening tests.

Table 2-10. Methods of Calculating Accuracy and Validity Measures of Screening Tests

Measure	Formula
Sensitivity	True Positive = TP + FP
Specificity	True Negative = TN + FP
Positive predictive value	True Positive = TP + FP
Negative predictive value	True Negative = TN + FN

TP = true positive test result; TN = true negative test result; FP = false positive test result; FN = false negative test result

Note. From "Issues in Determining Cancer Screening Recommendations: Who, What, and When," by A. Foltz, 2000, Oncology Nursing Forum, 27(Suppl. 9), p. 14. Copyright 2000 by the Oncology Nursing Press, Inc. Reprinted with permission.

Using Multiple Tests

Nurses who provide cancer screening also can help to minimize the existence of some false-negative and false-positive cases by using more than one cancer-screening test whenever possible. The American Cancer Society (ACS) (2001) recommended that both men and women who are 50 years of age should have a yearly fecal occult blood test combined with flexible sigmoidoscopy every 5 years, a double contrast barium enema every 5 years, or a colonoscopy every 10 years. The use of multiple tests for colorectal cancer screening is a good example of simultaneous testing. On baseline examination, such testing is performed all at once, and the person is considered positive for a disease if he or she has a positive result on any one or more of the tests (Gordis, 2000). Simultaneous testing provides a gain in net sensitivity because the case is considered positive for cancer based on previous testing.

Sequential testing is conducted in two stages and is less expensive and uncomfortable for patients. Sequential testing retests the patients who tested positive the first time, resulting in a loss in net sensitivity and a gain in net specificity. An example of sequential testing is used for the early detection of cervical cancer. ACS (2001) recommended that all women who are sexually active or older than 18 years of age have annual Pap tests and pelvic examinations, with less frequent testing performed among normal cases at the discretion of the physician. The Pap test and pelvic examination could be considered as stage one of the sequential testing.

If the results of the Pap test and pelvic examination are "abnormal," the healthcare provider will recommend additional diagnostic testing or will implement the sec-

Table 2-11. Measures That Improve Sensitivity and Specificity of Cancer Screening Tests

Measure	Examples
Certification of compliance with federal standards	Use Mammography Screening Quality Assurance Act for mammography and Clinical Laboratory Improvement Amendments for laboratories.
Quality assurance testing	Conduct periodic evaluation of examination techniques using direct observation, continuing education, patient satisfaction surveys, comparison of testing and disease outcome, surrogate patient feedback, or computerized or other outside review.
Standardized patient preparation	Ensure a documented, effective patient instruction procedure (e.g., avoidance of douching 24 hours prior to cervical cancer screening, avoidance of beef for three days before obtaining stool sample for occult blood testing).
Provider training	Ensure that clinical staff competency is supported and reviewed periodically (e.g., teaching clinical breast exam using national guidelines, continuing education for mammography technique).
Ongoing equipment evaluation	Have a mechanism to review new products or adoption of research on test equipment (e.g., use of cervical brushes in postmenopausal women).

Note. From "Issues in Determining Cancer Screening Recommendations: Who, What, and When," by A. Foltz, 2000, *Oncology Nursing Forum, 27*(Suppl. 9), p 15. Copyright 2000 by the Oncology Nursing Press, Inc. Reprinted with permission.

ond stage of the two-stage screening process. ACS supports the notion that because the Pap test is a screening test rather than a diagnostic test, patients with abnormal Pap test results should have additional tests (colposcopy and biopsy) to find out whether a precancerous change or cancer is present. The use of the colposcopy and biopsy then could be considered as the second stage of the two-stage process. Those cases of cervical cancer found during the Pap testing and pelvic examination screening and colposcopy and biopsy diagnosis would increase the net specificity.

Predictive Value of Screening Tests

Another way of determining the quality of available cancer screening and diagnostic tests is to evaluate the predictive value of the test. Understanding the proportion of a population that has cancer and correctly identifying it is important, particularly when screening large populations. However, in clinical settings, nurses must take into consideration the patients and families who are seeking information about screening and the likelihood that the patient actually has cancer. The consideration of the predictive value of a screening test may be helpful in answering the question as to the probability of a patient having cancer when the result of his or her cancer screening test is positive.

Positive predictive value (PPV) measures the proportion of people who test positive and have the condition in relation to all people who test positive (true positive in relation to true and false positives) (see Table 2-10). A test that is very sensitive will have a high percentage of people who correctly test positive and only a few who test positive but do not have the disease (Gordis, 2000). Thus, the PPV will be high. Negative predictive value measures the proportion of people who accurately test negative in relation to all people who test negative (true negatives in relation to true and false negatives) (Foltz, 2000). A test that is very specific will correctly identify the absence of disease in the majority of people who are healthy and rarely fails to identify the illness in people with the disease of interest.

Determining Test Reliability

A third consideration when determining the quality of cancer screening and diagnostic tests is its reliability. If repeated, does a screening test yield the same results? Although the sensitivity and specificity of a cancer-screening test is important, the repeatability or reliability of the same test is equally of value. A cancer-screening test is not helpful to the nurse or patient if differing or conflicting answers occur. Factors (i.e., intrasubject and interobserver variation) that can contribute to differences in screening test results will be reviewed.

Intrasubject and Interobserver Variation

Intrasubject variation refers to the changes in values that measure human characteristics (Gordis, 2000). Human characteristics (e.g., weight, blood count, health status) vary from minute to minute, day to day, and year to year and can be noted when measured by certain tests. Accordingly, when evaluating a cancer-screening test result, one must consider the conditions under which the test was performed. For example, how close was a premenopausal patient's mammogram scheduled to her menstrual cycle? What time of the day was Mr. Jones' prostate-specific antigen (PSA) drawn? Is Mrs. Davis currently on any medication that could affect the results of her fecal occult blood test?

Interobserver variation refers to differences in conclusions that may occur between two observers (Gordis, 2000). The observers (e.g., laboratory or healthcare professionals) may consider information gained from laboratory results, physical examinations, and related testing but do not come to the same results. To express the extent of agreement in quantitative terms, an overall percent agreement can be calculated. In the following formula, A refers to the positive cases that both observers (Observer 1 and Observer 2) agree upon; B refers to the cases that Observer 1 reports as negative and Observer 2 reports as positive; C refers to those cases that Observer 1 reports as positive and Observer 2 reports as negative; and D refers to those cases that both observers report as negative. (D is ignored in the formula because we only are concerned with potentially positive cases.)

$$\text{Percent agreement} = \frac{A \times 100}{A + B + C}$$

When the percent agreement is affected by the use of completely different criteria for calling cases positive or negative, the likelihood that two observers agree may be a function of chance (Gordis, 2000). To determine the extent of the agreement of two observers is beyond chance, a Kappa statistic should be used.

$$\text{Kappa} = \frac{\text{Percent observed agreement} - \text{Percent agreement expected by chance alone}}{100\% - \text{Percent agreement expected by chance alone}}$$

A Kappa statistic of 0.75 or greater suggests an excellent agreement beyond chance, between 0.40 and 0.75 suggests an intermediate to good agreement, and less than 0.40 suggests poor agreement. Further discussion of the use of Kappa statistics can be found in Gordis (2000) and Pagano and Gauvreau (2000).

Evaluating the Benefits of Screening

Nurses often are called upon to assist patients in deciding whether cancer screening is beneficial. The question of whether a patient would benefit from the early detection of cancer requires the consideration of the following (Gordis, 2000).
- Can the cancer in question be detected early?
- What are the sensitivity, specificity, and predictive value of the cancer-screening test?
- How significant is the problem of a false-positive test result?
- What is the cost of the early detection of cancer (e.g., monies, resources, emotional)?
- Can patients be harmed in any way by early testing?
- Does the individual benefit in any way from having her disease detected early?

Of these considerations, the major challenge is determining whether or not an individual would truly benefit from early detection. Determining individual benefit must be based on measurable outcomes. Nurses should promote cancer screening if the test will reduce the cancer mortality of that population screened, reduce the case-fatality rates of individuals who are screened, increase the percentage of cases detected at early stages, reduce cancer complications, prevent or reduce cancer recurrences or metastases, and improve the qualify of life of screened individuals (Gordis, 2000).

Types of Cancer Screening

Cancer screening can be rendered in several ways (Harkness, 1995). Mass screening is applied to entire populations. Selective screening is applied to specific high-risk populations An example of selective screening is the use of PSA. PSA screening is controversial primarily because of the absence of randomized trials documenting that early detection and aggressive treatment of prostate cancer can reduce mortality; however, it is offered to males as a way to monitor their risk for prostate cancer. Multiphasic screening applies to a variety of screening tests given to the same populations on the same occasion. Finally, case finding screening involves a clinician's search for illness as part of patients' periodic health examination.

Screening programs also must have certain characteristics to be of benefit in the fight against cancer. First, a screening program must focus on cancers that have a significant impact on the target population. According to Harkness (1995), the expenditure of resources for screening should result in positive health outcomes or be cost effective. In addition, for screening to be beneficial, the treatment given during the preclinical phase should result in a better prognosis for the individual than the treatment given after the symptoms have developed; therefore, the cancer screening should be effective in reducing both morbidity and mortality. Finally, screening programs should be cost effective when the prevalence of cancer is high in a certain population and should be efficacious for members of the population to use (Harkness).

Bias

When evaluating cancer testing, the nurse also must take into consideration biases that may influence the perception of screening benefit. These may involve selection bias, lead-time bias, length-time bias, lead-time and five-year survival, and over-diagnosis bias.

According to Gordis (2000), selection bias relates to a bias in assignment: How was the individual assigned to be screened or not screened for the disease under investigation? Were those assigned to be screened the same or different than those not screened? Ideally, when a screening test is offered or is under investigation, the population of people offered cancer-screening tests should be similar to individuals who do not partake in the screening. However, people do differ, and many screening programs or studies elicit volunteers. Health programs and research studies that use volunteers often are presented with individuals who have unique characteristics that make them "different" than the general population. These differences (e.g., more healthy, at greater risk, more eager to please) may introduce a bias, making tempered interpretation of any screening program or study results essential. To reduce selection bias, the use of a randomized experimental study that examines two groups that are similar in profile is warranted (Gordis, 2000).

Lead-time bias refers to the bias that arises by adding the time gained as a result of earlier diagnosis to the survival time (Evidence Based Medicine Working Group, 2001a). How much time can be gained in making a diagnosis if nurses screen for cancer in comparison to the usual timing of the diagnosis if cancer screening is not performed? Figure 2-6 illustrates how a lack of screening with and without effective treatment can affect the mortality. The lead-time of detecting a cancer early, along with the provision of effective treatment, may result in an extension at the end of life. In contrast, Clinical Example 2 describes how lead-time bias may uncover the lack of benefit of certain cancer screening. Finally, lead time can affect five-year survival in that the perception of longer survival may be an artifact of an earlier detection of cancer (see page 71 for a definition of five-year survival). Lead time must be considered when interpreting the results of nonrandomized studies (Gordis, 2000).

Length bias arises because of the preferential diagnosis of more indolent cases of cancer through the use of screening (Foltz, 2000). Some cancers have variable disease patterns. For example, breast and prostate cancers have subsets of both extremely aggressive and indolent diseases. The aggressive tumors progress rapidly from onset to symptoms and to death. Indolent cancers can remain localized

Figure 2-6. Interaction of Screening and Treatment on Disease Outcome

Disease Trajectory	Onset →	Subclinical Disease →	Clinical Disease →	End of Life
Without screening			Diagnosis X	
Screening without effec- tive treatment		Diagnosis X		
Screening with effective treatment		Diagnosis X		

Note. Based on information from Earle & Hobort, 1996. From "Issues in Determining Cancer Screening Recommendations: Who, What, and When," by A. Foltz, 2000, *Oncology Nursing Forum, 27*(Suppl. 9), p. 16. Copyright 2000 by the Oncology Nursing Press, Inc. Reprinted with permission.

Clinical Example 2

Lead-time bias is a major issue in the controversy surrounding testicular cancer screening, either by testicular clinical exam (TCE) or testicular self-exam (TSE). TCE and TSE are questioned as being true screening tests because, to be positive, the testicular mass must be large enough for palpation. Minimal clinical evidence has suggested that a mass found by incidental exam varies more in stage or treatment than one found by purposeful TCE of TSE. Treatment for testicular cancer found incidentally also is extremely effective, so treatment initiated at screening or at incidental discovery usually consists of the same regimen and has the same cure rate. The lack of clear benefit from screening and the costs for clinical time spent in examination or teaching TSE techniques underlie the decision of organizations that do not endorse routine screening for testicular cancer.

Note. From "Issues in Determining Cancer Screening Recommendations: Who, What, and When," by A. Foltz, 2000, *Oncology Nursing Forum, 27*(Suppl. 9), p. 16. Copyright 2000 by the Oncology Nursing Press, Inc. Reprinted with permission.

to the original organ for a long time. Some cancers remain in situ and never present a health threat. Because of the relatively long time of growth before symptoms appear, indolent cancers are much more likely to be detected by screening tests than are the aggressive forms. Thus, people whose cancers are found during screening may appear to have longer survival times, although the differences in survival lie more with tumor kinetics than with the screening process. Clinical Example 3 illustrates issues surrounding length bias and the decision to screen.

Overdiagnosis bias is the result of screening in excess. False-positive readings and overzealous screeners may inflate the actual detection and diagnosis of early-stage cancers as a result of the screening and may erroneously elevate the estimates

Clinical Example 3

Length bias and lead-time bias both are part of the controversy surrounding prostate cancer screening. The indolent nature of the majority of prostate cancers and its resulting length-time bias leads the U.S. Preventive Services Task Force to oppose routine prostate cancer screening. Many of the people diagnosed with prostate cancer found on screening have tumors that do not become a threat to health for years. Because standard prostate cancer treatment has significant morbidity, early screening and treatment may cause screenees to have a longer period of morbidity from treatment than they would have had by waiting until symptoms appeared. Concerns about lead bias in prostate cancer screening arise because cancers found during screening and those found when mild symptoms exist are treated the same and have the same outcome. In contrast, proponents of routine prostate cancer screening maintain that advances in treatment limit morbidity. Thus, treatment initiated at the time of screening may not threaten quality of life as much as delayed treatment. Moreover, the inability to accurately predict which tumors are indolent and which are aggressive leads these clinicians to treat all prostate cancers when they are found, rather than waiting. Both proponents and opponents of prostate screening have legitimate points. The decision to screen may depend on characteristics of the institution performing the screening as well as the population being served.

Note. From "Issues in Determining Cancer Screening Recommendations: Who, What, and When," by A. Foltz, 2000, *Oncology Nursing Forum, 27*(Suppl. 9), p. 17. Copyright 2000 by the Oncology Nursing Press, Inc. Reprinted with permission.

of cancer survival after screening cases who are thought to have cancer (Gordis, 2000). Nurses can assist in reducing overdiagnosis bias by ensuring that standard cancer diagnostic procedures be rigorously enforced.

No Benefit

The early detection of cancer often presents with the result of no benefit; that is, no differences exist in outcomes (e.g., morbidity, mortality) between patients who used the screening test and those who did not (Gordis, 2000). When such circumstances arise in practice, the nurse should consider that the lack of benefit could be because of the natural course of the cancer (no detectable or extremely short preclinical phase); that the current treatment available may not be more effective if provided earlier in comparison to a usual time of diagnosis; or the natural history and treatments that currently are available. However, limitations in the provision of care to those who tested positive may account for the observed lack of benefit (Gordis). Nursing efforts, therefore, should focus on assisting the patient in evaluating and making tailored informed choices about other treatment and quality-of-life options.

Cost-Benefit Analysis

Cost-benefit analysis calculates the trade-offs by measuring the cost of consumed resources but also by placing a dollar value on the years of life saved and other benefits (Petitti, 1994). It implies that if the monetary benefits exceed the costs, the screening program should be implemented. Although cost-benefit analysis is theoretically sound, offering a way to trade off all effects of an intervention using a dollar amount, techniques for quantifying health, and other benefits has fallen out of favor (Petitti). The cost-effectiveness analysis defines costs in a similar manner, but effectiveness may be defined simply based on nonfinancial costs, such as quality of life (Elliott & Harris, 2001).

Nurses must consider issues related to cost benefit and cost effectiveness when participating in cancer prevention and control activities. First, a cancer-screening intervention is not always more cost effective simply because it affects large numbers of people. The need for resources (e.g., manpower, facilities) may inflate the cost of providing screening but may yield little in the way of new cases. In addition, cost-effective interventions are not necessarily those screening and early-detection tests that are most effective. For example, cervical cancer has a long preclinical phase and well-defined precursor lesions that are readily detected, and widespread routine use of the Pap test has been a highly effective public health measure (Rubin, 2001). More recently, refinements such as computerized screening and fluid-based cytology have been introduced but with minor improvements that have significantly increased the cost of screening. As a result, Pap testing remains the gold standard for the early detection of cervical cancer. Finally, cost effectiveness does not always imply that the benefits of screening are consistently high or low. Rigel and Carucci (2000) noted that the annual screening for malignant melanoma could reduce the number of deaths from this disease, possibly making the benefits of screening high. The cost-benefit ratio of skin-cancer screening, as well as the feasibility of screening 280 million Americans for skin cancer, however, presents a major challenge. As an alternative, the authors recommend target screening for melanoma for those who are at highest risk.

Cancer Surveillance

Surveillance is the systematic collection of data pertaining to the occurrence of specific diseases, the analysis and interpretation of information, and the dissemination of the information to healthcare professions, the general public, and other consumers of public health data (Friis & Sellers, 1999). Surveillance is carried out to monitor changes in disease frequency or to monitor changes in the prevalence of risk factors (Gordis, 2000) and can provide "decision-making guidance" in the development and implementation of "best strategies" for disease prevention and control programs (Gordis; Pedersoli et al., 1998). For example, surveillance data can be used in modeling to better understand the impact of interventions (e.g., screening, treatment, primary prevention) on population-based cancer trends in the United States.

In response to the growing incidence, prevalence, and mortality of cancer in the United States, the National Cancer Act was passed in 1971. It mandated the collection, analysis, and dissemination of data essential to the prevention, detection, and control of cancer (NCI, 2001e). As a result, NCI established the SEER program to collect data on U.S. cancer incidence and survival (NCI, 2001e) (see Figure 2-7).

The SEER program is the most authoritative source of information on cancer incidence and survival in the United States and is the only comprehensive source of population-based information in the United States that includes stage of cancer at the time of diagnosis and survival rates within each stage. The SEER database includes information on more than 2.5 million in situ and invasive cancer cases, and approximately 160,000 new cases are accessioned each year within the SEER

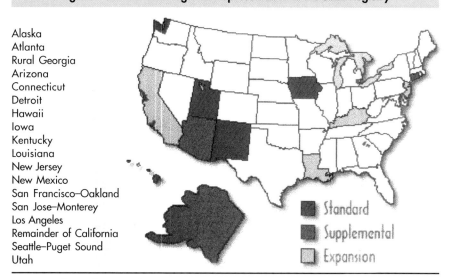

Figure 2-7. State and Regional Representation in the SEER Registry

Alaska
Atlanta
Rural Georgia
Arizona
Connecticut
Detroit
Hawaii
Iowa
Kentucky
Louisiana
New Jersey
New Mexico
San Francisco–Oakland
San Jose–Monterey
Los Angeles
Remainder of California
Seattle–Puget Sound
Utah

Standard
Supplemental
Expansion

Note. Based on information from NCI, 2001a.

catchment areas (NCI, 2001e). In addition to cancer cases, the SEER registries routinely collect data on patient demographics, primary tumor site, morphology, stage at diagnosis, first course of treatment, and follow-up for vital status (NCI, 2001e). The National Center for Health Statistics provides the mortality data that are reported by SEER.

SEER collects and publishes cancer incidence and survival data from 11 population-based cancer registries and three supplemental registries covering approximately 14% of the U.S. population (NCI, 2001e). The collection of SEER data began in early 1973, with seven SEER sites (Connecticut, Iowa, New Mexico, Utah, and Hawaii and the metropolitan areas of Detroit and San Francisco-Oakland). Since then, the SEER program gradually was expanded to increase the coverage of the diverse U.S. population, including predominantly African American rural counties in Georgia, Alaska Native populations in Alaska, Native Americans in Arizona, and Hispanics in California. In 2001, SEER coverage was expanded even further from 14% to 26% of the U.S. population, an increase from approximately 35 million to 65 million people (NCI, 2001b) through a collaboration with the CDC.

SEER data are updated each year and are provided as a public service in print (e.g., monographs, annual reports), electronic formats (e.g., public-use data file on CD-ROM), and various software packages (e.g., SEER*Stat, SEER*Prep) through the SEER Web site (http://seer.cancer.gov). The data are used by thousands of researchers, clinicians, public health officials, legislators, policymakers, community groups, and the general public. SEER data also are used in an ongoing program of special studies to address emerging cancer research questions, such as screening programs; passage of tobacco-related legislation; identification of populations at risk for higher rates of cancer; comparisons of cancer incidence, mortality, and risk factors in specific geographic areas; and studies of patterns of cancer care.

NCI also collaborates with a number of organizations that also are involved in cancer surveillance and related disciplines. For example, in a collaboration with the Census Bureau and CDC, the U.S. National Longitudinal Mortality Study has been expanded and extended to link with the National Death Index to add 60,000 cancer deaths. This will overcome the limited availability of individual-level sociodemographic information on death certificates, and self-reported racial/ethnic data will be obtained to allow an in-depth analysis of racial/ethnic, socioeconomic, and occupational differentials in cancer mortality for major cancer sites. These collaborations result in the development or improvement of standards for data collection by cancer registries, the interchange of ideas and tools for cancer surveillance, the training and provision of educational materials for the credentialing of cancer registrars, the provision of workshops for advanced training in data collection and coding, collaboration in the analysis and reporting of cancer rates, and support for efforts to expand existing cancer surveillance and to establish new cancer reporting systems. Figure 2-8 lists other cancer surveillance agencies that collaborate with the SEER program.

Figure 2-8. Select Cancer Registry Agencies and Health Professional Agencies That Collaborate With the SEER Program

• American Cancer Society
• American College of Surgeons
• Centers for Disease Control and Prevention
• International Association of Cancer Registries
• International Association for Research on Cancer
• National Cancer Registrars Association
• North American Association of Central Cancer Registries
• World Health Organization

Cancer Surveillance and Nursing Practice

Cancer surveillance commonly is used in nursing practice. Nurses use surveillance data in identifying those communities and populations most in need of provider outreach services (Harkness, 1995; Mulhull, 2000). Primary outreach services are primary prevention community interventions that are delivered in the patient's environment (e.g., home visits, school, church programs). See Section IV for examples of how nurses from around the country integrate cancer surveillance in practice. Cancer surveillance data also provide nurses with information on needed screening or secondary cancer prevention interventions. In addition, nurses engage in surveillance activities as they monitor the health of their patients (Harkness; Mulhull). Following-up on an adolescent female with a history of abnormal Pap tests to ensure that she receives a colposcopy or determining whether an elderly man has dependable transportation to and from his radiation therapy appointments are just a few examples of how nurses participate in cancer surveillance.

Expressing Cancer Prognosis and Outcomes

When screening for cancer is successful, determining one's prognosis or prospect for survival becomes paramount. How can the prognosis be expressed, and why is describing cancer prognosis important? Cancer prognosis can be expressed in terms of survival or mortality. Nurses should be proficient in quantitatively characterizing the natural history of cancer for several reasons. First, knowing the prognosis of patients diagnosed with specific cancers is essential to understanding the severity of their disease and aids in prioritizing clinical services and in the development of public health programs (Gordis, 2000; Valanis, 1986). Furthermore, understanding the natural history of cancer and its prognosis is necessary in determining the efficacy of new cancer treatments compared to current treatments (Chu & Kramer, 1995; Gordis).

Survival

Patient survival is one of the most important measures of the benefit of early detection through screening and of the effectiveness of patient care. Studies of survival of patients with cancer, using various data sources (e.g., medical records, population-based cancer registries), are essential for monitoring and evaluating the effectiveness of treatment of cancer in the population and in providing a vital perspective for nurses to plan cancer-control activities.

The difference in living 1 year or 10 years after diagnosis is important to both patients and healthcare professionals. How long patients survive after diagnosis is a function of their disease stage at diagnosis, clinical characteristics, other illnesses and conditions they may have, and the treatment they receive. Survival analyses are used to (a) estimate failure time distributions, (b) compare the experiences of different groups after their cancer diagnosis, (c) estimate the effects of treatment, (d) and evaluate the prognosis of different variables by themselves or in combination with other variables (Marubini & Valsecchi, 1996). Cancer survival rates differ from mortality rates in that they focus on the length of time that elapses between diagnosis and disease recurrence, death, or another event of interest rather than just the actual number of cancer deaths that occur among individuals in a particular population. Survival rates typically used in cancer prevention and control research include the observed, disease or recurrence free, cause or disease specific, and relative survival rates (see Table 2-12). Survival rates can be interpreted either as the proportion of patients who survive or the probability of surviving given the characteristics (e.g., type of cancer, stage, age) of the patients used to calculate the survival rate.

Because patients generally will have had cancer for varying lengths of time prior to diagnosis, survival analyses frequently are performed separately by stage. This is referred to as stratified analyses, and the resulting statistic is the stage-specific survival rate (Ries et al., 2000). The stage-specific survival rate provides a more accurate description of patient prognosis given the extent of disease at diagnosis than does a combined rate. Further, stage-specific survival rates are useful means of controlling for disease characteristics when examining the role of other

Table 2-12. Survival Definitions

Rate	Description
Survival time	Average (mean) or median time for a group of patients
Relative survival rate	The likelihood that a patient will not die from causes associated specifically with a given cancer before some specified time after diagnosis, usually five years
Observed (overall) survival rate	The likelihood of surviving **all causes** of death for a certain time after cancer diagnosis
Event-free, disease-free, relapse survival	The proportion of patients who did not have an event within a specified time period. Examples of events in cancer include a cancer recurrence after a period of remission and biochemical failure such as prostate-specific antigen elevation after treatment for prostate cancer.

Note. Based on information from Marubini & Valsecchi, 1996; Ries et al., 2000.

clinical or nonclinical characteristics such as tumor grade, histology, age, race, and gender. Stage-specific survival can be calculated for all survival rates.

Observed Survival Rate

The observed survival rate (also known as overall survival rate) is a measure of the proportion of patients who survive all causes of death after a cancer diagnosis during the period of study (Gordis, 2000). The observed survival can be easily calculated when the time of all deaths (events) is known. The observed survival rate provides information about the likelihood or rate of survival given the distribution of other diseases/conditions that might affect prognosis. The disadvantage of the observed survival rate is that it includes deaths from diseases or conditions other than the specific cancer under study (Friis & Sellers, 1999). As a consequence, differences in the number of events between two groups from causes not related to the specific cancer under study may be interpreted as differential prognosis between the two groups.

Cause-Specific/Disease-Specific Survival

The cause- or disease-specific survival rate is a measure of the proportion of patients who do not die from the specific disease (or cancer) under study during the study period (Friis & Sellers, 1999; Gordis, 2000). An important difference between the overall and disease-specific rate is that only patients who die from cancer under study are counted as failures. The cause- or disease-specific survival rate provides a more accurate measure of the prognosis from a specific cancer because it adjusts for other causes of death. This is especially important in studies of older populations where the likelihood of death from other noncancer related causes can be substantial.

Relative Survival Rate

The relative survival rate is a ratio of the observed survival rate to the expected survival rate for a patient cohort (Ries et al., 2000). The expected survival rate is based on the mortality experience of the total population after adjusting for age, sex, race, and year of diagnosis, as appropriate, and represents the "normal life expectancy" of the cohort during the period of observation. Thus, the relative survival is the observed survival rate of individuals with a specific cancer relative to the survival rate that is expected for people of similar age, race, and gender in the general population during the same period of observation.

Five-Year Survival

The five-year survival rate represents the proportion of patients who did not experience the event of interest during the five years after diagnosis or after cancer treatment begins (Friis & Sellers, 1999; Gordis, 2000). The selection of a five-year interval is arbitrary; there are no fast rules on what time interval should be used. Historically, a significant portion of cancer deaths occurred during the first five years after diagnosis; thus, health practitioners typically use this time period as an index of successful medical management (Friis & Sellers; Gordis).

Life Tables

Life tables can be used to calculate survival rates for individuals observed for varied lengths of time. Two major methods are available for calculating observed survival rates from life tables: the actuarial and the Kaplan-Meir methods. The major difference between the two methods is in the timing of the survival calculations. In the Kaplan-Meir method, a survival calculation is performed every time a death occurs in the cohort, providing a more exact description of the survival pattern. In contrast, with the actuarial method, survival calculations are performed at regular intervals (usually one year). Because of the more frequent calculations required for the Kaplan-Meir method, it is performed more frequently with a computer using statistical software such as Egret, SAS, or SPSS. For a more detailed discussion of survival analyses, see Klein and Moeschberger, 1997.

Table 2-13 provides an example of the actuarial life table calculations. To calculate survival using the actuarial life table method, determine the time intervals of interest (e.g., years, months, weeks) (A), the number of subjects that begin the interval (B), the number of subjects that failed during that interval (died or experienced the event of interest) (C), and the number of withdrawals (subjects that are lost to follow-up or withdrawn before experiencing the event) (D). Subjects that began the time interval in consideration but did not complete it are said to be censored. The effective number exposed to the risk of the dying (E) is calculated by subtracting one-half of the number of withdrawals (D) from the number of subjects who were alive at the beginning of the interval (B). The probability or proportion of subjects dying (F) is equal to the number of people who died (failed) during the interval (C) divided by the effective number exposed to the risk of dying/failing (E). The probability or proportion of people surviving (G) is equal to one minus the probability of proportion of people dying during the interval (F).

Surviving a later time interval is conditioned upon having survived all of the earlier intervals; this is measured by the cumulative survival. The cumulative survival can be obtained by multiplying the survival rate for the time period of interest by each of the preceding survival rates (percent surviving). Survival curves fre-

Table 2-13. Actuarial Method of Life Table Calculations

| (A) | (B) | (C) | (D) | (E) | Probability | | |
					(F)	(G)	(H)
Time at beginning of interval (years)	Number alive at beginning of interval	Died during interval	Last seen alive during interval "withdrawals"	Effective number exposed to the risk of dying	Dying during the interval	Surviving through interval	Cumulative survival rates*
				(B–½ D)	(C/E)	(1–F)	
0–< 1	41	5	6	38	0.132	0.868	0.868
1–< 2	30	2	2	29	0.069	0.931	0.808
2–< 3	26	0	1	25.5	0.00	1.00	0.808
3–< 4	25	2	7	21.5	0.093	0.907	0.733
4–< 5	16	2	1	15.5	0.129	0.871	0.638
5 or more	13	2	11				

* The cumulative survival is equal to G for the first row. For subsequent rows, the cumulative survival rate is equal to G* H from the row above it.

Note. Based on information from Shambaugh et al., 1994.

quently are used to provide a graphical representation of the cumulative survival. A survival curve is a graph of the number of events occurring over time or the chance of being free of these events over time. The events must be discrete, and the time at which they occur must be precisely known.

The survival rate can be approximated from survival curves by determining the proportion surviving at the end of the interval of interest (e.g., one year, five years). All people included in a survival curve are alive at point 0; thus, the survival curve always starts at 100% or 1.0. In most clinical situations, the chance of an event changes over time. Examples of a survival curves are provided in Figures 2-9 and 2-10. Figure 2-9 illustrates the five-year survival experiences of patients with pancreatic cancer who are treated with pancreaticoduodenectomy. The difference in the slope or steepness of the curve between two periods provides information about the rate of events, in this case, deaths during the interval or, conversely, survival. Between year 0 (the beginning of the observation period) and year 1, a sharper drop occurs in the survival curve than for other intervals. This indicates that the rate of death was higher during the first year after surgery than for the remaining four years. The survival curve levels off between years four and five, which indicates that few deaths occurred after year four. From this survival curve it can be concluded that the risk of death is highest during the period immediately after surgery, especially during the first year. The probability of surviving one year, that is the one-year survival rate, is about 55%, and the five-year survival rate is approximately 21%. The median survival rate, or the time at which the survival rate is equal to 50%, is approximately 1.3 years (this is typically given in months).

Figure 2-9. Example of a Survival Curve*

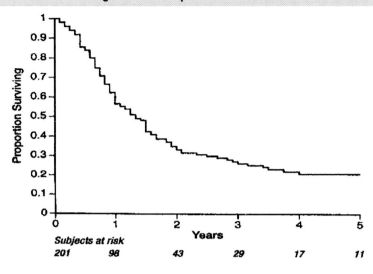

Note. From "Pancreatic Cancer: State of the Art Care," by K.D. Lillemoe, C.J. Yeo, and J.L. Cameron, 2000, *CA: A Cancer Journal for Clinicians, 50,* p. 258. Copyright 2000 by the American Cancer Society. Reprinted with permission.

*The actuarial survival curve (Kaplan-Meier) for 201 patients undergoing pancreaticoduodenctomy for pancreatic adenocarcinoma.

Figure 2-10. The Actuarial Survival Curve

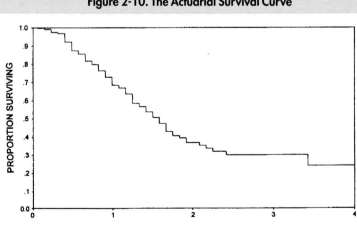

Note. From "Pancreaticoduodenectomy for Pancreatic Adenocarcinoma: Postoperative Adjunctive Chemoradiation Improves Survival. A Prospective, Single-Institution Experience," by C.J. Yeo, R.A. Abrams, L.B. Goochow, T.A. Sohn, S.E. Ord, R.H. Hruban, M.L. Zahurak, W.C. Dooley, J. Coleman, P.K. Sauter, H.A. Pitt, K.D. Lillemoe, and J.L. Cameron, 1997, *Annals of Surgery, 225,* p. 626. Copyright 1997 by Lippincott Williams & Wilkins. Reprinted with permission.

Figure 2-10 compares the three-year survival experiences of patients treated with adjuvant therapy to patients who were not treated with adjuvant therapy. The survival curve for patients treated with adjuvant therapy shows that they had a better three-year survival experience than did patients who did not receive this treatment. The difference in the width between the two curves represents the difference in the survival rates. The statistical significance of the difference between the two survival curves can be ascertained by the CIs or by the p-value obtained from hypothesis testing. The differences between the two survival curves in this example are statistically significant, with a p-value = 0.03. The difference in the width between the two survival curves is greatest during the interval after diagnosis and the first year than for subsequent periods. The one-, two-, and three-year survival rates are about 77%, 39%, and 35%, respectively, among patients treated with adjuvant chemotherapy compared to 68%, 30%, and 27% for patients not treated with adjuvant chemotherapy.

Summary and Conclusion

Epidemiology and nursing are interdependent disciplines. The integration of epidemiological concepts into nursing practice is an essential tool for combating cancer. Moreover, the use of nursing education, research, and practice perspectives that address cancer epidemiologic findings are urgently needed to reduce the national cancer epidemical. A recent call for expert nurses in epidemiology (Anonymous, 1994; Mulhull, 2000; Whitehead, 2000a, 2000b) directs attention to the need for nurses who are competent in epidemiology to become experts in cancer prevention, detection, and control. As nurses continue to fight the war against cancer, they must armor themselves with an understanding of concepts in epidemiology and increase the use of these concepts in practice. Moreover, nurses involved in cancer prevention and control must continue to evaluate usefulness of epidemiology within the profession via scientific and educational inquiry.

The authors would like to acknowledge the helpful insight on earlier drafts of the chapter of Vickie L. Shavers, PhD, epidemiologist, Health Services and Economics Branch, and Deirdre Lawrence, PhD, MPH, epidemiologist, Risk Factor Monitoring and Methods Branch, both of the Applied Research Program at the National Cancer Institute, National Institutes of Health in Bethesda, MD.

References

Abramson, J.H. (2001). *Making sense of data: A self-instruction manual on the interpretation of epidemiological data*. New York: Oxford University Press.

Aikin, J.L. (2000). Nursing roles in clinical trials. In A.D. Klimaszewski, J.L. Aikin, M.A. Bacon, S.A. DiStasio, H.E. Ehrenberger, & B.A. Ford (Eds.), *Manual for clinical trials nursing* (pp. 273–276). Pittsburgh: Oncology Nursing Press, Inc.

Althuis, M.D., Sexton, M., Langenberg, P., Bush, T.L., Tkaczuk, K., Magaziner, J., & Khoo, L. (2000). Surveillance for uterine abnormalities in tamoxifen-treated breast carcinoma survivors. *Cancer, 89*, 800–810.

American Cancer Society. (2001). *Colon and rectum cancer detection and symptoms.* Retrieved July 17, 2001 from the World Wide Web: http://www3.cancer.org/cancerinfo/

Anonymous. (1994). Epidemiology in nursing research and health policy. *National League of Nursing Research and Policy Prism, 2*(3), 1–2, 8.

Arthur, A., & McGarry, J. (1999). Epidemiology and nursing: The Melton Aowbray aging project. *Nursing Times, 95,* 56–57.

Bain, C., Willett, W., Hennekens, C.H., Rosner, B., Belanger, C., & Speizer, F.E. (1981). Use of postmenopausal hormones and risk of myocardial infarction. *Circulation, 64,* 42–46.

Buring, J.E., & Hennekens, C.H. (1996). Intervention studies. In D. Schottenfeld & J.F. Fraumeni, Jr. (Eds.), *Cancer epidemiology and prevention* (pp. 1422–1432). New York: Oxford University Press.

Cabriales, S. (2000a). Conflict of interest. In A.D. Klimaszewski, J.L. Aikin, M.A. Bacon, S.A. DiStasio, H.E. Ehrenberger, & B.A. Ford (Eds.), *Manual for clinical trials nursing* (pp. 221–223). Pittsburgh: Oncology Nursing Press, Inc.

Cabriales, S. (2000b). Nursing guidelines. In A.D. Klimaszewski, J.L. Aiken, M.A. Bacon, S.A. DiStasio, H.E. Ehrenberger, & B.A. Ford (Eds.), *Manual for clinical trials nursing* (pp. 225–226). Pittsburgh: Oncology Nursing Press, Inc.

Cardenas, V.M., Thun, M.J., Austin, H., Lally, C.A., Clark, W.S., Greenberg, R.S., & Heath, C.W. (1997). Environmental tobacco smoke and lung cancer mortality in the American Cancer Society's Cancer Prevention Study. *Cancer Causes and Control, 8*(1), 57–64.

Carmel, B., & Reid, M. (1997). Cancer control and epidemiology. In S.L. Groenwald, M.H. Frogge, M. Goodman, & C.H. Yarbro (Eds.), *Cancer nursing: Principles and practice* (4th ed.) (pp. 50–74). Boston: Jones and Bartlett.

Centers for Disease Control and Prevention. (2000). *CDC fact book 2000–2001.* Atlanta: Department of Health and Human Services.

Centers for Disease Control and Prevention. (2001). *Glossary of epidemiology terms.* Retrieved July 17, 2001 from the World Wide Web: http://www.cdc.gov/

Chu, K.C., & Kramer, B.S. (1995). Cancer patterns in the United States. In P. Greenwald, B.S. Kramer, & D.L. Weed (Eds.), *Cancer prevention and control* (pp. 9–22). New York: Marcel Dekker.

Cohen, J.H., Kristal, A.R., & Stanford, J.L. (2000). Fruit and vegetable intakes and prostate cancer risk. *Journal of the National Cancer Institute, 92,* 61–68.

Colditz, G.A., Hoaglin, D.C., & Berkey, C.S. (1997). Cancer incidence and mortality: The priority of screening frequency and population coverage. *Milbank Quarterly, 75,* 147–171.

Cookfair, D.L., & Cookfair, J.M. (1996). Epidemiology in community health nursing. In J.M. Cookfair (Ed.), *Nursing care in the community* (2nd ed.) pp. 125–142. St. Louis, MO: Mosby.

Correa, A. (1995). Nonexperimental methods. In P. Greenwald, B.S. Kramer, & D.L. Weed (Eds.), *Cancer prevention and control* (pp. 195–212). New York: Marcel Dekker.

DiGiulio, P., Arrigo, C., Gall, H., Molin, C., Neweg, R., & Strohbucker, B. (1996). Expanding the role of the nurse in clinical trials: The nursing summaries. *Cancer Nursing, 19,* 343–347.

Earle, C., & Hebert, P.C. (1996). A reader's guide to the evaluation of screening studies. *Postgraduate Medical Journal, 72,* 77–83.

Edens, T.R., & Safcsak, K. (1998). Issues in clinical trials management: Collaborating with colleagues. Part I: Staff nurse involvement: A necessity for successful clinical trials. *Research Nurse, 4*(4), 1, 4–9, 12–4.

Elliott, S.L., & Harris, A.H. (2001). *The methodology of cost-effective analysis: Avoiding common pitfalls.* Retrieved August 28, 2001 from the World Wide Web: http://pcdon.net

Ellison, L.F. (2000). Tea and other beverage consumption and prostate cancer risk: A Canadian retrospective cohort study. *European Journal of Cancer Prevention, 9*(2), 125–130.

Evidence Based Medicine Working Group. (2001a). Clinical epidemiology glossary. *Survival curves.* Retrieved August 28, 2001 from the World Wide Web: http://www.med.ualberta.ca/

Evidence Based Medicine Working Group. (2001b). Clinical epidemiology glossary. *Gold standard.* Retrieved August 28, 2001 from the World Wide Web: http://www.med.ualberta.ca/

Foltz, A. (2000). Issues in determining cancer screening recommendations: Who, what, and when. *Oncology Nursing Forum, 27* (Suppl. 9), 13–17.

Friedman, L.M., Furberg, C.D., & DeMets, D.L. (1998). *Fundamentals of clinical trials.* New York: Springer-Verlag.

Friis, R.H., & Sellers, T.A. (1999). *Epidemiology for public health practice* (2nd ed.). Gaithersburg, MD: Aspen Publishers.

Glantz, S.A. (1997). *Primer of biostatistics.* New York: McGraw-Hill.

Gordis, L. (2000). *Epidemiology* (2nd ed.). Philadelphia: W.B. Saunders.

Greenwald, P. (1995). Preventive clinical trials. An overview. *Annals of the New York Academy of Sciences, 768,* 129–140.

Greenwald, P. (1996). Cancer risk factors for selecting cohorts for large-scale chemoprevention trials. *Journal of Cellular Biochemistry, 25,* 29–36.

Harkness, G.A. (1995). *Epidemiology in nursing practice.* St. Louis, MO: Mosby.

Hennekens, C.H., & Buring, J.E. (1987). *Epidemiology in medicine.* Boston: Little, Brown and Co.

Hennekens, C.H., Speizer, F.E., Rosner, B., Bain, C.J., Belanger, C., & Peto, R. (1979). Use of permanent hair dyes and cancer among registered nurses. *Lancet, 111,* 301–308.

Institute of Medicine. (2001). *Mammography and beyond: Developing technologies for the early detection of breast cancer: A nontechnology summary.* Washington, DC: National Academy Press.

Jennings-Dozier, K., & Mahon, S.M. (2000). Introduction: Cancer prevention and early detection—From thought to revolution. *Oncology Nursing Forum, 27*(Suppl. 9), 3–4.

Jung, B.C. (2001). *Biostatistics and statistics sites.* Retrieved August 28, 2001 from the World Wide Web: http://www.geocities.com/bettycjung/statsites.htm

Kelsey, J.L., Whittemore, A.S., Evans, A.S., & Thompson, D.W. (1996). *Methods in observational epidemiology* (2nd ed.). New York: Oxford University Press.

Klein, J.P., & Moeschberger, M.L. (1997). *Survival analyses.* New York: Springer-Verlag.

Klimaszewski, A.D., Anderson, A., & Good, M. (2000). Informed consent. In A.D. Klimaszewski, J.L. Aikin, M.A. Bacon, S.A. DiStasio, H.E. Ehrenberger, & B.A. Ford (Eds.), *Manual for clinical trials nursing* (pp. 213–219). Pittsburgh: Oncology Nursing Press, Inc.

Malthaner, R., & Fenlon, D. (2001). *Preoperative chemotherapy for resectable thoracic esophageal cancer* (Cochrane Review). Hamilton, Ontario, Canada: Cochrane Databases Systematic Reviews.

Marubini, E., & Valsecchi, M.G. (1996). *Analyzing survival data from clinical trials and observational studies.* New York: John Wiley and Sons.

Morton, R.F., Hebel, J.R., & McCarter, R.J. (2000*). A study guide to epidemiology and biostatistics.* Gaithersburg, MD: Aspen Publishers.

Mulhull, A. (2000). The case for a more epidemiologically informed nursing profession . . . including commentary by Walker M. *NT Research, 5*(1), 65–74.

National Cancer Institute. (2001a). *Cancer trials.* Retrieved February 20, 2001 from the World Wide Web: http://cancertrials.nci.nih.gov/

National Cancer Institute. (2001b). *Dictionary of cancer terms.* Retrieved January 9, 2001 from the World Wide Web: http://www.cancernet.nci.nih.gov/

National Cancer Institute. (2001c). *Physician data query breast cancer.* Retrieved August 28, 2001 from the World Wide Web: http://cancernet.nci.nih.gov/

National Cancer Institute. (2001d). *Supportive care.* Retrieved July 17, 2001 from the World Wide Web: http://cancertrials.nci.nih.gov/

National Cancer Institute. (2001e). *Surveillence, Epidemiology, and End Results Program.* Retrieved January 9, 2001 from the World Wide Web: http://www.seer.cancer.gov/

Nelson, K.E. (2001). *Infectious disease epidemiology. Theory and practice.* Gaithersburg, MD: Aspen Publishers.

Newman, T.B., Browner, W.S., Cummings, S.R., & Hulley, S.B. (2000). Designing an observational study: Cross-sectional and case-control studies. In S.B. Hulley, W.S. Browner, & S.R. Cummings (Eds.), *Designing clinical research* (pp. 107–124). Baltimore: Williams & Wilkins.

Pagano, M., & Gauvreau, K. (2000). *Principle of biostatistics* (2nd ed.). Pacific Grove, CA: Duxbury Press.

Pastides, H. (2001). The descriptive epidemiology of cancer. In P.C. Nasca & H. Pastides (Eds.), *Fundamentals of cancer epidemiology* (pp. 1–22). Gaithersburg, MD: Aspen.

Pedersoli, C.E., Antonialli, E., & Vila, T.C.S. (1998). Nursing profession in epdemiolgic surveillance (ES) in Ribeirao Preto (1988–1996). *Revista Latino-Americicana de Enfermagem, 6*(5), 99–105.

Petitti, D.B. (1994). *Meta-analyses, decision analyses, and cost effectiveness analyses: Methods for quantitative synthesis in medicine.* New York: Oxford University Press.

Polit, F.P., & Hungler, B.P. (1999). *Nursing research: Principles and methods* (6th ed.). Philadelphia: J.B. Lippincott.

Potter, P.A., & Perry, A.G. (1998). Critical thinking and nursing judgment. In P.A. Potter & A.G. Perry (Eds.), *Fundamentals of nursing* (pp. 273–289). St. Louis, MO: Mosby.

Ries, L.A.G., Eisner, M.P., Kosary, C.L., Hankey, B.F., Miller, B.A., Clegg, L.X., & Edwards, B.K. (Eds). (2000). *SEER cancer statistics review, 1973–1997.* Bethesda, MD: National Cancer Institute.

Rigel, D.S., & Carucci, J.A. (2000). Malignant melanoma: Prevention, early detection, and treatment in the 21st century. *CA: A Cancer Journal for Clinicians, 50,* 215–236.

Rosner, B.A. (1995). *Fundamental of biostatistics* (4th ed.). Belmont, CA: Wadsworth Publishing Co.

Rubin, R.C. (2001). Guest editorial: Cervical cancer: Successes and failures. *CA: A Cancer Journal for Clinicians, 51,* 89–91.

Sadler, G.R., Lantz, J.M., Fullerton, J.T., & Dault, Y. (1999). Nurses' unique roles in randomized clinical trials. *Journal of Professional Nursing, 15*(2), 106–115.

Schwartz, G.G., Skinner, H.G., & Duncan, R. (1998). Solid waste and pancreatic cancer: An ecologic study in Florida, USA. *International Journal of Epidemiology, 127,* 781–787.

Shambaugh, E.M., Young, J.L., Sippin, C., Lum, D., Akers, C., & Weiss, M.A. (1994). *SEER Program self-instructional manula for cancer registars, Book 7: Statistics and epidemiology for cancer registries* (NIH Publication No. 94-3766). Bethesda, MD: National Cancer Institute, National Institutes of Health.

Shortridge, L., & Valanis, B. (1992). The epidemiological model applied in community health nursing. In M. Stanhope & J. Lancaster (Eds.), *Community health nursing: Process and practice for promoting health* (3rd ed.) (pp. 151–170). St. Louis MO: Mosby.

Smigel, K. (1998). Breast cancer prevention trial shows some benefit, some risk. *Journal of the National Cancer Institute, 90,* 647–648.

Speizer, F.E., Colditz, G.A., Hunter, D.J., Rosner, B., & Hennekens, C. (1999). Prospective study of smoking, antioxidant intake, and lung cancer in middle-aged women. *Cancer Causes and Control, 10,* 475–482.

United States Department of Health and Human Services. (1998, October 29). *Tamoxifen approved for reducing breast cancer incidence.* Press release.

Valanis, B. (1986). *Epidemiology in nursing and health care.* New Yorlu Appleton-Century-Crofts.

Whitehead, D. (2000a). The role of epidemiology in orthopaedic practice. *Journal of Orthopaedic Nursing, 4*(1), 33–38.

Whitehead, D. (2000b). Is there a place for epidemiology in nursing? *Nursing Standard, 14,* 35–39.

Willett, W.C., Bain, C., Hennekens, C.H., Rosner, B., & Speizer, F.E. (1981). Oral contraceptives and risk of ovarian cancer. *Cancer, 48,* 1684–1687.

CHAPTER 3

Human Behavior and Health Education

Cathy A. Coyne, PhD, and Janice V. Bowie, PhD, MPH

Introduction

In the past few decades of developing strategies to prevent and control cancer, there has been an increasing awareness of the need to understand human behavior. Doll and Peto (1981) attributed nearly 65% of cancer deaths to lifestyle behaviors, such as smoking and diet. Since that time, interventions aimed at changing human behavior to reduce cancer incidence and mortality have been designed and evaluated in various settings and with diverse populations. For example, population-based smoking control interventions have been tested in healthcare settings, worksites, and communities (Lichtenstein, 1997). These interventions have been aimed not only at smoking cessation but also at smoking prevention, particularly those interventions implemented in school settings that have targeted adolescents.

Research into human behavior has increased our understanding of the factors that are associated with cancer risk. These factors include both knowledge and health beliefs, social norms, self-efficacy, coping styles, motivation, and skills development. A keen understanding of these factors through behavioral research is critical for the development of effective cancer prevention and control interventions. A report of the National Cancer Institute's (NCI's) Working Group on Behavioral Research noted that research in human behavior and how it relates to cancer control needs to be enhanced and expanded. In this report, the Working Group identified several priorities in behavioral research in cancer control. These areas include efforts to improve cancer risk communication and comprehension to facilitate informed decision-making; identifying factors associated with youth smoking and planning interventions to reduce the prevalence of tobacco use among youth; designing and testing cancer control interventions in healthcare settings; examining behaviors associated with diet and exercise to develop effective interventions targeting those at risk; examining factors that are affected by the disclosure of genetic information; and designing effective interventions to improve the quality of life of cancer survivors (National Cancer Institute Working Group on Behavioral Research in Cancer Prevention and Control, 1996). The broad scope of these priority areas illustrates how important it is to understand human behavior when developing strategies to prevent and control cancer.

In 1996, NCI received similar recommendations from the NCI Cancer Control Review Group (1997). An increase in behavioral and social science research was encouraged by the Review Group to "develop theoretical models, identify underlying mechanisms and principles of behavior change, and conduct pre-intervention research to inform the next generation of cancer prevention and control interventions and social policies" (1997, p. 8). These recommendations led to the establishment of a unit within NCI focused on basic behavioral and social research.

As will be discussed at length in subsequent chapters within this text, numerous human behaviors are associated with cancer risk, incidence, and prognosis. These include personal behaviors, such as tobacco use, diet, sexual activity, sun protection, and cancer screening, as well as institutional behaviors, including the promulgation and enforcement of smoking policies at the workplace, pollution-control initiatives, and occupational hazard-control policies (see Table 3-1). Each of these behaviors is a complex action influenced by an array of social, psychological, and, in some cases, biological factors that are inter-related and vary with the individual or group they are affecting. It is this complex dynamic that challenges cancer control researchers and practitioners, encouraging their continued efforts in the critical area of cancer prevention and control.

Factors Influencing Human Behavior

Researchers and practitioners in human behavior and health education have assumed an ecological approach to intervention design and implementation. This

Table 3-1. Human Behaviors Associated With Risk of Cancer

Behaviors	Cancer Site/Type
Smoking or chewing tobacco	Lung, head and neck, cervix
Dietary intake of fiber, fat, alcohol, fruits and vegetables	Colon, rectum, stomach, breast, prostate, lung, liver, cervix
Multiple sexual partners, sexual intercourse at an early age	Cervix
Wearing sun-protective clothing and lotion	Melanoma, skin cancer
Obtaining screening tests on a regular basis	Breast, cervix, colon, prostate, skin, melanoma
Smoking policy promulgation and enforcement	Lung
Institution of pollution control initiatives	Lung, leukemia
Institution of occupational hazard control	Lung, mesothelioma, prostate

approach recognizes multiple levels of determinants that influence health behavior and takes into account the complexity of human behavior. McLeroy, Bibeau, Stecker, and Glanz (1988), drawing from the work of others, identified five levels of behavioral determinants that affect health: intrapersonal, interpersonal, institutional, community, and public policy. *Intrapersonal* determinants are those at the individual level, including knowledge, attitudes, personal behaviors and skills, and self-efficacy. Social networks and social support systems, both formal and informal, are *interpersonal* determinants. These include family, friends, coworkers, and others who influence behavior. As will be discussed later in this chapter, interpersonal determinants have become increasingly important in cancer control interventions. *Institutional* determinants are organizational characteristics that can influence behavior, including communication styles, workplace demands, job complexity, school policies and structures, and styles of management. These factors can be important supports for health behavior change and maintenance. *Community* determinants have been defined by McLeroy et al. as mediating structures that provide social resources and social identity, as relationships among organizations and groups within defined political or geographic areas that may serve as settings for health-education programs, and as power structures that have a role in defining problems and resources in the community. The last determinant of health behavior, *public policy*, can influence health behavior through regulations that restrict certain unhealthy behaviors and laws to improve environmental conditions. Interventions directed at this level of influence can greatly affect the health behaviors of large population groups and make a significant impact on a health problem.

Intrapersonal Determinants

Many intrapersonal determinants have been associated with various behaviors and behavioral intentions that affect cancer risk. Among African American female smokers, concern about the effects of smoking on health was found to be strongly correlated with the women's plans to quit smoking (Manfredi, Lacey, Warnecke, & Petraitis, 1998). Among Korean American women participating in focus groups conducted by Lee (2000), lack of knowledge about cervical cancer was related to poor compliance with yearly cervical cancer screening. In a cross-sectional telephone survey conducted by Bosompra et al. (2000) in Upstate New York, family history of cancer was found to be associated with the likelihood of undergoing genetic testing for cancer.

Interpersonal Determinants

Social support, an example of an interpersonal determinant, is associated with a number of health behaviors and health outcomes (Bandura, 1977; Berkman & Syme, 1979). This concept of support has been studied within the context of the workplace, the home, and the community. In a study conducted by Sorensen, Stoddard, and Macario (1998), coworker support was found to be significantly associated with readiness to increase consumption of fruits and vegetables among community health center workers. Plans to quit smoking among low income African American women were positively associated with having close friends who wanted them to quit (Manfredi et al., 1998). A number of interventions to increase mammography screening provide or build upon a woman's social support system. The American Cancer Society's "Tell-a-Friend" program involves women telephoning their friends to encourage them to have mammograms (Calle, Miracle-McMahill, Moss, & Heath, 1994). The "A Su Salud" program uses lay health workers from the community to provide role modeling and social support to encourage Hispanic women to have mammograms (Suarez, Nichols, & Brady, 1993). Physician recommendation, the most significant determinant of mammography use (Yabroff & Mandelblatt, 1999) is another example of an interpersonal determinant and underscores the importance of significant others in affecting individual behavior change.

Institutional Determinants

Many programs on the organizational level seek to affect behavior change to reduce cancer risk. These programs tend to be more effective at sustaining behavior change than those that do not direct any programmatic effort beyond the intrapersonal level. Many tobacco-control programs intervene through the implementation and enforcement of no-smoking policies at the workplace and in schools (Orleans & Cummings, 1999). Such policies spread the message that smoking should not be the norm and raise the public's awareness of the hazards of smoking. Nutrition programs aimed at reducing the amount of fat in people's diets often incorporate a component targeting school or workplace cafeterias (Biener et al., 1999; Glanz, 1999). These programs seek to change organizations' ways of serving meals by modifying recipes and providing healthful food choices, such as fresh fruits and vegetables, instead of high-fat foods. Mammography screening initiatives also have been targeted at organizations through the implementation of physician reminder systems (Burack & Gimotty, 1997; Preston, Scinto, Grady, Schulz, & Petrillo, 2000; Saywell et al., 1999) or by providing appointment times on weekends or during the evening.

Community Determinants

Cancer control interventions at the community level take into account the relationships among organizations within the community or the political and economic impact the interventions may have (McLeroy et al., 1988). For example, the COMMIT trial used community coalitions and community-wide interventions in an effort to reduce tobacco use (COMMIT Research Group, 1995). Although this large, community-based study did not generate high quitting rates among heavy smokers, it did have a modest impact on light and moderate smokers. One study targeting female smokers used community coalitions to affect smoking cessation (Secker-Walker et al., 2000). Community-wide support for the women's efforts helped them to succeed in quitting.

Public Policy Determinants

Public policy interventions can have a wide-ranging impact on health behaviors and cancer risk by affecting large segments of the population. Examples of such interventions include enforcement of youth access laws, advertising restrictions, smoking restrictions in public buildings, and increased state and federal taxes on tobacco products and alcohol (Orleans & Cummings, 1999; Toomey &

Wagenaar, 1999). Changes in health insurance regulations also have lead to changes in health behavior by covering the cost of mammograms and clinical breast examinations.

Theory and Health Education

Health education activities are developed based on a comprehensive understanding of human behavior that is drawn from the knowledge and strategies of various disciplines, including nursing, psychology, sociology, anthropology, epidemiology, statistics, medicine, communications, and marketing (Glanz, Lewis, & Rimer, 1997). These disciplines' diverse perspectives on health and human behavior have contributed to an improved understanding of individuals, communities, organizations, and the interactions among these groups. Indeed, the methods and strategies developed by these disciplines often are used by health-education professionals to design interventions directed at specific population groups. The complexity of human behavior requires that health-education practitioners integrate information and skills drawn from these various professions to develop interventions that effectively reduce cancer risk and improve overall health.

In the design of cancer control interventions, it is essential to use a theoretical approach drawn from these disciplines. Theory has been defined as "a set of interrelated propositions containing concepts that describe, explain, predict, or control behavior" (Glanz et al., 1997, p.22). Theory, thus, provides practitioners with a systematic way to approach a specific cancer risk in order to explain related behaviors and their interrelationships with other factors. The ability to describe a cancer risk through the identification of its various social, psychological, behavioral, biomedical, and environmental components gives intervention designers a better understanding of the causal factors on which to focus educational activities. This understanding helps in the development of strategies that specifically target the cancer risk. In addition, through the application of theory, an understanding of the mechanisms through which these causal factors effect cancer risk is obtained. This helps to define various aspects of the intervention, such as timing for implementation, possible barriers to implementation, and intermediate and outcome variables that are important for evaluation.

In a review of the health behavior and health promotion literature published from mid-1992 to 1994, Glanz et al. (1997) found that, of 497 articles that reported using theory, 66 different theories and models were used. The 10 most frequently cited were the Health Belief Model (HBM), Social Cognitive Theory, self-efficacy, Theory of Reasoned Action/Theory of Planned Behavior, community organization, Stages of Change/Transtheoretical Model, social marketing, social support/social networks, PRECEDE-PROCEED Model, and Diffusion of Innovation. Each of these theories or models can be used either to help to explain a particular health behavior related to cancer risk or to guide the development of interventions to change a behavior and reduce risk.

Selection of the appropriate theory for developing an intervention depends upon both the health behavior and the intervention's intended audience. In the following section, several theories or models commonly used in cancer control interventions will be defined and described through an example from cancer control research or practice.

Health Belief Model

The HBM is one of the most frequently used models in health education and cancer control. Its origins are in the discipline of psychology, where it initially was developed in the 1950s to explain why people were not participating in tuberculosis screening programs (Glanz et al., 1997; Rosenstock, 1960, 1974). Since that time, the HBM has been widely used both to explain numerous health behaviors and to design interventions to change or maintain them (Bosompra et al., 2000; Choudhry, Srivastava, & Fitch, 1998; Lee, 2000; McDonald, Thorne, Pearson, & Adams-Campbell, 1999; Mikanowicz, Fitzgerald, Leslie, & Altman, 1999). The components of the HBM are described in Table 3-2. This model takes into account a person's beliefs regarding susceptibility to a particular health problem, the severity of the health problem, and the likelihood that a particular behavior change will be beneficial. In addition, the model incorporates the individual's perceptions regarding barriers to behavior change and confidence in one's ability to make a change.

The HBM was used to design the Learn, Share and Live program, a breast cancer education program targeting low-income elderly women living in an urban area (Skinner et al., 1998). Learn, Share and Live, implemented through an existing peer network, educated peer leaders about breast cancer so they could disseminate this information to others in their networks. Core sessions of the educational program focused on components of the HBM, including benefits of screening, barriers to screening, and breast cancer risk, particularly among older women.

Table 3-2. Components of the Health Belief Model

Component	Description
Perceived susceptibility	The individual believes that he or she is at risk for the health problem.
Perceived severity	The individual believes that the health problem is serious, perhaps resulting in disability or death.
Perceived benefits	The individual believes that changing a behavior or taking a specific recommended action will reduce his or her risk of the health problem.
Perceived barriers	The individual identifies barriers to taking a recommended action to reduce the risk and weighs these barriers against the benefits of taking the action. Barriers may be tangible, such as expensive or time-consuming as well as intangible, such as painful or anxiety-provoking.
Cues to action	Events or strategies that motivate the individual to take action. Symptoms, information, and reminders all may be cues to action.
Self-efficacy	The individual's confidence that he or she can take the recommended action or behavior.

In a study conducted by Bosompra et al. (2000), the researchers used a survey based upon the HBM to examine the factors that influence participation in genetic testing for cancer among the general population. Telephone interviews were conducted with 622 adults; results indicated that an understanding of genetic testing was influenced by perceived susceptibility to cancer, perceived barriers, and perceived benefits. Information about factors that motivate a population's behavior, such as the uptake of genetic testing, can be used to design interventions to influence behavior change. Because the HBM seeks to explain behavior from the perspective of the individual's behaviors and beliefs, it is considered an individual-level theory of change or, as discussed earlier in this chapter, an intrapersonal determinant.

Theories of Reasoned Action and Planned Behavior

Two other intrapersonal theories are the Theory of Planned Behavior and its progenitor, the Theory of Reasoned Action (Fishbein, 1967; Fishbein & Ajzen, 1975). The Theory of Reasoned Action and Theory of Planned Behavior are cognitive theories that assume individuals rationally consider the costs and benefits of a certain behavior before engaging in it. The primary components of these theories are attitude and subjective norms that influence behavior by affecting behavioral intent. Therefore, the key determinant to engaging in a behavior is behavioral intent. The component of perceived behavioral control was added to the Theory of Reasoned Action by Ajzen (1991) to account for the individual's ability to engage in the behavior with consideration given to the conditions supporting or inhibiting, resulting in the development of the Theory of Planned Behavior. Each of the components of the theory (i.e., attitude, subjective norm, and perceived behavioral control) has two subcomponents, as presented in Table 3-3. Subcomponents of attitude are behavioral beliefs and evaluation of behavioral outcomes, and those of subjective norms are normative beliefs and the individual's motivation

Table 3-3. Components of the Theory of Reasoned Action and the Theory of Planned Behavior

Subcomponent	Description
Behavioral belief	Beliefs that certain outcomes are associated with a behavior.
Evaluation of behavioral outcome	Values attached to the outcome of the behavior.
Normative belief	Belief about whether important others think that the individual should perform the behavior.
Motivation to comply	The individual's motivation to do what important others think he or she should do.
Control belief	The individual's belief that he or she has control over the behavior, including resources or conditions that would inhibit or facilitate performance of the behavior.
Perceived power	The individual's perception that resources or certain conditions can inhibit or facilitate the behavior.

to comply with the beliefs of important others. Subcomponents of perceived behavioral control are control belief and perceived power, which is similar to the construct of self-efficacy.

Hillhouse, Adler, Drinnon, and Turrisi (1997) used the Theory of Planned Behavior to examine the factors that influence sunbathing, tanning salon use, and sunscreen use among university undergraduates. The study found that attitudes were more strongly associated with the subjects' intentions to engage in these high risk behaviors than were subjective norms, although subjective norms were also found to be important. For example, investigators found that positive attitudes towards sunbathing were predictive of the intention to sunbathe. Perceived behavioral control was found to be a moderator among attitudes, subjective norms, and behavioral intention. Information regarding the factors that influence behaviors that result in exposure of skin to ultraviolet radiation can be used to design a skin cancer prevention program targeting undergraduate students. A heuristic model that integrated elements of the Theory of Reasoned Action with the HBM and the Transtheoretical Model was used to examine factors associated with intentions to obtain mammograms among women who have not followed screening guidelines (Allen, Sorensen, Stoddard, Colditz, & Peterson, 1998). Factors examined included confidence in one's ability to ask healthcare providers about mammography and to obtain a mammogram (self-efficacy) and the woman's perception of others' approval of mammography screening (subjective norm).

The Transtheoretical Model

The Transtheoretical Model incorporates processes and change principles derived from a number of theories from the fields of psychotherapy and behavior change (Prochaska, Redding, & Evers, 1997). It suggests that behavior change follows a series of six stages that are essentially sequential (Prochaska & DiClemente, 1983). The first stage is *precontemplation*, during which the individual has no intention of changing. This lack of intention to change may be the result of lack of knowledge regarding the need to change a behavior or strategies to use to effect the desired change. Individuals at this stage need information regarding their behavior and reasons to change it before they can move into the next stage. The second stage is *contemplation*, in which the individual is aware of the benefits of and costs associated with changing his or her behavior and intends to change within the next six months. Progression from this stage into *preparation* requires additional information that helps the individual to weigh the benefits more favorably than the costs. During *preparation*, the individual intends to take action within the next 30 days (Thompson & Kinne, 1999). Generally, the individual knows what he or she needs to do to change the behavior and has made plans to do so. *Preparation* leads to *action*, the fourth stage in the Transtheoretical Model. During the *action* stage, the individual makes changes in his or her behavior, but these changes are not yet considered to be permanent. The possibility of relapse to one of the previous stages still exists. If the *action* stage is completed, the individual progresses into the *maintenance* stage, during which time the behavior change is maintained, although infrequent relapses may occur. The *maintenance* stage is estimated to last from six months to five years (Prochaska et al., 1997). The final stage is *termination*, during which time the behavior change is seen as permanent. Prochaska et al. pointed out that for some behaviors, such as cancer screening or dietary fat reduction, this stage is not appropriate.

The Transtheoretical Model, commonly referred to as the Stages of Change Model, has been used extensively in the management and relapse prevention of some cancer-related risk behaviors (e.g., dietary fat intake, obesity, smoking cessation). Additionally, it has been used to tailor messages to affect behavior change in women who are nonadherent for mammography screening. In a study conducted by Lipkus, Rimer, Halabi, and Strigo (2000), the impact of tailored telephone counseling and tailored print materials on the mammography screening behavior of women age 50 and older who were members of a large health-maintenance organization (HMO) was compared against the effect of usual care. Usual care within this HMO consisted of two reminder letters followed by a certified letter reminding the woman that she is overdue for a mammogram. Telephone counseling and print messages were tailored based on the woman's stage of change according to the Transtheoretical Model. Trained female counselors delivered the telephone counseling twice in two years, following a specific protocol based on the information and barriers identified by the women in the preintervention assessment. The tailored print message was delivered in two small booklets designed to look like greeting cards. The second card was sent to the women one year after the first card. The tailored telephone counseling in the first year of the study demonstrated stronger effects than did the tailored print material and the usual care in promoting mammography use among the HMO population. This effect was not seen in the second year of the intervention. The results do suggest, however, that tailored messages, guided by the Transtheoretical Model, may be effective in getting some nonadherent women to obtain mammograms. Unfortunately, the researchers did not report whether the tailored interventions resulted in women progressing from *precontemplation* to *contemplation*, which would be a positive result. It is important to be able to measure movement through the stages as well as actual behavior change when using stage theories to guide the design of an intervention because the premise of using such a theory is that individuals should progress through the stages to achieve final behavior change.

Recent intervention approaches by providers in primary care settings (Elder, Ayala, & Harris, 1999) have used the Transtheoretical Model in guiding the selection of effective patient education methods to achieve patient compliance to treatment regimens. The flexibility of the model allows for matching of the intervention to the cognitive stage exhibited by the patient. Similarly, applications in the prevention, treatment, and control of cancer through assessment of the individual's level of readiness to begin the process of change may lead to maintenance of the desired behavior (Kelaher et al., 1999; Ruggiero, 1999).

Social Cognitive and Social Learning Theories

The Social Cognitive Theory incorporates a number of different theoretical constructs derived from psychology, including observational learning, self-efficacy, behavioral capability, reinforcement, and reciprocal determinism. A key aspect of this theory is the interaction between the individual and the environment, which makes this theory quite relevant to health educators' desire to use a more ecological approach to intervention design. Many of the constructs of the Social Cognitive Theory have been used to better understand health problems and to develop effective interventions targeting specific health behaviors. Observational learning, for example, in which an individual learns a behavior through the observation of another person engaging in that behavior, has guided the use of role models in behavior change interventions. Role models have been used widely in Pap test and mammography screening programs targeted at noncompliant women (Suarez et al., 1997). Self-efficacy, a construct noted in other models of behavior change, encourages intervention planners to provide members of their program's intended audience with opportunities to practice a certain behavior, as through role-playing, to obtain confidence in their abilities to perform the behavior.

Role-playing was used in the Gimme 5 program to increase the self-efficacy of fourth and fifth-grade children to ask their parents to buy more fruits and vegetables (Baranowski et al., 2000). The Gimme 5 program, designed using many of the constructs of the Social Cognitive Theory, encouraged children to eat more fruits and vegetables and provided them with the knowledge and skills to do so. The program attempted to change the children's environment both at home and in school to increase the likelihood that they would change their behaviors. The influence of the environment is recognized as a very important construct within the Social Cognitive Theory.

Precede-Proceed Model

A commonly used framework for the planning of health education programs that incorporates a strong needs assessment component is the Precede-Proceed model developed by Green and Kreuter (1999). This model incorporates components of many health-behavior models and theories, including two previously described in this chapter, the Health Belief Model and the Social Learning Theory (progenitor of the Social Cognitive Theory) (Michielutte, Dignan, & Smith, 1999). The Precede-Proceed framework is comprised of nine phases that take the program planner through a systematic process in developing health education programs. Figure 3-1 illustrates the various phases of the model and how they are interrelated.

The model begins by focusing the program planner's attention on the outcome of interest and then works backwards to identify the determinants of the outcome, resulting in an intervention that addresses the factors that, indeed, have an impact on the outcome. Because the model was designed to be worked in reverse, novices to its use often initially are confused, as the tendency is to work forward. However, the systematic approach that the model walks the program planner through is quite rational and forces the focus to be on the quality-of-life outcome, asking why it exists, rather than on a specific intervention with which the program planner may be more comfortable.

The first phase of the model is the *social assessment*, in which the social problems or concerns of the target population are defined. These may include poverty, unemployment, crime, discrimination, or self-esteem. The second phase is the *epidemiological diagnosis*, in which the health problem is identified. During this phase,

Figure 3-1. Precede-Proceed Model

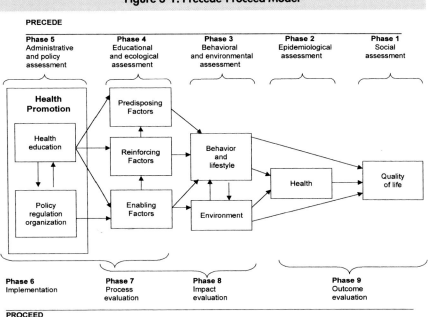

Note. From *Health Promotion Planning: An Educational and Environmental Approach* (3rd ed.) (p. 490), by L.W. Green and M.W. Kreuter, 1999, Mountain View, CA: Mayfield Publishing Co. Copyright 1999 by Mayfield Publishing Co. Reprinted with permission.

epidemiological data are collected and reviewed to identify the most salient health problems. This includes data on morbidity, mortality, and disability. The third phase of the model is the *behavioral and environmental assessment*, in which data are collected on the behavioral and environmental factors that may be related to the salient health problem identified in phase 2. Following phase 3, an *educational and ecological assessment* is conducted. Factors to be examined during this phase have been grouped into three categories: predisposing, enabling, and reinforcing. Predisposing factors are those characteristics that motivate a behavior, including knowledge, attitudes, beliefs, and perceptions. Enabling factors are characteristics of the environment that facilitate or inhibit a behavior, including resources, skills, and access. Examples of enabling factors relevant to cancer control include the availability of grocery stores that sell fresh fruits and vegetables at reasonable prices, mammography appointment slots during evening or weekend hours, and availability of non-smoking areas in restaurants. Reinforcing factors are the rewards received for engaging in a behavior, including the emotional support given by friends and family members. Phase 5 is the *administrative and policy assessment*, in which the organizational resources and capabilities to implement an intervention are assessed. These include staffing, time availability, and budget. Phase 6 is the *implementation* of the intervention, and phases 7–9 are the *evaluation*. Planning for the intervention's evaluation actually takes place at the beginning of the intervention planning process and continues throughout as the components of the intervention are developed and subsequently implemented. This is illustrated by the location of phases 7–9 on the diagram; they are identified below the components of the planning process that are integral for effective evaluation planning.

Michielutte et al. (1999) used the Precede-Proceed framework to classify psychosocial factors found to be associated with breast cancer screening behavior among women over age 60. The framework of predisposing, enabling, and reinforcing factors also was used in the design of a community-based intervention to help women quit smoking (Secker-Walker et al., 2000).

Recent articles have presented arguments that not all theories are relevant for every population (Ashing-Giwa, 1999; Jennings-Dozier, 1999). Most behavior-change theories used in health education have been developed and tested primarily on middle- to high-income White populations. Though these theories currently are being used in more diverse population groups, their relevance has not been adequately tested with these groups. Ashing-Giwa suggested that sociocultural factors, such as interconnectedness and religiosity, need to be incorporated into theories and models that examine the health behaviors of African Americans. In selecting a theory to use for designing a cancer control intervention, researchers and practitioners first must consider the nature of the question that they seek to answer and then consider the population that is to be studied. Does the theory incorporate constructs that are relevant to the population? Has the theory been tested with the population? Because few theories have been developed or tested with non-White, low-income populations, basic behavioral research likely will need to be conducted to better understand the health behaviors of certain ethnic minority and poor populations. Nurse researchers and clinicians are encouraged to contribute to this body of knowledge by conducting behavioral research within communities currently underserved by cancer control efforts.

Components of Health-Education Interventions: Strategies, Settings, and Audiences

Utilization of a program planning framework that has a strong needs assessment component, such as the Precede-Proceed model, assists intervention planners in identifying the determinants affecting health risk and leads to the selection of effective intervention strategies.

In her article describing trends in mammography use in the United States, Rimer (1994) proposed a typology that can be used to categorize intervention strategies used in cancer-control programs. Summarized in Table 3-4, this typology categorizes interventions found in the mammography literature into seven categories based on the channel and intended audience.

When selecting an intervention strategy, all of the findings from the needs assessment must be considered, including audience characteristics, determinants that may need to be modified (i.e., predisposing, reinforcing, and enabling factors), behavior(s) targeted, as well as the setting for the intervention and the program's budget (Burack et al., 1996) and resources.

Table 3-4. Typology of Interventions

Type of Intervention	Description
Media campaigns	Interventions designed to reach a large segment of the population; channels include television, radio, newspapers, billboards, and magazines.
Individual-directed	Interventions directed at the at-risk individual; may include tailored letters, telephone counseling, interactive computer programs, educational print material
System-directed	Interventions designed to affect change at the interpersonal or organizational level; may include changes in physician office practices, changes in roles and responsibilities of organizations and their staffs
Access-enhancing	Interventions designed to improve access to health care or public health services by reducing costs, modifying service hours, providing transportation
Policy level	Interventions designed to affect changes in or adoption of policies at the workplace, in schools, or at the community, state, or federal level
Social network	Interventions designed to utilize the target audience's social network in order to affect behavior change; examples include the use of peer leaders, lay health workers, and community organizations.
Multi-strategy	Interventions that utilize more than one strategy in their design

Note. Based on information from Rimer, 1994.

Audience Characteristics

The needs assessment will identify the segment of the population at risk for a certain cancer. This population may not necessarily be the intended audience of the intervention. Identification of the behavioral, social, and environmental determinants of a particular cancer risk may suggest that interventions at the interpersonal or organizational level may have a greater impact on the cancer risk than directing the intervention to the individual, or *intrapersonal*, level. For example, an intervention physicians were targeted by an intervention designed to increase screening mammography use by increasing utilization of physician and patient reminder systems (Burack & Gimotty, 1997; Preston et al., 2000). The intended audience for these programs is physicians and office staff rather than the at-risk population of women who are not compliant with routine mammography screening. Thus, the behavior of the at-risk population (i.e., women's mammography use) is indirectly affected by changing the behavior of others.

Regardless of the level of the intervention, it is critical to have a clear description of the intervention's intended audience as well as that of the at-risk population, which may or may not be the same as the intended audience. Important audience characteristics to consider include demographic variables such as age, race/ethnicity, gender, income, marital status, level of educational attainment, employment status, and health insurance coverage. These demographic data generally are gathered by governmental agencies such as the U.S. Census Bureau and can be obtained for a specific geographic area by researchers and program planners.

Literacy level is another audience characteristic that healthcare and health-education practitioners are addressing more frequently when communicating with patients or developing interventions. Although level of educational attainment may provide a guidepost as to the literacy level of an individual or a population, it does not always correlate directly with ability to read and comprehend a message. In 1992, the National Adult Literacy Survey (NALS) found that, overall, approximately 47% of the U.S. population (90 million people) demonstrated literacy skills in the lowest two levels assessed. Of those with literacy skills in the lowest level, 38% had completed high school (Kirsch, Jungeblut, Jenkins, & Kolstad, 1993). Five percent of the respondents who had completed four years of college were found to have literacy levels in the lowest two levels (Kirsch et al., 1993). Thus, one cannot always rely on grade of school completed to determine an individual's ability to read. A number of tools have been developed that practitioners can use to assess the literacy level of their intervention's intended audience. One such tool is the Rapid Estimate of Adult Literacy in Medicine (REALM) (Davis et al., 1993). The REALM uses word recognition to assess an adult's ability to read common medical and lay terms. The REALM has been positively correlated with other standardized literacy assessment tests, including the Peabody Individual Achievement Test-Revised, the Wide Range Achievement Test-Revised, and the Slosson Oral Reading Test-Revised (Davis et al.). This literacy test is appropriate for use in a clinical setting because of the terminology it uses to assess literacy level and the two- to three-minute administration time. The Test of Functional Health Literacy in Adults (TOFHLA) also is a useful tool in the clinical or health setting. This instrument is composed of two sections: the first section contains 50 items measuring reading comprehension, and the next section uses 17 items to assess a patient's ability to understand prescription labeling, appointment cards, blood glucose tests, and financial information forms (Williams et al., 1995). Scores are classified into three levels of functional health literacy: inadequate, marginal, and adequate. The TOFHLA takes significantly longer to administer than the REALM but provides useful information regarding an individual's literacy level regarding health information. It is important to know the literacy level of the audience to develop appropriate print material and intervention strategies.

Another important characteristic is the cultural background, including level of acculturation, of the intended audience. Understanding the culture of a population is essential for designing health messages that are relevant and sensitive to its cultural beliefs and actions. A cancer-control intervention that incorporates the culture of the intended audience as part of its foundation is more likely to engage the audience members and be effective in changing behavior (Brant, Fallsdown, & Iverson, 1999; Powe & Weinrich, 1999). Use of theory in designing interventions that target diverse cultural population groups is encouraged; however, few existing health-education and health-behavior theories and models have been adequately tested in cultural or ethnic minority populations. Intervention planners are encouraged to review the literature and be certain that use of a selected theory or model is appropriate for the intended audience.

Setting

The setting for the intervention also must be considered carefully. Setting refers to the location where the intervention is to be implemented. If the intervention is designed to reach inner-city women with nutrition information, program planners need to decide whether the women can best be reached through a community center, in their homes, at the grocery store, or in churches. The setting should be selected with the audience, the intervention's message, and implementation feasibility in mind. For example, a church may be an appropriate place to reach women over age 65 in some communities, but it may not be a good setting for an intervention seeking to reach men in their 30s. In addition, if the intervention's message includes information on safe sex and the use of condoms, some churches may not condone sharing such messages with their congregations. Examples of settings for cancer-control interventions include health clinics, senior centers, schools, workplaces, adult learning centers, churches, and beauty salons. Just about anywhere people congregate are possible intervention settings.

Budget and Resources

Program budget and administrative resources are very important considerations in the health-education intervention planning process. Insufficient funding can cause program planners to make unwise decisions in the effort to reduce expenditures and meet the budget. In addition, inadequate or inappropriate staffing can have deleterious effects on intervention outcomes. Thus, creating a realistic budget and identifying adequate resources are critical. Budget items to consider include personnel, office supplies, computer equipment, telephone, postage (including overnight delivery services), incentives for participation in the needs assessment or intervention, and healthcare service costs (e.g., mammography screening, fecal occult blood testing kits).

Evaluation

An often-neglected component of health-education programs that are not part of a research study is evaluation. The incorporation of a thorough evaluation component into the cancer-control intervention is essential for the program planners and funders to know that the intervention is having its intended effect, and if it is not, why. The three levels of evaluation that need to be incorporated into each intervention plan are *process*, *impact*, and *outcome*. *Process* evaluation informs the program planners that the intervention is being implemented as intended and if it has reached the intended audience. Questions that should be asked as part of the intervention's process evaluation include, What materials were developed? How were these materials distributed? What staff or volunteers were hired or trained? Did members of the intended audience participate in the intervention? Sources of data to answer these questions include program records, education and training materials, attendance logs, and media tracking. Process evaluation is important in establishing why a program did or did not work. If the process evaluation results indicate that the program was not implemented as intended (e.g., educational materials were not distributed at the correct location, staff were not well trained), then this could explain poor program outcomes.

The second level of evaluation, *impact* evaluation, answers the question, Did the intervention achieve the intended behavior change? Population surveys, participant interviews, and service delivery logs can be used to answer this question. Depending upon the intervention's objectives, specific questions may include What percentage of the intended audience quit smoking, had a mammogram, or reduced the amount of fat in their diet during the follow-up period of the intervention? In order to know whether the intervention actually helped to improve rates of quitting, mammography use, or dietary fat reduction in a population, it is important to have gathered this information prior to implementation of the intervention. This information should have been gathered during the needs assessment process, providing a baseline of behavior to compare with post-intervention rates of behavior.

Outcome evaluation assesses the long-term effects of the intervention, including cancer morbidity and mortality. Sources of data include vital records, cancer registries, hospital records, and population surveys. Because the effects of an intervention on morbidity and mortality take a long time to be seen in a population, this type of evaluation is not always performed when implementing an intervention to effect change in a behavior that is known to affect cancer morbidity and mortality, such as smoking. However, if an intervention for which the long-term outcomes are not known is being tested, the outcome evaluation must be conducted using the appropriate impact and outcome measures.

Sustainability of cancer prevention and control interventions is another reason to include evaluation as part of the planning and implementation phases. The concept of sustainability is defined as the continuation of the intervention or some of its components beyond the initial period of funding (Shediac-Rizkallah & Bone, 1998). Sustainable programs generally are characterized by having adequate resources of time, money, and personnel, along with administrative, community, and political support where indicated. In addition, the benefits of the sustainable program would cease if the program were eliminated. Good programs should be continued, and poorly implemented ones should not.

Conclusion

Although significant advances have been made in our understanding of human behavior as it relates to cancer risk, gaps still remain, particularly in regard to ethnic minorities and low-income populations. With the increasing diversity of the U.S. population, gaining a better understanding of the contribution of cultural and socioeconomic factors to behavior and cancer risk is essential. The investigation of these factors requires that researchers and practitioners work "with" the targeted communities, not merely "in" these communities. Collaboration among disciplines, including nursing, health education, psychology, anthropology, sociology, and the targeted communities, is critical for effective theories and models to be developed and tested. These theories then need to be used, along with existing theories, to develop cancer-control interventions. These interventions need to be targeted to specific communities and tailored to the needs of the individual at risk. The better we understand human behavior, the more accurate we will be in our targeting and tailoring efforts, and the more likely we will have an impact on decreasing cancer incidence and mortality.

References

Ajzen, I. (1991). The theory of planned behavior. *Organizational Behavior and Human Decision Processes, 50,* 179–211.

Allen, J.D., Sorensen, G., Stoddard, A.M., Colditz, G., & Peterson, K. (1998). Intention to have a mammogram in the future among women who have underused mammography in the past. *Health Education and Behavior, 25,* 474–488.

Ashing-Giwa, K. (1999). Health behavior change models and their socio-cultural relevance for breast cancer screening in African American women. *Women's Health, 28*(4), 53–71.

Bandura, A.T. (1977). Self-efficacy: Toward a unifying theory of behavior change. *Psychological Review, 84*(2), 191–215.

Baranowski, T., Davis, M., Resnicow, K., Baranowski, J., Doyle, C., Lin, L.S., Smith, M., & Wang, D.T. (2000). Gimme 5 fruit, juice, and vegetables for fun and health: Outcome evaluation. *Health Education and Behavior, 27,* 96–111.

Berkman, L.F., & Syme, S.L. (1979). Social networks, host resistance, and mortality: Nine-year follow-up study of Alameda County Residents. *American Journal of Epidemiology, 109,* 186–204.

Biener, L., Glanz, K., McLerran, D., Sorensen, G., Thompson, B., Basen-Engquist, K., Linnan, L., & Varnes, J. (1999). Impact of the Working Well trial on the worksite smoking and nutrition environment. *Health Education and Behavior, 26,* 478–494.

Bosompra, K., Flynn, B.S., Ashikaga, T., Rairikar, C.J., Worden, J.K., & Solomon, L.J. (2000). Likelihood of undergoing genetic testing for cancer risk: A population-based study. *Preventive Medicine, 30*(2), 155–166.

Brant, J.M., Fallsdown, D., & Iverson, M.L. (1999). The evolution of a breast health program for Plains Indian women. *Oncology Nursing Forum, 26,* 731–739.

Burack, R.C., & Gimotty, P.A. (1997). Promoting screening mammography in an inner-city setting: The sustained effectiveness of computerized reminders in a randomized controlled trial. *Medical Care, 35,* 921–931.

Burack, R.C., Gimotty, P.A., George, J., Simon, M.S., Dews, P., & Moncrease, A. (1996). The effect of patient and physician reminders on use of screening mammography in a health maintenance organization. Results of a randomized controlled trial. *Cancer, 78,* 1708–1721.

Calle, E.E., Miracle-McMahill, H.L., Moss, R.E., & Heath, C.W.H., Jr. (1994). Personal contact from friends to increase mammography usage. *American Journal of Preventive Medicine, 10,* 361–366.

Choudhry, U.K., Srivastava, R., & Fitch, M.I. (1998). Breast cancer detection practices of South Asian women: Knowledge, attitudes, and beliefs. *Oncology Nursing Forum, 25,* 1729–1736.

COMMIT Research Group. (1995). Community Intervention Trial for Smoking Cessation (COMMIT) I. Cohort results from a four-year community intervention. *American Journal of Public Health, 85*, 183–192.

Davis, T.C., Long, S.W., Jackson, R.H., Mayeaux, E.J., George, R.B., & Crouch, M.A. (1993). Rapid Estimate of Adult Literacy in Medicine: A shortened screening instrument. *Family Medicine, 25*, 391–395.

Doll, R., & Peto, R. (1981). The causes of cancer: Quantitative estimates of avoidable risks of cancer in the United States today. *Journal of the National Cancer Institute, 66*, 1191–1308.

Elder, J.P., Ayala, G.X., & Harris, S. (1999). Theories and intervention approaches to health-behavior change in primary care. *American Journal of Preventive Medicine, 17*, 275–284.

Fishbein, M. (Ed.). (1967). *Readings in attitude theory and measurement.* New York: Wiley.

Fishbein, M., & Ajzen, I. (1975). *Belief, attitude, intention, and behavior: An introduction to theory and research.* Reading, MA: Addison-Wesley.

Glanz, K. (1999). Progress in dietary behavior change. *American Journal of Health Promotion, 14*(2), 112–117.

Glanz, K., Lewis, F.M., & Rimer, B.K. (Eds.). (1997). *Health behavior and health education: Theory, research, and practice* (2nd ed.). San Francisco: Jossey-Bass.

Green, L.W., & Kreuter, M.W. (1999). *Health promotion planning: An educational and ecological approach* (3rd ed.). Mountain View, CA: Mayfield Publishing Company.

Hillhouse, J.J., Adler, C.M., Drinnon, J., & Turrisi, R. (1997). Application of Azjen's theory of planned behavior to predict sunbathing, tanning salon use, and sunscreen use intentions and behaviors. *Journal of Behavioral Medicine, 20*, 365–378.

Jennings-Dozier, K. (1999). Predicting intentions to obtain a Pap smear among African American and Latina women: Testing the theory of planned behavior. *Nursing Research, 48*, 198–205.

Kelaher, M., Gillespie, A.G., Allotey, P., Manderson, L., Potts, H., Sheldrake, M., & Young, M. (1999). The Transtheoretical Model and cervical screening: Its application among culturally diverse communities in Queensland, Australia. *Ethnicity and Health, 4*, 259–279.

Kirsch, I.S., Jungeblut, A., Jenkins, L., & Kolstad, A. (1993). *Adult literacy in America: A first look at the results of the National Adult Literacy Survey* (GPO 065-000-00588-3). Washington, DC: National Centre for Educational Statistics, U.S. Department of Education.

Lee, M.C. (2000). Knowledge, barriers, and motivators related to cervical cancer screening among Korean-American women. *Cancer Nursing, 23*, 168–175.

Lichtenstein, E. (1997). Behavioral research contributions and needs in cancer prevention and control: Tobacco use prevention and cessation. *Preventive Medicine, 26*(5 pt. 2), S57–S63.

Lipkus, I.M., Rimer, B.K., Halabi, S., & Strigo, T.S. (2000). Can tailored interventions increase mammography use among HMO women? *American Journal of Preventive Medicine, 18*, 1–10.

Manfredi, C., Lacey, L.P., Warnecke, R., & Petraitis, J. (1998). Sociopsychological correlates of motivation to quit smoking among low-SES African American women. *Health Education and Behavior, 25*, 304–318.

McDonald, P.A., Thorne, D.D., Pearson, J.C., & Adams-Campbell, L.L. (1999). Perceptions and knowledge of breast cancer among African-American women residing in public housing. *Ethnicity and Disease, 9*(1), 81–93.

McLeroy, K.R., Bibeau, D., Steckler, A., & Glanz, K. (1988). An ecological perspective on health promotion programs. *Health Education Quarterly, 15,* 351–377.

Michielutte, R., Dignan, M.B., & Smith, B.L. (1999). Psychosocial factors associated with the use of breast cancer screening by women age 60 years or over. *Health Education and Behavior, 26,* 625–647.

Mikanowicz, C.K., Fitzgerald, D.C., Leslie, M., & Altman, N.H. (1999). Medium-sized business employees speak out about smoking. *Journal of Community Medicine, 24,* 439–450.

National Cancer Institute Cancer Control Review Group. (1997). *A new agenda for cancer control research: Report of the Cancer Control Review Group.* Bethesda, MD: National Cancer Institute.

National Cancer Institute Working Group on Behavioral Research in Cancer Prevention and Control. (1996). *Report of working group: Priorities in Behavioral Research in Cancer Prevention and Control.* Bethesda, MD: National Cancer Institute.

Orleans, C.T., & Cummings, K.M. (1999). Population-based tobacco control: Progress and prospects. *American Journal of Health Promotion, 14*(2), 83–91.

Powe, B.D., & Weinrich, S. (1999). An intervention to decrease cancer fatalism among rural elders. *Oncology Nursing Forum, 26,* 583–588.

Preston, J.A., Scinto, J.D., Grady, J.N., Schulz, A.F., & Petrillo, M.K. (2000). The effect of a multifaceted physician office-based intervention on older women's mammography use. *Journal of the American Geriatric Society, 48,* 1–7.

Prochaska, J.O., & DiClemente, C.C. (1983). Stages and processes of self-change of smoking: Toward an integrative model of change. *Journal of Consulting and Clinical Psychology, 51,* 390–395.

Prochaska, J.O., Redding, C.A., & Evers, K.E. (1997). The Transtheoretical Model and stages of change. In K. Glanz, F.M. Lewis, & B.K. Rimer (Eds.), *Health behavior and health education* (2nd ed.) (pp. 60–84). San Francisco: Jossey-Bass.

Rimer, B.R. (1994). Mammography use in the U.S.: Trends and the impact of interventions. *Annals of Behavioral Medicine, 16,* 317–326.

Rosenstock, I.M. (1960). What research in motivation suggests for public health. *American Journal of Public Health, 50,* 295–301.

Rosenstock, I.M. (1974). Historical origins of the Health Belief Model. *Health Education Monographs, 2,* 328–335.

Ruggiero, L. (1999). Transtheoretical Model: Applications in the prevention and treatment of cancer. *Medical and Pediatric Oncology, 30* (Suppl. 1), 69–74.

Saywell, R.M., Champion, V.L., Skinner, C.S., McQuillen, D., Martin, D., & Maraj, M. (1999). Cost-effectiveness comparison of five interventions to increase mammography screening. *Preventive Medicine, 29,* 374–382.

Secker-Walker, R.H., Flynn, B.S., Solomon, L.J., Skelly, J.M., Dorwaldt, A.L., & Ashikaga, T. (2000). Helping women quit smoking: Results of a community intervention program. *American Journal of Public Health, 90,* 940–946.

Shediac-Rizkallah, M.C., & Bone, L.R. (1998). Planning for the sustainability of community-based health programs: Conceptual frameworks and future directions for research, practice, and policy. *Health Education Research, 13*(1), 87–108.

Skinner, C.S., Sykes, R.K., Monsees, B.S., Andriole, D.A., Arfken, C.L., & Fisher, E.B. (1998). Learn, share, and live: Breast cancer education for older, urban minority women. *Health Education and Behavior, 25,* 60–78.

Sorensen, G., Stoddard, A., & Macario, E. (1998). Social support and readiness to make dietary changes. *Health Education and Behavior, 25,* 586–598.

Suarez, L., Nichols, D.C., & Brady, C.A. (1993). Use of peer role models to increase Pap smear and mammography screening in Mexican-American and black women. *American Journal of Preventive Medicine, 9,* 290–296.

Suarez, L., Roche, R.A., Pulley, L.V., Weiss, N.S., Goldman, D., & Simpson, S.M. (1997). Why a peer intervention program for Mexican-American women failed to modify the secular trend in cancer screening. *American Journal of Preventive Medicine, 13,* 411–417.

Thompson, B., & Kinne, S. (1999). Social Change Theory. Application to community health. In N. Bracht (Ed.), *Health promotion at the community level: New advances* (2nd ed.) (pp. 29–46). Thousand Oaks, CA: Sage Publications.

Toomey, T.L., & Wagenaar, A.C. (1999). Policy options for prevention: The case of alcohol. *Journal of Public Health Policy, 20,* 192–213.

Williams, M.V., Parker, R.M., Baker, D.W., Parikh, N.S., Pitkin, K., Coates, W. C., & Nurss, J.R. (1995). Inadequate functional health literacy among patients at two public hospitals. *JAMA, 274,* 1677–1682.

Yabroff, K.R., & Mandelblatt, J.S. (1999). Interventions targeted toward patients to increase mammography use. *Cancer Epidemiology, Biomarkers, and Prevention, 8,* 749–757.

CHAPTER 4

Cancer Prevention, Screening, and Early Detection: Human Genetics

Ellen Giarelli, EdD, RN, CS, CRNP, Linda A. Jacobs, PhD, CRNP, AOCN®, BC, and Jean Jenkins, PhD, RN, FAAN

Introduction

"Genetics promises to give us a new vision on how to diagnose and treat virtually any illness. . . . Our challenge over the next few years is how to live in the interval where diagnostics are more advanced than therapeutics" (Collins, 1999).

Groundbreaking discoveries on the genetic nature of cancer promise to change oncology healthcare services. Practice issues related to cancer genetics have been introduced and discussed during the last 50 years. In response, nursing organizations such as the American Nurses Association (ANA) and the Oncology Nursing Society (ONS), along with the National Institute of Nursing Research (NINR), the National Cancer Institute (NCI), and the National Human Genome Research Institute (NHGRI) have identified the critical role nurses will play in clinical genetics. Professional nursing associations affirm that with appropriate education and experience, oncology nurses are ideal for "providing comprehensive care in the area of cancer genetics and for meeting the needs of the increased number of individuals requiring . . . counseling" (ONS, 1998, p. 463). Nurses are accustomed to helping patients to live in the interval where diagnostics are more advanced than therapeutics. The promise of genetics for nurses is that the diagnostic tools will help practitioners to identify those at increased risk to use this information during the "interval" to prevent the devastating effects of cancer.

NHGRI, NCI, and NINR share a threefold initiative: to incorporate genetics into research and training programs for nurse scientists; to integrate nursing research with research training programs for genetic scientists; and to provide opportunities for addressing the ethical, legal, and social implications of genetics research (NHGRI, 1998). Nurses who understand the concepts of genetics and the role it plays in the development of human disease will be able to incorporate this knowledge into practice and play a critical role in prevention, early detection, and disease control.

This chapter presents an overview of the relationship between clinical genetics and nursing care. Sections address historical landmarks in genetics research, the basic scientific concepts of genetics and inheritance, and the mechanisms of mutation and carcinogenesis of some common cancers. Figure 4-1 contains a glossary of common genetics terminology. Implications for health care from the perspective of professional practice in nursing is presented.

Figure 4-1. Glossary of Genetic Terms

Alkaptonuria—Excretion in the urine of homogentisic acid and its oxidation products as a result of a genetic disorder of phenylalanine

Alleles—Alternative forms of a genetic locus; a single allele for each locus is inherited separately from each parent.

Amino Acid—Any of a class of 20 molecules that are combined to form proteins in living things. The sequence of amino acids in a protein and then protein function are determined by the genetic code.

Autosome—A chromosome not involved in sex determination. The diploid human genome consists of 46 chromosomes; 22 pairs of autosomes and one pair of sex chromosomes.

Chromosomes—The self-replicating genetic structures of cells that contain DNA, which has a linear array of genes

Co-dominance—Two or more alleles making a positive contribution to a phenotype resulting in blending of characteristics

Crossing over—The breaking during meiosis of one maternal and one paternal chromosome, the exchange of corresponding sections of DNA, and the rejoining of the chromosomes

Diploid—Carrying two copies of each somatic chromosome and either one or two copies of the pair of sex chromosomes (xx or xy)

DNA (deoxyribonucleic acid)—The molecule that encodes genetic information. DNA is a double-stranded molecule held together by weak bonds between base pairs of nucleotides. The four nucleotides in DNA contain the bases: adenine (A), guanine (G), cytosine (C), and thymine (T). In nature, base pairs form only between A and T and G and C.

Drosophila melanogaster—The common fruit fly

Eukaryote—A cell or organization that contains a membrane bound nucleus with chromosomes, and undergoes mitosis and/or meiosis

Exon—The protein-coding DNA sequence of a gene

Gamete—The cells (egg or sperm) that fuse to form a zygote in sexual reproduction

Gene—A hereditary unit or region of DNA that occupies a specific site locus on a chromosome that contains genetic information that can be replicated, transcribed, and translated to produce a polypeptide

Gene expression—The process by which a gene's coded information is converted into the structures present and operating in a cell

Genetic code—The sequence of nucleotides, coded in triplets (codons) along the mRNA, that determines the sequence of amino acids in protein synthesis. The DNA sequence of a gene can be used to predict the mRNA sequence, and the genetic code can in turn be used to predict the amino acid sequence.

Genetic map (also known as a Linkage Map)—A map of the relative positions of genetic loci on a chromosome. Positions are determined on the basis of how often the loci are inherited together.

Gene product—The biochemical material, either RNA or protein, resulting from expression of a gene. The amount of gene product is used to measure how active a gene is. Abnormal amounts of gene product can be associated with disease-causing alleles.

(Continued on next page)

Figure 4-1. Glossary of Genetic Terms *(Continued)*

Genome—The complete DNA content of an organism

Genotype—The allelic composition of an individual for one or more genes

Germline—Specialized cells that give rise to gametes

Haploid—A single set of chromosomes (half of a full set of genetic material) present in the egg and sperm cells of animals; possessing only one complete copy of the genome

Heterozygosity—The presence of different alleles at one or more loci on homologous chromosomes

Homologous chromosomes—A pair of chromosomes containing the same linear gene sequences, each derived from one parent

Human gene therapy—Insertion of normal DNA directly into cells to correct a genetic defect

Intron—The DNA base sequences that interrupt the protein-coding sequences of a gene. These sequences are transcribed into RNA but are cut out of the message before it is translated into protein.

Locus—A site or position on a chromosome as determined by combinational mapping

Marker—An identifiable physical location on a chromosome whose inheritance can be monitored

Meiosis—Cell division that occurs in sexually reproducing organisms. Diploid cells produce haploid gametes. One chromosome replication is followed by two nuclear divisions, called Meiosis I and Meiosis II.

Meiosis I—Cellular division that creates two haploid daughter cells with 23 chromosomes each; one-half the original cell

Meiosis II—A haploid cell replicates to produce two identical daughter cells, each with 23 chromosomes

Messenger RNA—RNA that serves as a template for protein synthesis

Mitosis—The process by which cells divide to produce two identical daughter cells. Each daughter cell contains the same number of chromosomes as the parents. Diploid mitosis creates daughter cells with 46 chromosomes. Haploid mitosis creates daughter cells with 23 chromosomes.

Mutation—A stable and heritable change in the base sequence of a DNA molecule.

Pedigree—A table, chart, diagram, or list of an individual's ancestor's used in genetics in the analysis of Mendelian inheritance; from the French *peid du gru*, meaning "foot of the crane"

Penetrance—The degree to which a genotype is correlated with a phenotype

Phenotype—The actual physical manifestation of a trait that is determined by genes (e.g., height, hair color, disease)

Physical map—A map of the locations of identifiable landmarks on DNA regardless of inheritance. Distance on the map is measured in base pairs.

Polygenic disorders—Genetic disorders resulting from the combined action of more than one gene

Polymorphism—Difference in DNA sequence among individuals

Polypeptide—A string of amino acids linked by peptide bonds formed during the process of gene translation

Protein—Molecules that do the work of cells. They perform enzymatic reactions, produce energy. Sequences of amino acids form the building blocks of proteins. Amino acids are coded by genes.

Punnet square—A method used to determine the probabilities of allele combinations in a zygote

Recombination—The assortment of parental genes to form new combinations of chromosomes in the offspring as a result of crossing-over

Somatic cell—Any cell in a eukaryote that is not in the germ cell line

Translation—The process by which the genetic code carried by mRNA directs protein formation. Translation occurs in the ribosome.

Transcription—The synthesis of an RNA copy from a sequence of DNA (a gene). This is the first step of gene expression. Information contained in a sequence of DNA (gene) is used to direct the production of a sequence of amino acids in a polypeptide.

Zygote—A fertilized egg

Heredity, Disease, and Environment

The scientific community has long known of the relationships among heredity, disease, and environment. The relative impact of environment and genetics on health and certain illnesses, and the interaction of the two factors, are apparent but not well understood. The interactions are believed to be commonplace, and few diseases are uniquely caused by environment alone (Rimoin, Connor, & Pyeritz, 1997). Therefore, the relationship between environmental contributions and genetic predisposition are under investigation, and findings will have an impact on disease-prevention strategies.

Many common disorders have a genetic component, including cardiovascular disease, diabetes mellitus, mental illness, neurological diseases, and cancer. Multifactorial disorders, such as hypertension and rheumatoid arthritis, are caused by the interaction of one or more genes with one or more environmental agents. Genetic factors make an individual more susceptible to the effect of the environmental factors. Yet, even the manifestation of single gene disorders, such as hereditary colorectal cancer (Lynch, 1997) and familial breast cancer may be mediated by environmental factors, such as ionizing radiation (Boice, Harvey, Blettner, Stovall, & Flannery, 1992) and the use of hormone replacement therapy (Colditz et al., 1995). In the case of cancer predisposition, the form and magnitude of the interaction of environmental and genetic factors may be impossible to separate, and specific contributions of each may be indeterminate, but some investigators think that 80% of all cancers are caused by various environmental and lifestyle factors. (Cohen, 1987; Spitz, Wei, Li, & Wu, 1999; Trichopoulos, Li, & Hunter, 1996).

At one time, environmental influences were believed to be largely modifiable, while hereditary factors were considered to be largely absolute. However, in light of recent advances in human genome scientific research and technology, both factors may be alterable through human intervention. When environment along with genetic factors can be modified, diseases such as cancer may become preventable, and early detection may equal cure. Knowledge of genetic predisposition to the development of disease can lead to effective screening and early-detection programs for individuals and groups in populations who are at increased risk. Utilization of this information by the Office of Genetics and Disease Prevention of the Centers for Disease Control and Prevention (CDC) contributes to their mission of integrating advances in human genetics into public health research, policy and program development, and evaluation. To help to accomplish this mission, the public health force, including nurses, is being educated in the genetics of disease prevention and the scientific basis of public health action (CDC, 1999).

Historical Landmarks

Genetics is the branch of biology that deals with the phenomenon of heredity and its governing laws. The subspecialty of medical genetics is the science of human biologic variation as it applies to health and disease. Clinical genetics applies most specifically to patient care and is concerned with the health of individuals and their families, addressing the causes, diagnosis, prevention, and management of health disorders related to genetic alterations. Genes are found in deoxyribonucleic acid (DNA); as the carriers of hereditary information in human chromosomes, they often are described as the biologic blueprints or recipes for life (McKusick, 1997). Because cancer may arise from either acquired or inherited changes in cellular DNA, and genes are sections of DNA, cancer may be diagnosed using genetic technology and has been labeled a genetic disorder (Vogelstein & Kinzler, 1993). Even though cancer is considered a "genetic disease," in that carcinogenesis is mediated by genetic mutations, most mutations that predispose to carcinogenesis are acquired (Offit, 1998).

Early Discoveries

DNA

DNA was discovered accidentally by Friedrich Miescher in 1867 (McKusick, 1997). Thought to be one of the most significant scientific achievements of the 19th century, this discovery was part of the quest in the scientific community for an answer to the question of what causes a cell to live. Theories on the nature of life included life as the unknown transformation of lifeless matters to spontaneous generation, with life as a result of the movement and interaction of cellular components (Lagerkvist, 1998). The key observation that led to the discovery of DNA was made after denaturing pus cells. In an experiment on weakly alkaline fluids, Miescher noted that precipitates were obtained from the solutions by neutralization and that these precipitates were not soluble in water, acetic acid, hydrochloric acid, or sodium chloride. He concluded that the precipitates could not be any of the protein substances then known to exist in the cell (Greenstein, 1943) The new substance, called "nuclein," also was found in other cells, such as yeast, kidney, liver, and nucleated red blood cells (Portugal & Cohen, 1977). In subsequent decades, the precipitates were identified, renamed amino acids, and linked to proteins. The early studies on the chemistry of these materials illustrated that the nucleus of the cell is composed of two important substances: proteins and nucleic acids (Mange & Mange, 1999).

Chromosomes

Rod-like structures in the nucleus of cells were seen and reported in 1842 by Karl Nägeli. Chromosomes first were observed in plant cells and later in sperm. Wilhelm Hofmeister noted that before a cell divides into two new cells, its nucleus first divides to produce two daughter nuclei. With the addition of staining techniques, these rod-like structures could be selectively stained different colors, depending on their content and electrical charge (Jenkins, 1998). The structures were named *chromosomes* from the Greek *chromo*, meaning "color," and *soma*, meaning "body" (McKusick, 1997). By the mid-1870s, staining techniques were improved, microscopic technology was enhanced, mitosis (cell division) was reported, and the relationship between chromosomes and various stages of cell division was described (Flemming, 1879). Cyto-biologists described the nucleus as separate from the cytoplasm, as having specific chemical properties, and having an important role in the process of cell division (Baker, 1955). By the late 1880s, biologists were on the track of understanding the relationship between chromosomes and cellular division (McKusick, 1997).

Mendel's Discoveries

Principles of inheritance and the foundations of clinical genetics are traced to the 19th century to the contributions of Gregor Johann Mendel, an Austrian monk with a multidisciplinary education in physics, mathematics, biology, chemistry, and logic. In the greenhouse and garden of an Augustinian monastery at Moravia, Mendel experimented with pea and other plants to discover how simple physical traits were passed on to successive generations of offspring (Mendel, 1865/1966).

Mendel started by pure-breeding species of plants. All pure-bred progeny resembled the parents in all successive generations. The offspring had no variation; they were genetically identical. He then cross-bred different pure-bred lines to produce hybrid offspring. These offspring possessed genetic material from two separate pure-bred parent lines. He kept descendants separate and bred them at least four generations through self-fertilization. He noticed that different classes of offspring resulted from specific matings at regular frequencies that seemed to be mathematically predictable. He also noted that traits such as height stayed pure, such that tall plants bred with short plants produced tall and short plants, but never medium-height plants (Mange & Mange, 1999; McKusick 1997).

After Mendel described the steps necessary to isolate pure-bred lines of a species, he developed a mathematical formula to predict frequencies of offspring. In 1865, he reported and published his findings and conclusions. His observations became known as Mendel's Laws of Inheritance, and these laws identified the units of inheritance as "factors." Traits that were passed on in a straightforward way from one generation to another were called simple Mendelian traits. Description of patterns of inheritance evolved nearly concurrently with knowledge of chromosomes but preceded description of the process of meiosis, which was not described until 1887 (McKusick, 1997) (see Figure 4-2).

Development of Gene Theory

Mendel's conclusions were largely forgotten, but not dismissed. In 1892, August Weismann, a German physiologist, described his observations of the process of cell division. Before a cell divides, thread-like structures named chromosomes appear in the nucleus of the cell. The chromosomes line up in matched pairs, double, then split apart, producing identical sets of daughter cells. He also observed that germ cells, sperm and ovum, have only one-half the number of chromosomes. He concluded that at fertilization, the male and female parents contribute equally but give only half of the total hereditary material to the offspring. The new individual receives a full set of paired chromosomes, or two copies of each chromosome. One copy of each chromosome comes from the male and the other from the female parent. "Germ plasm" was the name given to the material in eggs

Figure 4-2. Selected Events and Medical Advances Associated With the Development of Genetics

1665—Robert Hooke described living cells.

1700—Antoni van Leeuwenhoek described the nucleus of a cell.

1780—Lazzari Spallanzani demonstrated that sperms are needed to fertilize eggs.

1839—Theodor Schwann and Matthias Jakob Schleiden confirmed that the cell is the basic unit of life.

1865—Gregor Johann Mendel identified factors as traits that are dominant or recessive in pattern of inheritance.

1866—Down syndrome was first described.

1869—Friedrich Miescher discovered nucleic acids.

1881—Edouard Balbiani first described giant chromosomes in the salivary glands of *Drosophila melanogaster.*

1882—Walther Flemming described the process of mitosis.

1887—August Weismann predicted the basic steps of meiosis.

1888—Waldeyer introduced the term "chromosome."

1888—Weismann developed the theory that chromosomes carry determinants of heredity and development.

1897—Weismann proposed the process of recombination, the shuffling of inherited characteristics during sperm and egg cell formation.

1900—Hugo de Vries, Carl Correns, and Erich Tschermak rediscovered the work of Mendel and its significance.

1903—Walter Sutton suggested that chromosomes carry genetic information.

1905—Crundall Punnet invented the Punnet square, a method to predict the outcomes of genetic crosses.

1907—William Bateson coined the word "genetics."

1908—Sir Archibald Garrod suggested that genetic factors make enzymes; Wilhelm Johannsen coined the word "gene."

1910—Aaron Theodor Levene identified ribose and deoxyribose sugars in nucleic acids.

1911—Edward B. Wilson was the first to assign a specific gene to a specific chromosome: color blindness to chromosome X.

1916—Calvin B. Bridges proved that genes were associated with chromosomes.

1924—Robert Feulgen established that DNA is confined to chromosomes.

1927—Herman J. Muller demonstrated that x-radiation produces an increase in the rate of mutation in *Drosophila melanogaster.*

1928—Frederick Griffith demonstrated that genetic material could be passed from one bacterium to another.

1929—Boveri proposed that cancer might result from alterations in the genetic material of cells.

1933—Thomas Hunt Morgan received the Nobel Prize for Medicine and Physiology for discovering sex-linked genes in *Drosophila.*

1934—Genes were measured in nanometers (nm=0.000.000/cm) for the first time by Hermann J. Muller and colleagues.

1937—George W. Beadle and Edward L. Tatum showed that genes have a chemical effect on the development of organisms.

1947—Erwin Chargaff analyzed DNA and determined the relative amounts of its four nucleotide bases.

1949—Linus Pauling introduced the concept of molecular disease.

1950—Linus Pauling and Robert Brainard Corey discovered the helical nature of some protein molecules.

1952—Alexander Lathan Dounce predicted the three-base codon in DNA.

1953—James Watson and Francis Crick described the structure of DNA as a double helix.

(Continued on next page)

Figure 4-2. Selected Events and Medical Advances Associated With the Development of Genetics (Continued)

1958—Beadle and Tatum received the Nobel Prize for Medicine and Physiology for showing that one gene controls the production of one enzyme.
1959—Arthur Kornberg received the Nobel Prize for Medicine and Physiology for showing that DNA can self-replicate.
1969—Li Fraumeni genetic disease was identified at the National Institutes of Health.
1972—First patent on life was given to Amanda Chakrabarty for genetically engineered bacteria that breaks down crude oil.
1977—The Dounreay nuclear power station explosion occurred, and research was done in the possible effects of radiation on genes.
1978—First tumor suppressor gene, p53, was found.
1978—First genetically engineered version of insulin was created.
1982—The first automatic gene sequencer was created.
1983—HIV was isolated and identified as causative agent of AIDS.
1985—The first extensive human gene maps were made.
1985—Viral oncogenes were first described.
1985—Polymerase chain reaction was developed by Karry B. Mullis.
1986—Chernoble nuclear power station disaster occurred, alerting health officials to the potential for massive increases in the frequency of gene mutation in local populations.
1987—Gene associated with familial adenomatous polyposis (Gene APC) is located on Chromosome 5.
1988—Bert Vogelstein and others linked p53 with tumorogenesis.
1990—Gene associated with cystic fibrosis was discovered.
1990—BRCA1 gene localized to chromosome 17.
1990—The Human Genome Project began.
1993—The exact position of the gene for Huntington's chorea was discovered.
1994—BRCA2 gene localized to chromosome 13
1997—First transgenic (cloned) sheep, "Dolly," is created.
1997—First primate cloning took place.
1999—Abnormalities in chromosome 8 were linked to prostate cancer
2000—Completed sequencing of the genome of *Drosophila melanogaster*
2000—Successful cloning of multiple offspring (piglets) occurred.
2003—Human Genome Project is expected to be completed.

and sperm that transported heritable traits from parents to progeny. In his book *Das Keimplasma (The Germ-Plasm)*, Weismann suggested that sexual reproduction generated new combinations of hereditary factors, and chromosomes carried these factors from parent to offspring (Judson, 1992; Weismann, 1893). This process was later termed "recombination." During the last years of the 1890s, several biologists associated cellular development with activity within the nucleus (Muller, 1951; Wilson, 1899).

Genes

The term "gene" first was used in 1909 by Wilhelm Johannsen to describe a particle, as yet unseen, that was carried on chromosomes to mediate inheritance. The gene was equated to the atom. In the same sense as atoms and electrons are described as invisible but essential to chemistry and physics, genes were described as invisible elements that are essential to heredity (Morgan, 1926).

Thomas Hunt Morgan studied genetic mutations caused by chemicals and radiation in *Drosophila melanogaster,* the fruit fly. This work led to cytological empiric evidence of the exchange of genetic materials among chromosomes during early stages of meiosis. Morgan (1911) wrote,

> There is good evidence to support the view that . . . when chromosomes separate the split is in a single plane. . . . In consequence, the original material will, for short distances, be more likely to fall on the same side as the last, as on the opposite side. . . . We find coupling in certain characteristics, and not in others . . . the difference depending on the linear distance apart of the chromosomal materials that represent the factors. . . . Instead of random segregation in Mendel's sense, we find 'associations of factors' that are located close together in the chromosomes. (p. 384)

This process later was called "crossing over" and was associated with genetic mutation and the appearance of genetic variation and variety in the physical expression of genes (Morgan, Sturtevant, Muller, & Bridges, 1915).

Studies conducted by Archibold Garrod on inherited errors of metabolism, such as alkaptonuria, led to descriptions of the connection between a specific gene and its product (a protein) (Garrod, 1928). Soon after, the concepts of phenotype and genotype also were described (Muller, 1951). Phenotype is the outward manifestation or appearance of a trait. Genotype is the genetic basis for the physical expression. In 1910, the difference between the two concepts was demonstrated when several genes or factors were shown to be present for a single physical trait or appearance. The relationship between genotype and phenotype provided a theoretical connection between hereditary factors and the development of disease (East, 1910).

DNA Linked to Heredity

The first linkage of a gene to a specific chromosome was credited to E.B. Wilson in 1911. Color blindness was assigned to the X chromosome (McKusick, 1997). During the first half of the 20th century, scientific medical research was under way at Rockefeller Institute in New York. Oswald Avery investigated the relationship between the bacteria *Pneumococci* and disease (Avery, MacLeod, & McCarty, 1944). In a series of experiments with collaborators in the United States and the United Kingdom, Avery showed that *Pneumococci* could change from one serological type to another in an infected organism. He proposed that the transformational activity was controlled by DNA. This was an original idea that was received skeptically in the scientific community because it contradicted the common belief that the entire genetic material of an organism (genome) was carried in proteins, not nucleic acids. Later, results from a separate investigation by Alfred Hershey and Martha Chase (1952) on *Escherichia coli* supported the claim. Now there was empiric evidence that DNA was the molecular basis of heredity.

During the mid-20th century, other important contributions were made to the overall gene theory. DNA was shown to have base complementarity by Erwin Chargaff (1950), who reported that DNA contained equal amounts of guanine and cytosine nuclei acids and adenine and thymine nucleic acids. In the 1950s, James Watson and Francis Crick, two biologists with backgrounds in chemistry and physics, were investigating the three-dimensional structure of DNA. They used the concept of the helix, first proposed by Linus Pauling, as the structure of macromolecules (Lagerkvist, 1998). Watson and Crick integrated the concepts of base complementarity with helical structure of macromolecules and proposed DNA as a double helical coil. In 1953, Watson, an American, and Crick, an Englishman, conceptualized the DNA molecule as two polynucleotide strands linked to each other by weak hydrogen bonds. Each one nucleotide can pair with only one other. Cytosine bonds with guanine and adenine bonds with thymine to form a sequential strand of base pairs. The backbone of the strand is made of macromolecules of sugar and phosphoric acid. The base pairs are stacked on each other between strands, creating a stable macromolecular helical coil (Crick, 1988; Watson, 1968; Watson & Crick, 1953). This is the popular and universally accepted simple model of the DNA molecule.

Modern Medical Genetics

From 1950 to the present, advances in medical genetics have rapidly progressed. Contemporary science represents a cumulative history of complementary multidisciplinary discoveries in cytogenetics, immunogenetics, and population genetics. Cytobiologists, physicists, and chemists systematically linked nucleic acids with chromosomes. Chromosomes were linked with heredity, and meiosis and mitosis were linked with principles of inheritance. Work in the field of cytogenetics contributed discoveries that led to the understanding of mitosis and meiosis (McKusick, 1997). Discoveries in molecular genetics contributed to the understanding of the relationship between genes and gene products and the concept of the biochemical basis of disease. Research in immunogenetics illustrated the role of Mendelian inheritance in humans when ABO blood types in the population were assigned to chromosomal alleles inherited from only one parent (Levine & Stetson, 1939). Work in population genetics provided a method to quantify the probability of an individual inheriting a specific genetic trait (Hardy, 1908; McKusick, 1997). The progressive development of modern medical genetics illustrates the complex interdependence of scientific disciplines in the quest to more fully understand human inheritance.

Gene Mapping

The discovery that genes carry information for the production of molecular genetics and that proteins are responsible for all cellular functions provided the impetus to fully understand the human genome by using genetic mapping. The aims of genetic mapping are (a) to assign specific genes to specific chromosomes, (b) to assign specific proteins to specific genes, and (c) to associate genes with phenotypical expression (Collins & Galas, 1993). The mapping results in the graphic representation of the human genome. Sometimes referred to as genetic linkage maps, they lay out the arrangement of genes and DNA markers along the chromosomes. The layout is determined by patterns of inheritance of distinctive cytological features on chromosomes. Markers are found in several generations of a family. Markers tend to be inherited together because they are physically close (linked) together on the chromosome. The physical closeness and tendency to be inherited together is called linkage. Markers inherited independently are far apart on the mapped chromosomes. Linkage mapping has clinical value when markers associated with a specific disease can be identified in an individual's cellular DNA, predicting the likelihood of developing that disease (Mange & Mange, 1999; White & Lalouel, 1988). See Figure 4-3 for an illustration of how genes are pinpointed on chromosomes.

Another way to fully understand the human genome and inheritance is by creating a physical map (Collins & Galas, 1993). This kind of map shows physical landmarks along measured distances between markers on chromosomes. Landmarks can be stainable bands, break points, deletions, or a sequence of nucleotide base pairs. An important part of the process of physical mapping of the genome is to identify the sequential line-up of base pairs along the DNA molecule and then search for variations. When variations are found, they can be associated with physical expression and labeled as normal or abnormal. Abnormal variations may be associated with disease (Mange & Mange, 1999).

Human Genome Research

The Human Genome Project (HGP) is a worldwide initiative to describe the structure of human DNA, locate all the genes, and sequence more than three billion nucleotides of the haploid genome. The Project originated from initiatives taken in the mid-1980s by Robert Sinsheimer, a molecular biologist at the University of California at Santa Cruz, and Charles DeLisi, a physicist at the U.S. Department of Energy (DOE) in Washington, DC. The DOE had sponsored research in

Figure 4-3. Pinpointing Genes

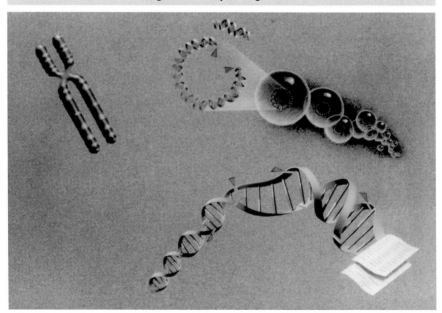

There are three key techniques for identifying the location of disease-causing genes in chromosomes: (1) chromosome staining (top left), (2) identifying inherited markers (top right), and (3) DNA cloning (bottom right).

Note. Figure courtesy of the National Cancer Institute of the National Institutes of Health, Bethesda, MD. Reprinted with permission.

the biological effects of radiation, especially genetic mutations, and recognized the importance of studying the variety of genetic defects. The DOE established a major database called "Genbank" for DNA sequence information in 1983, and in 1985, Sinsheimer invited a dozen American and European molecular biologists to Santa Cruz for a workshop on the technical prospects of determining the details of the human genome (Kevles, 1992). Between 1985 and 1990, the HGP was conceptualized and developed (McKusick, 1980; Organization for Economic Co-Operation and Development, 1995).

The formal project began on October 1, 1990, with federal funding provided jointly through the DOE and the National Institutes of Health (NIH). James G. Watson (of the Watson and Crick team) led the HGP for the first three years, during which time he also directed the National Center for Human Genome Research (NCHGR).

In 1993, Francis Collins became the director of the NCHGR. He developed a medical genetics program that made gene identification a central focus. In 1998, genetic scientists began building a catalogue of human genetic variation and correlating variation with disease susceptibility. Of the six million potential variations, some may affect gene expression or change protein sequences that are encoded by genes. Some portion of these variations will affect disease susceptibility. Human genome technology has developed in tandem with the process of linking specific genes with diseases and has contributed to the growing body of knowledge on health-related benefits of genetics research (McKusick, 1980; Organisation for Economic Co-Operation and Development, 1995).

The HGP evolved into a collaborative effort between an international public consortium and the efforts in the private sector. Each took a different approach to the sequencing of the human genome. On June 26, 2000, U.S. President Bill Clinton and British Prime Minister Tony Blair credited both the International Human Genome Project and Celera Genomics Corporation with the landmark achievement of completing an initial sequence of the human genome. The announcement was described as the starting point for a new era of genetic medicine ("President Clinton Announces," 2000).

Genes and Cancer

Understanding variation in the human genome is expected to lead to understanding of disease. During the 1980s, researchers made discoveries about the role of genes in the development of cancer. One such gene was the proto-oncogene; when altered at the molecular level, the gene becomes an oncogene, which promotes deregulation, indiscriminant cell reproduction, and the development of neoplasias (Krontiris, 1995). In a 1987 editorial published in the journal *Science*, Nobel Laureate in physiology and medicine Ranato Dulbecco (1986) asserted that cancer research would progress further and faster if scientists had a complete sequence of the DNA in the human genome. Thus, one aim of the HGP and genetics research is to better understand the nature of cancer and carcinogenesis and to develop preventative strategies, diagnostic technologies, and treatment options.

To accomplish this aim, NCI formed the Cancer Genome Anatomy Project (CGAP), an interdisciplinary program to develop databases, available to the public, and technologies to help researchers to understand the molecular anatomy of the cancer cell. The project's goals are to describe the molecular genetics of normal, precancerous, and malignant cells (National Center for Biotechnology Information, 2000). One initiative under the CGAP is the Human Tumor Gene Index (HTGI), which was set up to catalogue human genes. Another initiative is the Cancer Chromosome Aberration Project (CCAP) which is designed to develop ways to define and characterize distinct chromosomal alterations that are associated with the development of malignancy. It is the hope of the NCI that this information can be used by clinicians to diagnose, classify, and treat cancer based on the cancer's distinct genetic "fingerprint" (National Center for Biotechnology Information, 2001). Of the more than 73,000 genes already catalogued, more than 40,000 are active, directly or indirectly, associated with one or more cancers (NCI, 1999).

Fundamental Concepts

Some important theoretical statements evolved over the last 150 years from the study of genetics. The organization of apparently simple ideas formed the foundation for future discoveries. The fundamental concepts have been important to students of medicine and nursing, and ultimately to health care.

First is the distinction made between separation of the inherited and noninherited human characteristics. The identification of these two components of biologic change has led to debates regarding the variable impact of heredity and environment (Goldschmidt, 1951). The concepts of nature and nurture infuse the discussion of human development, health, and illness. Clinicians and scientists may debate the variable impact of each factor. Nurses are aware that certain environmental carcinogens, such as tobacco, ionizing radiation, ultraviolet radiation, and industrial products, have been attributed to the development of lung, thyroid, skin, and bladder cancers (Armstrong & Kricker, 1993; Barrett & Huff, 1991; Jablon & Kato, 1970; Doll, 1993; Doll & Peto, 1987; Jourand, 1991; Lieber, 1993; Shields & Harris, 1993; Shimizu, Schull, & Kato, 1990; Tomatis et al., 1978). It also is known that certain gene mutations have been linked to the development of specific cancers. For example, several known mutations to the BRCA1 gene have been associated with the development of breast and ovarian cancers (Easton, Narod, Ford, & Steel, 1994; Hall et al., 1990; Li & Fraumeni, 1969), and alteration of the RET proto-oncogene may predispose an individual to the development of endocrine gland tumors (Sipple, 1961; Szabo, Heath, & Hill, 1995; Wermer, 1954).

The second basic consequence of genetics is the notion that heredity is localized in the chromosomes (Goldschmidt, 1951), the delicately connected network of biologic structures in the nucleus of cells that are composed of DNA and proteins and contain sets of linked genes. Chromosomes have a constant polar organization, and they are different from end to end along their length. This means that chromosomes are both different from each other and along their length. The polar organization has a role in their self-replication. Following this concept is the assumption that there is a tendency for pairs of chromosomes (one paternal and one maternal copy) to exchange sections during self-replication. This process, called crossing over, permits the recombination of genetic materials between parents and the possibility of producing offspring with an infinite variety of genetic and physical traits.

Another main concept of genetics is the establishment of a mutation as the only proven means of hereditary change (Goldschmidt, 1951). A mutation is a heritable change in structural or chemical makeup of a gene. Changes may be large or small, visible or invisible, and nonpathological or pathological. Genetic abnormalities may take the form of gross chromosomal alterations, such as changes in chromosome number, shape, and size. Gross chromosomal abnormalities are associated with diseases, such as Down's syndrome, in which affected people have an extra chromosome 21, or three copies of chromosome 21 (Trisomy 21). People with chronic myelogenous leukemia have gross abnormalities in chromosomes 9 and 22. Genetic aberrations associated with disease also may be micromolecular. At the molecular level, minute sections of DNA can be deleted, gained, or translocated. In the cases of some cancers, changes as small as a single base pair can precede predisposition to tumor development (see Figure 4-4 and Figure 4-5 for illustrations on the translocations of sections of DNA). From these basic observations has come specific explanations about the principles of inheritance, the process of genetic mutation, and the origin and nature of inherited diseases.

Figure 4-4. Translocation of Chromosomes

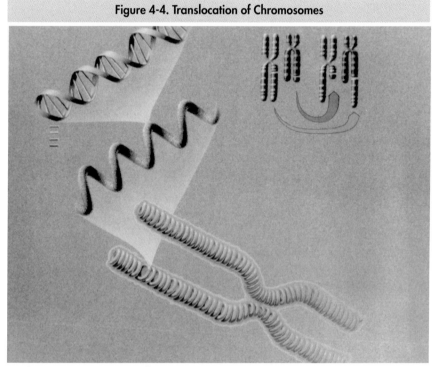

Translocation, or the breaking off and replacement, of parts of whole chromosomes may cause some kinds of cancer.

Note. Figure courtesy of the National Cancer Institute of the National Institutes of Health, Bethesda, MD. Reprinted with permission.

Figure 4-5. Translocation of Chromosomes, Close Up

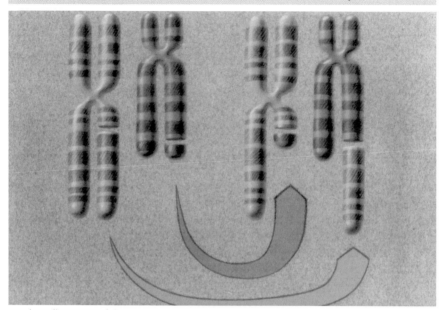

Up-close illustration of the translocation of chromosomes

Note. Figure courtesy of the National Cancer Institute of the National Institutes of Health, Bethesda, MD. Reprinted with permission.

Structure and Function of Genetic Material: A Review

Chromosomes

Our bodies are made of billions of cells, and the human genome is contained in the nucleus of each cell. A single DNA molecule is too small to be visible, but a large quantity of DNA molecules together appear as a clean, white string and viscous mass. DNA, in condensed form, is found in chromosomes. A chromosome is a long stretch of DNA that is tightly coiled and surrounded by certain proteins. The chromosomes are arranged in pairs, and the two members of a pair are nearly identical, or "homologous," copies of each other. Sites along the chromosome are called loci. Specific genes are found at specific loci on a specific chromosome. Eukaryotes have two copies (alleles) of each gene. The copies may be identical or different versions of the same gene. The entire complement of genetic material of a human is the human genome and is identified as 46 chromosomes (23 pairs). Every cell nucleus has 22 pairs of somatic chromosomes and 1 pair of sex chromosomes. Males have 22 pairs of autosomes and one set of xy sex chromosomes. Females have 22 pairs of autosomes and a set of xx sex chromosomes to bring the total to 46.

DNA

DNA is composed of two strands of sugar and phosphate molecules that coil around each other in a double-helix configuration. Each of these skeletal strands is notched with molecules called nucleotides (bases), which are themselves composed of one of four molecules: adenine, guanine, thymine, and cytosine. The nucleotides are lined up in a sequence along one side and matched with a complementary sequence along the other. Once the sequence of nucleotide bases on one strand is known, the sequence on the opposing strand is also known. The sequence of base pairs contains the genetic information in sections, of variable length, called genes (Mehlman & Botkin, 1998) (see Figure 4-6).

Whole strands of DNA may separate for the purpose of self-replication, as is done in cellular reproduction (mitosis) and in gamete formation during oogenesis

Figure 4-6. Cellular DNA

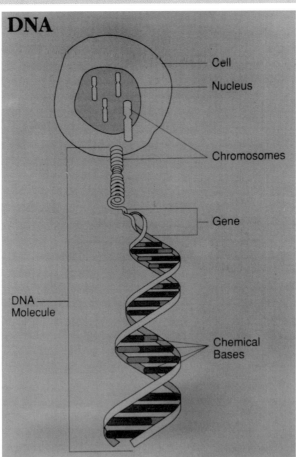

DNA is made up of four chemical bases. Coiled strands of DNA are packed into chromosomes in the nucleus of cells. DNA carries instructions that allow cells to make proteins. The protein coding regions of DNA are called genes.

and spermatogenesis for sexual reproduction (meiosis). Replication of DNA requires the presence of enzymes called DNA helicase and DNA polymerase. DNA helicase opens up the double helix, exposing stranded sequences to be copied. DNA polymerase is an exzyme that travels along the exposed DNA strand and aids in the selection, placement, and matching of new nucleotides to exposed complimentary bases. Another enzyme, DNA ligase, rejoins the single strands to reconstitute the DNA double helix at the completion of self-replication. After they separate, each single strand of DNA acts as a template for the construction of another double helix. Complementary bases match up with the exposed bases to reconstruct the original double strand. Thus, one double helix splits, and the replication process forms two identical double helices of DNA (Mange & Mange, 1999).

Genes and Proteins

The segments of DNA that contain biochemical messages are called genes. Genes are made of specific sequences of nucleotide base pairs that contain the codes that regulate the cellular production of proteins, such as structural proteins, hormones, hemoglobin, and enzymes. Structural proteins form muscle, hair, and tendons. Hemoglobin is a protein that transports oxygen, hormones deliver biochemical messages to organs, and enzymes catalyze biochemical reactions. At any time, thousands of protein-mediated chemical reactions take place in the body. Proteins are constructed with amino acids that join to polypeptide chains. A protein is fully formed when it assumes a unique spatial shape. Both the content and form of the protein molecule are essential to its ultimate biochemical purpose. Small sections of the double helix of DNA may separate along the length of DNA at a site that contains biochemical information that codes for a specific protein. The exposed sequences of base pairs serve as templates for the reproduction of biochemical messages contained in the gene.

Each gene contains a message for the construction of a string of amino acids (polypeptide) that becomes a protein. Along the gene, which can be many thousand base pairs long, are regions called exons and introns. Exons are sections that contain coding information. Introns are sections of the gene that do not contain information used for protein production. Codons, a group of three base pairs, are associated with specific amino acids. There are 64 possible triplets of nucleotide bases that specify, or code, for the 20 amino acids found in the polypeptide chains and in other genetic signals. The relationship between a specific codon and a specific amino acid is called the genetic code. Changes in the order of base pairs in a gene is the molecular basis of mutation because a change in a base pair has the potential to change the biochemical message.

Only a small percentage of human DNA codes for protein. Presently, the function of the majority of DNA that does not code for protein is largely unknown. It sometimes is called "junk" DNA, even though geneticists believe that it may, in fact, serve an important, as yet unknown, function in the cell (Mehlman & Botkin, 1998). The genetic code mediates gene expression through transcription and translation. Transcription is the process of reading DNA, and translation is the process of transforming that message to the biochemical product.

Transcription: Copying the Genetic Code

Messages contained in DNA must be transcribed and processed, and messenger ribonucleic acid (mRNA) performs this task. Strands of mRNA, made up of nucleotide base pairs that are complementary to those on the DNA strand, read the code. Decoding of the information contained in genes proceeds in two steps. A section of DNA containing a genetic code for a specific protein, called the template, is exposed. The beginning point of the gene has a sequence of bases that promotes reading (promoter sequence), and the end has a sequence that stops the reading (terminator sequence). When the cell requires the production of a certain protein, the double helix of DNA unravels at the loci where the gene that codes for the needed protein is located. The enzyme RNA polymerase, like DNA polymerase, travels along the exposed length of DNA, attracting and linking ribonucleotides that are complementary to the DNA bases. When RNA polymerase reaches the termination sequence, the single strand of RNA breaks off. Messenger RNA has "read" and rewritten the coded message by matching complementary bases to the sequential base pairs along the strand of DNA. In the process of transcription, mRNA splices and removes the noncoding regions of DNA called introns. It then assembles the regions (exons) to form a complete message. The final strand of mRNA contains only exons that contain codons for specific amino acids. Then, the mRNA carries the genetic information across the nuclear membrane into the cytoplasm for protein production.

Translation: Interpreting the Genetic Code

The second stage of gene expression occurs in cytoplasmic structures called ribosomes. Here, the information contained in the mRNA is translated by transfer RNA (tRNA), which uses the genetic information that was delivered to the cytoplasm. Another kind of RNA, called ribosomal RNA (rRNA), facilitates the formation of the ribosome-tRNA complex, on which protein synthesis occurs. Each of the 20 amino acids has a tRNA. The rRNA forms the workbench on which protein molecules are constructed. tRNA attracts its signature amino acids from the cytoplasm according to the decoded message, transports them to the ribosome, and assists in assembling the collected amino acids into a polypeptide chain. From 12 to more than a thousand amino acids are linked to form a linear polypeptide. One or several linked polypeptides will coil, fold, or intertwine to form the unique three-dimensional structure (Mange & Mange, 1999). Figure 4-7 provides an illustration of the processes of transcription and translation.

The main difference between RNA and DNA is found in the chemical base pairs. It is known that DNA matches adenine to guanine and cytosine to thymine. Base pairing differs for RNA, which complements adenine to guanine but replaces thymine with uracil to complement cytosine (see Figure 4-8).

The sequence of complementary base pairs is the chemical basis for virtually all interactions between nucleic acids. Complementary base pairing occurs between DNA strands in DNA replication, between DNA and mRNA in transcription, and between mRNA and tRNA in the process of translation. The two steps of transcription and translation represent how genetic information becomes a biologic product. This is called gene expression.

Figure 4-7. Transcription and Translation

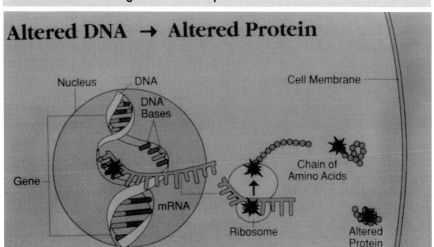

When genes contain a mutation, the protein encoded by the gene will be abnormal.

Note. Figure originally created for the National Cancer Institute. Reprinted with permission of the artist Jeanne Kelly. Copyright 1996.

Figure 4-8. Complementary Base Pairs

Complementary Base Pairs in Deoxyribonucleic Acid
Adenine = Guanine
Cytosine = Thymine
Complementary Base Pairs in Ribonucleic Acid
Adenine = Guanine
Thymine = Uracil

The central dogma of molecular biology is that genetic information flows from DNA to RNA to polypeptides. Therefore, it is a prevailing belief that transcription and translation are unidirectional in the human genetic code. One known exception is found in retroviruses, where RNA may code for DNA in a host organism in the process called reverse transcription.

Meiosis

Like most plants and animals, human organisms are formed by the proliferation of a single cell into 2, then 4, 8, 16, and so on. The cells gradually differentiate into tissues, organs, and organ systems. The first step in the process of cellular reproduction occurs at the molecular level. Egg and sperm formation occur as a result of a type of cell division called meiosis. This process produces cells that contain only one-half the total number of chromosomes of a cell. Female eggs and sperm each contain the haploid number of chromosomes. When an egg and male sperm unite, they create the full complement of genetic material comprising the human genome (Murray & Kirschner, 1991).

117

Genetic variety in offspring is the result of independent assortment of chromosomes and crossing-over during meiosis. Independent assortment is the random and independent distribution of each of the pair of chromosomes or each of the pair of unlinked alleles during sperm and egg formation. Independent assortment is Mendel's second law of inheritance (Mange & Mange, 1999). Crossing over results in the shifting of genes from one chromosome to the other during gamete formation. These two events are responsible for infinite genetic variety and unpredictability of the genotype of offspring.

Mendelian Inheritance

Mendel's study of garden peas, combined with the work of other genetics researchers, produced the main premises of inheritance. The concepts of Mendelian inheritance are limited and apply only to organisms that reproduce sexually, perform normal meiosis, and have more than one chromosome. Many patterns of inheritance in humans can be explained in terms of Mendelian genetics. The rules of inheritance are (a) the principle of dominance, (b) the law of segregation, and (c) the law of independent assortment (Mange & Mange, 1999).

Diseases inherited in Mendelian pattern are categorized according to whether the gene is on an autosome or a sex chromosome and according to whether the inherited trait is dominant or recessive (Mueller & Cook, 1997). The first rule of inheritance is Mendel's principle of dominance. The principle describes the relationship between the two alleles in a pair. When parents differ in a characteristic, their offspring will be genetic hybrids of that trait. The offspring will have a copy, however different from each parent, but will not necessarily show a blend of the two copies of a trait. Rather, the trait from one parent will be dominant over the trait of the other parent. The other form of the trait will be recessive. Although the other trait is not visible, it is still present. Some human characteristics that obey the principle of dominance are hair color (dark dominant to light), hair texture (curly hair dominant to straight), and eye color (brown dominant to blue or grey).

At meiosis, during gamete formation, the pair of alleles in the parent cell separate from each other, and the offspring cells (gametes) have only one of the alleles. As a result, a gamete has an equal probability of obtaining either copy of a gene pair. This is Mendel's law of segregation. When a hybrid reproduces, its egg or sperm will be of two types. Half will carry the dominant trait provided by one parent, and half will have the recessive trait from the other parent. A parent that is homozygous for brown eyes (BB) will produce gametes that all contain one allele for brown eyes (B). The parent that is homozygous for blue eyes (bb) will produce gametes with one allele for blue eyes (b). A parent that is heterozygous (Bb) will produce one gamete with an allele for brown (B) and one with an allele for blue (b) (DeVries, 1900/1966).

Last, when parents differ in two or more characteristics, the occurrence of any characteristic in the next generation will be independent of any other characteristic. The separation of pairs of alleles during meiosis is independent, such that the alleles migrate to daughter cells independently to produce an assortment of alleles. This is the law of independent assortment (Mueller & Cook, 1997; Peters,

1959). A parent heterozygous for brown eyes and black hair (Bb Ll) may produce gametes with a mixture of alleles as follows:

	B	b
L	BL	bL
l	Bl	bl

The Punnett square, named for R.C. Punnett who was an early geneticist, shows the independent assortment of pairs of alleles and is used as a simple model to calculate the results of genotypic crosses. It is used to account for the genotypic makeup of all offspring in the right proportions. The grid is used to represent the genetic combinations of offspring with one or more pairs of alleles.

Simple Mendelian inheritance patterns are dominant or recessive. However, inheritance patterns may be complex and follow different sets of rules. The principle of co-dominance describes the condition in which the heterozygote has a phenotype intermediate between the two homozygous phenotypes, much like what occurs when two colors are blended together to create a different color. Co-dominance may be observed when a heterozygote shows a phenotype with characteristics of both alleles expressed equally. Non-Mendelian patterns of inheritance are associated with complex disorders. These disorders show incomplete or reduced penetrance and late age of onset of symptoms. Recurrence risks are lower than seen for traits that follow simple Mendelian inheritance patterns. These disorders may be multigenic or multifactorial and involve gene-to-gene, or gene-to-environment interactions. Many kinds of cancers and cancer syndromes may be categorized as complex disorders (Shields & Harris, 1993).

Mechanisms of Mutation and Carcinogenesis

A mutation is a stable, heritable alteration in the DNA sequence that can be passed from a cell to its progeny during cell division and replication. Mutations can affect either somatic or germline cells. Somatic mutations are alterations of DNA sequence in cells of the body other than those that give rise to germ cells. Somatic alterations are transmitted only through the affected cell line during self-replication. Because somatic cells do not give rise to gametes, somatic mutations cannot be inherited by offspring. Somatic mutations that lead to the development of cancer may be induced by environmental agents such as ionizing radiation and exposure to certain chemicals (see Figure 4-9). Germline genetic alterations, also called hereditary mutations, occur in the cells that give rise to eggs and sperm. If a mutation occurs in germ cell DNA, it will be transmitted to all the cells that differentiate from the original zygote- both germ and somatic cells (see Figure 4-10). Therefore, mutations can arise spontaneously, or they may be inherited. Very small amounts (alteration of one or a few bases in DNA) or very large amounts of genetic material (chromosomal abnormalities, as seen in translocation) may constitute the mutation.

DNA sequences encode proteins, so an alteration or mutation in the sequence may alter the function of a gene and its protein product. However, not all mutations have a deleterious affect on gene expression, and not all are associated with disease. The effect of a gene mutation depends upon how the protein product is affected and the protein's biological function. As a result of mutation, genetic sequences

Figure 4-9. Oncogenes

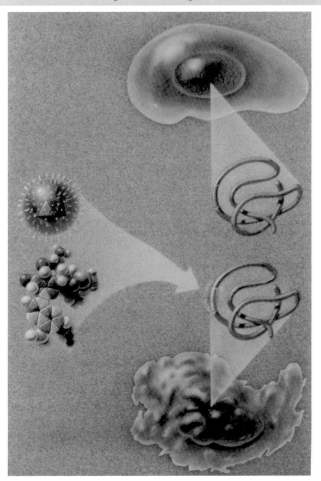

A normal cell (top right) is converted to a cancer cell (bottom right) when an oncogene (highlighted region of the coil) is activated.

Note. Figure courtesy of the National Cancer Institute of the National Institutes of Health, Bethesda, MD. Reprinted with permission.

may differ among individuals. The presence in the population of two or more relatively common forms of a gene is called polymorphism. The more copies or versions of a gene, the greater the polymorphism. Variations are common in the human genome, and some polymorphisms are normal, such as the variable forms of the gene that encodes for blood type or eye color. The different forms of genes are referred to as alleles, and the location of a gene on a chromosome is referred to as a locus. Each person has two copies of each gene. If an individual has the same allele on both members of a chromosome pair, he or she is said to be a homozygote. If the alleles differ in DNA sequence, the individual is heterozygote. Some individuals have a mutated copy that may predispose them to the development of cancer.

Figure 4-10. Oncogene Activation

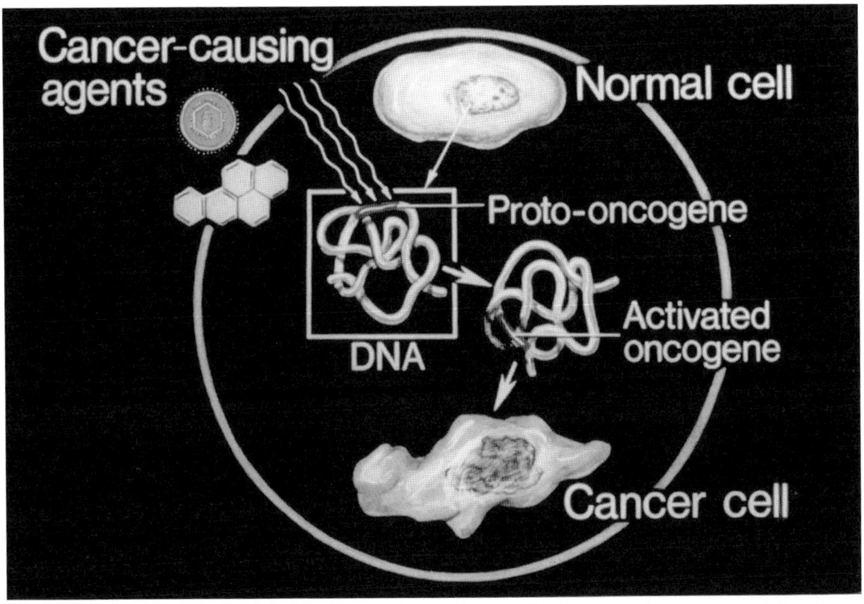

A proto-oncogene in a normal cell appears to regulate and influence cell growth and division. When a cancer-causing agent affecting a cell's DNA and the proto-oncogene is converted to an oncogene, a cancer cell develops.

Note. Figure courtesy of the National Cancer Institute of the National Institutes of Health, Bethesda, MD. Reprinted with permission.

Different alleles of a gene can result in the formation of different gene products. Because the codons are read as triplets, an addition or deletion of only one nucleotide shifts the entire reading frame for transcription and can cause changes in the amino acids, premature chain termination, or chain elongation, resulting in a defective biological product.

Types of Mutations

A gene may become altered in several ways, all of which involve the changing of the sequence of DNA nucleotide bases. One or more bases may be inserted, deleted, substituted, or shifted in the linear sequence. Long strands of unstable trinucleotide repeats also may occur. The change in the order of bases changes the genetic message. A single nucleotide substitution is the most frequent kind of mutation. One base pair is substituted for another. Most often, these alterations occur during the vulnerable multistage process of DNA replication (Antonarakis, 1997). These mutations also are known as point mutations and can result in a change in the amino acid sequence. A base substitution in one codon may or may not change the amino acid because it may change it to another codon that still codes for the specified amino acid. However, because the genetic code is redundant, many of these mutations do not change the amino acid sequence and, thus, have no consequence. Single gene mutations that have no consequence are known as silent mutations because they have no significant effect on structure or function of the protein product. The majority of point mutations are corrected by the DNA repair system.

There are two types of nonsilent base pair substitutions: missense and nonsense mutations. Missense mutations change the reading frame of the genetic code with the exchange of one base pair for another. A triplet that originally coded for alanine (GCU, or guanine, cytosine, uracil) may by changed to GGU (guanine, guanine, uracil), which now codes for glycine. The message is still transcribed, but the changed sequence of amino acids contains inaccurate information and may result in the production of the defective protein product by replacing one amino acid for another in the polypeptide.

Nonsense, or chain termination mutations, comprise a small percent of random base substitutions. They change the message to prematurely stop translation with one of the stop codons. The result is a shortened chain of amino acids or a truncated polypeptide. When a stop codon is altered so that it encodes an amino acid, an abnormally elongated polypeptide is produced. These alterations of the sequence of amino acids can have profound consequences. Many of the serious genetic diseases arise as a result of these kinds of base pair substitutions.

Gene deletion can occur from mistakes in the DNA repair system after extensive damage. Because codons consist of groups of three bases, insertions and deletions of one or more bases may be especially harmful when a number of missing or extra base pairs is not a multiple of three. These types of mutations are known as frameshifts because all of the downstream codons will be shifted and the reading frame will be incorrect.

Other types of mutations can alter the regulation of transcription and translation. A promoter mutation can decrease the affinity of RNA polymerase for a promoter site, resulting in a decrease in the production of a particular protein. Enhancer mutations can have similar effects. Splice site mutations alter the splicing signal necessary for proper removal of a section of a noncoding nucleotide (intron). Excision often takes place within the next exon at a splice site located in the next coding region. Several types of DNA sequences also are capable of propagating copies of themselves. These copies are then inserted into other locations on chromosomes. The insertion of these transpositions can cause frameshift mutations. Chromosomal translocation occurs when broken ends of DNA from two different chromosomes are joined incorrectly, resulting in pieces of each chromosome being exchanged. This process disrupts the genes near the breakpoint on each chromosome with the potential for loss of gene regulation.

The final type of mutation that will be discussed affects tandem repeated DNA sequences that occur within or near certain disease genes. A normal individual will have a relatively small number of repeat segments that lie next to each other. For reasons not yet understood, the number of repeats can dramatically increase during meiosis or possibly during early fetal development, so that a newborn may have hundreds or even thousands of repeats. When this occurs in certain regions of the genome, it causes genetic disease.

In summary, mutations are the source of genetic variation. Some mutations result in genetic disease, while others have no physical effect. The principal types of mutations include missense, nonsense, frameshift, promoter, and splice site mutations.

Evidence also exists to show that random insertion of repeat sections of DNA causes mutations, and several genetic diseases are known to be caused by expanded repeats.

Carcinogenesis

Cancer is a multistep process involving loss of control by the malignant cell, failure of DNA repair, and loss of back-up systems for preventing abnormal cell growth. A number of etiologic factors that cause cancer have been identified. These include genetic and environmental components. Carcinogenesis occurs at the molecular level. This process involves a point mutation in DNA, gene deletion, or chromosomal translocation resulting in gene rearrangement, failure of DNA repair, activation of oncogenes, and loss of tumor suppresser function.

Mechanisms for Development of a Malignancy

Carcinogenic radiation, chemical exposure, and a number of other factors may cause a malignant transformation; however, cancer growth may not occur until many generations of descendants of the affected cell have passed. The time from the first insult to cancer expression is termed latency. Cancers seem to result from a progressive series of events that incrementally increase the extent of deregulation within a cell lineage. This process also interferes with apoptosis, the programmed death of abnormal or damaged cells, and a cell eventually emerges whose descendants multiply without restraints.

The multi-hit concept of carcinogenesis explains the requirement for more than one mutation to occur before a cancer will manifest. Initiation is the first step in this process, when the cell is transformed so that it or its progeny is capable of behaving as cancer. The second event, causing initiated cells to begin the unregulated proliferation leading to tumor formation, is called promotion. In most cases, multiple mutations occurring over decades drive the neoplastic process. The timing of tumor genesis stimulated Knudson (1971) to propose his now well- accepted model for neoplastic development. This model invokes two important principles. First, in childhood tumors of the eye and kidney, only two mutations are rate-limiting for cancer formation. Second, either the two mutations can develop somatically, or one can be inherited and the other acquired somatically. In the latter case, every eye and kidney cell of the individual has a "head start" on the neoplastic process, and such individuals have a high risk of developing these specific cancers. Thus, the number of hits required is likely to vary in different cell types for all types of tumor development.

The pattern of growth and the nature of cell function are genetically regulated. A significant aspect of carcinogenesis is the alteration of specific genes regulating growth and function. Proto-oncogenes are genes whose protein product is involved in the regulation of cell growth. Oncogenes are growth-control genes present in the human genome and virtually all multicellular organisms. They are necessary for normal cell growth. However, incorrect expression of an oncogene or proto-oncogene can result in unregulated cell growth, as seen in a malignant cell. The first oncogenes to be identified came from a study of retroviruses that cause cancer in animal systems. Retroviruses were identified that invaded new cells, transformed oncogenes into the genome of the ncw host, and transformed healthy cells into tumor-producing cells. Most oncogenes, however, originate from proto-oncogenes, and when a mutation occurs in a proto-oncogene, it can become an oncogene. When an oncogene causes a cell to proceed from regulated to unregulated growth, the cell is said to have transformed. Some oncogenes have been identified in which specific rearrangements of chromosomal material were found to be associated with certain cancers. The translocation of material in these cases is thought to have disrupted specific genes that are vital to growth control in those cell types (see Table 4-1 and Figures 4-9 and 4-10).

Table 4-1. Selected Human Oncogenes and the Associated Neoplasms

Oncogene	Chromosome	Neoplasms
ABL1	9	Chronic myelogenous leukemia
GLI1	12	Glioblastoma
LYL1	19	Acute T-cell leukemia
MYC	8	Burkitt's lymphoma
RET	10	Medullary thyroid cancer Pheochromocytoma

Note. Based on information from National Center for Biotechnology Information, 1999.

Tumor suppressor genes regulate or stop the growth of damaged cells. If a suppressor gene is defective, a cell is allowed to proliferate wildly. The mechanisms by which these genes halt the development of malignancy are not fully known. Mutant tumor suppressor alleles seem to have a primarily recessive phenotype at the cellular level.

Knudson (1971) hypothesized that a set of recessively acting genes might play a role in carcinogenesis. He suggested that these genes normally would inhibit cell proliferation, that a single intact allele would be sufficient for this function, and that homozygous inactivation would be required to release cells from their growth-suppressive effects. This hypothesis helped to conceptualize the familial predisposition to cancer. In cancer, germ-line inactivation of one allele could be inherited, leaving every cell in the body with one wild-type or nonmutated and one mutated copy of the gene. Somatic events, such as mutations occurring in a nongerm cell, would be required to inactivate the wild-type allele, leaving the cell with no normal copies of the gene (see Table 4-2).

Errors in DNA replication normally are repaired immediately after mitosis. Certain genes are involved in mismatch repair (MMR) (Boland, 1996). DNA MMR proteins repair base pair mismatches that develop during new DNA synthesis. This repair is achieved in humans by a complex of proteins; a loss of any of these proteins results in a total loss of the MMR mechanism, allowing the process of carcinogenesis to occur (see Table 4-3).

Mutations may occur in any of the steps involved in cell growth and differentiation. When such mutations accumulate within a cell lineage, the progressive deregulation of growth eventually produces a cell whose progeny form a tumor.

Table 4-2. Selected Human Tumor Suppressor Genes and Associated Neoplasms

Gene	Chromosome	Neoplasm
APC	5	Familial adenomatous polyposis
BRCA1	17	Breast cancer, ovarian cancer
BRCA2	13	Breast cancer, ovarian cancer
NF1	17	Neurofibromatosis type 1
VHL	3	von Hippel-Lindau syndrome
P53	17	Li-Fraumeni syndrome

Note. Based on information from National Center for Biotechnology Information, 1999.

Table 4-3. Selected DNA Repair Genes and Associated Neoplasms

Gene	Chromosome	Neoplasm
MLH2, MLH1	2, 3	Hereditary nonpolyposis colon
ATM	11	Gliomas, breast
BLM	15	Bloom's syndrome; leukemia, gastrointestinal
FACA	16	Fanconi's anemia; leukemia

Note. Based on information from National Center for Biotechnology Information, 1999.

Cancers form when the growth and differentiation of cells are deregulated. During the past two decades, researchers have identified cancer-causing genes that encode substances that normally regulate the cellular processes of growth and differentiation. Cancer-susceptibility genes for colon cancer, breast cancer, retinoblastoma, Li-Fraumeni syndrome, von Hippel-Lindau syndrome, multiple endocrine neoplasia syndrome, and neurofibromatosis have been cloned and can be used for direct screening of cancer susceptibility. The availability of these genetic tests raises challenging ethical, legal, and social questions that must be investigated if clinicians are to keep pace with scientific advances in molecular genetics.

Genetics Applied to Cancer Care

Some disorders are caused by chromosomal aberrations, while others are caused by mutations at the molecular level. All cancers develop as a consequence of a series of genetic changes in a single cell that causes that cell to reproduce indiscriminately. Whereas some mutations are acquired over a lifetime, others may be inherited.

When human hereditary factors were implicated in the development of diseases once thought to be acquired, the understanding of the detection and management of these diseases was transformed. Breast cancer, colon cancer, medullary thyroid carcinoma, pheochromocytoma, ovarian cancer, and other cancers have been linked to inherited genetic alterations. Moreover, more than 20 cancer syndromes are known to exist, and nearly every organ system in the body can manifest a neoplasm associated with a genetic alteration (Offit, 1998). Using data from NCI's Surveillance, Epidemiology, and End Results (SEER) Program, the American Cancer Society anticipates the diagnosis of 1,220,100 new cases of invasive cancer in 2000 (Greenlee, Murray, Bolden, & Wingo, 2000). Between 5% and 10% of this number are believed to be linked to inherited genetic alterations, which calculates to the potential for 6,100–12,200 new cases in one year that can be traced to inherited susceptibilities.

Presently, no therapeutic interventions can correct the defects that predispose one to the development of acquired or inherited cancers. The heritability of genetic mutations constitutes a risk factor that may be identified early in life, presymptomatically, and before the development of disease. When individuals are aware of their genetic risk, they may work with health professionals to define and implement cancer-specific or cancer syndrome–specific risk-reduction strategies. Although individuals who carry inherited susceptibility have a higher-than-average lifetime risk of developing cancer, early diagnosis leads to early treatment.

Genetic technology in humans has resulted in two major practical applications with respect to clinical genetics. They are molecular genetic testing and gene therapy.

Molecular Genetic Testing

Molecular genetic testing (MGT) for human inheritable disease is used in the diagnosis of symptomatic individuals, carrier screening, prenatal and newborn screening, in tests for factors that may be associated with adult onset of disease, and to predict susceptibility to chronic disease. Several hundred tests are currently offered by clinical laboratories (Children's Health Care System, Seattle, 1999; NIH, 1999), and more will be developed over the next decade. As new genes are identified, the clinical significance of MGT will increase. The number of applications in testing is expected to rise and continue to be developed and improved. Tests that currently are in use soon will be obsolete. MGT has been under comprehensive evaluation by the Public Health Practice Program of the CDC (Williams et al., 1999). Although genetic tests can be used in several ways, at this time the most clinically useful way is as a diagnostic tool or to confirm a diagnosis in a symptomatic individual. Genetic tests in the future will provide limited predictive information about the course of a disease, severity, or expected age of onset. There is evidence that some genetic features of breast tumors indicate a higher likelihood that the cancer will metastasize early in the course of the disease (Marx, 1989). Therefore, the clinical application and usefulness of genetic testing is apparent and emerging.

General recommendations for quality assurance of MGT have been prepared using input from clinicians, researchers, and laboratory scientists (Williams et al., 1999). The accuracy and reliability of MGT must be assured to realize its clinical potential. Validity and reliability are affected by the variety of applications, regional differences in tests offered and population tested, low-volume testing, and the lack of industry standards. The availability of commercial test kits has made quality assurance a priority goal. Accuracy of tests depends on types, volume and variety of samples received by the laboratory, laboratory experience, test volume, procedure/method used, technician training, and the level of sensitivity required.

In addition, MGT should be evaluated for its effectiveness and usefulness. A test that is analytically valid measures the property or characteristic it is intended to measure. It must produce the same results repeatedly and in different laboratories. A test that is clinically valid accurately predicts a clinical condition by successfully detecting the predisposition. Many genetic tests are under investigation and only should be administered to subjects with known disease to establish clinical validity. Both analytic and clinical validity should be established before a genetic test is used for presymptomatic or predictive purposes (NIH, 1999).

MGT involves the analysis of chromosomes, genes, and gene products (proteins and enzymes) to determine if a genetic alteration is related to a specific disease in a patient. For patients with cancer, genetic tests may be performed for several reasons:

- To determine if an individual is a carrier of a copy of a mutated gene for a cancer that is known to be transmitted in a recessive or dominant pattern (germline mutation). The purpose is to assess the person's risk of passing the mutation to an offspring. This is called carrier testing.
- To determine if an individual with a family history of a kind of cancer, but without current symptoms, is a carrier of a copy of a germline mutation that predisposes that individual to the development of cancer. This is called presymptomatic testing.
- To determine the probability that a healthy individual with or without a family history of a certain cancer might develop the disease. This is called predictive testing (American College of Medical Genetics, 1996).

Detecting a genetic mutation helps to confirm a medical diagnosis and guide management options. Confirmation of an inherited genetic alteration may be used to help individuals and family members understand their altered risk for developing cancer and enable them to make informed decisions with regard to prevention strategies, risk management, treatment options, and future family planning. Even in the absence of specific preventative or treatment options, individuals may find that knowing one's genetic risk may help them to be prepared emotionally for treatment choices and for planning future healthcare needs (Holtzman & Watson, 1997).

Susceptibility testing or screening is intended to identify individuals who are at risk for future illness. Testing is conducted on those who are at higher-than-average risk of being carriers of a genetic alteration that has been associated with the cancer in question. Identification of a genetic mutation may enable implementation of specific preventative or risk management strategies. However, identification of a genetic mutation does not necessarily mean that disease will develop. In other cases, there may not be known treatment or prevention options. Screening is performed on a wider cohort of the public, including those who may be at low risk. Because genetic testing is a highly specific process, relatively expensive, and aims to identify minute alterations, screening for cancer predisposition using genetic technology is not yet widely available as a diagnostic tool.

Testing Methods

MGT can be conducted in three ways: direct analysis, linkage analysis, and functional analysis. Direct analysis involves sequencing of the base pairs of a patient's DNA sample to identify mutations that are known to be associated with a disease. In linkage analysis, a known region of DNA located close (linked) to a target gene is used as a marker. The marker is followed, and predictions are made about the state of the target gene. Linkage analysis depends on the tendency of sections of DNA to remain connected to each other during gamete formation (Zallen, 1997). Functional gene tests, or functional analysis, detect protein rather than DNA to demonstrate that an altered gene is responsible for coding for an abnormal protein product.

Applications Most Commonly Used

Four technologies currently are used in MGT: nucleic acid amplification, DNA sequencing, Southern Blot analysis (SBA), and fluorescence in situ hybridization (FISH). Sometimes, two different MGTs are used to corroborate findings. All techniques rely on the ability of single-stranded DNA to reanneal, or recombine, with a complementary strand to reform a double helix.

Nucleic acid amplification (NAA) creates a large quantity of target probe or signal of a sample to analyze. Polymerase chain reaction (PCR) often is used to amplify the sample, which can be obtained from whole blood, frozen cell pellets, or tissues. NAA can be used for DNA or RNA (American College of Medical Genetics, 1996).

DNA sequencing determines the exact order of bases along a single strand of DNA. The sequence of a human gene is compared to the sequence in the sample gene to detect for a known mutation. To find a target gene mutation in a sample of DNA, a length of single-stranded DNA that matches the target section is labeled with a radioactive isotope. This treated section of nucleotide bases is called a probe because it seeks and binds to the gene. Radioactive signals are then recorded by x-ray, showing where the probe and gene match (American College of Medical Genetics, 1996).

The SBA technique begins with the extraction of DNA from a patient's cells. DNA fragments of varying length are then separated according to size by electrophoresis. Small fragments move quickly through a gel substrate, whereas large fragments move more slowly. The fragments are then blotted onto filter paper and overlaid with a labeling probe. The probe aligns with complementary sequencing DNA. The technique is used to detect unique DNA sequences in a large background of unrelated sequences. Critical steps in all techniques include sample collection, DNA extraction without contamination, use of controls, and interpretation of results (American College of Medical Genetics, 1996).

FISH locates a target gene with a probe that is treated with a fluorescent chemical. It aids in the visualization, under a microscope, of the chromosomal abnormalities and gene sequences associated with particular regions of a chromosome (American College of Medical Genetics, 1996).

Gene Therapy

Gene therapy involves identifying specific genes, removing them, or adding them into chromosomes. Gene therapy is the technology that aims to alter the genes that are responsible for certain disorders—the insertion or removal of target genes for therapeutic purposes. The basic approach is to insert a functional gene into an individual's DNA to replace the gene that is nonfunctional. The altered cellular DNA will then produce the proper protein in the proper quantities. Even a low level of a normal protein may be able to produce therapeutic effects (Mulligan, 1993). Several diseases are under investigation for potential treatment through gene therapy. These include AIDS, lung cancer, cystic fibrosis, glioblastoma, and kidney cancer. The *Journal of Human Gene Therapy* publishes updated lists of approved studies biannually.

Gene therapy also may be used to augment the antitumor potential and activity of white blood cells. White blood cells have been isolated from a patient's tumor, altered with the addition of a gene that produces tumor necrosis factor (TNF), and reinfused into the subject to secrete TNF and destroy tumors (Rosenberg, 1992; Wivel & Wilson, 1998). These methods of somatic cell gene therapy promise to be effective cancer treatments.

In October 1999, a patient who was a subject in a gene therapy clinical trial died unexpectedly. This event raised concerns about the safety of gene therapy using genetically modified adenoviruses as vectors to carry the therapeutic genetic material into the target cell. Research using gene therapy presently is under intensive oversight by the Recombinant DNA Advisory Committee of the NIH (Stolberg, 1999). The scrutiny will include an exhaustive review of past research for similar or related problems associated with using viral vectors, such as unexpected or severe side effects. The review also will evaluate ongoing research for conditions that compromise patient safety to ensure that there is adequate control of risks and that the process of informed consent is stringently followed. Careful record keeping and skillful observation are important responsibilities of research nurses caring for patients receiving gene therapy. In the future, genetic therapy may be utilized as a preventative or a therapeutic intervention along with other risk-management strategies, such as prophylactic surgery, surveillance, and chemoprevention.

Implications for Nursing and Health Care

Basic scientific discoveries about genetic contributions to the development of disease and the understanding of changes that occur within the genetic structure of cells as disease occurs provide a foundation for opportunity within health care. The enhanced understanding of molecular changes that predict, promote, or result in cancer opens a window of opportunity for nurses who dedicate their practice to finding better ways to provide cancer care. The application of cancer genetics technology in the clinical setting is in its infancy, but nurses recognize that the technology offers challenge and possibility. The challenge is to understand the structural, functional, and applied science of genetics. The possibility is the design of models of care that integrate genetic knowledge, improve current patient care, and ameliorate the health and well-being of future generations.

New Directions for Nursing

Few nurses currently recognize the potential value of genetics tools to transform available health care. Therefore, responsibility is placed on nursing leaders and professional organizations to envision and prepare for the future. Professional nursing societies, such as ANA, the International Society of Nurses in Genetics (ISONG), and specialty organizations, such as ONS, have accepted this responsibility by supporting educational and research initiatives.

NIH funded a research study, implemented by the ANA Center for Ethics and Human Rights, that assessed ways in which nurses in the United States were managing genetic information (Scanlon & Fibison, 1995). The survey of 1,000 nurses examined attitudes and experiences with genetic testing, counseling, and referral. This study also evaluated the current legal, ethical, and social concerns of nurses regarding the collection and use of genetic information. Survey outcomes revealed knowledge gaps within the profession. It showed that nurses are sensitive to the ethical, legal, and social issues that may arise from the clinical issues of genetic technology. Results showed that most nurses (68%) did not feel knowledgeable in genetics, even though the majority had seen clients who requested genetic information. Overall, the survey provided evidence of interest in and need for genetics education for all nurses. Educators can use results from these surveys to craft student centered educational programs.

Educational needs for all healthcare professionals, including nurses, are being addressed through a coalition of which the ANA Center is a leading member. ANA, along with the American Medical Association and NHGRI, created the National Coalition for Health Professional Education in Genetics (NCHPEG) (Collins, 1997). This coalition is comprised of representatives from more than 150 diverse healthcare professional organizations, consumer groups, government agencies, private industry, and professional societies. It aims to provide an organized, systematic, and national approach to genetics education.

ISONG is a member of NCHPEG and is recognized as the specialty group of nurses involved with human genetics. Educational outreach efforts have been led by members of ISONG since 1987. ISONG members believe that genetics is integral to all nursing practice. Members of ISONG and ANA cooperated to develop the Statement on the Scope and Standards of Genetics Clinical Nursing Practice (International Society of Nurses in Genetics & American Nurses Association, 1998). This statement offers guidance for organizations that are evaluating how genetics can be integrated into specialized practice and continuing educational programs. ONS was one of the first specialty groups to recognize the implications of genetics for individuals and families cared for by nurses.

ONS has responded in several ways to begin to prepare the membership for the future needs of consumers of cancer care. A Genetics Project Team was established in 1995 to formulate a plan to address clinical, educational, and research needs. In 1996, an invitational conference was held to establish the scope and responsibilities of nurses regarding genetics knowledge and practice. Position statements were developed to clarify the role and responsibilities of nurses regarding cancer genetic testing, risk assessment, and cancer genetic counseling (ONS, 1997a, 1997b). The Cancer Genetics Special Interest Group was established within ONS; the group offers education and networking opportunities. ONS and ISONG collaborated and jointly sponsored a survey that assessed member concerns and experiences with ethical issues related to genetics technology (Cassels, Gaul, Lea, Calzone, & Jenkins, 1999; Gaul, Cassels, Lea, Calzone, & Jenkins, 1999). Additionally, ONS partially funded a survey to measure ONS members' genetics knowledge and needs (Rieger & Peterson, 1999). Survey results highlighted the need for accurate and comprehensive educational programs that are timely and easily accessed. One method offered by ONS to begin the preparation of oncology nurses is a video titled *Basic Genetics for the Oncology Nurse* (ONS, 1999). Other methods should be explored and developed. Nurses, in general, will need ongoing help to integrate genetics into clinical practice and to sufficiently expand their roles to keep pace with expanding knowledge.

Demands of the Future
Practice

Although discoveries in genetics eventually will have an impact on all healthcare practice, nurses already are beginning to experience the effects of this new knowledge. Increasingly, individuals and families are turning to oncologists and nurses to answer questions about hereditary cancer risk factors. They also may be asking questions about information they have heard on the news concerning risks and benefits of genetic testing. Or, they may be seeking details about screening, surveillance, or prevention practices that should be considered based on their individual cancer risk profile. General information is becoming readily available to the public. This is placing the demand on nurses to determine how to expand current practice skills to keep up with the constant influx of information from various media. In addition, genetic information is most useful in individualized care when nurses have comprehensive understanding and can accurately interpret the data.

ISONG and ANA (1998) have described guidelines that clarify expectations of basic and advanced nurses in the provision of care. The organizations agree that "all licensed registered nurses, regardless of their practice setting, have a role in the delivery of genetics services and the management of genetic information" (p. 2). However, role ambiguity may be present, and guidelines are needed to further distinguish and define the roles and responsibilities of basic and advanced nurses. The challenge for nurses is to become informed about the clinical, physical, and emotional effects of genetics technology. Nurses must be prepared to integrate genetics into the assessment, plan of care, education, and evaluation of all clients. Models of practice that offer this type of visionary nursing role must consider economic demand, patient and family outcomes, and role delineation to ensure competency in future cancer care.

Education

As nurses aim to integrate genetics with clinical services, they must overcome a significant barrier created by insufficient educational preparation. Several sources document the inadequacy of both higher and continuing-education programs to provide suitable learning experiences for basic students and practicing nurses (Anderson, 1996; Hetteberg, Prows, Deets, Monsen, & Kenner, 1999; Monsen & Anderson, 1999). Most conspicuous is the lack of training programs that provide didactic along with practice components in clinical genetics. Few programs are available, and these include limited content on communication methods for complex information, such as absolute and relative risks (Lipkus & Hollands, 1999); cancer preventive options versus intervention (Lippman, Lee, & Sabichi, 1998); and pharmacogenetics or tailored therapy (Prows & Prows, 1998). This content, in addition to concepts of basic human and population genetics, are essential for clinical competency (Jenkins, 1999).

Academic nursing programs also must integrate other aspects of genetics into the curricula. The ethical, legal, and social implications of new and emerging genetic technology are fundamental to practitioners in a socially responsive profession. Nurses will be called upon to design and implement interventions to modify risk factors and promote healthy lifestyles. With adequate educational preparation and through discussion and analysis of complex issues, nurses can influence public policy. Informed nurses can channel the force and direction of health promotion in healthcare culture and in society.

Currently, healthcare practices focus mainly on treatment and tertiary prevention. Through increased understanding of the interactive effects of environment, lifestyle, and genetics on the manifestation of disease, nurses may shift their focus to primary and secondary prevention strategies. The public may be encouraged to view cancer in a different way and be persuaded to choose behaviors that maintain health and prevent disease.

Research

Much remains to be learned about the human genome and effects of advances in genetic technology on the experiences of individuals and families (Sigmon, Grady, & Amende, 1997). Opportunities abound for nurse researchers to study the physical, emotional, and social consequences of learning about the contributions of genetics to the development of cancer. Furthermore, genetic factors may increase cancer susceptibility, affect prognosis, and influence treatment choices. Little is known of the relative importance of genetic information to patients and their families. Even less is known about how patients and families make decisions after receiving genetic information. Lifestyle and behavior decisions will be affected in part by an individual's perception of their risk (Rimer & Glassman, 1999; Vernon, 1999).

As more is learned about specific factors that predict those at increased risk for cancer, more nurses will be involved in communicating health risks to their patients. Several questions require answers before nurses can perform this service in an ethical and responsible way. Nurses are beginning to investigate how people perceive cancer risk information and how to enhance patients' understanding. For example, one study of patient participation in prostate cancer screening identified predictors as perceived benefits, being White, being married, and having at least a high-school education (Tingen, Weinrich, Heydt, Boyd, & Weinrich, 1998). The patient's perception of the relative impact of genetic predisposition on the development of disease is, as yet, unknown. A patient's choice to undergo molecular genetic testing and to participate in cancer screening that may lead to earlier detection of cancer may be influenced by recommendations from healthcare professionals (Daly, 1999; McCaul & Tulloch, 1999). Thus, nurses must expand their knowledge base on methods to help people to understand the relationship between genetic risk and risk-reduction options.

Factors that influence informed decision making for changes in behavior are the focus of priority research. Nurses need to know what interventions facilitate informed decision making (Bekker et al., 1999). For example, despite common knowledge about the cause and effect of the relationship between tobacco and the development of cancers, the current rate of smoking has increased among certain subsamples of the population. Research is needed on the process and content of patients' perceptions and on how they may best use the information that will be available as a result of genetic technology. Through scientific inquiry, nurses can objectively evaluate the impact of technology on healthcare services and contribute to quality genetics cancer care.

Policy

Recent policy debates have considered plans of action regarding issues related to genetics. The policy statements, when adopted by the various healthcare and governmental organizations, have the potential to influence and determine future decisions or actions on matters related to the use of genetics technology. Decisions about the role nurses will have in genetic counseling, testing, and follow-up care will be affected by guidelines and standards set by nursing, other professions, and governmental bodies. Recognition and acceptance of the professional nurse as a provider of genetic services will, in turn, facilitate policy-driven regulations that mandate training programs and provide sufficient resources to meet future demands.

Recent research supports the assertion that both genetic counselors and nurses can effectively provide pretest education to women contemplating genetic testing (Bernhardt, Geller, Doksum, & Metz, 2000). The counselor must include sufficient information for the individual to make an informed decision (Rieger & Pentz, 1999). The process of informed consent is complex and heavily dependent on the counselor's depth and breadth of knowledge, as well as his or her sensitivity to interpersonal dynamics. Nurses are well trained in interpersonal dynamics, which equips them for counseling services. A nurse counselor's ability to ascertain the patient's reality contributes to the integrity of the process (Giarelli, 1999).

In addition, genetic counselors should have up-to-date knowledge of actuarial trends and indemnification rules within the insurance industry. Currently, genetic predisposition to disease may be considered an uninsurable liability. Therefore, the possibility of lost coverage or increased insurance premiums for individuals with a known genetic disorder are considered to be potential risks of knowing (Johnson, Wilkinson, & Taylor-Brown, 1999). Proactive nurses may influence policy decisions in this arena (Wilfond, Rothenberg, Thomson, & Lerman, 1997).

Healthcare Culture and Genetics

Genetic discrimination is a concern voiced by potential consumers of genetic technology. Fear that what is learned about their genetic status will be used against them has historical overtones as well as concerns about abuse in the future. Accounts of past stigmatization of individuals or communities with disabilities has intensified concerns about how genetic information will be interpreted and used. This has caused clinicians to move cautiously in the use of genetic predisposition testing. During the process of informed consent applicants are advised that genetic information is personal but there is a chance that it may become known to third parties, such as insurers and employers. One may speculate that as consumers learn about the potential benefits to be gained from the use of genetic technology they may request genetic testing of predisposition to disease. Thus, consumers' wants may drive industry to increase the availability and use of genetic technology. It is unclear how consumer-driven accessibility of genetics healthcare services will affect dissemination of information (Jacobs, 1998).

Consumer access to genetics services may well be determined by healthcare providers who base referrals on empiric models and test availability. However, genetic tests are available for conditions that have no current treatment options, such as Huntington's disease. Perhaps interventions are not modifiable, regardless of genetic status (Holtzman & Watson, 1997). Before evidenced-based use of a new genetic test enters clinical practice, it may be evaluated by a panel of experts or a consortium of experts and consumers. Nurses have a unique perspective to offer to this process and can make significant, meaningful contributions as members of a decision-making body that determines the availability, safety, and effectiveness of new genetic tests (ISONG, 2000).

In addition to availability, cost is another factor that will influence utilization of genetics technology in the clinical setting. The public may wish to know their risk for disease to guide health-promoting behavior and family planning. Costs of genetics services may be determined by test methods, types of facilities providing services, insurance regulations, and whether genetic tests are considered to be an integral part of public health care (Kutner, 1999). However, if cost is prohibitive, certain individuals will not be able to purchase the services. The exclusion of potential consumers on the basis of ability to pay, although a common social phenomenon, is a form of discrimination in healthcare culture. The extraordinary public potential of genetic information to contribute to the prediction and prevention of disease may be the justification to exclude it as a simple healthcare commodity to be allocated based on ability to pay.

Commercialization of human genetics by companies that are patenting genetic materials may lead to increased availability of affordable products from genetic research (Reynolds, 2000). If genetic testing becomes consumer-driven, the public's understanding of genetics science may have a profound effect on the utilization of services. Current recommendations for models of care include patient education and counseling as necessary components of predictive screening services (Cunningham, 1997). However, if the general public is afraid of potential financial and emotional costs without seeing the value of the genetic test, consumers may not fully benefit from the advances in genetic technology. The potential for improved screening, surveillance, and risk management interventions may be realized if consumers clearly see the value of genetic services along with realistically portrayed limitations. Public education about genetics may become the most important determinant of the use of services for the prevention, early detection, and control of cancer (see Figure 4-11).

Figure 4-11. Selected Internet Sources on Human Genetics and Related Issues

Healthcare Provider Sites
Blazing a genetic trail: www.hhmi.org/Genetictrail/
Helix: http://healthlinks.washington.edu/helix/
List of biochemical genetics tests by disease: http://biochemgen.ucsd.edu/wbgtests/dx-tst.htm
Online Mendelian inheritance in man: www3.ncbi.nlm.nih.gov/omim/searchomim.html
A gene map of the human genome: www.ncbi.nlm.nih.gov/science96
Cancer genome anatomy project: www.ncbi.nlm.nih.gov/ncicgap
GeneCards: http://bioinformatics.weizmann.ac.il/cards
Genomic medicine: www.ama-assn.org/sci-pubs/journals/archive/jama/vol_278/no_15/jjn71002.htm
Medsite navigator: www.MedsiteNavigator.com

Sites for Patients and the General Public
Alliance of Genetic Support Groups: http://medhlp.netusa.net/www/agsg.htm
Genetic conditions and rare conditions information: www.kumc.edu/gen/support/groups.html
March of Dimes genetics site: www.modimes.org/pub/genetics.html
Genetics Information—National Cancer Institute: http://cancernet.nci.nih.gov/p_genetics.html
Genomics: A global resource: www.phrma.org/genomics
Understanding gene testing: www.gene.com/ae/AE/AEPC/NIH/index.html
U.S. Department of Energy—Human genome information: www.ornl.gov/TechResources/Human_Genome/publicat/publications.html

Conclusion

In conclusion, modern medical genetics represents a cumulative history of multidisciplinary contributions. Similarly, clinical genetics has been formed by interdisciplinary contributions from the healthcare and scientific communities. Advances in genetic technology undoubtedly will continue to have an impact on a wide spectrum of healthcare policy, services, and professional education. The greatest promise is in its potential as a diagnostic tool for clinical use by healthcare professionals to prevent, screen for, and detect cancer before it has a devastating effect on an individual's quality of life. Cancer is a genetic disease. From a nursing perspective, the principles of molecular, population, and clinical genetics are part of the repertoire of comprehensive cancer care. Nursing's roles in cancer genetics care are just beginning to take shape.

References

American College of Medical Genetics. (1996). *Standards and guidelines: Clinical genetic laboratories.* Bethesda, MD: Author.

Anderson, G. (1996). The evolution and status of genetics education in nursing in the United States 1983–1995. *Image, 28*(2), 101–106.

Antonarakis, S.E. (1997). Mutation in human disease: Nature and consequences. In D. Rimoin, J. Connor, and R. Pyeritz (Eds.), *Emery and Rimoin's principles and practice of medical genetics* (Vol. I, 3rd ed.) (pp. 53–66). New York: Churchill Livingstone.

Armstrong, B.K., & Kricker, A. (1993). How much melanoma is caused by sun exposure? *Melanoma Research, 3,* 395–401.

Avery, O.T., MacLeod, C.M., & McCarty, M. (1944). Studies on the chemical nature of the substance inducing transformation of pneumococcal types. *Journal of Experimental Medicine, 79,* 137–158.

Baker, J.R. (1955). The cell theory: A restatement, history and critique. Part V. The multiplication of nuclei. *Quarterly Journal of Microscopial Science, 96,* 449–481.

Barrett, J.C., & Huff, J.E. (1991). Cellular and molecular mechanisms of chemically induced renal carcinogenesis. In P.H. Bach, N.J. Gregg, M.F. Wilks, & L. Delacruz (Eds.), *Nephrotoxicity* (pp. 287–306). New York: Marcel Dekker, Inc.

Bekker, H., Thornton, J., Airey, C., Connelly, J., Hewison, J., Robinson, M., Lilleyman, J., MacIntosh, M., Maule, A., Michie, S., & Pearman, A. (1999). Informed decision making: An annotated bibliography and systematic review. *Health Technology Assessment, 3*(1), 1–56.

Bernhardt, B., Geller, G., Doksum, T., & Metz, S. (2000). Evaluation of nurses and genetic counselors as providers of education about breast cancer susceptibility testing. *Oncology Nursing Forum, 27,* 33–39.

Boice, J.D, Harvey, E.B, Blettner, M., Stovall, M., & Flannery, J.T. (1992). Cancer in the contralateral breast after radiotherapy for breast cancer. *New England Journal of Medicine, 326,* 781–785.

Boland, C.R. (1996). Roles of the DNA mismatch repair genes in colorectal tumorogenesis. *International Journal of Cancer, 69*(1), 47–49.

Cassels, J., Gaul, A., Lea, D., Calzone, K., & Jenkins, J. (1999). An ethical assessment framework: Oncology nurses evaluate usefulness for clinical practice. *Cancer Genetics Special Interest Group Newsletter, 3*(2), 4–5, 8.

Centers for Disease Control and Prevention. (1999). *Office of Genetics and Disease Prevention 1999 highlights.* Retrieved January 10, 1999 from World Wide Web: http://www.cdc.gov/genetics/publications/hightlights.htm

Chargaff, E. (1950). Chemical specificity of nucleic acids and mechanisms of their enzymatic degradation. *Experientia, 6,* 201–209.

Children's Health Care System, Seattle. (1999). *GeneTests: Genetic testing resource.* Retrieved January 25, 2000 from the World Wide Web: http://www.genetests.org

Cohen, L.A. (1987). Diet and cancer. *Scientific American, 257,* 42–48.

Colditz, G.A., Hankinson, S.E, Hunter, D.J., Willett, W.C., Manson, J.E., Stampfer, M.J., Hennekens, C., Rosner, B., & Speizer, F.E. (1995). The use of estrogens and progestins and the risk of breast cancer in postmenopausal women. *New England Journal of Medicine, 332,* 1589–1593.

Collins, F. (1997). Preparing health professionals for the genetic revolution. *JAMA, 278,* 1285–1286.

Collins, F. (1999). *Keynote address: Overview of advances in human genetics.* Second National Conference of Genetics and Disease Prevention, December 6, 1999, Baltimore, MD.

Collins, F., & Galas, D. (1993). A new five-year plan for the U.S. Human Genome Project. *Science, 262,* 43–46.

Crick, F. (1988). *What mad pursuit: A personal view of scientific discovery.* New York: Basic Books.

Cunningham, G.C. (1997). A public health perspective on the control of predictive screening for breast cancer. *Health Matrix, 7*(1), 31–48.

Daly, M. (1999). NCCN practice guidelines: Genetics/familial high-risk cancer screening. *Oncology, 13*, 161–183.

Delbecco, R. (1986). A turning point in cancer research: Sequencing the human genome. *Science, 231*, 1055–1056.

DeVries, H. (1900/1966). The law of segregation of hybrids. In C. Stern & E.R. Sherwood (Eds.), *The origin of genetics: A Mendel source book* (pp. 107–117). San Francisco: W.H. Freeman.

Doll, R. (1993). Health and the environment in the 1990s. *American Journal of Public Health, 82*, 933–941.

Doll, R., & Peto, R. (1987). Epidemiology of cancer. In D.J. Weatherall, J.G.G. Ledingham, & D.A. Warrell (Eds.), *Oxford textbook of medicine* (Vol. 1., 2nd ed.) (pp. 4.95–4.123). New York: Oxford University Press.

East, E.M. (1910). The Mendelian interpretation of variation that is apparently continuous. *American Naturalist, 44*, 65–82.

Easton, D., Narod, S., Ford, D., & Steel, C. (1994). The genetic epidemiology of BRCA1. *Lancet, 344*, 761.

Flemming, W. (1879). Contributions to the knowledge of the cell and its life phenomena. *Archiv fur Mikroskopische Anatomie, 16*, 302–404.

Garrod, A. (1928). The lessons of rare diseases. *Lancet, 1*, 1055–1060.

Gaul, A., Cassels, J., Lea, D., Calzone, K., & Jenkins, J. (1999). Issues of ethical concern frequently encountered in oncology nursing: A survey funded by a grant from ONS. *Cancer Genetics Special Interest Group Newsletter, 3*(2), 2–3.

Giarelli, E. (1999 February). Prophylactic thyroidectomy for patients with MEN2A: When parents must decide. *New Jersey Medicine*, pp. 37–42.

Goldschmidt, R. (1951). The impact of genetics upon science. In C.L. Dunn (Ed.), *Genetics in the 20th century. Essays on the progress of genetics during its first 50 years* (pp. 1–23). New York: Macmillan.

Greenlee, R.T., Murray, T., Bolden, S., & Wingo, P.A. (2000). Cancer statistics, 2000. *CA: A Cancer Journal for Clinicians, 50*, 7–11.

Greenstein, J.P. (1943). Friedrich Miescher, 1844–1895. *Science Monthly, 57*, 34.

Hall, J.M, Lee, M.K., Newman, B., Morrow, J.E., Anderson, L.A., Huey, B., & King, M.C. (1990). Linkage of early onset breast cancer to chromosome 17q21. *Science, 250*, 1684–1689.

Hardy, G.H. (1908). Mendelian proportions in a mixed population. *Science, 28*, 49–50.

Hershey, A.D., & Chase, M. (1952). Independent functions of viral protein and nucleic acid in growth of bacteriophage. *Journal of General Physiology, 36*, 39–56.

Hetteberg, C., Prows, C., Deets, C., Monsen, R., & Kenner, C. (1999). National survey of genetics content in basic nursing preparatory programs in the United States. *Nursing Outlook, 47*, 168–180.

Holtzman, N., & Watson, M. (Eds.). (1997). *Promoting safe and effective genetic testing in the United States.* Washington, DC: Task Force on Genetic Testing.

International Society of Nurses in Genetics. (2000, January). *Comments on the secretary's Advisory Committee on Genetic Testing.* Presented at the public meeting, A Consultation on Genetic Testing, Baltimore, MD.

International Society of Nurses in Genetics & American Nurses Association. (1998). *Statement on the scope and standards of genetics clinical nursing practice.* Washington, DC: Author.

Jacobs, L. (1998). At-risk for cancer: Genetic discrimination in the workplace. *Oncology Nursing Forum, 25,* 475–480.

Jenkins, J. (1999). Diffusion of innovation: Genetics nursing education. (Doctoral dissertation, George Mason University, Virginia). *Dissertation Abstracts International-B, 60/06,* 9934809.

Jenkins, M. (1998). *Genetics.* London: Hodder & Stoughton.

Jablon, S., & Kato, H. (1970). Childhood cancer in relation to prenatal exposure to atomic-bomb radiation. *Lancet, 2,* 1000–1003.

Johnson, A., Wilkinson, D., & Taylor-Brown, S. (1999). Genetic testing: Policy implications for individuals and their families. *Families, Systems and Health, 17*(1), 49–61.

Jourand, M.C. (1991). Observations on the carcinogenicity of asbestos fibers. *Annals of the New York Academy of Sciences, 643,* 258–270.

Judson, H.F. (1992). A history of the science and technology behind gene mapping and sequencing. In D. Kevles & L. Hood (Eds.), *The code of codes: Scientific and social issues in the Human Genome Project* (pp. 37–80). Cambridge, MA: Harvard University Press.

Kevles, D. (1992). Out of Eugenics: The historical politics of the human genome. In D. Kevles & L. Hood (Eds.), *The code of codes: Scientific and social issues in the Human Genome Project* (pp. 18–19). Cambridge, MA: Harvard University Press.

Knudson, A.G. (1971). Mutation and cancer: Statistical study of retinoblastoma. *Proceedings of the National Academy of Sciences, 68,* 820–823.

Krontiris, T.G. (1995). Oncogenes. *New England Journal of Medicine, 333,* 303–306.

Kutner, S. (1999). Breast cancer genetics and managed care. *Cancer, 86,* 2570–2574.

Lagerkvist, U. (1998). *DNA pioneers and their legacy.* New Haven, CT: Yale University Press.

Leiber, C.S. (1993). Herman Award Lecture, 1993: A personal perspective on alcohol, nutrition and the liver. *American Journal of Clinical Nutrition, 58,* 430–442.

Levine, P., & Stetson, R. E. (1939). An unusual case of intragroup agglutination. *JAMA, 113,* 126–127.

Li, F.P., & Fraumeni, J.F (1969). Soft tissue sarcomas, breast cancer and other neoplasms: A familial syndrome. *Annals of Internal Medicine, 71,* 747–752.

Lipkus, I., & Hollands, J. (1999). The visual communication of risk. *Journal of the National Cancer Institute Monographs, 25,* 149–163.

Lippman, S., Lee, J., & Sabichi, A. (1998). Cancer chemoprevention: Progress and promise. *Journal of the National Cancer Institute, 90,* 1514–1528.

Lynch, J. (1997). The genetics and natural history of hereditary colon cancer. *Seminars in Oncology Nursing, 13,* 91–98.

Mange, E.J., & Mange, A.P. (1999). *Basic human genetics* (2nd ed.). Sunderland, MA: Sinauer Associates.

Marx, J.L. (1989). Gene signals relapse of breast, ovarian cancers. *Science, 244,* 654–655.

McCaul, K., & Tulloch, H. (1999). Cancer screening decisions. Cancer risk communication: What we need to learn. *Journal of the National Cancer Institute Monographs, 25,* 52–58.

McKusick, V.A. (1980). The anatomy of the human genome. *American Journal of Medicine, 69,* 267–276.

McKusick, V.A. (1997). History of medical genetics. In D.L. Rimoin, J.M. Connor, & R.E. Pyeritz (Eds.), *Emery and Rimoin's principles and practice of medical genetics* (3rd ed.) (pp. 1–30). New York: Churchill Livingstone.

McNeil, C. (1999). Using HER2 to choose chemotherapy in breast cancer: Is it ready for the clinic? *Journal of the National Cancer Institute, 91*, 110–112.

Mehlman, M.J., & Botkin, J.R. (1998). *Access to the genome: The challenge of equality.* Washington, DC: Georgetown University Press.

Mendel, G. (1865/1966). Experiments on plant hybrids. In C. Stern & E.R. Sherwood (Eds.), *The origin of genetics: A Mendel source book* (pp. 1–48). San Francisco: W.H. Freeman.

Monsen, R., & Anderson, G. (1999). Continuing education for nurses that incorporates genetics. *Journal of Continuing Education in Nursing, 30*(1), 20–24.

Morgan, T.H. (1911). Random segregation versus coupling in Mendelian inheritance. *Science, 34,* 384.

Morgan, T.H. (1926). *The theory of the gene.* New Haven: Yale University.

Morgan, T.H., Sturtevant, A.H., Muller, H.J., & Bridges, C.B. (1915). *The mechanism of Mendelian heredity.* New York: Henry Holt & Company.

Mueller, R.F., & Cook, J. (1997). Mendelian inheritance. In D. Rimoin, J.M. Connor, & R.E. Pyeritz (Eds.), *Emery and Rimoin's principles and practice of medical genetics* (3rd ed.) (pp. 87–102). New York: Churchill Livingstone.

Muller, H.J. (1951). The development of the gene theory. In L.C. Dunn (Ed.), *Genetics in the 20th century: Essays on the progress of genetics during its first 50 years* (pp. 77–100). New York: Macmillan.

Murray, A., & Kirschner, M.W. (1991). What controls the cell cycle? *Scientific American, 264,* 56–61.

National Cancer Institute. (1999, August 10). *NCI's Tumor Gene Index reaches its two-year mark.* Retrieved January 25, 2000 from the World Wide Web: http://rex.nci.nih.gov/massmedia/pressreleases/tumor.html

National Center for Biotechnology Information. (1999). *OMIM—Online Mendelian inheritance in man.* Retrieved January 25, 2001 from the World Wide Web: http://www3.ncbi.nlm.nih.gov/omim

National Center for Biotechnology Information. (2000). The *Cancer Genome Anatomy Project.* Retrieved January 25, 2001 from the World Wide Web: http://www.ncbi.nlm.nih.gov/cgap

National Center for Biotechnology Information (2001). The Cancer Chromosome Aberration Project (CCAP). Retrieved February 4, 2001 from the World Wide Web: http://www.ncbi.nlm.nih.gov/CCAP/

National Human Genome Research Institute. (1998). Linking nursing and genetics research—Individual post-doctoral and senior fellowships. *NIH Guide, 26*(6), pp. 1–6. Retrieved January 25, 2001 from the World Wide Web: http://www.nhgri.nih.gov/Grant_Info/funding/Training/linking.html

National Institutes of Health. (1999). *A public consultation on oversight of genetic tests, December 1, 1999–January 31, 2000. Secretary's Advisory Committee on Genetic Testing.* Retrieved December 1, 1999 from the World Wide Web: http://www.nih.gov/od/orda/sacgtdocs.htm

Offit, K. (1998). *Clinical cancer genetics: Risk counseling and management.* New York: Wiley-Liss.

Oncology Nursing Society. (1997a). *Position statement: Cancer genetic testing and risk assessment counseling.* Pittsburgh: Author.

Oncology Nursing Society. (1997b). *Position statement: The role of the oncology nurse in cancer genetic counseling.* Pittsburgh: Author.

Oncology Nursing Society. (1998). Position statement: The role of the oncology nurse in cancer genetic counseling. *Oncology Nursing Forum, 25,* 463.

Oncology Nursing Society. (1999). *Basic genetics for the oncology nurse* [Video no. 1]. Pittsburgh: Author.

Organisation for Economic Co-Operation and Development. (1995). *The global Human Genome Programme.* Paris: Author.

Peters, J. (1959) *Classical papers in genetics.* Englewood Cliffs, NJ: Prentice-Hall.

Portugal, F.H., & Cohen, J.S. (1977). *A century of DNA: A history of the discovery of the structure and function of the genetic substance.* Cambridge, MA: MIT Press.

President Clinton announces the completion of the first survey of the entire human genome. (2000, June 26). Retrieved August 25, 2000 from the World Wide Web: http://www.whitehouse.gov/WH/new/html/20000626.html

Prows, D., & Prows, C. (1998). Optimizing drug therapy based on genetic differences: Implications for the clinical setting. *AACN Clinical Issues, 9,* 499–512.

Reynolds, T. (2000). Pricing human genes: The patent rush pushes on. *Journal of the National Cancer Institute, 92,* 96–97.

Rieger, P., & Pentz, R. (1999). Genetic testing and informed consent. *Seminars in Oncology Nursing, 15,* 104–115.

Rieger, P., & Peterson, S. (1999). The on-genes study: Oncology nurses' knowledge of genetics and genetic testing. *Oncology Nursing Forum, 26,* 411.

Rimer, B., & Glassman, B. (1999). Is there a use for tailored print communication in cancer risk communication? *Journal of the National Cancer Institute Monographs, 25,* 140–148.

Rimoin, D.L., Connor, J.M., & Pyeritz, R.E. (1997). Nature and frequency of genetic disease. In D. Rimoin, J. Connor, & R. Pyeritz (Eds.), *Emery and Rimoin's principles and practice of medical genetics* (3rd ed.) (pp. 31–34). New York: Churchill Livingstone.

Rosenberg, S. (1992). Gene therapy for cancer. *JAMA, 268,* 2416–2419.

Scanlon, C., & Fibison, W. (1995). *Managing genetic information: Implications for nursing practice.* Washington, DC: American Nurses Association.

Shields, P.G., & Harris, C.C. (1993). Principles of carcinogenesis: Chemicals. In V.T. DeVita, Jr., S. Hellman, & S.A. Rosenberg (Eds.), *Cancer: Principles and practice of oncology* (4th ed.) (pp. 200–221). Philadelphia: J.B. Lippincott.

Shimizu, Y., Schull, W.J., & Kato, H. (1990). Cancer risk among atomic bomb survivors: The RERF Life Span Study. *JAMA, 264,* 601–604.

Sigmon, H., Grady, P., & Amende, L. (1997). The National Institutes of Nursing Research explores opportunities in genetics research. *Nursing Outlook, 45,* 215–219.

Sipple, J.H. (1961). The association of pheochromocytoma with carcinoma of the thyroid gland. *American Journal of Medicine, 31,* 163–166.

Spitz, M., Wei, Q., Li, G., & Wu, X. (1999). Genetic susceptibility to tobacco carcinogenesis. *Cancer Investigation, 17,* 645–659.

Stolberg, S. (1999, November 4) A death puts gene therapy under increasing scrutiny. *The New York Times,* p. A21.

Szabo, J., Heath, B., & Hill, V.M. (1995). The hereditary hyperparathyroidism jaw tumor syndrome: A new endocrine tumor gene maps to chromosome 1q21-q31. *American Journal of Human Genetics, 56,* 944–950.

Tingen, M.S., Weinrich, S.P., Heydt, D.D., Boyd, M.D., & Weinrich, M.C. (1998). Perceived benefits: A predictor of participation in prostate cancer screening. *Cancer Nursing, 21*, 349–357.

Tomatis, L., Agthe, C., Bartsch, H., Huff, J., Montesano, R., Saracci, R., Walker, E., & Wilbourn, J. (1978). Evaluation of the carcinogenicity of chemicals: A review of the monograph program of the International Agency for Research on Cancer. *Cancer Research, 38*, 877–885.

Trichopoulos, D., Li, F.P., & Hunter, D.J. (1996). What causes cancer? *Scientific American, 275*, 80–88.

Vernon, S. (1999). Risk perception and risk communication for cancer screening behaviors: A review of cancer risk communication: What we need to learn. *Journal of the National Cancer Institute Monographs, 25*, 101–119.

Vogelstein, B., & Kinzler, K. (1993). The multistep nature of cancer. *Trends in Genetics, 9*(4), 138–141.

Watson, J.D. (1968). *The double helix.* London: Weidenfeld & Nicolson.

Watson, J.D., & Crick, F.H.C. (1953). Molecular structure of nucleic acids. A structure for deoxyribose nucleic acid. *Nature, 171*, 737–738.

Weismann, A. (1893). *The germ-plasm: A theory of heredity.* London: Walter Scott.

Wermer, P. (1954). Genetic aspects of adenomatosis of the endocrine glands. *American Journal of Medicine, 16*, 363–371.

White, R., & Lalouel, J. (1988). Chromosome mapping with DNA markers. *Scientific American, 258*, 40–48.

Wilfond, B., Rothenberg, K., Thomson, E., & Lerman, C. (1997). Cancer genetic susceptibility testing: Ethical and policy implications for future research and clinical practice. Cancer Genetics Consortium, National Institutes of Health. *Journal of Law, Medicine, and Ethics, 25*, 243–251.

Williams, L.O., Cole, E.C., Iglesius, N.I., Jordan, R.L., Lubin, I.M., Elliot, L.E., & Boone, D.J. (1999, August 31). *General recommendations for quality assurance programs for laboratory molecular genetic tests* (Contract #200-98-0011). Atlanta: Centers for Disease Control and Prevention.

Wilson, E.B. (1899). *The cell in development and heredity.* New York: Macmillan.

Wivel, N.A., & Wilson, J.M. (1998). Methods of gene delivery. *Gene Therapy, 12*, 483–501.

Zallen, D.T. (1997). *Does it run in the family? A consumer's guide to genetic testing for genetic disorders* (pp. 66–76). New Brunswick, NJ: Rutgers University Press.

CHAPTER 5

Pathology and the Clinical Laboratory in Cancer Control

Linda J. Trapkin, DO

Introduction

"Your test came back from the laboratory, and it is normal."

"Your biopsy has been sent to the pathology laboratory, and it will take four days to get the report back."

Nurses very often are the healthcare professionals who convey important diagnostic information to patients. While the first-hand reports on significant findings usually are given by physicians, patients frequently need the information reinforced in terms that they can easily grasp. Can the nurse interpret the pathologist's report when the patient wants to know what "small cell carcinoma of the lung" means? What is small about it? Is that good or bad? For reasons such as this, nurses need to have a very clear understanding of clinical laboratory testing to be able to accurately answer patients' questions. By knowing why the test was ordered, basic laboratory methods, and how to interpret the result, nurses can do much to allay patients' anxieties as well as to help them to cope with whatever treatment is next. This chapter will give nurses a better understanding of these issues.

Modern medicine, and certainly oncologic medicine, could not function without reliance on the laboratory for screening, diagnosing, treating, and monitoring diseases. So, what, exactly, is "the laboratory?" In many hospitals, if one wants the patient's hematocrit, one calls "the lab," but if the results of the transbronchial biopsy are needed, one calls another number to reach "pathology." Both areas are overseen by pathologists—physicians who have taken their specialty medical boards in clinical pathology (the clinical laboratory) or anatomic pathology. Most pathologists are board certified in both anatomic and clinical pathology.

In addition to the obvious role of analyzing specimens, the laboratory is very much involved with cancer prevention and control. Technologists perform the tests on blood, urine, or other body substances that are used to screen for disease risk, detect early disease, confirm a diagnosis, and then monitor disease progression or remission. Most clinical laboratories include, at a minimum, the subdivisions of hematology, chemistry, and microbiology. Hospital laboratories also will have a blood bank. Esoteric tests, such as cytogenetic tests, most likely are sent to university or commercial reference laboratories.

The other, sometimes less well known, division of laboratory medicine is anatomic pathology with its cytology and histology laboratories. The laboratories of anatomic pathology, also known as surgical pathology, are where the biopsies, needle aspirates, and resection specimens are sent so that the pathologist may render a definitive diagnosis of the disease process and give it an exact name, such as infiltrating ductal carcinoma of the left breast.

In the arena of cancer pathology, the traditional boundaries between clinical and anatomic pathology are eroding. Although the main goal of the anatomic pathologist remains to classify malignant tumors based on their gross and microscopic appearances and to give prognostic information based on the tumor's stage (e.g., size, extent of invasion, status of regional lymph nodes), the field of molecular pathology is no longer solely the research tool of academic institutions. Molecular oncology is being applied to patients being treated in community hospitals in ways that help to further define risk and to refine cancer treatments and prognosis.

The Clinical Laboratory: Basics of Laboratory Test Interpretation

Reference Ranges

"Your lab test is normal." Everyone who is undergoing testing hopes to hear these words, but what exactly is "normal"? By looking at a patient report from any clinical laboratory, one can see that the patient's results are tagged as abnormal (e.g., with asterisks) if they are outside the values listed in the reference range column. Reference ranges reflect values that are most likely seen in a population of healthy individuals, but rarely does a "normal" value guarantee health, or does an "abnormal" value necessarily indicate that something is wrong. Even the phrase "reference range" has replaced "normal range" as an acknowledgment that normalcy is difficult to define and that normalcy, or health, cannot be guaranteed by any specific laboratory test result. Table 5-1 presents some examples of reference ranges.

When asked to define what a reference range is, many laboratorians will draw an example of a bell-shaped curve, also known as Gaussian distribution (Pincus, 1996). The peak of this curve represents the mean (or average value) and the mean plus or minus two standard deviations is defined to encompass the middle 95% of all values under the curve. Under the idealized example, one could take any measurable trait (e.g., age, height, weight, serum sodium), and if enough individuals were measured for that trait, the accumulated data of test values would sort into a bell-shaped curve. By convention, the central 95% of values from the curve (i.e.,

Table 5-1. Examples of Reference Ranges for Commonly Used Tests

Test	Adult Reference Range for Blood Serum Levels
Albumin	3.1–4.3 g/dl
Anti-mitochondrial antibodies	Negative
Calcium, total	8.9–10.7 mg/dl
Hemoglobin	13.5–18.0 g/dl (males) 12.5–16.0 g/dl (females)
Prostate-specific antigen	< 4.0 ng/ml (males)

Note. Based on information from Wallach, 1996.

the mean plus or minus two standard deviations) become the reference range for that substance. In other words, the highest 2.5% of values and the lowest 2.5% of values, although still obtained from the test population of similar individuals, are excluded. However, reality rarely is so cooperative, and most biological data are not symmetrical (Solberg, 1999). In fact, rather arbitrary decisions sometimes are made to define cut-off values (Pincus).

To simplify the explanation of how reference ranges are made, three general approaches can be described. Each approach has specific advantages, depending on the substance being measured and the circumstances affecting the values expected in healthy people versus values possibly indicating disease. In some instances, reference ranges may need to come from specific populations relevant to the patient being tested for the test to be interpreted in its proper context. Examples of specific reference ranges are those defined by age, gender, or race.

The first of the three basic approaches for reference ranges will cover the majority of medical tests because these tests measure substances present in individuals who, for all intents and purposes, are healthy. In other words, the utility of the test (e.g., serum sodium) comes from the fact that disease will cause a decrease or increase in the substance outside of the range usually seen in healthy individuals. The relevant reference range may be defined by those values seen in a tested healthy population or a subset of those values (e.g., the central 95% of values from all values obtained from the reference population).

In the second approach, the reference range indicates that the substance in question normally is not present in healthy individuals (e.g., antibodies to hepatitis C). The question that the medical test will answer is whether the substance is present or absent. Additional information sometimes is obtained from titers, as rising or falling levels can indicate the time course of the infection or disease. Third, if disease is associated with abnormal production of a substance (e.g., the hemoglobin in sickle cell anemia or an aberrant oncogene associated with high risk for breast cancer), then the test method must be able to distinguish between normal and abnormal forms of the substance being analyzed. In some cases, the mere presence of the abnormal substance may not necessarily indicate disease, and the reference range might indicate the relative value of various levels of the substance for predicting or diagnosing true disease.

Cholesterol testing has been a case study of the pitfalls of the population-based Gaussian curve method for obtaining reference ranges. Using age-based population data, a cholesterol level of 240 mg/dl once was considered perfectly "normal" for otherwise healthy 40-year-old men. However, it is now recognized that these men are at higher risk for atherosclerosis and ischemic heart disease; therefore, the currently used reference range for total cholesterol is based on long-term population studies and is aimed at preventing ischemic heart disease ("Summary of the Second Report," 1993). Similarly, genetic tests that better define risk for certain cancers will change the definition of "normal" in the absence of detectable disease.

Sensitivity and Specificity

Sensitivity and specificity reflect additional challenges in medical testing. A perfect test for cancer would have 100% sensitivity, meaning that everyone with cancer would have abnormal results (see Table 5-2). The perfect test would also have 100% specificity, meaning that everyone who did not have cancer would have results within the reference range. Unfortunately, such a test has yet to be invented. Many substances used to diagnose and monitor cancer can also be present in cancer-free individuals. An example of such a substance is prostate-specific antigen (PSA); although PSA usually becomes elevated in men with prostate cancer, there is a large overlap of values between the prostate cancer-free and diseased populations.

When medical personnel refer to false-positive and false-negative results (e.g., the patient with prostate cancer with a PSA level within the reference range is a false-negative), often the implication is that such results are due to mistakes made by laboratory personnel. However, the true meaning of these terms relates to the inherent characteristics of the test. A realistic example would be a test that should be positive (i.e., outside the reference range) when disease is present, but population studies have shown that this test displays 95% sensitivity (5% of patients with disease have a negative result) and 60% specificity (40% of individuals with a positive result do not have disease). One can immediately see the problem of confidently interpreting a positive or negative result if this test were to be used as a screening test on random, asymptomatic individuals.

Errors in sensitivity are termed false-negative results. Negative results (i.e., within the reference range) can be divided into two classes: true negatives from nondiseased patients and false negatives from patients who really do have disease. Because no cancer tests with 100% sensitivity are available, there will be patients with cancer who will have a falsely negative test result. If this is because of low

Table 5-2. Hypothetical New Test for Cancer: Sensitivity and Specificity

Group	Normal Test	Abnormal Test	Sensitivity of Text	Specificity of Test
100 people with colon cancer	5 people (false-negative result)	95 people (true-positive result)	95/100 x 100 = 95%	not applicable
100 people without colon cancer	60 people (true-negative result)	40 people (false-positive result)	Not applicable	60/100 x 100 = 60%

levels of the substance, increased levels may be detected with repeat testing after a suitable time period. At other times, the cancer in a given patient may act in an idiosyncratic manner and not produce the substance.

Errors in specificity are termed false-positive results. Positive results (i.e., outside the reference range) also can be divided into two classes: true positives from patients with disease and false-positive results from nondiseased patients. For many substances used to detect or monitor cancer, results for the healthy and diseased populations overlap; therefore, the placement of the cut-off value for the reference range will affect sensitivity and specificity. Using PSA again as a typical example, placing the cut-off of the reference range at a lower value will increase sensitivity (it will pick up more patients with prostate cancer) at the expense of decreased specificity (it will yield more false-positive results). Conversely, raising the cut-off value will decrease sensitivity (increase the number of false-negative results) while improving specificity (decrease the number of false-positive results).

One way to overcome the problem of balancing sensitivity and specificity is to use two tests. The first is the screening test, which has very high sensitivity at the expense of specificity. An example of such a screening test is the Pap smear test for cervical cancer. Screening tests by their very nature err on the side of maximizing sensitivity, thereby sacrificing specificity. Whenever possible, positive screening tests are followed by a confirmatory test chosen for its high specificity. In this case, an abnormal Pap test is usually followed by a cervical biopsy. A positive confirmatory test, by virtue of its high specificity, is much more likely to be a true positive test. Similarly, many sensitive serologic tests for infections (e.g., Lyme disease) are confirmed with the more specific Western blot assay.

Predictive Values

An understanding of the concepts of sensitivity and specificity is important, but these concepts need to be turned into predictive values if they are to be clinically useful. When a female patient wants to know what her elevated CA 125 means, one needs to know the likelihood that the elevation indicates ovarian cancer (a true positive) or a benign condition (a false-positive). In the final analysis, no test can be interpreted in a vacuum; one must know something about the patient to interpret the result and make a prediction about the meaning of the test result. In this example, a young patient with pelvic pain, no palpable pelvic masses, and a slightly elevated CA 125 likely has benign disease (e.g., endometriosis), while an elevated result in a postmenopausal woman is much more ominous. Of course, other factors, such as family history and the findings of a physical exam, also will influence the positive predictive value of any test. One also may be in a situation in which a negative test, and its negative predictive value, is called into question.

Disease prevalence affects predictive values. Appropriate testing performed on a high-risk population has a high predictive value. Inappropriate testing can yield misleading information and the need for further, and often expensive or invasive, clinical investigation. An example of the impact of disease prevalence on predictive value and test interpretation is commonly seen in emergency departments, where medical personnel are assessing traffic accident victims with chest pain.

The serum creatine kinase (CK) might seem a reasonable test to aid in excluding myocardial infarction. The positive predictive value of an elevated result is going to be high in an elderly patient with a history of angina but very low in the athlete returning from a track meet. In the latter case, the chest pain and the elevated CK are most likely caused by chest wall and myocardial contusions. In other words, all medical tests must be ordered and then interpreted in the context of the individual patient's medical history, physical examination, and personal risk factors.

Many of the controversies concerning the use of tumor markers as screening tests in the asymptomatic population concern the low predictive values of these tests in these situations. Prostate-specific antigen and CA 125 are two examples of tests that some feel should be performed as mass screening tests for the purpose of identifying those with prostate cancer and ovarian cancer, respectively. But in the general population, the prevalence of many cancers is low, and the specificity of the corresponding tumor marker tests also is low, leading to situations where most people with a "positive" test result will not have disease but likely will undergo expensive and invasive tests to rule out the possibility.

Table 5-3 shows an example of a hypothetical cancer test that has 95% sensitivity (5% of patients with cancer will have a negative test) and 60% specificity (40% of patients without cancer will have a positive test). In a mass screening situation in which the hypothetical prevalence of disease in the general population is 14%,

Table 5-3. Positive Predictive Value and Disease Prevalence

Hypothetical cancer test used in random population with 14% disease prevalence

Test Result[a]	Number of Patients With Cancer[b]	Number of Patients Without Cancer[c]	Predictive Value of Test
Positive test result	133 (true positives)	344 (false positives)	28% positive predictive value (133/477)
Negative test result	7 (false positives)	516 (true negatives)	99% negative predictive value (516/523)

Hypothetical cancer test used in high-risk population with 75% disease prevalence

Test Result[a]	Number of Patients With Cancer[d]	Number of Patients Without Cancer[e]	Predictive Value of Test
Positive test result	712 true positives	50 false positives	93% positive predictive value
Negative test result	38 false negatives	150 true negatives	80% negative predictive value

[a] Test has 95% sensitivity and 60% specificity.
[b] For this example, 14% of 1,000 random individuals, n = 140.
[c] For this example, 86% of 1,000 random individuals, n = 860.
[d] For this example, 75% of 1,000 high-risk individuals, n = 750.
[e] For this example, 25% of 1,000 high-risk individuals, n = 250.

random screening of an unselected population will yield a positive predictive value of only 28%, meaning that 72% of all individuals with a positive test will not have cancer but will surely be worried as the follow-up studies are performed. A better use of this test would be in a selected population at high risk for cancer because of a strong family history. In this second scenario, the prevalence of cancer is 75% and the same test, when given to this population, will yield a positive predictive value of 93%.

Variables in Medical Testing

Testing errors that result from incorrect detection of the test substance generally fall into two error classes: analytical and preanalytical. Analytical errors include errors that are a result of the limitations of the test method. The substance being measured may be in amounts too low to be detected by the current test method, leading to a false negative report. For example, viral infections (e.g., HIV) will have "window periods" when the virus or a serologic response cannot yet be detected.

Other reasons for erroneous laboratory results are preanalytical in nature. This category includes anything that influences the reliability of the specimen to be tested, such as patient preparation, phlebotomy technique, and specimen storage. For example, a patient may not have been properly instructed about fasting prior to glucose testing. Likewise, proper phlebotomy technique is paramount. Tests performed on blood specimens collected after prolonged tourniquet times, from veins receiving IV fluids, or from squeezed fingersticks often are occult sources of medical testing error.

Finally, physiologic variation may occur. Although the body regulates some analytes (e.g., potassium) very closely, other substances (e.g., PSA) can vary quite dramatically on a daily or weekly basis without regard to changes in diet, exercise, or medical treatment. Therefore, significant changes are not always related to therapy (or its failure), and correlation with clinical assessment is always appropriate, and repeat testing may be needed.

Anatomic Pathology: General Concepts of Cancer Pathology

Although the surgeon may remove the diseased tissue or the radiologist may perform the fine-needle aspiration, the anatomic pathologist renders the definitive diagnosis based upon the microscopic examination of the submitted tissue or cells. Anatomic pathology covers surgical pathology, cytopathology, and autopsy pathology.

If clinical pathology is the essence of medical science, then anatomic pathology very much represents the art of medicine. The most basic issues in the diagnosis of cancer remain: is it malignant, and if so, what type of cancer is it? These questions still are answered at the microscope by pathologists who are trained in the visual recognition of malignant tumors. Molecular pathology is aiding, but not replacing, this very human intellectual endeavor.

Cytopathology

Cytopathology plays an important role in the diagnosis and management of cancer, as cytologic material often can be obtained with relatively simple and noninvasive techniques. The pathologist renders diagnoses from the microscopic examination of body fluids, aspirates from tissue that can be reached by a needle, or material gathered from brushings or washings of body cavities. The most common cytology test is the cervical Pap test.

Regardless of tissue origin or procurement technique, all cytology specimens are eventually placed on glass slides, stained, and screened by cytotechnologists, who mark what appear to be abnormal cells. The screened slides are then taken to the pathologist, who renders the actual diagnosis seen on the final report. The only exception to this arrangement is cervical Pap tests; if the cytotechnologist finds no abnormal cells, he or she is allowed to release the report as normal or benign without the review of a pathologist.

Surgical Pathology

Surgical pathology is the gold standard for the definitive diagnosis, classification, and staging of cancer. After the office biopsy or surgical specimen is received in the histology laboratory and its relevant attributes with regard to size and gross appearance are recorded, appropriate samples are removed for microscopic analysis. The chosen tissue samples usually are fixed in formalin, treated to a variety of chemical baths, embedded in paraffin, thinly sliced, mounted on a glass slide, and stained with hematoxylin and eosin (H&E) by histotechnologists who then bring the slides to the pathologist. If ancillary studies are needed, more tissue is cut from the paraffin block. Finally, the pathologist issues a pathology report detailing the histologic diagnosis as well as additional information needed for staging of the tumor. The modern surgical pathology report contains important treatment and prognostic information.

Basic Nomenclature and Classification of Malignant Tumors

As commonly used, the terms *neoplasm* and *tumor* have become nearly synonymous, and both often refer to abnormal growths although neither denotes malignancy. The term *cancer,* however, is the general term for all malignant tumors, and there are many different types of malignant neoplasms, reflective of their diverse cells of origin (Cotran, Kuman, & Collins, 1999) (see Table 5-4).

Benign tumors often are designated by the use of the suffix "-oma" to the cell of origin. Examples from mesenchymal tissues include lipoma (benign tumor of fat cells), fibroma (benign tumor of fibroblasts), and osteoma (benign tumor of bone cells). When naming benign tumors derived from epithelial tissue, the term *adenoma* is usually incorporated into the name, such as tubular adenoma of the colon. However, there are striking exceptions to these rules, including melanoma, which is a malignant tumor of melanocytes, and hepatoma, which is also known by the more accurate name of hepatocellular carcinoma.

Malignant tumors also have a nomenclature that indicates the cell of origin. Malignant neoplasms arising from mesenchymal elements are usually called sarcomas. Examples of malignant mesenchymal tumors include liposarcoma, fibro-

Table 5-4. Nomenclature of Benign and Malignant Tumors: Common Examples

Cell of Origin	Benign Neoplasm	Malignant Neoplasm
Squamous epithelial cell	Squamous papilloma	Squamous carcinoma
Glandular epithelial cell	Adenoma	Adenocarcinoma
Fat cell	Lipoma	Liposarcoma
Bone cell	Osteoma	Osteosarcoma
Blood vessel cell	Hemangioma	Hemangiosarcoma
Smooth muscle cell	Leiomyoma	Leiomyosarcoma
Lymphocytes	Not applicable	Lymphoma

sarcoma, and osteosarcoma. Malignant fibrous histiocytoma, the most common sarcoma in adults, is another exception to these nosologic rules.

Malignant neoplasms arising from epithelial tissues are called carcinomas. Carcinomas derive from the epithelial component of all three embryonic germ cell layers: endodermis, mesodermis, and ectodermis; hence, malignant epithelial tumors, or carcinomas, can arise in the skin, internal organs, and the gastrointestinal and respiratory tracts. Many carcinomas have the organ or tissue of origin incorporated into the name (e.g., renal cell carcinoma, ductal carcinoma of the breast, prostate carcinoma). Carcinomas are much more common than sarcomas, which are rare tumors.

Carcinomas are often classified further as to whether they show glandular or squamous differentiation. The malignant cells of adenocarcinomas make glands and the cancer cells of squamous carcinomas show squamous differentiation. For example, a diagnosis of esophageal carcinoma needs to be further defined as to whether it is an adenocarcinoma or a squamous carcinoma. In general, if no further designation is made (e.g., renal cell carcinoma), the cancer is likely to be an adenocarcinoma.

Mixed tumors, both benign and malignant, show features of both mesenchymal and epithelial origin. These tumors have a variety of names reflecting the cellular appearance, the presumed precursor cells, and idiosyncratic tradition (how else to explain the name *cystosarcoma phyllodes* to describe a usually benign mixed tumor of the breast). Among the most interesting of neoplasms showing both mesenchymal and epithelial differentiation are the teratomas, which are tumors often made up of all three germ layers. The most common is the benign, cystic teratoma (dermoid cyst) of the ovary, which can show mixtures of skin and related structures, gastrointestinal tissue, cartilage, and brain.

Malignant tumors of blood cells, such as lymphocytes, are technically mesenchymal tumors but have come down to us as leukemias (when the malignant cells circulate in the peripheral blood) and lymphomas (usually primary to lymph nodes).

Premalignant Lesions

The fight against cancer usually is spoken of in terms of preventing cancer (e.g., smoking cessation initiatives) or early detection (e.g., breast self-examinations, mammography). Early detection usually is meant to be synonymous with detection of cancer in its earliest stages, when it is most easily treated and most likely to be curable. However, several of the mass screening programs (including for colon, breast, and cervical cancers) are most successful when they detect premalignant disease.

The term *premalignant*, or precursor, signifies that these lesions have no ability for metastasis but, if left untreated, might progress to fully malignant cancers with such abilities. Atypical hyperplasia, dysplasia, carcinoma in situ, and intraepithelial neoplasia are types of premalignant conditions. Examples of premalignant lesions include atypical hyperplasia of the endometrium, ductal carcinoma in situ of the breast, and intraepithelial neoplasia of the prostate. All denote increased risk for invasive, or fully malignant, tumors if left untreated.

The uterine cervix has had an evolving series of terms for premalignant disease, reflecting improved understanding of the underlying biological processes and attempts to improve communication between the pathologist and clinician. Premalignant disease in the cervix may be referred to as dysplasia, cervical intraepithelial neoplasia (CIN), and squamous intraepithelial lesion (SIL).

Histologic Grading of Malignant Tumors

One of the important pieces of information provided by the pathologist's assessment of the malignant neoplasm is a statement about tumor grade. Most tumors are given one of three grades. Malignant tumors that very closely mimic the benign condition (e.g., the presence of glands in an adenocarcinoma) are said to be well-differentiated, low-grade, or grade I. Tumors that retain little resemblance to their tissue of origin and show aggressive features such as necrosis or high mitotic activity are said to be poorly differentiated, high-grade, or grade III. On occasion, these poorly differentiated tumors are so bizarre that they are called anaplastic. Between these two extremes are the moderately differentiated, intermediate-grade, or grade II tumors. Two common cancers with unique grading systems are adenocarcinomas of the breast and prostate; their specific grading criteria are shown in Tables 5-5 and 5-6, respectively.

Tumor Staging

Staging is used to stratify patients into treatment protocols as well as to assess prognosis. Research comparing the efficacy of differing treatment protocols could not reach meaningful conclusions unless results were stratified for stage (e.g., all patients with tumor confined to the prostate, or all patients with colon cancer that has metastasized to the liver). Although numerous organ-specific staging systems exist, the TNM staging protocols of the American Joint Committee on Cancer (Fleming et al., 1997) are commonly employed. The TNM system assesses the primary tumor (T), metastatic disease to regional lymph nodes (N), and metastasis to distant sites (M). Although clinical staging can be done by clinical assessment and imaging techniques, the notation pTNM is used when pathologic staging has been performed from tissue specimens. Pathologic staging can be the most accurate method. As an example, it is not uncommon for men with prostate carcinoma to have their tumors increased in stage once a pathologist has examined the pros-

Table 5-5. Grading of Breast Cancer Using the Elston and Ellis Approach to the Scarff-Bloom-Richardson Method

Histologic Element	Description	Number of Points
Tubule formation by malignant glands	> 75% of tumor	1 point
	10%–75% of tumor	2 points
	< 10% of tumor	3 points
Nuclear pleomorphism of malignant cells	Mild	1 point
	Moderate	2 points
	Marked	3 points
Number of mitotic figures among malignant cells per 10 high power fields (hpf)	< 10/10 hpf	1 point
	10–20/10 hpf	2 points
	> 20/10 hpf	3 points

Final grade of breast carcinoma determined by adding the points from each of the above 3 categories: 3–5 total points = Grade 1; 6–7 total points = Grade 2; 8–9 total points = Grade 3.

Note. Based on information from Henson et al., 1997.

Table 5-6. Grading of Prostate Adenocarcinoma Using the Gleason System

Histologic Appearance of Tumor	Gleason Grade
Single, uniform glands in closely packed masses	Gleason grade = 1
Single, slightly less uniform glands in loosely packed masses	Gleason grade = 2
Cribriform pattern	Gleason grade = 3
Fused glands with ragged infiltrative pattern	Gleason grade = 4
Anaplastic carcinoma	Gleason grade = 5

Final Gleason score for prostate adenocarcinoma equals the addition of the two most common Gleason grades in the tumor (double the single score if only one pattern is present). Examples of final Gleason scores: Grades 3 + 3 = Gleason score of 6; Grades 3 + 4 = Gleason score of 7.

Note. Based on information from Rosai, 1996.

tatectomy specimen and microscopically proven that the tumor has extended outside the prostate—a level of invasion that may not have been clinically evident with presurgical imaging.

The T portion of the TNM staging system refers to characteristics of the primary tumor, such as size, level of invasion into the underlying benign tissue, and direct extension into adjacent organs or structures. Histologic grade is not taken into consideration, but the definitions for each T level can be organ-specific, such as lung versus colon.

The N portion of the TNM staging system refers to the assessment of metastasis to regional lymph nodes (e.g., ipsilateral axillary nodes for breast carcinoma). The various N levels define either the number of affected lymph nodes (as with colon carcinoma) or the location of the affected lymph nodes (as with lung carcinoma).

The M portion of TNM staging refers to the presence or absence of distant metastasis. These sites include nonregional lymph nodes or hematogenous spread to distant sites, such as bone marrow or liver. There are usually three M designations: unknown, absent, or present.

The information from the assessment of the primary tumor (T), regional lymph nodes (N), and distant metastasis (M) is used to place the patient with cancer into one of several tumor-specific stages, with higher stages indicating increasingly more advanced disease. As expected, stage I tumors usually are small, localized tumors without lymph node or distant metastasis, and stage IV tumors are defined by the presence of distant metastasis, regardless of tumor size or local lymph node metastasis.

The Role of the Laboratory in Cancer Prevention and Control: A Look at Five Cancers

The American Cancer Society (ACS) publishes annual statistics on the occurrence of cancer in the United States. In its 2000 report, ACS estimated that approximately 1,200,000 new cases of invasive cancer would be diagnosed during the year and that an average of 1,500 Americans would succumb daily to cancer (Greenlee, Murray, Bolden, & Wingo, 2000). Between 1996 and 1997, total cancer deaths among American men declined. This was the first such decrease in 79 years and was attributed to decreased mortality from lung, prostate, and colon cancers. Unfortunately, the total cancer deaths among women continued to increase as a result of the climbing number of deaths associated with lung cancer.

The effort to decrease cancer incidence continues to be aimed at early detection, as the means to prevent most cancers is still unknown. One of the most striking exceptions, however, is lung cancer. Although lung cancer kills approximately 150,000 Americans each year and is the number-one cancer killer for both men and women, the means for its prevention is known: abolish cigarette smoking.

Recommendations for mass population screening in asymptomatic individuals are largely limited to cancers of the breast, colon, prostate, and cervix. The sensitivity and specificity of most tumor markers or imaging techniques for the remaining cancers cannot justify their use in the general population; the positive predictive value is unacceptably low. Therefore, most cancers are detected in individuals being evaluated for symptoms, which unfortunately means that many tumors cannot be detected at the very earliest—and most easily curable—stages.

Tumor markers, by convention, refer to substances secreted by the malignant cells into the peripheral blood. Currently, the only tumor marker with acceptable mass screening utility is prostate-specific antigen (PSA). Other tumor markers, such as alpha-fetoprotein (AFP), CA 15-3, CA 19-9, CA 125, and carcinoembryonic antigen (CEA), are used to monitor patients with known malignancies (Wu, 1996). Often the tumor marker will start to rise in the blood before there is clinical evidence of recurrence.

Molecular markers, defined as substances related to DNA, include DNA, mRNA, cell-surface receptors, and related protein products. Testing for molecular markers in cancer requires the actual malignant cells. Although hormone receptor analysis in breast cancer has been performed for several decades, the field of molecular pathology is in its infancy at the dawn of the 21st century. One of the approaches that will be refined during the early portions of this century is the multivariate approach, in which algorithms will seek to look at a number of tumor and molecular markers to reach significant and reliable conclusions about diagnosis, treatment, and prognosis.

Lung Cancer
Screening for Lung Cancer

Although lung cancer is the second most commonly diagnosed invasive cancer in the United States (behind prostate cancer in men and breast cancer in women), it has the dubious distinction of being the number-one cancer killer of both sexes, accounting for approximately 30% of cancer deaths in men and 25% of cancer deaths in women (Greenlee et al., 2000). Approximately 8% of American men and almost 6% of American women develop invasive carcinomas of the lungs and bronchi, but lung cancer remains a largely preventable disease because most cases can be attributed to cigarette smoking (Smith, Mettlin, Davis, & Eyre, 2000).

Given the poor survival statistics of lung cancer and the current lack of a test suitable for the screening of the population at risk, the major thrust of public health policy has been toward disease prevention. Efforts are aimed at preventing children and young adults from starting cigarette smoking and convincing current smokers to quit.

Lung cancer has a grim overall five-year survival rate of approximately 14% (Greenlee et al., 2000). One general strategy for reducing mortality from any type of cancer is to detect the cancer at earlier, potentially curable, stages. However, the two mainstays of screening tests for lung cancer, sputum cytology and chest x-rays, have failed to affect overall morbidity and mortality, reflecting the poor sensitivity of these tests for early-stage disease. Newer technology, such as low-radiation dose computed tomography and fluorescence bronchoscopy, currently are being evaluated in the hope that more effective screening procedures may be offered in the future. At this time, there are no recommended routine screening tests for lung cancer in asymptomatic but high-risk populations (Smith et al., 2000).

Diagnosing Lung Cancer

When a lung lesion is detected, the first objective is to determine benignity versus malignancy (see Figure 5-1). If malignant, is it a primary lung lesion or a metastatic lesion? And if it is a primary lung lesion, is it a small cell carcinoma or a non-small cell carcinoma?

Lesions within or close to the bronchus often can be reached by bronchoscopy. Sampling methods include bronchial brushings and washings and transbronchial biopsy. Peripheral lesions may still be accessible for needle sampling, avoiding the need for thoracotomy for diagnostic purposes.

Once a diagnosis of a primary lung cancer has been reached, the second diagnostic concern of the pathologist is whether the tumor is a small cell carcinoma or a non-small cell carcinoma. This differential diagnosis has major treatment and prognostic implications. Small cell carcinomas are classified as poorly differentiated neuroendocrine malignancies, and the term small cell simply refers to the cell size as compared to other common malignancies. Non-small cell carcinomas include the epithelial tumors adenocarcinoma, squamous carcinoma, and their variants. Other, unusual lung cancers account for a minority of pulmonary tumor cases.

Approximately one-quarter of lung cancers are small cell cancers. The aggressive nature of these tumors is reflected in the short survival time after diagnosis even when treated (Ihde, Pass, & Glatstein, 1997). As with the non-small cell carcinomas of the lung, there is a clear relationship

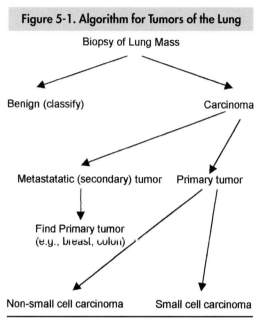

Figure 5-1. Algorithm for Tumors of the Lung

between cigarette smoking and the development of small cell lung cancer (Ihde et al.) The typical presentation is that of a hilar mass on chest x-ray; metastatic disease at the time of diagnosis is common. The sites of dissemination can include other intrapulmonary sites, adrenal glands, bone, liver, lymph nodes, and the central nervous system (Ihde et al.). The importance of differentiating small cell carcinomas from the non-small cell carcinomas of the lung relates to both treatment and prognosis. These tumors usually are not surgically resected because of tumor extent, but their rapid growth characteristics makes them responsive to both radiotherapy and chemotherapy (Ihde et al.).

Non-small cell carcinomas cover a broader spectrum of tumors. Three major carcinomas fall under this heading: adenocarcinoma, squamous cell carcinoma, and large cell carcinoma. Variants include bronchioloalveolar carcinomas, adenosquamous carcinomas, and clear cell carcinoma. Rare tumors will demonstrate both carcinomatous and sarcomatous elements; the name *carcinosarcoma* reflects this dual expression. If caught in an early stage, surgical resection offers the hope of cure, but the overall curability of lung cancer remains low. If resectable, surgical treatment is regarded as the most effective method of control. Radiotherapy can be palliative, and chemotherapy usually is an adjunct to surgery.

Non-small cell carcinomas of the lung are histologically graded based on nuclear and cytologic pleomorphism. Adenocarcinomas that are low-grade (i.e., well differentiated) will make obvious glands, and low-grade squamous carcinomas will have obvious squamous differentiation. It is sometimes difficult to determine if a poorly differentiated, non-small cell lung carcinoma is glandular or squamous in origin, but fortunately, this does not make a difference in the current therapy.

The pathologist's report of a lung malignancy will include the histologic type of the tumor and its grade. The surgical pathology report from a resection specimen will note tumor size and location and whether any of the following are present: vascular or lymphatic invasion, involvement of the overlying visceral pleura, adherence to or direct extension into adjacent structures, and metastasis to regional lymph nodes. Currently, no molecular methods are routinely employed for diagnostic purposes.

The TNM staging system for lung carcinoma (Fleming et al., 1997) includes assessment of the tumor (T) for size, invasion of the main bronchus, invasion of visceral pleura, direct invasion into adjacent structures (e.g., diaphragm, mediastinal pleura, parietal pericardium), or presence of a malignant pleural effusion. Evidence of metastatic disease is sought in regional lymph nodes (N), including the ipsilateral peribronchial, hilar, subcarinal, or mediastinal lymph nodes. The presence or absence of distant metastasis is noted in the M component of staging. The accumulated data from the T, N, and M levels will yield the final stage for treatment and prognostic purposes.

Prostate Cancer
Screening for Prostate Cancer

Up to 40% of men over age 50 have prostate cancer, yet only 8% of these cancers will become clinically significant (Dugan et al., 1996). In other words, most men have prostate carcinomas that are clinically insignificant, and these men will die with, not of, their prostate cancer.

Despite these statistics, prostate adenocarcinoma is a major public health problem. Prostate cancer is the second leading cancer killer of men in the United States, accounting for approximately 32,000 deaths annually (Greenlee et al., 2000). African American men have higher rates of prostate cancer and have twice the mortality rate of White American men (von Eschenbach, Ho, Murphy, Cunningham, & Ling, 1997).

Current screening guidelines from the ACS call for all men over age of 50 to have an annual digital rectal exam (DRE) and PSA test (Smith et al., 2000). Some suggest that screening begin at age 40 for men from high-risk groups (Polascik, Oesterling, & Partin, 1999). Men at increased risk include African Americans and anyone with two or more first-degree relatives (i.e., father or brother) with prostate cancer. Nodules detected with DRE or elevated blood levels of PSA are further investigated with transrectal ultrasonography (TRUS) and needle biopsy.

The widespread use of PSA has been given credit for the improved detection of and the increased incidence of prostate cancer documented in the 1990s. As expected, the use of PSA testing resulted in detection of many of these additional cancers at earlier stages, and there is now evidence that mortality has been reduced as a result (Smith et al., 2000). However, the use of PSA as a screening test is not without controversy, and there are concerns that this test detects and consequently leads to the treatment of clinically insignificant tumors (Polascik et al., 1999). Arguments have been put forth that small, low-grade tumors in elderly men need not be aggressively treated, but controversy exists as to how to define clinically insignificant tumors (Dugan et al., 1996).

The PSA reference range for all men is generally accepted to be less than 4.0 ng/ml. When PSA is used as a screening test in the general population, it has a reported sensitivity for the detection of prostate cancer of up to 80%. However, because many men with benign conditions (e.g., benign prostatic hypertrophy [BPH]) have elevated PSA levels, the test loses specificity and yields numerous false-positive results. When used in a mass screening situation, the PSA has an overall positive predictive value of probably no more than 35% (Woolf, 1995). This means that up to 65% of men with an elevated result will not have prostate cancer. As a result, many of these men may be subjected to unnecessary prostate needle biopsy to rule out the possibility of prostate cancer. Conversely, there are also problems with the negative predictive value of a normal range result, and up to 25% of men with prostate cancer will have a PSA within the reference range (i.e., less than 4.0 ng/ml) (von Eschenbach et al., 1997).

The search is on to improve the predictive value of the PSA test (Brawer, 1999), and studies have looked at PSA density (PSA corrected for prostate volume), PSA velocity (changes of PSA with time), age-specific PSA reference ranges (PSA increases with age), and percent free PSA (unbound PSA divided by total PSA). Only the percent free PSA test has shown real clinical utility.

Most of the PSA present in the blood circulates bound to plasma proteins; however, the percentage of free PSA has been shown to be lower in men with prostate cancer than in men with benign prostatic conditions. If the goal of using the percent free PSA is to increase both the sensitivity and the specificity of the PSA test, then the percent free PSA measurement is most useful for those men with a total PSA between 4 and 10 ng/ml and a negative DRE. For men in this "gray zone," the overall probability of prostate cancer is 25%, but the risk can be further stratified by measuring the percentage of free PSA. Those with a percent free PSA of less than 10% may have seven times the probability of harboring prostate cancer as those men with a percent free PSA greater than 25% (probability of cancer 56% versus 8%) (Catalona et al., 1998).

The results of the DRE and the PSA screening tests for prostate cancer should be interpreted in conjunction with the patient's age, medical history, and risk factors. Men with slightly elevated PSA, a negative DRE, no risk factors, and high percent free PSA may not require a prostate biopsy (Polascik et al., 1999). However, if there is sufficient clinical suspicion, the urologist will proceed with ultrasonography and prostate biopsy.

Premalignant Prostate Lesions

A nodule on digital rectal exam, elevated blood levels of PSA, or abnormalities on ultrasound can lead to the clinical suspicion that prostate cancer is present. In these instances, transrectal needle biopsy of the prostate gland is performed under TRUS guidance. The biopsied tissue is sent to the histology laboratory for the pathologist's diagnostic examination.

Prostate intraepithelial lesion (PIN) is considered a premalignant condition; a diagnosis of PIN on the prostate biopsy is associated with an increased incidence of concurrent prostate adenocarcinoma. Approximately 85% of PIN cases coexist with carcinoma; therefore, if no cancer is identified in the biopsy tissue, close follow-up with repeat biopsy within an appropriate time frame is recommended (Bostwick, 1997). PIN is divided into low-grade and high-grade forms, and high-grade PIN has the strongest association with prostatic adenocarcinoma. Low-grade PIN is not always reported by the pathologist, as its significance is not known with certainty.

Diagnosing Prostate Cancer

Multiple prostate biopsies often are taken, and each will be individually labeled as to location (e.g., right, left, base, apex). The pathologist's report will include important preliminary data, including the histologic diagnosis and grading information. Often a statement is made about the percentage of biopsy tissue involved by tumor (e.g., cancer involves 25% of the needle biopsy of the left base), and although this is an inexact attempt to estimate tumor size, it can be correlated by the urologist's clinical assessment of tumor size.

The majority of prostate cancers are adenocarcinomas. A minority of adenocarcinomas will show histologic variations, such as mucinous or signet ring patterns. Other, less common, tumors include transitional cell carcinoma and squamous carcinoma, both of which represent tumors of the epithelial lining of the urethra (urothelium) or direct extension of such tumors from the urinary bladder.

A diagnosis of prostatic adenocarcinoma always is accompanied by a histologic grade. Several grading schemes are used, but the most widely accepted is the Gleason grading system (see Table 5-6). The Gleason system is specific for prostatic adenocarcinomas and is unusual in that the malignant cells are assessed against five histologic patterns ranging from the lowest grade (grade 1) to the highest grade (grade 5). The grades of the two predominant patterns are added to arrive at a Gleason score, which can range from a low score of 2 (grades 1 + 1) to a high score of 10 (grades 5 + 5). The exact Gleason grades are included in the pathologist's report.

Based upon the physical examination of the patient, imaging studies, and the biopsy report, the patient is clinically staged. If there is evidence that the prostate cancer has metastasized to distant sites (e.g., bone), palliative measures usually are offered. If the prostate cancer clinically appears to be restricted to the prostate, a prostatectomy often is performed. A standard operative scenario is for a preliminary lymph node dissection of the regional pelvic lymph nodes with immediate evaluation by the pathologist at the time of surgery. If the pathologist calls the nodes negative for metastatic disease (N0 in the TNM staging system), the surgeon immediately proceeds with a radical prostatectomy (removal of the prostate and seminal vesicles).

The pathologist's evaluation of the regional lymph nodes and prostatectomy will yield a definitive tumor stage. It is not uncommon for the pathologic staging to be higher than the presurgical clinical staging. The pathology report will document where tumor was found (one lobe versus both lobes), the extent of any invasion beyond the prostate capsule or into the seminal vesicle, and the Gleason grade. Most reports also will comment on tumor size, multifocality, perineural or vascular invasion, and the surgical margins (Amin et al., 1996).

Using the TNM system (Fleming et al., 1997), the tumor (T) is assessed as to whether it was found incidental to a transurethral resection or on random biopsies (T1), palpable but confined to the prostate (T2), or associated with extracapsular extension (T3 and T4, depending on extent). The lymph node (N) assessment concerns the number of nodes with metastatic disease. Distant metastases (M) can be to nonregional lymph nodes, bones, or other sites. The various combinations of the T, N, and M levels will yield a specific tumor stage for treatment and prognostic purposes (see Figure 5-2).

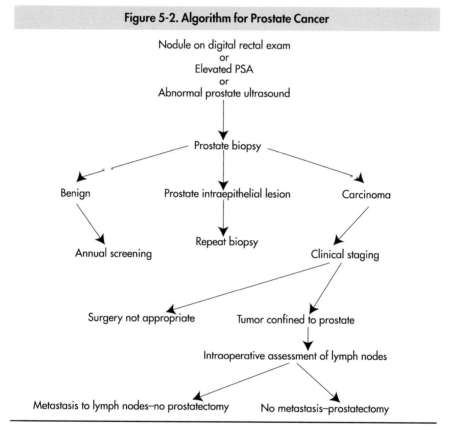

Figure 5-2. Algorithm for Prostate Cancer

Nodule on digital rectal exam
or
Elevated PSA
or
Abnormal prostate ultrasound

Prostate biopsy

Benign

Prostate intraepithelial lesion

Carcinoma

Annual screening

Repeat biopsy

Clinical staging

Surgery not appropriate

Tumor confined to prostate

Intraoperative assessment of lymph nodes

Metastasis to lymph nodes–no prostatectomy

No metastasis–prostatectomy

Breast Cancer
Screening for Breast Cancer

Breast cancer is the most commonly occurring malignancy among American women (excluding skin cancers) and is the number-two cancer killer in the same population, accounting for more than 41,000 deaths per year, or approximately 15% of all cancer deaths in women. Approximately 1 in 8 women will develop invasive breast cancer (Greenlee et al., 2000).

No blood tumor marker has been found that effectively screens for the disease; therefore, screening programs for the detection of early- stage breast cancer center on breast examination and mammography. ACS's screening recommendations suggest that monthly breast self-examinations begin at age 20 and that clinical breast examination by the woman's primary care physician be performed every three years between the ages of 20 and 39. Beginning at age 40, women should perform monthly breast examinations and schedule annual clinical breast examinations and mammography (Smith et al., 2000).

The importance of beginning screening procedures at a young age is emphasized by the fact that breast cancers that start in premenopausal women are likely to be more aggressive and grow at a faster rate than tumors in postmenopausal women (Smith et al., 2000). The earlier these tumors are found, the better the likelihood that the patients will have low-stage tumors. Screening guidelines also suggest that the clinical breast examination should precede the mammography by a short interval to facilitate communication between the woman's physician and the radiologist and correlation of their respective findings (Smith et al.). Palpable masses not detected by mammography should be further investigated by alternative means.

Molecular tests exist for the assessment of hereditary susceptibility to breast cancer. Approximately 7% of breast carcinomas are the result of inherited genetic mutations; therefore, women with a family history of breast or ovarian cancer have an increased likelihood for harboring mutations in the BRCA1 and BRCA2 genes (Frank, 1999). These mutations are associated with significantly increased risk of breast (and ovarian) cancer. A woman without either of these inherited genetic mutations has a 2% risk of developing breast carcinoma before the age of 50, whereas a woman with either one of these mutations has a risk of 33%–50% (Frank). For women with increased risk for breast cancer because of the genetic mutation, the management options include heightened surveillance, prophylactic surgery, and chemoprevention (Frank). The use of tamoxifen, a selective estrogen-receptor modulator, has shown promising results in decreasing the occurrence of breast cancer in this high-risk population (Fisher et al., 1998).

If, during screening examinations, a suspicious lump or mammographic abnormality is found, there are several options for obtaining material for the pathologic assessment. Fine needle aspiration techniques can be performed on palpable lesions. Needle biopsies can be done under imaging guidance. If a larger excision is desirable, the preoperative preparation can involve ultrasound-guided placement of a localization needle to aid the surgeon in locating the suspicious area.

Premalignant Breast Conditions

Several conditions within breast tissue are associated with increased risk for the development of invasive breast carcinoma. The most obvious premalignant lesions of the breast are ductal carcinoma in situ (DCIS, intraductal carcinoma) and lobular carcinoma in situ. Although this division implies that DCIS originates in the ducts and that lobular carcinoma in situ arises from the breast lobules (where the lactational activity of the glands occurs), this is not necessarily true. It is now accepted that both histologic types of in situ breast carcinoma, and their corresponding invasive tumors, arise from the terminal duct-lobular unit despite the histologic appearance of the tumors (Tavassoli, 1997). This also explains why some breast carcinomas will show both lobular and ductal differentiation. Although ductal carcinoma in situ and lobular carcinoma in situ lesions are considered the direct precursors to invasive disease, a variety of benign, proliferative lesions also are associated with increased relative risk for invasive tumors (see Figure 5-3).

Figure 5-3. Relative Risk for Invasive Breast Carcinoma Based on Pathologic Examination of Benign Breast Tissue

No increased risk
Women with the following lesions are at no greater risk for invasive breast carcinoma than women who have not had a breast biopsy:
• Adenosis (other than sclerosing adenosis)
• Duct ectasia
• Fibroadenoma with complex features
• Fibrosis
• Mastitis
• Mild hyperplasia without atypia
• Ordinary cysts (gross or microscopic)
• Simple apocrine metaplasia (no associated hyperplasia or adenosis)
• Squamous metaplasia

Slightly increased risk (1.5–2.0)
Women with the following lesions have a slightly increased risk for invasive breast carcinoma compared with women who have not had a breast biopsy:
• Fibroadenoma with complex features
• Moderate or florid hyperplasia without atypia
• Sclerosing adenosis
• Solitary papilloma without coexistent atypical hyperplasia

Moderately increased risk (4.0–5.0)
Women with the following lesions have a moderately increased risk for invasive breast carcinoma compared with women who have not had a breast biopsy:
• Atypical ductal hyperplasia
• Atypical lobular hyperplasia

Markedly increased risk (8.0–10.0)
Women with the following lesions have a high risk for invasive breast carcinoma compared with women who have not had a breast biopsy:
• Ductal carcinoma in situ (DCIS) (This category refers to small, low-grade, noncomedo DCIS lesions. The relative risk of high-grade or extensive DCIS is difficult to determine because most patients are subsequently treated by wider surgical excision, which reduces the risk of recurrence.)
• Lobular carcinoma in situ

Note. From "Benign Breast Changes and the Risk for Subsequent Breast Cancer: An Update of the 1985 Consensus Statement," by P.L. Fitzgibbons, D.E. Henson, and R.V.P. Hutter, 1998, *Archives of Pathology and Laboratory Medicine, 122,* p. 1054. Copyright 1988 by the College of American Pathologists. Adapted with permission.

Relative risk does not connote absolute risk to the individual patient but represents comparisons with age-matched women in the general population. For example, a 40-year-old woman with no risk factors has a 1 in 67 probability of developing invasive breast cancer during the next decade. A 60-year-old woman has a 1 in 29 chance of developing invasive breast cancer during the same period of time. If either of these women develops a suspicious lesion, and atypical ductal hyperplasia is found in the biopsy, a corresponding fourfold increase in the risk for developing invasive breast cancer during the next ten years will occur—an increase to 1 in 17 for the 40-year-old woman and to 1 in 7 for the 60-year-old woman (Fitzgibbons, Henson, & Hutter, 1998). These estimates of relative risk are meant to provide guidance for clinical management.

The presence of either DCIS or lobular carcinoma in situ is associated with a markedly increased risk for invasive cancer. DCIS lesions are graded using the characteristics of histologic pattern, nuclear grade (degree of pleomorphism), and presence or absence of necrosis. Comedocarcinoma (DCIS with intraluminal necrosis and poorly differentiated tumor cells) is a high-grade DCIS lesion. Lobular carcinoma in situ generally is not graded. In situ lesions can occur with or without concurrent invasive tumor at the time of the biopsy.

Often, a breast biopsy is done because of the mammographic identification of calcifications in the absence of any palpable mass or other radiologic lesion. In this case, the pathologist will make a comment as to whether calcification or birefringent material (seen with polarized light microscopy) is present and whether such material is within tumor or benign breast tissue. The important issue is to be satisfied that the lesion detected by mammography has been adequately sampled for histologic examination.

Diagnosing Breast Carcinoma

The pathologist's diagnostic report of a breast biopsy showing invasive breast cancer will include a histologic classification, a tumor grade, and a series of other attributes that will define the tumor's stage and guide the cancer therapy. Infiltrating ductal carcinoma and infiltrating lobular carcinoma are the two main categories of invasive breast cancer. The majority of invasive carcinomas are ductal carcinomas, and a minority of these tumors can be further classified as to subtype, such as medullary, mucinous (colloid), papillary, or tubular. The various types of invasive breast cancers are associated with differing risks for lymph node metastasis, recurrence, or pattern of distant metastasis. For example, infiltrating ductal carcinoma, tubular type, is always a low-grade neoplasm. Lobular carcinomas are associated with increased risk of bilateral breast disease. Unusual breast malignancies include malignant cystosarcoma phyllodes, which is a biphasic tumor showing both epithelial and sarcomatous elements.

The infiltrating ductal carcinomas also are graded (see Table 5-5). Although several grading schemes exist, the Elston and Ellis modification of the Scarff-Bloom-Richardson breast tumor grading system is the most widely used (Henson, Oberman, & Hutter, 1997). This system takes into account three histologic elements: extent of tubule (glandular) formation, degree of nuclear pleomorphism, and the number of mitoses per 10 high-power fields. Each of these elements is given a score between 1 and 3. The three scores are then added to arrive at a total score, which is then translated into one of three grades (grades I, II, or III).

Additional information in the pathologist's report will depend on the type of specimen that was received. Diagnoses from fine needle aspirates may only be able to state whether malignant cells are present, without any further information. Core needle biopsies will be inadequate to make a determination of gross tumor size and, of course, will be limited by sampling artifact; important elements may not have been included in the small sampling of a large tumor. Surgical pathology reports from excisional biopsies will detail tumor size, the presence or absence of vascular or lymphatic invasion, and the status of margins.

Based upon the findings of the aspirate or biopsy, the surgeon and patient may elect to proceed with lumpectomy or mastectomy, and either can be done in conjunction with an axillary node dissection. The examination of the axillary lymph nodes will detail the number of nodes present and the number with metastatic breast cancer (Henson et al., 1997).

The TNM staging system for breast cancer assesses the tumor (T) for tumor size and presence of local extension into surrounding structures (T1 through T4). Regional lymph nodes (N) are assessed for the number of involved nodes, micrometastasis (foci less than 0.2 cm), or extension of tumor beyond the lymph node capsule. Assessment of distant metastasis (M) includes spread to ipsilateral supraclavicular lymph nodes. The various combinations of the T, N, and M elements will yield the final stage for treatment and prognostic purposes.

Monitoring Therapy for Breast Cancer

Breast cancer represents a common cancer for which molecular markers are used to assess prognosis and guide therapy. Hormone receptor assays have been used for several decades, and a completely different molecular marker, for the overexpression of the breast cancer-related oncogene HER2/neu, is now in common use, too. The tumor markers (substances shed by the tumor into the peripheral blood) CA 15-3 or CA 27.29 sometimes are used for monitoring patients with metastatic breast cancer (Wu, 1996).

Hormonal manipulation (e.g., oophorectomy, tamoxifen) has been used for several decades in treating women with metastatic breast cancer. It has long been standard protocol for the pathologist to assess the presence of estrogen and progesterone receptors in the malignant tumor cells. Currently, a common means of hormone receptor analysis is by immunohistochemistry performed on paraffin-embedded tissue, a technique that allows for direct visualization of the tumor cells. Two immunohistochemical assays routinely are performed—one for estrogen receptors and one for progesterone receptors. If the hormone receptors are present on the malignant cells, they attract the specific antibodies in the staining solution (the "immuno" part of the term *immunohistochemistry*) and the reaction is visualized as a "brown stain" (the "histochemistry" portion of the test name). Lack of staining indicates the absence of the respective hormone receptor. The pathologist's report will document the presence or absence of estrogen and progesterone receptors, as the lack of these receptors indicates a tumor that may not respond to hormonal manipulation therapy.

Recent decades have seen a variety of prognostic factors investigated for their utility for guiding treatment options or predicating outcomes. Few are in routine use. However, the expression of the oncogene HER2/neu is correlated with a specific therapy, and its assessment (by immunohistochemistry or other means) might become routine (see Figure 5-4).

Colorectal Carcinoma
Screening for Colorectal Carcinoma

Colorectal carcinoma ranks as the third cancer killer in both men and women in the United States, accounting for approximately 55,000 annual deaths, or about 10% of all cancer deaths in men and 11% in women. Almost 6% of Americans, or

Figure 5-4. Algorithm for Breast Cancer

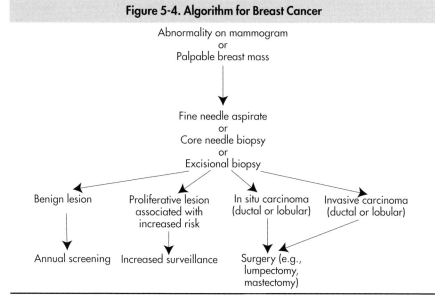

1 in 18, will develop colorectal carcinoma during their lives (Greenlee et al., 2000). No current tumor marker blood test is suitable for screening purposes.

Known risk factors for colorectal carcinoma include familial syndromes such as familial adenomatous polyposis and hereditary nonpolyposis colorectal cancer syndromes. Molecular testing for the mutation in the APC gene associated with familial adenomatous polyposis is currently available, and the routine application of molecular assays for other mutations is likely to be possible in the near future (Hamilton, 1999).

The ACS screening recommendations for the general population suggest that adults begin annual fecal occult blood testing at age 50 (Smith et al., 2000). A flexible sigmoidoscopy should be obtained at age 50 and then every five years. An alternative protocol is to obtain a double-contrast barium enema at age 50 and, thereafter, every 5–10 years. A third option is to undergo colonoscopy every 10 years starting at age 50.

The goal of screening is to decrease the morbidity and mortality from colon and rectal cancers in two important ways: to detect early-stage carcinomas of the bowel and to detect and remove adenomatous polyps. Such polyps are visible on the mucosal surfaces as elevated lesions and are believed to be precursors to invasive cancers.

The efficacy of the fecal occult blood (stool guaiac) test is contingent on the fact that cancer and large polyps may bleed, and products of that blood can be detected in the patient's stool. Although this test has both low sensitivity for cancer and low specificity (many conditions will give a positive stool guaiac result), it is a very convenient screening test because it allows the patient to discreetly collect fecal specimen samples at home over a three-day period and return the cards to the physician's office or laboratory. To increase the accuracy of the test, the patients must be instructed to avoid red meats, poultry, fish, raw vegetables, vitamin C and iron supplements, and nonsteroidal anti-inflammatory drugs and aspirin. Positive tests are followed by either double-contrast barium enema or colonoscopy. If any of the screening or follow-up examinations reveal mucosal lesions, biopsies are taken and sent to the pathologist for diagnostic examination.

Premalignant Colorectal Lesions

The natural history of colorectal carcinoma is believed to follow a sequence of epithelial dysplasia, adenomatous polyp, and adenocarcinoma. By the ninth decade of life, colorectal adenomas are present in more than 50% of the population, although colorectal cancer develops in only 5% of the population (Hamilton, 1999). The identification and removal of colorectal polyps therefore plays an important role in the prevention of colorectal cancer.

For patients with inflammatory bowel diseases (i.e., Crohn's disease or ulcerative colitis), the risk for colorectal carcinoma is higher, and surveillance protocols with random biopsies of the entire colon are done at appropriate intervals. The finding of high-grade dysplasia may lead to total colectomy, as the risk of subsequent invasive carcinoma is high (Fenoglio-Preiser et al., 1999).

Diagnosing Colorectal Carcinoma

By definition, all adenomatous polyps have at least low-grade dysplasia. Those polyps with high-grade dysplasia, carcinoma in situ, or invasive carcinoma confined to the superficial portions of the polyp may be cured by the polypectomy alone (Fenoglio-Preiser et al., 1999). Larger colon cancers often have overgrown the precursor polyp.

The pathologist's report of either the polyp or colectomy specimen with cancer will detail the histologic type and the tumor grade. Colectomy specimens also will be assessed for the depth of invasion into the underlying bowel wall, including any direct extension into surrounding structures, and the presence or absence of metastatic carcinoma to regional lymph nodes will be noted (Compton, Henson, Hutter, Sobin, & Bowman, 1997).

The most common carcinoma of the bowel is adenocarcinoma. Two of the more common variants of adenocarcinoma include mucinous (colloid) carcinoma and signet ring cell carcinoma. Less common are squamous cell, adenosquamous, and small cell carcinomas. The histologic classification is important, as some types are associated with a poorer prognosis (e.g., signet ring cell carcinoma, small cell carcinoma).

The Dukes staging system is an older system that largely has been replaced by the TNM staging protocol. Both systems are based on the depth of tumor invasion into the bowel wall, extension into adjacent structures, and metastasis to regional lymph nodes and distant sites. Staging is best completed after the pathologic examination of the surgically removed colon.

In the TNM staging system (Fleming et al., 1997), invasive cancer that is confined to the lamina propria or muscularis mucosae is considered the equivalent of in situ disease and is given the T designation of Tis. As the tumor invades deeper structures of the bowel wall, the T level is increased to reflect the greater risks of adverse outcome. The regional lymph nodes (N) are assessed for the number of regional lymph nodes with metastatic disease. Metastasis to four or more lymph nodes warrants the highest N level (N2). Distant metastasis is either unknown, absent (M0), or present (M1). Abdominal seeding is considered equivalent to M1. The T, N, and M results are combined to arrive at a tumor stage for treatment and prognostic purposes.

The tumor marker carcinoembryonic antigen (CEA) is a substance secreted into the peripheral blood by many cancers, including colorectal carcinoma. Although not useful as a screening test, CEA does have utility in postoperative surveillance (Wu, 1996) (see Figure 5-5).

Uterine Cervical Cancer
Screening for Cervical Cancer

Cervical cancer is the eighth leading cause of cancer deaths in the United States (Grennlee et al., 2000). Its fall from the leading cause of cancer deaths in the mid-20th century to its current status is due, in part, to the cervical Pap test. Invasive cervical cancer currently accounts for approximately 4,600 deaths per year, which contrasts with the 62,000 annual deaths among American women resulting from lung cancer and the 42,000 annual deaths from breast cancer (Greenlee et al.).

ACS screening recommendations call for annual pelvic examinations and Pap tests in all women who are, or have been, sexually active or have reached the age of 18 years (Smith et al., 2000). These recommendations state that after a woman has had three or more consecutive annual normal Pap tests, the test may be performed less frequently at the discretion of the physician. The College of American Pathologists disagrees and has issued a policy statement encouraging annual Pap tests for all women throughout their lives (College of American Pathologists, 1997).

The current reporting system for the Pap test is the Bethesda system (Kurman & Solomon, 1994). The Bethesda system recommends that the Pap test report contain a statement as to whether endocervical cells are present in the smear. Most cervical dysplasia and carcinomas arise at the squamocolumnar junction, or the transformation zone, where the glandular epithelium of the endocervical canal meets the squamous epithelium of the ectocervix; the lack of endocervical cells can signify inadequate sampling of this area of the cervix.

Abnormal cervical Pap tests may be followed by repeat Pap

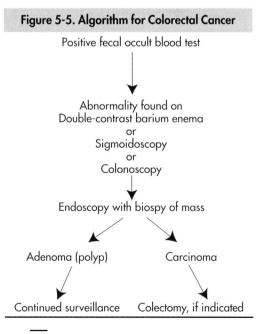

Figure 5-5. Algorithm for Colorectal Cancer

Positive fecal occult blood test

↓

Abnormality found on Double-contrast barium enema or Sigmoidoscopy or Colonoscopy

↓

Endoscopy with biospy of mass

Adenoma (polyp) / Carcinoma

Continued surveillance / Colectomy, if indicated

tests or colposcopy with cervical biopsy. It is generally agreed that up to 90% of squamous cervical cancers, and their precursor lesions, are associated with human papillomavirus (HPV) infections, the most common being types 16 and 18. HPV typing is not routinely performed, but as test methods improve, such typing may play a role in prognosis and treatment options (Smith et al., 2000).

Premalignant Cervical Lesions

Under the Bethesda system for cervical Pap tests, abnormal tests with findings of either premalignant and malignant lesions are placed in the category of "epithelial cell abnormality." The pathologist will then attempt to further classify the lesion. Most of the premalignant, or dysplastic, lesions of the cervix involve squamous cells, and these lesions are further categorized as either low-grade squamous intraepithelial lesions (SIL) or high-grade SIL. Fortunately, there is usually a long period of time (years) between the appearance of SIL and the onset of invasive squamous carcinoma. This long lead time contributes to the effectiveness of the annual Pap smear—most women have ample time to discover the premalignant lesions and be adequately treated.

A Pap test diagnosis of SIL usually is investigated with colposcopy and cervical biopsy to confirm the diagnosis. Dysplasia in the cervical biopsy is commonly diagnosed using the cervical intraepithelial neoplasia (CIN) system. Table 5-7 discusses the correlation between Pap smear and cervical biopsy diagnostic terms (Crum, Cibas, & Lee, 1997).

Traditionally, it was thought that an orderly progression occurred from CIN I through to CIN III, then onto carcinoma in situ, and finally to invasive cancer—a process that could take decades. This assumption has been challenged: probably depending on the HPV type, lesions can start out at any point in the spectrum and then either regress or progress, although the progression to invasive carcinoma in most instances can still take significant time (Crum, 1999).

Diagnosing Cervical Cancer

Although squamous carcinoma usually is diagnosed in women who have not had a Pap test in the preceding five years, approximately 1 in 500 women who have been treated for CIN III eventually develops an invasive carcinoma (Crum, 1999). As with all malignancies, the prognosis depends on the stage at diagnosis.

Table 5-7. Correlation Between Pap Test and Cervical Biopsy Diagnoses for Premalignant Lesions

Pap Test Diagnoses for Premalignant Lesions	Cervical Biopsy Diagnoses for Premalignant Lesions	
Squamous intraepithelial lesion, low-grade	Low-grade dysplasia	Cervical intraepithelial lesion (CIN) I
Squamous intraepithelial lesion, high-grade	Moderate-grade dysplasia High-grade dysplasia	CIN II CIN III (includes carcinoma in situ)

The pathologist's report will give the histologic type of the tumor, usually squamous carcinoma or, less often, adenocarcinoma. Grading is considered optional, but most pathologists will grade carcinomas (Kurman & Amin, 1999). The utility of HPV typing is uncertain, and such testing currently is not routinely performed.

The TNM staging system for cervical cancer (Fleming et al., 1997) assesses the extent of tumor spread, such as cervical carcinoma confined to the uterus (T1) or invasion of the mucosa of the bladder or rectum (T4). The status of the regional lymph nodes is noted by either N0 (no regional metastasis) or N1 (regional metastasis present). Distant metastasis also is either absent (M0) or present (M1). The T, N, and M results are combined to arrive at a tumor stage for treatment and prognostic purposes (see Figure 5-6).

Figure 5-6. Algorithm for Cervical Cancer

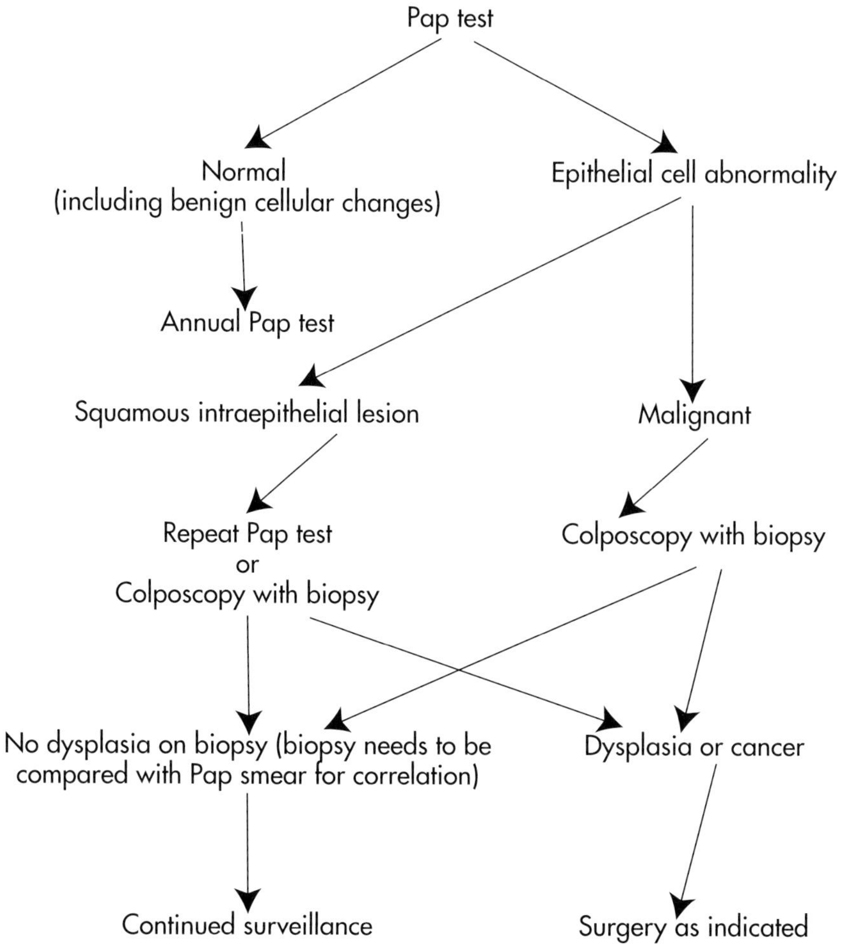

Nursing and Laboratory Medicine

As the role of nurses in the healthcare system evolves, there can be little doubt that their relationship with all patients, not just those with cancer, will be enhanced by a better appreciation of laboratory medicine. By understanding the limitations of laboratory testing, the nurse is in a better position to correlate the clinical expectations with the laboratory result and counsel the patient regarding appropriate medical care. An understanding of the principles of clinical laboratory testing leads to a greater willingness to take responsibility for comprehensive patient teaching, proper specimen collection, and then appropriate handling of the specimen during transport to the laboratory. Those performing the actual testing in the laboratory often cannot determine if a test result is an accurate reflection of the patient's condition or has been biased by inappropriate collection or handling. They rely on physicians and nurses to interpret the test results with knowledge of the patient's condition and an understanding of testing limitations. An understanding of the principles of screening leads to knowledge that can be communicated to patients who may be confused about tests that were "wrong." Enhanced understanding of each other's roles and improved communication between nursing and laboratory personnel can only improve the quality, and cost-effectiveness, of medical care to the patient.

Nurses who treat patients with cancer have additional reasons to understand the role of pathologists in the care of their patients. If there is a diagnosis of cancer, nurses who understand the wealth of information in the pathologist's report are in a position to help patients to understand their diagnosis, prognosis, and treatment options. As new tumor markers and molecular tests are incorporated into routine medical practice, those nurses who establish a collaborative relationship with pathologists will be in a better position to evaluate the true significance of these tests. From this enhanced knowledge, better communication between the nurse and the attending physician about their patients will lead to better use of laboratory tests to improve cancer control

References

Amin, M.B., Grignon, D., Bostwick, D., Reuter, V., Troncoso, P., Ro, J.Y., & Ayala, A.G. (1996). Recommendations for the reporting of resected prostate carcinomas. *Human Pathology, 27,* 321–323.

Bostwick, D.G. (1997). Neoplasms of the prostate. In D.G. Bostwick & J.N. Eble (Eds.), *Urologic surgical pathology* (pp. 342–421). St. Louis, MO: Mosby.

Brawer, M.K. (1999). Prostate-specific antigen: Current status. *CA: A Cancer Journal for Clinicians, 49,* 264–281.

Catalona, W.J., Partin, A.W., Slawin, K.M., Brawer, M.K., Flanigan, R.C., Patel, A., Richie, J.P., deKernion, J.B., Walsh, P.C., Scardino, P.T., Lange, P.H., Subong, E.N.P., Parson, R.E., Gasior, G.H., Loveland, K.G., & Southwick, P.C. (1998). Use of the percentage of free prostate-specific antigen to enhance differentiation of prostate cancer from benign prostatic disease: A prospective multicenter clinical trial. *JAMA, 279,* 1542–1547.

College of American Pathologists. (1997). Frequency of Pap tests. In *College of American Pathologists policies and guidelines manual* (Appendix FF). Northfield, IL. Author.

Compton, C.C., Henson, D.E., Hutter, R.V.P., Sobin, L.H., & Bowman, H.E. (1997). Updated protocol for the examination of specimens removed from patients with colorectal carcinoma. *Archives of Pathology and Laboratory Medicine, 121*, 1247–1254.

Cotran, R.S., Kuman, V., & Collins, T. (1999). Neoplasia. In R.S. Cotran, V. Kuman, & T. Collins (Eds.), *Robbins pathologic basis of disease* (6th ed.) (pp. 260–327). Philadelphia: W.B. Saunders.

Crum, C.P. (1999). The female genital tract. In R.S. Cotran, V. Kuman, & T. Collins (Eds.), *Robbins pathologic basis of disease* (6th ed.) (pp. 1035–1091). Philadelphia: W.B. Saunders.

Crum, C.P., Cibas, E.S., & Lee, K.R. (1997). *Pathology of early cervical neoplasia.* New York: Churchill Livingstone.

Dugan, J.A., Bostwick, D.G., Myers, R.P., Qian, J., Bergstralh, E.J., & Oesterling, J.E. (1996). The definition and preoperative prediction of clinically insignificant prostate cancer. *JAMA, 275*, 288–294.

Fenoglio-Preiser, C.M., Noffsinger, A.E., Stemmermann, G.N., Lantz, P.E., Listrom, M.B., & Rilke, F.O. (1999). *Gastrointestinal pathology: An atlas and text* (2nd ed.). Philadelphia: Lippincott-Raven.

Fisher, B., Costantino, J.P., Wickerham, D.L., Tedmond, C.K., Kavanah, M., Cronin, W.M., Vogel, V., Robidoux, A., Dimitrov, N., Atkins, J., Daly, M., Wieand, S., Tan-Chiu, E., Ford, L., & Wolmark, N. (1998). Tamoxifen for prevention of breast cancer: Report of the National Surgical Adjuvant Breast and Bowel Project P-1 study. *Journal of the National Cancer Institute, 90*, 1371–1388.

Fitzgibbons, P.I., Henson, D.E., & Hutter, R.V.P. (1998). Benign breast changes and the risk for subsequent breast cancer: An update of the 1985 consensus statement. *Archives of Pathology and Laboratory Medicine, 122*, 1053–1055.

Fleming, I.D., Cooper, J.S., Henson, D.E., Hutter, R.V.P., Kennedy, B.J., Murphy, G.P., O'Sullivan, B., Sobin, L.H., & Yarbro, J.W. (1997). *AJCC cancer staging manual* (5th ed.). Philadelphia: Lippincott-Raven.

Frank, T.S. (1999). Laboratory determination of hereditary susceptibility to breast and ovarian cancer. *Archives of Pathology and Laboratory Medicine, 123*, 1023–1026.

Greenlee, R.T., Murray, T., Bolden, S., & Wingo, P.A. (2000). Cancer statistics, 2000. *CA: A Cancer Journal for Clinicians, 50*, 7–33.

Hamilton, S.R. (1999). Colon cancer testing and screening. *Archives of Pathology and Laboratory Medicine, 123*, 1027–1029.

Henson, D.E., Oberman, H.A., & Hutter, R.V.P. (1997). Practice protocol for the examination of specimens removed from patients with cancer of the breast. *Archives of Pathology and Laboratory Medicine, 121*, 27–33.

Ihde, D.C., Pass, H.I., & Glatstein, E. (1997). Small cell lung cancer. In V.T. DeVita, S. Hellman, & S.A. Rosenberg (Eds.), *Cancer: Principles and practice of oncology* (5th ed.) (pp. 911–918). Philadelphia: Lippincott-Raven.

Kurman, R.J., & Amin, M.B. (1999). Protocol for the examination of specimens from patients with carcinomas of the cervix: A basis for checklists. *Archives of Pathology and Laboratory Medicine, 123*, 55–61.

Kurman, R.J., & Solomon, D. (1994). *The Bethesda system for reporting cervical/vaginal cytologic diagnoses: Definitions, criteria, and explanatory notes for terminology and specimen adequacy.* New York: Springer-Verlag.

Pincus, M.R. (1996). Interpreting laboratory results: Reference values and decision making. In J.B. Henry (Ed.), *Clinical diagnosis and management by laboratory methods* (19th ed.) (pp. 74–91). Philadelphia: W.B. Saunders.

Polascik, T.J., Oesterling, J.E., & Partin, A.W. (1999). Prostate specific antigen: A decade of discovery—What we have learned and where we are going. *Journal of Urology, 162,* 293–306.

Rosai, J. (1996). *Ackerman's surgical pathology* (8th ed.). St. Louis, MO: Mosby.

Smith, R.A., Mettlin, C.J., Davis, K.J., & Eyre, H. (2000). American Cancer Society Guidelines for the early detection of cancer. *CA: A Cancer Journal for Clinicians, 50,* 34–49.

Solberg, H.E. (1999). Establishment and use of reference values. In C.A. Burtis & E.R. Ashwood (Eds.), *Tietz textbook of clinical chemistry* (3rd ed.) (pp. 336–356). Philadelphia: W.B. Saunders.

Summary of the second report of the National Cholesterol Education Program (NCEP) Expert Panel on Detection, Evaluation, and Treatment of High Blood Cholesterol in Adults (Adult Treatment Panel II). (1993). *JAMA, 269,* 3015–3023.

Tavassoli, F.A. (1997). *Pathology of the breast.* New York: Appleton & Lange.

von Eschenbach, A., Ho, R., Murphy, G.R., Cunningham, M, & Ling, N (1997). American Cancer Society guideline for the early detection of prostate cancer: Update 1997. *CA: A Cancer Journal for Clinicians, 47,* 261–264.

Wallach, J. (1996). *Interpretation of diagnostic tests* (6th ed.). Boston: Little, Brown & Co.

Woolf, S.H. (1995). Screening for prostate cancer with prostate-specific antigen: An examination of the evidence. *New England Journal of Medicine, 333,* 321–323.

Wu, J.T. (1996). Diagnosis and management of cancer using serologic tumor markers. In J.B. Henry (Ed.), *Clinical diagnosis and management by laboratory methods* (19th ed.) (pp. 74–91). Philadelphia: W.B. Saunders.

CHAPTER 6

An Overview of Bioethical Issues and Approaches in Cancer Prevention, Detection, and Control

Jennifer Flach, BS

Introduction

All areas of healthcare practice and research demand ethical scrutiny. Traditionally, ethical discussions in oncology have focused on issues related to end-of-life care, management of pain and other sequelae of cancer and its treatment, obtaining consent for research participation from patients with cancer, access to novel cancer therapies, and other treatment-centered concerns. In the field of cancer prevention, detection, and control, moral concerns also must be confronted (Flach & Jennings-Dozier, 2000; Weed & Coughlin, 1995). Many of the ethical challenges in this growing field of oncology are different from those found in the cancer treatment arena, while others are similar but more pronounced. As caregivers, researchers, educators, policy makers, and program administrators, nurses encounter ethical conflicts from a variety of perspectives. Nurses should be aware of ethical issues they are likely to face when working in all areas of oncology. This chapter discusses some of the prominent ethical considerations in cancer prevention, detection, and control research and practice and presents methods and theories that can assist nurses in addressing these issues.

Evolution of Bioethics

Ethics, the study of morality, involves the examination and determination of the rightness or wrongfulness of conduct, character attributes, and social policies. Ethics generally is divided into three main branches: normative, descriptive, and metaethics. Normative ethics seeks to determine what people should do (or not do) to act morally. Descriptive ethics is the study of what behavior is considered moral in a society. Insofar as descriptive ethics is not concerned with the "ought" or "should", it differs in focus from normative ethics. The third branch, metaethics, examines morality at a higher, more abstract level. It is concerned with the nature and grounds of systems of beliefs about ethics. Metaethics analyzes the language and concepts of ethical reasoning and examines theories of moral knowledge. In this chapter, the term "bioethics" will primarily relate to the normative branch of ethics.

The study of moral issues in health care, medicine, biomedical research, and related disciplines is called bioethics. Societies and individuals have discussed and debated moral issues related to health since ancient times, although bioethics has emerged as a discipline of its own relatively recently. The Hippocratic Oath, the first known code of medical ethics, is thought to have originated in the fifth century BC (Veatch, 1997). The contemporary bioethics movement started in the 1970s in response to the rapid development of new medical technologies and strides in civil rights resulting from the social reform movements of the 1960s (Arras, Steinbock, & London, 1999). The examination of moral considerations in medical research also was an integral part of the birth of modern bioethics. Gross mistreatment of individuals in Nazi medical experiments and other outrages in human subjects research prompted ethical guidelines. The Nuremberg Code of 1947, the Declaration of Helsinki of 1964 and the United States' Belmont Report of 1979 were promulgated to prevent further misconduct in biomedical research (National Commission for the Protection of Human Subjects of Biomedical and Behavioral Research, 1979). In the 21st century, bioethics remains at the forefront of the public's conscience. The creation of the National Bioethics Advisory Commission (NBAC) in 1995 demonstrates the federal government's increased attention to the ethics of healthcare practice and research (Federal Register, 1995). Ethical decision making is part of the daily lives of healthcare professionals and their clients and families as much as it is a focus of discussion for government bodies, professional associations, and ethics committees. In fact, ethical problems and solutions faced by individual physicians, nurses, researchers, and patients have the potential to create and drive social movements and policies related to the ethics of health care and biological sciences.

In all areas of professional and personal life, human relationships often are the key sources of moral conflict. In bioethics, interactions between nurses and physicians, clients and healthcare professionals, patients and family members, governments and healthcare insurers, and researchers and practitioners can all generate ethical tension. Nurses are well aware that each case and every client involves a different set of concerns, values, and ethical considerations.

Well-intentioned individuals from diverse backgrounds or disciplines are likely to draw different conclusions with respect to patient management or public health planning. Nurses frequently find themselves in ethical struggles stemming from multiple allegiances, such as to the client, client's family, physician, other health team members, society, third-party payors, government, and one's self (Case, 1999).

Changes in technology, economics, and society have an impact on our views of health-related values and priorities as well as modify our definitions of health, family, and other concepts central to discussions of bioethics. Thus, these forces alter the focus and application of ethical methods and theories to science and health care. This is illustrated by the regular updating of guides to ethical conduct for healthcare professionals in response to changing environments and professional duties. The American Nurses Association (ANA) has modified its code of ethics and added interpretative statements several times since its adoption in 1950 (ANA, 1985). The ANA and the Oncology Nursing Society collaborated to publish the *Statement on the Scope and Standards of Oncology Nursing Practice* in 1987 (Fowler, 1993). International guides for ethical conduct, such as the Declaration of Helsinki, have been revised periodically since 1964 (World Medical Association, 1997, 2000) Currently, U.S. regulations and policies regarding human subjects research are being re-examined (Department of Health and Human Services, 2000; Federal Register, 1995; NBAC, 2001).

Sources of Ethical Considerations in Cancer Prevention, Detection, and Control

The field of cancer care has undergone its own changes over time. Strides in the science of cancer prevention, detection, and control, as well as increased cancer survival rates, have reshaped our definition of cancer and its management and created new ethical questions in oncology. Other sources of moral conflicts and concerns have emerged from the larger environment in which oncology care and research reside, namely the managed care system (see Figure 6-1). In cancer prevention, detection, and control, ethical issues are generated by economic, political, social, and scientific and technological forces (Flach & Jennings-Dozier, 2000). While the scope of ethical issues in cancer prevention, detection, and control is vast (Weed & Coughlin, 1995), several of the prominent issues are discussed here and arranged loosely in the categories of economic and political, social, and scientific and technological influences, although these influences certainly overlap. Figure 6-2 contains a larger list of bioethical considerations for nurses working in these areas of oncology. Political and economic influences include the evolution of managed healthcare systems and policies related to the allocation of resources with respect to cancer prevention and detection research. Consumer movements, the increasing cultural and ethnic diversity of the United States, and the growing population of cancer survivors represent some of the social trends affecting the ethics of cancer prevention, detection, and control. Finally, moral questions and concerns result from the expansion of information technologies and biomedical technologies that guide cancer practice and research. A brief overview of ethical implications of cancer risk assessment and screening, genetic testing, the collection and use of human biological specimens for research, and cancer chemoprevention clinical trials is given.

Economic and Political Influences

Managed Health Care

Managed health care has been built on the underlying principles of controlling the escalating costs of care and promoting preventive strategies, but it has been marked by a host of problems, including ethical concerns. Healthcare profession-

Figure 6-1. General Sources of Bioethical Issues for Nurses

• Definitions of health and disease
• Client and family conflict
• Religious and cultural values
• Capacity and competence
• Legal versus ethical issues
• Informed consent
• Right to assent to or refuse care or participation in research
• Confidentiality
• Professional codes and standards
• Institutional policies
• Conflicts of interest
• Dual roles of researcher and healthcare practitioner
• Government policies and priorities
• Insurance coverage for care and research
• Managed health care
• Biotechnology and pharmaceutical activities
• Nurse-client relationships
• Nurse-physician relationships
• Rationing, allocation, and access to health care
• Care for special populations (age, ethnicity, race, gender, education, economic level)
• Minority representation in clinical trials
• Consumerism
• Patient advocacy
• Scientific knowledge and medical technology
• Information technology
• Tissue banking and research
• Human subjects protection
• Institutional review boards
• Complementary and alternative approaches
• Quality of life
• Reproductive issues

Note. From "Ethical Issues in Oncology Nursing Practice: An Overview of Topics and Strategies," by G. Winters, E. Glass, and C. Sakurai, 1993, *Oncology Nursing Forum, 20*(Suppl. 10), p. 26. Copyright 1993 by the Oncology Nursing Press, Inc. Adapted with permission.

als, public policymakers, and consumers have criticized managed-care systems that focus on cost reduction and increased profits rather than on providing high-quality health care (Council on Ethical and Judicial Affairs, American Medical Association, 1995). Managed-care organizations are diverse in terms of financial structure, size, focus, clinician participation, and ethical aspects. Barriers to ethical care are more likely to be found in managed-care organizations that are for-profit, provide strong financial incentives for healthcare professionals to control costs, and have direct capitation arrangements (Christensen, 1999). These elements create conflicts of interest that place nurses and physicians in competing roles of trying to provide quality care to their clients while also reducing medical costs. Patient care and autonomy may be compromised when physicians have diminished autonomy and benefit in some way from withholding services to save resources. Professional integrity, the need to prevent harm to clients, and the desire for the respect of peers often direct healthcare professionals away from

---

Figure 6-2. Sources of Bioethical Issues for Nurses Working in Cancer Prevention, Detection, and Control

- Conception of cancer
- Early detection technology
- Screening programs
- Risk assessment and notification
- Biomarker risk testing
- Genetic screening
- Genetic risk for cancer
- Genetic components of behavior
- Genetic counseling
- Environmental causes of cancer
- Employment or insurance discrimination based on risk or cancer detection
- Stigmatization based on genetic risk
- High-risk families
- Risk assessment in children and adolescents
- Gene transfer
- Cancer vaccines
- Prophylactic surgeries
- Chemoprevention
- Behavioral and lifestyle interventions
- Survivorship
- Second cancers
- Priorities in research and care among treatment, prevention, detection, and control
- Competition for research and care resources among types of cancer and conditions

---

incentives in managed care. External forces that can reduce negative forces of financial incentives and promote quality care include medical practice guidelines, peer review, fear of malpractice, patient/member involvement, and regulation and legislation (Christensen, 1999). If properly structured and focused, managed-care organizations can lead to improved healthcare services for individuals and society. Some health-maintenance organizations have claimed to expand cancer-control programs, such as breast cancer screening, by breaking down barriers to services and by positioning such programs as healthcare priorities (Mandelson & Thompson, 1998). When Kaiser Permanente introduced BRCA1 and BRCA2 testing to practice, it developed a program of practice guidelines, health-professional education and training, and genetic counseling (Kutner, 1999). While some managed care organizations may raise obstacles to quality and ethical care, persons without medical insurance may experience greater barriers. Issues related to delivering cancer prevention, detection, and control services to the uninsured and underinsured are discussed in the sections on special populations.

Allocation of Cancer Research Costs

The costs and potential benefits of research programs are prime considerations when setting priorities in the healthcare agenda. Policymakers have to determine who in society will benefit and who will bear the burdens associated with decisions about health research and care. Controlled, randomized clinical trials of cancer prevention and screening with cancer incidence and/or mortality endpoints often are highly expensive because they tend to require large sample sizes, the participation of multiple research centers, and long-term interventions and follow-up for study subjects (Prentice, 1995; Prorok, 1995). Often, funding for and enrollment in clinical research must rely on insurance reimbursement for the costs of routine medical examinations and other procedures. Invasive procedures that are not medically indicated but are needed to assess cancer biomarker endpoints add to the costs and risks associated with prevention studies; conversely, in treatment studies, most invasive treatments stipulated by the research also may be considered part of standard care. Insurance companies are less likely to pay for medical procedures and clinical visits that are required of research protocol but fall outside of the standard of care. For these reasons, leaders of research and public health organizations may find it difficult to dedicate heavy resources to prevention and screening research; however, the long-term rewards of developing and implementing cancer prevention strategies compel society to pursue research in this arena.

Research establishments, investigators, healthcare professionals, insurance organizations, governments, and the public grapple with questions of moral and social responsibilities for the support of medical research. Increasingly, members of the research community, the public, and government officials are urging medical insurance companies to help support clinical research (Chemoprevention Working Group to the American Association for Cancer Research, 1999; National Cancer Institute [NCI], 1999a). Insurance organizations are better positioned to create scientifically sound and ethically justified coverage plans when they possess evidence from clinical research that can inform them about prudent medical practice. Thus, third-party payors have a stake in the progress of research. In addition, advances in medical knowledge and technology in cancer prevention and early detection can lead to reduced insurance costs in the long run by allowing payors to avoid the high costs of cancer treatment and supportive care. Advocates for insurance coverage of clinical studies argue these benefits of research should compel them to reimburse clients for participation in clinical studies. Some states have begun to pass legislation requiring insurance companies to provide coverage for clinical trials. The state of Maryland passed a bill that demands coverage for some clinical trials for cancer and other life-threatening diseases (General Assembly of Maryland, 1998). NCI, the federal government's leading institute for cancer research, is seeking agreements with insurance organizations for support of some of the costs incurred by patients participating in clinical trials (NCI, 1999b). The Health Care Financing Administration now provides coverage for certain clinical trials for medicare recipients (HCFA, 2000). While these efforts have focused primarily on expenses related to promising experimental therapies, research sponsors and study participants often must continue to pay for additional costs required by prevention and screening trials. Clinical trial nurses frequently interact with third-party payors and healthcare professionals from cooperating practices to arrange for the coverage of research expenses that otherwise would be paid by the research participants. Nurses also are well positioned to inform about and influence policies and programs for funding clinical trial research in cancer prevention, detection, and control.

Social Trends

Consumer Movements

Consumer movements, such as those dealing with women's rights and patient advocacy, can promote shifts in public health priorities, access to medical care, and biomedical research agendas and alter the nature of health professional-client relationships. Civil rights movements and increased consumerism also have sparked an increased awareness of bioethical issues. In particular, these events have led to an emphasis on patient autonomy that supplanted the paternalistic paradigm of the doctor-patient relationship, which dominated the era of modern medicine until recently (Thomasma, 2000). In the past, the clinician's perception of the patient's best interest was the major determinant of ethical medical care. Today in the United States, medical ethics demands that patients be provided with the opportunity to participate in decisions about their care. In addition, patient advocacy movements, such as those related to AIDS and breast cancer, have shown how consumers can shape healthcare priorities and perceptions of rights to care by raising questions about ethical healthcare rationing and individual rights (McCabe, Varricchio, Padberg, & Simpson, 1995).

As healthcare users have become more sophisticated, and in some cases more skeptical about the medical research establishment, a greater emphasis has been placed on consumer input into decisions about medical research. This trend is illustrated by a report issued by the Office of Inspector General, Department of Health and Human Services (1998), which called for greater consumer representation on institutional review boards, the independent bodies that review research proposals for the protection of human subjects. In cancer research, consumer movements have increased support for cancer prevention trials that previously may have been considered dangerous because of risks to "healthy" volunteers. In addition, formal participant advisory boards have emerged to give research volunteers input into the design and conduct of clinical studies, such as the National Surgical Adjuvant Breast and Bowel Project's (NSABP's) Breast Cancer Prevention Trial (BCPT) (Psillidis, Flach, & Padberg, 1997). In the BCPT, the selective estrogen receptor modulator tamoxifen reduced the risk of developing breast cancer by almost 50% in women who were at increased risk for the disease (Fisher et al., 1998). Tamoxifen is now an option for many women who have an elevated risk for breast cancer.

Population Diversity and Cancer Control

The U.S. population is becoming progressively more multicultural and is characterized by large differences in age and socioeconomic status. The diversity of society carries important implications for healthcare access, delivery, and priorities. The dilemma of equitable allocation of limited health resources is exacerbated in such a heterogeneous society, posing a serious ethical challenge. In the United States, considerable discussion revolves around questions of moral responsibility for lessening the disparity of health care among special populations. Questions about the equitable distribution of health care, such as cancer prevention and screening programs, touch on a more encompassing issue that relates to how well-being is defined in a society. When resources are scarce, efforts to address social inequalities involve the prioritization of values and rights in a community, such as those related to food and shelter in addition to various aspects of health care.

Wide disparities in the burden of cancer exist between the general population and a variety of special populations. Special populations carrying greater burden may include the working poor, homeless, and others with low incomes; people with limited education, literacy, and language ability; elderly, adolescents, and children; women; the geographically isolated; people with diverse cultural backgrounds and lifestyles; racial and ethnic minorities; and the medically uninsured and underinsured (Facione & Facione, 1997; NCI, 1999b). People from ethnic minority populations often have worse cancer outcomes than their counterparts in the general population, as do economically disadvantaged people from all ethnic backgrounds (Haynes & Smedley, 1999). Special populations have a higher incidence of cancer, lower survival rates, and a greater chance of dying from cancer. There is considerable evidence that this imbalance is usually the result of differences in detection, treatment, and preventive care rather than biological reasons (NCI, 1999b).

Disparities in the accessibility of health care can be greater in the preventive setting than in the treatment environment. When a person has no obvious signs of illness, he or she is less motivated to seek medical care, pay medical expenses, and follow healthcare recommendations than are those who are suffering from disease. On top of these challenges, distributing the benefits of state-of-the-art prevention and detection to special populations requires breaking down financial, social, cultural, educational, and other barriers (Freeman, 1989; Mandelblatt, Yabroff, & Kerner, 1999; Olsen & Frank-Stromborg, 1993; Underwood, 1995). Racial differences between healthcare providers and patients can create barriers to cancer control. Cultural, socioeconomic, and age differences that affect perceptions and attitudes about prevention and screening practices are important considerations in delivering proven prevention and detection techniques to diverse communities. Moral conflicts result when cultural values and personal beliefs conflict with optimal healthcare practices (Case, 1999). Nurses delivering cancer prevention and detection interventions are likely to encounter instances when the medical benefit to the client may be at odds with the individual's spiritual or cultural beliefs. In addition, the ramifications of introducing screening and related control programs to underserved communities should be considered prior to embarking on such an effort. Psychological and social harm can be caused when screening programs are brought to communities whose members do not have the means to pay for proper medical care if problems are detected.

Cancer Survivors

Progress in early detection and cancer therapies has led to a growing number of long-term survivors of cancer, who represent another population with special cancer prevention and detection needs. Survivors experience a wide range of negative physical (Loescher et al., 1989) and psychosocial effects (Welch-McCaffrey, 1989) for years after successful treatment (Dow, Ferrell, Haberman, & Eaton, 1999; Ferrell & Dow, 1997; Meadows et al., 1998).

Long-lasting symptoms, such as fatigue and depression, can cause survivors to experience problems in the workplace, with relationships, and in other areas of life. They may experience financial hardship resulting from treatment costs and time away from work during therapy. Cancer survivors often are at higher risk for second cancers, which carries implications to privacy, confidentiality and discrimination, and economic considerations related to increased monitoring. When caring for cancer survivors, from diagnosis through long-term survival, physicians and nurses will need to identify and address ethical issues related to the unmet needs and concerns of individuals from this special population. Fostering survivors' skills in personal and public advocacy can empower cancer survivors (Clark & Stovall, 1996). Government representatives and investigators are increasingly paying attention to survivorship concerns when designing research programs and public policies. Cancer survivors have special experiences that give them the unique ability to reach and educate the public about cancer control and prevention (Haynes & Smedley, 1999). By participating in educational activities in the community and advisory roles in health policy and research planning, they may assist healthcare providers in reaching less accessible populations and lessening the burden of cancer. Survivors have the potential to benefit society by strengthening efforts in prevention, detection, and control practice and research. They often are selected as the study population in prevention studies because they are at higher risk for cancer than the general population because of the risk of recurrence or second primaries (Kelloff et al., 1997). Survivors who elect to participate in these efforts may receive personal rewards, such as satisfaction from acting on altruistic motives or improved outlook and self-esteem that may result from fighting back against the disease.

Research Involving Special Populations

Participation in clinical studies by members of special populations is necessary for applying research results to these groups (NCI, 1999a). While ethnic minorities and special populations generally are represented proportionately in cancer treatment studies, their enrollment in cancer prevention and control trials tends to fall short in this respect (Haynes & Smedley, 1999; NCI, 1999a). Reasons for this disparity are numerous. People who are cancer-free are less motivated to enroll and remain in research studies as compared to people with cancer and are willing to accept only minimal toxicity (Dunn et al., 1998). Randomized, controlled cancer prevention and screening trials expect heavy commitments of study participants because of the long duration of trials with cancer endpoints. Also, the potential benefits of trial participation may seem more subtle and distant in prevention and screening studies than in cancer treatment studies (McCabe, Varricchio, & Padberg, 1994). In special populations, limited health-related education, lack of medical insurance, lower incomes, cultural beliefs, low literacy and/or proficiency in the English language, and distrust of the medical research establishment add to these barriers to prevention study participation (Good, 2000; Millon-Underwood, Sanders, & Davis, 1993).

Attention and resources increasingly are being dedicated to research on and care of special populations. Traditionally, women and children have been viewed as "vulnerable" populations and were systematically excluded from participation in clinical studies to protect them from research risks. The scientific community and the public have now acknowledged that enrollment of both genders, racial and ethnic minorities, children, and other special populations in clinical research is essential for translating research findings to these populations. The National Institutes of Health (NIH) has created policies, guidelines, and funding programs to stimulate the inclusion of special populations to NIH-sponsored clinical studies (Federal Register, 1994; NIH, 1998).

For example, when the results of NSABP's BCPT were released, concerns were voiced about generalizing the potential benefits and risks because the overwhelming majority of participants in the BCPT were educated, middle- to upper-class White women, despite intense efforts to recruit women from special populations (Haynes & Smedley, 1999). Recently, a meta-analysis using data from breast cancer adjuvant therapy studies showed no significant difference in tamoxifen effects in White and African American women (McCaskill-Stevens et al., 2000). These data were only available for examination because tamoxifen was used initially in the adjuvant setting. Investigators could not have gleaned that information from prevention studies alone.

Promoting representation of special populations in cancer prevention, detection, and control studies carries ethical considerations for the participants in the research. Many believe that members of special populations should be afforded greater protection from research risks than those in the general population because they are more likely to be harmed or wronged. Measures that can be undertaken to achieve this end include modifying informed-consent procedures for people who do not speak English or have low literacy skills and counseling women of childbearing potential about pregnancy prevention when participating in studies of potentially teratogenic drugs. Reducing the potential harms of research can make trials more difficult and expensive and interfere with progress in science that can benefit individuals in the future. Protections such as protocol-specific restrictions on the types of contraceptives that can be used can conflict with individual values and autonomous decision making of individuals considering participation in the study.

Recruitment strategies for cancer prevention and control studies should be respectful and considerate of the members of the community (Good, 2000). To reduce potential harms and respect the rights of individuals in special populations, many advocate for input from community representatives in designing clinical studies and forming research policies. Offering healthcare resources and education that can improve decision making about health practices and clinical research participation also have been touted to help to foster mutually-beneficial relationships between researchers and the community.

Scientific and Technological Sources

Information Technology

The growth of information technologies is creating new ethical concerns in the field of health care. Modern computer science has significantly increased our ability to store, analyze, and transfer large amounts of data. As a result, healthcare professionals, institutions, and governments must pay greater attention to privacy and confidentiality issues in both practice and biomedical research (National Research Council, Computer Science and Telecommunications Board, 1997). In addition, the World Wide Web and other modern forms of communication have provided consumers access to increasing amounts of health information, which is largely unmonitored. Because monitoring and ensuring the accuracy of health claims appearing on the Internet is simply not possible, consumers, government officials, and healthcare professionals worry about the consequences of misinformation. Lack of access to electronic communications and other modern forms of communication may lead to wider gaps in knowledge and health care among members of society (NCI, 1999a). Factors such as cultural background, age, and socioeconomic status may influence one's ability and inclination to use electronic communications. Finally, there are fears that if mass media pushes aside other important forms of health communication, such as one-on-one conversations between healthcare professionals and clients, the quality of health care will be compromised. Accurate and understandable information is critical to delivering the benefits of cancer prevention and detection strategies and to facilitating autonomous patient decision making. Nurses should be cognizant of both the potential benefits and drawbacks of using electronic forms of communication in health care and research activities.

Biomedical Technology

Any new medical intervention has ramifications in a number of realms, including physical, psychological, economic, and social; therefore, potential harms are associated with releasing new interventions to the public (see Figure 6-3). This is especially true when interventions are disseminated before the risks of long-term or widespread use of the new technology have been well studied. Moral concerns often are raised when advances in technology supercede our understanding of the

Figure 6-3. Cartoon Depiction of Public Fears Concerning New Biomedical Technology

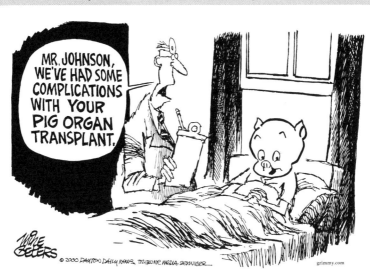

impact that technology has on individuals and society. Also, the release of clinically proven but expensive medical technologies to the general public raises ethical questions relating both to equitable access and to cost/benefit considerations. When state-of-the-art medical procedures only are available to people of higher socioeconomic status, disparities in access to quality health care are increased. Insurers, governments, and institutions often are faced with difficult decisions about how and to whom new technologies should be offered. These are only some of the many ethical considerations that are driven by progress in scientific knowledge and technology in biomedicine. The expansion of cancer prevention, detection, and control practice and research has provoked ethical discussion in such areas as cancer prevention clinical trials, genetic testing and other methods of cancer risk assessment, and the use of human tissue specimens for cancer prevention and detection research.

Cancer Prevention Research

The field of prevention science involves investigation of the causes and sequence of events in the process of cancer development, with the ultimate goal of evaluating interventions to stop or reverse the initiation or progression of changes leading to cancer (Chemoprevention Implementation Group, 1999). Chemoprevention studies test synthetic and natural agents for their effectiveness in preventing or prolonging cancer occurrence. Clinical research is important for confirming or dismissing promising laboratory results and epidemiological data (Chemoprevention Working Group, 1999). Only through studies involving humans can researchers properly test the effectiveness and toxicities (or other potential harms) of potential preventive interventions.

Clinical trials of cancer prevention involve a host of ethical considerations in terms of study design and implementation and interpretation and communication of scientific findings (Dunn, Kramer, & Ford, 1998). Ethical questions also revolve around issues such as determining acceptable risk-to-benefit ratios for "healthy" research participants, achieving appropriate representation of special populations in prevention trials, and setting research priorities when resources are limited. Research nurses and other investigators are bound to encounter novel ethical concerns as they move from traditional studies of cancer therapy into clinical cancer prevention research. Emanuel, Wendler, and Grady (2000) proposed seven requirements for deciding whether a clinical research study is ethical (see Table 6-1). Several of these requirements—including a favorable risk-benefit ratio, scientific validity, and fair selection of subjects—often are more difficult to fulfill in cancer prevention studies than in cancer treatment studies. Besides the issues related to the enrollment of special populations in cancer prevention and the costs of prevention studies that were discussed earlier in this chapter, other issues are highlighted here.

In general, prevention studies target populations who are symptom free but at increased risk for developing cancer because of biological, clinical, and/or epidemiological factors. When a study involves people who are not presenting clinical disease, a lower level of physical and psychosocial risk is tolerable as compared to studies involving people with serious disease (Dunn et al., 1998; Nayfield, 1996). Mechanisms for monitoring and reducing toxicity are crucial aspects of chemoprevention study design. Prevention studies may require participants to

Table 6-1. Seven Requirements for Determining Whether a Research Trial Is Ethical

Requirements	Explanation	Justifying Ethical Values
Social or scientific value	Evaluation of a treatment, intervention, or theory that will improve health and well-being or increase knowledge	Scarce resources and nonexploitation
Scientific validity	Use of accepted scientific principles and methods, including statistical techniques, to produce reliable and valid data	Scarce resources and nonexploitation
Fair subject selection	Selection of subjects so that stigmatized and vulnerable individuals are not targeted for risky research and the rich and socially powerful are not favored for potentially beneficial research	Justice
Favorable risk-benefit ratio	Minimization of risks; enhancement of potential benefits; risks to the subject are proportionate to the benefits to the subject and society	Nonmaleficence, beneficence, and nonexploitation
Independent review	Review of the design of the research trial, its proposed subject population, and risk-benefit ratio by individuals unaffiliated with the research	Public accountability; minimizing influence or potential conflicts of interest
Informed consent	Provision of information to subjects about purpose of the research, its procedures, potential risks, benefits, and alternatives so that the individual understands this information and can make a voluntary decision whether to enroll and continue to participate	Respect for subject autonomy
Respect for potential and enrolled subjects	Respect for subjects by (1) Permitting withdrawal from the research (2) Protecting privacy through confidentiality (3) Informing subjects of newly discovered risks or benefits (4) Informing subjects of results of clinical research (5) Maintaining welfare of subjects	Respect for subject autonomy and welfare

Note. From "What Makes Clinical Research Ethical?" by R.J. Emanuel, D. Wendler, and C. Grady, 2000, *JAMA, 283*, p. 2703.

undergo invasive procedures that are not medically indicated to obtain tissue specimens for the analysis of biomarkers that may be precursors to cancer or to detect early cancers (Dunn et al.). Such invasive procedures unfavorably shift the study's risk-to-benefit ratio, as well.

Prevention studies usually target populations at increased risk for developing cancer. In addition to physical risks and discomfort, prevention trials may entail psychological and social risks associated with having an increased risk for cancer. Individuals may be identified as having an increased risk prior to seeking enrollment in a cancer prevention trial, at trial entry according to risk assessments needed to determine eligibility, or during the conduct of the trial through the evaluation of tissue samples or other means. Prevention research studies may ask that individuals with a family history of cancer undergo genetic testing so investigators can better understand the individual's level and type of risk. Potential harms are associated with the release of information about individuals' risk for developing cancer, such as the potential for inappropriate discrimination in insurance or employment based on risk status. A third party could label the individual at high risk based on knowledge of the individual's participation in a prevention study in which the entry criteria require an elevated cancer risk. Measures to protect the confidentiality of research records are critical to respecting the privacy of participants as well as preventing harm resulting from disclosure. Risk assessments used in prevention trials may be considered suitable for the research context but have not been validated for clinical use. In some studies, the investigators may be able decide whether participants or their physicians should be given the opportunity to receive individual test results at all. If participants are informed of risk assessment results, the limitations of such tests should be communicated to the participants and, if appropriate, to their healthcare providers or insurers. Genetic counseling should be provided if individuals are given access to test results (ASCO Subcommittee on Genetic Testing for Cancer Susceptibility, 1996). An informed-consent process that conveys the risks and purposes of the study is important to facilitating autonomous decision making about participation.

Compared to research into cancer treatment, cancer prevention research is in its infancy. The validity of many of these newer scientific approaches is not as well established as the long-standing methods used in treatment trials. Randomized controlled chemoprevention trials that have endpoints of cancer incidence are considered to provide a higher level of scientific evidence than noncontrolled or other forms of investigation (CancerNet, 2000b). However, because of the high costs of and time required for these studies, alternative designs may be implemented (Kelloff et al., 1997). One approach uses biological markers, such as modulation of precursor lesions, as surrogate endpoints for cancer. The advantages to science, society, and research participants of biomarker studies as alternatives to large prevention trials include that they are shorter in duration, require fewer numbers of participants, and generally are less expensive than prevention trials with cancer endpoints. In theory, answers about potential chemoprevention agents may be discovered faster at less cost, allowing promising agents to be made available to the public sooner. Also, ineffective or unacceptably toxic agents can be dismissed before exposing larger populations to the agent. Biomarker studies can also be conducted during or following studies of incidence or mortality to refine our understanding of the chemopreventive agent (Prentice, 1995). Large studies often are necessary to confirm studies of biomarkers and assess the intervention's impact on cancer incidence and its long-term effects. The scientific validity of many cancer biomarkers remains to be established, and investigators must choose study biomarkers carefully and interpret research results cautiously (Kelloff et al., 1997; Prentice, 1995). Using biomarker endpoints is often more complex than endpoints of tumor response and survival used in cancer therapeutic trials. Thus, participant risk, benefits and costs to society, and questions of scientific validity and value must be analyzed in ethical decision making about chemoprevention studies.

A fair selection of participants in chemoprevention research involves defining the study population and employing participant recruitment methods that are unlikely to lead to the enrollment of people who will be harmed by the investigational agent, procedures, and associated costs. Populations of individuals who are at increased risk for cancer and are generally healthy usually are targeted for chemoprevention studies. Although this approach may reduce risks and increase potential benefits to study participants, questions may remain about the use of new chemopreventive agents in less healthy individuals or in people with lower risk for cancer, if the agent is found to be effective in the study. Participant recruitment and retention is more difficult and resource-intensive in prevention trials than in treatment trials because healthy individuals are less motivated to enroll in and continue in research than are patients with cancer or other diseases (Good, 2000). In response, researchers may entertain creative recruitment approaches. A controversial practice is offering monetary payments to participants in an attempt to compensate them for the potential discomfort of study agents and procedures associated with some cancer prevention studies. Ethical concerns are associated with offering payments to subjects for research participation (Dickert & Grady, 1999). Payments to participants or the offer of free monitoring can sound enticing enough to interfere with the individual's careful deliberation about study participation. For the medically underserved, these perceived benefits may act as even higher incentives to study participation. When economically disadvantaged people agree to accept additional risks and physical discomfort to obtain services or income that most of society can access readily, an ethical standard of fairness in the selection of research participants is not achieved.

Cancer Detection and Risk Assessment

The goals of improving technologies to detect cancer, precancerous conditions, or predisposition to cancer more accurately and earlier in the carcinogenic process are to increase survival and decrease the burden associated with the disease. New cancer-detection technologies and greater knowledge about environmental and behavioral risk factors offer individuals the opportunity to make more informed decisions about medical choices, family planning, and lifestyles. Carcinogenesis is a continuum. Detection and prevention of cancer are functions of technology and our understanding of the carcinogenic process.

Complexity of Risk

Nurses involved in cancer risk assessment, counseling, and follow-up care for people at risk must be aware of a variety of ethical considerations. These include concerns related to the interpretation and communication of risk information, the potential for negative psychosocial and physical outcomes, the costs and access to risk assessment and related care, and privacy and confidentiality rights of clients.

Because of the complexities of cancer risk and the multitude of interpretations of the term "risk," information about cancer risk often is difficult to communicate to clients and their families, as well as to society and public policy makers. Personal values, experiences, cultural backgrounds, and opinions of significant others may influence how individuals perceive and react to risk information. "Risk" refers to something different across disciplines such as nursing, medicine, epidemiology, and anthropology and for the lay public (Jacobs, 2000). The probabilistic nature of risk also is a difficult concept to communicate. Cancer risk may include many components—behavioral, environmental, and/or genetic—of which there are varying levels of control and understanding. Assessing cancer risk is, therefore, a challenging endeavor that includes detecting biological predisposition to cancer, recognizing epidemiological contributors, and discerning how various gene-gene and gene-environment interactions occur in different individuals.

Furthermore, the interpretation of risk-assessment techniques for cancer predisposition and precursors is fraught with challenges. The interpretation of biological tests is susceptible to ambiguity as a result of the technical limitations such as false-positive results, false-negative results, and unclear results. This can be compounded by an incomplete understanding of the clinical significance of the results for individuals because of a lack of consensus of the predictability of the test or the medical management of risk or early stages for that particular cancer. The potential harms associated with identifying biological risk factors for cancer development can be great when little is known about the clinical implications of having those risk factors, the limitations of the testing results, and strategies for reducing the risk associated with those factors. The acquisition of medical risk information should increase autonomy by promoting informed decision making; however, decision making may not be facilitated when medical options are unchanged despite greater knowledge.

Risk-Benefit Considerations

The balance between the costs and benefits of screening tests and novel risk-assessment tools for individuals and groups is dependent upon the pace of related advances in cancer detection, prevention, and treatment science. While chemoprevention and nutritional science are evolving, risk management options such as "watchful waiting" and prophylactic surgeries continue to be the leading alternatives. For many precancerous conditions and some early-stage, slow-growing cancers (e.g., prostate cancer), a reasonable option is a "watchful waiting" approach that includes increased monitoring to detect early cancers or progression of the existing cancer. Although medically justified, wait-and-see approaches to cancer management elicit feelings of a loss of control and fatalism. In addition, psychological sequelae, such as anxiety and feeling helpless, are associated with being at increased risk for a disease that has no or limited preventive options. Such psychological distress may, in turn, lead to decreased compliance with monitoring recommendations. Lack of finances or medical insurance can increase the negative psychosocial effects of the diagnosis and decrease compliance with monitoring guidelines. Removal of precursor lesions or prophylactic surgery may be options for the management of increased cancer risk when there are no accepted alternate preventive strategies, such as lifestyle changes, diet modifications, or chemoprevention interventions. With some types of prophylactic surgeries, the adverse physical outcomes for someone identified as at increased risk for cancer may not be significantly less than the treatment options. For a woman who is at increased risk for breast cancer because of a strong family history, prophylactic mastectomy may offer a slightly decreased risk, but the physical and psychological sequelae are significant (Hartmann et al., 1999).

Prostate-specific antigen (PSA) testing for the detection of prostate cancer has generated extensive ethical discussion. The use of PSA screening became widespread before the medical community had reached agreement about whether the results of PSA screening and the detection and treatment of prostate cancer at earlier stages were associated with greater benefit or harm to patients (Chan & Sulmasy, 1998; Godley, 1999). In addition, the target population for this screening test is not defined. Patients, their families, and healthcare providers must wrestle with conflicting recommendations by medical associations until further investigations provide answers to the question of PSA screening. Recommendations for screening programs should be based on the accuracy of the screening technology, identification of the appropriate population and testing intervals, and understanding of the safety and cost of screening (Foltz, 2000).

Even when safe and effective monitoring or preventive interventions are available for individuals in a particular risk category, those at risk may face psychosocial harms. Patients identified as having an increased risk of developing cancer may have concerns about privacy and confidentiality. Notification to third parties of cancer risk results may lead to inappropriate discrimination in employment and health and life insurance, for instance (see Figure 6-4). All of these considerations should be taken in account as nurses educate patients about risk assessment, risk management, and early detection for cancer. In genetic testing for cancer risk, many of these issues are amplified.

Genetic Testing

Advances in technology for identifying genes and genetic variations can be used to increase our understanding of the genetic causes of a variety of diseases as well as to identify possible genetic influences on behavior, race, and other sociological aspects of the human population. Society can benefit immensely from research to identify genetic influences on disease and health that can lead to more effective screening, prevention, and treatment of inherited diseases, such as cancer. Genetic information also carries the potential for great psychosocial harm such as stigmatization and inappropriate discrimination (Clayton et al., 1995). Privacy and confidentiality are primary components in genetic testing practice. These risks not only apply to the individuals whose DNA is being studied but also to his or her relatives and others with whom genetic information is shared. Perceptions of genetic determinism can amplify an individual's adverse psychological reactions to finding out he is at increased risk for disease (NBAC, 1999). Managing information about risk when there are not yet any clinical interventions for the condition carries a host of ethical considerations, and this often is the case with genetic screening. The identification of genes and mutations associated with cancer development is occurring faster than the development of methodologies for the prevention and treatment of cancers caused by such genetic mutations (Bove, Fry, & MacDonald, 1997).

Tests for genetic variation associated with a predisposition to cancer may become commercially available before the medical community adequately understands limitations to interpreting test results or has reached sufficient agreement about the clinical management of people who are carrying the genetic variation. Ideally, genetic tests should not be introduced to the public until health professionals have determined who should be offered testing and who is likely to be helped or harmed by testing (Holtzman & Watson, 1997). However, genetic testing does not always follow this path, as seen in the case of BRCA1 and BRCA2 screening. The uncertainties and limitations of BRCA1 and BRCA2 testing have posed challenges for nurses and other care providers (Baron & Borgen, 1997). The bulk of research on BRCA1 and BRCA2 has been conducted in studies of families at high-risk for breast and ovarian cancer. Members of these families may have significantly different risk profiles than people in the general population. Therefore, researchers are unsure of the probability cancer developing in people in the general population who test positive for BRCA1 or BRCA2 variation (CancerNet, 2000a). Deciding whether to undergo testing is a hard question for women with clinical risk factors or family history of breast or ovarian cancer. In addition, women who are BRCA positive have little information to help them with the decision of whether to start tamoxifen for reduction of risk for breast cancer (Dunn et al., 1998). The BCPT determined breast cancer risk using the Gail model, a risk assessment tool based on clinical and epidemiological factors (Fisher et al., 1998). Tamoxifen's effectiveness in women testing positive for BRCA1 or BRCA2 variations, however, is unknown because genetic tests for these mutations were not available at the initiation of BCPT.

Informed consent in genetic testing and genetic counseling are key components in the ethical care of people who are considering undergoing genetic testing to determine disease predisposition and preventing harm to their offspring. Several organizations have released statements concerning genetic testing, counseling, and informed consent. The American Society of Clinical Oncology (ASCO) has recommended that several elements be conveyed during the consent process for genetic testing (see Figure 6-4). Movements toward state and federal legislation for genetic privacy and against genetic discrimination have begun, as well (Clinton, 2000; Gostin, 1995; Rothenberg et al., 1997). Nurses may have responsibilities in educating clients and obtaining consent for genetic testing, and nurses are one of the leading groups of professionals entering the field of genetic counseling (Mahon & Casperson, 1995). They also can advocate for legal and social policies that protect from infringement of individual rights and from wrongs or harms that may stem from genetic information.

Additional moral questions surface when genetic testing for cancer predisposition is introduced in the pediatric setting. The ethical implications of genetic testing in asymptomatic children and adolescents includes conflicts in preferences and values among family members; uncertainties in the medical community about the psychosocial risks and potential clinical benefits of genetic testing for adult-onset disease; and questions of children's ability to process information and cope with fears, guilt, and other potential negative emotional reactions. The American Society of Human Genetics Board of Directors and the American College of

---

Figure 6-4. ASCO Recommendations on Informed Consent for Genetic Testing

- Information on the specific test being performed
- Implications of a positive and negative result
- Possibility that the test will not be informative
- Options for risk estimation without genetic testing
- Risk of passing a mutation to children
- Technical accuracy of the test
- Fees involved in testing and counseling
- Risks of psychological distress
- Risks of insurance or employer discrimination
- Confidentiality issues
- Options and limitations of medical surveillance and screening following testing

---

Note. From "Statement of American Society of Clinical Oncology: Genetic Testing for Cancer Susceptibility," by ASCO Subcommittee on Genetic Testing for Cancer Susceptibility, 1999, *Journal of Clinical Oncology, 14,* p. 1732. Copyright 1999 by Lippincott Williams and Wilkins. Reprinted with permission.

Medical Genetics Board of Directors (1995) developed points for healthcare professionals and others to address when contemplating genetic testing in children and adolescents (see Figure 6-5).

Human Tissue Banking and Research

Genetic research often is conducted on stored DNA samples, which may be gathered through regular medical care or clinical research studies and later given to researchers for genetic studies. In the past, this practice frequently occurred without the knowledge and consent of the person from whom the tissue came. This approach carries ethical concerns about the respect for autonomy and for privacy, confidentiality, and other rights of the individuals whose samples are used for research (Clayton et al., 1995; NBAC, 1999). Additional ethical concerns relate to the potential for psychosocial harms that are associated with the use of human DNA specimens and the information that can be derived from them. Biological samples containing genetic code hold an immeasurable and unpredictable amount of information that may be tapped into in the future; thus, the potential for wrongs associated with the release or misuse of genetic samples is great (Giarelli & Jacobs, 2000). The potential for wrongs or harms applies to the source of the sample and related groups of people. Even when genetic materials are not present in the sample, moral questions about control of one's body parts are raised by using human tissue samples without permission from the source (NBAC).

As a result, medical professionals, the public, and policy makers have turned their attention to the ethics and policies related to the collection, storage, and use of human tissue for genetic and other kinds of research. NBAC (1999) developed recommendations related to the use of biological specimens in research that will have an impact on cancer prevention, detection, and control practice. Recommendations that are particularly relevant to nurses are presented in Figure 6-6. Nurses may be involved in the collection and handling of human tissue samples. They may administer the informed-consent process for the storage of specimens for future

Figure 6-5. ASHG/ACMG Points to Consider	

The Impact of Potential Benefits and Harms on Decisions About Testing
• Timely medical benefit to the child should be the primary justification for genetic testing in children and adolescents.
• Substantial psychosocial benefits to the competent adolescent also may be a justification for genetic testing.
• If the medical or psychosocial benefits of a genetic test will not accrue until adulthood, as in the case of carrier status or adult-onset diseases, genetic testing generally should be deferred.
• If the balance of benefits and harms is uncertain, the provider should respect the decision of competent adolescents and their families.
• Testing should be discouraged when the provider determines that potential harms of genetic testing in children and adolescents outweigh the potential benefits.

The Family's Involvement in Decision Making
• Education and counseling for parents and the child, depending on the maturity of the child, should precede genetic testing.
• The provider should obtain the permission of the parents and, as appropriate, the assent of the child or consent of the adolescent.
• The provider is obligated to advocate on behalf of the child when he or she considers a genetic test to be or not to be in the best interest of the child.
• A request by a competent adolescent for the results of a genetic test should be given priority over parents' requests to conceal information.

Considerations for Future Research
• As genetic testing for children and adolescents becomes increasingly feasible, research should focus on the effectiveness of proposed preventive and therapeutic interventions and on the psychosocial impact of tests.

Note. From "ASHG/ACMG Report Points to Consider: Ethical, Legal, and Psychosocial Implications of Genetic Testing in Children and Adolescents," by American Society of Human Genetics Board of Directors and American College of Medical Genetics Board of Directors, 1995, *American Journal of Human Genetics, 57,* pp. 1233–1234. Copyright 1995 by the University of Chicago Press. Adapted with permission.

research. Therefore, they have an important role in guarding the rights and interests of people from whom samples are obtained, while also facilitating potentially beneficial research that may be conducted using these samples.

Approaches to Bioethics

Ethical problems, such as those alluded to in the previous section, are complex. Intuition, experience, and advice from colleagues may provide sufficient guidance for working through many of the moral issues that arise in the healthcare and research environment; however, the use of a formal problem-solving framework and a greater understanding of bioethical theories can be useful in tackling the more complicated or unusual ethical dilemmas. Bioethical methods and theories also can improve the consistency and quality of decisions about "ordinary" ethical situations. An overview of several leading contemporary bioethical theories is given here.

Figure 6-6. Selected Recommendations From the National Bioethics Advisory Commission Report on the Use of Human Biological Specimens

Obtaining Informed Consent
- When informed consent to the research use of human biological materials is required, it should be obtained separately from informed consent to clinical procedures.
- The person who obtains informed consent in clinical settings should make it clear to potential subjects that their refusal to consent to the research use of biological materials will in no way affect the quality of their clinical care.
- To facilitate collection, storage, and appropriate use of human biological materials in the future, consent forms should be developed to provide potential subjects with a sufficient number of options to help them understand clearly the nature of the decision they are about to make. Such options might include
  - Refusing use of their biological materials in research
  - Permitting only unidentified or unlinked use of their biological materials in research
  - Permitting coded or identified use of their biological materials for one particular study only, with no further contact permitted to ask for permission to do further studies
  - Permitting coded or identified use of their biological materials for one particular study only, with further contact permitted to ask for permission to do further studies
  - Permitting coded or identified use of their biological materials for any study relating to the condition for which the sample was originally collected, with further contact allowed to seek permission for other types of studies
  - Permitting coded use of their biological materials for any kind of future study.

Waiver of Informed Consent
- Institutional review boards (IRBs) should operate on the presumption that research on coded samples is of minimal risk to the human subject if
  - The study adequately protects the confidentiality of personally identifiable information obtained in the course of research
  - The study does not involve the inappropriate release of information to third parties
  - The study design incorporates an appropriate plan for whether and how to reveal findings to the sources or their physicians should the findings merit such disclosure.
- In determining whether a waiver of consent would adversely affect subjects' rights and welfare, IRBs should be certain to consider
  - Whether the wavier would violate any state or federal statute or customary practice regarding entitlement to privacy or confidentiality
  - Whether the study will examine traits commonly considered to have political, cultural, or economic significance to the study subjects
  - Whether the study's results might adversely affect the welfare of the subject's community.

Reporting Research Results to Subjects
- IRBs should develop general guidelines for the disclosure of the results of research to subjects and require investigators to address these issues explicitly in their research plans. In general, these guidelines should reflect the presumption that the disclosure of research results to subjects represents an exceptional circumstance. Such disclosure should occur only when all of the following apply.
  - The findings are scientifically valid and confirmed.
  - The findings have significant implications for the subject's health concerns.
  - A course of action to ameliorate or treat these concerns is readily available.
- The investigator in his or her research protocol should describe anticipated research findings and circumstances that might lead to a decision to disclose the findings to a subject, as well as plan for how to manage such a disclosure.
- When research results are disclosed to a subject, appropriate medical advice or referral should be provided.

(Continued on next page)

> ## Figure 6-6. Selected Recommendations From the National Bioethics Advisory Commission Report on the Use of Human Biological Specimens *(Continued)*

Considerations of Potential Harms to Others

- Research using stored human biological materials, even when not potentially harmful to individuals from whom the samples are taken, may be potentially harmful to groups associated with the individual. To the extent that such potential harms can be anticipated, investigators should to the extent possible plan their research so as to minimize such harm and should consult, when appropriate, representatives of the relevant groups regarding study design. In addition, when research on unlinked samples that pose a significant risk of group harms is otherwise eligible for exemption from IRB review, the exemption should not be granted if IRB review might help the investigator to design the study in such a way as to avoid those harms.
- If it is anticipated that a specific research protocol poses a risk to a specific group, this risk should be disclosed during any required informed-consent process.

Professional Education and Responsibilities

- The National Institutes of Health, professional societies, and healthcare organizations should continue to expand their efforts to train investigators about the ethical issues and regulations regarding research on human biological materials and to develop exemplary practices for resolving such issues.

Use of Medical Records in Research on Human Biological Materials

- Because many of the same issues arise in the context of research on both medical records and human biological materials, when drafting medical records privacy laws, state and federal legislators should seek to harmonize rules governing both types of research. Such legislation, while seeking to protect patient confidentiality and autonomy, should also ensure that appropriate access for legitimate research purposes is maintained.

Categories of Human Biological Materials

- Repository Collections
  - *Unidentified specimens:* For these specimens, identifiable personal information was not collected or, if collected, was not maintained and cannot be retrieved by the repository.
  - *Identified specimens:* These specimens are linked to personal information in such a way that the person from whom the material was obtained could be identified by name, patient number, or clear pedigree location (i.e., his or her relationship to a family member whose identity is known).
- Research Samples
  - *Unidentified samples:* Sometimes termed "anonymous," these samples are supplied by repositories to investigators from a collection of unidentified human biological specimens.
  - *Unlinked samples:* Sometimes termed "anonymized," these samples lack identifiers or codes that can link a particular sample to an identified specimen or a particular human being.
  - *Coded samples:* Sometimes termed "linked" or "identifiable," these samples are supplied by repositories to investigators from identified specimens with a code rather than with personally identifying information, such as a name or Social Security number.
  - *Identified samples:* These samples are supplied by repositories from identified specimens with a personal identifier (such as a name or patient number) that would allow the researcher to link the biological information derived from the research directly to the individual from whom the material was obtained.

Note. From "Research Involving Human Biological Materials: Ethical Issues and Policy Guidance—Final Report," by National Bioethics Advisory Commission, 1999, retrieved August 12, 1999 from the World Wide Web: http://bioethics.gov/hbm.pdf

Bioethical Theories

Today, no single theory or method is widely accepted as representing a full account of bioethics. Contemporary bioethics thought has been dominated by a principle-based account of bioethics, in which certain norms are the primary guides for moral decisions and justifications for moral action (Arras, Steinbock, & London, 1999). In later years, numerous other bioethical accounts have entered the discussion. Some of the theories are claimed to refute the principle-oriented account, and others are said to complement it. In general, ethical theories differ in their focus with respect to the moral event. Depending upon the theory, the emphasis may be on the act, virtues of the moral agent, consequences, or particulars of the case at hand. Theories that differ mainly in emphasis may not be mutually exclusive. They can, and perhaps should, be used in conjunction with each other to more completely and effectively tackle ethical concerns. Some theories, however, are philosophically incompatible and cannot be used in tandem in moral decision making. In addition, fundamental questions can be argued within theories as well as between them.

Bioethicists continue to debate over moral theory, and healthcare professionals still grapple with interpreting and applying these theories in their professional lives. Nevertheless, a basic understanding of the prominent approaches to bioethics can help nurses and other healthcare professionals to identify, analyze, and work through ethical problems. Following is an overview of a broad range of theories and methods in bioethics: principle-based moral reasoning, casuistry, utilitarianism, obligation-based theories, rights-based theories, virtue ethics, an ethic of care, and communitarian ethics (see Table 6-2).

Principle-Based Moral Reasoning

The **principle-based account** of bioethics maintains that principles, rules, or obligations are central guides to moral acts. The most widely known form of principle-based bioethics was proposed by Tom Beauchamp and James Childress. In their account, principles are based on a theory of common morality as derived from the ordinary (nonphilosophical) moral traditions and beliefs shared by members of society (Beauchamp & Childress, 1994). Beauchamp and Childress listed four primary (or fundamental) principles—respect for autonomy, nonmaleficence, beneficence, and justice—and the secondary (or derivative) principles of veracity, fidelity, and privacy and confidentiality (Childress, 1997).

Respect for autonomy (self-determination) is the duty to respect an individual's capability to make decisions and act as a free agent. Nonmaleficence is the duty to avoid causing harm. Beneficence is the duty to prevent harm, repair harm, promote good, and balance benefits against potential harms for individuals and society. Justice is the duty to treat others fairly and to distribute benefits and burdens in an equitable manner. The secondary principles are sometimes called rules because they are more specific than the primary principles. Their justification is found in the primary principles. Veracity is the duty to tell the truth. Fidelity is the duty to maintain trust in relationships, keep promises, and uphold contracts. Privacy and confidentiality relate to the duty to respect the privacy of others and to prevent disclosing private information about others.

Table 6-2. Prominent Contemporary Bioethical Approaches

Bioethical Account	Emphasis
An ethic of care	Caring, relationships
Casuistry	Cases, circumstances
Communitarianism	Community values
Kantian ethics	Obligations
Principlism	Principles
Rights-based theories	Moral rights
Utilitarianism	Utility, consequences
Virtue theory	Moral agent

Other bioethicists reframe or add to the principles developed by Beauchamp and Childress. For example, Robert Veatch lists beneficence, contract-keeping, autonomy, honesty, avoiding killing, and justice in his account (Childress, 1997). In nursing ethics, **advocacy** often is cited as a central ethical principle (Winters, Glass, & Sakurai, 1993). Advocacy refers to the helping of clients to gain a sufficient understanding to make decisions and to enable them to make those decisions.

Because Beauchamp and Childress do not place the primary principles in a hierarchy that commands us to choose one over the others in all situations. These principles can conflict with each other in an ethical dilemma. Each case must be evaluated individually and a determination made about which principle has a higher moral position. Some critics view the lack of prioritization among principles as a serious detriment to this principle-based approach (Clouser & Gert, 1997).

The principle-based approach to bioethics has also been challenged on practical and philosophical grounds. It has been argued that principles often are used mechanically without meaningful reflection, causing the moral agent to lose sight of a deeper moral vision (Jonsen, 1995). The argument is similar to not being able to see the forest for the trees. Some ethicists believe that this weakness is more than a problem of application. Rather, the principles are missing a real moral foundation and do not provide a solid theory of bioethics that would allow the principles to provide moral guidance (Clouser & Gert, 1997). Beauchamp and Childress (1994) countered these arguments by contending that the principles are meaningful if they are "interpreted, analyzed, specified, and connected to other norms."

These criticisms of "principlism" have led to an increase in support for alternative and complementary theories of bioethics, which are the focus of the next sections of this chapter. Exponents of casuistry have argued that principles and rules based on general norms lack the precision needed for making judgments in a particular case. Virtue ethicists think the principle-centered account undervalues the role of character attributes and virtues. According to an ethic-of-care perspective, the principle-based approach neglects the morality of caring and compassion in relationships. Utilitarianism, obligation-based theories, rights-based theories, and communitarianism are some of the other leading approaches in contemporary bioethics that will be described in this chapter. Despite the criticism, the principles of respect for autonomy, nonmaleficence, beneficence, and justice remain in the forefront of ethical discussions in modern medicine and public health.

Casuistry

Case-based reasoning, called casuistry, is a traditional mode of reasoning that resurfaced in contemporary times as an alternative to the principle-based method (Arras, 1997; Jonsen, 1995). In casuistry, the determinants of a moral course of action are the particulars of the case, not abstract principles. One approaches a case by reviewing a previous, similar case (or set of similar cases). A conclusion can be made through examination of the details, ethical judgments, and solutions of the current case and comparing and contrasting them with previous cases. An analogy often is drawn between casuistry and the practice of case law, in which legal precedents of previous court cases are used as a basis for judging new, similar cases. Over time, rules and principles may be used to describe norms that are seen across cases. Principles, of sorts, are said to grow out of specific cases, not the other way around.

There is disagreement as whether case-based reasoning is a complement or alternative to principle-based reasoning (Jonsen, 1995). Some believe that casuistry operates at a more detailed level than principlism, but it is not a fundamentally distinct method of reasoning (Arras, 1997; Arras, Steinbock, & London, 1999). Defendants of principle-oriented bioethics claim that these opponents are actually using principles and rules but are not acknowledging it (Childress, 1997).

Both principle-based and case-based approaches often are called forms of moral reasoning rather than full-blown ethical theories. A revival of traditional ethical theories and an emergence of new theories recently have occurred in response to perceived shortcomings of principle- and case-based approaches to bioethics.

Utilitarianism

Utilitarianism is the theory that morality is achieved by maximizing good and preventing bad to the greatest number of members of a society. The writings of Jeremy Bentham (1748–1832) and John Stuart Mill (1806–1873) are some of the first sources of this philosophy (Arras, Steinbock, & London, 1999). Utilitarianism is consequence-based (or teleological), which means that moral focus is the outcome produced by an action rather than the action itself, the motivations behind it, or the virtues of the moral agent. The only criterion of morality is the utility principle, which focuses on producing the greatest net benefit for the largest numbers. If good cannot be achieved, then the utility principle seeks to minimize the net harm produced. The good in utilitarianism is human happiness, usually defined as pleasure versus pain. Utilitarianism comes in two main forms: act utilitarianism and rule utilitarianism. Rule utilitarians use the utility principle to create and justify rules that maximize happiness. Act utilitarians only consider the consequences of the act and do not factor rules in the equation.

Several objections to utilitarianism have been raised. First, some question the focus of happiness as the moral goal (Arras et al., 1999). For most utilitarian philosophers, happiness does not include such goods as health and friendship. Its role in bioethics then comes into question. Second, the utility principle has been called an impossible moral standard to follow. It requires challenging calculations to be made for every action. The third common criticism is against teleology as a moral theory. Most agree that our intuitions seem to tell us that the result is not the only object of moral significance in a moral event. For instance, our intentions seem to matter. Also, the outcome of our actions depends on many factors that are out of our control. So, critics ask how morality can rest on these factors. Finally, utilitarianism is associated with the problem of "unjust social distribution" because the utility principle allows the majority's interests to outweigh the minority's rights (Beauchamp & Childress, 1994). Feminist writers, in particular, have criticized utilitarianism for counting the preferences of dominant groups the same as those of oppressed groups (Sherwin, 1997).

One of the strengths of utilitarianism is that, in a loose sense, it seeks to promote human welfare, which is valued in other ethical accounts such as principlism in the form of beneficence. It also forces us to look beyond the immediate issues at hand to consider the overall effects of action. Last, the theory relies on one criteria for moral determination (i.e., net happiness), which can possibly be measured empirically. This is seen as an advantage in public policy decision making (Arras et al., 1999). Utilitarian theory has a greater presence in the area of public health and research policies and program planning than in other areas of bioethics.

Obligation-Based (Kantian) Theories

Most obligation-based ethical theories have their origins in the writings of Immanuel Kant (1724–1804) and are sometimes called Kantian ethics. Contemporary versions of Kantian-based ethics have been proposed by Alan Donagan with a Judeo-Christian orientation and by John Rawls in the form of a social contract-theory (Arras et al., 1999).

In contrast to consequence-based utilitarianism, obligation-based ethical theories are deontological (act-focused). In deontological theories, some elements of actions, other than or in addition to consequences, make the actions morally right or wrong (Beauchamp & Childress, 1994). Kant claimed that the rationality (ability to think abstractly) of human beings gives them moral status. This status entails a moral obligation to respect people as autonomous beings. What Kant means by autonomy is deeper and more significant than the principle in Beauchamp and Childress' bioethical account. It is at the heart of humanity and morality. Some of the key tenants of Kant's ethics include (a) never act in a morally wrong manner to produce good outcomes (b) do not use people only as means to an end, and (c) consequences may only matter if the act is considered to be morally acceptable (Beauchamp, 1999; Feldman, 1997).

Ethicists have identified some weaknesses of obligation-based theories. The theory has trouble handling the conflicting obligations, often overestimates legal considerations while underestimating human relationships, and has been said to have abstractness without substance (Arras et al., 1999; Beauchamp & Childress, 1994). Perhaps the greatest strength of Kantian ethics is its consistency as a moral theory. It demands that all persons are consistently treated and that a consistent rationale must be consistently applied to justifying actions.

Rights-Based Theory

In **rights-based theories,** moral actions are those that uphold and protect the rights of individuals. The concept of rights has appeared in moral philosophy in the writings of Hobbes, Locke, Bentham, and many others. Like obligation-based ethics, rights theories are deontological. A good outcome cannot justify an action that violates or compromises a human right. A right entitles an individual to something basic to human life. Moral rights are justified on moral (rather than social) grounds. For example, an informed-consent process that communicates the procedures, risks, and subject rights in a clinical study to the potential participants plays a key role in honoring the right of a person to choose whether to participate in research.

Philosophers have differentiated between negative and positive rights (Beauchamp, 1999). A negative right refers to an obligation *to not do* something to someone. A positive right involves an obligation *to do* something for someone else. Libertarians only acknowledge negative rights. Positive rights, they believe, interfere with rights to have the freedom to pursue personal interests. Honoring a positive right requires individuals to release their resources to others.

The focus of rights-centered ethics is the individual rather than society or the community. Rights-based theorists have attacked utilitarianism for an inadequate account of rights and neglect of individual interests. Libertarianism, however, also may lead to the disadvantage of persons who, because of reasons out of their control, are born into weaker social, economic, and health positions (Arras et al., 1999). In the libertarian account, no positive rights exist to level the playing field by compelling individuals to tend to the needs of those who are less fortunate.

Like most of the theories presented in this chapter, rights-based theories primarily are criticized for incompleteness (e.g., in terms of virtues, communal goods). Rights do not determine everything that is moral. Because the emphasis of the rights-based theories is the individual rather than society, they have also been criticized for not giving the needs and concerns of society sufficient moral weight. Additional criticisms are that rights-based theories do not provide sufficient guidance for resolving conflicts between rights (Beauchamp & Childress, 1994) nor can they usually answer questions about whether one should exercise a right. This question speaks to other moral considerations such as obligations and virtues, not just rights.

Nevertheless, one cannot deny the positive impact that rights have had in protecting individuals throughout history. The serious threats to humanity faced by individuals in communities where rights are few or are not enforced further illustrate the significance of rights to morality (Beauchamp & Childress, 1994).

Virtue Ethics

Virtue ethics stresses the character, intentions, and motives of the moral agent over his or her acts and their consequences. Ethical theories in which virtues played a prominent role have existed since the days of Aristotle. In general, virtue ethics became less popular in modern times but has found a home in some professional ethics, especially in bioethics (Pellegrino, 1995).

In this theory, the virtues of importance are those that are morally valued rather than socially valued, as we commonly think of virtues. An individual who has morally virtuous attributes is more inclined to do the right thing and less likely do the wrong thing. A virtuous healthcare professional will be better able to help clients to achieve health than one who lacks virtuous character. According to virtue theory, however, possessing moral virtues is not sufficient for acting morally. Virtues must be accompanied by the proper motives, as well (Beauchamp, 1999). If one of virtuous character acts on improper motives, a key component of morality is lacking even if the morally right action was taken. When applying virtue ethics to the practice of cancer prevention, the intention of the healthcare professional should be interpreted to include helping individuals to maintain and improve health as well as treating illnesses and healing patients. In addition, some virtue ethicists argue that the moral agent must feel the proper emotions along with having moral character traits and the right motives.

As in principle-based bioethics, there is no consensus about what virtues belong in a bioethical account and how they should be categorized and prioritized. Edmund Pellegrino, one of the leading proponents of virtue ethics, includes the following in his account: fidelity, nonmalevolence, benevolence, effacement of self-interest, compassion and caring, intellectual honesty, justice, and prudence (Beauchamp & Childress, 1994; Pellegrino, 1995).

A primary criticism of virtue ethics is that virtues alone are not sufficient for promoting moral behavior and outcomes. Having virtuous attributes may increase the likelihood that an individual will act in a moral way, but by themselves, virtues cannot provide the individual with the guidance needed for taking moral action. Principles or other elements are needed to inform the moral act (Beauchamp & Childress, 1994).

Similarities between the principles and virtues are apparent. The virtues respectfulness, nonmalevolence, benevolence, and fairness correspond to the principles respect for autonomy, nonmaleficence, beneficence, and justice, respectively (Beauchamp & Childress, 1994). Many consider virtue and principle-based theories not only compatible but complementary. The debate between principle-oriented and virtue ethics then becomes a matter of emphasis. It is possible that in some cases virtues are more relevant, whereas in others principles are more relevant.

An Ethic of Care

An ethic of care places caring (or compassion) at the forefront of morality. Caring means "to care for, emotional commitment to, and willingness to act on behalf of persons with whom one has a significant relationship" (Beauchamp & Childress, 1994, p. 85). The delivery of technical care to the client is seen as the other main component of caring in health care (Reich, 1995). While the former relates more to the moral nature of caring, the latter is seen as critical for carrying the moral component of caring to the clinical setting.

For the most part, an ethic of care has evolved from the work of feminine ethicists that have criticized traditional ethical theories centered on obligations, rights, and principles as being based on limited, male perspectives (Beauchamp & Childress, 1994; Fry, 1995; Reich, 1995). Feminine ethicists have primarily criticized other theories for imposing a standard of impartiality to moral reflection (Sherwin, 1997). This impartiality asks us to view relationships with detachment that allows for fairness in deliberations. Supporters of an ethic of care believe that this impartiality may be acceptable when people in a relationship are equals, but it prevents the formation of moral relationships between those with unequal power. People who are vulnerable or weak deserve special concern about and care for their needs rather than impartial judgment about their rights or about principles of justice.

The nursing profession has been closely associated with an ethic of care more than most other areas of bioethics (Beauchamp & Childress, 1994). Codes of ethics for professional nursing have promoted caring as a key of nursing (Taylor, 1998). Recently, the association between nursing and an ethic of care has caused some uneasiness among ethicists and nursing theorists. One concern is that this association will prevent an ethic of care from entering other areas of bioethics. Feminists worry that it reinforces ideas that the woman's tendency toward caring is connected to her lesser status in society, and it perpetuates traditional gender-bias in professional roles in health care (Arras et al., 1999). Others question the appropriateness of a focus on an ethic of care in nursing while the professional duties and functions of nursing are expanding. Additional moral responsibilities may be demanded of roles such as healthcare administrator, researcher, and policy planner that do not involve direct patient care (Taylor). The care perspective in nursing may be inadequate for including the duty of nurses to be advocates for patients (Jecker & Reich, 1995). Regardless of these concerns, nursing remains closely aligned with an ethic of care.

Communitarianism

Communitarianism is a theory that morality is based on the traditions, shared values, virtues, and ideals of the community (Clouser, 1995). Moral conduct is that which supports the goals of society and the common good. This is in contrast to the utilitarian goal of maximizing the good of the sum of the individuals in society. Communitarians differ in their conception of community. Community has been defined as society as whole, smaller communities, institutions, professional associations, or family. Another struggle for communitarian theorists can be defining common values in a community. In bioethics, communitarianism is more prominent in public policy deliberations than in clinical decision making (Arras et al., 1999).

Summary

Although often presented as incompatible, many believe that no one method or theory provides a complete system of bioethics. Several of the country's leading bioethicists advocate for a pluralist approach that incorporates aspects of different methods and theories whereby they can be coherently and appropriately used together. When examining moral problems from different ethical perspectives, we are more likely to take into account the values of those other than ourselves and to identify a wider spectrum of ethical issues and solutions. Even evaluating a problem using philosophically incongruent theories, such as deontological accounts and moral teleology, can help us to understand opposing viewpoints and make better decisions.

Decision-Making Framework

Often, ethical problems are not easily solved. Even if one subscribes to a particular moral theory or group of theories, employing it in a particular situation can be challenging. Several frameworks have been proposed to help individuals and groups to solve ethical problems. The model presented in this chapter includes the key components of several contemporary decision-making tools that have been developed to assist nurses and other healthcare professionals in approaching ethical problems encountered in their daily professional lives (Case, 1999; Thomasma, 2000; Winters et al., 1993) (see Figure 6-7). This framework is intended to be of use no matter which bioethical theories the decision-maker chooses to apply to the situation and can help to compare differences between theories in a given case.

A Framework for Ethical Decision Making

1. **Gather the facts of the case.** Research relevant medical information and situational facts that are impacting the problems or limiting possible solutions.

2. **Identify the involved parties.** The relevant people in the case include the person(s) making the decision as well as those who will be affected by the decision, such as the client, family, physicians, nurses, researchers, institution, community, society as a whole, and you. Identify conflicts between individuals and between individuals and groups. Who is involved directly or indirectly? Do some people, groups, or institutions have more of a stake in the decision than others do? What is the relationship between interested parties? What is your relationship with them? Who are the decision makers?

3. **Explore the values at risk for each of the involved parties.** What values and interests are at stake for each of the parties involved? What values are shared?

4. **Determine the conflicts between values, professional norms, and**

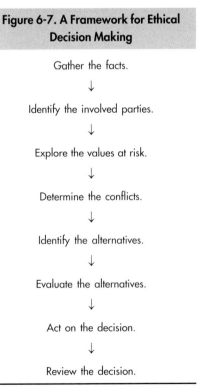

Figure 6-7. A Framework for Ethical Decision Making

Gather the facts.

↓

Identify the involved parties.

↓

Explore the values at risk.

↓

Determine the conflicts.

↓

Identify the alternatives.

↓

Evaluate the alternatives.

↓

Act on the decision.

↓

Review the decision.

ethical rules and principles. Conflicts may occur between these elements or within them. Several conflicts may occur in a single case.

5. **Identify the possible alternatives to the ethical problem.**
6. **Evaluate the alternatives in terms of bioethical approaches.** Look at the alternatives from various moral theories and ethical viewpoints. Determine whether any of the values or principles is absolute (necessary to uphold in any situation) or whether there are reasons to uphold them in this situation in particular. Refer to similar cases and determine the similarities and differences between the cases. For each alternative, weigh the benefits and burdens to the involved parties in the short-term and long-term. Consult others. Choose the best alternative.
7. **Act on the decision.** This step encompasses implementing, supporting, and defending the decision. You should be able to explain why the alternative is better than the others.
8. **Review the decision.** Evaluate the action and outcome of the decision on the involved parties. How does this decision relate to your daily life? If you or someone else encountered a similar situation, should it be handled the same way, and why? On what moral theory or theories did you base your decision, and why? Did certain principles and values take precedence in the decision? What nonmoral factors affected your decision?

In addition to moral theory, other elements are critical to individual decision making about moral problems (Callahan, 1995). Self-knowledge is important because our feelings, attitudes, and interests can illuminate or cloud moral decision making. An awareness of one's social environment and an understanding of the cultural context of our choices also are needed for good ethical decision making. Further, a conception of the human good will provide direction in ethical struggles. The definition of a good human life has been and always will be a source of discussion and debate, but the desire to seek this understanding is crucial to bioethics and ethics in general. Only in the company of these other elements can moral theories effectively contribute to ethical decision making.

Conclusion

Nurses working in the area of cancer prevention, detection, and control regularly face ethical concerns stemming from a broad range of sources. In particular, they encounter ethical questions when delivering new cancer prevention and detection information and technologies to various members of society; conducting research in the area of cancer prevention, detection, and control; and participating in the creation of administrative, social, and economic policies related to the practice and study of cancer prevention and detection science. Identifying and handling ethical conflicts can be difficult and overwhelming tasks. Contemporary theories and decision-making models in bioethics can provide assistance to nurses as they take on ethical challenges. Clients, colleagues, and society all benefit when nurses effectively make ethical decisions.

The author gratefully acknowledges Mary S. McCabe, RN, MA, director, Office of Education and Special Initiatives, National Cancer Institute (NCI), and Barbara K. Dunn, MD, PhD, medical officer, Basic Prevention Science Research Group, Division of Cancer Prevention (DCP), NCI, for helpful comments on this manuscript.

References

American Nurses Association. (1985). *Code for nurses with interpretative statements* (Publication No. G-56, 17.5, 6/9R). Washington, DC: Author.

American Society of Human Genetics Board of Directors and the American College of Medical Genetics Board of Directors. (1995). ASHG/ACMG Report points to consider: Ethical, legal, and psychosocial implications of genetic testing in children and adolescents. *American Journal of Human Genetics, 57,* 1233–1241.

ASCO Subcommittee on Genetic Testing for Cancer Susceptibility. (1996). Statement of American Society of Clinical Oncology: Genetic testing for cancer susceptibility. *Journal of Clinical Oncology, 14,* 1730–1736.

Arras, J.D. (1997) Getting down to cases: The revival of casuistry in bioethics. In N.S. Jecker, A.R. Jonsen, & R.A. Pearlman (Eds.), *Bioethics: An introduction to the history, methods, and practice* (pp. 175–183). Boston: Jones and Bartlett.

Arras, J.D., Steinbock, B., & London, A.J. (1999). Moral reasoning in the medical context. In J.D. Arras & B. Steinbock (Eds.), *Ethical issues in modern medicine* (5th ed.) (pp. 1–40). Mountain View, CA: Mayfield Publishing Co.

Baron, R.H., & Borgen, P.I. (1997). Genetic susceptibility for breast cancer: Testing and primary prevention options. *Oncology Nursing Forum, 24,* 461–486.

Beauchamp, T.L. (1995). Principlism and its alleged competitors. *Kennedy Institute of Ethics Journal, 5*(3), 181–197.

Beauchamp, T.L. (1999). Ethical theory and bioethics. In T.L. Beauchamp & L. Walters (Eds.), *Contemporary issues in bioethics* (5th ed.) (pp. 1–32). Belmont, CA: Wadsworth Publishing Co.

Beauchamp, T.L., & Childress, J.F. (1994). *Principles of biomedical ethics* (4th ed.). New York: Oxford University Press.

Bioethics Advisory Commission. (2001). *Ethical and policy issues in research involving human participants* [Fact sheet]. Retrieved March 8, 2001 from the World Wide Web: www.bioethics.gov

Bove, C.M., Fry, S.T., & MacDonald, D.J. (1997). Presymptomatic and predisposition genetic testing: Ethical and social considerations. *Seminars in Oncology Nursing, 13,* 135–140.

Callahan, D. (1995). Bioethics. In W.T. Reich (Ed.), *Encyclopedia of bioethics* (pp. 247–256). New York: Simon & Schuster Macmillan.

Callahan, D. (1997). Bioethics as a discipline. In N.S. Jecker, A.R. Jonsen, & R.A. Pearlman (Eds.), *Bioethics: An introduction to the history, methods, and practice* (pp. 87–92). Boston: Jones and Bartlett.

CancerNet. (2000a). *Genetic testing for cancer risk (PDQ): Screening/detection—Health professionals.* Retrieved July 7, 2000 from the World Wide Web: http://cancer.nci.nih .gov

CancerNet. (2000b). *Prevention of cancer (PDQ): Prevention—Health professionals.* Retrieved July 7, 2000 from the World Wide Web: http://cancer.nci.nih.gov

Case, N.K. (1999). Philosophical and ethical perspectives. In J.E. Hitchcock, P.E. Schubert, & S.A. Thomas (Eds.), *Community health nursing: Caring in action* (pp. 91–110). Albany, NY: Delmar Publishers.

Chan, E.C.Y., & Sulmasy, D.P. (1998). What should men know about prostate-specific antigen screening before giving informed consent? *American Journal of Medicine, 105,* 266–274.

Chemoprevention Implementation Group. (1999). *New directions for chemoprevention research at the National Cancer Institute: Report of the Chemoprevention Implementation Group, National Cancer Institute.* Retrieved March 14, 2001 from the World Wide Web: http://dcp.nci.nih.gov/rpts/cig

Chemoprevention Working Group to the American Association for Cancer Research. (1999). Prevention of cancer in the next millennium: Report of the Chemoprevention Working Group to the American Association for Cancer Research. *Cancer Research, 59,* 4743–4758.

Childress, J.F. (1997). The normative principles of medical ethics. In R.M. Veatch (Ed.), *Medical ethics* (2nd ed.) (pp. 29–55). Boston: Jones and Bartlett.

Christensen, K.T. (1999). Ethically important distinctions among managed care organizations. In J.D. Arras & B. Steinbock (Eds.), *Ethical issues in modern medicine* (5th ed.) (pp. 103–108). Mountain View, CA: Mayfield Publishing Co.

Clark, E.J., & Stovall, E.L. (1996). Advocacy: The cornerstone of cancer survivorship. *Cancer Practice, 4,* 239–244.

Clayton, E.W., Steinberg, K.K., Khoury, M.J., Thomson, E., Andrews, L., Kahn, M.J., Kopelman, L.M., & Weiss, J.O. (1995). Informed consent for genetic research on stored tissue samples. *JAMA, 274,* 1786–1792.

Clinton, W.J. (2000, February 8). *Executive Order 13145 to prohibit discrimination in federal employment based on genetic information.* Retrieved February 9, 2001 from the World Wide Web: http://frwebgate.access.gpo.gov/cgi-bin/getdoc.cgi?dbname=2000_register&docid=fr10fe00-165.pdf

Clouser, K.D. (1995). Common morality as an alternative to principlism. *Kennedy Institute of Ethics Journal, 5,* 219–236.

Clouser, K.D., & Gert, B. (1997). A critique of principlism. In N.S. Jecker, A.R. Jonsen, & R.A. Pearlman (Eds.), *Bioethics: An introduction to the history, methods, and practice* (pp. 147–151). Boston: Jones and Bartlett.

Council on Ethical and Judicial Affairs, American Medical Association. (1995). Ethical issues in managed care. *JAMA, 273,* 330–335.

Department of Health and Human Services (2000). Secretary Shalala bolsters protections for human research subjects [Press release]. Retrieved November 5, 2000 from the World Wide Web: http://www.hhs.gov/news.

Dickert, N., & Grady, C. (1999). What's the price of a research subject? Approaches to payment for research participation. *New England Journal of Medicine, 341,* 198–203.

Dow, K.H., Ferrell, B.R., Haberman, M.R., & Eaton, L. (1999). The meaning of quality of life in cancer survivorship. *Oncology Nursing Forum, 26,* 519–528.

Dunn, B., Kramer, B.S., & Ford, L.G. (1998). Phase III, large-scale chemoprevention trials. *Hematology/Oncology Clinics of North America, 12,* 1019–1036.

Emanuel, E.J., Wendler, D., & Grady, C. (2000). What makes clinical research ethical? *JAMA, 283,* 2701–2711.

Facione, N.C., & Facione, P.A. (1997). Equitable access to cancer services in the 21st century. *Nursing Outlook, 45,* 118–124.

Federal Register. (1994, March 28). 59 (59), 14508–14513.

Federal Register. (1995, October 5). 60 (193), 52063–52065.

Feldman, F. (1997). Kantian ethics. In N.S. Jecker, A.R. Jonsen, & R.A. Pearlman (Eds.), *Bioethics: An introduction to the history, methods, and practice* (pp. 131–140). Boston: Jones and Bartlett.

Ferrell, B.R., & Dow, K.H. (1997). Quality of life among long-term cancer survivors. *Oncology, 11,* 565–571.

Fisher, B., Costantino, J.P., Wickerham, D.L., Redmond, C.K., Kavanah, M., Cronin, W.M., Vogel, V., Robidoux, A., Dimitrov, N., Atkins, J., Daly, M., Wieand, S., Tan-Chiu, E., Ford, L., & Wolmark, N., and other National Surgical Adjuvant Breast and Bowel Project Investigators. (1998). Tamoxifen for prevention of breast cancer: Report of the National Surgical Adjuvant Breast and Bowel Project P-1 Study. *Journal of the National Cancer Institute, 90,* 1371–1388.

Flach, J., & Jennings-Dozier, K. (2000). Bioethical considerations in cancer prevention and early detection practice and research. *Oncology Nursing Forum, 27*(Suppl. 9), 37–45.

Foltz, A.T. (2000). Issues in determining cancer screening recommendations: Who, what, and when. *Oncology Nursing Forum, 27*(Suppl. 9), 13–17.

Fowler, M.D.M. (1993). Professional associations, ethics, and society. *Oncology Nursing Forum, 20*(Suppl. 10), 13–20.

Freeman, H. (1989). Cancer in the socioeconomically disadvantaged. *CA: A Cancer Journal for Clinicians, 39,* 266–288.

Fry, S.T. (1995). Nursing ethics. In W.T. Reich (Ed.), *Encyclopedia of bioethics* (pp. 1822–1827). New York: Simon & Schuster Macmillan.

General Assembly of Maryland. (1998). *Health insurance—Medical clinical trials—Coverage, S. 137/ H.R. 43.* Retrieved February 12, 2001 from the World Wide Web: http://mlis.state.md.us/1998rs/billfile/sb0137.htm

Giarelli, E., & Jacobs, L.A. (2000). Issues related to the use of genetic material and information. *Oncology Nursing Forum, 27,* 459–467.

Godley, P.A. (1999). Prostate cancer screening: Promise and peril—A review. *Cancer Detection and Prevention, 23*(4), 316–324.

Good, M. (2000). Cancer prevention and control study considerations. In A.D. Klimaszewski, J.L. Aikin, M.A. Bacon, S.A. DiStasio, H.E. Ehrenberger, & B.A. Ford (Eds.), *Manual for clinical trials nursing* (pp. 79–84). Pittsburgh: Oncology Nursing Press, Inc.

Gostin, L.O. (1995). Genetic privacy. *Journal of Law, Medicine and Ethics, 23,* 320–30.

Hartmann, L.C., Schaid, D.J., Woods, J.E., Crotty, T.P., Myers, J.L., Arnold, P.G., Petty, P.M., Sellers, T.A., Johnson, J.L., McDonnell, S.K., Frost, M.H., & Jenkins, R.B. (1999). Efficacy of bilateral prophylactic mastectomy in women with a family history of breast cancer. *New England Journal of Medicine, 340,* 77–84.

Haynes, M.A., & Smedley, B.D. (Eds.). (1999). *The unequal burden of cancer: An assessment of NIH research and programs for ethnic minorities and the medically underserved.* Institute *of Medicine, Committee on Cancer Research Among Minorities and the Medically Underserved, Health Sciences Policy Program, Health Sciences Section, Institutes of Medicine.* Washington, DC: National Academy Press.

Health Care Financing Administration. (2000). *Medicare Coverage Policy—Clinical Trials. Final National Coverage Decision.* Retrieved March 13, 2001 from the World Wide Web: www.hcfa.gov/coverage/8d2.htm

Holtzman, N.A., & Watson, M.S. (Eds.). (1997). *Promoting safe and effective genetic testing in the United States.* Final report of the Task Force on Genetic Testing. Retrieved on March 12, 2000 from the World Wide Web: http://www.nhgri.nih.gov/ELSI/TFGT_final/

Jacobs, L.A. (2000). An analysis of the concept of risk. *Cancer Nursing, 23,* 12–19.

Jecker, N., & Reich, W.T. (1995). Contemporary ethics of care. In W.T. Reich (Ed.), *Encyclopedia of bioethics* (pp. 336–344). New York: Simon & Schuster Macmillan.

Jonsen, A. (1995). Casuistry: An alternative or complement to principles? *Kennedy Institute of Ethics Journal, 5,* 237–251.

Kelloff, G.J., Hawk, E.T., Karp, J.E., Crowell, J.A., Boone, C.W., Steele, V.E., Lubet, R.A., & Sigman, C.C. (1997). Progress in clinical chemoprevention. *Seminars in Oncology, 24,* 241–252.

Klausner, R.D., Bravo, N.R., Chapell, J., Feigal, E., Hartinger, J., Kramer, B.S., Knudson, A., Liu, E., Rimer, B., Tucker, M., & Van Evel, P. (1999). *The Nation's investment in cancer research: A budget proposal for fiscal year 2001* (NIH Publication 99-4373). Bethesda, MD: National Institutes of Health.

Kutner, S.E. (1999). Breast cancer genetics and managed care: The Kaiser Permanente experience. *Cancer, 86,* 2570–2582.

Loescher, L.J., Welch-McCaffrey, D., Leigh, S.A., Hoffman, B., & Meyskens, F.L., Jr. (1989). Surviving adult cancers. Part 1. Physiologic Effects. *Annals of Internal Medicine, 111,* 411–432.

Mahon, S., & Casperson, D. (1995). Hereditary cancer syndromes: Part 1—Clinical and education issues. *Oncology Nursing Forum, 22,* 763–771.

Mandelblatt, J.S., Yabroff, K.R., & Kerner, J.F. (1999) Equitable access to cancer services: A review of barriers to quality care. *Cancer, 86,* 2378–2390.

Mandelson, M.T., & Thompson, R.S. (1998). Cancer screening in HMOs: Program development and evaluation. *American Journal of Preventive Medicine, 14*(3S), 26–32.

McCabe, M.S., Varricchio, C.G., & Padberg, R.M. (1994). State of the art care: Efforts to recruit the economically disadvantaged to national clinical trials. *Seminars in Oncology Nursing, 10,* 123–129.

McCabe, M.S., Varricchio, C.G., Padberg, R.M., & Simpson, N. (1995). Women's health advocacy: As growth and development in oncology. *Seminars in Oncology Nursing, 11,* 137–142.

McCaskill-Stevens, W., Bryant, J., Costantino, J., Wickerham, D.L., Vogel, V., & Wolmark, N. (2000). Incidence of contralateral breast cancer (CBC), endometrial cancer (EC), and thromboembolic events (TE) in African American (AA) women receiving tamoxifen for treatment of primary breast cancer. *Proceedings of American Society of Clinical Oncology, 19,* A269.

Meadows, A.T., Varricchio, C., Crosson, K., Harlan, L., McCormick, P., Nealon, E., Smith, M., & Ungerleider, R. (1998). Research issues in cancer survivorship: Report of a workshop sponsored by the Office of Cancer Survivorship, National Cancer Institute. *Cancer Epidemiology, Biomarkers, and Prevention, 7,* 1145–1151.

Millon-Underwood, S., Sanders, E., & Davis, M. (1993). Determinants of participation in state-of-the-art cancer prevention, early detection/screening, and treatment trials among African-Americans. *Cancer Nursing, 16,* 25–33.

National Bioethics Advisory Commission. (1999). *Research involving human biological materials: Ethical issues and policy guidance—Final report.* Retrieved August 12, 1999 from the World Wide Web: http://bioethics.gov/hbm.pdf

National Bioethics Advisory Commission. (2001). "Ethical and policy issues in research involving human participants." Fact sheet. Retrieved March 8, 2001 from the World Wide Web: http://bioethics.gov

National Cancer Institute. (1999). *Clinical trials and insurance coverage: A resource guide.* Retrieved August 12, 1999 from the World Wide Web: http://cancertrials.nci.nih.gov/NCI_CANCER_TRIALS/zones/TrialInfo/Deciding/insurance.html

National Commission for the Protection of Human Subjects of Biomedical and Behavioral Research, Office of the Secretary, Department of Health, Education, and Welfare. (1979, April 18). *The Belmont Report: Ethical principles and guidelines for the protection of human subjects of research.* Bethesda, MD: National Institutes of Health.

National Institutes of Health. (1998, March 6). *NIH policy and guidelines on the inclusion of children as participants in research involving human subjects.* Bethesda, MD: Author.

National Research Council, Computer Science and Telecommunications Board. (1997). *For the record: Protecting electronic health information.* Washington, DC: National Academy Press.

Nayfield, S.G. (1996). Ethical and scientific considerations for chemoprevention research in cohorts at genetic risk for breast cancer. *Journal of Cellular Biochemistry, 25*(Suppl.), 123–130.

Office of Inspector General, Department of Health and Human Services. (1998, June). *Institutional review boards: A time for reform.* Washington, DC: U.S. Department of Health and Human Services.

Olsen, S.J, & Frank-Stromborg, M. (1993). Cancer prevention and early detection in ethnically diverse populations. *Seminars in Oncology Nursing, 9,* 198–209.

Pellegrino, E.D. (1995). Toward a virtue-based normative ethics for the health professions. *Kennedy Institute of Ethics Journal, 5,* 253–277.

Prentice, R. (1995). Experimental methods in cancer prevention research. In P. Greenwald, B. Kramer, & D. Weed (Eds.), *Cancer prevention and control* (pp. 213–224). New York: Marcel Dekker, Inc.

Prorok, P.C. (1995). Screening studies. In P. Greenwald, B. Kramer, & D. Weed (Eds.), Cancer prevention and control (pp. 225–242). New York: Marcel Dekker, Inc.

Psillidis, L., Flach, J., & Padberg, R.M. (1997). Participants strengthen clinical trial research: The vital role of participant advisors in the breast cancer prevention trial. *Journal of Women's Health, 6,* 227–232.

Reich, W.T. (1995). Historical dimensions of an ethic of care in health care. In W.T. Reich (Ed.), *Encyclopedia of bioethics* (pp. 331–336). New York: Simon & Schuster Macmillan.

Rothenberg, K., Fuller, B., Rothstein, M., Duster, T., Kahn, M.J.E., Cunningham, R., Fine, B., Hudson, K., King, M.C., Murphy, P., Swergold, G., & Collins, F. (1997).

Genetic information and the workplace: Legislative approaches and policy challenges. *Science, 275*, 1755–1757.

Sherwin, S. (1997). Gender, race, and class in the delivery of health care. In N.S. Jecker, A.R. Jonsen, & R.A. Pearlman (Eds.), *Bioethics: An introduction to the history, methods, and practice* (pp. 392–401). Boston: Jones and Bartlett.

Taylor, C. (1998). Reflections on "Nursing considered as moral practice." *Kennedy Institute of Ethics Journal, 8*, 71–82.

Thomasma, D.C. (2000). Ethical issues in cancer nursing practice. In C.H. Yarbro, M.H. Frogge, M. Goodman, & S.L. Groenwald (Eds.), *Cancer nursing: Principles and practice* (5th ed.) (pp. 1741–1759). Boston: Jones and Bartlett.

Underwood, S.M. (1995). Enhancing the delivery of cancer care to the disadvantaged: The challenge to providers. *Cancer Practice, 3*(1), 31–36.

Veatch, R.M. (1997). Medical ethics: An introduction. In R.M. Veatch (Ed.), *Medical ethics* (2nd ed.) (pp. 1–27). Boston: Jones and Bartlett.

Weed, D.L., & Coughlin, S.S. (1995). Ethics in cancer prevention and control. In P. Greenwald, B. Kramer, & D. Weed (Eds.), *Cancer prevention and control* (pp. 497–507). New York: Marcel Dekker, Inc.

Welch-McCaffrey, D., Hoffman, B., Leigh, S.A., Loescher, L.J., & Meyskens, F.L., Jr. (1989). Surviving adult cancers. Part 2: Psychosocial Implications. *Annals of Internal Medicine, 111*, 517–524.

Winters, G., Glass, E., & Sakurai, C. (1993). Ethical issues in oncology nursing practice: An overview of topics and strategies. *Oncology Nursing Forum, 20*(Suppl. 10), 21–34.

World Medical Association. (1997). Declaration of Helsinki: Recommendations guiding physicians in biomedical research involving human subjects. *JAMA, 277*, 925–926.

World Medical Association. (2001). *Declaration of Helsinki: Ethical principles for medical research involving human subjects.* Retrieved February 19, 2001 from the World Wide Web. www.wma.net/e/policy/17-c_e.html

SECTION II

Cancer Prevention

OVERVIEW

Section II

Suzanne M. Mahon, RN, DNSc, AOCN®, APNG(c)

The words cancer prevention and early detection often are used interchangeably. These two words, however, have very different meanings and implications for clinical practice. When thinking about cancer control, most clinicians focus on the early detection aspect. The early detection of cancer is a form of secondary cancer prevention and focuses on finding small cancers in asymptomatic people by using techniques such as mammography or prostate-specific antigen testing. The focus of this section is primary prevention. Primary prevention refers to the prevention of disease through certain measures to minimize carcinogen exposure. Examples of primary prevention might include avoiding tobacco products or reducing exposure to ultraviolet rays. More recently, chemoprevention has been added to the spectrum of primary prevention.

Primary prevention measures for malignancy reduce the risk of developing cancer but do not guarantee that the person will not develop a malignancy. Primary prevention is an important and often neglected component of the cancer prevention trajectory.

For many years, the benefits of primary prevention by avoiding carcinogen exposure have been well known. This is particularly true of exposure to tobacco, ultraviolet light, dietary fat, radon, chemicals, and alcohol. Clearly, many cancers could be prevented through the consistent implementation of primary-prevention measures. An estimated 75%–85% of all cancers are lifestyle-related and possibly could be prevented or delayed by avoiding these behaviors (American Cancer Society [ACS], 2001). An understanding of these statistics may be the first step to help both public and healthcare professionals be aware of the importance of primary-prevention efforts. In Chapter 9, Cataldo and Cooley examine issues related to tobacco use and cancer in great detail. They discuss the many roles that nurses should consider when implementing smoking cessation programs.

Primary prevention, however, involves more than just avoidance of carcinogen exposure. Physical activity plays a role in cancer prevention. Intentional weight loss by people who are overweight may reduce cancer risks. Up to one-third of the 563,000 cancer deaths annually are related to nutrition (Willett, 1999). Primary-prevention education should include a discussion of how important diet and exercise are in helping to reduce cancer incidence and mortality. In Chapter 7, Nebeling and Van Duyn give a detailed review of nutrition and the prevention of cancer. Oncology nurses need to consider these concepts when implementing primary-prevention programs into their practice.

Chemoprevention holds immense promise for primary cancer prevention and is an ever-growing area of cancer control. Chemoprevention is defined as the use of specific natural or synthetic agents to reverse or suppress the progression of premalignancy to invasive malignancy. Chemoprevention agents do not include compounds ingested in food. The fundamental premise of chemoprevention is that the development of cancer is a multistep process involving at least two mutations in the same location of DNA within a cell and is reversible in it early stages. In 1998, the U.S. Food and Drug Administration approved the use of Nolvadex® (Zeneca Pharmaceuticals, Wilmington, DE) in reducing the incidence of breast cancer in healthy women. This represents a new era in primary prevention.

Currently, more than 35 open clinical chemoprevention trials are taking place in the United States (www.nci.nih.gov). Chemoprevention trials seek to determine whether the agent actually prevents cancer and is safe. The National Surgical Adjuvant Breast and Bowel Project trial with tamoxifen demonstrated the complicated logistics of conducting large-scale chemoprevention trials (Fisher et al., 1998). First, potential agents must be identified from a research perspective. Agents selected for chemoprevention must not cause unnecessary harm or other side effects. Successful chemoprevention trials require a large number of healthy participants willing to take a medication or placebo for a number of years. As with many other aspects of cancer control, maintaining the commitment necessary to continue with the trial takes a highly motivated person. Oncology nurses who are actively involved in clinical trials and, more particularly, chemoprevention trials need to continue to devise ways to keep patients motivated to take part in a trial for a number of years, especially when the end results are not immediately obvious. Oncology nurses now have the challenge of counseling patients about taking a pharmacologic agent to reduce the incidence of cancer. In Chapter 8, Aikin provides a detailed discussion of the oncology nurse's role in educating patients about chemoprevention and participating in chemoprevention clinical trials.

Getting people to change lifelong habits is more difficult than it appears. It is especially difficult to motivate people to change habits or adopt healthier behaviors when the benefits of such actions will not be obvious for many years. Oncology nurses often speak of the importance of primary prevention but, in reality, little time is spent putting these actions into place. Patients are instructed that they should exercise more, eat less fat, increase fiber consumption, and decrease exposure to ultraviolet light. Less effort is spent teaching patients the behavioral tools they need to make these important changes in their lives. More importantly, oncology nurses need to role model these healthy practices for their patients to see.

Primary cancer prevention is an area where the impact of the efforts and long-term benefits are not completely clear but probably are substantial. Ideally, these practices begin early in childhood. Primary prevention efforts, in particular, should be targeted at children and young adults who stand to reap the most long-term benefits. Nurses who focus on cancer-control issues need to look for ways to partner with fellow nurses who have expertise in pediatrics to deliver this message to parents and their young children.

Nurses also need to help adult patients and their families understand that implementing primary-prevention strategies is important, even into adulthood. Smoking cessation has been shown to have both immediate and long-term benefits. The proper and consistent use of sunscreen and avoidance of ultraviolet rays can substantially reduce the risk of second primary skin cancers. Primary-prevention activities also help patients have some sense of control over their destiny. Individuals who consistently implement these actions have the satisfaction of knowing they have tried their best to prevent malignancy.

The papers in this section represent the scope and depth of the dilemmas and challenges of primary cancer prevention. Nurses are challenged not only to understand the complex physiologic information but also interpret this information to patients in an understandable format. Even more challenging is helping patients to make the necessary behavioral changes to consistently implement primary-prevention practices into their lives. This is truly an exciting era in nursing that will continue to expand and offer new challenges to nurses.

References

American Cancer Society. (2001). *Cancer facts and figures, 2001*. Atlanta: Author.

Fisher, B., Constantino, J.P., Kavanah, M., Cronin, W.M., Vogel, V., Robidoux, A., Dimitrov, N., Atkins, J., Daly, M., Wieand, S., Tan-Chiu, E., Ford, L., & Wolmark, N. (1998). Tamoxifen for prevention of breast cancer: Report of the National Surgical Adjuvant Breast and Bowel Project P-1 study. *Journal of the National Cancer Institute, 90*, 1371–1388.

Willett, W.C. (1999) Goals for nutrition in the year 2000. *CA: A Cancer Journal for Clinicians, 49*, 331–352.

CHAPTER 7

Diet and Cancer Prevention: Why Fruits and Vegetables Are Essential Players

Linda C. Nebeling, PhD, MPH, RD, FADA, and
Mary Ann S. Van Duyn, PhD, MPH, RD

Introduction

Mounting scientific evidence supports that a diet rich in fruits and vegetables may help to reduce the risk of some cancers and other chronic diseases such as heart disease and cataracts (Cooper, Eldridge, & Peters, 1999; van't Veer, Jansen, Klerk, & Kok, 1999). Doll and Peto (1991) estimated that up to 35% of all cancers in the United States might be attributed to diet. The European School of Oncology Task Force on Diet, Nutrition, and Cancer made similar estimates in 1994 (Miller et al., 1994), as did the World Cancer Research Fund (WCRF) and the American Institute of Cancer Research (AICR) in 1997 (WCRF/AICR, 1997).

Current U.S. dietary recommendations intended to reduce cancer risk are based upon extensive data that examine the relationship between diet and cancer incidence (American Cancer Society [ACS] Advisory Committee on Diet, Nutrition, and Cancer Prevention, 1996; WCRF/AICR, 1997). In the United States, cancer is the second leading cause of death after cardiovascular disease and is responsible for one out of four deaths (Ries, 2000). Figures 7-1–7-4 present the 1987–1991 U.S. age-adjusted cancer incidence rates for the 10 most common cancer sites by gender and race. Epidemiological studies, using case-control or cohort designs, provide the most significant data. Overall, findings from observational studies support the conclusion that a diet high in fruits and vegetables is associated with lower risks of cancer for many sites, especially the gastrointestinal tract (e.g., oral, esophageal, gastric, colorectal) and the respiratory tract (e.g., lung, laryngeal) (ACS; WCRF/AICR). Understandably, these estimates may be imprecise when one considers the complexity of the role of dietary factors and dietary assessment method-

Figure 7-1. Age-Adjusted Cancer Incidence Rates[a], 1987–1991; 10 Most Common Sites for White Males

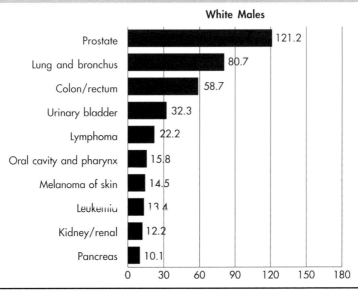

White Males

Site	Rate
Prostate	121.2
Lung and bronchus	80.7
Colon/rectum	58.7
Urinary bladder	32.3
Lymphoma	22.2
Oral cavity and pharynx	15.8
Melanoma of skin	14.5
Leukemia	13.4
Kidney/renal	12.2
Pancreas	10.1

[a] Incidence rates per 100,000 (age-adjusted to 1970 U.S. standard)
Note. Based on information from Ries, 2000.

Figure 7-2. Age-Adjusted Cancer Incidence Rates[a], 1987–1991; 10 Most Common Sites for African American Males

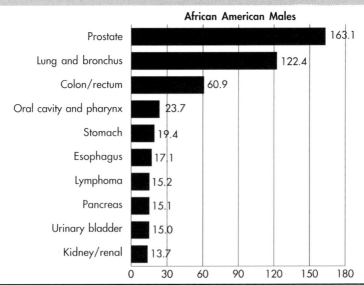

African American Males

Site	Rate
Prostate	163.1
Lung and bronchus	122.4
Colon/rectum	60.9
Oral cavity and pharynx	23.7
Stomach	19.4
Esophagus	17.1
Lymphoma	15.2
Pancreas	15.1
Urinary bladder	15.0
Kidney/renal	13.7

[a] Incidence rates per 100,000 (age-adjusted to 1970 U.S. standard)
Note. Based on information from Ries, 2000.

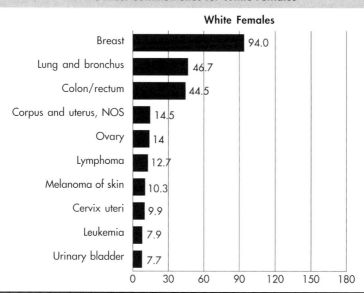

Figure 7-3. Age-Adjusted Cancer Incidence Rates[a], 1987–1991; 10 Most Common Sites for White Females

White Females

Site	Rate
Breast	94.0
Lung and bronchus	46.7
Colon/rectum	44.5
Corpus and uterus, NOS	14.5
Ovary	14
Lymphoma	12.7
Melanoma of skin	10.3
Cervix uteri	9.9
Leukemia	7.9
Urinary bladder	7.7

[a]Incidence rates per 100,000 (age-adjusted to 1970 U.S. standard)
Note. Based on information from Ries, 2000.

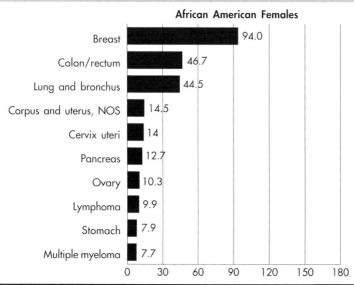

Figure 7-4. Age-Adjusted Cancer Incidence Rates[a], 1987–1991; 10 Most Common Sites for African American Females

African American Females

Site	Rate
Breast	94.0
Colon/rectum	46.7
Lung and bronchus	44.5
Corpus and uterus, NOS	14.5
Cervix uteri	14
Pancreas	12.7
Ovary	10.3
Lymphoma	9.9
Stomach	7.9
Multiple myeloma	7.7

[a]Incidence rates per 100,000 (age-adjusted to 1970 U.S. standard)
Note. Based on information from Ries, 2000.

ology. Despite such limitations, the data consistently provide evidence to support the fact that diets high in fruits and vegetables are associated with lower risks for select cancers (ACS; WCRF/AICR).

Purpose of Chapter

The purpose of this chapter is to review and summarize recent evidence on the relationship between a diet rich in fruits and vegetables and the risk for select cancers (e.g., breast, prostate, colon/rectal, lung) and to summarize strategies for dietary change to prevent cancer. A combination of bibliographic sources was used for this review. In an effort to synthesize and highlight the evidence regarding effective epidemiological data and dietary interventions, the design and findings of many individual studies are not summarized here.

Instead of summarizing the design and findings of many individual studies, the evidence related to the effectiveness of dietary interventions to decrease cancer risk has been synthesized.

Readers are encouraged to refer to the cited review articles on diet and cancer associations and the original research articles for more detail. No attempt was made to summarize the evidence with respect to vitamins, minerals, and other components of the diet.

Why Are Fruits and Vegetables a Major Part of a Healthy Diet?

Evidence suggesting that vegetables and fruits are protective against select cancers and other diseases has been seen in population studies that track a group of people over a defined period of time (Steinmetz & Potter, 1996). In a prospective cohort study, a large group of healthy people provides information on a risk factor of interest, such as diet. The subjects are followed for a period of time, typically several years or more, to determine which people contract specific diseases. The data gathered allow scientists to determine whether specific dietary patterns are related to the risk of getting a specific disease. In a case-control study, people with a specific disease are identified and asked about past diets or other possible risk factors for the disease. Control subjects, who do not have the specific disease, are asked the same kinds of questions. The diets of both groups are compared to identify possible differences that may have influenced the development of the disease. Studies like these have helped scientists to identify food intake patterns that may have potential health benefits. In the case of fruits and vegetables, hundreds of studies have been conducted to explore the relationship between consumption patterns and disease risk (Steinmetz & Potter, 1996). The majority of these findings report that consuming five to nine servings of fruits and vegetables daily provides people with better protection against developing disease when compared to those who eat fewer amounts (WCRF/AICR, 1997).

Led by population studies, laboratory scientists seek to identify the nutritive and non-nutritive ingredients that are present in fruits and vegetables, such as phytochemicals, to better isolate how they provide health benefits. Phytochemicals are part of the many substances found in vegetables and fruits that do not have nutritional value but are involved with critical physiologic activities such as cellular repair and enzymatic processes. On the other hand, essential nutrients (e.g., vitamin C, folic acid, iron) cannot be manufactured in the body and must be obtained from the diet. A diet lacking essential vitamins and minerals may lead to specific nutrient deficiencies that could have negative health consequences.

The accumulated scientific evidence shows that certain varieties of brightly colored fruits and vegetables may reduce a person's disease risk because of the phytochemicals they contain (Cooper et al., 1999; Lampe, 1999; Pavia & Russell, 1999; Serdula et al., 1996). High concentrations of vitamin C, folic acid, and carotenoids are found in brightly colored red, orange, yellow, and green fruits and vegetables. Carotenoids such as lutein in green leafy vegetables, lycopene in bright-red fruits and vegetables, and beta-carotene in orange-yellow fruits and vegetables have been shown to have antioxidant effects. Antioxidants enable cells to repair themselves more effectively, bind with free radicals to prevent further cell damage, and help to keep cell proliferation in check. Carotenoids work in partnership with one another and with other phytochemicals to produce these effects (Pavia & Russell). Other phytochemical-rich fruits and vegetables are onions and garlic, which contain allium compounds; flavonoid-rich berries such as grapes, strawberries, and blueberries; cruciferous vegetables such as cabbage and brussels sprouts, which contain a variety of isothiocyanates and indoles; and soybeans and soy products, which contain phytoestrogens and isoflavones (Lampe). These compounds can boost a cell's ability to prevent the growth of premalignant cancer cells or further cellular damage, reducing future risk for disease. Tables 7-1 and 7-2 identify common phytochemicals and other potential anticarcinogenic compounds, first by their function and presence in fruits and vegetables (Table 7-1) and then by their presence in specific types of fruits and vegetables (Table 7-2).

Why Whole Fruits and Vegetables Are a Better Choice Than Supplements

Epidemiological studies have shown weaker relationships between cancer and nutrients taken as supplements than for nutrients absorbed from eating whole fruits and vegetables (ACS, 1996; Serdula et al., 1996; WCRF/AICR, 1997). Consuming a diet that contains plenty of colorful fruits and vegetables, approximately five to nine servings a day, will provide a rich assortment of phytochemicals and nutrients the body can use to prevent oxidative damage, maximize cellular repair and integrity, and protect against the development of chronic diseases. A supplement cannot match all the benefits found in whole fruits and vegetables, no matter how many nutrients the pill contains. Relying on supplements instead of consuming a diet rich in fruits and vegetables will shortchange possible health benefits (Alpha-Tocopherol, Beta-Carotene Cancer Prevention Study Group [ATBCSG], 1994). People who rely too heavily on supplements miss out on the synergistic effects of the nutrients present in food. Finally, the effects of diet and nutritional

Table 7-1. Phytochemicals: Functions and Presence in Fruits and Vegetables

Phytochemicals	Function	Fruits	Vegetables
Sulfides (allium)			
Diallyl sulfide	Stimulates anticancer enzymes, detoxifies carcinogens; antibacterial activity may serve to inhibit conversion of nitrate to nitrite, reducing formation of nitrosamines, which are thought to be carcinogenic.		X
Allyl methyl trisulfide	Stimulates anticancer enzymes, detoxifies carcinogens; antibacterial activity may serve to inhibit conversion of nitrate to nitrite, reducing formation of nitrosamines, which are thought to be carcinogenic.		X
Dithiolthiones	Increases activity of enzymes involved in detoxification of carcinogens and other foreign compounds		X
Carotenoids			
Alpha-carotene	Antioxidant, vitamin A precursor, inhibits cell proliferation		X
Beta-carotene	Antioxidant; precursor to vitamin A that helps in differentiation of normal epithelial cells; inhibits cell proliferation	X	X
Lutein	Antioxidant, protects against cataracts, macular degeneration	X	X
Lycopene	Antioxidant		
Flavonoids			
Quercetin	Antioxidants; may reduce cell proliferation; extends action of vitamin C; inhibits blood clot formation; anti-inflammatory action	X	X
Kaempferol	Antioxidants; may reduce cell proliferation; extends action of vitamin C; inhibits blood clot formation; anti-inflammatory action	X	X
Tangeretin	Antioxidants; may reduce cell proliferation; extends action of vitamin C; inhibits blood clot formation; anti-inflammatory action	X	
Nobiletin	Antioxidants; may reduce cell proliferation; extends action of vitamin C; inhibits blood clot formation; anti-inflammatory action	X	
Rutin	Antioxidants; may reduce cell proliferation; extends action of vitamin C; inhibits blood clot formation; anti-inflammatory action	X	
Glucosinolates/ indoles			
Glucobrassicin	Forms indoles		X
Sinigrin			X
Indoles	Protects against estrogen-promoted cancers, induces protective enzymes		X
Phytoestrogens			
Genistein	Antioxidant; inhibits cancer cell growth; lowers blood cholesterol and platelet aggregation		X

(Continued on next page)

222

Table 7-1. Phytochemicals: Functions and Presence in Fruits and Vegetables *(Continued)*

Phytochemicals	Function	Fruits	Vegetables
Phytoestrogens *(continued)*			
Biochanin A	Antioxidant; inhibits cancer cell growth; lowers blood cholesterol and platelet aggregation		X
Lignans	Antioxidant; may block or suppress cancerous changes	X	X
Isothiocyanates			
Sulphorophane	Exceptionally potent inducer of detoxification enzyme		X
D-Limonene	Increases activity of glutathione transferase, a detoxification enzyme	X	
Phytosterols	Protects against hormone-dependent cancers, slows colon cancer growth		X
Protease inhibitors	Anticancer agent, suppresses cancer cell enzyme action		X
Saponins	Anticancer activity, possibly by preventing tumor cell division; binds bile acids and cholesterol to help reduce cholesterol level.		X
Phenols			
Chlorogeric acid	Prevents cancer-causing nitrosamines	X	X
Ellagic acid	Antioxidant; protects against DNA damage by carcinogens	X	
Caffeic acid	Prevents formation of carcinogens and blocks reaction of carcinogens with cells	X	
Coumarins	Increases activity of glutathione transferase, a detoxification enzyme	X	X
Catechins	Antioxidant	X	
Capsaicin	Antioxidant; prevents carcinogens from binding to DNA		X
Resveritrol	Antioxidant; protects against heart disease	X	
Anthocyanins	Antioxidant	X	X
Tannins	Prevents carcinogens from binding to target sites	X	X
Terpenes	Produces enzymes that deactivate carcinogens; prevents carcinogens from reacting with target sites; possible inhibition/blocking of hormones that promote tumor growth	X	X
Dietary fiber	Binds to and dilutes carcinogenic substances; speeds carcinogens through digestive tract; helps to control diabetes and high serum cholesterol; may prevent diverticulosis	X	X
Vitamins/minerals			
Vitamin C	Antioxidant; also reduces nitrite, thereby reducing formation of nitrosamines	X	X

(Continued on next page)

Table 7-1. Phytochemicals: Functions and Presence in Fruits and Vegetables *(Continued)*

Phytochemicals	Function	Fruits	Vegetables
Vitamins/minerals *(continued)*			
Vitamin E	Antioxidant that protects polyunsaturated fatty acids in cell membranes from oxidation; assists with antioxidant capacity of selenium	X	X
Folic acid	Inadequate intake may lead to chromosomal damage at sites relevant to specific cancers and also may lead to reduced methylation of DNA, which may permit a loss of normal controls on the expression of genes.	X	X
Potassium	May help to prevent or control hypertension and reduce the subsequent risk of stroke and heart disease	X	X
Selenium	A cofactor for glutathione peroxidase, an enzyme that protects against oxidative tissue damage	X	X

Note. Based on information from Beecher, 1999; Coughlin & DeBusk, 1998; Mangels et al., 1993; Produce Marketing Association, 1991; Steinmetz & Potter, 1991; Steinmetz & Potter, 1996.

supplements can be complicated by behaviors such as physical activity, smoking, alcohol consumption, food choices and preparation, and illness symptoms such as cachexia or anorexia, which may confound any associations that may be noted among diet, supplement use, and cancer risk (Byers, 1999; Hill, 1999).

The reader is encouraged to use this chapter as a review of current scientific evidence and leading health recommendations regarding fruit and vegetable consumption and cancer prevention. The data document a beneficial and more-or-less universal effect of vegetable consumption and, perhaps less definitively, a similar effect of fruit consumption. Potentially protective factors include various carotenoids, folic acid, vitamin C, flavonoids, phytoestrogens, isothiocyanates, and fiber. The identification of specific protective compounds, or their appropriate combination, is challenging and may never be completely defined. Additional data on the types and amounts of fruits and vegetables that are particularly protective could provide better guidance for those wanting to select an optimally healthy diet. Other reviews more detailed than this can provide an excellent summary of the effects of animal protein, fat, and fiber (WCRF/AICR, 1997). The chapter concludes with practical applications on diet and cancer prevention for the allied health practitioner.

Scientific Review of the Literature

Breast Cancer

Breast cancer is the third leading cause of death in U.S. women, following heart disease and lung cancer (Ries, 2000). In 2001, an estimated one in eight American women may be diagnosed with breast cancer. If survival rates remain consistent

Table 7-2. Phytochemicals in Specific Vegetables and Fruits

Vegetable/Fruit	Sulfides	Carotenoids	Flavonoids	Glucosinolates/ Indoles	Phytoestrogens	Isothiocyanates	Phenols	Other
Vegetables								
Allium vegetables								
Onions	X		X				X	Saponins
Garlic	X		X				X	Saponins
Green onions	X		X				X	
Leeks	X		X				X	
Chives	X		X				X	
Artichokes			X				X	
Asparagus		X	X				X	
Beans								
Lima beans			X		X	X	X	Saponins, phytosterols
Pinto beans			X		X	X	X	Saponins, phytosterols
Chickpeas			X		X	X	X	Saponins, phytosterols
Kidney beans			X		X	X	X	Saponins, phytosterols
Lentils			X		X	X	X	Saponins, phytosterols
Split peas			X		X	X	X	Saponins, phytosterols
Soy beans			X		X	X	X	Phytosterols, saponins, lignans, protease inhibitors
Tofu					X	X	X	Saponins
Beets			X				X	
Belgian endive			X				X	
Bell peppers		X	X				X	Terpenes
Carrots		X	X				X	Terpenes
Celery		X	X				X	
Corn		X	X					Dithiolthiones, tannins, terpenes

(Continued on next page)

225

Table 7-2. Phytochemicals in Specific Vegetables and Fruits (Continued)

Vegetable/Fruit	Sulfides	Carotenoids	Flavonoids	Glucosinolates/ Indoles	Phytoestrogens	Isothiocyanates	Phenols	Other
Vegetables								
Cruciferous vegetables								
Broccoli		X		X		X	X	Dithiolthiones, tannins, terpenes
Bok choy			X	X		X	X	Dithiolthiones, tannins, terpenes
Cauliflower		X	X	X		X	X	Dithiolthiones, anthoxanthins
Brussels sprouts		X	X	X		X	X	Dithiolthiones, anthoxanthins
Green cabbage		X	X	X		X	X	Dithiolthiones, anthoxanthins
Kale			X	X		X	X	Terpenes
Cucumbers			X			X		Phytosterols, terpenes
Eggplant			X					Terpenes, anthocyanins
Ginger root			X					Gingerol
Green leafy vegetables								
Collards		X	X				X	
Endive		X	X				X	
Iceberg lettuce		X	X				X	
Leaf lettuce		X	X				X	
Mustard greens		X	X	X			X	
Parsley		X					X	Terpenes
Romaine lettuce		X	X				X	
Spinach		X	X				X	
Green snap beans		X	X				X	
Hot chili peppers			X					Capsaicin
Mushrooms			X					Terpenes
Okra			X					
Potato			X				X	

(Continued on next page)

Table 7-2. Phytochemicals in Specific Vegetables and Fruits (Continued)

Vegetable/Fruit	Sulfides	Carotenoids	Flavonoids	Glucosinolates/ Indoles	Phytoestrogens	Isothiocyanates	Phenols	Other
Vegetables								
Pumpkins		X	X				X	
Radishes		X	X				X	Anthocyanins
Rutabagas			X	X			X	
Summer squash		X	X				X	Terpenes
Sweet potatoes		X	X				X	Terpenes
Tomatoes		X	X				X	Terpenes
Turnips			X	X			X	
Winter squash			X				X	
Fruits								
Apples			X				X	
Apricots			X					
Avocados			X					
Bananas			X					
Berries								
Blueberries			X				X	Lignans, catechins, tannins
Cranberries			X				X	Catechins
Raspberries			X				X	Lignans, catechins, tannins
Blackberries			X				X	Lignans, catechins, tannins
Strawberries			X				X	Saponins, lignans, catechins, tannins
Cantaloupe			X					
Carambola			X					
Cherries			X					
Citrus								
Grapefruit			X			X		Terpenes

(Continued on next page)

Table 7-2. Phytochemicals in Specific Vegetables and Fruits (Continued)

Vegetable/Fruit	Sulfides	Carotenoids	Flavonoids	Glucosinolates/ Indoles	Phytoestrogens	Isothiocyanates	Phenols	Other
Fruits								
Red grapefruit		X	X			X	X	Terpenes
Lemons			X			X	X	Terpenes
Limes			X			X	X	Terpenes
Oranges			X			X	X	Terpenes
Tangerines			X			X	X	Terpenes
Dates			X					
Figs			X					
Grapes			X				X	Anthocyanins, resveritrol
Honeydew melon			X					
Kiwifruit		X	X					
Mangos		X	X					
Nectarines			X					
Papayas			X				X	
Peaches		X	X					
Pears			X					
Pineapples			X				X	
Plums		X	X					
Prunes		X	X					
Raisins			X					
Rhubarb		X	X					
Watermelon		X	X					

Note. Based on information from Beecher, 1999; Coughlin & DeBusk, 1998; Mangels et al., 1993; Produce Marketing Association, 1991; Steinmetz & Potter, 1991; Steinmetz, & Potter, 1996.

with the present rate, approximately 69% of patients will survive after 10 years, and 57% will survive after 15 years (Ries).

For this reason, breast cancer is the most intensively studied human neoplasm with respect to possible nutritional causes. Scientific studies have documented the potential protective effects of diets high in fruits and vegetables. Adequate fruit and vegetable intakes have been associated with lower breast cancer risk in many studies, although the degree of the association is less than has been reported for colorectal or lung cancers (Howe, 1997; Hunter & Willett, 1996; Serdula et al., 1996). Additionally, conclusions about dietary effects are not entirely clear because individuals who report eating fewer fruits and vegetables typically report other health-related risk factors, such as greater levels of body weight, above-average alcohol use, and less physical activity. Combined, these factors confound the weak relationship with fruits and vegetables (Fisher et al., 1998). Other risk factors may include age; family history; atypical hyperplasia (i.e., irregular cells in benign breast lumps) confirmed by biopsy; never having given birth or having had the first live birth at a late age; early age at first menstrual period; late menopause; recent use of oral contraceptives or postmenopausal estrogens; and higher educational and socioeconomic status (Serdula et al., 1996).

Data suggest that breast cancer risk may be modified by the phytoestrogenic compounds found in certain fruits and vegetables (Davis, Dalais, & Simpson, 1999). The beneficial endocrine effects of these compounds, together with essential vitamins and minerals, may account for reduced breast cancer risk. Recently reported studies on the effects of tamoxifen to reduce breast cancer risk have spurred an interest in natural antiestrogens that can be obtained from foods (Fisher et al., 1998). Soybean products, which contain high levels of phytoestrogens, have been of particular interest. Soy plant foods could reduce breast cancer risk because they act as antiestrogens; however, soy also may exert pro-estrogenic effects, especially in postmenopausal women, when taken in high doses (Cline & Huges, 1998). This may result in increased breast cancer incidences among women carrying estrogen receptor-positive breast tumors (Petrakis et al., 1996).

Although the relationship between dietary fat intake and breast cancer has been examined repeatedly, it remains controversial (Glanz, 1994; Hankin, 1993; Hunter et al., 1996; Willett et al., 1992). In a pooled analysis of studies with more than 2,000 cases of breast cancer, no overall association was observed for total fat intakes ranging from 15% to more than 45% of energy from fat (Hunter et al.). A similar lack of association was seen in analyses restricted to postmenopausal women. Among the small number of women consuming less than 15% of energy from fat, breast cancer risk was elevated twofold (Hunter et al.). Although total fat intake has been unrelated to breast cancer risk in prospective epidemiologic studies, some evidence suggests that the type of fat, primarily animal fat rather than vegetable fat, may be important (Hopkins & Carroll, 1979; Hopkins, Kennedy, & Carroll, 1981). The Women's Health Initiative, a large trial involving thousands of women who were randomly assigned to a mixed dietary intervention, features a diet containing 20%–25% of calories from fat along with high fruit and vegetable consumption (Greenwald, Sherwood, & McDonald, 1997). The results of this trial are still pending.

Does the type of fat, vegetable versus animal, make a difference? Previously, animal models suggested that the tumor-promoting effect of fat intake was primarily caused by polyunsaturated fats (Hopkins & Carroll, 1979; Hopkins et al., 1981), but such an association has not been supported by the pooled data analysis from large cohort studies (Hunter et al., 1996). Notably, case-control studies conducted in Spain and Greece indicated that women who used greater amounts of olive oil, instead of animal fats, had reduced risks of breast cancer (Martin-Moreno et al., 1994; Trichopoulou et al., 1995). Animal studies suggest that olive oil may be protective when compared to other sources of fat (Welsh, 1992). This effect may be because of olive oil's high content of monounsaturated fat and antioxidants. Still, not all of the evidence points to a significant role for fat. The Nurses' Health Study, one of the largest cohort studies to test the dietary fat-breast cancer hypothesis, did not find an association between total fat intake or saturated fat intake and breast cancer incidence (Willett et al., 1992).

Given the balance of epidemiologic evidence to date, increased consumption of fruits and vegetables possibly may reduce breast cancer risk, whereas the effect of decreased dietary fat intake is less evident.

Prostate Cancer

Prostate cancer has emerged as an important health concern in the United States. According to 2000 estimates, more than 170,000 new cases were diagnosed and more than 37,000 men may die of prostate cancer (Parker, Tong, Bolden, & Wingo, 1997; Ries, 2000). Rates of diagnosed prostate cancers have increased dramatically in the United States since 1988, when prostate-specific antigen screening became commonplace (Parker et al.). Prostate cancer occurs primarily in older men and rarely is seen prior to age 40. African American men have a greater risk than Whites or other ethnic groups living in the United States and have one of the highest overall rates of prostate cancer in the world (Ries). Adjustments for lower socioeconomic and education levels have not accounted for the greater incidence rates observed in African American men. The underlying cause of the racial differences in risk remains speculative (Clinton & Giovannucci, 1998; Giovannucci & Clinton, 1998; Mills, Beeson, Phillips, & Fraser, 1989).

Although a causal relationship for any specific dietary factor and prostate cancer risk remains to be defined, a number of hypotheses are considered possible. Prostate cancer is common in nations with an affluent dietary pattern characterized by excessive calorie intake, high fat concentrations, excessive saturated fats, and highly refined carbohydrates, whereas the proportion of the diet from fruits, vegetables, and whole grains is comparably low (Clinton & Giovannucci, 1998). Inverse associations have not been seen between overall fruit and vegetable consumption and risk of prostate cancer (Cohen, Kristal, & Stanford, 2000). Intake of tomato products, the primary source of the carotenoid lycopene, has been linked to lower risk in case-control and prospective studies (Denis, Morton, & Griffiths, 1999; Giovannucci et al., 1995; Giovannucci & Clinton, 1998).

In a cohort study of 14,000 Seventh-Day Adventist men, a religious group consuming a vegetarian diet, participants completed a dietary questionnaire in 1976 and were monitored for cancer incidence through 1982 (Mills et al., 1989).

During the six-year follow-up, 180 histologically confirmed prostate cancers were detected. The dietary instrument was designed to examine food intake, not specific nutrients. As part of a multivariate analysis, only tomato intake and the consumption of beans, lentils, and peas were significantly related to lower prostate cancer risk. Specifically, the consumption of tomatoes one to four times per week, compared to less than one serving per week, was associated with a relative risk (RR) of 0.64 (confidence interval [CI] 95%: 0.42–0.97). Consumption of tomatoes more than five times per week was associated with an RR of 0.60 (CI 95%: 0.37–0.97). These relationships were independent of other dietary factors (Mills et al.).

The largest comprehensive study to date is the Health Professionals Follow-Up Study, which involves a large cohort of U.S. male healthcare professionals (Giovannucci et al., 1995). Dietary intake was assessed using a validated 131-item food frequency questionnaire with 47,894 healthcare professionals who were cancer free in 1986. Based on the specific carotenoid content of foods (Mangels, Holden, Beecher, Forman, & Lanza, 1993) and the self-reported intake of fruits and vegetables, estimated individual intake for specific carotenoids was calculated. Between 1986 and 1992, 812 new cases of prostate cancer were diagnosed in these participants. Greater lycopene intake was related to a statistically significant (21%) reduction in risk of prostate cancer.

Researchers assessed specific food items that were the major contributors of dietary carotenoids. Of 46 vegetables and fruits or related products, four (raw tomatoes, tomato juice, tomato sauce, and pizza) were significantly associated with lower prostate cancer. Tomato sauce, tomatoes, and pizza were the primary sources of lycopene (approximately 82%) in the diet. A combined intake of tomatoes and tomato products was associated with a 35% lower risk of prostate cancer (consumption frequency > 10 versus < 1.5 servings/week). The protective effect was stronger (a 53% lower risk) for the more advanced or aggressive prostate cancers (Giovannucci et al., 1995). Additionally, follow-up data collected in 1990 and again during 1991–1993 revealed that higher intakes of tomato sauce were strongly related to a lower risk of prostate cancer (Giovannucci & Clinton, 1998). Inverse associations observed with tomatoes and pizza were weaker, and no relationship was observed between tomato juice and the risk of prostate cancer.

Two other studies have addressed the tomato and prostate cancer relationship. A case-control study conducted in Minnesota found a nonsignificant inverse association between tomato intake and risk of prostate cancer (Schulman, Mandel, Radke, Seal, & Halberg, 1982). Another case-control study of 452 prostate cancer cases and 899 population controls conducted in a multi-ethnic population in Hawaii (Le Marchand, Hankin, Kolonel, & Wilkins, 1991) reported no association with consumption of tomatoes. However, the intake levels were not indicated, and it did not appear that tomato-based products, such as tomato sauce, were specifically accounted for.

Recent reports have suggested that the noted cancer-protective effects may be because of natural sex hormone modulators (phytoestrogens) that are found in nuts, vegetables, and legumes, including peas, beans, and lentils but especially in soy (Kolonel, 1996; Montironi, Mazzucchelli, Marshall, & Bartels, 1999).

The incidences of breast cancer in women and prostate cancer in men have been increasing in Western societies. Until recently, no satisfactory explanation has been available. Increased use of screening tests that has led to higher rates of detection provides a partial explanation; however, mortality rates have increased along with the incidence of early-stage diagnosis. People of ethnic origins from Asian countries who migrate to the United States show trends over time for increased risk and incidence of breast and prostate cancer compared to rates of U.S. Whites (Stephens, 1999). The prime factor appears to be related to diet. The most significant change has been from a diet high in plant foods, soy, and legumes, with little animal fat, to a reverse situation (Stephens; Yip, Heber, & Aronson, 1999). Thus, diet remains a probable factor influencing the risk of breast and prostate cancer. Further research is needed to confirm this assumption.

Colorectal Cancer

Colorectal cancer is the second leading cause of cancer-related deaths in the United States. The two most important considerations for avoidance of this disease are early detection and prevention (Ries, 2000). If metastasis has occurred to distant sites, such as the liver and lung, the five-year survival rate is less than 10% but will increase to greater than 90%, when the cancer is detected at an early stage (Dashwood, 1999). The causes of colorectal cancer still are under investigation. A family history increases the likelihood of developing colorectal cancer, and individuals who know that polyps or colorectal cancer run in their family are advised to obtain regular medical screening (i.e., sigmoidoscopy, colonoscopy).

Colon and rectal cancer rates differ by gender but exhibit similar incidences between the sexes for colon cancer, with a predominance for males (see Figures 7-1–7-4). Although cancers of the colon and rectum differ somewhat in their descriptive epidemiology, they will be reviewed together for the reader's convenience.

The epidemiological data on the association of vegetables and fruits and colorectal cancer are fairly consistent. In a review of 22 epidemiological studies (20 case-control, 2 cohort) that investigated the association of vegetables and fruits and incidence of colon and rectal cancers, the case-control studies reported protective associations (15 were statistically significant), and the cohort studies were in the direction of increased risk (Steinmetz, Kushi, Bostick, Folsom, & Potter, 1994; Steinmetz & Potter, 1991). A meta-analysis of six case-control studies found a combined odds ration of 0.48 (CI 95%: 0.41–0.57) (Trock, Lanza, & Greenwald, 1990).

The Iowa Women's Health Study is the only prospective study to report combined vegetable and fruit findings in relation to colon cancer incidence (RR 0.73; CI 95%: 0.47–1.13) (Steinmetz & Potter, 1991). The Iowa study also found an RR of 0.68 (CI 95%: 0.46–1.02) with high garlic intake. Among the case-control studies, specific categories of vegetables showed inverse associations with cruciferous vegetables, carrots, cabbage, and green vegetables (Steinmetz & Potter, 1991; Verhoeven, Goldbohm, van Poppel, Verhagen, & van den Brandt, 1996). Intake of fruit was less strongly associated with decreased risk, whereas intake of legumes was positively associated in two of three studies that were reviewed (Steinmetz & Potter, 1991).

Formation of colorectal adenomatous polyps can be conveniently studied with randomized clinical trials because healthcare professionals use a standard clinical protocol to assess discrete neoplastic endpoints that are part of the causal change of cancer development (Byers, 1999). The possible protective role of nutrients in the later phases of the transition of adenomas to cancer cannot be easily studied in these polyp trial designs as they focus on the first few years of new polyp growth following the removal of a metachromous polyp. Studying earlier phases of polyp development in individuals who were found to be polyp-free at baseline would require a larger number of subjects over longer periods of time. Additionally, it is difficult to study later phases of colorectal cancer development when large adenomatous polyps potentially develop into cancer (Bostick, 1999).

Effects of a whole-diet intervention on adenoma formation was tested by the National Cancer Institute (NCI) Polyp Prevention Trial, a randomized controlled trial investigating the effects of a low-fat diet that includes seven daily servings of fruits and vegetables on polyp formation (Schatzkin & Kelloff, 1995). Unfortunately, this intervention is reported to have no effect on polyp recurrence rates (Schatzkin et al., 2000). Although this study features a whole-diet intervention, it is weakened by the fact that it is being conducted only during the three-year period between initial polypectomy and repeated colonoscopic examination. Consequently, as in other polyp prevention trials, the NCI Polyp Prevention Trial does not test the effects of fruits and vegetables on later stages of cancer development.

One cannot fully review the effect of diet on colorectal cancer risk without mentioning dietary fiber. Fiber is hypothesized to reduce the risk of colorectal cancer in several ways: diluting potential carcinogens and speeding their transit through the colon; binding carcinogenic substances; altering the colonic flora; reducing the pH; or serving as the substrate for the generation of short-chain fatty acids that are the preferred substrate for colonic epithelial cells (Lipkin, Reddy, Newmark, & Lamprecht, 1999; Reddy, 1999). Recently published evidence suggested that the importance of dietary fiber in reducing the risk of colorectal cancer is less clear (Alberts et al., 2000). Populations with high fiber consumption and low colorectal cancer rates also are more likely to consume less meat, be less obese, and be more physically active (WCRF/AICR, 1997). The evidence suggests that each of these confounding factors reduces risk and is possibly part of the ecological associations noted between low intakes of dietary fiber and colorectal cancer rates.

In case-control studies, intake of cereal products or fiber from grains has not been associated with reduced risk of colon cancer, in contrast to the better support for a protective effect from fruits and vegetables (Alberts et al., 2000; Potter, 1996; Willett, 1989). In several large prospective studies, overall fiber intake has not been significantly associated with lower risk of colon cancer incidence after adjustment for other risk factors (Fuchs et al., 1999; Giovannucci et al., 1994; Goldbohm et al., 1994; Thun et al., 1992; Willett, Stampfer, Colditz, Rosner, & Speizer, 1990). In these studies, higher grain fiber intake has been associated with a lower risk of coronary heart disease, which suggests that dietary fiber provides physiologically important effects (Rimm et al., 1996). Thus, fiber intake does not appear to account for the protective effect of fruits and vegetables against colon cancer, and available evidence does not support the idea that higher grain or fiber consumption will reduce colon cancer risk.

In summary, epidemiologic evidence suggests that diets rich in vegetables may protect against cancers of the colon and rectum. Data on fruit consumption are more limited and less consistent. Data on dietary fiber intake show that it does not appear to reduce colon cancer risk. Components found in vegetables (e.g., phytochemicals, fiber, folic acid, calcium, antioxidant enzyme-associated micronutrients) support the biological plausibility of this protective association between increased vegetable consumption and reduced risk (Dashwood, 1999; Eastwood, 1999). This is supported by published analytical, observational, epidemiological literature (WCRF/AICR, 1997). Overall, the findings of recent trials (Alberts et al., 2000; Schatzkin et al., 2000) suggest that more prospective data are needed.

Lung Cancer

Lung cancer is the leading cause of cancer deaths in males, accounting for approximately 150,000 deaths per year (Ries, 2000). Statistics show that cigarette smoking is the primary cause of deaths from lung cancer in the United States, with approximately 90% of cases in men and 79% of cases in women (Shopland, Eyre, & Pechacek, 1991). Other risk factors in lung cancer incidence include occupational exposure to asbestos, arsenic, radon, and pollution and behavioral factors such as physical activity, alcohol consumption, and diet (especially fruit and vegetable intakes) (Du, Zhou, & Wu, 1998).

Reported epidemiological studies consistently suggest that diets high in fruits and vegetables are associated with lower risk for cancer of the lung and larynx, even after adjustment for the observation that smokers tend to eat less-healthy diets than nonsmokers (Ziegler, Mayne, & Swanson, 1996). A significant inverse association by racial subgroups was reported between the intake of vegetables, fruits, and carotenoids (e.g., green leafy, bright red, orange-yellow vegetables) and the number of lung cancer cases in White females, suggesting a protective effect (Dorgan et al., 1993). African American males showed only a weak inverse association between lung cancer and vegetables. In both groups, an increasing risk associated with decreasing fruit and vegetable intake was limited to smokers. Neither smoking patterns nor lung cancer history explained the discrepancy between African Americans and Whites.

In a case-control study on lung cancer among nonsmoking women, the results of analysis, after adjustment for age, education, and total calories, indicated that a strong protective effect was associated with consuming above-average quantities of vegetables, especially those containing carotene (Candelora, Stockwell, Armstrong, & Pinkham, 1992). Vegetable intake has been reported to protect against the adverse effects of lung cancer caused by smoking and occupational exposure to pollutants (Forman et al., 1992). Among heavy-smoking (e.g., cigarette, pipe) male residents of a Chinese mining community, where radon and arsenic exposure further compound their risk factors, dark green vegetable intake was significantly associated with inverse lung cancer risk (Forman et al.). Consumption of fresh green fruits also was associated with a significant dose-dependant reduction in lung cancer risk in U.S. nonsmokers (Mayne et al., 1994). A study of postmenopausal women from Iowa showed that lung cancer risk was doubled in women with a low intake of all vegetables and fruits, all vegetables, or green leafy vegetables. Comparable effects were not observed for provitamin A carotenoid or vitamin C intake or for foods rich in beta-carotene, lutein, or lycopene (Steinmetz, Potter, & Folsom, 1993).

Reviews of numerous prospective studies of diet and lung cancer indicate stronger inverse trends with vegetable and fruit intake than with estimated provitamin A carotenoid intake (WCRF/AICR, 1997; Ziegler et al., 1996). Studies suggest that vegetables, especially dark-green and yellow-orange vegetables rich in beta-carotene, reduce lung cancer risk; similar but less significant patterns have been noted with fruit intake (Ziegler et al.).

Use of nutritional supplements has been less effective in reducing lung cancer risk. Both the Alpha-Tocopherol Beta-Carotene Study and the Carotene and Retinol Efficacy Trial found an increased risk of lung cancer when high doses of beta-carotene were taken (ATBCSG, 1994; Omenn et al., 1996). The results of the Physicians Health Study were neutral; thus, beta-carotene did not alter lung cancer risk in either direction (Hennekens et al., 1996). The reason for these unanticipated adverse effects remains unclear (Cooper et al., 1999).

Overall, evidence is strong that certain factors in fruits and vegetables inhibit the initiation or promotion of lung cancer (Ziegler et al., 1996). What is potentially important for both public health application and determining the mode of action is the possible interaction of smoking and dietary substances that are cancer protective (ATBCSG, 1994). Future studies should include stratification of the results by smoking status and gender. Current data support general dietary recommendations to decrease ingestion of fat to less than 30% of caloric intake and to increase the daily number of fruit and vegetable servings in the diet to at least five. No specific dietary supplements are recommended at this time.

Summary of Evidence for Fruits and Vegetables

Extensive review of the research on the health benefits of fruits and vegetables and cancer risk have resulted in several major reports. WCRF and AICR commissioned the first report, and the second was the report of the Chief Medical Officer's Committee on Medical Aspects of Food and Nutrition Policy (COMA) by the British Department of Health (COMA, 1998; WCRF/AICR, 1997). The majority of the research reviewed by COMA and WCRF/AICR is drawn from epidemiological studies.

Table 7-3 summarizes the epidemiological evidence related to vegetable and fruit intakes and cancer as assessed by AICR and COMA. AICR's panel classified the strength of evidence as convincing, probable, possible, or insufficient evidence to base a judgment. The COMA working group used classifications of strongly consistent, moderately consistent, and weakly consistent. In general, the COMA working group tended to be more conservative in its judgment of the evidence than the AICR panel.

AICR and COMA found the science base convincing (AICR) or strongly consistent (COMA) for a protective effect of vegetables and fruits against stomach and

Table 7-3. Summary of Epidemiological Evidence Related to Fruits and Vegetables and Cancer

Cancer	Vegetables		Fruits	
	WCRF/AICR[a]	COMA[b]	WCRF/AICR	COMA
Mouth and pharynx	⇓ convincing	inconsistent	⇓ convincing	⇓ weakly convincing
Larynx	⇓ probable	⇓ moderately consistent, limited data	⇓ probable	⇓ moderately consistent, limited data
Esophagus	⇓ convincing	⇓ strongly consistent	⇓ convincing	⇓ strongly consistent
Lung	⇓ convincing	⇓ weakly consistent	⇓ convincing	⇓ moderately consistent
Stomach	⇓ convincing	⇓ moderately consistent	⇓ convincing	⇓ moderately consistent
Pancreas	⇓ probable	⇓ strongly consistent, limited data	⇓ probable	⇓ strongly consistent, limited data
Liver	⇓ possible			
Colon, rectum	⇓ convincing	⇓ moderately consistent		⇓ inconsistent, limited data
Breast	⇓ probable	⇓ moderately consistent	⇓ probable	⇓ weakly consistent
Ovary	⇓ possible	insufficient	⇓ possible	insufficient
Endometrium	⇓ possible	insufficient	⇓ possible	insufficient
Cervix	⇓ possible	⇓ strongly consistent, limited data	⇓ possible	⇓ strongly consistent, limited data inconsistent
Prostate	⇓ possible	⇓ moderately consistent, especially raw and salad type		
Thyroid	⇓ possible		⇓ possible	
Kidney	⇓ possible			
Bladder	⇓ probable	⇓ moderately consistent, limited data	⇓ probable	⇓ moderately consistent, limited data

Note. No evidence reviewed by either WCRF/AICR or COMA for nasopharynx or gallbladder cancers.

[a] WCRF/AICR—World Cancer Research Fund/American Institute for Cancer Research, 1997
[b] COMA—Committee on Medical Aspects of Food and Nutrition Policy, 1998
⇓ — decreasing risk

esophageal cancers. For a number of other site-specific cancers, AICR and COMA tended to differ somewhat in their assessments of the science base. For colorectal cancer, the evidence was judged convincing (AICR) or moderately consistent (COMA) for vegetables but inconsistent (COMA) or insufficient (AICR) for fruits.

For cancers of the lung and mouth/pharynx, the AICR panel found the evidence convincing for a protective effect of high intakes of vegetables and fruits. However, the COMA Working Group determined the evidence to be moderately consistent for vegetables in lung cancer, weakly consistent for fruits in cancers of the mouth and pharynx and for vegetables in lung cancer, and inconsistent for vegetables in cancers of the mouth and pharynx. For laryngeal cancer, the science base was determined to be moderately consistent (COMA) or probable (AICR) for a protective effect of both fruits and vegetables.

The AICR panel judged the evidence to be probable for a protective effect of vegetables and fruits in breast cancer. The evidence is stronger and more consistent for a protective effect of vegetables, particularly green vegetables. COMA's assessment of the evidence was similar to AICR's for vegetables in breast cancer but determined that the evidence is only weakly consistent for fruits. The evidence is less strong for cancers of the prostate, ovary, endometrium, cervix, thyroid, kidney, bladder, and liver (COMA, 1998; WCRF/AICR, 1997).

Despite some differences in their assessments of the underlying science base, summary recommendations by AICR and COMA for vegetable and fruit intakes and cancer risk focus on variety. AICR promoted the year-round consumption of a variety of vegetables and fruits, which provide 7% or more of a person's total energy intake. COMA recommended increasing vegetable and fruit intakes (COMA, 1998; WCRF/AICR, 1997).

Dietary Behavioral Change Counseling and Intervention: Translating the Science Into Practice

The weight of the scientific evidence linking fruit and vegetable consumption with cancer prevention and control, including the ever-increasing understanding of the biological mechanisms in action, provides a solid knowledge base for nurses and other healthcare professionals to encourage individuals to increase their fruit and vegetable consumption.

Vegetables and Fruits: Quantity

The evidence reviewed in this chapter supports the intake of five servings of vegetables and fruits daily as a minimum goal for all Americans. In the recent report commissioned by WCRF and AICR (1997), an exhaustive collection of relevant worldwide research on this topic was reviewed. The report set 400 grams per day (g/d), or five servings, of vegetables and fruits as the lower limit of the recommended range, and it estimated that diets high in vegetables and fruits (> 400 g/d) could prevent at least 20% of all cancer incidences (WCRF/AICR). Five servings of vegetables and fruits also are the minimum number estimated to ensure adequacy of select nutrients among individuals with low energy needs, regardless if they are fresh, cooked, dried, canned, frozen, or juice form. This is based on a system designed to provide dietary guidance for individuals with low or high energy needs (Cronin, Shaw, Krebs-Smith, Marsland, & Light, 1987). For those with greater total energy needs, the intake of larger or additional servings is encouraged.

The AICR panel recommends up to 10 servings daily as the upper intake level of fruits and vegetables for cancer risk reduction (WCRF/AICR, 1997); the Food Guide Pyramid encourages up to nine servings of fruits and vegetables daily for general good health, consisting of two to four servings of fruit and three to five servings of vegetables (U.S. Department of Agriculture, 1992). More research still is warranted, however, to enhance understanding of threshold levels for increased fruit and vegetable intake and to assess the relationship between quantity and quality of fruit and vegetable intake.

Vegetables and Fruits: Quality

In addition to a focus on quantity, the evidence reviewed in this chapter supports increased consumption of a wide variety of vegetables, particularly dark-green leafy, cruciferous, and yellow-orange ones, and fruits, particularly citrus and deep yellow-orange ones, for cancer risk reduction and health promotion. Microconstituents in vegetables and fruits that are likely to protect against cancers and other diseases and health conditions (e.g., cardiovascular disease, stroke) are antioxidants, such as carotenoids, flavonoids, and vitamin C. Other micro-constituents that may help to explain the protective effect in cancer and heart disease are the sulfur-containing compounds in the allium family vegetables. For cancer, the dithiothiones, indoles, and isothiocyanates in cruciferous vegetables and folic acid found in most fruits and vegetables, particularly in green leafy vegetables and some citrus fruits, may play additional protective roles.

Current Vegetable and Fruit Intakes

Recent national surveys suggest that Americans have made modest, yet important, improvements in meeting the minimum of five daily fruit and vegetable servings. Using data from the Continuing Survey of Food Intake of Individuals (CSFII), American adults in 1994 consumed an average of 4.4 servings of fruits and vegetables daily, a slight increase from 3.9 servings in 1991 (Krebs-Smith, Cleveland, Ballard-Barbash, Cook, & Kahle, 1997). Although these gains are encouraging, further improvements in dietary practices are critical to better ensure a reduction in the risk for cancer and other chronic diseases. This is particularly true for children, as children are reported to eat a full serving less than adults (Krebs-Smith et al., 1996, 1997).

Fruit and vegetable intake is not uniform across various subpopulations. Consumption of fruits and vegetables is lower among African Americans compared to Whites (Serdula et al., 1995). Hispanics also consume fewer fruits and vegetables than non-Hispanic Whites (Serdula et al., 1995). An examination of motivations, as well as barriers, to increase fruit and vegetable consumption in these groups is an important aid to developing targeted nutrition messages, which, in turn, enhance the likelihood of effecting positive behavior changes within these populations.

The public health benefits of good dietary habits would be enormous. Hypertension, heart disease, stroke, cancer, diabetes mellitus, obesity, and osteoporosis all have dietary links. Combined, these seven health-related conditions cost an estimated $250 billion each year in medical costs and lost productivity—a significant portion of which might be saved by improved nutritional habits ("ADA Testifies," 1998).

Clinical Applications of the Science

Applications of current research findings to clinical settings by healthcare professionals have several advantages. First, the counseling of patients on increasing fruit and vegetable intakes is facilitated by the fact that people already know what fruits and vegetables are, whereas some dietary sources of sodium or fat may be less evident. Second, the addition of a behavioral criterion, such as eating five or more fruits and vegetables, facilitates goal setting and self-monitoring of whether a goal is reached. Additional behavioral strategies can help to ensure effective dietary change by patients. These include employing a lifestyle approach, which includes focusing on skill building (e.g., how to select and prepare vegetables, how to pack healthy lunches); emphasizing the natural good taste of fruits and vegetables; problem solving (e.g., determine what raw vegetables cause indigestion and solve problem by cooking them); increasing fruit and vegetable availability (e.g., keeping a supply in the house) and accessibility (e.g., keeping cut-up fruits and vegetables in a bowl in the refrigerator, placing washed fruits in a bowl on the kitchen table); and a trial-and-error approach with feedback from the nurse. A smaller step might be to add fruit to cereal in the morning (goal); the individual finds that the bananas he bought are now over-ripe, so he adds sliced strawberries to the cereal instead, after discussion with the nurse. Education on the importance of increased fruit and vegetable consumption alone, even if it includes a discussion on the associated health benefits of increased fruit and vegetable intake, does not appear to be enough. Third, counseling to increase fruit and vegetable intake is a positive message that can capture patients' attention and provide them with information about adding more healthy food to their daily intake. Thus, it shifts the focus in the counseling to something people *can* do rather then something they should avoid or limit. Finally, it is useful to inform patients that meeting the recommendations for fruit and vegetable intake can help reduce dietary fat intake. When the fruit recommendation was met in a recent analysis of the diets of individuals participating in the 1989–1991 CSFII, the percentage of energy from fat was at or below the population average (Krebs-Smith et al., 1997).

Effecting Behavioral Change at the Individual Level

Food choices, including those for fruits, vegetables, fiber, and fat content, are influenced by a host of psychosocial, demographic, and environmental factors. People report taste, cost, convenience, weight control, and, to a lesser extent, nutrition as important influences on food choices (Glanz, Basil, Maibach, Goldberg, & Snyder, 1998). Knowledge and beliefs also influence food choices. However, the belief that dietary factors may play a role in preventing cancer is not widespread among Americans, although most Americans (83%) in a recent national survey reported a belief that eating well may reduce their chance of developing major diseases (Harnack, Block, Subar, Lane, & Brand, 1997). Foods and nutrient categories mentioned most often as recognized to reduce cancer risk were fiber (72%), fruits and vegetables (66%), and less fat (60%). For breast cancer, in particular, there is a limited belief among women that diet plays a role in cancer risk reduction. Only 20% of women in 1991 and 23% of women in 1995 cited a relationship between dietary factors and reducing cancer risk (Barnard & Nicholson, 1997). These findings suggest a need to counsel patients and plan interventions to increase awareness of the link between diet and disease and, in particular, diet and cancer.

A unilateral focus on disseminating nutritional information about the importance of diet to promote health and reduce disease risk is unlikely to effect positive dietary change. Although attitudes, knowledge, and beliefs about diet and disease are associated consistently with healthy dietary behavior (Dittus, Hillers, & Beerman, 1995; Eisner, Loughrey, Hadley, & Doner, 1992; Harnack et al., 1997; Patterson, Kristal, Lynch, & White, 1995), perceived barriers to healthy eating (e.g., increased intake of fruits and vegetables) generally are cited as stronger predictors of intake (Dittus et al.; Harnack et al.). These findings challenge nurses and other healthcare professionals to address not only the importance of diet to health but also to discover ways of reducing perceived barriers to healthy eating by counseling patients and planning interventions.

The most frequently cited barriers to eating more fruits and vegetables are taste, cost, and availability (Eisner et al., 1992; Treiman, Freimuth, & Damron, 1996). Time and perceived inconvenience of preparation also have been reported (Office of Communications, NCI, 1998). Low-income individuals, in particular, report cost, availability, perishability/short shelf life, and difficulties with preparation and storage as barriers to eating more fruits and vegetables (Dittus et al., 1995; Reicks, Randall, & Haynes, 1994; Treiman et al.). This corresponds with several studies that have identified a relationship between people with low income/low education and low fruit/vegetable intakes (Laforge, Greene, & Prochaska, 1994; Serdula et al., 1995). Cited in the literature as additional barriers to healthful eating are difficulties in changing one's existing dietary behaviors (Reicks et al.), a preference for one's current diet and belief that one's diet is already a "good" one (Cotugna, Subar, Heimendinger, & Kahle, 1992), and a belief that too many diet-related recommendations exist (Cotugna et al.). Evidence also suggests that barriers are different for fruits than vegetables. Individuals participating in a focus group cited expense and perishability as barriers for increasing fruit consumption, whereas preparation time and taste were barriers to eating more vegetables (Office of Communications, NCI, 1992).

Overcoming barriers to eating more fruits and vegetables can be addressed with patients in a variety of ways. Table 7-4 lists educational and promotional activities to encourage dietary behavior change. Building self-confidence (also known as self-efficacy) in one's abilities to make healthy choices is associated with eating more fruits and vegetables (Havas et al., 1998). Demonstrating techniques for easy-to-prepare recipes and menus that incorporate fruits and vegetables and providing opportunities for practicing new skills also may enhance self-efficacy and consumption. Providing practical tips on how to choose fresh produce and serve it in appetizing ways can help people to practice healthy eating habits. Parents should be encouraged to welcome their children into the kitchen during meal preparations to not only enjoy a little togetherness and individualized attention but also to share some nutrition lessons.

Table 7-4. Educational and Promotional Activities to Encourage Dietary Behavior Change

Level of Intervention	Type of Activity	Examples
Individual	Create awareness.	Conduct media events or activities emphasizing the need to eat "5 a day" for better health. • Make educational messages simple and easy to understand. Materials should be developed for a sixth-grade reading level and include plenty of pictures to illustrate examples.
	Provide motivation.	• Tailor educational messages to each patient's needs, resources, cultural or ethnic background, and food preferences. The more relevant the message is to the patient's interest, the better the opportunity to motivate for long-term behavior changes. • Include messages about the association between diet and cancer or between eating a healthy diet and looking and feeling better. • Include incentive-based activities, such as contests involving fruits and vegetables or coupons for purchasing them.
	Develop skills.	Offer preparation and cooking demonstrations. • Show patients concerned with time constraints or complex recipes that vegetables are delicious when cooked in the microwave. They retain their bright color, fresh taste, crisp texture, and nutrients when cooked with a minimum amount of water. • Lead a tour of the produce section at a local grocery store to help relieve consumer anxiety about identifying and selecting fruits and vegetables. Be sure to tell patients about the variety of precut vegetables (packaged and from the salad bar) that are available for brown bag lunches or a fast salad with dinner.
	Develop social support.	Include suggestions on how to use peer influence by adopting "buddies" at work or home to reinforce healthful eating habits.
Environmental	Promote food system and environmental support.	Increase the availability, appeal, and variety of fruits and vegetables served in hospital cafeterias. • Label fruit and vegetable dishes served in cafeterias that meet the "5 A Day" criteria. • Modify food service menus. • Develop catering policies that include fruit and vegetable options at all company-sponsored events such as picnics and conferences.

Focusing counseling and intervention efforts on personal motives for healthy eating may be necessary to effect positive dietary behavior change (Kristal et al., 1995; Trudeau, Kristal, Li, & Patterson, 1998). Internal motivators, such as the desire to stay healthy, feel better, prevent cancer, and control one's weight, have been strongly associated with healthy eating (Trudeau et al.). Conversely, external factors, such as a physician's recommendation to eat a healthful diet or family and friends who generally eat healthy and encourage people to do the same, do not appear to affect dietary change to the same extent and, consequently, may be a less-important focus (Trudeau et al.). Given the positive association between internal motivators and healthy eating, a promising strategy might be to stress with patients how eating more fruits and vegetables can help one to stay healthy, feel better, prevent cancer, and control weight.

Studying cultural factors also can provide insight into how to encourage positive behavioral change. For example, traditional foods such as collard, kale, sweet potatoes, and watermelon have been identified as an important part of the African American diet. Effective educational efforts among this group should allow for the enjoyment of traditional African American dishes by teaching how to prepare healthier versions of these recipes (Office of Communications, NCI, 1995). Taking a patient-centered approach can help to ensure that realistic goals, compatible with the patient's physical and cognitive makeup, are established and that newly adopted behaviors will be culturally supported.

Assessment of adherence to new dietary behaviors may be aided by an acknowledgment that relapse to a former behavior is not a failure but rather the successful maintenance of a behavior previously held (Bouton, 2000). This approach puts the emphasis on the prior behavior and encourages a closer examination of the context of those prior behaviors, prompting a reexamination of the personal, environmental, and physical factors influencing behavioral change. The tendency in counseling and intervention is not to acknowledge these former behaviors, which can result in the setting of unrealistic goals.

A popular new approach to individual counseling and intervention is the use of tailored plans that use technologic strategies to deliver intervention messages designed especially for a particular individual. Two strategies that have received increased attention are tailored print communications (Rimer & Glassman, 1999) and tailored telephone counseling (Campbell et al., 1994). These interventions use computer-based programs that match algorithms from a large library of messages to patients' wants and needs, packaging specific messages and graphics into personal interventions.

Effecting Behavioral Change at the Community Level

Community-level interventions target populations in healthcare settings, workplaces, recreational centers, churches, and schools. These population-based interventions have the advantage of potentially reaching a much larger number of people than individually based interventions, although the community-based approach typically is much less intensive than the individually targeted one. Intervention results may be smaller as a result, but, because they are applied to larger audiences, the overall effect is greater. Some community-based interventions have yielded no intervention effects (Luepker et al., 1994), whereas others have generated effects for only some of the targeted behaviors (Sorensen, Stoddard, & Ockene, 1996). A number of reasons have been postulated regarding the results of these trials. Secular trends, in particular, have been cited as a plausible reason for why it is so challenging to achieve strong positive effects from community trials.

Recent community-based interventions targeting increased fruit and vegetable intake for cancer risk reduction have yielded encouraging results. In 1993, NCI funded nine four-year research projects with randomized designs; five were adult-focused and four were youth-focused projects. These community-based projects were conducted in a variety of community channels—four were based in schools, three at worksites, one in a church, and one in a food assistance program. Eight of the nine research projects significantly increased fruit and vegetable intakes pre- and postintervention in the intervention versus control groups. Mean fruit and vegetable intakes, across studies, increased from 0.2 to 1.7 servings daily (Potter et al., 2000; Stables, Van Duyn, Heimendinger, Nebeling, & Berkowitz, 2001).

These projects used multidisciplinary teams of investigators with expertise in a variety of fields, including nutrition, public health, health education, and communication, to develop theory-driven, multilevel interventions that use simple, positive behavioral nutrition messages to capture the attention of their target audiences (Havas et al., 1994). Several of the projects also included family members as part of the target audience and were aimed at changing individual, environmental, and community levels. Both the High-5-Alabama and Minnesota's 5 A Day Power Plus projects consisted of a classroom curriculum, parent intervention, and an environmental component. Georgia's Gimme 5 Fruits and Vegetables sought to increase fruit and vegetable availability in the cafeteria, preferences (e.g., via food tasting sessions to "introduce" new fruits and vegetables), and children's skills (e.g., fruit and vegetable preparation, cooking skills) through a behavioral modification approach. Gimme 5 in Louisiana used workshops and complementary activities, in addition to school meal and snack modification, a school-wide media and marketing campaign, and a parental component to increase fruit and vegetable intakes among teens in New Orleans. In Maryland, the Women, Infants, and Children (WIC) 5 A Day promotion used educational programs, WIC staff-delivered messages, lay counseling, trained peer group discussion leaders, and a farmer's market campaign to encourage women from minority groups to change their fruit and vegetable eating habits. Arizona's 5 A Day Worksite Wellness Project used motivational techniques and a health peer program to influence the fruit and vegetable intakes of men in the blue-collar Hispanic population. In Massachusetts, the Treatwell 5 A Day Project influenced employee advisory boards to conduct education and taste-test programs at worksites, and some added a program targeted toward workers' families. Using a theory-driven stages-of-change model with environmental-level and individual-level intervention(s), Seattle's 5 A Day Worksite program incorporated education and behavior change strategies among primarily white-collar employees to increase fruit and vegetable intakes.

One of the strengths of several of the "5 A Day" community projects was the focus on environmental and organizational variables. Frequently, studies aimed at changing health behavior focus strongly on the individual level, with only a limited focus on the environment and organization. Even though studies conducted in organizational settings have the advantage of being able to influence organizational environment and policies, few have fully utilized this advantage. The positive results of the "5 A Day" community projects suggest that including a focus on environmental and organizational variables, in addition to individual-level interventions, is a key component to successful interventions. Moreover, efforts to emphasize the implementation and evaluation of environmental and organizational strategies may be important considerations in developing the next generation of behavioral change studies.

Theoretical Issues in Effecting Behavioral Change

Use of behavior change theory can strengthen counseling and intervention strategies to encourage healthy eating. The social-ecological model is a prominent theoretical framework for guiding the design and implementation of multilevel behavioral interventions. In this model, five levels of influence for health education are postulated: intrapersonal/individual, interpersonal/group, institutional/organization, community, and public policy. Although programs often are targeted at one or, perhaps, two levels, a multilevel approach using a combination of different strategies is thought to be most effective. At the intrapersonal level, educators might try motivational interventions, skill-building opportunities, and tailored intervention materials. At the interpersonal level, appropriate interventions are those that target social norms or social networks, such as implementing healthy eating catering policies. At the organizational or environmental level, interventions are aimed at various settings, such as healthcare systems, workplaces, and food-assistance programs, and include involving key organizational groups, such as employee advisory boards, to support targeted healthy practices and policies. Implementing reduced relative prices to promote low-fat snack choices through school vending machines is another example of an environmental strategy that has been found to be effective in promoting healthier food choices (French, Jeffery, Story, Hannan, & Snyder, 1997). At the community level, interventions are aimed at networking with community resources and structural and environmental changes in the broader community, such as influencing key community leaders to support and promote healthy behavior efforts. Food assistance or surplus food distribution programs would be an example. Finally, at the policy level, interventions focus on influencing social norms and laws, including regulatory practices.

Transtheoretical Model

Identifying a patient's readiness to change may be helpful in planning counseling and interventions. The Transtheoretical Model proposed by DiClemente and Prochaska (1992) assumes that people will be at different points in their readiness to adopt a specific health-related behavior, such as increasing fruit and vegetable intake. Prochaska and DiClemente postulated that behavior can be divided into five basic stages of change: precontemplation (when an individual has no intention to change), contemplation (when an individual is seriously thinking about changing), preparation (when an individual actually is planning to change), action (when an individual actively is involved in behavior change), and maintenance (when an individual is sustaining a behavior change). The process of behavior adoption is seen as cyclical rather than linear, in which individuals may relapse and reenter at various points in the change process.

Applications of the model to increase fruit and vegetable intake demonstrate that people can be classified by their readiness to eat more fruits and vegetables. Stages of change have been associated, in a stepwise manner, with fruit and vegetable consumption (Glanz et al., 1994; Van Duyn et al., 1998), and studies have predicted dietary intake better than demographic characteristics (Campbell et al., 1998; Glanz et al., 1994; Van Duyn et al.). More advanced stages of change have been positively associated with self-efficacy (Campbell et al., 1998), knowledge (Campbell et al., 1998; Van Duyn et al.), female gender, and having more education (Campbell et al., 1998; Van Duyn et al.). This is important because the matching of individuals at different points of readiness to make a dietary change with tailored messages has been shown to be effective in improving dietary behavior (Campbell et al., 1994).

Taken altogether, these findings suggest that using the Transtheoretical Model to classify people by their readiness to make a targeted behavior change to increase fruit and vegetable intake may enable program planners and implementers to identify subgroups of individuals who would be most likely to benefit from an intervention. Changes in dietary stage by subgroup following program implementation then could be tracked. Although a growing body of literature exists related to the application of the Transtheoretical Model to dietary behavior, passage through the stages is poorly understood for nutrition-related behaviors. Detection of change in dietary stages from stage-based strategies could be used to assess the process by which individuals in subgroups move from awareness of the need to increase fruit and vegetable intake to positive behavior change. In a recently reported intervention, the most usual pattern of change was no change initially, followed by forward movement, and, finally, backward movement to an earlier stage (Kristal, Glanz, Tilley, & Li, 2000). Stage of change at follow-up, but not baseline, was associated with positive dietary change. This finding suggests that dietary interventions can be relevant and effective regardless of stage of change at baseline, and even people who already eat a healthy diet still can make additional dietary changes. Thus, counseling should emphasize continued dietary change and behavior goal attainment even for those at higher stages.

Public Policy Supports

Role of Public Nutrition Education: 5 A Day for Better Health Program

Since 1991, the "5 A Day for Better Health Program," a nationwide nutrition initiative sponsored in partnership by NCI and the Produce for Better Health Foundation, has combined research with a national dietary guidance program to work toward increasing fruit and vegetable consumption to a daily minimum of five servings (Heimendinger, Van Duyn, Chapelsky, Foerster, & Stables, 1996). This goal is supported by ACS's 1996 nutrition guidelines (ACS Advisory Committee on Diet, Nutrition, and Cancer Prevention 1996).

Designed to improve the health of Americans, the "5 A Day" program operationalizes its message through partnerships among the health community, government agencies, the fruit and vegetable industry, and other private sectors. The program consists of four components: (a) industry, which develops retail and point-of-purchase programs, (b) media, consisting of a national campaign developed jointly by NCI and Produce for Better Health as a way to spread program messages, (c) community, which incorporates state-based efforts to target different ages, ethnic groups, schools, and worksites at the local community level, and (d) research, funded by NCI to determine the effectiveness of nutrition and behavioral change interventions to promote increased consumption of fruits and vegetables as part of a healthy diet.

The "5 A Day" program is the framework for individual-level counseling by nutritionists, nurses, and other healthcare professionals that is supported and reinforced through a nationwide research and public health initiative. Program objectives are intended to (a) increase public awareness of the importance of eating five or more servings of fruits and vegetables every day, and (b) provide consumers with specific information about how to include more servings of fruits and vegetables into daily eating patterns. To meet these objectives, the program incorporates a combination of awareness and skill-building strategies to challenge individuals, families, schools, and communities to increase fruit and vegetable consumption to reduce disease risk and promote good health. For more information about the "5 A Day" program and ideas on how to add more fruits and vegetables into a daily diet, visit the "5 A Day" Web site at http://www.5aday.gov.

National Health Promotion and Disease Prevention Objectives

The message to eat more fruits and vegetables is echoed in the nation's health promotion and disease prevention objectives in *Healthy People 2010* (U.S. Department of Health and Human Services, 2000) and also keeps within its broader message that a healthful diet is low in fat and high in fiber. Table 7-5 provides a summary of current dietary recommendations for intakes of fruits and vegetables in the U.S. population. Primary instruments for nurses and other healthcare professionals to encourage increased intake of fruits and vegetables are the Food Guide Pyramid (U.S. Department of Agriculture, 1992) and *Nutrition and Your Health: Dietary Guidelines for Americans* (U.S. Department of Agriculture and U.S. Department of Health and Human Services, 2000). The dietary guidelines published in *Healthy People 2010* provide healthcare professionals with a powerful tool that reflects the science behind the recommendations. If the *Dietary Guidelines for Americans*, as a cornerstone of the national nutrition policy, placed a greater emphasis on fruits and vegetables, it could have far-reaching effects in efforts by healthcare professionals, in federal nutrition programs such as school lunch programs, and in further refinement of educational tools such as the Food Guide Pyramid.

Dietary Supplements

In light of the varied and often confusing information about diet and health in the media, nurses can play an important role in helping patients to understand and

Table 7-5. Current Dietary Recommendations for Intakes of Fruits and Vegetables in the U.S. Population

Source	Recommendation
U.S. Department of Agriculture & U.S. Department of Health and Human Services, 2000	Choose a variety of fruits and vegetables daily: • Eat at least two servings of fruits and at least three servings of vegetables each day. • Choose fresh, frozen, dried, or canned forms and a variety of colors and kinds. • Choose dark-green leafy vegetables, orange fruits and vegetables, and cooked dry beans and peas.
U.S. Department of Health and Human Services, 2000	Objective 19-5: • Increase the proportions for people who are two years of age and older who consume at least two daily servings of fruit. Objective 19-6: • Increase the proportions for people who are two years of age and older who consume at least three daily servings of vegetables, with at least one-third being dark-green or deep-yellow vegetables.
World Cancer Research Fund/American Institute for Cancer Research, 1997	Promote year-round consumption of a variety of vegetables and fruits, providing 7% or more of a person's total energy. • Eat 400–800 grams (15–30 ounces) or five or more portions (servings) a day of a variety of vegetables and fruits, all year round.
American Cancer Society Advisory Committee on Diet, Nutrition, and Cancer Prevention, 1996	Choose most of the foods you eat from plant sources. Eat five or more servings of fruits and vegetables each day. • Include fruits or vegetables in every meal. • Choose fruits and vegetables for snacks.

interpret this information. The science in this area can be difficult to interpret because hypotheses based on case studies and observational findings are not always borne out when studied in a more controlled setting, such as a randomized controlled trial. The general public, when presented with these seemingly conflicting or varying results, often views the findings, and consequently, the science underpinning these results, with skepticism. Impatient for answers, the public frequently is drawn to unproven diets and nutritional supplements.

Although dietary supplements are sometimes used as substitutes for increased fruit and vegetable consumption, science suggests using some caution with this approach (Radimer, Subar, & Thompson, 2000). Healthcare professionals need to reassure patients that a diet low in fat with plenty of fruits, vegetables, and grains is still the optimal choice to make to reduce the risk of chronic diseases.

Clinical dietary supplement trials to date have not successfully replicated the beneficial effects of fruit and vegetable intake. Three large clinical supplementation trials have shown either no or detrimental effects of supplements of beta-carotene, vitamin A, and vitamin E (ATBCSG, 1994; Gaziano & Hennekens,

1993; Omenn et al., 1994). NCI, in collaboration with the National Public Health Institute of Finland, conducted the Alpha-Tocopherol Beta Carotene (ATBC) trial among 29,000 male Finnish smokers. The trial demonstrated 18% more cases of lung cancer and 8% more deaths among treatment subjects receiving beta-caro- tene compared with controls. Following on the heels of ATBC, the Beta-Carotene and Retinol Efficacy Trial (CARET) found that after an average of four years into the trial, 28% more cases of lung cancer and 17% more deaths among participants taking beta-carotene and vitamin A supplements, respectively, were reported com- pared with controls (Omenn et al., 1996). Based on the lack of benefits resulting from supplements and the possibility of a detrimental effect, CARET was termi- nated 21 months early. The 18,000 study participants were advised to stop taking their supplements. Earlier results from the Physicians' Health Study, involving 22,000 male physicians taking either beta-carotene or a placebo every other day for 12 years, showed no significant effect—either positive or negative—on cancer or cardiovascular risk reduction from beta-carotene supplements (Gaziano & Hennekens; Hennekens et al., 1996).

Nonvitamin, nonmineral supplement usage also is growing. Research suggests that people do not routinely inform their physicians about the use of alternative medical therapies, including dietary supplements (Radimer et al., 2000). Supple- ment use increases with age and more healthy lifestyles; however, a link also exists with people who use alcohol and are obese. Use of garlic and lecithin is reportedly more frequent than for any other product, which may be related to the numerous claims made about them. Garlic is promoted for its antibiotic properties for such conditions as colds, sore throats, and ear, fungus, and yeast infections. It also is used to treat chronic diseases, including cancer; boost the immune system; lower blood sugar; enhance the flow of urine; and aid in the production of bile. Manufac- turers promote lecithin to prevent cardiovascular disease, increase brain function, promote energy, repair liver damage caused by alcoholism, purify the kidneys, increase the immune system, and distribute body weight (Austin Nutritional Re- search, 1998; Nutri-Mart, 1998).

Consumers, as well as many healthcare professionals, may be well advised to view dietary supplements as drugs rather than foods, given the fact that they fre- quently are used for disease prevention or treatment purposes. Although supple- ment usage may be appropriate in some individuals, the current open-market environment can increase the potential for problems. At this time, manufacturers have limited legal requirements to prove they are selling effective products or to identify the active components within the supplements. Evidence for the efficacy of some supplements exists but often is based on studies conducted in other coun- tries or on reported use over the centuries. This evidence may not pertain to the particular plant species, supplement form, potency of the given product, or the claim being made. Quality control is questionable, raising the concern about the safety and purity of supplements. Nurses and other healthcare professionals can play an important role in helping to safeguard patients' health by asking about supplement use when taking history information. They also can educate consum- ers that these supplements do have drug-like properties and can interact or inter- fere with prescription and over-the-counter drug compounds.

Conclusion

The evidence is positive for the relationship between a diet rich in fruits and vegetables and a reduced risk for cancer at several sites: breast, prostate, colorectal, and lung. Overall, certain factors (e.g., phytochemicals, nutrients) found in fruits and vegetables are recognized to help to reduce the risk for developing select cancers. Current data support general dietary guidelines to increase the number of daily fruit and vegetable servings in the diet and decrease ingestion of fat to 30% of caloric intake. Substituting specific dietary supplements for whole fruits and vegetables is not recommended at this time.

The weight of the scientific knowledge linking fruit and vegetable consumption with cancer prevention and control and an ever-increasing understanding of relevant behavior mechanisms can empower nurses and other healthcare professionals to encourage individuals to successfully increase their fruit and vegetable intake. Current strategies for changing eating habits identify ways to overcome barriers, build self-efficacy, and tailor interventions and communications to best motivate and meet the needs of the patient. Effective behavioral change strategies exist that target the individual and also work at the community level, potentially reaching a large number of people. Ideas for practical application and dissemination by various channels are given. Public initiatives, such as the "5 A Day for Better Health Program," provide the larger context into which individual teaching and counseling efforts can grow. The continuing efforts of nutritionists, nurses, and other healthcare professionals to teach good nutrition truly can make a difference in the prevention of cancer.

References

ADA testifies on value of nutrition education as Congress considers reauthorization of child nutrition programs. (1998). *Journal of the American Dietetic Association, 98*, 633.

Alberts, D.S., Martinez, M.E., Roe, D.J., Guillen-Rodriguez, J.M., Marshal, J.R., van Leeuwen, J.B., Reid, M.E., Ritenbaugh, C., Vargas, P.A., Bhattacharya, A.B., Earnest, D.L., Sampliner, R.E., & the Phoenix Colon Cancer Prevention Physicians' Network. (2000). Lack of effect of a high-fiber cereal supplement on the recurrence of colorectal adenomas. *New England Journal of Medicine, 342*, 1156–1162.

Alpha-Tocopherol, Beta-Carotene Cancer Prevention Study Group. (1994). The effect of vitamin E and beta carotene on the incidence of lung cancer and other cancers in male smokers. *New England Journal of Medicine, 330*, 1029–1035.

American Cancer Society Advisory Committee on Diet, Nutrition, and Cancer Prevention. (1996). Guidelines on diet, nutrition, and cancer prevention: Reducing the risk of cancer with healthy food choices and physical activity. *CA: A Cancer Journal for Clinicians, 46*, 325–341.

Austin Nutritional Research. (1998). *Research guide for other nutrients*. Retrieved December 14, 1998 from the World Wide Web: http://www.realtime.net/anr/utreint.html

Barnard, N.D., & Nicholson, A. (1997). Beliefs about dietary factors in breast cancer prevention among American women. *Preventive Medicine, 26*, 109–113.

Beecher, G.R. (1999). Phytonutrients' role in metabolism: Effects on resistance to degenerative process. *Nutrition Review, 57*(9 Pt. 2), 53–56.

Bostick, R.M. (1999). Diet and nutrition in the etiology and primary prevention of colon cancer. In A. Bendich & R.J. Deckelbaum (Eds.), *Preventive nutrition: The comprehensive guide for health professionals* (pp. 57–95). Totowa, NJ: Humana Press, Inc.

Bouton, M.E. (2000). A learning theory perspective on lapse, relapse, and the maintenance of behavior change. *Health Psychology, 19*(Suppl. 1), 57–63.

Byers, T. (1999). What can randomized controlled trials tell us about nutrition and cancer prevention? *CA: A Cancer Journal for Clinicians, 49*, 353–361.

Campbell, M.K., DeVellis, B.M., Strecher, V.J., Ammerman, A.S., DeVellis, R.F., & Sandler, R.S. (1994). Improving dietary behavior: The effectiveness of tailoring messages in primary care settings. *American Journal of Public Health, 84*, 783–787.

Campbell, M.K., Reynolds, K.D., Havas, S., Curry, S., Bishop, D., Nicklas, T., Palombo, R., Buller, D., Feldman, R., Topor, M., Johnson, C., Beresford, S.A., Motsinger, B.M., Morrill, C., & Heimendinger, J. (1998). Stages of change for increasing fruit and vegetable consumption among adults and young adults participating in the national 5-A-Day for Better Health community studies. *Health Education and Behavior, 26*, 513–534.

Candelora, E.C., Stockwell, H.G., Armstrong, A.W., & Pinkham, P.A. (1992). Dietary intake and risk of lung cancer in women who never smoked. *Nutrition and Cancer, 17*, 263–270.

Cline, J.M., & Huges, C.L. (1998). Phytochemicals for the prevention of breast and endometrial cancer. *Cancer Treatment and Research, 94*, 107–134.

Clinton, S.K., & Giovannucci, E. (1998). Diet, nutrition, and prostate cancer. *Annual Review Nutrition, 18*, 413–440.

Cohen, J.H., Kristal, A.R., & Stanford, J.L. (2000). Fruit and vegetable intakes and prostate cancer risk. *Journal of the National Cancer Institute, 92*, 61–68.

Committee on Medical Aspects of Food and Nutrition Policy. (1998). *Nutritional aspects of the development of cancer*. London, England: Stationery Office.

Cooper, D.A., Eldridge, A.L., & Peters, J.C. (1999). Dietary carotenoids and certain cancers, heart disease, and age-related macular degeneration: A review of recent research. *Nutrition Review, 57*, 201–214.

Cotugna, N., Subar, A.F., Heimendinger, J., & Kahle, L. (1992). Nutrition and cancer prevention knowledge, beliefs, attitudes, and practices: The 1987 National Health Interview Survey. *Journal of the American Dietetic Association, 92*, 963–968.

Coughlin, C.M., & DeBusk, R.M. (1998). *Integrative medicine: Your quick reference guide*. Tallahassee, FL: Integrative Medicine, Inc.

Cronin, F.J., Shaw, A.M., Krebs-Smith, S.M., Marsland, P.M., & Light, L. (1987). Developing a food guidance system to implement the dietary guidelines. *Journal of Nutritional Education, 19*, 281–302.

Dashwood, R.H. (1999). Early detection and prevention of colorectal cancer. *Oncology Reports, 6*, 277–281.

Davis, S.R., Dalais, F.S., & Simpson, E.R. (1999). Phytoestrogens in health and disease. *Recent Progress in Hormone Research, 54*, 185–210.

Denis, L., Morton, M.S., & Griffiths, K. (1999). Diet and its preventive role in prostatic disease. *European Urology, 35*, 377–387.

Dittus, K.L., Hillers, V.N., & Beerman, K.A. (1995). Benefits and barriers to fruit and vegetable intake: Relationship between attitudes and consumption. *Journal of Nutritional Education, 27,* 120–126.

Doll, R., & Peto, R. (1991). *The causes of cancer.* New York: Oxford University Press.

Dorgan, J.F., Ziegler, R.G., Schoenberg, J.B., Hartge, P., McAdams, M.J., Falk, R.T., Wilcox, H.B., & Shaw, G.L. (1993). Race and sex differences in association of vegetables, fruit, and carotenoids with lung cancer risk in New Jersey (United States). *Cancer Causes and Control, 4,* 273–281.

Du, Y.X., Zhou, B.S., & Wu, J.M. (1998). Lifestyle factors and human lung cancer: An overview of recent advances. *International Journal of Oncology, 13,* 471–479.

Eastwood, M.A. (1999). Interaction of dietary antioxidants in vivo: How fruits and vegetables prevent disease. *Quarterly Journal of Medicine, 92,* 527–530.

Eisner, E., Loughrey, K., Hadley, L., & Doner, L. (1992). *Understanding benefits and barriers to fruit and vegetable consumption.* Bethesda, MD: National Cancer Institute.

Fisher, B., Costantino, J., Wickerham, D.L., Redmond, C.K., Kavanah, M., Cronin, W.M., Vogel, V., Robidoux, A., Dimitrov, N., Atkins, J., Daly, M., Wieand, S., Tan-Chiu, E., Ford, L., & Wolmark, N. (1998). Tamoxifen for prevention of breast cancer: Report of the National Surgical Adjuvant Breast and Bowel Project P-1 Study. *Journal of the National Cancer Institute, 90,* 1371–1388.

French, S.A., Jeffery, R.W., Story, M., Hannan, P., & Snyder, M.P. (1997). A pricing strategy to promote low-fat snack choices through vending machines. *American Journal of Public Health, 87,* 849–851.

Forman, M.R., Yao, S.X., Graugard, B.L., Qiao, Y.L., McAdams, M., Mao, B.L., & Taylor, P.R. (1992). The effect of dietary intake of fruits and vegetables on the odds ratio of lung cancer among Yunan tin miners. *International Journal of Epidemiology, 21,* 37–44.

Fuchs, C.S., Giovannucci, E.L., Colditz, G.A., Hunter, D.J., Stampfer, M.J., Rosner, B., Speizer, F.E., & Willett, W.C. (1999). Dietary fiber and the risk of colorectal cancer. *New England Journal of Medicine, 340,* 169–176.

Gaziano, J.M., & Hennekens, C.H. (1993). The role of beta-carotene in the prevention of cardiovascular disease. *Annals of the New York Academy of Science, 691,* 148–155.

Giovannucci, E., Ascherio, A., Rimm, E.B., Stampfer, M.J., Colditz, G.A., & Willett, W.C. (1995). Intake of carotenoids and retinol in relation to risk of prostate cancer. *Journal of the National Cancer Institute, 87,* 1767–1776.

Giovannucci, E., & Clinton, S.K. (1998). Tomatoes, lycopene, and prostate cancer. *Proceedings of the Society for Experimental Biology and Medicine, 218,* 129–139.

Giovannucci, E., Rimm, E.B., Stampfer, M.J., Colditz, G.A., Ascherio, A., & Willett, W.C. (1994). Intake of fat, meat, and fiber in relation to risk of colon cancer in men. *Cancer Research, 54,* 2390–2397.

Glanz, K. (1994). Reducing breast cancer risk through changes in diet and alcohol intake: From clinic to community. *Annals of Behavioral Medicine, 16,* 334–346.

Glanz, K., Basil, M., Maibach, E., Goldberg, J., & Snyder, D. (1998). Why Americans eat what they do: Taste, nutrition, cost, convenience, and weight control concerns and influences on food consumption. *Journal of the American Dietetic Association, 98,* 1118–1126.

Glanz, K., Patterson, R.E., Kristal, A.R., DiClemente, C.C., Heimendinger, J., & Linnan, L. (1994). Stages of change in adopting healthy diets: Fat, fiber, and correlates of nutrient intake. *Health Education Quarterly, 21,* 499–519.

Goldbohm, R.A., van den Brandt, P.A., van't Veer, P., Brants, H.A., Dorant, E., & Sturmans, F. (1994). A prospective cohort study on the relation between meat consumption and the risk of colon cancer. *Cancer Research, 54,* 718–723.

Greenwald, P., Sherwood, K., & McDonald, S.S. (1997). Fat, caloric intake, and obesity: Lifestyle risk factors for breast cancer. *Journal of the American Dietetic Association, 97*(Suppl. 7), S24–S30.

Hankin, J.H. (1993). Role of nutrition in women's health: Diet and breast cancer. *Journal of the American Dietetic Association, 93,* 994–999.

Harnack, L., Block, G., Subar, A., Lane, S., & Brand, R. (1997). Association of cancer prevention-related nutrition knowledge, beliefs, and attitudes to cancer prevention dietary behavior. *Journal of the American Dietetic Association, 97,* 957–965.

Havas, S., Anliker, J., Damron, D., Langenberg, P., Ballesteros, M., & Feldman, R. (1998). Final results of the Maryland WIC 5-A-Day Promotion Program. *American Journal of Public Health, 88,* 1161–1167.

Havas, S., Heimendinger, J., Reynolds, K., Baranowski, T., Nicklas, T.A., Bishop, D., Buller, D., Sorensen, G., Beresford, S.A., Cowan, A., & Damron, D. (1994). 5 A Day for Better Health: A new research initiative. *Journal of the American Dietetic Association, 94,* 32–36.

Heimendinger, J., Van Duyn, M.A., Chapelsky, D., Foerster, S., & Stables, G. (1996). The national 5 A Day for Better Health Program: A large-scale nutrition intervention. *Journal of Public Health Management Practice, 2,* 27–35.

Hennekens, C.H., Buring, J.E., Manson, J.E., Stampfer, M., Rosner, B., Cook, N.R., Betanger, C., La Motte, F., Gaziano, J.M., Ridker, P.M., Willett, W., & Peto, R. (1996). Lack of effect of long-term supplementation with beta-carotene on the incidence of malignant neoplasms and cardiovascular disease. *New England Journal of Medicine, 334,* 1145–1149.

Hill, M.J. (1999). Diet, physical activity, and cancer risk. *Public Health Nutrition, 2,* 397–401.

Hopkins, G.J., & Carroll, K.K. (1979). Relationship between amount and type of dietary fat in promotion of mammary carcinogenesis induced by 7,12-dimethylbenz[a]anthracene. *Journal of the National Cancer Institute, 62,* 1009–1012.

Hopkins, G.J., Kennedy, T.G., & Carroll, K.K. (1981). Polyunsaturated fatty acids as promoters of mammary carcinogenesis-induced Sprague-Dawley rats by 7,12-dimethylbenz[a]anthracene. *Journal of the National Cancer Institute, 66,* 517–522.

Howe, G.R. (1997). Nutrition and breast cancer. In A. Bendich & R.J. Deckelbaum (Eds.), *Preventive nutrition: The comprehensive guide for health professionals* (pp. 97–109). Totowa, NJ: Humana Press Inc.

Hunter, D.J., Speigelman, D., Adami, H.O., Beeson, L., van den Brandt, P.A., Folsom, A.R., Fraser, G.E., Goldbohm, R.A., Graham, S., Howe, G.R., Kushi, L.H., Marshall, J.R., McDermott, A., Miller, A.B., Speizer, F.E., Wolk, A., Yaun, S.S., & Willett, W.C. (1996). Cohort studies of fat intake and risk of breast cancer: A pooled analysis. *New England Journal of Medicine, 334,* 356–361.

Hunter, D.J., & Willett, W.C. (1996). Nutrition and breast cancer. *Cancer Causes and Control, 7,* 56–68.

Kolonel, L.N. (1996). Nutrition and prostate cancer. *Cancer Causes and Control, 7,* 83–94.

Krebs-Smith, S.M., Cleveland, L.E., Ballard-Barbash, R., Cook, D.A., & Kahle, L.L. (1997). Characterizing food intake patterns of American adults. *American Journal of Clinical Nutrition, 65*(Suppl. 4), 1264S–1268S.

Krebs-Smith, S.M., Cook, A., Subar, A.F., Cleveland, L., Friday, J., & Kahle, L.L. (1996). Fruit and vegetable intakes of children and adolescents in United States. *Archives of Pediatric Adolescent Medicine, 150*, 81–86.

Kristal, A.R., Glanz, K., Tilley, B.C., & Li, S. (2000). Mediating factors in dietary change: Understanding the impact of a worksite nutrition intervention. *Health Education and Behavior, 27*(1), 112–125.

Kristal, A.R., Patterson, R.E., Glanz, K., Heimendinger, J., Hebert, J.R., Feng, Z., & Probart, C. (1995). Psychosocial correlates of healthful diets: Baseline results from the Working Well Study. *Preventive Medicine, 24*, 221–228.

Laforge, R.G., Greene, G.W., & Prochaska, J.O. (1994). Psychosocial factors influencing low fruit and vegetable consumption. *Journal of Behavioral Medicine, 17*, 361–374.

Lampe, J.W. (1999). Health effects of vegetables and fruits: Assessing mechanisms of action in human experimental studies. *American Journal of Clinical Nutrition, 70*(Suppl. 3), 475S–490S.

Le Marchand, L., Hankin, J.H., Kolonel, L.N., & Wilkins, L.R. (1991). Vegetable and fruit consumption in relation to prostate cancer risk in Hawaii: A re-evaluation of the effect of dietary beta-carotene. *American Journal of Epidemiology, 133*, 215–219.

Lipkin, M., Reddy, B., Newmark, H., & Lamprecht, S.A. (1999). Dietary factors in human colorectal cancer. *Annual Review of Nutrition, 19*, 545–586.

Luepker, R.V., Murray, D.M., Jacobs, D.R., Mittelmark, M.B., Bracht, N., Carlaw, R., Crow, R., Elmer, P., Finnegan, J., & Folsom, A.R. (1994). Community education for cardiovascular disease prevention: Risk factor changes in the Minnesota Heart Health Program. *American Journal of Public Health, 84*, 1383–1393.

Mangels, A.R., Holden, J.M., Beecher, G.R., Forman, M., & Lanza, E. (1993). Carotenoid content of fruits and vegetables: An evaluation of analytic data. *Journal of the American Dietetic Association, 93*, 284–296.

Martin-Moreno, J.M., Willett, W.C., Gorgojo, L., Banegas, J.R., Rodriguez-Artalejo, F., Fernandez-Rodriguez, J.C., Maisonneuve, P., & Boyle, P. (1994). Dietary fat, olive oil intake, and breast cancer risk. *International Journal of Cancer, 58*, 774–780.

Mayne, S.T., Janeirich, D.T., Greenwald, P., Chorost, S., Tucci, C., Zaman, M.B., & Melamed, M.R. (1994). Dietary beta-carotene and lung cancer risk in U.S. nonsmokers. *Journal of the National Cancer Institute, 86*, 3–38.

Miller, A., Berrino, F., Hill, M., Pietinen, P., Riboli, E., & Wahrendorf, J. (1994). Diet in the etiology of cancer: A review. *European Journal of Cancer, 30A*, 207–220.

Mills, P.K., Beeson, W.L., Phillips, R.L., & Fraser, G.E. (1989). Cohort study of diet, lifestyle, and prostate cancer in Adventist men. *Cancer, 64*, 598–604.

Montironi, R., Mazzucchelli, R., Marshall, J.R., & Bartels, P.H. (1999). Prostate cancer prevention: Review of target populations, pathological biomarkers, and chemopreventive agents. *Journal of Clinical Pathology, 52*, 793–803.

Nutri-Mart. (1998). *Herbs and specialty foods and their uses.* Retrieved December 14, 1998 from the World Wide Web: http://www.nutrimart.com/herbinfo.html

Office of Communications, National Cancer Institute. (1992). *Message test of the 5 A Day campaign theme line.* Bethesda, MD: National Cancer Institute.

Office of Communications, National Cancer Institute. (1995). *Focus groups with African Americans on nutrition and cancer.* Bethesda, MD: National Cancer Institute.

Office of Communications, National Cancer Institute. (1998). *5 A Day visual approach: A comparison of illustrated and photographic styles.* Bethesda, MD: National Cancer Institute.

Omenn, G.S., Goodman, G.E., Thornquist, M.O., Balmes, J., Cullen, M.R., Glass, A., Keogh, J.P., Meyskens, F.L., Valanis, B., Williams, J.H., Barnhart, S., & Hammar, S. (1996). Effects of a combination of beta-carotene and vitamin A on lung cancer and cardiovascular disease. *New England Journal of Medicine, 334,* 1150–1155.

Omenn, G.S., Goodman, G.E., Thornquist, M.O., Grizzle, J., Rosenstock, L., Barnhart, S., Balmes, J., Cherniack, M., Cullen, M., Glass, A., Geogh, J., Meyskens, F., Valanis, B., & Williams, J. (1994). The beta-carotene and retinol efficacy trial (CARET) for chemoprevention of lung cancer in high-risk populations: Smokers and asbestos-exposed workers. *Cancer Research, 54*(Suppl. 7), 2038S–2043S.

Parker, S.L., Tong, T., Bolden, S., & Wingo, P.A. (1997). Cancer statistics, 1997. *CA: A Cancer Journal for Clinicians, 47,* 5–27.

Patterson, R.E., Kristal, A.R., Lynch, J., & White, E. (1995). Diet—Cancer-related beliefs, knowledge, norms, and their relationship to healthful diets. *Journal of Nutritional Education, 27,* 86–92.

Pavia, S.A.R., & Russell, R.M. (1999). Beta-carotene and other carotenoids as antioxidants. *American Journal of Clinical Nutrition, 18,* 426–433.

Petrakis, N.L., Barnes, S., King, E.B., Lowenstein, J., Wiencke, J., Lee, M.M., Miike, R., Kirk, M., & Coward, L. (1996). Stimulatory influence of soy protein isolate on breast secretion in pre- and postmenopausal women. *Cancer Epidemiology, Biomarkers, and Prevention, 5,* 785–794.

Potter, J.D. (1996). Nutrition and colorectal cancer. *Cancer Causes and Control, 7,* 127–146.

Potter, J.D., Finnegan, J.R., Guinard, J.X, Huerta, E., Kelder, S.H., Kristal, A.R., Kumanyikas, S., Lin, R., Mostinger, B.M., Prendergast, F.G., Sorensen, G., & Callahan, K.M. (2000). *5 A Day for Better Health Program evaluation report* (NIH Publication No. 01-4904). Bethesda, MD: National Institutes of Health, National Cancer Institute.

Prochaska, J.O., & DiClemente, C.C. (1992). Stages of change in the modification of problem behaviors. In M. Hersen, R.M. Eisler, & P.M. Miller (Eds.), *Progress in behavior modification* (pp. 184–218). New York: Sycamore Publishing.

Produce Marketing Association. (1991). *Nutrient data bank for fresh fruits and vegetables.* Newark, DE: Author

Radimer, K.L., Subar, A.F., & Thompson, F.E. (2000). Nonvitamin, nonmineral dietary supplements: Issues and findings from NHANES III. *Journal of the American Dietetic Association, 100,* 447–454.

Reddy, B.S. (1999). Role of dietary fiber in colon cancer: An overview. *American Journal of Medicine, 106*(Suppl. 1A), 16S–19S.

Reicks, M., Randall, J.L., & Haynes, B.J. (1994). Factors affecting consumption of fruits and vegetables by low-income families. *Journal of the American Dietetic Association, 94,* 1309–1311.

Ries, L.A.G. (2000). *NCI cancer risks and rates.* Retrieved May 8, 2000 from the World Wide Web: http://rex.nci.nih.gov/NCI_Pub_interface/

Rimer, B.K., & Glassman, B. (1999). Is there a use for a tailored print communications in cancer risk communication? *Journal of the National Cancer Institute Monographs, 25,* 140–148.

Rimm, E.B., Ascherio, A., Giovannucci, E., Spiegelman, D., Stampfer, M.J., & Willett, W.C. (1996). Vegetable, fruit, and cereal fiber intake and risk of coronary heart disease among men. *JAMA, 275*, 447–451.

Schatzkin, A., & Kelloff, G. (1995). Chemo- and dietary prevention of colorectal cancer. *European Journal of Cancer, 31*, 1198–1204.

Schatzkin, A., Lanza, E., Corle, D., Lance, P., Iber, F., Caan, B., Shike, M., Weissfeld, J., Burt, R., Cooper, M.R., Kikendall, J.W., Cahill, J., & the Polyp Prevention Trial Study Group. (2000). Lack of effect of a low-fat, high-fiber diet on the recurrence of colorectal adenomas. *New England Journal of Medicine, 342*, 1149–1155.

Schulman, L.M., Mandel, J.S., Radke, A., Seal, U., & Halberg, F. (1982). Some selected features of the epidemiology of prostate cancer: Minneapolis-St. Paul, case-control study, 1976–1979. In K. Magnes (Ed.), *Trends in cancer incidence: Causes and implications* (pp. 345–354). Washington, DC: Hemisphere Publishing Corp.

Serdula, M.K., Byers, T., Mokdad, A.H., Simoes, E., Mendlein, J.M., & Coates, R.J. (1996). The association between fruit and vegetable intake and chronic disease risk factors. *Epidemiology, 7*, 161–165.

Serdula, M.K., Coates, R.J., Byers, T., Simoes, E., Mokdad, A.H., & Subar, A.F. (1995). Fruit and vegetable intake among adults in 16 states: Results of a brief telephone survey. *American Journal of Public Health, 85*, 236–239.

Shopland, D.R., Eyre, H.J., & Pechacek, T.F. (1991). Smoking-attributed cancer mortality in 1991: Is lung cancer now the leading cause of death among smokers in the United States? *Journal of the National Cancer Institute, 83*, 1142–1148.

Sorensen, G., Stoddard, A., & Ockene, J. (1996). Worksite-based cancer prevention: Primary results from the Working Well Trial. *American Journal of Public Health, 86*, 939–947.

Stables, G., Van Duyn, M.A., Heimendinger, J., Nebeling, L., & Berkowitz, S. (2001). 5 A Day Program evaluation research. In G. Stables (Ed.), *5 A Day For Better Health Program monograph* (NIH Publication No. 01-5019) (pp. 99–111). Bethesda, MD: National Cancer Institute, National Institutes of Health.

Steinmetz, K.A., Kushi, L.H., Bostick, R.M., Folsom, A.R., & Potter, J.D. (1994). Vegetables, fruits and colon cancer in the Iowa Women's Health Study. *American Journal of Epidemiology, 139*, 1–15.

Steinmetz, K.A., & Potter, J.D. (1991). Vegetables, fruit, and cancer. I. Epidemiology. *Cancer Causes and Control, 2*, 325–357.

Steinmetz, K.A., & Potter, J.D. (1996). Vegetables, fruits, and cancer prevention: A review. *Journal of the American Dietetic Association, 96*, 1027–1039.

Steinmetz, K.A., Potter, J.D., & Folsom, A.R. (1993). Vegetables, fruits, and lung cancer in the Iowa's Women's Health Study. *Cancer Research, 53*, 536–543.

Stephens, F.O. (1999). The rising incidence of breast cancer in women and prostate cancer in men. Dietary influences: A possible preventive role for nature's sex hormone modifiers—The phytoestrogens. *Oncology Reports, 6*, 865–870.

Thun, M.J., Calle, E.E., Namboodiri, M.M., Flanders, W.D., Coates, R.J., Byers, T., Boffette, P., Garfinkel, L., & Heath, C.W. (1992). Risk factors for fatal colon cancer in a large prospective study. *Journal of the National Cancer Institute, 84*, 1491–1500.

Treiman, K., Freimuth, V., & Damron, D. (1996). Attitudes and behaviors related to fruits and vegetables among low-income women in the WIC program. *Journal of Nutritional Education, 28*, 149–156.

Trichopoulou, A., Katsouyanni, K., Stuver, S., Tzala, L., Gnardellis, C., Rimm, E., & Trichopoulos, D. (1995). Consumption of olive oil and specific food groups in relation to breast cancer in Greece. *Journal of the National Cancer Institute, 87,* 110–116.

Trock, B., Lanza, E., & Greenwald, P. (1990). Dietary fiber, vegetables, and colon cancer: A critical review and meta-analyses of the epidemiologic evidence. *Journal of the National Cancer Institute, 82,* 650–661.

Trudeau, E., Kristal, A., Li, S., & Patterson, R. (1998). Demographic and psychosocial predictors of fruit and vegetable intakes differ: Implications for dietary interventions. *Journal of the American Dietetic Association, 98,* 1412–1417.

U.S. Department of Agriculture. (1992). *Food Guide Pyramid: A guide to daily food choices* (Home and Garden Bulletin No. 252). Washington, DC: Author.

U.S. Department of Agriculture and U.S. Department of Health and Human Services. (2000). *Nutrition and your health: Dietary guidelines for Americans* (5th ed.). Washington, DC: Author.

U.S. Department of Health and Human Services. (2000). *Healthy People 2010.* Washington, DC: Author.

The use and abuse of vitamin A. (1971). *Canadian Medical Association Journal, 104,* 521–522.

Van Duyn, M.A.S., Heimendinger, J., Russek-Cohen, E., DiClemente, C., Sims, L.S., Subar, A.F., Krebs-Smith, S.M., Pivonka, E., & Kahle, L.L. (1998). Use of the transtheoretical model of change to successfully predict fruit and vegetable consumption. *Journal of Nutritional Education, 30,* 371–380.

van't Veer, P., Jansen, M.C., Klerk, M., & Kok, F. (1999). Fruits and vegetables in the prevention of cancer and cardiovascular disease. *Public Health Nutrition, 3*(1), 103–107.

Verhoeven, D.T., Goldbohm, R.A., van Poppel, G., Verhagen, H., & van den Brandt, P.A. (1996). Epidemiological studies on brassica vegetables and cancer risk. *Cancer Epidemiology, Biomarkers, and Prevention, 5,* 733–748.

Welsh, C.W. (1992). Relationship between dietary fat and experimental mammary tumorigenesis: A review and critique. *Cancer Research, 52*(Suppl. 7), 2040S–2048S.

Willett, W.C. (1989). The search for the causes of breast and colon cancer. *Nature, 338,* 389–394.

Willett, W.C., Hunter, D.J., Stampfer, M.J., Colditz, G., Manson, J.E., Spiegelman, D., Rosner, B., Hennekens, C.H., & Speizer, F.E. (1992). Dietary fat and fiber in relation to risk of breast cancer. An 8-year follow-up. *JAMA, 268,* 2037–2044.

Willett, W.C., Stampfer, M.J., Colditz, G.A., Rosner, B.A., & Speizer, F.E. (1990). Relation of meat, fat, and fiber intake to the risk of colon cancer in a prospective study among women. *New England Journal of Medicine, 323,* 1664–1672.

World Cancer Research Fund/American Institute for Cancer Research. (1997). *Food, nutrition, and the prevention of cancer: A global perspective.* Washington, DC: American Institute for Cancer Research.

Yip, I., Heber, D., & Aronson, W. (1999). Nutrition and prostate cancer. *Urologic Clinics of North America, 26,* 403–411.

Ziegler, R.G., Mayne, S.T., & Swanson, C.A. (1996). Nutrition and lung cancer. *Cancer Causes and Control, 7,* 157–177.

CHAPTER 8

Chemoprevention

Jennifer Aikin, RN, MSN, AOCN®

Introduction

Traditionally, primary cancer prevention strategies have focused on making lifestyle changes and avoiding exposure to carcinogens. Healthcare professionals have encouraged people to eliminate cancer risk factors by modifying their diet, abstaining from smoking, avoiding exposure to the sun, and limiting alcohol consumption (Greenwald, 1992; Loescher, 1993). Although these approaches are reasonable and have led to the prevention of some cancers, additional methods of cancer prevention are required because the problem of cancer persists. One of the most promising methods is chemoprevention. During the past two decades, this approach has demonstrated the ability to disrupt the process of carcinogenesis, thereby preventing the appearance of invasive cancer.

This chapter presents an overview of chemoprevention: the design and goals of chemoprevention trials, a discussion of nutrients and pharmacologic agents used for cancer prevention, and a summary of landmark studies. Implications for nursing practice such as identifying high-risk populations, recruiting patients for chemoprevention studies, the risks and benefits of chemopreventive agents, ways to encourage patient compliance with prevention regimens, and symptom management strategies also are highlighted.

Chemoprevention: Definition and Rationale

The most widely accepted definition of chemoprevention is "the use of specific natural or synthetic chemical agents to reverse, suppress, or prevent carcinogenic progression to invasive cancer" (Lippman, Benner, & Hong, 1994, p.

851). Chemoprevention generally involves the ingestion of a pharmacologic agent in pill form and therefore is different from diet therapy, in which chemical substances known to decrease cancer risk are obtained from food. To illustrate this distinction, obtaining beta-carotene through the ingestion of fruits and vegetables is *not* considered chemoprevention; however, when this nutrient is concentrated and administered in pill form, it becomes chemoprevention (Lippman et al.; Swan & Ford, 1997).

The principles of chemoprevention are based on the knowledge of carcinogenesis, a step-wise process that involves the initiation, promotion, and progression of disease (see Figure 8-1). During *initiation*, exposure to carcinogens, such as chemicals, viruses, or ultraviolet light, can cause changes in cellular DNA (Olsen & Love, 1986). These genetic changes are *promoted* when the exposure to carcinogens continues over a long period of time. Finally, premalignant cells *progress* to malignancy. According to Lippman et al. (1994), the initiation phase is rapid and irreversible, the promotion stage is prolonged and generally reversible, and the progression period is prolonged but irreversible.

Generally, there is an extended period of time from the initiation of carcinogenesis to the point where invasive disease is diagnosed, offering the opportunity for intervention and disruption of the process (Alberts & Garcia, 1995; Greenwald, Kelloff, Burch-Whitman, & Kramer, 1995). Chemopreventive agents can block the initiation of carcinogenesis or halt the progression of premalignant cells (Sporn, 1993). However, intervention at the initiation phase is thought to be difficult because specific initiators have not been identified for most cancers and the initiation step may occur many years before intervention is considered (Garewal & Meyskens, 1991). Thus, the most effective agents

Figure 8-1. Steps in the Process of Carcinogenesis

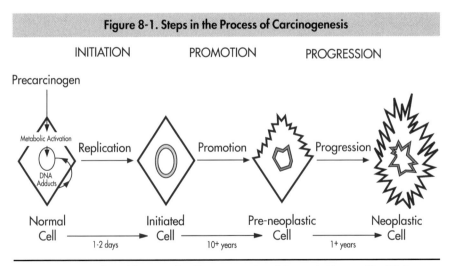

Note. From "Rationale and Strategies for Chemoprevention of Cancer in Humans," by J.S. Bertram, L.N. Kolonel, and F.L. Meyskens, 1987, *Cancer Research, 47,* p. 3013. Copyright 1987 by the American Association of Cancer Research, Inc. Reprinted with permission.

likely will be those that work to circumvent the promotion and progression phases.

The Design of Chemoprevention Trials

Study Aims

As in studies of cancer treatment, chemopreventive agents are evaluated by an orderly process. Phase I chemoprevention studies identify the highest dose of an agent that can be administered with the least possible toxicity. Phase II trials are randomized, double-blind studies in which toxicities associated with the intervention are measured and further examined. Phase III studies are large, randomized, placebo-controlled trials (Alberts & Garcia, 1995). According to Greenwald et al. (1995), phase III trials are the best means of determining whether chemopreventive agents actually do reduce cancer risk. The primary goal for phase III studies is to determine whether a chemopreventive agent lowers the incidence of cancer. To evaluate this endpoint, thousands of participants must be followed over long periods of time, often at great expense (Greenwald et al., 1995; Lippman et al., 1994; Loescher & Meyskens, 1991).

Alternately, researchers may choose more intermediate endpoints such as premalignant lesions (e.g., oral leukoplakia, dysplastic nevi, adenomatous colon polyps) or biomarkers (e.g., oncogene activation, inactivation of tumor suppressor genes) (Greenwald et al., 1995; Morse & Stoner, 1993). When biomarkers are used as intermediate endpoints, the impact of the chemopreventive agent can be evaluated in a shorter period of time and with fewer study subjects (Alberts & Garcia, 1995).

Some prevention trials use a unique factorial design that permits multiple interventions to be evaluated at the same time. With a "2 x 2" design (i.e., a four-arm study), researchers evaluate two agents (A and B) in a number of different combinations: A alone, B alone, A and B together, and placebo. Some studies use a modified version of this design (2^3 or 2^4 factorial design) to evaluate a larger number of agents (Greenwald et al., 1990; Nixon, 1994).

Target Populations

Participants in phase III prevention trials generally are either at high risk for the cancer in question or have been treated for cancer and are disease-free (Nixon, 1994). These individuals may (a) be engaging in high-risk behaviors (e.g., smoking, using snuff), (b) have occupational exposure to known carcinogens (e.g., asbestos), (c) have a genetic predisposition to cancer (e.g., familial adenomatous polyposis, BRCA mutations), (d) have premalignant lesions (e.g., oral leukoplakia, atypical hyperplasia of the breast), or (e) be survivors of primary cancers who are disease free but at high risk for recurrence (Morse & Stoner, 1993). According to Alberts and Garcia (1995), when study participants are from high-risk populations, the number of participants required to observe a significant reduction in cancer incidence is decreased. In addition, these individuals are more likely to be more compliant with study medications because they perceive themselves to be at high risk for developing cancer.

Chemopreventive Agents

According to Morse and Stoner (1993), the ideal chemopreventive agent has five favorable characteristics: (a) effectiveness, (b) few untoward side effects, (c) oral administration, (d) known mechanism of action, and (e) low cost. In chemoprevention studies, high-risk populations generally are made up of healthy individuals who will take a drug for an extended period of time. Therefore, ease of administration and low toxicity are essential to help to maintain long-term compliance with the chemopreventive regimen (Nixon, 1994).

According to Lippman et al. (1994), more than 2,000 natural and synthetic chemicals have been shown to have chemopreventive activity in the laboratory. Figure 8-2 provides a list of agents that have been evaluated in human chemoprevention studies.

Retinoids

Retinoids are the most common class of drugs studied as chemopreventive agents. In animal models, retinoids have been shown to inhibit carcinogenesis in epithelial cells, including those of the breast, bladder, oral cavity, lungs, pancreas, cervix, liver, colon, esophagus, skin, and prostate (Lippman et al., 1994). The term "retinoid" includes both natural and synthetic forms of vitamin A. Natural vitamin

Figure 8-2. Chemopreventive Agents Evaluated in Humans

Retinoids (Vitamin A)
Natural retinoids
• Retinol esters
• Carotenoids (e.g., beta-carotene)
Synthetic retinoids
• Etretinate
• 13-*cis*-retinoic acid (isotretinoin [Accutane®, Roche Laboratories, Nutley, NJ])
• All-*trans*-retinoic acid (ATRA, retinoic acid, tretinoin [Vesanoid®, Roche Laboratories])
• N-(4-hydroxyphenyl) retinamide (4-HPR, fenretinide)
Other micronutrients
• Vitamin C
• Alpha-tocopherol (vitamin E)
• Calcium
• Vitamin D
• Selenium
• Folic acid
• Oltipraz
Nonsteroidal anti-inflammatory agents
• Aspirin
• Sulindac
• Piroxicam
• Ibuprofen
• Celecoxib
Other agents
• Tamoxifen citrate
• Finasteride
• Alpha-difluoromethylornithine

A is found in animal tissues (in the form of retinol esters) and in fruits and vegetables (as carotenoids) (Olsen & Love, 1986); synthetic retinoids include etretinate,
13- *cis*-retinoic acid, all-*trans*-retinoic acid, and N-(4-hydroxyphenyl) retinamide
(also called 4-HPR or fenretinide). The latter may be the most promising synthetic
retinoid used in chemoprevention studies to date (Lippman et al.; Swan & Ford,
1997).

Although they offer potential as chemopreventive agents, retinoids are not without side effects. Toxicities that have been reported with their use include cheilitis,
dry or peeling skin, pruritus, headache, arthralgia, abnormal liver function tests,
hypertriglyceridemia, visual disturbances, lethargy, malaise, weakness, and gastrointestinal complaints (Alberts & Garcia, 1995; deKlerk et al., 1998; Loescher
& Meyskens, 1991; Swan & Ford, 1997).

Other Micronutrients

Vitamin C, another micronutrient that has been studied in chemoprevention, is
thought to prevent the formation of nitrosamines, thereby inhibiting tumor formation (Olsen & Love, 1986). A number of studies explored the ingestion of vitamin C
to lower the risk for cancers of the stomach, colon, larynx, bladder, cervix, and
esophagus; however, data as to its effectiveness are contradictory (Alberts & Garcia,
1995; Lippman et al., 1994; Olsen & Love; Roncucci et al., 1993; Taylor et al., 1994).

Alpha-tocopherol, the functional form of vitamin E, has been studied in the
chemoprevention of colon, lung, and esophageal cancer (Roncucci et al., 1993;
Taylor et al., 1994), and, similar to vitamin C, it inhibits carcinogenesis by blocking the formation of carcinogenic nitrosamines (Padberg, 1994).

Epidemiological studies suggest that an inverse relationship exists between
dietary calcium intake, especially that ingested from milk products, and colorectal
cancer (Schatzkin & Kelloff, 1995). Calcium has been studied with and without
vitamin D for the chemoprevention of this cancer (Lippman et al., 1994; Olsen &
Love, 1986; Schatzkin & Kelloff). In a small study, Duris et al. (1996) found that
calcium enhanced survival after colorectal cancer surgery and reduced the recurrence of adenomatous polyps after polypectomy.

Selenium is a trace element that has been studied as a chemopreventive agent in
skin, esophageal, and lung cancers (Loescher & Meyskens, 1991; Taylor et al.,
1994; Yu et al., 1990). Recently, Clark et al. (1998) reported that although selenium did not protect against squamous and basal cell carcinomas of the skin,
selenium did reduce the incidence of prostate cancer. According to Bertram,
Kolonel, and Meyskens (1987), a fine line exists between effective and toxic doses
of selenium. Toxicities such as weight loss, liver cirrhosis, paresthesias, nausea and
vomiting, lassitude, and skin rashes have been reported (Loescher & Meyskens).

Folic acid (folate) also may be useful as a chemopreventive agent in a number of
different cancers. An inverse relationship appears to exist between dietary folate
and colorectal cancer; however, other studies have shown mixed results in women
with cervical dysplasia (Butterworth et al., 1992; Childers et al., 1995; Schatzkin &
Kelloff, 1995).

Oltipraz (4-methyl-5-[2-pyrazinyl]-1,2-dithiole-3-thione) is another new agent
that shows promise in preclinical testing (Lippman et al., 1994). This synthetic

dithiolethione appears to increase the activity of detoxicating enzyme gene expression, providing protection against colon cancer. Natural dithiolethiones are found in certain vegetables such as cabbage, cauliflower, and broccoli (O'Dwyer et al., 1996). In animal studies, oltipraz protected rats from developing lung and forestomach cancers following exposure to alkylating agents and protected them against hepatotoxicity associated with exposure to acetaminophen and carbon tetrachloride (O'Dwyer et al.).

Nonsteroidal Anti-Inflammatory Drugs

The anti-inflammatory action of nonsteroidal anti-inflammatory drugs (NSAIDs) results from their inhibition of prostaglandin synthesis. Because prostaglandins may play a role in carcinogenesis, NSAIDs are promising chemopreventive agents for colorectal cancer (Ahnen, 1998; Sandler, 1996; Schatzkin & Kelloff, 1995; Turner & Berkel, 1993). Aspirin, sulindac, piroxicam, and ibuprofen have been studied for this purpose. In 1996, Sandler published a detailed review of studies of aspirin and other NSAIDS conducted from 1985–1995. This review included studies in laboratory animals, epidemiological studies, and randomized trials. He concluded that "the literature on aspirin and NSAIDs makes it clear that these agents can prevent colorectal cancer and precursor adenomas" (p. 134). However, he cautioned that it was too soon to make recommendations about dose and duration of therapy because potential toxicities such as gastrointestinal hemorrhage and hemorrhagic stroke also must be considered.

Since Sandler's review, another promising NSAID has emerged. In animal studies, celecoxib (Celebrex®, G.D. Searle & Co., Skokie, IL) decreased the incidence of colon tumors by 93%, suppressing overall colon tumor burden by more than 87% (Kawamori, Rao, Seibert, & Reddy, 1998). Celecoxib's ability to reduce the number of adenomatous colorectal polyps was evaluated later in 83 patients with familial adenomatous polyposis (FAP). In that study, a 28% reduction occurred in the number of colorectal polyps in patients who received celecoxib, compared to a 5% reduction for those who received a placebo (G.D. Searle & Co., 1999). Based on these results, the U.S. Food and Drug Administration (FDA) approved celecoxib in 1999 for use in patients with FAP.

Other Agents

Tamoxifen citrate, a selective estrogen receptor modulator, has been prescribed for the treatment of breast cancer since the 1970s (Aikin, 1996). In treatment trials, this drug not only reduced the recurrence of cancer in the affected breast but also decreased its occurrence in the contralateral breast (Early Breast Cancer Trialists' Collaborative Group, 1998; Fisher et al., 1989). This preventive effect in the opposite breast and the known reasonable toxicity profile of the drug provided the rationale for studying tamoxifen as a preventive agent in the National Surgical Adjuvant Breast and Bowel Project (NSABP) Breast Cancer Prevention Trial (BCPT). Based on positive results from the BCPT, the FDA approved tamoxifen in 1998 for the reduction of breast cancer incidence in high-risk women (Aikin, 1999).

The hormonal agent finasteride, approved in 1992 for the treatment of benign prostatic hyperplasia, inhibits the enzyme 5-alpha reductase, which, in turn, decreases androgenic stimulation of the prostate gland, thereby blocking the conversion of testosterone to dihydrotestosterone (DHT) (Thompson, Feigl, & Coltman, 1995). Low levels of DHT are associated with a decreased risk of prostate cancer (Greenwald et al., 1995; Padberg, 1994; Swan & Ford, 1997). The most common side effects seen with finasteride are decreased libido, decreased volume of ejaculate, and impotence. The Southwest Oncology Group is evaluating finasteride in the Prostate Cancer Prevention Trial (PCPT), a large, randomized clinical trial that began recruitment in 1993.

In animal models, alpha-difluoromethylornithine (DFMO) is a potent inhibitor of carcinogenesis, particularly in epithelial cancers (Meyskens et al., 1998). DFMO currently is being evaluated in phase II studies as a chemopreventive agent for colorectal cancer and Barrett's esophagus and may have activity in the chemoprevention of prostate cancer. Unfortunately, DFMO is associated with thrombocytopenia and reversible ototoxicity, which may limit its clinical usefulness (Thompson et al., 1995).

Landmark Chemoprevention Trials

According to Greenwald et al. (1995), large-scale, randomized phase III clinical trials are the best way to test the effectiveness of chemopreventive agents. A number of such trials conducted in the 1980s and 1990s yielded important insights into cancer prevention. Other studies are ongoing.

The Breast Cancer Prevention Trial

The BCPT may be one of the most important large, randomized phase III chemoprevention studies that has been conducted to date. From 1992–1997, NSABP randomly assigned 13,388 healthy women at high risk for developing breast cancer to receive either 20 mg of tamoxifen or placebo daily for five years. Women who were at least 35 years old and at increased risk for developing breast cancer were eligible if they had a history of lobular carcinoma in situ (LCIS) or if they were 35–59 years old and had a 1.66% five-year risk of breast cancer, as calculated by the Gail Model (Fisher et al., 1998). All women older than age 60 were eligible. The study participants were followed with annual mammograms and gynecologic examinations and semiannual breast examinations and blood work.

After a median follow-up of 69 months, study results demonstrated that the group of women who received tamoxifen had a 49% reduction in the incidence of invasive breast cancer and a 50% reduction in the incidence of noninvasive cancer (e.g., ductal carcinoma in situ, LCIS). The BCPT also provided further insight into the known toxicities of tamoxifen. Side effects such as hot flashes and vaginal discharge were more prevalent in the tamoxifen-treated group, and these women also were more likely to develop endometrial cancer and thromboembolic events, such as deep vein thrombosis, pulmonary embolus, and stroke (Fisher et al., 1998).

The Linxian Trial

Linxian County, China, exhibits some of the world's highest rates of esophageal and stomach cancers. From 1985–1991, Blot et al. (1993) recruited 29,584 people ages 40–69 to participate in a study designed to determine whether dietary supplementation with vitamins and minerals could lower cancer incidence and mortality. The trial used a 2^4 factorial design, randomizing patients to one of four different combinations of nutrients: (a) retinol and zinc, (b) riboflavin and niacin, (c) vitamin C and molybdenum, or (d) beta-carotene, vitamin E, and selenium. Results of this study demonstrated a 9% reduction in overall mortality and a 13% reduction in cancer mortality for those who received beta-carotene, vitamin E, and selenium. This reduction in cancer mortality was primarily because of a lower incidence of stomach cancer (Blot et al.). Overall compliance in taking the nutrients during the six-year period was 93% for all participants, which is excellent support for the study's validity. According to Greenwald et al. (1995), these results are encouraging but may not be applicable to a Western population, so further study of these agents is needed.

The Alpha-Tocopherol Beta-Carotene Cancer Prevention Study

From 1985–1993, 21,133 male cigarette smokers in Finland participated in the Alpha-Tocopherol Beta-Carotene (ATBC) Cancer Prevention Study. Using a 2 x 2 factorial design, study participants randomly were assigned to receive one of four chemopreventive regimens daily for five years: (a) 20 mg beta-carotene, (b) 50 mg alpha-tocopherol (vitamin E), (c) both beta-carotene and alpha-tocopherol, or (d) placebo (Albanes et al., 1995; ATBC Cancer Prevention Study Group, 1994). The trial yielded unexpected results: a small (2%) but not statistically significant reduction in lung cancer incidence occurred in men who received vitamin E, and an 18% *higher* incidence of lung cancer occurred in the group of men who received beta-carotene. (Those who received both vitamin E and beta-carotene showed the same higher incidence of lung cancer that was seen in the beta-carotene alone group). Vitamin E also reduced the incidence of prostate cancer by 34% (which was statistically significant) and colorectal cancer by 16% (which was not statistically significant) but increased the incidence of stomach cancer by 25% (Albanes et al.; ATBC Cancer Prevention Study Group). The investigators on this trial concluded that their "results provide no evidence of a beneficial effect of supplemental vitamin E (alpha-tocopherol) or beta-carotene in terms of the prevention of lung cancer. In fact, men who received beta-carotene were found to have lung cancer more frequently than those who did not receive beta-carotene" (ATBC Cancer Prevention Study Group, p. 1032). Huttunen (1996) hypothesized that three reasons were possible for the negative results of this study: (a) incorrect doses were used, (b) characteristics of the study population were inappropriate, or (c) the study duration was too short. He concluded that further information about the beneficial or harmful effects of these antioxidant vitamins on lung cancer would be gained from the results of other ongoing clinical trials.

The Beta-Carotene and Retinol Efficacy Trial

The Beta-Carotene and Retinol Efficacy Trial (CARET) evaluated the efficacy of the combination of retinol (vitamin A) and beta-carotene in 18,314 individuals from two high-risk groups: men and women who were heavy smokers or former heavy smokers and men with occupational asbestos exposure (Goodman et al., 1998; Omenn et al., 1996). The primary endpoint for this placebo-controlled trial was the incidence of lung cancer. CARET was stopped 21 months earlier than planned because an interim analysis showed that the active treatment group had a 28% greater incidence (a 1.28 relative risk) of lung cancer than did the placebo group. Furthermore, participants who received retinol and beta-carotene had a 17% higher mortality rate than did the placebo group. No evidence of systemic toxicity was observed with use of beta-carotene, except for skin yellowing. The investigators concluded that this trial confirmed the results of the ATBC trial and that until other chemopreventive agents are identified for lung cancer, healthcare professionals should focus on smoking cessation, prevention of smoking, and avoidance of exposure to carcinogens (Omenn et al.).

Ongoing Trials

The Prostate Cancer Prevention Trial

From 1993–1996, the PCPT recruited 18,059 men, age 55 and older, to receive either 5 mg of finasteride or placebo daily for seven years (Padberg, 1994). To be eligible, participants were required to have a negative digital rectal exam (DRE) and a prostate-specific antigen (PSA) level of 3.0 ng/ml or less. Participants were asked to take a placebo during a three-month run-in phase so that compliance, side effects, and commitment to the trial could be assessed. Those who were eligible for the next phase had an 80%–120% compliance with the dosing schedule and then were randomized to receive finasteride or placebo (Thompson et al., 1995). Participants undergo a DRE and serum PSA on a yearly basis (Brawley & Thompson, 1996). The primary endpoint of this double-blind study, the occurrence of prostate cancer, will be determined by prostate biopsy at the end of seven years of treatment (Feigl et al., 1995; Swan & Ford, 1997; Thompson et al.).

Other Ongoing Phase III Chemoprevention Trials

In 1999, NSABP began the follow-up study to the BCPT, the Study of Tamoxifen and Raloxifene (STAR). In STAR, postmenopausal women are randomly assigned to receive either tamoxifen or another selective estrogen-receptor modulator, raloxifene. Raloxifene is approved for the prevention of osteoporosis. When the drug was evaluated in a landmark osteoporosis study, a secondary finding was a 76% reduction in breast cancer incidence in those receiving raloxifene compared to placebo (Cummings et al., 1999; Ettinger et al., 1999). Thus far, raloxifene has not been shown to cause endometrial hyperplasia or endometrial cancer, making it a promising new agent.

In the near future, the Southwest Oncology Group will launch the next large randomized prostate prevention trial, the Selenium and Vitamin E Chemoprevention Trial (SELECT). Using a 2 x 2 factorial design, more than 32,000 men will be recruited for this study.

Nursing Roles and Responsibilities

Nurses have an important role in the conduct of chemoprevention trials. Some work as research nurses who coordinate large, randomized chemoprevention studies such as BCPT, PCPT, STAR, and SELECT. In this role, they recruit study participants, participate in the informed-consent process, ensure compliance with study medications, and manage side effects associated with chemopreventive agents. They also contribute to continuity of care as they interact with participants during the many years of study follow-up.

Nurses who work in high-risk clinics will interact with healthy individuals at increased risk for cancer. Two specific groups that may be targeted for preventive interventions include women with breast cancer and those who have been diagnosed with familial adenomatous polyposis. Because tamoxifen and celecoxib have been approved for these indications, nurses need to support patients who are considering chemoprevention by helping them to weigh the risks and benefits of the agents and by monitoring side effects and toxicities. Thus, nurses are crucial in recruiting high-risk populations for chemoprevention trials, in discussing risks and benefits of chemopreventive agents, and in encouraging compliance in symptom management and long-term follow-up.

Recruiting High-Risk Populations for Chemoprevention Studies

Unique challenges are inherent in recruiting participants to chemoprevention trials. Most individuals who are at high risk for a particular cancer generally are not seen in oncology settings, so proactive recruitment approaches are required. In addition, participants in chemoprevention studies are healthy volunteers who may be less motivated to accept a rigorous medication schedule or bothersome side effects (Swan & Ford, 1997). Chemoprevention studies also require large numbers of healthy subjects who are followed for many years. Poor recruitment or high dropout rates can jeopardize the successful completion of these trials (Goodman et al., 1998; Kinney, Richards, Vernon, & Vogel, 1998). Another consideration is the successful recruitment of adequate numbers of minority populations so that study results can be generalized to the entire population.

Large, randomized chemoprevention trials such as CARET, BCPT, and PCPT have employed a number of different strategies in meeting their recruitment goals. To be successful, recruitment must be an ongoing priority and must involve a variety of approaches.

Direct Mailings

Investigators in the CARET lung cancer prevention trial mailed study information and eligibility questionnaires directly to health-insurance subscribers. Eligible individuals received a telephone call to clarify information on the survey, and, subsequently, an appointment was scheduled at the study center (Goodman et al., 1998). More than 1,200,000 people were contacted, resulting in 12,184 patients being randomized to the study (a yield of about 1%). CARET centers also contacted the national office of the American Association of Retired Persons, military bases, and the American Lung Association and sent targeted mailings to the constituents of these groups.

Physician Referral

Because healthy volunteers are needed for chemoprevention studies, primary-care physicians (PCPs) are referral sources for potential study participants. Kinney et al. (1998) evaluated the effect of physicians' recommendations on patients' enrollment in the BCPT. This study showed that physicians' recommendations strongly influenced the likelihood that a woman would enter the study. In addition to acting as referral sources, many PCPs also conduct the clinical examinations required by a given study, which is important for follow-up of participants. PCPs may be educated about available trials by direct mailings, presentations at local scientific meetings, and meeting individually with study staff.

Participant-to-Participant Recruitment

Individuals who already are enrolled in a trial may help to recruit others because they can give a personalized, first-hand description of what is involved. In the BCPT, participants assisted study coordinators in educating potential participants about the study, acted as spokespersons at regional meetings and events, were involved in programs to increase the number of participants from different racial and ethnic groups, and participated in local and national media interviews (Psillidis, Flach, & Padberg, 1997).

Other Recruitment Strategies

Nurses involved in recruiting individuals from high-risk populations for the BCPT targeted the family members of patients with cancer. These people are familiar with the devastating effects of cancer and are likely to be more motivated to participate in a chemoprevention trial than are those without first-hand experience of the disease.

Some trials target individuals with premalignant conditions such as atypical ductal hyperplasia of the breast, LCIS, or adenomatous polyps. For these studies, research nurses may identify potential participants by reviewing pathology reports, notifying physicians that these individuals have a pathology diagnosis that may render them eligible for a particular study, and encouraging those physicians to discuss the study with possible candidates.

Another effective recruitment strategy used in breast care clinics is the risk assessment questionnaire. While individuals are waiting to see the doctor, they answer questions about their own risk factors for breast cancer. Their responses may be used to help to quantify breast cancer risk and to set the stage for further discussion about chemoprevention strategies and trial participation.

For the BCPT, study coordinators worked with NSABP to promote the study in the media. The group operations office issued regular press releases that prompted a number of radio, television, and newspaper reports about the study. As a result, coordinators received many telephone calls from potential participants.

Discussing Risks and Benefits of Chemopreventive Agents

The drugs used in prevention studies have side effects and toxicities. Some, like vitamin E, have relatively few side effects, and the potential benefits clearly outweigh any risks associated with the intervention. Others, like tamoxifen, may cause serious toxicities that must be considered carefully by those who will use the agent for disease prevention. Oncology nurses who are familiar with the risks and benefits of chemopreventive agents can effectively educate patients and support them in their decision making.

Although the risks and benefits of many chemopreventive agents are not completely understood, tamoxifen has been studied extensively for both the treatment and prevention of breast cancer. Therefore, women must consider a great deal of information before deciding to use this agent for breast cancer prevention. First, women must understand their own risk for developing breast cancer. After the BCPT results were announced, the National Cancer Institute and the NSABP developed a risk-assessment tool, the "Risk Disk," bringing the Gail Model to the clinical setting (Aikin, 1999) The next challenge is to compare the expected benefits and risks of tamoxifen. In 1999, Gail et al. outlined the absolute risks from tamoxifen for endometrial cancer, stroke, pulmonary embolus, and deep vein thrombosis as a function of age and race and presented them alongside the benefits of tamoxifen according to age, race, and level of breast cancer risk. Tables from their published paper can be used as decision aids when physicians discuss the risks and benefits of tamoxifen with women who are considering this drug for chemoprevention. For some older women, the risks from tamoxifen outweigh the expected benefits. Gail et al. concluded that "tamoxifen is most beneficial for younger women with an elevated risk of breast cancer" (p. 1829).

For NSABP's second prevention study, STAR, women who complete a risk assessment form receive an individualized risk profile based on their age, level of breast cancer risk, and race (see Table 8-1). This profile presents the risks and benefits of tamoxifen in specific terms: how many cases of invasive breast cancer, endometrial cancer, stroke, pulmonary embolus, deep vein thrombosis, and in situ breast cancer will occur in 10,000 women who are untreated, and then how many cases are likely to be prevented or caused with tamoxifen therapy? This information assists clinicians as they discuss the potential risks and benefits of the study medications with women who are considering participating in STAR.

When women weigh the risks and benefits of tamoxifen for chemoprevention or consider participation in the STAR trial, nurses assist them by providing education and support. Some will assign greater weight to certain risks or benefits; for example, a woman whose mother had a stroke is more likely to be concerned about this risk when compared to a woman whose sister recently died from breast cancer, whose concern is more likely to be her own risk for developing breast cancer. Whether or not individuals choose chemoprevention, nurses need to respect their decisions and provide information about other primary prevention strategies, such as exercise, low-fat diet, avoidance of hormone replacement therapy, and the need for regular mammograms and breast examinations.

Table 8-1. Example of Benefit/Risk Summary Projecting Among 10,000 Women

Severity of Event	Type of Event	Expected Number of Cases in Five Years Among 10,000 Untreated Women	Potential Effect Among 10,000 Women if Treated for Five Years
Life-threatening events	Invasive breast cancer	358	**Potential Benefits** 174 of these cases may be prevented.
	Hip fracture	50	22 of these cases may be prevented. **Potential Risks**
	Uterine cancer	40	120 more cases may be caused.
	Stroke	27	16 more cases may be caused.
	Blood clot in lung	12	25 more cases may be caused.
Other severe events	In situ breast cancer	111	**Potential Benefit** 55 of these cases may be prevented. **Potential Risk**
	Blood clot in large vein	27	16 more cases may be caused.
Other events	–	–	**Potential Benefit** Treatment may reduce the yearly rate of wrist fractures and fractures of the spine. For age and race group, the reduction in the rate would be approximately one case for every 1,000 women treated. **Potential Risk** Treatment may increase the yearly rate of cataract development. For age and race group, the increase in the rate would be approximately two cases for every 1,000 women treated.

Encouraging Compliance

Nurses play a key role in encouraging adherence to chemopreventive regimens. Compliance is important for a number of reasons. To gain the greatest benefit, individuals must take their medication as prescribed and comply with their follow-up examinations so that toxicities and side effects can be identified and managed as soon as they occur.

Compliance can be assessed in several ways. Participants may be required to return pill bottles to the study center at regular intervals so that pill counts can be performed. They also may keep calendars, indicating the days they took their study medication and any side effects they experienced, and present them at subsequent follow-up visits. In the CARET and PCPT, a three- to six-month run-in phase was used to assess the likelihood of compliance.

When working with a healthy population, healthcare professionals should make study participation as convenient as possible. Individuals are more likely to comply with clinical examinations if flexible appointment schedules are available, including early morning or evening appointment times, and if study participation costs are kept to a minimum (Aikin, 1999).

Finally, nurses who display a personal interest in study participants and maintain close follow-up also encourage compliance. In the BCPT, program coordinators telephoned study participants at intervals, planned social events for them, and provided reminders to enhance compliance with study medication (e.g., pill boxes, mugs with the BCPT logo) (Aikin, 1999). According to Swan and Ford (1997), "Participants are volunteers, and the more contact they have with the research staff, the greater the compliance" (p. 726).

Symptom Management

In addition to providing comfort, symptom management is important for enhancing compliance. Healthy individuals without a cancer diagnosis are more likely to discontinue chemopreventive agents if side effects are not addressed. General symptom management strategies are outlined in Figure 8-3.

Figure 8-3. General Symptom Management Strategies

- Obtain a baseline history.
- Educate participants about possible side effects.
- Develop a relationship with the participant based on trust, caring, and open communication.
- Initiate discussion about symptoms at each follow-up visit.
- Start with the intervention that is most cost effective and has the fewest side effects.
- Evaluate and document the effectiveness of interventions.
- Maintain a positive attitude and emphasize that every effort will be made to alleviate symptoms.
- Consider a drug holiday.

Before study medication is begun, the nurse should conduct an assessment of symptoms that will serve as a baseline for comparison in the future. For example, it is important to determine at baseline whether women beginning tamoxifen have menopausal symptoms and to assess sexual function in men who will be taking finasteride. Patients should be encouraged to keep a diary or study calendar, and side effects should be assessed at each follow-up visit.

Proactive symptom management is essential. In addition to pharmacologic and nonpharmacologic interventions, a drug holiday may be an appropriate option for relieving symptoms. During a drug holiday, oral chemopreventive agents are temporarily discontinued for a few weeks or longer. This serves two purposes: to determine whether symptoms were directly related to the medication and to give the individual a brief rest. Sometimes symptoms are less severe when the agent is resumed.

Long-Term Follow-Up

Long-term follow-up is important to help to maintain compliance, monitor toxicities, and ensure early detection of cancer. In most chemoprevention trials, participants are followed for 5–10 years, and information about adverse events and cancer diagnoses must be submitted to the study sponsor at regular intervals. According to Loescher and Meyskens (1991), maintaining compliance over a long period of time is challenging because of "outside" influences, including the media, family and friends, and other healthcare professionals not involved in the trial.

Regardless of whether a person participates in a prevention study, nurses need to have regular contact with those who take chemopreventive agents. Ideally, this contact will be "face-to-face" so that a physical assessment can be performed. When this is not feasible, telephone contact is essential. During these contacts, nurses should assess compliance with both the chemopreventive agent and clinical examinations, initiate discussion about side effects, inquire about any new medications, and review the goals of the study. As long as women are taking chemopreventive agents, they also should be counseled to avoid pregnancy because many of these agents are teratogenic (Loescher & Meyskens, 1991).

Opportunities for Nursing Research

Given the nursing roles and responsibilities, opportunities are available for nursing research related to chemoprevention. Research is needed to explore factors that enhance both recruitment to chemoprevention trials and compliance with chemopreventive agents. Another research question relates to the optimal method for communicating risk. Finally, research is needed to identify what level of cancer risk is necessary for an individual to accept the toxicities associated with a particular chemopreventive agent.

Conclusion

According to Greenwald et al. (1995), "Chemoprevention has progressed to the point where [it] is now considered to be an extremely promising approach to the prevention of invasive cancer" (p. 45). With these advances come new responsibilities for oncology nurses, who have an important role to play in recruiting people at high risk for cancer for chemoprevention studies, educating individuals about the risks and benefits of chemopreventive agents, encouraging compliance, and helping with the management of symptoms associated with these interventions.

The author would like to thank Barbara Good, PhD, for her editorial assistance with this chapter.

References

Ahnen, D.J. (1998). Colon cancer prevention by NSAIDs: What is the mechanism of action? *European Journal of Surgery, 164*, 111–114.

Aikin, J.L. (1996). Tamoxifen in perspective: Benefits, side effects, and toxicities. In K.H. Dow (Ed.), *Contemporary issues in breast cancer* (pp. 59–68). Boston: Jones and Bartlett.

Aikin, J.L. (1999). The role of tamoxifen in breast cancer prevention: Nursing implications. *Innovations in Breast Cancer Care, 4(2)*, 45–49.

Albanes, D., Heinonen, O.P., Huttunen, J.K., Taylor, P.R., Virtamo, J., Edwards, B.K., Haapakoski, J., Rautalahti, M., Hartman, A.M., Palmgren, J., & Greenwald, P. (1995). Effects of alpha-tocopherol and beta-carotene supplements on cancer incidence in the Alpha-Tocopherol Beta-Carotene Cancer Prevention Study. *American Journal of Clinical Nutrition, 62*(Suppl. 6), 1427S–1430S.

Alberts, D.S., & Garcia, D.J. (1995). An overview of clinical cancer chemoprevention studies with emphasis on positive phase III studies. *Journal of Nutrition, 125*(Suppl. 3), 692S–697S.

Alpha-Tocopherol, Beta-Carotene Cancer Prevention Study Group. (1994). The effect of vitamin E and beta-carotene on the incidence of lung cancer and other cancers in male smokers. *New England Journal of Medicine, 330*, 1029–1035.

Bertram, J.S., Kolonel, L.N., & Meyskens, F.L. (1987). Rationale and strategies for chemoprevention of cancer in humans. *Cancer Research, 47*, 3012–3031.

Blot, W.J., Li, J., Taylor, P.R., Wande, G., Dawsey, S., Guo, W., Yang, C.S., Zheng, S., Gail, M., Li, G., Yu, Y., Liu, B., Tangrea, J., Sun, Y., Liu, F., Fraumeni, J.F., Zhang, Y., & Li, B. (1993). Nutrition intervention trials in Linxian, China: Supplementation with specific vitamin/mineral combinations, cancer incidence, and disease-specific mortality in the general population. *Journal of the National Cancer Institute, 85*, 1483–1492.

Brawley, O.W., & Thompson, I.M. (1996). The chemoprevention of prostate cancer and the prostate cancer prevention trial. *Diagnosis and Treatment of Genitourinary Malignancies, 88*, 189–200.

Butterworth, C.E., Jr., Hatch, K.D., Soong, S.J., Cole, P., Tamura, T., Sauberlich, H.E., Borst, M., Macalust, M., & Baker, V. (1992). Oral folic acid supplementation for cervical dysplasia: A clinical intervention trial. *American Journal of Obstetrics and Gynecology, 166*, 803–809.

Childers, J.M., Chu, J., Voigt, L.F., Feigl, P., Tamimi, H.K., Franklin, E.W., Alberts, D.S., & Meyskens, F.L. (1995). Chemoprevention of cervical cancer with folic acid: A phase III Southwest Oncology Group Intergroup Study. *Cancer Epidemiology, Biomarkers, and Prevention, 4*, 155–159.

Clark, L.C., Dalkin, B., Krongrad, A., Combs, G.F., Turnbull, B.W., Slate, E.H., Witherington, R., Herlong, J.H., Janosko, E., Carpenter, D., Borosso, C., Falk, S., & Rounder, J. (1998). Decreased incidence of prostate cancer with selenium supplementation: Results of a double-blind cancer prevention trial. *British Journal of Urology, 81*, 730–734.

Cummings, S.R., Eckert, S., Krueger, K.A., Grady, D., Powles, T.J., Cauley, J.A., Norton, L., Nickelson, T., Bjarnason, N.H., Morrow, M., Lippman, M.E., Black, D., Glusman, J.E., Costa, A., & Jordan, V.C. (1999). The effect of raloxifene on risk of breast cancer in postmenopausal women: Results from the MORE randomized trial. *JAMA, 281,* 2189–2197.

deKlerk, N.H., Musk, A.W., Ambrosini, G.L., Eccles, J.L., Hansen, J., Olsen, N., Watts, V.L., Lund, H.G., Pang, S.C., Beilby, J., & Hobbs, M.S.T. (1998). Vitamin A and cancer prevention II: Comparison of the effects of retinol and beta-carotene. *International Journal of Cancer, 75,* 362–367.

Duris, I., Hruby, D., Pekarkova, B., Huorka, M., Cernakova, E., Bezayova, T., & Ondrejka, P. (1996). Calcium chemoprevention in colorectal cancer. *Hepatogastroenterology, 43*(7), 152–154.

Early Breast Cancer Trialists' Collaborative Group. (1998). Tamoxifen for early breast cancer: An overview of the randomised trials. *Lancet, 351,* 1451–1467.

Ettinger, B., Black, D.M., Mitlak, B.H., Knickerbocker, R.K., Nickelsen, T., Genant, H.K., Christiansen, C., Delmas, P.D., Zanchetta, J.R., Stakkestad, J., Glüer, C.C., Krueger, K., Cohen, F.J., Eckert, S., Ensrud, K.E., Avioli, L.V., Lips, P., & Cummings, S.R. (1999). Reduction of vertebral fracture risk in postmenopausal women with osteoporosis treated with raloxifene. *JAMA, 282,* 637–645.

Feigl, P., Blumenstein, B., Thompson, I., Crowley, J., Wolf, M., Kramer, B.S., Coltman, C.A., Brawley, O.W., & Ford, L.G. (1995). Design of the Prostate Cancer Prevention Trial (PCPT). *Controlled Clinical Trials, 16,* 150–163.

Fisher, B., Costantino, J., Redmond, C., Poisson, R., Bowman, D., Couture, J., Dimitrov, N.V., Wolmark, N., Wickerham, D.L., Fisher, E.R., Margolese, R., Robidoux, A., Shibata, H., Terz, J., Paterson, A.H.G., Feldman, M.I., Farrar, W., Evans, J., Lickley, H.L., & Ketner, M. (1989). A randomized clinical trial evaluating tamoxifen in the treatment of patients with node-negative breast cancer who have estrogen-receptor-positive tumors. *New England Journal of Medicine, 320,* 479–484.

Fisher, B., Costantino, J.P., Wickerham, D.L., Redmond, C.K., Kavanah, M., Cronin, W.M., Vogel, V., Robidoux, A., Dimitrov, N., Atkins, J., Daly, M., Wieand, S., Tan-Chiu, E., Ford, L., & Wolmark, N. (1998). Tamoxifen for prevention of breast cancer: Report of the National Surgical Adjuvant Breast and Bowel Project P-1 Study. *Journal of the National Cancer Institute, 90,* 1371–1388.

Gail, M.H., Costantino, J.P., Bryant, J., Croyle, R., Freedman, L., Helzlsouer, K., & Vogel, V. (1999). Weighing the risks and benefits of tamoxifen treatment for preventing breast cancer. *Journal of the National Cancer Institute, 91,* 1829–1846.

Garewal, H.S., & Meyskens, F.L. (1991). Chemoprevention of cancer. *Hematology/Oncology Clinics of North America, 5,* 69–77.

Goodman, G.E., Valanis, B., Meyskens, F.L., Williams, J.H., Metch, B.J., Thornquist, M.D., & Omenn, G.S. (1998). Strategies for recruitment to a population-based lung cancer prevention trial: The CARET experience with heavy smokers. *Cancer Epidemiology, Biomarkers, and Prevention, 7,* 405–412.

Greenwald, P. (1992). Keynote address: Cancer prevention. *Journal of the National Cancer Institute Monographs, 12,* 9–14.

Greenwald, P., Kelloff, G., Burch-Whitman, C., & Kramer, B.S. (1995). Chemoprevention. *CA: A Cancer Journal for Clinicians, 45,* 31–49.

Greenwald, P., Nixon, D.W., Malone, W.F., Kelloff, G.J., Stern, H.R., & Witkin, K.M. (1990). Concepts in cancer chemoprevention research. *Cancer, 65,* 1483–1490.

Huttunen, J.K. (1996). Why did antioxidants not protect against lung cancer in the Alpha-Tocopherol, Beta-Carotene Cancer Prevention Study? *IARC Scientific Publications, 136,* 63–65.

Kawamori, T., Rao, C.V., Seibert, K., & Reddy, B.S. (1998). Chemopreventive activity of celecoxib, a specific cyclooxygenase-2 inhibitor, against colon carcinogenesis. *Cancer Research, 58,* 409–412.

Kinney, A.Y., Richards, C., Vernon, S.W., & Vogel, V.G. (1998). The effect of physician recommendation on enrollment in the Breast Cancer Prevention Trial. *Preventive Medicine, 27,* 713–719.

Lippman, S.M., Benner, S.E., & Hong, W.K. (1994). Cancer chemoprevention. *Journal of Clinical Oncology, 12,* 851–873.

Loescher, L.J. (1993). Strategies for preventing breast cancer. *Innovations in Oncology Nursing, 9,* 2–6.

Loescher, L.J., & Meyskens, F.L. (1991). Chemoprevention of human skin cancers. *Seminars in Oncology Nursing, 7,* 45–52.

Meyskens, F.L., Gerner, F.W., Emerson, S., Pelot, D., Durbin, T., Doyle, K., & Lagerberg, W. (1998). Effect of alpha-difluoromethylornithine on rectal mucosal levels of polyamines in a randomized, double-blinded trial for colon cancer prevention. *Journal of the National Cancer Institute, 90,* 1212–1218.

Morse, M.A., & Stoner, G.D. (1993). Cancer chemoprevention: Principles and prospects. *Carcinogenesis, 14,* 1737–1746.

National Surgical Adjuvant Breast and Bowel Project. (1999). *The Study of Tamoxifen and Raloxifene (STAR) procedures manual and information handbook.* Pittsburgh, PA: Author.

Nixon, D.W. (1994). Special aspects of cancer prevention trials. *Cancer, 74*(Suppl. 9), 2683–2686.

O'Dwyer, P.J., Szarka, C.E., Yao, K., Halbherr, T.C., Pfeiffer, G.R., Green, F., Gallo, J.M., Brennan, J., Frucht, H., Goosenberg, E.B., Hamilton, T.C., Litwin, S., Balshem, A.M., Engstrom, P.F., & Clapper, M.L. (1996). Modulation of gene expression in subjects at risk for colorectal cancer by the chemopreventive dithiolethione oltipraz. *Journal of Clinical Investigations, 98,* 1210–1217.

Olsen, S.J., & Love, R.R. (1986). A new direction in preventive oncology: Chemo prevention. *Seminars in Oncology Nursing, 2,* 211–221.

Omenn, G.S., Goodman, G.E., Thornquist, M.D., Balmes, J., Cullen, M.R., Glass, A., Keogh, J.P., Meyskens, F.L., Valanis, B., Williams, J.H., Barnhart, S., & Hammar, S. (1996). Effects of a combination of beta-carotene and vitamin A on lung cancer and cardiovascular disease. *New England Journal of Medicine, 334,* 1150–1155.

Padberg, R.M. (1994). Chemoprevention trials. *Cancer Practice, 2,* 154–156.

Psillidis, L., Flach, J., & Padberg, R.M. (1997). Participants strengthen clinical trial research: The vital role of participant advisors in the Breast Cancer Prevention Trial. *Journal of Women's Health, 6,* 227–232.

Roncucci, L., Di Donato, P., Carati, L., Ferrari, A., Perini, M., Bertoni, G., Bedogni, G., Paris, B., Svanoni, F., Girola, M., & Ponz de Leon, M. (1993). Antioxidant vitamins or lactulose for the prevention of the recurrence of colorectal adenomas. *Diseases of the Colon and Rectum, 36,* 227–234.

Sandler, R.S. (1996). Aspirin and other nonsteroidal anti-inflammatory agents in the prevention of colorectal cancer [Review]. In V.T. Devita, S. Hellman, & S.A. Rosenberg (Eds.), *Important advances in oncology* (pp. 123–137). Philadelphia: Lippincott-Raven.

Schatzkin, A., & Kelloff, G. (1995). Chemo- and dietary prevention of colorectal cancer. *European Journal of Cancer, 31,* 1198–1204.

G.D. Searle Co. (1999). Celebrex (celecoxib capsules) [Package insert]. Skokie, IL: Author.

Sporn, M.B. (1993). Chemoprevention of cancer. *Lancet, 342,* 1211–1213.

Swan, D.K., & Ford, B. (1997). Chemoprevention of cancer: Review of the literature. *Oncology Nursing Forum, 24,* 719–727.

Taylor, P.R., Li, B., Dawsey, S.M., Li, J., Wang, C.S., Guo, W., Blot, W.J., & the Linxian Nutrition Intervention Trials Study Group. (1994). Prevention of esophageal cancer: The nutrition intervention trials in Linxian, China. *Cancer Research, 54*(Suppl. 7), 2029S–2031S.

Thompson, I., Feigl, P., & Coltman, C. (1995). Chemoprevention of prostate cancer with finasteride [Review]. In V.T. Devita, S. Hellman, & S.A. Rosenberg (Eds.), *Important advances in oncology* (pp. 57–76). Philadelphia: Lippincott-Raven.

Turner, D., & Berkel, H.J. (1993). Nonsteroidal anti-inflammatory drugs for the prevention of colon cancer. *Canadian Medical Association Journal, 149,* 595–602.

Yu, S., Mao, B., Xiao, P., Yu, W., Wang, Y., Huang, C., Chen, W., & Xuan, X. (1990). Intervention trial with selenium for the prevention of lung cancer among tin miners in Yunan, China: A pilot study. *Biological Trace Element Research, 24,* 105–108.

CHAPTER 9

Smoking and Cancer

*Janine K. Cataldo, PhD, RN, CS, Mary E. Cooley, PhD, CRNP, AOCN®,
and Ellen Giarelli, EdD, RN, CS, CRNP*

Introduction

Cigarette smoking is the most preventable cause of illness, disability, and premature death, and, paradoxically, the practice is damaging health on a global scale. Approximately 1.15 billion people smoke worldwide, each consuming an average of 14 cigarettes per day (World Bank, 1999). Tobacco usage fell between 1981 and 1991 in most high-income countries. However, tobacco consumption is increasing in developing countries by approximately 3.4% per year. Overall, smoking prevalence among men in developing countries is approximately 48% (World Health Organization [WHO], 1999). Given current smoking patterns, by 2030, smoking is expected to kill 10 million people annually worldwide. More than 70% of these deaths will be in the developing world (WHO).

This chapter provides information about nicotine dependence and the health consequences associated with tobacco use across the lifespan and within special populations. Because cancer is a major risk associated with tobacco use, the affiliation between cigarette smoking and various cancers is highlighted. The benefits associated with smoking cessation are discussed, and interventions to promote smoking cessation and tobacco control are provided. Tobacco legislation and policy also will be reviewed.

Smoking Prevalence

In the United States, the prevalence of smoking reached a peak in 1964 when 40% of all adult Americans, including 60% of men, smoked. By 1997, the smoking prevalence among adult Americans had decreased to 23% (WHO, 1999). An estimated 48 million (24.7%) adults in the United States currently smoke (27.6% of men and 22.1% of women). The prevalence of adult cigarette smoking essentially has remained unchanged in the 1990s (25% in 1993 and 24.7% in 1997) and has fallen short of the nation's public health goal of reducing smoking to no more than 15% by 2000. In 1997, an estimated 44 million adults were former smokers, which remained unchanged from 1995 (Centers for Disease Control and Prevention [CDC], 1999a). Previously, smokers 25–44 years old had the highest smoking prevalence; however, smokers age 18–24 and age 25–44 were smoking at equal rates in 1997 (28.7% and 28.6%, respectively) (CDC, 1994a). These prevalence rates of current smoking highlight the increase in the number of younger adults choosing to use tobacco. Recent trend analyses indicate that the prevalence of smoking among high school students has increased significantly from 27.5% in 1991 to 36.4% in 1997 (Wingo et al., 1999). Although overall cigar usage in the United States declined during the 1970s and 1980s, it has been increasing steadily in the 1990s, and total cigar consumption in the United States was approximately 5.3 billion cigars in 1998 (National Cancer Institute [NCI], 1998).

Smoking prevalence among various racial and ethnic populations has remained stable in recent years, showing higher trends among American Indians/Alaska Natives (34.1%), African Americans (26.7%), and Whites (25.3%) than among Hispanics (20.4%) and Asian/Pacific Islanders (16.9%) (CDC, 1999a). From 1978–1995, the prevalence of cigarette smoking declined among African American, Asian American/Pacific Islander, and Hispanic adults. However, among American Indians and Alaska Natives, current smoking prevalence did not change for men from 1983–1995 or for women from 1978–1995 (United States Department of Health and Human Services [USDHHS], 1998).

The current prevalence of smoking among adults in the United States varies by state. In 1998, Kentucky had the highest smoking prevalence in the United States for adults (33.3% males and 28.1% females). Utah had the lowest adult smoking rates for males (15.9%) and females (12.5%) (CDC, 1999a).

Although social awareness of the adverse effects of tobacco smoking has increased since the U.S. Surgeon General warned of the hazards, the prevalence of smoking remains unacceptably high (U.S. Department of Health, Education, and Welfare, 1964). Oncology nurses can make important contributions to health promotion and cancer control through interventions that are directed toward smoking prevention and cessation and tobacco control.

Nicotine Dependence

Nicotine is a poisonous alkaloid derived from tobacco that is rapid acting with diverse neuroregulatory effects, making it a perfect substance for abuse. Nicotine is available on demand, and its effects rarely outlast the circumstances that prompt its use (Pomerleau & Pomerleau, 1984). Only recently has nicotine dependence resulting from tobacco use been classified as drug abuse, in part because the harm to health was not widely recognized and because the habit was not associated with obvious intoxication or socially deviant behavior (Pomerleau, 1997). In 1988, the U.S. Surgeon General's report on the health consequences of smoking (USDHHS, 1988) summarized the cumulative findings of more than 2,500 scientific papers, which led to the unequivocal conclusion that cigarettes and other forms of tobacco are addicting. The report identified nicotine as the drug in tobacco that causes addiction and that the pharmacological and behavioral processes that determine tobacco addiction are similar to those that determine addiction to other drugs, such as heroin and cocaine (USDHHS, 1988).

Neurobiology of Tobacco Smoking

Nicotine is a potent drug that affects the central nervous system and activates the mesolimbic dopamine system. Nicotine is known to stimulate dopamine release in the nucleus accumbens, which is a neurobiologic hallmark of addiction. Most, if not all, drugs abused by humans have this same effect (Ascher et al., 1995). The mesolimbic dopaminergic system can play an important role in mediating the reinforcing effects of natural rewards as well as those of various drugs that are abused (Fibiger & Phillips, 1987).

Nicotine dependence involves a pattern of heavy consumption that is resistant to change, which includes nicotine tolerance and the regulation of nicotine intake within relatively narrow limits (Pomerleau, Fertig, & Shanahan, 1983). Abstinence from nicotine produces withdrawal symptoms, including dysphoria, depressed mood, insomnia, irritability, frustration, anger, anxiety, difficulty concentrating, restlessness, decreased heart rate, and increased appetite (Patten & Martin, 1996). Although withdrawal symptoms usually peak in two to three days and dissipate over a few months, intensity and duration of symptoms vary (Pomerleau, 1997).

The primary reasons people give for smoking are stimulation (increased energy), sensorimotor stimulation (handling the cigarettes), relaxation, habit (smoking automatically), reduction of negative affect (e.g., tension, anxiety, anger, boredom, frustration), and addiction (smoking to avoid withdrawal symptoms) (Pomerleau, 1997). The behavioral and subjective effects of smoking correlate strongly with the neuroregulatory actions of nicotine (see Figure 9-1). Nicotine

Figure 9-1. The Relationship of the Behavioral and Subjective Effects of Smoking and Neuroregulatory Actions

Positive Reinforcement	Negative Reinforcement
Pleasure/enhancement of pleasure	Reduction of anxiety and tension
Dopamine	ß-Endorphin
Norepinephrine	Pain reduction
ß-Endorphin	Acetylcholine
Facilitation of task performance	ß-Endorphin
Acetylcholine	Reduction of hunger
Norepinephrine	Dopamine
Improvement of memory	Norepinephrine
Acetylcholine	Serotonin
Norepinephrine	Relief from nicotine withdrawal
Arginine vasopressin	Acetylcholine
	Cortisol

Note. From "Nicotine Dependence" (p. 125) by O.F. Pomerleau in C.T. Bolliger and K.O. Fagerstrom (Eds.), *The Tobacco Epidemic,* 1997, New York: S. Karger AG. Copyright 1997 by S. Karger AG. Reprinted with permission.

alters the bioavailability of numerous behaviorally and physiologically active neuroregulators, producing a variety of transient effects in smokers (Breslau, 1995; Pomerleau; Pomerleau & Pomerleau, 1984).

Earlier theories of nicotine addiction focused on negative reinforcement, with the relief from withdrawal as the force driving nicotine consumption. These early theories conceptualized smoking as an escape-avoidance response to aversive consequences caused by nicotine abstinence. Although this evidence was supported, the analysis of recidivism and retrospective examination of factors related to cravings and the situations that cue smoking revealed factors independent of nicotine dependence that control smoking behaviors (Pomerleau & Pomerleau, 1984). Smokers also reported that some cigarettes are smoked for pleasure and perceived improvement in affect and performance. Therefore, cognitive perceptions and affective states can be viewed in a favorable or adaptive way and serve as prompts for smoking. A vast number of external and internal events unrelated to the nicotine addiction cycle serve as cues for smoking, explaining how the habit can become so thoroughly woven into the patterns of daily living (Pomerleau & Pomerleau).

Genetics of Tobacco Smoking

Several studies have investigated genetic influences on the age at onset of tobacco use (smoking initiation) and smoking persistence (Koopmans, Slutske, Heath, Neale, & Boomsma, 1999; Madden et al., 1999; Stallings, Hewitt, Beresford, Heath, & Eaves, 1999). A growing body of literature suggests that initiation of substance use is influenced primarily by environmental rather than genetic factors. Findings suggest that the familial resemblance for age at first use of tobacco is largely the result of shared environmental factors, whereas the latencies between first use and regular patterns of use are more genetically influenced (Stallings et al.).

In a study of the genetics of smoking initiation and quantity smoked in Dutch adolescent and young adult twins, the findings showed smoking initiation was influenced more by shared environmental influences than by genetic factors; once smoking is initiated, genetic factors determine to a large extent the quantity that is smoked (Koopmans et al., 1999).

Health Consequences of Tobacco

Tobacco-Related Mortality
International

Research during the last five decades has left no doubt that prolonged smoking is an important cause of premature mortality and disability worldwide. The nature of the smoking epidemic varies across nations. In developed countries, cardiovascular disease is the most common smoking-related cause of death. In populations where cigarette smoking has been common for several decades, approximately 90% of lung cancer and 15%–20% of other cancers are attributable to tobacco use (WHO, 1999). Tobacco-related cancer constitutes 16% of the total annual incidence of cancer cases and 30% of cancer deaths in developed countries and 10% in developing countries (Parkin, 1994). In the near future, the epidemic will expand to include more developing countries and a larger number of women (WHO).

United States
Tobacco smoking is the single most preventable cause of premature death in the United States (CDC, 1999a). One in every five deaths in the United States is smoking-related; 430,000 Americans die every year from smoking (CDC, 1999a). Approximately 10 million people in the United States have died from causes attributed to smoking since the Surgeon General's first report on smoking and health in 1964, with 2 million of these deaths being from lung cancer alone (CDC, 1993a). Men who smoke increase their risk of death from lung cancer by more than 22 times and from bronchitis and emphysema by nearly 10 times. Women smokers increase their risk of dying from lung cancer by nearly 12 times and the risk of dying from bronchitis and emphysema by more than 10 times. Smoking triples the risk of dying from heart disease among middle-aged men and women (CDC, 1993a). On average, smokers die nearly seven years earlier than nonsmokers (CDC, 1993b).

Tobacco-Related Morbidity
Cigarette smokers have greater morbidity than nonsmokers. Current smokers have more acute and chronic illness, restricted activity days, bed disability days, and school and work absenteeism than former smokers or those who have never smoked (American Thoracic Society [ATS], 1996).

Coronary Heart Disease
Heavy smoking increases coronary heart disease risk by a factor of 3–10 (USDHHS, 1988; Willett, Green, & Stampfer, 1987). The cardiovascular effects of tobacco smoke are attributable to more than one mechanism. Smoking reduces blood levels of high-density lipoprotein cholesterins, increases the aggregation of platelets and levels of fibrinogen, and accelerates atherogenesis (Weibel, 1997).

Pulmonary Disease
Tobacco inhalation alters both the structure and function of central and peripheral airways, alveoli and capillaries, and the immune system of the lung (Wyser & Bolliger, 1997). Chronic cigarette smoke exposure stimulates bone marrow and contributes to leukocytosis, which plays a large role in the pathogenesis of chronic lung inflammation seen in cigarette smokers (Terashima, Wiggs, & English, 1997). Exposure of bronchial epithelial cells to cigarette smoke augments interleukin-8 release, which assists in the inflammation of the lower respiratory tract of smokers and thereby contributes to the pathogenesis of smoking-related lung diseases (Wyser & Bolliger).

Smoking-induced changes in airway epithelium include loss of cilia, mucous gland hypertrophy, and increase in the number and permeability of goblet cells. These changes are responsible for increased respiratory symptoms among cigarette smokers, such as chronic cough, phlegm production, wheeze, and dyspnea (ATS, 1996). Cigarette smoking has been shown to be a major environmental risk factor predisposing to the development of chronic obstructive pulmonary disease (COPD); 15% of one-pack-per-day and 25% of two-pack-per-day cigarette smokers develop COPD (Wyser & Bolliger, 1997). COPD also is a key factor that increases individual risk for lung cancer (Biesalski et al., 1998).

Lung Cancer

The association between cigarette smoking and cancer has been established through retrospective and prospective investigations that conclusively have shown that cigarette smoking causes lung cancer of each of the principal histologic types (i.e., epidermoid, small cell, large cell, and adenocarcinoma) in both men and women (Wyser & Bolliger, 1997). Several prospective studies have reported a multistep transformation from normal pseudostratified ciliated epithelium to squamous metaplasia, carcinoma in situ, and eventually invasive bronchogenic carcinoma (Yesner, 1993).

Lung cancer is among the most commonly occurring malignancies in the world. The lung is the number-one cancer mortality site overall and is one of the top four incidence sites for each racial and ethnic group in the United States (Wingo et al., 1999). From 1990–1996, a statistically significant decline occurred in male lung cancer incidence and death rates (–2.6% and –1.6% per year, respectively). Lung cancer incidence rates peaked in 1981 for men age 50–59 at diagnosis, in 1985 for men age 60–79, and in the early 1990s for men age 80 and older. Declines occurred in histologic types most associated with cigarette smoking: squamous cell carcinoma and small cell carcinoma. Rates of adenocarcinoma of the lung, which is associated with using "low-tar" cigarettes, peaked in the early 1990s in males (Wingo et al.). Overall female lung cancer incidence and death rates, however, have been increasing. In 1987, lung cancer surpassed breast cancer as the leading cause of cancer death in women (Wingo et al.). From 1990–1996, the average annual percent increase was +0.1% for incidence and +1.4% for mortality (Wingo et al.). Since 1994, female lung cancer incidence rates have been decreasing an average of –1.3% per year (not statistically significant). However, incidence rates for women older than age 69 continue to increase, resulting in the increased statistic for female lung cancer death rates (Wingo et al.).

Smoking is the major risk factor, accounting for 90% of lung cancer incidence (Biesalski et al., 1998). Research consistently provides clear evidence for a dose-response relationship between smoking tobacco and lung cancer (Wyser & Bolliger, 1997). The amount and duration of smoking determine the risk of lung cancer for individual smokers. The risk of lung cancer increases with the number of lifetime cigarettes smoked, years of smoking duration, level of nicotine dependence, earlier age at onset of smoking, degree of inhalation, tar and nicotine content, and use of unfiltered cigarettes. The rate decreases in proportion to the number of years after smoking cessation (Jacobs et al., 1999). Men or women who smoke more than 40 cigarettes a day have twice the lung cancer risk of those who smoke less than 20 cigarettes a day. Those who start smoking before the age of 15 are four times more likely to develop lung cancer than those who begin after age 25 (Parkin, 1989).

Lifetime smoking exposure affects the distribution of specific histologic sub-types of lung cancer, especially in women. Analysis of female lung cancer by histologic type revealed that rates of squamous cell lung cancer have been level since the mid-1980s; rates of small cell lung cancer decreased from 1991–1996; and rates of adenocarcinoma of the lung continued to increase (Wingo et al., 1999). Adenocarcinoma is related to smoking low-tar cigarettes. Declines by histologic type in males also were remarkable. Large declines occurred among men who had histologic types most strongly associated with cigarette smoking, namely squamous cell carcinoma and small cell carcinoma (Morabia & Wynder, 1991; Sridhar & Raub, 1992; Wingo et al.).

Characteristics of older adults with lung cancer include predominantly males, squamous cell and small-cell type, advanced stages of disease, poor prognosis (median survival time is seven months and the three-year survival rate is only 6.3%), and undergoing fewer surgeries (Antonia, Robinson, Ruckdeschel, & Wagner, 1998; Mitzushima, Kashii, Yoshida, Sugiyama, & Kobayashi, 1996). Older African Americans are at higher risk for lung cancer than Whites in the United States. Schwartz and Swanson (1997) explained this difference in lung carcinoma incidence by differences in smoking habits among those 55–84 years of age.

Lung cancer screening: Although several breakthroughs have occurred in lung cancer screening (e.g., spiral computed tomography [CT], biomarker assessment), no proven detection strategy exists for lung cancer. Primary prevention remains the best strategy in the fight against lung cancer.

The Early Lung Cancer Action Project evaluated baseline and annual repeat screening by low-radiation-dose CT (spiral CT) in people at high risk of lung cancer. The findings suggested that spiral CT can greatly improve the likelihood of detection of small noncalcified nodules and, thus, of lung cancer at an earlier and potentially more curable stage (Henschke et al., 1999). However, a large-scale longitudinal study is needed to further explore the effectiveness of this method.

The rapid increase in knowledge about the molecular events leading to lung cancer may make it possible to use biomarkers to identify the early clonal phase of progression of lung cancer in high-risk populations, thus enabling cancers to be detected earlier than is possible with spiral CT. The use of biomarkers also might be valuable as a complementary test to spiral CT, because the latter is not as sensitive for small central cancers as it is for small peripheral cancers (Mulshine & Henschke, 2000).

Other Cancers

In addition to lung cancer, it also is well established that smoking is causally associated with cancers in other sites, including the oral cavity, pharynx, larynx, esophagus, prostate, bladder, pancreas, and cervix (Jacobs et al., 1999; Shopland, Eyre, & Pechacek, 1991).

The overall effects of smoking on cancer development include mutations in tumor-suppressor genes (cell growth control) and dominant oncogenesis (overexpression causes unregulated cell growth) and impairment of mucocilliary clearance in the lungs, with decreased immunologic responsiveness, which is associated with a predisposition to cancer (Carbone, 1992). (See Chapter 4 for an in-depth discussion of genetic mutations and cancer.)

Head and neck cancer: The largest, single, most irrefutable causative factor in head and neck carcinogenesis is tobacco use (Endicott, 1998). Esophageal cancer is the most common nonrespiratory cancer associated with cigarette smoking. Contact carcinogenesis is the most likely mechanism for this cancer. Tobacco constituents that condense in the pharynx and in mucus cleared from the lungs are swallowed and directly expose the esophageal mucosa to high concentrations of carcinogenic material, producing cellular changes that result in neoplasia (Newcomb & Carbone, 1992). A study of 200 male patients with esophageal cancer found that the effects of drinking and smoking appear to be independent of one another (Mashberg, Garfinkle, & Harris, 1981). Nondrinking smokers are at two to four times the risk of developing carcinoma as abstainers from alcohol and tobacco (Feldman, Hazan, Nagarajan, & Kissin, 1975).

There is a four- to sixfold increase in oral and oropharyngeal cancer risk among subjects with medium or high tobacco consumption; an increasing risk is associated with greater duration of usage and with earlier age at onset (Merletti, Boffetta, Ciccone, Mashberg, & Terracine, 1989). Heavy alcohol consumption combined with cigarette smoking is synergistic in causing an increased incidence of cancer of the upper aerodigestive tract (Kabat, Chang, & Wynder, 1994).

The presence of a first cancer in the upper aerodigestive tract signifies an increased risk of having or developing a second cancer elsewhere in the upper aerodigestive tract. With this phenomenon, called field cancerization, significant dysplastic changes occur throughout a wide epithelial field in high-risk patients, such as heavy smokers. An initial lesion heralds a general susceptibility to other squamous carcinomas. It is not uncommon for a patient to be confronted with synchronous or metachronous multiple primaries (Mashberg & Samit, 1995).

Squamous cell carcinoma of the glottic larynx is the most common head and neck cancer and is strongly related to cigarette smoking and excessive ethanol intake (Mendenhall, Million, Stringer, & Cassisi, 1999). In a case referent study to identify the role of tobacco use in the etiology of head and neck cancer, Lewin et al. (1998) found an almost multiplicative effect for tobacco smoking and alcohol consumption. Among those who were tobacco smokers, the relative risk of head and neck cancer was 6.5% (95% confidence interval, 4.4%–9.5%). After cessation of smoking, the risk gradually declined, and no excess risk was found after 20 years. Patients with head and neck cancer who continue to smoke during radiation therapy have lower rates of response and survival than patients who stop smoking before radiation (Browman et al., 1993).

Prostate cancer: The prostate is the leading cancer site for men in the United States, accounting for 29% of new cancer cases (Landis, Murray, Bolden, & Wingo, 1998). The incidence and mortality rates among African American men are the highest in the world. Prostate cancer has become the second leading cause of cancer deaths in men, second only to lung cancer (Landis et al.). Conflicting reports exist about whether tobacco is a factor that influences the development of prostate cancer. Some reports indicate that no association exists between tobacco use and prostate cancer (Moon, 1998; Wynder, Mabuchi, & Whitmore, 1971). However, other evidence suggests that tobacco use may influence either the onset or progression of prostate cancer (Boyle, Hsieh, & Maisonneuve, 1989; Murr, Sarr, & Oishi, 1994). Certain nitrosamines that induce prostatic cancer in laboratory rats are found in the urine of cigarette smokers. Smokers have elevated levels of serum testosterone and androstenedione, two steroids that may contribute to the progression of prostate cancer (Dai, Gutai, Kuller, & Cauley, 1988). Three large prospective mortality studies found higher prostate cancer death rates in smokers than in nonsmokers (Coughlin, Neaton, & Sengupta, 1996; Hsing, McLaughlin, & Hrubec, 1991; Hsing, McLaughlin, & Schuman, 1990). In a prospective mortality study of 450,279 men, those who were cigarette smokers at the time of enrollment in the study had a 34% higher death rate from prostate cancer than men who never smoked during the nine years of follow-up (Rodriguez, Tatham, Thum, Calle, & Heath, 1997). The association was seen between both African American and White current cigarette smokers but not among former smokers of any type of tobacco.

Bladder cancer: Bladder cancer ranks as the fourth leading cause of cancer and seventh leading cause of cancer death in men and is the eighth leading cause of cancer and 10th leading cause of cancer death in women in the United States (Droller, 1998). Arylamines are known bladder carcinogens and are a significant component of tobacco smoke (Taylor et al., 1998). Over the years, many studies have found cigarette smoking to be a risk factor that is linked to bladder cancer (Engeland, Andersen, Haldorsen, & Tretli, 1996; Morrison, Buring, & Verhoeck, 1984; Probert, Persad, Greenwood, Gillatt, & Smith, 1998; Taylor et al., 1998). An increased risk of at least two- to fourfold of bladder cancer exists among smokers (Droller).

Transitional cell carcinoma (TCC) is the most common carcinoma of the bladder in the United States, accounting for 90% of the cases. The most common cause of TCC in the United States is tobacco smoke (Pow-Sang, Friedland, & Einstein, 1998). Significant linear trends exist in terms of dose response for cigarette consumption; no difference in risk was found between the use of filtered or unfiltered cigarettes (Probert et al., 1998). Some reports have suggested that 50% of bladder cancers in men would not occur if they did not smoke cigarettes (Clavel, Cordier, & Boccon-Gibod, 1989).

Pancreatic cancer: Although conflicting findings exist, the most consistently observed exogenous risk factor for pancreatic cancer is cigarette smoking (Tominaga & Kuroishi, 1998). This disease is approximately twice as common in heavy smokers as in nonsmokers (Engeland et al., 1996; Gold & Goldin, 1998; MacMahon, 1982; Tominaga & Kuroishi). However, Shibata, Mack, Paganini-Hill, Ross, and Henderson (1994), in a nine-year study of 13,979 residents of a retirement community, found no strong or consistent association between either smoking or alcohol consumption and risk of pancreatic cancer.

Leukemia: The overall risk of leukemia is only modestly associated with smoking in the overall population. The smoking-related risk for leukemia is estimated to account for approximately 14% of all leukemia cases in the United States (Brownson, Novotony, & Perry, 1993). However, among those age 60 and older, smoking is associated with a twofold increase in risk for acute myeloid leukemia and a threefold increase in risk for acute lymphocytic leukemia (Brownson et al.).

The mechanism by which smoking promotes leukemia is uncertain. Cigarette smoke contains benzene, which has been linked with leukemia in the past; a typical smoker inhales 10 times more benzene than a nonsmoker (Wyser & Bolliger, 1997).

Gynecologic cancers: Cigarette smoking is a known factor for increasing a woman's risk for cervical cancer (Sasson, Halley, & Hoffman, 1985). An association has been found consistently between uterine cervical cancer and smoking (Engeland, Bjorge, Haldorsen, & Tretli, 1997). Sasagawa et al. (1997), in a case control study of 178 women, found that smoking was the only human papillomavirus (HPV) infection-independent factor for cervical cancer, suggesting that smoking may have a direct carcinogenic effect on the cervix. Smoking also has been found to be a cofactor in the progression from infection with HPV to high-grade precursors and cancer (Chichareon et al., 1998; Daling et al., 1996).

Health Effects of Passive Smoking

Passive smoking is defined as breathing in airborne tobacco smoke and is used synonymously with the term "second-hand smoking" (Weibel, 1997). Active smokers usually are closest to the smoke coming off their cigarette, cigar, or pipe, making them the heaviest passive smokers as well (Weibel). Environmental tobacco smoke (ETS) consists of the side stream smoke emitted from smoldering tobacco between puffs and mainstream smoke that is exhaled by the smoker. Side stream smoke provides 80%–90% of ETS. Active and passive smokers inhale the same toxins and suffer from the same health effects (Weibel). Passive smoking has been linked to deleterious health effects on both children and adults. Research demonstrates a link between ETS and lung damage in children (U.S. Environmental Protection Agency [EPA], 1993), fetal toxicity and low birth weight (Saito, 1991), and sudden infant death syndrome (SIDS). Infants exposed to ETS have an increased risk of SIDS by a factor of 2.5–3.5, as compared to nonexposed infants (Klonoff-Cohen et al., 1995).

In the adult population, several studies show the risk of coronary heart disease increased by approximately 20% among nonsmokers exposed to ETS (Steenland, Thun, Lally, & Heath, 1996). Considering the toxicological evidence that the chemical composition and biological effects of mainstream and second-hand smoke are similar, ETS apparently is a human lung carcinogen (EPA, 1993). Therefore, the central issue, and current hot topic of debate, is not whether ETS increases the risk of lung cancer but by how much. Using highly sensitive biomonitoring, several investigators have shown that the mutagenicity of urine is significantly increased in nonsmokers exposed to ETS (Bartsch et al., 1990). During the last few decades, 32 epidemiological studies have focused on the lung cancer risk of non-smoking spouses of smokers, and the annual lung cancer deaths in Germany and the United States associated with passive smoking have been estimated to be 40 and 3000, respectively (Weibel, 1997). Taken together, the toxicological and epidemiological evidence give confidence to the conclusion that ETS is a human lung carcinogen.

Benefits of Smoking Cessation

Decreased Mortality

A significant reduction in mortality occurs after successful smoking cessation. Relative risk of mortality from cancer increases with the number of cigarettes smoked per day and with a decreasing number of years since cessation of smoking (Paganini-Hill & Hsu, 1994). A model that relates clinical risk factors to subsequent mortality was used to simulate the impact of smoking cessation (Russell et al., 1998). Researchers found that five years after baseline, the number of cumulative deaths and annual deaths per 1,000 people were 15% lower with smoking cessation than they would have been in its absence. Twenty years after baseline, the number of deaths was 11% less. In a 25-year follow-up on the Seven Countries Study of cigarette smoking and mortality risk, 625 subjects who had quit smoking 10 years or more before baseline had a 2% higher total death rate than that of people who never smoked (Jacobs et al., 1999). Recent quitters had a death rate equivalent to that of current smokers of five to nine cigarettes per day, 9% greater than the rate in people who never smoked. The Seven Countries Study, with data pooled from many nations, provides striking evidence about the risk of death attributed to smoking. If the participants had never smoked, 64% of men who were 40–59 years old in the early 1960s still would have been alive after 25 years (Jacobs et al.). However, if everyone had been a pack-a-day smoker, only about 47% would have been alive after 25 years. Jacobs et al. also found that after 10 or more years of smoking cessation, total risk of death is attenuated to almost the same level as that of never smokers. The researchers concluded that former smokers had a 24% reduction in risk for cardiovascular disease mortality within two years of quitting compared with continuing smokers. They also found that the excess risk for total mortality, cardiovascular disease, and total cancer mortality among former smokers approached the level of that for never smokers after 10–14 years of abstinence (Jacobs et al.). An important message to convey to the general public is that the relative risk of mortality from cancer and other diseases decreases with each pack of cigarettes not smoked.

Health Benefits

Those who achieve smoking cessation reap numerous health benefits, especially to the pulmonary and cardiovascular systems (CDC, 1991; Hermanson, Omenn, Kronmal, & Gersh, 1988; Jajich, Ostfeld, & Freeman, 1984; LaCroix, Lang, & Scherr, 1991; Salive et al., 1992). The greatest benefits from smoking cessation occur when people stop smoking before the age of 40. However, within all age groups, those who stop smoking show an increase in lung function compared with those who continue to smoke (Higgins et al., 1993). Some effects of smoking can be reversed within days or weeks of cessation, such as increased platelet activation that contributes to atherosclerosis and thrombosis, high carbon monoxide levels that inhibit oxygen availability, coronary artery spasm, and increased susceptibility to ventricular dysrhythmia (Hecht et al., 1994; USDHHS, 1990). The health benefits of smoking cessation are impressive. Carbon dioxide levels can be decreased within 24 hours. Pulmonary cilia beating begins to improve within several days, and sputum volume may decrease within several weeks of cessation (Pearce & Jones, 1984). Improvements to the immune and metabolic systems may begin six to eight weeks postcessation. Kawachi, Coditz, and Stampfer (1993, 1994) have found that clear health benefits exist from smoking cessation regardless of the age of smoking initiation or cessation and daily number of cigarettes smoked.

A major benefit of cessation may be the fewer total packs smoked/years of smoking, which translates into shorter exposure to carcinogens. Smoking cessation or less lifetime smoking exposure affects the distribution of specific histologic subtypes of lung cancer, especially for women, and cessation may postpone the age at which lung cancer occurs (Cook, Shaper, Procock, & Kussick, 1986; Tong, Spitz, Fueger, & Amos, 1996).

Decreased Medical Costs

The economic impact of smoking and tobacco use almost is beyond measure. It was estimated in the 1990s that $50 billion was being spent annually for healthcare costs associated with tobacco use (CDC, 1994a). This figure is most likely conservative because the medical costs attributable to burn care from smoking-related fires, perinatal care for low birth weight infants of mothers who smoke, and treatment of disease caused by second-hand smoke exposure were not included in this calculation. The Office of Technology Assessment used these 1994 projections to further estimate what they believed were the smoking-related costs to Americans, which they projected to be at $68 billion annually (Beheney & Hewitt, 1997). This figure does not include an estimated $21 billion in costs for providing health care to people with smoking-related illnesses, more than $7 billion in costs for lost productivity by people disabled with smoking-attributable diseases, and $40 billion in indirect costs for forfeited earnings for those dying from premature deaths related to smoking-attributable diseases (Beheney & Hewitt). The CDC (1994a) reported that smoking is responsible for approximately 7% of total U.S. healthcare costs. According to the Center for the Advancement of Health (1996), even people who quit after the age of 70 are estimated to avoid up to 50% of their direct medical costs.

Assessment

The most important thing nurses can do to decrease morbidity and mortality caused by smoking is to incorporate the assessment of tobacco use into everyday clinical practice (Sarna, 1999). Assessments are multifaceted and include smoking history, readiness to change, nicotine dependence, and motivators and barriers for quitting.

Smoking History

All patients should be asked about their current and past patterns of tobacco use and over-the-counter nicotine use, including the amount and type of product (Ziedonis, Wyatt, & George, 1998). A complete assessment includes smoking cessation history; the number, types, and lengths of prior attempts; the reasons for quitting; any changes in functioning during abstinence; and cause(s) of relapse.

Readiness to Change

The assessment of readiness to change and motivation to quit smoking is essential. Smokers who are not considering quitting need different approaches than smokers who are either ambivalent about stopping or who presently are interested in stopping (Fiore, Bailey, & Cohen, 1996). The Contemplation Ladder (Bierner & Abrams, 1991) is a tool to assess the level of motivation that is based on the Prochaska and DiClemente (1992) stages of change model (precontemplation, contemplation, preparation, action, and maintenance). The tool's reliability of measuring readiness to consider smoking cessation has been validated in adults. The scores are significantly predictive of reported intention to quit, number of quit attempts, and subsequent participation in smoking cessation programs. In the Fiore et al. (1996) study, approximately 40% of smokers were not considering stopping in the near future (precontemplation); it was speculated that they were either misinformed, demoralized about their ability to change, or defensive and resistant to change. Another 40% were ambivalent about quitting (contemplation); these smokers had given quitting serious thought but were not yet ready to abstain. Approximately 20% of smokers were intending to quit in the next few months (preparation). From a counseling and educational standpoint, each type of smoker requires a different type of treatment (Fiore et al., 1996).

Nicotine Dependence

Quantifying a smoker's degree of nicotine dependence is essential because highly nicotine-dependent smokers require more intensive treatment. Within a few years of daily smoking, most smokers begin to develop dependence (USDHHS, 1994). Nicotine dependence is associated with heavy consumption, tolerance, and unpleasant withdrawal symptoms. These signs of addiction are the basis for two approaches in the treatment of nicotine dependence: assess the appropriateness of nicotine replacement therapy to overcome the physical symptoms of addiction, and identify emotional distress and impairment in social and occupational functioning caused by nicotine dependence as a psychiatric disorder using the criteria in the *Diagnostic and Statistical Manual of the American Psychiatric Association* (APA) (DSM-IV) (APA, 1994).

Models for Assessing and Treating Nicotine Dependence
Nicotine Replacement

This approach was developed based on the need to identify smokers who would benefit from nicotine replacement. The most widely used instruments for this purpose are the Fagerstrom Tolerance Questionnaire and the Fagerstrom Test for Nicotine Dependence (Pomerleau, Carton, Lutzke, Flessland, & Pomerleau, 1994). Dependence is characterized as a continuous variable, and a score of five or higher is indicative of nicotine dependence, suggesting the need for higher intensity psychosocial treatment and higher dose nicotine replacement (Ziedonis et al., 1998) (see Table 9-1).

Psychiatric Disorder

Another assessment and treatment approach, using the DSM-IV, conceptualizes nicotine dependence as a psychiatric disorder, taking into account lifetime smoking to determine number or severity of symptoms (Pomerleau, 1997). Smokers are classified as nondependent, mildly dependent, or highly dependent (see criteria listing in Figure 9-2).

Nicotine dependence and withdrawal can develop with all forms of tobacco use (e.g., cigarettes, chewing tobacco, snuff, pipes, cigars) and can be maintained with nicotine replacement (e.g., nicotine gum, patch, nasal spray) (Fiore et al., 1996). The essential feature of nicotine dependence is a cluster of cognitive, behavioral,

Table 9-1. Items and Scoring for Fagerstrom Test for Nicotine Dependence

Questions	Answers	Points
How soon after you wake up do you smoke your first cigarette?	Within 5 minutes	3
	6–30 minutes	2
	31–60 minutes	1
	After 60 minutes	0
Do you find it difficult to refrain from smoking in places where it is forbidden, such as in church, at the library, or in the cinema?	Yes	1
	No	0
Which cigarette would you hate most to give up?	The first one in the morning	1
	All others	0
How many cigarettes per day do you smoke?	10 or fewer	0
	11–20	1
	21–30	2
	31 or more	3
Do you smoke more frequently during the first hours of waking than during the rest of the day?	Yes	1
	No	0
Do you smoke even if you are so ill that you are in bed most of the day?	Yes	1
	No	0

Scores range from 0 (no dependence) to 10 (high dependence). A score of 8 or more is considered to be an indication of high dependence and 4–7 moderate dependence.

Note. Based on information from Fagerstrom et al., 1996.

and physiological symptoms indicating that the individual continues the use of nicotine despite significant nicotine-related problems.

Motivators For and Barriers to Quitting

Assessment of motivators and barriers is helpful in motivating patients. Identifying what the individual perceives as the roadblocks to success can lead to confronting those issues and dealing with them. Once the barriers have been moved, the individual can focus more on the benefits to be gained. The most common reasons individuals give for trying to stop smoking are to improve health and in response to social pressure. The most common barriers are weight gain, fear of withdrawal, and fear of failure (Orleans, 1993). Along with teaching about the health risks of smoking, nurses can tap into the patient's unique set of barriers and motivators to affect behavioral change.

Nicotine Withdrawal

Approximately 50% of adults who attempt to stop smoking will meet DSM-IV criteria for nicotine withdrawal (Glassman, 1993) (see Figure 9-2). Traditional theories of smoking relapse emphasize the significance of physiological dependence in the maintenance of smoking behavior and general failure of treatment interventions (Benowitz, 1992). The need to decrease or eliminate withdrawal symptoms is only one of the complex factors that serve to maintain smoking behavior, and it remains unknown if nicotine withdrawal is the primary reason why individuals persist in their smoking behavior (Shiffman, 1982). Patten and Martin (1996) reviewed 16 prospective studies to examine the relationship of nicotine withdrawal to unsuccessful smoking cessation and relapse and concluded that the research to date does not appear to strongly implicate nicotine withdrawal in adversely affecting smoking cessation or maintenance of abstinence.

Figure 9-2. DSM-IV Diagnostic Criteria for Nicotine Withdrawal

A. Daily use of nicotine for at least several weeks
B. Abrupt cessation of nicotine use or reduction in the amount of nicotine used followed within 24 hours by four (or more) of the following signs
1. Dysphoric or depressed mood
2. Insomnia
3. Irritability, frustration, or anger
4. Anxiety
5. Difficulty concentrating
6. Restlessness
7. Decreased heart rate
8. Increased appetite or weight gain
C. The symptoms in criterion B cause clinically significant distress or impairment in social, occupational, or other important areas of functioning.
D. The symptoms are not caused by a general medical condition and are not better accounted for by another mental disorder.

Note. From *Diagnostic and Statistical Manual of Mental Disorders* (4th ed.) (pp. 244–245), from American Psychiatric Association, 1994, Washington, DC: Author. Copyright 1994 by the American Psychiatric Association. Reprinted with permission.

Although the role of nicotine withdrawal in smoking cessation is debatable, negative affect states (e.g., frustration, anger, depression) are cited as precipitants of relapse by a majority of ex-smokers (Patten & Martin, 1996; Shiffman, 1982). However, research has yielded inconclusive results. In some studies, depressed mood is reported to be predictive of unsuccessful smoking cessation and relapse (Covey, Glassman, & Stetner, 1990; Glassman, 1993). However, other research has failed to demonstrate that a relationship between depressed mood with smoking withdrawal and increases in depressed mood during smoking abstinence is not reliably associated with smoking relapse (Gritz, Carr, & Marcus, 1991; Hughes, Gust, Skoog, Keenan, & Fenwick, 1991; Norregaard, Tonnesen, & Petersen, 1993).

Demographics, Psychosocial Factors, and Comorbid Conditions

Smoking is becoming the habit of the less affluent and less educated (Pomerleau, 1997). Adults with 9–11 years of education had higher smoking prevalence (35.4%) than adults with 16 or more years of education (11.6%) (Fiore et al., 1996). Rates are higher among adults living below the poverty level (33.3%) than those living at or above the poverty level (24.6%). Social support is a major predictor of smoking cessation. The smoking status (e.g., never smoked, ex-smoker, current smoker) of others in the household and close friends should be assessed (Fiore et al., 1996) because of the importance of environmental cues and the health impact of second-hand smoke.

Several comorbid conditions are associated with smoking, including substance abuse, affective disorders, and eating disorders. Among these comorbid conditions, a history of depression has the strongest association. This linkage persists even after other comorbid conditions such as alcoholism and anxiety disorders are factored out (Glassman, 1993). Glassman found that 60% of patients volunteering for a clinic smoking-cessation trial had a history of major depression (though they were not depressed at the time); these patients failed at more than twice the rate of those without a history of depression.

Intervention

Public Health Service-Sponsored Clinical Practice Guidelines

In 1996, the Agency for Health Care Policy and Research (AHCPR) produced the first set of guidelines for smoking cessation (Fiore et al., 1996). *Treating Tobacco Use and Dependence*, a Public Health Service-sponsored Clinical Practice Guideline, was published in June 2000 (Fiore et al., 2000). This guideline is the result of a partnership among federal government and nonprofit organizations—the Agency for Healthcare Research and Quality (AHRQ, previously AHCPR), CDC, NCI, and others. It was designed to assist clinicians, tobacco-dependence treatment specialists, and healthcare administrators and insurers in providing effective treatments for tobacco use and dependence. The recommendations are based on a meta-analysis of the existing scientific literature. The major conclusions of this clinical practice guideline are as follows: (a) tobacco dependence is a chronic condition that requires repeated intervention until long-term permanent abstinence is achieved; (b) effective tobacco dependence treatments are available, and every patient who uses tobacco should be offered those treatments; (c) clinicians and all healthcare delivery systems need to institutionalize a consistent method to identify, document, and treat every tobacco user; (d) three types of counseling have been found to be effective (e.g., practical counseling, social support as part of treatment, social support arranged outside of treatment); (e) five first-line pharmacotherapies have been proven to be effective and should be prescribed in the absence of contraindications (e.g., sustained release bupropion hydrochloride, nicotine gum, nicotine inhaler, nicotine nasal spray, nicotine patch); and (f) tobacco dependence treatments are cost effective relative to other medical and disease prevention interventions and should be a reimbursed benefit in all health insurance plans (Fiore et al., 2000).

National Cancer Institute's "4A's" Becomes the "5A's"

The most widely used initial intervention and the one recommended by AHCPR was NCI's 4A's. The recently published Public Health Service's (PHS's) Clinical Practice Guidelines (Fiore et al., 2000) proposes a 5A's program consisting of five steps. These strategies are designed to be brief, requiring three minutes or less of direct clinician time.

1. **Ask**—Systematically identify all tobacco users at every visit. Implement an office-wide system that ensures that at every clinic visit, tobacco-use status is queried and documented for every patient.
2. **Advise**—Strongly urge all tobacco users to quit. In a clear and personalized manner, convey the health risks of tobacco use and the benefits of curbing or stopping the habit.
3. **Assess**—Determine users' willingness to make a quit attempt. Ask every tobacco user if he or she is willing to make a timely (i.e., within the next 30 days) attempt to quit.
4. **Assist**—Aid the patient in quitting. Help the patient develop a plan. Elicit a commitment to quit with a specific quit date. Provide practical counseling (problem solving/skills training). Stress the importance of social support and refer to a smoking cessation support group. Provide supplementary materials like books, pamphlets, videos, or Web sites.
5. **Arrange**—Schedule follow-up contact. Follow-up contact can be in person or by phone and should occur soon after the quit date, preferably during the first week. A second follow-up contact is recommended within the first month.

Interventions for Smokers Unwilling to Quit

As clinicians follow PHS's "5 A's" guidelines during routine office visits, relevant patient information will be gathered. A brief intervention designed to promote the motivation to quit should be used for smokers who are not yet ready to make a quit attempt (Fiore et al., 2000).

Patients currently not motivated to quit may lack information about the harmful effects of tobacco, lack the financial resources needed for intervention, have fears or concerns about quitting, or be demoralized because of previous relapse.

PHS's guidelines recommend a motivational intervention called the "5 R's": relevance, risks, rewards, roadblocks, and repetition (Fiore et al., 2000) (see Figure 9-3). Motivational interventions are most likely to be successful when the clinician is empathic, promotes patient autonomy (i.e., choice among options), avoids arguments, and supports the patient's self-efficacy by identifying previous successes in behavior change efforts (Fiore et al., 2000).

Figure 9-3. Enhancing Motivation to Quit Tobacco Use: The "5 R's" for the Patient Unwilling to Quit

Relevance
Encourage the patient to indicate why quitting is personally relevant (e.g., disease status or risk, health concerns, family or social situation).

Risks
Ask the patient to identify potential negative consequences of tobacco.

Examples of risks
Acute risks: shortness of breath, exacerbation of asthma, harm to pregnancy, impotence, infertility, increased carbon monoxide levels
Long-term risks: myocardial infarction and stroke, lung and other cancers (larynx, oral cavity, pharynx, esophagus, bladder, cervix), chronic obstructive pulmonary disease, long-term disability and need for extended care
Environmental risks: increased risk of lung cancer and heart disease in spouse; higher rates of smoking by children of tobacco users; increased risk for low birth weight, sudden infant death syndrome, asthma, middle-ear disease, and respiratory infections in children of smokers.

Rewards
Ask the patient to identify potential benefits of stopping tobacco use and suggest and highlight those that are most relevant to the patient.

Examples of rewards
Improved health, food will taste better; improved sense of smell; save money; feel better about yourself; home, car, clothing, and breath will smell better; stop worrying about quitting; set a good example for children; have healthier babies; stop worrying about exposing others to smoke; feel better physically; perform better in physical activities; reduced wrinkling/aging of skin

Roadblocks
Ask the patient to identify barriers or impediments to quitting and note elements of treatment (problem solving, pharmacotherapy) that could address barriers.

Examples of barriers
Withdrawal symptoms, fear of failure, weight gain, lack of support, depression, enjoyment of tobacco

Repetition
The motivational intervention should be repeated every time an unmotivated patient visits the clinical setting. Tobacco users who have failed in previous quit attempts should be told that most people make repeated quit attempts before they are successful.

Note. From *Treating Tobacco Use and Dependence: A Clinical Practice Guideline,* by M.C. Flore, W.C. Bailey, S.J. Cohen, et al., 2000, Rockville, MD: U.S. Department of Health and Human Services, Public Health Service.

Interventions for Smokers Willing to Quit

The science of treating nicotine addiction is rapidly changing. In the past few years, guidelines for treating smokers have been revised, numerous over-the-counter and prescription medications have been approved, and more drugs currently are being tested (Hughes, Goldstein, Hurt, & Shiffman, 1999). Today's remaining smokers are the more heavily dependent and require more intensive treatment (Fagerstrom, Kunze, & Schoberberger, 1996). As with chronic diseases, the most effective treatment of tobacco dependence requires the use of multiple modalities. Although great interest exists for the new pharmacotherapy options, treatment of smokers with severe nicotine dependence and comorbidity requires psychosocial treatments in addition to pharmacotherapy. Combining pharmacotherapies and psychosocial interventions leads to improved outcomes (Sarna, 1999; Ziedonis et al., 1998).

Psychosocial Interventions

APA guidelines (1996) provide an excellent overview of specific psychosocial treatments for smoking cessation (see Table 9-2). All smoking cessation psychosocial treatments are similar in using motivational interviewing or motivational enhancement therapy approaches and relapse prevention (i.e., identifying cues or triggers to tobacco use and developing coping techniques to manage those cues and triggers) (Ziedonis et al., 1998). Social support and skill training for problem solving are essential components of cessation (Fiore et al., 1996; Sarna, 1999).

Matching, stepped care, and tailored approaches to interventions are gaining attention, but more research is needed to ascertain whether these approaches are efficacious (Lichtenstein, 1997; Orleans et al., 1998; Prochaska, DiClemente, Velicer, & Rossi, 1993). Matching interventions are when the smokers' stage of readiness to quit is assessed and cessation materials are "matched" to their motivation to quit. Stepped care approaches are similar to matching interventions in that the intensity of the intervention is matched to the level of the smoker's addiction. In this model, interventions are provided on a continuum of care, beginning with self-help materials, progressing through brief counseling in medical settings, and moving into group interventions and nicotine replacement therapies. Finally, tailored interventions are those that are directed toward a particular group of smokers. The interventions within this approach are directed toward unique benefits and barriers that this group may experience. Moreover, cessation strategies are tailored to the special needs of the group. Specific suggestions for tailoring cessation interventions for older adults, women, racial and ethnic minority groups, adults with cancer, and children and adolescents are provided later in this chapter.

Pharmacotherapies

The pharmacological approaches to smoking cessation that the U.S. Food and Drug Administration (FDA) approved and the PHS guideline panel (Fiore et al., 2000) identified as first-line medications include nicotine replacement therapies (i.e., patch, gum, spray, and inhaler) and bupropion sustained release.

Table 9-2. Specific Psychosocial Treatments

Treatments	Goals	Efficacy	Techniques	Implementation
Behavioral therapies— Based on the theory that learning processes operate in the development, maintenance, and cessation of smoking.	To change the antecedents to smoking, to reinforce non-smoking, and to teach skills to avoid smoking in high-risk situations	Six-month quit rates are 20%–25% Increases quit rates twofold over control groups	Skills training/relapse prevention Stimulus control Aversive therapy Social support Contingency management Cue exposure Nicotine fading Relaxation Physiological feedback	Individual or group Patient preference of group or individual is important.
Self-help materials	To increase motivation and cessation skills	More effective patients who are less nicotine dependent and more motivated	Tailor materials to the specific needs and concerns of each patient.	Written materials plus phone or personal contact Use as part of a behavioral package
Educational and supportive groups	To teach patients the harms of smoking and the benefits of cessation	Efficacy without behavioral technique is debatable.	Social support is very important for some patients.	Group
Hypnosis	To implant nonconscious suggestions that will deter smoking	Mixed reports	Hypnosis	Individual

Note. Based on information from American Psychological Association, 1996.

Nicotine Replacement Therapy

Nicotine replacement therapy (NRT) is based on the principle that nicotine is the dependence-producing constituent of cigarette smoking and that smoking cessation can be achieved by replacing nicotine without the toxins in cigarette smoke (Ziedonis et al., 1998). The goal is to relieve the symptoms of withdrawal, allowing the patient to focus on personal conditioning factors that will help to break the habit. After the acute phase of NRT, the dosage gradually is reduced. Available products that aid in smoking cessation include slow-acting (nicotine patch), intermediate-acting (nicotine gum and inhaler), and fast-acting (spray) delivery systems. However, all of these methods are much less efficient than cigarettes in delivering nicotine. Because the nicotine patch and gum now are available over the counter, these are the first-line medication choice of many smokers who are attempting to quit on their own. Given that NRT has been deemed safe and effective and that major side effects are very rare, all smokers, except those who are pregnant, should be encouraged to use it. Although NRT has been proposed for use in pregnant women who are heavy smokers, formal clinical trials are needed to determine safety and efficacy (Benowitz, 1991; Kendrick & Merritt, 1996).

The nicotine transdermal patch provides ready absorption of nicotine through the skin but does not allow for self-titrated dosing for withdrawal symptoms. The patch is convenient and produces less fluctuation in plasma nicotine levels. The available brands begin at 15, 21, and 22 mg doses, and lower doses of 7 and 14 mg are used for tapering the patch after eight weeks of abstinence. A substantial number of well-designed placebo-controlled clinical trials of the nicotine patch have been conducted, with excellent short-term (six week) abstinence rates (40% versus 20% for placebo) but more modest long-term (one year) rates (19% versus 10%) (Balfour & Fagerstrom, 1996; Ziedonis et al., 1998).

Nicotine polacrilex gum is available in doses of 2 mg and 4 mg. Recommended dosing is in the range of 9–16 pieces per day, and heavy smokers (> 20 cigarettes a day) require the 4 mg dose. The gum is effective in reducing cravings but is less effective in reducing nicotine withdrawal symptoms. Three recent control trials indicate using nicotine gum (2 mg) in addition to a nicotine patch, over either therapy used alone, to increase quit rates without significantly increasing side effects (APA, 1996).

Nicotine nasal spray is the most recent NRT modality to be approved by the FDA. The spray is a prescription drug, and smokers are advised to use it as needed to control symptoms. A single dose of the spray delivers 0.5 mg to each nostril, and it can be used one to three times an hour. The suggested effective daily dose is 15–20 sprays (Balfour & Fagerstrom, 1996). Onset of action of the spray is the most rapid of all NRTs; the drug is absorbed through the nasal mucosa into the arterial circulation and reaches the brain within 10 seconds (Balfour & Fagerstrom). The placebo-controlled studies to date support the efficacy of spray in long-term treatment of smoking cessation; quit rates with the spray are double those with placebo spray (Jones, Nguyen, & Man, 1998; Schneider, 1995).

A nicotine vapor inhaler mimics the upper airway stimulation derived by smokers; however, absorption is mostly buccal and not respiratory (APA, 1996). The amount of nicotine delivered is only 0.013 mg, significantly less than the spray, and produces lower plasma nicotine levels than other NRTs (Ziedonis et al., 1998).

Bupropion

Bupropion is the first FDA approved non-nicotine replacement therapy for treating nicotine dependence. This is a heterocyclic, atypical antidepressant that blocks the reuptake of both dopamine and norepinephrine. Clinical trials have demonstrated bupropion's efficacy in both depressed and nondepressed populations. In a study of 615 smokers, bupropion significantly enhanced smoking cessation rates after seven weeks of treatment (Hurt, 1997). The effects were dose dependent, and bupropion was most effective at 300 mg per day, with an abstinence rate of 44.2% (Hurt). Hayford, Patten, Rummans, Schroeder, and Offord (1999) found a significant dose-response effect of bupropion for smoking cessation that was independent of a history of major depression or alcoholism. Further, it has been found that abstinence rates are improved further with a combination treatment of bupropion and nicotine patch (Ziedonis et al., 1998).

Non-U.S. Food and Drug Administration-Approved Medications

Several medications currently are undergoing clinical trials. Clonidine is an antihypertensive and sympatholytic agent that has been used extensively in the management of opiate and alcohol withdrawal. Some studies suggest it is effective in reducing nicotine withdrawal and craving (Gourlay, 1994). Buspirone is a nonsedating, nonbenzodiazepine, anxiolytic agent indicated for the treatment of generalized anxiety. Limited evidence shows that buspirone can reduce nicotine withdrawal and craving (Cinciripini, 1995).

Other than bupropion, the most promising antidepressants for smoking cessation are nortriptyline (Hall, Reus, Munoz, Lees, & Humfleet, 1998) and doxepine (Edwards, Murphy, Downs, Ackerman, & Rosenthal, 1989). Moclobemide is a reversible inhibitor of monoamine oxidase that has been approved in Canada and Europe for treatment of major depression and has been effective in smoking cessation in highly dependent smokers (Ziedonis et al., 1998). The PHS guideline panel (Fiore et al., 2000) listed clonidine and nortriptyline as second-line medications.

Relapse Prevention

Relapse prevention efforts are necessary because of the chronic relapsing nature of tobacco dependence. When clinicians encounter a patient who has quit tobacco use recently, they should reinforce the decision to quit, review the benefits of cessation, and assist in resolving any residual problems arising from quitting (Fiore et al., 2000). Although most relapse occurs within weeks of the quitting process, some relapse occurs months or even years after the initial quit date (Fiore et al.).

Relapse prevention interventions can be delivered by means of scheduled clinic visits, telephone calls, or any time a clinician encounters an ex-tobacco user. Relapse prevention interventions can be divided into two categories: minimal practice for all quitters and prescriptive interventions for patients with problems maintaining abstinence.

Minimal practice interventions should be part of every encounter with a patient who recently has quit. Every ex-tobacco user should receive congratulations on any success and strong encouragement to remain abstinent.

Prescriptive relapse prevention components are based individually on information obtained about problems the patient has encountered in maintaining abstinence. These interventions need to be delivered during dedicated follow-up contact (in person or by telephone) or through a specialized clinic or program.

Tobacco Use and Cessation Interventions in Special Populations

Older Adults

Nationally, approximately 13% of people age 65 and older are smokers, and approximately 26% of people age 50–64 are smokers (an estimated 9 million people total) (Husten et al., 1997). Today's generation of older people (those who are now age 50 and older) in the United States had smoking rates among the highest of any U.S. generation. In the mid-1960s, approximately 54% of adult males smoked and another 21% were former smokers; more than 34% of adult females were smokers and another 8% were former smokers (Husten et al.). Today's epidemic of smoking-related deaths is the result of these high smoking rates.

Adverse Consequences for Older Adults Associated With Smoking

According to the Center for Social Gerontology (1999a), one in three smokers in the United States dies prematurely, losing an average of 12–15 years of life and eliminating their retirement years. Worldwide trends in mortality attributable to smoking tobacco are mostly increasing in women and almost universally in old age (Peto et al., 1996).

Regardless of the advances in cancer prevention and treatment during the last two decades for younger and middle-aged adults, cancer mortality has not improved for the aged (Hoel, Davis, & Miller, 1992). The number of cancer deaths in the United States peaks between the ages of 65 and 75 and then decreases because of competing risks for mortality in the declining population that is at risk. Cancer incidence and mortality rates continue to increase throughout life (Kennedy, 1998). Most of the increase in cancer mortality rates in people age 65 and older has been because of tobacco-related cancers. These cancers include lung and oral cancer and, to a lesser degree, genitourinary cancer and hematologic malignancies (Kennedy). In fact, lung cancer is the leading cause of death from cancer in both men and women older than 75 (Kennedy). Oral and oropharyngeal squamous carcinoma is predominantly a disease of men age 50–70 and women age 60–80; smoking is the largest single most irrefutable causative factor for head and neck cancer (Endicott, 1998; Mashberg & Samit, 1995). The incidence of transitional cell carcinoma (TCC), the most common carcinoma of the bladder, increases with age; more than 50% of all cases of TCC occur in people older than 65 (Pow-Sang et al., 1998).

Aging is associated with molecular changes (e.g., DNA hypomethylation), which are seen in early carcinogenesis. These changes prime the tissue to the effects of late-stage carcinogens. In several animal studies, older tissues were found to be more prone than younger tissues to develop cancer after exposure to late-stage carcinogens (Balducci & Barry, 1994). Older people are more likely to develop lung cancer after exposure to an environmental carcinogen (Barbone, Bovenzi, & Cavalleri, 1995). This suggests that older individuals would benefit from a smoke-free environment in which environmental carcinogens are decreased. Therefore, smoking cessation, in the global sense, is a critical element of cancer prevention for older adults.

Benefits of Smoking Cessation

An enhanced focus on smoking behaviors and smoking cessation is evident during the past few decades; however, older smokers have been excluded. Even though nonsmoking status can provide older smokers with a chance for increased quality as well as quantity of life, they are asked less often to quit, given fewer resources, and provided less guidance than their younger counterparts. A limited effort is being made toward developing and delivering effective smoking cessation interventions for older adults. The explanation for the absence of an empirical and clinical focus on smoking cessation for the older adult is, in part, because of healthcare providers' beliefs in myths rather than reality (Cataldo, in press). A majority of the current care practices for older smokers are based on inaccurate information about the health consequences of smoking behaviors and the benefits of smoking cessation. In reality, older adults benefit from smoking cessation; it is never too late to quit smoking.

Smoking cessation, even in the frail elderly, produces objective benefits in terms of decreased mortality, health benefits, increased quality of life, and decreased cost of care. Regardless of age, those who stop smoking show an increase in lung function compared with those who continue to smoke (Higgins et al., 1993). Kawachi et al. (1993, 1994) found that clear health benefits exist from smoking cessation despite the age of smoking initiation, the age of smoking cessation, and daily number of cigarettes smoked.

The major benefit of cessation may be because of fewer total packs smoked/years of smoking (Cook et al., 1986; Tong et al., 1996), which translates into shorter exposure to carcinogens. Smoking cessation for older adults means less exposure to carcinogens during the period of life when one has less resistance to carcinogens, an alteration of antitumor defenses, and defects in tumor suppressor genes (Kennedy, 1998). Smoking cessation or less lifetime smoking exposure affects the distribution of specific histologic subtypes of lung cancer, especially for women, and cessation may postpone the age at which lung cancer occurs.

Barriers to Smoking Cessation for Older Adults

In public surveys, 85%–90% of older smokers verbalize an interest in smoking cessation; most either do not attempt to quit or they try to stop on their own and do not succeed (Grabowski & Hall, 1985; Rustin, 1991). However, when older adults do participate in smoking cessation programs, they are successful. Increased age consistently has proven to be positively related to successful smoking cessation (Davis et al., 1994; Stapleton et al., 1995). In general, barriers to the older person using cancer prevention services regularly or at all are numerous, including personal characteristics, demographic barriers, healthcare provider-patient communication, knowledge gaps, attitudinal barriers, and community barriers (Boyd, 1996; Fox, Roetzheim, & Kington, 1998). Older smokers tend to be less educated, are from a lower socioeconomic status, are heavy smokers (more than 20 cigarettes a day), and are more heavily addicted to nicotine (Fiore et al., 1990; Rimer, Orleans, & Slade, 1993). They are less likely to believe in the health consequences of smoking and that impaired functioning, such as shortness of breath, is related to smoking (Boyd; USDHHS, 1990). Older smokers are more likely to use smoking as a coping strategy for stress and weight control (Rimer, Orleans, & Keintz, 1990). One demographic barrier is insufficient income to purchase services. Nicotine replacement systems have been approved for over-the-counter sales and are no longer covered by third-party reimbursement. Medicare does not cover bupropion, an effective smoking cessation treatment. Older smokers have more frequent contact with their healthcare providers, making an average of 6.3 visits each year (Boyd). However, numerous studies have shown that physicians' recommendations for smoking cessation for older people have been significantly less than for younger patients (Balducci & Lyman, 1997; CDC, 1991; Cox, 1993; Ockene et al., 1987a; Senore et al., 1999; Thorndike, Rigotti, Stafford, & Singer, 1998). Only about 50% of older smokers reported that their doctor had asked about their smoking habits (USDHHS, 1990). In 1999, Senore et al. studied smokers' characteristics that influence their likelihood of being offered smoking cessation advice in the context of routine clinical activity and found that the likelihood of being recruited into a smoking cessation program was less for smokers older than 29. The chance of being considered also was reduced for smokers who had been smoking for more than 10 years.

When both patients and providers let the myths stand in the way of the realities, poor healthcare decisions are made. Several myths that interfere with the promotion of smoking cessation for older adults include (a) smoking may provide a protective factor in cognitive decline; (b) the damage that is done by a lifetime of smoking is no longer reversible after the age of 40; (c) smoking cessation decreases the quality of life; and (d) increased age results in decreased ability to successfully quit smoking (Cataldo, in press). Knowledge deficits are major factors that interfere with the assessment and treatment of smokers, such as how to efficiently identify smokers, which interventions are effective, how to implement the interventions, and relative efficacies of different smoking cessation strategies (Fiore et al., 1996).

A significant community barrier is the lack of smoking cessation programs available for older adults. Community-based interventions to promote smoking cessation in older adults should be developed, with attention to the specific needs of this population.

An important barrier to cancer prevention efforts in the older adult population is the belief, discussed previously, that by old age, carcinogenic exposures already have been accrued and that the benefits of adopting risk-reducing behaviors do not outweigh the difficulties involved in changing lifelong habits. It bears repeating that it is never too late to adopt a healthier lifestyle. Primary prevention of cancer in old age begins in youth and continues throughout life (Blesch, 1998). Smoking cessation is a critical aspect of cancer prevention in older adults. Although adoption of risk-reducing behaviors early in life has the most powerful impact on cancer prevention, the adoption of these behaviors by older adults still is beneficial (Blesch). Nurses play an important role in disseminating these facts and encouraging smoking cessation in older adults.

Women

An estimated 22 million women older than age 18 currently smoke tobacco, and quit rates have decreased more slowly in women than men (Wingo et al., 1999). Prevalence of smoking decreases as education rises and is highest among women of reproductive ages (18–44) and those who are poor, unemployed, and lack social support (CDC, 1994b). Smoking is a critical issue for women. More than 150,000 women die each year from smoking-related diseases (Husten, 1998). Heart disease, pulmonary disease, and lung cancer are among the most common causes of smoking-related mortality (Husten). Since 1987, lung cancer has killed more women each year than breast cancer.

Moreover, cigarette smoking affects the reproductive system, has adverse effects during pregnancy, and has deleterious effects on infants and children. Studies consistently have shown that women smokers experience menopause one to two years earlier than women who do not smoke (USDHHS, 1990). Maternal smoking is associated with miscarriage, premature delivery, and increased risk of having a low-weight baby (USDHHS, 1990). An estimated 17%–26% of low-weight births could be prevented by not smoking during pregnancy. Unfortunately, 70% of women who stop smoking during pregnancy resume smoking within one year after delivery. This places their children at risk for SIDS, increased respiratory infections, and middle ear disease (USDHHS, 1990).

Although the prevalence of smoking has decreased over time, it remains unacceptably high. Clearly, a need exists to increase public awareness of the negative effect of cigarette smoking on women's health. Healthcare providers should be aware of specific smoking cessation and relapse issues related to gender so that successful intervention programs can be developed and tested.

Gender-Related Factors Affecting Smoking Cessation and Relapse

Most women want to quit smoking; however, only 2.5% successfully quit each year (Royce, Corbett, Sorensen & Ockene, 1997). Several studies identified that women have a more difficult time quitting smoking as compared to their male counterparts (Ockene et al., 1987b; Osler, Prescott, Godtfredsen, Hein, & Schnohr, 1999; Royce et al., 1997). Differences in patterns of tobacco use, stress responses and coping strategies, and concerns about weight gain may account for the disparity in smoking cessation and relapse rates.

Men and women differ in their patterns of tobacco use. Women tend to be light to moderate smokers (less than 24 cigarettes per day), smoke filtered cigarettes that are lower in tar (less than 15 mg), and rarely use other forms of tobacco (Solomon & Flynn, 1993). Although these patterns suggest that women smokers are less dependent on cigarettes than men, Royce et al. (1997) reported that women were more likely to smoke their first cigarette within 10 minutes of awakening. This is an indicator of increased physiologic addiction to nicotine. In an attempt to explain these differences, Solomon and Flynn suggested that women may require a lower level of nicotine to achieve dependency because of their lower body weight.

Several studies have identified that women smoke to reduce emotional discomfort and stress (Gritz et al., 1998; Pomerleau, Adkins, & Pertschuk, 1978; Sorensen & Pechacek, 1987). Borland (1990) examined gender differences in smoking cessation relapse and found that women were more likely to slip up during negative emotional situations, whereas men lapsed under pressure from external sources, such as work. Competing family, social, and work roles may compound difficulties with smoking cessation, because evidence suggests that women are using cigarettes to cope with stress (Ockene, 1993). Poor, less educated women are at highest risk for smoking because of the stresses associated with their lives (Osler et al., 1999; Stewart et al., 1996). Stewart et al. interviewed 386 disadvantaged women about their smoking behaviors and the barriers and supports to smoking cessation. In this study, disadvantaged women were defined as those who had one of the following characteristics: poor, unemployed, low occupational status, low level of education, single parent status, and geographic isolation or lack of social support. Results of this study revealed that smoking was used to cope with poverty, isolation, and care giving. Traditional smoking cessation programs were identified to be of little value. Community-based programs that had social support as an integral part of the program were identified as desirable.

Another barrier to smoking cessation among women is fear of weight gain. Pirie, Murray, and Luepker (1991) found that women were more likely than men (57.9% versus 26.3%) to report concerns related to postcessation weight gain. Most people who quit smoking have some weight gain, but women are more likely to experience this. The average weight gain, however, is only five pounds (USDHHS, 1990; Pirie et al.). Postcessation weight gain is related to increases in food intake and a decrease in metabolic rate. Although dietary advice and exercise should be helpful adjuncts to prevent postcessation weight gain, studies conducted to date have not confirmed any benefit (Hall, 1990; Mermelstein, 1987). Similarly, although early studies examining the effect of nicotine replacement on postcessation weight gain were promising, more recent studies have suggested that nicotine replacement delays rather than prevents postcessation weight gain (Emont & Cummings, 1987; Gross, Stitzer, & Maldonado, 1989). Therefore, the best advice is to inform women about this issue and suggest that they avoid snacking on foods high in fat and sugar. The average postcessation weight gain poses minimal health risks, but the health benefits associated with quitting smoking are enormous.

Implications for Interventions

Women experience unique issues related to smoking cessation and relapse. Stress reduction and weight control were identified as issues of particular concern for women and should be addressed within the context of interventions (Ockene, 1993). Evidence suggests that women benefit from interventions that use social support in the form of individual or group assistance. Coppotelli and Orleans (1985) found that a postcessation measure of partner facilitation was a primary predictor of abstinence for women six to eight weeks after they quit smoking. Moreover, women who remained abstinent for eight weeks were more likely to have partners who were ex-smokers or partners who successfully quit smoking with them as compared to those who were nonabstinent. Group intervention methods also are useful for women (Pohl & Caplan, 1998). In particular, same gender groups (all women) appear to be more effective for women as compared to mixed gender groups (Delarue, 1973).

Because women use healthcare benefits frequently, healthcare providers can play an important role in motivating change in smoking behavior (Ockene, 1993). Although improvements have been made in physicians providing advice about smoking cessation, 50% of all patients still report that their smoking never has been addressed (Frank, Winkleby, Altman, Rockhill, & Fortmann, 1991). Each healthcare encounter provides an opportunity to identify women who smoke and provide them with information about the benefits of quitting. Future research should address whether gender-specific interventions improve cessation and maintenance rates.

Racial and Ethnic Minority Groups

Race and ethnicity are important factors that influence individuals' perceptions of their health and illness states and also their smoking behaviors. To date, cultural factors have not received the same attention in health care as biopsychosocial factors (Germain, 1992). Because smoking is a complex behavior, providing culturally relevant interventions has been recommended as a potentially promising strategy in the development and implementation of smoking cessation programs. Special challenges exist for researchers and clinicians to develop culturally relevant programs because of the diversity that exists within cultural groups.

The prevalence of smoking varies not only by gender but by race and ethnicity (Wingo et al., 1999). Understanding the overall patterns of smoking behavior are important so that high-risk groups can be targeted for smoking cessation interventions. Smoking prevalence declined among African Americans, Hispanics, Whites, and Asian and Pacific Islanders from 1978–1995, whereas smoking prevalence remained unchanged among American Indians and Alaska Natives. Because Asian and Pacific Islanders have the lowest rates of smoking prevalence (16.6%), this group will not be highlighted (Wingo et al.).

Within each cultural group, a wide range of diversity exists regarding smoking behaviors. For example, King, Poledenak, and Bendel (1999) noted that gender and region are significant factors in understanding smoking behavior in African Americans. They examined a large national sample of African Americans and found that residents in the West had the lowest unadjusted smoking prevalence and those in the Midwest the highest. Further analyses revealed that African American women in the South were less likely to smoke as compared with any other region or men. The number of people who smoke was higher among African Americans living in urban areas, even after adjusting for several sociodemographic covariates. Several other authors have noted differences in smoking prevalence among certain segments of African Americans (King, Bendel, & Delaronde, 1998; Resnicow et al., 1996; Taylor, Kerner, Gold, & Mandelblatt, 1997). Using data from the National Health Interview Survey for 1990–1993, King et al. (1998) assessed the effects of sociodemographic variables on smoking behavior among African Americans. Results from this study identified that middle-aged, African American men were more likely to smoke than women. In another study, smoking rates as high as 60% have been reported for African American men living in Harlem, NY (Resnicow et al.).

Heterogeneity in smoking behaviors also exists among Hispanic populations. Similar to African Americans, Hispanic men are more likely to smoke as compared to Hispanic women (Haynes, Harvey, Montes, Nickens, & Cohen, 1990; Markides, Coreil, & Ray, 1987). Haynes et al. examined patterns of cigarette smoking among Mexican Americans, Puerto Ricans, and Cuban Americans and found significant differences. Smoking prevalence was high among all groups of men: Mexican American (42.5%), Puerto Rican (39.8%), and Cuban American (41.6%). Cuban American men who were 20–34 years old, however, had the highest overall prevalence of smoking (50%). Puerto Rican and Cuban American men were found to be heavy smokers (52.3% and 64.1%, respectively, smoking a pack or more a day) as compared with Mexican American men (33.8%). Hispanic women smoked significantly less than men, and similar patterns were found among various ethnic groups, such that Mexican American women were lighter smokers (18.8% smoking a pack or more a day) as compared with Puerto Rican and Cuban American women (35.1% and 48.6%, respectively). Given the rapid growth of the Hispanic population, these smoking prevalence rates underscore the need for smoking prevention and cessation programs.

Smoking prevalence rates among American Indians and Alaska Natives also are high (36.2%) and have not changed over time (Wingo et al., 1999). In contrast to other racial and ethnic groups, no significant gender differences exist in smoking prevalence among American Indian and Alaska Native men and women (37.3% versus 35.4%). Differences in tobacco use do exist, however, according to geographic area and among various American Indian tribes. Alaska Natives have very high rates of tobacco use (39%–50%) as compared to Alaska non-Natives (25%) and American Indians and Alaska Natives who reside outside of Alaska (39%). Tobacco use is particularly high among rural (68%) versus urban (43%) Alaskan women (Kaplan, Lanier, Merritt & Siegel, 1997). Higher rates of tobacco use exist among northern American Indian tribes and lower rates among southwestern tribes (Michalek & Mahoney, 1994).

Factors Affecting Smoking Cessation and Relapse

Because of the disparity in smoking prevalence, African Americans, American Indians, and Alaska Natives suffer from a disproportionate burden of tobacco-related illnesses. Future disparities in these illnesses are expected to occur within Hispanic Americans because of the increasing numbers who are choosing to smoke. Therefore, smoking prevention and treatment programs targeted toward these groups are essential. To develop appropriate programs, however, knowledge about unique cultural influences on smoking cessation and relapse behaviors is needed. Certain sociodemographic factors, such as lower income and educational and occupational levels, male gender, unemployment, and single status, are associated with increased risk of smoking among all racial and ethnic groups (Cooley & Jennings-Dozier, 1998). Other factors such as differences in patterns of tobacco use, level of acculturation, stress and coping behaviors, limited access to health care, and targeted tobacco marketing are unique influences that may affect smoking cessation and relapse among these racial and ethnic groups. Because African Americans and Hispanics comprise the largest racial and ethnic minority groups, more information is available about the factors that influence smoking cessation and relapse within these groups.

Differences in patterns of tobacco use have been noted among African Americans and Hispanics. African Americans smoke fewer cigarettes and tend to begin smoking later in life than Whites, yet their smoking-related mortality is higher (Cooley & Jennings-Dozier, 1998). Royce et al. (1997) analyzed differences in smoking patterns between them. As compared to their counterparts, African Americans were more likely to be light to moderate smokers, were highly motivated to quit smoking, and made serious quit attempts. Although African Americans smoke fewer cigarettes as compared to their counterparts, quitting often is more difficult for them. Several reasons may account for these differences. First, the brands African Americans choose to smoke are high in nicotine and are mentholated. Second, those who are light to moderate smokers are more likely to smoke within 10 minutes of awakening (Ahijevych & Gillespie, 1997; Royce, Hymowitz, Corbett, Hartwell, & Orlandi, 1993). This tendency to "wake up" smoking indicates an increased level of nicotine addiction, making abstinence difficult for even light smokers. Finally, several studies evaluated cotinine levels in African American and White smokers and found that African Americans had higher levels of cotinine, suggesting differences in nicotine metabolism and cotinine excretion (Ahijevych & Gillespie; Wagenknecht et al., 1990). Wynder and Hoffman (1994) postulated that ethnic differences in nicotine metabolism might account for higher lung cancer mortality among African Americans.

Data from the Hispanic Health and Nutrition Examination Survey (HHANES) revealed that Hispanics smoke more cigarettes per day than African Americans or Whites (Haynes et al., 1990). They usually choose high tar and nicotine brand cigarettes (e.g., Marlboro, Winston) and tend to smoke more during social activities and on weekends but less often when they are by themselves (Haynes et al.; Ramirez & Gallion, 1993). Cotinine levels were checked with the HHANES, and a disparity existed between reported smoking status and cotinine levels: one in five reported light smokers may, in fact, be heavy smokers (Perez-Stable, Marin, Marin, Brody, & Benowitz, 1990). Thus, prevalence of smoking among some subgroups of Hispanics may be even higher than estimated.

Level of acculturation has been identified as a potential explanation for differences in smoking prevalence among the various racial and ethnic groups. Acculturation is defined as "the degree of social integration of a culture into the dominant social order" (Ramirez & Gallion, 1993, p. 353). Some authors hypothesize that cultural norms may offer a protective function against behaviors such as smoking and drinking, but research findings are contradictory. Some studies found that as the level of acculturation increases, smoking behaviors increase; whereas another study found no association between acculturation and smoking when education and income levels were controlled (Haynes et al., 1990; Scribner & Dwyer, 1989; Sorlie, Garcia-Palmieri, Costas, Cruz-Vidal, & Havlik, 1982).

For many African American and Hispanic groups, quitting and relapse problems are compounded by stresses and coping strategies associated with poverty and life hardships (Waldron & Lye, 1989). Romano, Bloom, and Syme (1991) found that urban African Americans reporting high stress were more likely to smoke than those reporting low stress. In particular, women with poor social networks were three times more likely to smoke. In another study, Ahijevych and Wewers (1993) tested a model of nicotine dependence among African American women and found that smoking to cope was the major contributor to nicotine dependence. Because a disproportionate number of African Americans and Hispanics have lower socioeconomic status and higher rates of unemployment, limited access to healthcare resources and smoking cessation programs also may contribute to lower levels of cessation.

In the recent past, extensive outdoor media campaigns and sponsorship of major sporting and cultural events created formidable barriers to tobacco control among African Americans and Hispanics (Robinson, Barry, & Bloch, 1993). Tobacco companies have spent millions of dollars on advertising in low income, minority neighborhoods. Davis (1987) estimated that 35% of all urban billboard spending occurred in African American neighborhoods. Moreover, 62% of all billboards within these neighborhoods featured tobacco ads as compared to only 36% in other neighborhoods. Although the Universal Tobacco Settlement prohibits outdoor advertising and sponsorship of events, tobacco advertising in many African American and Hispanic magazines continues to be a problem.

Implications for Interventions

Innovative strategies are needed to promote smoking cessation among racial and ethnic minority groups. Because smoking is a complex behavior, providing cessation programs that are tailored to unique cultural norms of a community may be an important avenue to improve long-term cessation rates. Given that many racial and ethnic minority groups have restricted access to healthcare and smoking cessation resources, community-based interventions are needed.

Several innovative strategies have been tested in African Americans that show promising results. Boyd et al. (1998) evaluated whether a targeted communication program in combination with community outreach could induce African Americans to call the Cancer Information Service, an information and education program sponsored by NCI, for advice related to smoking cessation. Radio and television advertising was used in combination with videos that were distributed among various community organizations within the African American community. Results of this study demonstrated that the call rate from African Americans was significantly greater among the community that received the targeted advertising. Moreover, radio seemed to be an effective way to reach an underserved population. Orleans et al. (1998) did a follow-up intervention targeting African Americans who called the Cancer Information Service. This study compared the standard Cancer Information Service intervention (self-help materials and brief telephone counseling) with a tailored intervention that combined a culturally relevant self-help guide with personalized counseling. Results from this study demonstrated a greater number of prequitting strategies, more quit attempts six months after calling, and a significantly higher 12-month quit rate among those subjects who received the tailored intervention. Even among the nonquitters at 12 months, those who received a tailored intervention reported greater progress through the stages of change.

In another study, Voorhees et al. (1996) evaluated a church-based smoking cessation intervention on readiness to quit in urban African Americans. Twenty-two churches were randomly assigned to either an intensive culturally relevant intervention or a minimal self-help group. Smokers were interviewed at entry into the study and at a one year follow-up. Results from the study suggested that the culturally specific intervention was more likely than a self-help intervention to positively influence smoking behavior. Interestingly, Baptists in the intervention group were three times more likely to make positive progress along the stages of change continuum than all other denomination groups. The researchers suggested that perhaps the strong social norms and sanctions against smoking, alcohol, and drug use in Baptist religions may explain why the intervention was more effective in this group.

These studies suggest that culturally relevant interventions may enhance interventions for smoking cessation. Therefore, healthcare professionals should consider whether the materials are culturally relevant and written at the appropriate reading level when planning interventions for various groups. Culturally appropriate smoking cessation materials have been developed for African Americans, Hispanics, and American Indians (Michalek & Mahoney, 1994; Orleans et al., 1998; Perez-Stable, Sabogal, Marin, Marin, & Oster-Sabogal, 1991).

Adults With Cancer

Although ongoing tobacco use is an important issue for many adults with cancer, limited information is available that addresses this topic. Several studies have examined the prevalence of smoking after the diagnosis of lung cancer (Davison & Duffy, 1982; Dresler, Bailey, Roper, Patterson, & Cooper, 1996; Sarna, 1995; Sridhar & Raub, 1992). Prevalence rates for smoking after lung cancer diagnosis and treatment have ranged from 8%–48%. Most patients who started smoking again relapsed within the first year. The reason for the disparity in prevalence rates among the studies is not clear. The time lapse between the studies may have contributed to an increased societal awareness about the negative effects of smoking. One of the limitations of the studies discussed, however, is that smoking status was obtained by self-report. The use of a self-report system is likely to give a substantial underestimation of the true prevalence of smokers, especially among adults with cancer (Jarvis, Tunstall-Pedoe, Feyerabend, Vesey, & Saloojee, 1987). Biochemical verification of smoking status is an important adjunct in tobacco studies. Cotinine levels in urine and saliva discriminate between smokers and nonsmokers and are the marker of choice in clinical research (Jarvis et al.).

Although smokers who have developed cancer may think that the damage already has been done, smoking cessation can yield significant health benefits. The few studies that have been conducted in this area suggest that smoking cessation is associated with a decrease in second primary cancers and even may enhance survival. Davison and Duffy (1982) examined the smoking habits and rate of second primary cancers in 52 long-term survivors who received surgery for lung cancer. Six of the 52 adults developed second primary cancers, and all of these patients had continued smoking after their surgery. Richardson et al. (1993) examined the relationship of smoking cessation and the development of second primary cancers in patients with small cell lung cancer and found that those who stopped smoking at the time of diagnosis had a relative risk of a second primary cancer of 11% (CI, 4.4%–23%) as compared with 32% (CI, 12%–69%) in those who continued to smoke. Survival from small cell lung cancer also was linked to smoking cessation. Johnston-Early et al. (1980) found that patients who had quit smoking before diagnosis or shortly after had significant improvements in their survival rate as compared with those who continued to smoke.

Smoking cessation also may affect symptoms and health-related quality of life. Smoking cessation was associated with a decrease in respiratory symptoms and improved lung function in adults (Buist, Sexton, Nagy, & Ross, 1976). Only one study examined the relationships of symptom distress, functional status, and smoking status with weight change over time in adults with lung cancer (Sarna, Lindsey, Dean, Brecht, & McCorkle, 1994). Results of the study indicate that smoking has an indirect effect on symptom distress and functional status such that the combination of chemotherapy and smoking predicted weight loss from entry into the study to eight months, and that weight loss was related to increased respiratory/gastrointestinal symptom distress and decreased total body functional status.

In summary, although these studies suggest that smoking is related to decreased quality of life, increased second primary cancers, and decreased survival in adults with lung cancer, further studies are needed in adults with cancer.

Implications for Interventions

Patients are more likely to comply with advice to quit smoking at the time of an acute illness (Schwartz, 1987). Therefore, the time surrounding the diagnosis of a life-threatening illness presents a unique opportunity to impact upon smoking behaviors. Surprisingly, few intervention studies have been conducted in adults with cancer and their family members (Gritz, 1991; Schilling et al., 1997). Griebel, Wewers, and Baker (1998) evaluated the effectiveness of a minimal smoking cessation intervention among hospitalized adults with cancer. Twenty-eight adults with cancer were assigned to either a minimal cessation intervention group (n = 14) or a usual care group (n = 14) and were evaluated for abstinence six weeks later. Results of the study indicated that only 21% of the intervention group and 14% of the usual care group were abstinent. Another study used biochemical verification with cotinine levels after an intervention for smoking cessation among adults newly diagnosed with lung cancer. Wewers, Jenkins, and Mignery (1997) found that although 93% of patients attempted at least one cessation effort, only 40% of patients were confirmed as nonsmokers six weeks after the intervention through saliva tests of cotinine levels. One study evaluated a smoking cessation intervention for family members of adults with cancer. Only 9% of relatives quit smoking for six months after receiving written advice and materials from physicians (Schilling et al.). As a whole, these studies suggest that maintaining smoking cessation in heavily nicotine-dependent adults presents a challenge, and more intensive interventions may be necessary (Griebel et al.). Whether all adults with cancer should be targeted for intensive cessation efforts still is not clear (Sarna, 1998; Wewers et al.). Although it is critical for adults with cancer who are undergoing curative treatments to quit smoking, questions surround whether smoking cessation advice in those with advanced or terminal illness is appropriate. The physical and psychological symptoms associated with nicotine withdrawal may be distressing to patients with advanced illness and cause unnecessary suffering (Sarna, 1998). Further studies in adults with cancer need to clarify what interventions are best and who should be targeted for these interventions.

Children and Adolescents
Overview of the Public Health Problem

Although selling cigarettes and smokeless tobacco to minors is illegal, young people continue to buy and use these products. More than three million American children younger than age 18 are estimated to use tobacco products (DiFranza & Tye, 1990). Research on youth buying and smoking patterns shows that minors purchase more than 256 million packs of cigarettes per year, amounting to almost $500 million in sales (Cummings, Pechacek, & Shopland, 1994). The CDC (1996) reported that 67% of 12- to 17-year-old smokers bought their own tobacco products, and 45% never had been asked for proof of age. They purchased products in a variety of ways: 89% typically made purchases from small stores, 37% bought cigarettes from large stores, and 13% used vending machines.

Recent behavioral studies confirm the ability of nicotine in tobacco to induce in adolescents both the tolerance and abstinence phenomena typical of other addicting substances that is well documented in the adult population (Woolf, 1997). Measures of behavioral and psychological aspects of smoking support using the DSM-IV criteria for tobacco dependence among young smokers to point to the need for treatment programs for addiction (Stanton, 1995).

The National Center for Chronic Disease Prevention and Health Promotion (NCCDPHP) data from the Youth Risk Behavior Survey (1996) indicated that the prevalence of tobacco use among high school students in 1995 was approximately 35% higher than in 1993 and 30% higher than in 1991. In addition, special segments of the youth population are affected differently. The number of African American male smokers almost doubled during this time period. In general, White non-Hispanics and U.S.-born Hispanics have the highest lifetime and past year prevalence rates of substance use (Khoury, Warheit, Zimmerman, Vega, & Gil, 1996), and the number of girls who use tobacco products often exceeds that of boys. NCCDPHP data match recent studies showing that tobacco use remains consistently high or is increasing among all groups, including Whites, Hispanics, and African Americans, in both boys and girls (Wills & Cleary, 1997). More than 70% of adults who smoke started before the age of 18 (Gold, Wang, Wypij, Speizer, Ware, & Dockery, 1996).

Tobacco Marketing to Youth

Tobacco imagery has been created specifically to appeal to potential young users. Perception of advertising messages is known to be higher among young smokers, and changes in market share as a result of advertising occurred mainly in the young (Pierce et al., 1991). Historical evidence shows that the tobacco industry has maintained marketing campaigns directed toward young users since the 19th century. Significant increases in smoking occurred in males under 18 years of age who were born before 1890, when marketing focused only on males (Pierce & Gilpin, 1995). Smoking use by males increased from 1910–1919 when the Camel brand was introduced to consumers. Use by females increased in the 1920s when women's marketing campaigns featured Chesterfield and Lucky Strike and increased significantly in the 1960s with the introduction of Virginia Slims (Pierce & Gilpin). More recently, billboards with "Joe Camel" have been used to target youth. Most brands have special campaigns to appeal to the younger market. After a 1995 study of usage patterns, investigators attributed the initiation of adolescent smoking to marketing efforts over that of the influence of peers and family (Evans, Farkas, Gilpin, Berry & Pierce, 1995).

Images of people using tobacco products are ubiquitous and integral with popular culture, including mass mediums such as film, television, and music videos. Nationally televised sporting events are sponsored by the tobacco industry, and written advertisements support tennis, car racing, and other sporting, visual, and performance arts events (Tobacco Talks, 1999). Even though public displays of tobacco products on billboards and television and other means of advertising have been restricted, the industry is able to continue to make tobacco products visible to the youth market in easily accessible literature, like magazines (Kuczynski, 1999), displays in retail stores, and through the more subtle means of role modeling by media personalities.

Impact on Health

Besides the overwhelming evidence that tobacco use is linked to several kinds of cancer, lung disease, and heart disease, a growing body of literature identifies young users as especially vulnerable to the negative health effects. Gold et al. (1996) found a gender-specific physiologic effect of smoking. Girls who smoked were found to have a lower mean level of the ratio of forced expiratory volume in one second of forced vital capacity, as well as a reduced forced expiratory flow. Investigators concluded that cigarette smoking is associated with evidence of mild airway obstruction and slowed growth of lung function in both adolescent girls and boys (Gold et al.).

Physical activity promotes well-being in adolescents and children, and early lifestyle choices have a lasting impact on health. Physical activity is positively associated with good health and the reverse is true for tobacco use. Winnail, Valois, McKeown, Sanders, and Pate (1995) reported that White males in high school who used cigarettes or smokeless tobacco were substantially less physically active than those who did not use tobacco products. These results suggested that a synergistic effect of limited physical activity and tobacco use may exist that is not yet understood but should be investigated.

A significant association has been drawn between tobacco use and other unhealthy lifestyle choices. Whiteman, Fowkes, Deary, and Lee (1997) found an affiliation between tobacco use and hostility. An increased level of smoking was found to be the strongest predictor of subsequent alcohol use in ninth graders (Parra-Medina, Talavera, Elder, & Woodruff, 1995). Kokotailo, Adger, Duggan, Repke, and Joffe (1992) found that cigarette, alcohol, and drug use were positively correlated with early sexual activity, and early sexual activity may lead to adolescent pregnancy. The dangers to a group already at high risk are compounded with potential risk to developing fetuses. In addition, children of males who smoke more than five packs a year prior to conception have a significantly elevated risk of childhood cancers, such as leukemia and lymphoma (Ji et al., 1997).

Adolescents who are cancer survivors face the same decisions as other adolescents but appear to be more at risk for the adverse health effects of tobacco use because of the previous effects of cancer treatment (Hollen, Hobbie, & Finley, 1999). The needs of this population merit specialized attention.

In summary, the impact of tobacco product use on health is extensive. This problem is systematic and serious. It persists as a significant health problem that has a negative impact and is directly proportional to duration, intensity, and frequency of tobacco use. The younger the age when one begins to smoke, the more likely he or she is to smoke heavily as an adult and suffer serious health consequences. The evidence is overwhelming and disturbing. Young people who use tobacco place themselves at significant health risk by establishing this negative behavior pattern.

Initiatives for Screening, Prevention, and Cessation

Standing on the threshold of adulthood, adolescents face a complex time of growth and experimentation, and they often experiment with tobacco. Because the age of onset of tobacco use and history of smoking are important determinants of cancer and other disease risk, a need exists for healthcare professionals to intervene at all levels of prevention. Oncology nurses may impact the health of youth in several ways. They may identify young people at increased risk, implement tobacco prevention programs, and develop age-specific cessation activities to reduce the number of youth who eventually will suffer the health problems associated with tobacco use.

Predicting Tobacco Use

More than a decade of research studies have shown that the strongest predictor of tobacco use is previous experimentation (Kelder, Perry, Klepp, & Lytle 1994; McNeill et al., 1988; Pederson & Lefcoe, 1987). Seventy-one percent of people in the United States who smoke tried their first cigarette during adolescence (Gold et al., 1996), and two-thirds of the smokers in ninth grade (15 years old) were still smoking at age 28 (Paavola, Vartiainen, & Puska, 1996). The relative risk for adult smoking is increased by an early onset of use (Chassin & Presson, 1990). Further, nicotine dependence develops quickly among young users (McNeill, 1991).

Peer Use and Pressure

Significant predictors of tobacco use are peer use and the pressures associated with the need for social acceptability and group identity. Bertrand and Abernathy (1993) identified interpersonal factors as key determinants of use. However, this may vary among subgroups, such that African American adolescents are impacted more by intrapersonal factors than by interpersonal influences (Botvin, Botvin, Dusenbury, Cardwell, & Diaz, 1993).

Reasons given by young people for smoking included "imitating others' behaviors," "seeing what it was like," beliefs that it makes one "look elegant, cool, or fashionable," and pressure from peers (Bertrand & Abernathy, 1993; Zhu, Liu, Shelton, Liu, & Giovino, 1996; Zhu et al., 1992). In a study by Elder, Molgaard, and Gresham (1988), the investigators pointed out a pattern of tobacco use such that the habits of one's best friend predicted both smoking and chewing tobacco experimentation and prevalence. White males were more likely to chew tobacco, whereas African Americans and Mexican Americans were more likely to smoke (Elder et al., 1988).

Furthermore, experiences that lead to a decision to start smoking may be different for males and females and affected by variables such as school achievement, family-peer orientation, psychogenic orientations, and health attitudes and behaviors (Brunswick & Messeri, 1983–1984). Evidence supports the claim that complex social processes are critical in the development of this behavior.

Moreover, girls may be motivated by different factors. McDermott et al. (1992) found that important predictors of cigarette use in adolescent girls include attitudes toward females who smoke, close friends or best friends who smoke, concurrent use of marijuana, and low levels or little need for higher levels of self-esteem. Age of onset at puberty also has been linked to cigarette smoking. Girls with early onset of puberty reported cigarette use 0.6 years earlier than those who started later (Wilson et al., 1994).

Parental and Family Influences

An early study of smoking among high school students found that the percentage of smokers was highest among children of families in which both parents smoked; smoking behaviors of boys conformed more closely to the patterns of the fathers, whereas girls conformed more closely to that of the mothers; and each successive grade had a higher percentage of smokers (Horn, Courts, Taylor, & Solaman, 1959). McGee and Stanton (1993) associated adolescent smoking with family disadvantage. These statements are supported by other literature that confirms the strong predictive potential of parental substance use on adolescent substance use across racial and ethnic groups (Moreno et al., 1994; Murphy & Price, 1988; Wills, Schreibman, Benson, & Vaccaro, 1994). DiStefan, Gilpin, Choi, and Pierce (1998) examined parental influences on two transitions of adolescent smoking uptake: (a) from never having smoked to experimentation and (b) from experimentation to established smoking. Of significance is that lack of parental concern or distress about tobacco use contributed to progression of established smoking habits. The important message is that parents who smoke or condone the use of tobacco are more likely to have children who smoke. A surprising finding was that family involvement in the tobacco industry was significantly associated with the intention to smoke but not smoking behaviors (Murphy & Price). Mixed findings exist with regard to the influence of parents and friends. van Reek, Knibbe, and van Iwaarden (1993) reported no association between adolescent and parent smoking behaviors.

Even though no clear causal relationship exists between tobacco use and other variables, tobacco use likely is not merely a consequence of environmental influences but rather linked more closely to interpersonal relationships. Research confirms the prediction that peer pressure, self-image, and self-esteem affect children's decisions to begin to smoke. Complex social processes critically influence a young person's decision to begin to use and continue to use tobacco products.

Prevention

The best way to achieve public health initiatives is to work toward modifying patterns of tobacco use, concentrating on control through prevention, and by developing effective cessation programs. Most adolescents who can avoid using tobacco will not use it during their adult life. Because cigarette smoking cessation programs have a low success rate (Meijer, Branski, Knoll, & Kerem, 1996), prevention programs should be initiated as early as possible.

Tobacco Use Prevention Programs

Because the use of tobacco products among school-age children is becoming increasingly widespread, attempts are being made to reach out to youngsters and teach them the ill effects at an early age. Programs may start as early as kindergarten and continue through grade 12. Curriculum content begins with messages to students to choose behaviors that maintain health. Each year, messages are reinforced and expanded.

Some evidence shows that school-based programs have a significant impact on preventing substance abuse. Early investigations by Bangert-Drowns (1988) found little information to support this. Usual programs are educative, with an emphasis on presenting the health risks associated with tobacco use. Few studies report the successful use of methods to influence attitudinal changes or teach the psychosocial skills to resist use (Bowen, Kinne, & Orlandi, 1995).

However, several studies have documented the success of school-based programs. A study of middle school students in Kentucky demonstrated that school-based interventions focusing on social influences lowered smoking rates in tobacco-producing regions (Noland et al., 1998). Interventions that are peer led and have high parental involvement have been associated with lower use of and intention to use tobacco (Murray, Davis-Hearn, Goldman, Pirie, & Luepker, 1988).

Giarelli (1999) suggested that the complexity of the interpersonal and intrapersonal phenomenon of tobacco use in this age group requires a combined theoretical approach to school-based programs. Integration and application of concepts from the Health Beliefs Model, Social Learning Theory, and Cognitive Theory may be used to develop prevention services that are meaningful and tailored to this special population.

Even without evidence of efficacy, school-based programs have been strongly advocated as the best way to bring the abstinence message to large groups. Peer educators, as young as fifth grade, can be trained to instruct and model resistance skills (Reding, Fischer, Lappe, & Gunderson, 1996).

Adolescents and children at risk may be difficult to influence through systematic approaches in public institutions. However, the same individuals are accessible through mass media. Videotaped instructional sessions have been designed and effectively used with African American adolescents (Sussman et al., 1995). Flynn et al. (1997) demonstrated that smoking prevention messages presented through the mass media can have a large and durable impact on high-risk teens who have had lower rates of smoking following a mass media and school intervention. A strategy that combines school interventions with messages presented via mass media has the greatest potential for positive impact (Flynn et al., 1992; Worden et al., 1996).

Prevention Services in Healthcare Agencies

Healthcare services traditionally are delivered in healthcare agencies, such as physician offices, clinics, and hospitals, where nurses may provide prevention and early detection and tobacco cessation services. However, these environments may not be suitable as the primary source of preventive health for older children and adolescents. A recent analysis of pre- and adolescent use of primary care showed that the number of visits made by adolescents (ages 11–21) to nonfederal, nonhospital physician offices has remained low since the early 1980s (Ziv, Boulet, & Slap, 1999). Visits have been disproportionately lower for those who are African American, Hispanic, or male and lowest in early adolescents (ages 11–14) (Ziv et al.). The increasing rates of substance abuse among this cohort and the low rate of nonemergency healthcare services support an age-stratified approach to health promotion by way of an alternative public agency.

A variety of means can be employed to reach out to children. One method, reported by Skjoldebrand and Gahnberg (1997), occurred in a public dental health clinic in Sweden, where a successful intervention was conducted by dental care staff and resulted in a reduction of tobacco use over three years. Another successful program employed college and undergraduate change agents and direct one-on-one telephone interventions to provide cost-effective behavior modification (Elder et al., 1993).

Considerable evidence shows that children acquire tobacco use habits in their homes and within the context of complex interpersonal relationships. Health promotion programs that integrate family, school, and community health are recommended (see Figure 9-4). Preventive efforts should increase the density of antitobacco messages and consequences in the environment by nontraditional means and by way of a medium that appeals to the young.

Figure 9-4. Guidelines for School Health Programs to Prevent Tobacco Use

1. Develop and enforce a school policy on tobacco use by minors and adults.
2. Provide instruction about the short-term and long-term negative psychological and social consequences of tobacco use.
3. Provide instruction on social influences of tobacco use.
4. Provide instruction on peer norms and refusal skills.
5. Establish curriculum content in K–12 on prevention education.
6. Provide program-specific training for teachers.
7. Involve parents or families in support of school-based programs.
8. Support cessation efforts among students and all staff who use tobacco.
9. Assess tobacco use prevention programs at regular intervals.

Note. Based on information from the Centers for Disease Control and Prevention, 1994c.

Tobacco Use Cessation Initiatives

The incidence of tobacco use by adolescents has increased while adult use steadily has decreased. This apparent failure of adolescent tobacco use cessation and prevention programs highlights the need for more research on the content and process of programs. Stanton and Silva (1992) reported that the source of the influence to smoke was more powerful than the extent of the influence. Interventions aimed at reducing adolescent tobacco use should encourage cessation for parents who smoke and help parents communicate strong antismoking norms to their children (DiStefan et al., 1998). They also should aim to involve peers in the intervention.

Community as Partners

Reducing access to tobacco is a responsibility of the community at large. Research shows that the most effective way to reduce underage access is to implement merchant compliance with comprehensive prevention strategies. Compliance would involve merchant refusal to sell tobacco products to minors, restricted access to vending machines, and a limitation or removal of visual prompts to use the products. There is a need to educate retailers and strictly enforce laws that are already in place that prohibit sales to minors, and new laws are needed to prohibit minors from smoking in public places.

In summary, besides the known risks (e.g., lung cancer, heart disease, pulmonary disease, disorders of teeth and skin, early aging) of cigarette smoking to the general public, specific evidence suggests that smoking poses special health hazards to children and adolescents. These include loss of lung function, risk of alcohol abuse, early sexual activity, and teenage pregnancy, with subsequent risks to the developing fetus. Previous smoking status and smoking by friends and family are the most important predictors of adult use (Paavola et al., 1996). The continuity of smoking from adolescence to adulthood supports the importance of prevention programs during childhood. Research highlights the need to reach out to children and teach them early in their development, as well as during the vulnerable years of adolescence, about the risks of tobacco use.

Prevention strategies for children should address the complex dynamics of interpersonal relationships during this period of psychological and physical development. Interventions should be cognitively appropriate and reach out to those at increased risk. Parents, adult role models, and peer counselors should participate. All evidence considered, the most effective intervention likely will combine media-school interventions, involve parents and peers who use tobacco in the intervention strategy, and stratify the adolescent smoking populations by age, ethnicity, and developmental milestones.

Tobacco Control Issues

Tobacco Legislation

The legal battle among consumers, healthcare professionals, and the tobacco industry has been waged in the courts for decades. Consumers claim the right to compensation from the tobacco industry for physical harm caused by years of tobacco use. Healthcare systems claim the right to reimbursement as compensation from the tobacco industry for the healthcare costs accrued from cessation programs and treatment for those affected by tobacco use. An ongoing debate in Congress focuses on the issue of tobacco as an addictive substance whose distribution should be controlled by the FDA and also the call to identify a cigarette as a drug delivery device.

To partially resolve the differences, the tobacco industry agreed to a monetary settlement, called the Universal Tobacco Settlement, that distributes $206 billion to state governments in allotments over 25 years (Center for Social Gerontology, 1999b). The initial expectation was that most of the money would support health programs, especially antismoking campaigns and treatment programs. Individual states may determine how to allocate the funds; however, no overriding legislation exists to ensure that funding is spent on health programs related to tobacco use. Some states are distributing the revenue to support college scholarships, deficit reduction, school construction, and capital outlays (Crary, 1999).

Legislative Efforts to Protect the Public

There continues to be a need to lobby for legislation that advocates for the health of consumers. Current and pending legislation that addresses tobacco control-related issues is continually evolving and can be accessed using LEXIS, an online legal research database, and by using NCI's State Cancer Legislative Database (SCLD) (Shelton et al., 1995).

Legislative efforts needed to protect the public from harmful effects of tobacco include (a) passing state laws that prohibit the sale of products to minors; (b) prohibiting the general use of tobacco products in public areas and facilities; (c) imposing excise taxes on the sale of tobacco products; and (d) passing local ordinances that prohibit public possession and use of tobacco products by minors. In general, those who advocate restrictions should urge the passage of federal legislation that mandates that all states develop programs to reduce accessibility of tobacco products (see Figure 9-5).

More than 1,238 state laws address tobacco control-related issues. Most laws either enact restrictions or strengthen current legislation that restricts tobacco use, sales to minors, or advertising. Some laws preempt stronger measures by local ordinances.

Restriction of Sales to Minors

Minors' access to tobacco is an important public health issue. The most common suppliers for youth users are grocery stores, convenience stores, gas station mini-marts, liquor stores, and drug stores. Some data reveal a moderate support of restrictive policies by merchants. Little is known, however, about the attitudes and beliefs of people in business who sell the products, beyond their underestimation of the extent of use and ill effects (Altman et al., 1992). In the late 1980s, Woodridge,

---

Figure 9-5. Recommended Components of an Enforcement Program to Limit Access to Tobacco Products

Products
1. An agency in the state with clear responsibility
2. Adequate, guaranteed funding for enforcement of laws
3. Licensing of vendors by the enforcing agency; licensing should be self-reporting
4. Frequent and realistic compliance checks, aiming for 95% compliance
5. Penalties for noncompliance that include graduated fines and, ultimately, license suspension
6. No preemption of local ordinances
7. Educational programs for merchants and the public

Note. Based on information from Campaign for Tobacco-Free Kids, 1999; Tobacco Control Resource Center, 1999.

IL, was the first U.S. town to demonstrate a significant reduction in the ability of youth to purchase cigarettes, a clear-cut case where purchasing power was curtailed and the incidence of smoking ultimately was reduced (Jason, Berk, Schnopp-Wyatt, & Talbot, 1999). Currently, all U.S. states prohibit the sale of tobacco to minors. Five states and Washington, DC, may suspend or revoke a retailer's tobacco products license for violation of youth access laws. In addition, 41 states and Washington, DC, have restrictions on the presence of cigarette vending machines in areas accessible to minors. In an effort to control the impact of second-hand smoke on minors, as well as other adults, 28 states and Washington, DC, limit smoking in commercial daycare facilities (CDC, 1999a, 1999b). Model laws that restrict access, such as those in Washington, DC, also include a requirement for a warning sign at the point of sale and a reward for individuals reporting violators of vending laws (DiFranza, Norwood, Garner, & Tye, 1987).

Restriction of Public Use

Most states require smoke-free indoor air to some degree or in some public places. At the local level and in environments that may serve youth populations, such as schools, no one may use tobacco products on the premises. Some local governments have imposed ordinances that prohibit the use of tobacco products by minors. If minors are found possessing and using a tobacco substance, they may be issued a summons and be required to participate in a smoking cessation program. Local town councils have expressed the intention to collaborate with parents and youth in their communities to enforce the message of the ills of tobacco. Penalties may include an issuance of a warning on first offence, parental notification and participation in community service projects for repeat offenders, and a combination of these plus entry into an educational program determined by the health officer of the municipality (Township of Lawrence, 1998). To date, no evidence shows that this kind of intervention is having a positive impact.

Taxing Tobacco Products

Many health professional organizations support the use of economic interventions to discourage the illegal sale and use of tobacco products. All U.S. states have placed an excise tax on cigarette sales that averages 3.89 cents per pack. Taxes range from 2.5 cents per pack in Virginia, a tobacco growing state, to $1.00 per pack in Alaska. Yet only 42 states have a tax on smokeless tobacco products (CDC, 1999c). Cigarette sales to minors are considered a significant source of revenue to retailers, representing $39.5 million in annual sales. Based on this estimate, Cummings, Pechacek, and Sciandra (1992) advocated levying an illegal drug profit tax on the cigarette industry to recover the millions in profits derived annually from the illegal sales to minors. State laws vary in relation to the extent of restrictions, enforcement and penalties, pre-emptions, and exceptions.

Recommendations of Healthcare Organizations

Prevention is the gold standard strategy in health promotion. Prevention of the use of harmful substances can lead to prevention of the ultimate harmful effects.

Because substances often are used in tandem, such as alcohol along with tobacco, prevention of tobacco has secondary benefits. The CDC has developed guidelines for the use of school health programs to prevent tobacco use and addiction in consultation with experts from many healthcare organizations, including the American Academy of Pediatricians, the American Medical Association, the National Association of School Nurses, and the American Cancer Society (CDC, 1994c). Educational programs should incorporate interventions that help students make formal commitments not to use tobacco, point out the social and physical consequences of use, and recommend alternative behaviors. The force of peer pressure should be factored into the interventions, along with assistance in assertiveness training.

Nursing organizations have joined tobacco opponents and help lead the fight on public health issues. Many healthcare associations have developed position statements or endorsed position statements in relation to tobacco, smoking, and health. These associations include the World Health Organization, the Oncology Nursing Society (ONS), the American Medical Association, the American Cancer Society, and the International Society of Nurses in Cancer Care (ISNCC). All of these organizations cite that tobacco use or exposure to second-hand smoke increases the occurrence of cancer as well as other serious diseases, leading to increased morbidity and mortality. All statements advocate control of tobacco use and endorse antismoking policies (AHCPR, 1996; Elders, Perry, Eriksen, & Giovino, 1994; ISNCC, 1999).

In 1997, ONS developed a position paper on proposals for U.S. tobacco policies that was future-oriented, protective, and reflects organizational consensus. Some of the proposed options have become policy and law, whereas others have just begun to receive legislative consideration. ONS proposed that international, national, state, and local policies should

1. Ensure complete ability of the FDA to regulate nicotine and other constituents and ingredients used in tobacco products.
2. Promote and facilitate treatment for adults and children who are addicted to tobacco.
3. Discourage adults and children from initiating smoking behaviors and/or the use of tobacco products.
4. Prohibit the sale and distribution of tobacco products to people under age 18.
5. Protect nonsmokers from involuntary exposure to tobacco smoke.
6. Ensure adequate funding needed to carry out regulatory, enforcement, public education, and research activities within appropriate agencies.
7. Promote global tobacco control and the prevention of tobacco-related illnesses.
8. Apply advertising and marketing restrictions to all tobacco products, as outlined by the Kessler-Koop Advisory Committee and the American Cancer Society.
9. Underwrite costs of clinical research trials on tobacco-related cancers that contribute to curative or preventive new therapies.
10. Promote research that explores factors relating to tobacco use and cessation behaviors.

11. Maintain the right of individuals and states to recover damages associated with tobacco-related illnesses and death.

In addition, ONS supports an increase in the federal and state excise tax on cigarettes of at least $2.00 per pack to act as a deterrent and to provide funding that can be directed toward health services.

ISNCC (1999) actively supports prevention and restriction efforts and has called upon members to take an active role in initiating and supporting national and international tobacco-control policy and legislation, while becoming nonsmoking role models.

Conclusion

Smoking accounts for the vast majority of lung cancer, numerous other cancers, heart disease, and pulmonary disease. Specific evidence suggests that smoking poses special health hazards to children and adolescents, including loss of lung function, risk of alcohol abuse, early sexual activity, and subsequent risks to the developing fetus in teenage pregnancy. Although the prevalence of smoking has decreased over time, it remains unacceptably high. The recent trend in increased prevalence of smoking among children and adolescents is alarming and must be addressed if future morbidity is to be avoided. Nurses can play an important role in health promotion and cancer control by participating in initiatives that address smoking prevention, cessation, and tobacco control; these specific interventions have been provided in this chapter. For interventions to be effective, however, a multipronged approach is needed. In addition to individual, family, and community-based interventions, an approach that includes healthcare delivery systems and legislative change is critical.

Helpful Web Sites

Addressing Tobacco in Managed Care: www.aahp.org/atmc.htm
Agency for Healthcare Research and Quality: www.ahrq.gov
American Academy of Family Physicians: www.aafp.org
American Cancer Society: www.cancer.org
American Legacy Foundation: www.americanlegacy.org
American Psychological Association: www.apa.org
National Cancer Institute: www.nci.nih.gov
National Center for Tobacco-Free Kids: www.tobaccofreekids.org
National Guideline Clearinghouse: www.guideline.gov
National Heart, Lung, and Blood Institute: www.nhlbi.nih.gov/index.htm
National Institute on Drug Abuse: www.nida.nih.gov/NIDAHome1.html
Office on Smoking and Health at the Centers for Disease Control and Prevention: www.cdc.gov/tobacco
Society for Research on Nicotine and Tobacco: www.srnt.org
World Health Organization: www.who.int

References

Agency for Health Care Policy Research. (1996). *Smoking cessation clinical practice guidelines* (Publication No. 96-0692). Rockville, MD: Author.

Ahijevych, K., & Gillespie, J. (1997). Nicotine dependence and smoking topography among black and white women. *Research in Nursing and Health, 20,* 505–514.

Ahijevych, K., & Wewers, M.E. (1993). Factors associated with nicotine dependence among African American women cigarette smokers. *Research in Nursing and Health, 16,* 283–292.

Altman, D.G., Linzer, J., Kropp, R., Descheemaeker, N., Feighery, E., & Fortmann, S.P. (1992). Policy alternatives for reducing tobacco sales to minors: Results from a national survey of retail chain and franchise stores. *Journal of Public Health Policy, 13,* 318–331.

American Psychiatric Association. (1994). *Diagnostic and statistical manual of mental disorders* (4th ed.). Washington, DC: Author.

American Psychiatric Association. (1996). *Practice guidelines for the treatment of patients with nicotine dependence.* Washington, DC: Author.

American Thoracic Society. (1996). Cigarette smoking and health. *American Journal of Respiratory Critical Care Medicine, 153,* 861–865.

Antonia, S.J., Robinson, L.A., Ruckdeschel, J.C., & Wagner, H. (1998). Lung cancer. In L. Balducci, G.H. Lyman, & W.B. Ershler (Eds.), *Comprehensive geriatric oncology* (pp. 611–628). Amsterdam, The Netherlands: Harwood Academic Publishers.

Ascher, J.A., Cole, J.O., Colin, J.N., Feighner, J.P., Ferris, R.M., Fibiger, H.C., & Golden, R.N. (1995). Bupropion: A review of its mechanism of antidepressant activity. *Journal of Clinical Psychiatry, 56,* 395–401.

Balducci, L., & Barry, P.P. (1994). A practical approach to the screening of asymptomatic older persons for cancer. *Cancer Control: Journal of the Moffitt Cancer Center, 1,* 126–131.

Balducci, L., & Lyman, G.H. (1997). Cancer in the elderly: Epidemiologic and clinical implications. *Clinics in Geriatric Medicine, 13,* 1–14.

Balfour, D.J., & Fagerstrom, K.O. (1996). Pharmacology of nicotine and its therapeutic use in smoking cessation and neurodegenerative disorders. *Pharmacology Therapeutics, 72,* 51–81.

Bangert-Drowns, R.L. (1988). The effects of school based substance abuse education—A meta-analysis. *Journal of Drug Education, 18,* 243–264.

Barbone, F., Bovenzi, M., & Cavalleri, F. (1995). Air pollution and lung cancer in Trieste, Italy. *American Journal of Epidemiology, 141,* 1161–1169.

Bartsch, H., Caporaso, N., Coda, M., Kadlubar, F., Malaveille, C., Skipper, P., Talaska, G., & Tannenbaum, S.R. (1990). Carcinogen hemoglobin adducts, urinary mutagenicity, and metabolic phenotype in active and passive cigarette smokers. *Journal of the National Cancer Institute, 82,* 1826–1831.

Beheney, C., & Hewitt, M. (1997). *Smoking-related deaths and financial costs: Office of Technology Assessment Estimates for 1990.* Atlanta: Centers for Disease Control, Office on Smoking and Health.

Benowitz, N.L. (1991). Nicotine replacement therapy during pregnancy. *JAMA, 266,* 3174–3177.

Benowitz, N.L. (1992). Cigarette smoking and nicotine addiction. *Medical Clinics of North America, 76*, 415–437.

Bertrand, L.D., & Abernathy, T.J. (1993). Predicting cigarette smoking among adolescents using cross-sectional and longitudinal approaches. *Journal of School Health, 63*, 100–105.

Bierner, L., & Abrams, D. (1991). The contemplation ladder: Validation of a measure of readiness to consider smoking cessation. *Health Psychologist, 10*, 360–365.

Biesalski, H.K., de Mesquita, B.B., Chesson, A., Chutil, F., Grimble, R., Hermus, R.J., & Kohrle, J. (1998). European consensus statement on lung cancer: Risk factors and prevention. *CA: A Cancer Journal for Clinicians, 48*, 167–176.

Blesch, K.S. (1998). Principles of cancer nursing. In L. Balducci, G. Lyman, & W. Ershler (Eds.), *Comprehensive geriatric oncology* (pp. 351–361). Baltimore, MD: Harwood Academic Publishers.

Borland, R. (1990). Slip ups and relapse in attempts to quit smoking. *Addictive Behavior, 15*, 235–245.

Botvin, B.J., Botvin, E.M., Dusenbury, L., Cardwell, J., & Diaz, T. (1993). Factors promoting cigarette smoking among black youth: A causal modeling approach. *Addictive Behaviors, 18*, 397–405.

Bowen, D.J., Kinne, S., & Orlandi, M. (1995). School policy in COMMIT: A promising strategy to reduce smoking by youth. *Journal of School Health, 65*, 140–144.

Boyd, N.R. (1996). Smoking cessation: A four-step plan to help older patients quit. *Geriatrics, 51*, 52–57.

Boyd, N.R., Sutton, C., Orleans, C.T., McClatchey, M.W., Bingler, R., Fleisher, L., Heller, D., Baum, S., Graves, C., & Ward, J. (1998). Quit today! A targeted campaign to increase use of the cancer information service by African American smokers. *Preventive Medicine, 27*(5 Pt. 2), S50–S60.

Boyle, P., Hsieh, C.C., & Maisonneuve, P. (1989). Epidemiology of pancreas cancer. *International Journal of Pancreatology, 5*, 327–346.

Breslau, N. (1995). Psychiatric comorbidity of smoking and nicotine dependence. *Behavior Genetics, 25*, 95–101.

Browman, G.P., Wong, G., Hodson, I., Sathya, J., Russell, R., & McAlpine, L. (1993). Influence of cigarette smoking on the efficacy of radiation therapy in head and neck cancer. *New England Journal of Medicine, 328*, 159–163.

Brownson, R.C., Novotony, T.E., & Perry, M.C. (1993). Cigarette smoking and adult leukemia: A meta-analysis. *Archives of Internal Medicine, 153*, 469–475.

Brunswick, A.F., & Messeri, P. (1983–1984). Causal factors in onset of adolescents' cigarette smoking: A prospective study of urban black youth. *Advances in Alcohol and Substance Abuse, 391*, 35–52.

Buist, A.S., Sexton, G.J., Nagy, J.M., & Ross, B.B. (1976). The effect of smoking cessation and modification on lung function. *American Review of Respiratory Disease, 114*, 115–122.

Campaign for Tobacco-Free Kids. (1999). *Enforcing laws prohibiting tobacco sales to minors reduces youth smoking.* Retrieved June 13, 2001 from the World Wide Web: http://tobaccofreekids.org/research/factsheets/pdf/0049.pdf

Carbone, D. (1992). Smoking and cancer. *American Journal of Medicine, 93*(Suppl. 1A), 13S–17S.

Cataldo, J.K. (in press). Smoking and aging: Clinical implications. *Journal of Gerontological Nursing.*

Center for the Advancement of Health. (1996). *Tobacco control and prevention: Performance indicators for managed care.* Retrieved February 7, 2000 from the World Wide Web: http://www.cfah.org

Center for Social Gerontology. (1999a). *Tobacco and the elderly.* Retrieved November 15, 1999 from the World Wide Web: http://www.csg.org/toba

Center for Social Gerontology. (1999b). *Tobacco settlement funds: State updates.* Retrieved November 6, 1999 from the World Wide Web: http://www.tcsg.org/tobacco/settlement/updates/htm

Centers for Disease Control and Prevention. (1991). Smoking-attributable mortality and years of potential life lost—United States, 1988. *Morbidity and Mortality Weekly Report, 40,* 62–63, 69–71.

Centers for Disease Control and Prevention. (1993a). Smoking-attributable mortality and years of potential life lost—United States. *Morbidity and Mortality Weekly Report, 42,* 645–648.

Centers for Disease Control and Prevention. (1993b). Mortality trends for selected smoking-related and breast cancer—United States, 1950–1990. *Morbidity and Mortality Weekly Report, 42,* 857, 863–866.

Centers for Disease Control and Prevention. (1994a). Cigarette smoking among adults—United States. *Morbidity and Mortality Weekly Report, 43,* 925–930.

Centers for Disease Control and Prevention. (1994b). Cigarette smoking among women of reproductive age—United States, 1987–1992. *Morbidity and Mortality Weekly Report, 43,* 789–797.

Centers for Disease Control and Prevention. (1994c). Guidelines for school health programs to prevent tobacco use and addiction. *Journal of School Health, 64,* 353–360.

Centers for Disease Control and Prevention. (1996). Accessibility of tobacco products to youths aged 12–17 years—United States, 1989 and 1993. *Morbidity and Mortality Weekly Report, 45,* 125–130.

Centers for Disease Control and Prevention. (1999a). State-specific prevalence of current cigarette and cigar smoking among adults—United States, 1998. *Morbidity and Mortality Weekly Report, 48,* 1034–1039.

Centers for Disease Control and Prevention. (1999b). Tobacco report on state laws shows moderate progress. *Cancer Practice, 7,* 218.

Centers for Disease Control and Prevention. (1999c). State laws on tobacco control—1998. *Morbidity and Mortality Weekly Report, 48*(SS-3). Retrieved June 13, 2001 from the World Wide Web: http://www.cdc.gov/mmwr/PDF/SS/SS4803.pdf

Chassin, L., & Presson, C.C. (1990). The natural history of cigarette smoking: Predicting young adult smoking outcomes from adolescent smoking patterns. *Health Psychology, 9,* 701–716.

Chichareon, S., Herrero, R., Munoz, N., Bosch, F.X., Jacobs, M.V., Deacon, J., & Santamaria, M. (1998). Risk factors for cervical cancer in Thailand: A case control study. *Journal of the National Cancer Institute, 90,* 50–57.

Cinciripini, P.M. (1995). A placebo-controlled evaluation of the effects of buspirone on smoking cessation: Differences between high- and low-anxiety smokers. *Journal of Clinical Psychopharmacology, 15,* 182–191.

Clavel, J., Cordier, S., & Boccon-Gibod, L. (1989). Tobacco and bladder cancer in males: Increased risk for inhalers and smokers of black tobacco. *International Journal of Cancer, 44*, 605–610.

Cook, D.G., Shaper, A.G., Procock, S.J., & Kussick, S.J. (1986). Giving up smoking and the risk of heart attacks: A report from the British Regional Heart Study. *Lancet, 2*, 1376–1380.

Cooley, M.E., & Jennings-Dozier, K. (1998). Lung cancer in African-Americans: A call for action. *Cancer Practice, 6*, 99–102.

Coppotelli, H., & Orleans, C. (1985). Partner support and other determinants of smoking cessation maintenance among women. *Journal of Clinical Psychology, 53*, 455–460.

Coughlin, S.S., Neaton, J.D., & Sengupta, A. (1996). Cigarette smoking as a predictor of death from prostate cancer in 348,874 men screened for the Multiple Risk Factor Intervention Trial. *American Journal of Epidemiology, 143*, 1002–1006.

Covey, L., Glassman, A., & Stetner, F. (1990). *Comprehensive Psychiatry, 31*, 350–354.

Cox, J.L. (1993). Smoking cessation in the elderly patient. *Clinical Chest Medicine, 14*, 423.

Crary, D. (1999, November 19). Smoking foes fume over use of payouts: Health campaigns often take a back seat. *The Trenton Times*, pp. A1, B4.

Cummings, K.M., Pechacek, T., & Sciandra, E. (1992). Economic interventions to discourage the illegal sale of cigarettes to minors. *New York State Journal of Medicine, 92*, 521–524.

Cummings, K.M., Pechacek, T., & Shopland, D. (1994). The illegal sale of cigarettes to U.S. minors: Estimates by state. *American Journal of Public Health, 84*, 300–302.

Dai, W.S., Gutai, J.P., Kuller, L.H., & Cauley, J.A. (1988). Cigarette smoking and serum sex hormones in men. *American Journal of Epidemiology, 128*, 796–805.

Daling, J.R., Madeline, M.M., McKnight, B., Carter, J.J., Wipf, G.C., Ashley, R., & Schwartz, S.M. (1996). The relationship of human papillomavirus-related cervical tumors to cigarette smoking, oral contraceptive use, and prior herpes simplex virus type 2 infection. *Cancer Epidemiology, Biomarkers and Prevention, 5*(7), 541–548.

Davis, L.J., Hurt, R.D., Offord, K.P., Lauger, G.G., Morse, R.M., & Bruce, B.K. (1994). Self-administered nicotine dependence scale (SANDS): Item selection, reliability estimation, and initial validation. *Journal of Clinical Psychology, 50*, 918–930.

Davis, R.M. (1987). Current trends in cigarette advertising and marketing. *New England Journal of Medicine, 316*, 725–735.

Davison, G., & Duffy, M. (1982). Smoking habits of long term survivors of surgery for lung cancer. *Thorax, 37*, 331–333.

Delarue, N.C. (1973). A study in smoking withdrawal. The Toronto Smoking Withdrawal Study Centre: Description of study activities. *Canadian Journal of Public Health, 64*(Suppl.), S5–S19.

DiFranza, J.R., Norwood, B.D., Garner, D.W., & Tye, J.B. (1987). Legislative efforts to protect children from tobacco. *JAMA, 257*, 3387–3389.

DiFranza, J.R., & Tye, J.F. (1990). Who profits from tobacco sales to children? *JAMA, 263*, 2784–2787.

DiStefan, J.M., Gilpin, E.A., Choi, W.S., & Pierce, J.P. (1998). Parental influences predict adolescent smoking in the United States—1989–1993. *Journal of Adolescent Health, 22*, 466–474.

Dresler, C.M., Bailey, M., Roper, C.M., Patterson, G.A., & Cooper, J.D. (1996). Smoking cessation and lung cancer resection. *Chest, 110*, 1199–1202.

Droller, M.J. (1998). Bladder cancer: State-of-the-art-case. *CA: A Cancer Journal for Clinicians, 48,* 269–284.

Edwards, N.B., Murphy, J.K., Downs, A.D., Ackerman, B.J., & Rosenthal, T.L. (1989). Doxepin as an adjunct to smoking cessation: A double-blind pilot study. *American Journal of Psychiatry, 146,* 373–376.

Elder, J.P., Molgaard, C.A., & Gresham, L. (1988). Predictors of chewing tobacco and cigarette use in a multiethnic public school population. *Adolescence, 23,* 689–702.

Elder, J.P., Wiley, M., de Moor, C., Sallis, J.F., Elkhart, L., Edwards, C., Erickson, A., Golbeck, A., Hovell, M., & Johnston, D. (1993). The long term prevention of tobacco use among junior high school students: Classroom and telephone interventions. *American Journal of Public Health, 83,* 1239–1244.

Elders, M.J., Perry, C.L., Eriksen, M.P., & Giovino, G.A. (1994). The report of the Surgeon General: Preventing tobacco use among young people. *American Journal of Public Health, 84,* 543–547.

Emont, S.L., & Cummings, K.M. (1987). Weight gain following smoking cessation: A possible role for nicotine replacement in weight management. *Addictive Behavior, 12,* 151–155.

Endicott, J.N. (1998). Head and neck oncology. In L. Balducci, G. Lyman, & W. Ershler (Eds.), *Comprehensive geriatric oncology* (pp. 673–678). Baltimore: Harwood Academic Publishers.

Engeland, A., Andersen, A., Haldorsen, T., & Tretli, S. (1996). Smoking habits and risk of cancers other than lung cancer: 28 years' follow-up of 26,000 Norwegian men and women. *Cancer Causes and Control, 7,* 497–506.

Engeland, A., Bjorge, T., Haldorsen, T., & Tretli, S. (1997). Use of multiple primary cancers to indicate associations between smoking and cancer incidence: An analysis of 500,000 cancer cases diagnosed in Norway during 1953–1993. *International Journal of Cancer, 70*(4), 401–407.

Evans, N., Farkas, A., Gilpin, E., Berry, C., & Pierce, J.P. (1995). Influence of tobacco marketing and exposure to smokers on adolescent susceptibility to smoking. *Journal of the National Cancer Institute, 87,* 1538–1545.

Fagerstrom, K.O., Kunze, M., & Schoberberger, J.C. (1996). Nicotine dependence versus smoking prevalence. *Tobacco Control, 5,* 52–56.

Feldman, J.G., Hazan, M., Nagarajan, M., & Kissin, B. (1975). A case control investigation of alcohol, tobacco, and diet in head and neck cancer. *Preventive Medicine, 4,* 444–463.

Fibiger, H.C., & Phillips, A.G. (1987). Role of catecholamine transmitters in brain reward systems; Implications for the neurobiology of affect. In J. Engel & L. Oreland (Eds.), *Brain reward systems and abuse* (pp. 61–74). New York: Raven Press.

Fiore, M.C., Bailey, W.C., & Cohen, S.J. (1996). *Smoking cessation clinical practice guideline No. 18* (AHCPR Publication No. 96–0690). Rockville, MD: U.S. Department of Health and Human Services.

Fiore, M.C., Bailey, W.C., Cohen, S.J., et al. (2000). *Treating tobacco use and dependence: Clinical practice guideline.* Rockville, MD: U.S. Department of Health and Human Services, Public Health Service.

Fiore, M.C., Novotny, T.E., Pierce, J.P., Giovino, G.A., Hatziandreu, E.J., Newcomb, P.A., Surawicz, T.S., & Davis, R.M. (1990). Methods used to quit smoking in the United States. *JAMA, 263,* 2760–2766.

Flynn, B.S., Worden, J.K., Secker-Walder, R.H., Badger, G.J., Geller, B.M., & Costanza, M.C. (1992). Prevention of cigarette smoking through mass media and school programs. *American Journal of Public Health, 82*, 827–834.

Flynn, B.S., Worden, J.K., Secker-Walder, R.H., Pirie, P.L., Badger, G.J., & Carpenter, J.H. (1997). Long term responses of higher and lower risk youths to smoking prevention interventions. *Preventive Medicine, 26*, 389–394.

Fox, S.A., Roetzheim, R.G., & Kington, R.S. (1998). Barriers to cancer prevention in the older person. *Clinics in Geriatric Medicine, 13*(1), 79–75.

Frank, E., Winkleby, M.A., Altman, D.G., Rockhill, B., & Fortmann, S.P. (1991). Predictors of physician cessation advice. *JAMA, 266*, 3139–3144.

Germain, C.P. (1992). Cultural care: A bridge between sickness, illness, and disease. *Holistic Nursing Practice, 6*, 1–9.

Giarelli, E. (1999). Smoking prevention in adolescent girls: Health promotion strategies for nurses. *Journal of School Nursing, 15*, 23–28.

Glassman, A.H. (1993). Cigarette smoking: Implications for psychiatric illness. *American Journal of Psychiatry, 150*, 546–553.

Gold, D.R., Wang, X., Wypij, D., Speizer, F.E., Ware, J.H., & Dockery, D.W. (1996). Effects of cigarette smoking on lung function in adolescent boys and girls. *New England Journal of Medicine, 335*, 931–937.

Gold, E.B., & Goldin, S.B. (1998). Epidemiology of and risk factors for pancreatic cancer. *Surgical Oncology Clinics of North America, 7*(1), 67–91.

Gourlay, S. (1994). A placebo-controlled study of three clonidine doses for smoking cessation. *Clinical Pharmacology Therapies, 55*, 64–69.

Grabowski, J., & Hall, S.M. (1985). Tobacco use, treatment strategies, and pharmacological adjuncts: An overview. *NIDA Research Monograph, 53*, 1–14.

Griebel, B., Wewers, M.E., & Baker, C.A. (1998). The effectiveness of a nurse managed minimal smoking cessation intervention among hospitalized patients with cancer. *Oncology Nursing Forum, 25*, 897–902.

Gritz, E.R. (1991). Smoking and smoking cessation in cancer patients. *British Journal of Addiction, 86*, 549–554.

Gritz, E.R., Carr, C.R., & Marcus, A.C. (1991). The tobacco withdrawal syndrome in unaided quitters. *British Journal of Addiction, 86*, 57–69.

Gritz, E.R., Thompson, B., Emmons, K., Okene, J.K., McLerran, D.F., & Nelson, I.R. (1998). Gender differences among smokers and quitters in the Working Well Trial. *Preventive Medicine, 27*, 553–561.

Gross, J., Stitzer, M.L., & Maldonado, J. (1989). Nicotine replacement: Effects on post cessation weight gain. *Journal of Consulting and Clinical Psychology, 57*, 87–92.

Hall, S.M. (1990). *Weight gain prevention after smoking cessation: A cautionary note.* Paper presented at the National Heart, Lung and Blood Institute and Body Weight Conference, Memphis, TN.

Hall, S.M., Reus, V.I., Munoz, R.F., Lees, K.L., & Humfleet, G. (1998). Nortriptyline and cognitive-behavioral therapy in the treatment of cigarette smoking. *Archives of General Psychiatry, 55*, 683–690.

Hayford, K.E., Patten, C.A., Rummans, D.R., Schroeder, K.P., & Offord, I.T. (1999). Efficacy of bupropion for smoking cessation in smokers with a former history of major depression or alcoholism. *British Journal of Psychiatry, 174*, 173–178.

Haynes, S.G., Harvey, C., Montes, H.M., Nickens, H., & Cohen, B.H. (1990). Patterns of cigarette smoking among Hispanics in the United States: Results from HHANES 1982–1984. *American Journal of Public Health, 80*(Suppl.), 47–54.

Hecht, J.P., Emmons, K.M., Brown, R.A., Everett, K.D., Farrell, N.C., Hitchcock, P., & Sales, S.D. (1994). Smoking interventions for patients with cancer: Guidelines for nursing practice. *Oncology Nursing Forum, 21,* 1657–1666.

Henschke, C.I., McCauley, D.I., Yankelevitz, D.F., Naidich, D.P., McGuinness, G.M., Olli, S., Libby, D.M., Pasmantier, M., Koizumi, J., Altorki, N.K., & Nasser, K. (1999). Early Lung Cancer Action Project: Overall design and findings from baseline screening. *Lancet, 354,* 99–105.

Hermanson, B., Omenn, G.S., Kronmal, R.A., & Gersh, B.J. (1988). Beneficial six-year outcome of smoking cessation in older men and women with coronary artery disease: Results from the CASS Registry. *New England Journal of Medicine, 310,* 1365–1369.

Higgins, M.W., Enright, P.L., Kronmal, R.A., Schenker, M.B., Anton-Culver, H., & Lyles, M. (1993). Smoking and lung function in elderly men and women. *JAMA, 269,* 2741–2748.

Hoel, D.G., Davis, D.L., & Miller, A.B. (1992). Trends in cancer mortality in 15 industrialized countries, 1969–1986. *Journal of the National Cancer Institute, 84,* 313–320.

Hollen, P.J., Hobbie, W.L., & Finley, S. (1999). Testing the effects of a decision-making and risk reduction program for cancer-surviving adolescents. *Oncology Nursing Forum, 26,* 1475–1486.

Horn, D., Courts, A.F., Taylor, M.R., & Solaman, S.E. (1959). Cigarette smoking among high school students. *American Journal of Public Health, 49,* 1497.

Hsing, A.W., McLaughlin, J.K., & Hrubec, Z. (1991). Tobacco use and prostate cancer: 26-year follow-up of U.S. veterans. *American Journal of Epidemiology, 133,* 437–441.

Hsing, A.W., McLaughlin, J.K., & Schuman, L.M. (1990). Diet, tobacco use, and fatal prostate cancer: Results from the Lutheran Brotherhood Cohort Study. *Cancer Research, 50,* 6836–6840.

Hughes, J.R., Goldstein, M.G., Hurt, R.D., & Shiffman, S. (1999). Recent advances in the pharmacotherapy of smoking. *JAMA, 281,* 72–76.

Hughes, J.R., Gust, S., Skoog, K., Keenan, R., & Fenwick, J. (1991). Symptoms of tobacco withdrawal: A replication and extension. *Archives of General Psychiatry, 48,* 52–59.

Hurt, R.D. (1997). A comparison of sustained-release bupropion and placebo for smoking cessation. *New England Journal of Medicine, 337,* 1195–1202.

Husten, C.G. (1998). Cigarette smoking. In E.A. Blechman & K.D. Brownell (Eds.), *Behavioral medicine and women* (pp. 425–430). New York: Guilford Press.

Husten, C.G., Shelton, D.M., Chrimson, J.H., Lin, Y.C., Mowery, P., & Powell, F.A. (1997). Cigarette smoking and smoking cessation among older adults: United States, 1965–1994. *Tobacco Control, 6*(3), 175–180.

International Society of Nurses in Cancer Care. (1999). Tobacco use and health: Position statement. *International Cancer Nursing News, 11,* 5.

Jacobs, D.R., Adachi, H., Mulder, I., Kromhout, D., Menotti, A., Nissinen, A., & Blackburn, H. (1999). Cigarette smoking and mortality risk: Twenty-five year follow-up of the Seven Countries Study. *Archives of Internal Medicine, 159,* 733–740.

Jajich, C.J., Ostfeld, A.M., & Freeman, D.H. (1984). Smoking and coronary heart disease mortality in the elderly. *JAMA, 252*, 2831–2834.

Jarvis, M.J., Tunstall-Pedoe, H., Feyerabend, C., Vesey, C., & Saloojee, Y. (1987). Comparison of tests used to distinguish smokers from non-smokers. *American Journal of Public Health, 77*, 1435–1438.

Jason, L.A., Berk, M., Schnopp-Wyatt, D.L., & Talbot, B. (1999). Effects of enforcement of youth access laws on smoking prevalence. *American Journal of Community Psychology, 27*, 143–160.

Ji, B., Shu, X., Linet, M., Zheng, W., Wacholder, S., Gao, Y., Ying, D., & Jin, F. (1997). Parental cigarette smoking and the risk of childhood cancer among offspring of non-smoking mothers. *Journal of the National Cancer Institute, 89*, 238–244.

Johnston-Early, A., Cohen, M.H., Minna, J.D., Paxton, L.M., Fossieck, B.E., Ihde, D.C., Bunn, P.A., Matthews, M.J., & Makuch, R. (1980). Smoking abstinence and small cell lung cancer survival: An association. *JAMA, 244*, 2175–2179.

Jones, R.L., Nguyen, A., & Man, S.F. (1998). Nicotine and cotinine replacement when nicotine nasal spray is used to quit smoking. *Psychopharmacology, 137*, 345–350.

Kabat, G.C., Chang, C.J., & Wynder, E.L. (1994). The role of tobacco, alcohol use, and body mass index in oral and pharyngeal cancer. *International Journal of Epidemiology, 23*, 1137–1144.

Kaplan, S.D., Lanier, A.P., Merritt, R.K., & Siegel, P.Z. (1997). Prevalence of tobacco use among Alaska Natives: A review. *Preventive Medicine, 26*, 460–465.

Kawachi, I., Coditz, G.A., & Stampfer, M.J. (1993). Smoking cessation and decreased risk of stroke in women. *JAMA, 269*, 232–236.

Kawachi, I., Coditz, G.A., & Stampfer, M.J. (1994). Smoking cessation and time course of decreased risks of coronary heart disease in middle-aged women. *Archives of Internal Medicine, 154*, 169–175.

Kelder, S.H., Perry, C.L., Klepp, L.I., & Lytle, L.L. (1994). Longitudinal tracking of adolescent smoking, physical activity, and food choice behaviors. *American Journal of Public Health, 84*, 1121–1126.

Kendrick, J.S., & Merritt, R.K. (1996). Women and smoking: An update for the 1990s. *American Journal of Obstetrics and Gynecology, 175*, 528–535.

Kennedy, B.J. (1998). Aging and cancer. In L. Balducci, G. Lyman, & W. Ershler (Eds.), *Comprehensive geriatric oncology* (pp. 1–6). Baltimore: Harwood Academic Publishers.

Khoury, E.L., Warheit, G.J., Zimmerman, R.S., Vega, W.A., & Gil, A.G. (1996). Gender and ethnic differences in the prevalence of alcohol, cigarette, and illicit drug use over time in a cohort of young Hispanic adolescents in South Florida. *Women & Health, 24*, 21–40.

King, G., Bendel, R., & Delaronde, S.R. (1998). Social heterogeneity in smoking among African Americans. *American Journal of Public Health, 88*, 1081–1085.

King, G., Poledenak, A.P., & Bendel, R. (1999). Regional variation in smoking among African Americans. *Preventive Medicine, 29*, 126–132.

Klonoff-Cohen, H.S., Edelstein, S.L., Lefkowitz, E.S., Srinivasan, I.P., Kaegi, D., Chang, J.C., & Wiley, K.J. (1995). The effect of passive smoking and tobacco exposure through breast milk on sudden infant death syndrome. *JAMA, 273*, 795–798.

Kokotailo, P.K., Adger, H., Duggan, A.K., Repke, J., & Joffe, A. (1992). Cigarette, alcohol, and other drug use by school age pregnant adolescents: Prevalence, detection, and associated risk factors. *Pediatrics, 90*, 328–334.

Koopmans, J.R., Slutske, W.S., Heath, A.C., Neale, M.C., & Boomsma, D.I. (1999). The genetics of smoking initiation and quantity smoked in Dutch adolescent and young adult twins. *Behavior Genetics, 29*, 383–393.

Kuczynski, A. (1999, December 12). Tobacco's newest billboards are the pages of its magazine. *The New York Times*, pp. A1, C1.

LaCroix, A.Z., Lang, J., & Scherr, P. (1991). Smoking and mortality among older men and women in three communities. *New England Journal of Medicine, 324*, 1619–1625.

Landis, S.H., Murray, T., Bolden, S., & Wingo, P.A. (1998). Cancer statistics, 1998. *CA: A Cancer Journal for Clinicians, 48*, 6–29.

Lewin, F., Norell, S.E., Johansson, H., Gustavsson, P., Wennerberg, J., Biorklund, A., & Rutqvist, L.E. (1998). Smoking tobacco, oral snuff, and alcohol in the etiology of squamous cell carcinoma of the head and neck: A population-based case-referent study in Sweden. *Cancer, 82*, 1367–1375.

Lichtenstein, E. (1997). Behavioral research contributions and needs in cancer prevention and control: Tobacco use prevention and cessation. *Preventive Medicine, 26*, 57–63.

MacMahon, B. (1982). Risk factors for cancer of the pancreas. *Cancer, 50*, 2676–2680.

Madden, P.A., Heath, A.C., Pedersen, N.L., Kaprio, J., Kosdenvuo, M.J., & Martin, N.G. (1999). The genetics of smoking persistence in men and women: A multicultural study. *Behavior Genetics, 29*, 423–431.

Markides, K.S., Coreil, J., & Ray, L.A. (1987). Smoking among Mexican Americans: A three generation study. *American Journal of Public Health, 77*, 708–711.

Mashberg, A., Garfinkle, A., & Harris, S. (1981). Alcohol as a primary risk factor in oral squamous carcinoma. *CA: A Cancer Journal for Clinicians, 31*, 146–155.

Mashberg, A., & Samit, A. (1995). Early diagnosis of asymptomatic oral and oropharyngeal squamous cancers. *CA: A Cancer Journal for Clinicians, 45*, 328–351.

McDermott, R., Sarvela, P., Hoalt, P., Bajracharya, S., Marty, P., & Emery, E. (1992). Multiple correlates of cigarette use among school students. *Journal of School Health, 62*, 146–150.

McGee, R., & Stanton, W.R. (1993). A longitudinal study of reasons for smoking in adolescents. *Addiction, 88*, 265–271.

McNeill, A.D. (1991). The development of dependence on smoking in children. *British Journal of Addiction, 86*, 589–592.

McNeill, A.D., Jarvis, M.J., Stapleton, J.A., Russel, M.S., Eiser, J.R., Gammage, P., & Gray, E.M. (1988). Prospective study of factors predicting uptake of smoking in adolescents. *Journal of Epidemiology and Community Health, 43*, 72–78.

Meijer, B., Branski, D., Knoll, K., & Kerem, E. (1996). Cigarette smoking habits among school children. *Chest, 110*, 921–926.

Mendenhall, W.M., Million, R.R., Stringer, S.P., & Cassisi, N.J. (1999). Squamous cell carcinoma of the glottic larynx: A review emphasizing the University of Florida philosophy. *Southern Medical Journal, 92*, 385–393.

Merletti, F., Boffetta, P., Ciccone, G., Mashberg, A., & Terracine, B. (1989). Role of tobacco and alcoholic beverages in the etiology of cancer of the oral cavity/oropharynx in Torino, Italy. *Cancer Research, 49*, 4919–4924.

Mermelstein, R.J. (1987). *Preventing weight gain following smoking cessation.* Paper presented at the Society of Behavioral Medicine Eighth Annual Scientific Session, Washington, DC.

Michalek, A.M., & Mahoney, M.C. (1994). Provision of cancer control services to Native Americans by state health departments. *Journal of Cancer Education, 9,* 145–147.

Mitzushima, Y., Kashii, T., Yoshida, Y., Sugiyama, S., & Kobayashi, M. (1996). Characteristics of lung cancer in the elderly. *Anticancer Research, 16,* 3181–3184.

Moon, T. (1998). Prostate cancer in the elderly. In L. Balducci, G. Lyman, & W. Ershler (Eds.), *Comprehensive geriatric oncology* (pp. 679–695). Baltimore, MD: Harwood Academic Publishers.

Morabia, A., & Wynder, E.L. (1991). Cigarette smoking and lung cancer cell types. *Cancer, 68,* 2074–2078.

Moreno, C., Laniado-Laborin, R., Sallis, J.F., Elder, J.P., de Moor, C., Castro, F.G., & Deosaransingh, K. (1994). Parental influence to smoking in Latino youth. *Preventive Medicine, 23,* 48–53.

Morrison, A.S., Buring, J.E., & Verhoeck, W.G. (1984). An international study of smoking and bladder cancer. *Journal of Urology, 131,* 650–654.

Mulshine, J.L., & Henschke, C.I. (2000). Prospects for lung cancer screening. *Lancet, 355,* 592–593.

Murphy, N.T., & Price, C.J. (1988). The influence of self-esteem, parental smoking, and living in a tobacco production region on adolescent smoking behaviors. *Journal of School Health, 58,* 401–405.

Murr, M.M., Sarr, M.G., & Oishi, A.J. (1994). Pancreatic cancer. *CA: A Cancer Journal for Clinicians, 44,* 304–318.

Murray, D.M., Davis-Hearn, M., Goldman, A.J., Pirie, P., & Luepker, R.V. (1988). Four and five year follow-up results from four seventh grade smoking prevention strategies. *Journal of Behavioral Medicine, 11,* 395–405.

National Cancer Institute. (1998). *Cigars: Health effects and trends.* Rockville, MD: U.S. Department of Health and Human Services.

National Center for Chronic Disease Prevention and Health Promotion. (1996). Tobacco use and usual sources of cigarettes among high school students—United States, 1995. *Journal of School Health, 66,* 222–224.

Newcomb, P.A., & Carbone, P.P. (1992). The health consequences of smoking: Cancer. *Medical Clinics of North America, 76,* 305–331.

Noland, M.P., Kryscio, R.J., Riggs, R.S., Linville, L.H., Ford, V.Y., & Tucker, T.C. (1998). The effectiveness of a tobacco prevention program with adolescents living in a tobacco-producing region. *American Journal of Public Health, 88,* 1862–1865.

Norregaard, J., Tonnesen, P., & Petersen, L. (1993). Predictors and reasons for relapse in smoking cessation with nicotine and placebo patches. *Preventative Medicine, 22,* 261–271.

Ockene, J.K. (1993). Smoking among women across the lifespan: Prevalence, interventions, and implications for cessation research. *Annals of Behavioral Medicine, 15,* 135–148.

Ockene, J.K., Hosmer, D.W., Williams, J.W., Goldberg, R.J., Ockene, I.S., & Biliouris, T. (1987a). The relationship of patient characteristics to physician delivery of advice to stop smoking. *Journal of General Internal Medicine, 2,* 337–340.

Ockene, J.K., Hosmer, D.W., Williams, J.W., Goldberg, R.J., Ockene, I.S., & Raia, T.J. (1987b). Factors related to patient smoking status. *American Journal of Public Health, 77,* 356–357.

Oncology Nursing Society. (1997). *Position paper on proposals for United States tobacco policies*. Pittsburgh, PA: Oncology Nursing Society.

Orleans, C.T. (1993). Treating nicotine dependence in medical settings: A stepped-care model. In C.T. Orleans & J.D. Slade (Eds.), *Nicotine addiction: Principles and management* (pp. 145–161). New York: Oxford Press.

Orleans, C.T., Boyd, N.R., Bingler, R., Sutton, C., Fairclough, D., Heller, D., McClatchey, M., Ward, M., Ward, J., Graves, C., Fleishner, L., & Baum, S. (1998). A self-help intervention for African American smokers: Tailoring Cancer Information Service counseling for a special population. *Preventive Medicine, 27*(5 Pt. 2), S61–S70.

Osler, M., Prescott, E., Godtfredsen, N., Hein, H.O., & Schnohr, P. (1999). Gender and determinants of smoking cessation: A longitudinal study. *Preventive Medicine, 29*, 57–62.

Paavola, M., Vartiainen, E., & Puska, P. (1996). Predicting adult smoking: The influence of smoking during adolescence and smoking among family and friends. *Health Education Research, 11*, 309–315.

Paganini-Hill, A., & Hsu, G. (1994). Smoking and mortality among residents of a California retirement community. *American Journal of Public Health, 84*, 992–995.

Parkin, D.M. (1989). Trends in lung cancer worldwide. *Chest, 96*(Suppl. 1), 5–8.

Parkin, D.M. (1994). At least one in seven cases of cancer is caused by smoking. Global estimates for 1985. *International Journal of Cancer, 59*, 494–504.

Parra-Medina, D., Talavera, G., Elder, J., & Woodruff, S.I. (1995). Role of cigarette smoking as a gateway drug to alcohol use in Hispanic junior high school students. *Journal of the National Cancer Institute Monograph, 18*, 83–86.

Patten, C.A. & Martin, J.E. (1996). Does nicotine withdrawal affect smoking cessation? Clinical and theoretical issues. *Annals of Behavioral Medicine, 18*, 190–200.

Pearce, A.C., & Jones, R.M. (1984). Smoking and anesthesia: Preoperative abstinence and perioperative morbidity. *Anesthesiology, 61*, 576–584.

Pederson, L.L., & Lefcoe, N. (1987). Short and long term prediction of self reported cigarette smoking in a cohort of late adolescents: Report of an 8-year follow-up of public school students. *Preventative Medicine, 16*, 432–447.

Perez-Stable, E.J., Marin, B.V., Marin, G., Brody, D.J., & Benowitz, N.L. (1990). Apparent under-reporting of cigarette consumption among Mexican American smokers. *American Journal of Public Health, 80*, 1057–1061.

Perez-Stable, E.J., Sabogal, F., Marin, G., Marin, B.V., & Oster-Sabogal, R. (1991). Evaluation of "Guia para dejar de fumar," a self-help guide in Spanish to quit smoking. *Public Health Reports, 106*, 564–570.

Peto, R., Lopez, A.D., Boreham, J., Thun, M., Heath, C., & Doll, R. (1996). Mortality from smoking worldwide. *British Medical Bulletin, 52*, 12–21.

Pierce, J.P., & Gilpin, E. (1995). A historical analysis of tobacco marketing and the uptake of smoking by youth in the United States: 1870–1977. *Health Psychology, 14*, 500–508.

Pierce, J.P., Gilpin, E., Burns, D.M., Whalen, E., Rosbrook, B., Shopland, D., & Johnson, M. (1991). Does tobacco advertising target young people to start smoking? Evidence from California. *JAMA, 266*, 3154–3158.

Pirie, P., Murray, D., & Luepker, R. (1991). Gender differences in cigarette smoking and quitting in a cohort of young adults. *American Journal of Public Health, 81*, 324–327.

Pohl, J.M., & Caplan, D. (1998). Smoking cessation: Using group intervention methods to treat low-income women. *The Nurse Practitioner, 23,* 13–37.

Pomerleau, C.S., Carton, S.M., Lutzke, M.L., Flessland, K.A., & Pomerleau, O.F. (1994). Reliability of the Fagerstrom Tolerance Questionnaire and the Fagerstrom Test for Nicotine Dependence. *Addictive Behaviors, 19,* 33–39.

Pomerleau, O.F. (1997). Nicotine dependence. In C.T. Bolliger & K.O. Fagerstrom (Eds.), *The tobacco epidemic* (pp. 122–131). New York: Karger.

Pomerleau, O.F., Adkins, D., & Pertschuk, M. (1978). Predictors of outcome and recidivism in smoking cessation treatment. *Addictive Behaviors, 3,* 65–70.

Pomerleau, O.F., Fertig, J.B., & Shanahan, S.O. (1983). Nicotine dependence in cigarette smoking: An empirically based, multivariate model. *Pharmacological Biochemical Behavior, 19,* 291–299.

Pomerleau, O.F., & Pomerleau, C.S. (1984). Neuroregulators and the reinforcement of smoking: Towards a biobehavioral explanation. *Neuroscience Biobehavioral Review, 8,* 503–513.

Pow-Sang, J., Friedland, J., & Einstein, A.B. (1998). Transitional cell carcinoma of the bladder. In L. Balducci, G. Lyman, & W. Ershler (Eds.), *Comprehensive geriatric oncology* (pp. 697–702). Baltimore: Harwood Academic Publishers.

Probert, J.L., Persad, R.A., Greenwood, R.P., Gillatt, D.A., & Smith, P.J. (1998). Epidemiology of transitional cell carcinoma of the bladder: Profile of an urban population in the south-west of England. *British Journal of Urology, 82,* 660–666.

Prochaska, J.O., & DiClemente, C. (1992). Stages of change in the modification of problem behaviors. *Program Behavior Modification, 28,* 183–218.

Prochaska, J.O., DiClemente, C.C., Velicer, W.F., & Rossi, J.S. (1993). Standardized, individualized, interactive, and personalized self-help programs for smoking cessation. *Health Psychology, 12,* 399–405.

Ramirez, A.G., & Gallion, K.J. (1993). Nicotine dependence among blacks and Hispanics. In C.T. Orleans & J. Slade (Eds.), *Nicotine addiction: Principles and management* (pp. 350–364). New York: Oxford University Press.

Reding, D., Fischer, V., Lappe, K., & Gunderson, P. (1996). Peer educators say no to smokeless tobacco [Abstract]. *Proceedings of the Annual Meeting of the American Society of Clinical Oncologists, 15,* 1609.

Resnicow, K., Futterman, R., Weston, R.E., Royce, J., Parms, C., Freeman, H.P., & Orlandi, M.A. (1996). Smoking prevalence of Harlem residents: Baseline results from the Harlem Health Connection Project. *American Journal of Health Promotion, 10,* 343–346.

Richardson, G.E., Tucker, M.A., Venzon, D.J., Linnoila, I., Phelps, R., Phares, J.C., Edison, M., Ihde, D.C., & Johnson, B.E. (1993). Smoking cessation after successful treatment of small cell lung cancer is associated with fewer smoking-related second primary cancers. *Annals of Internal Medicine, 119,* 383–390.

Rimer, B.K., Orleans, C.T., & Keintz, M.K. (1990). The older smoker: Status, challenges, and opportunities for intervention. *Chest, 97,* 547–553.

Rimer, B.K., Orleans, C.T., & Slade, J. (1993). *Nicotine addiction: Principles and management.* New York: Oxford University Press.

Robinson, R., Barry, M., & Bloch, M. (1993). Report of the Tobacco Policy Research Group on marketing and promotions targeted at African Americans, Latinos, and women. *Tobacco Control, 1*(Suppl.), 524–530.

Rodriguez, C., Tatham, L.M., Thum, M.J., Calle, E.E., & Heath, C.W. (1997). Smoking and fatal prostate cancer in a large cohort of adult men. *American Journal of Epidemiology, 145*, 466–475.

Romano, P.S., Bloom, J., & Syme, S.L. (1991). Smoking, social support, and hassles in an urban African American community. *American Journal of Public Health, 81*, 1415–1422.

Royce, J.M., Corbett, K., Sorensen, G., & Ockene, J. (1997). Gender, social pressure, and smoking cessation: The community intervention trial for smoking cessation (COMMIT) at baseline. *Social Science and Medicine, 44*, 359–370.

Royce, J.M., Hymowitz, N., Corbett, K., Hartwell, T.D., & Orlandi, M.A. (1993). Smoking cessation factors among African Americans and Whites. *American Journal of Public Health, 83*, 220–226.

Russell, L.B., Carson, J.L., Taylor, W.C., Milan, E., Dey, A., & Jagannathan, R. (1998). Modeling all-cause mortality: Projections of the impact of smoking cessation based on the NHEFS. *American Journal of Public Health, 88*, 630–636.

Rustin, T. (1991). *Quit and stay quit: A personal program to stop smoking.* Center City, MN: Hazelden.

Saito, R. (1991). The smoking habits of pregnant women and their husbands, and the effect on their infants. *Japanese Journal of Public Health, 38*, 124–131.

Salive, M.E., Cornoni-Huntley, J., Ostfeld, A.M., LaCroix, A.Z., Ostfeld, A.M., Wallace, R.B., & Hennedens, C.H. (1992). Predictors of smoking cessation and relapse in older adults. *American Journal of Public Health, 82*, 1268–1271.

Sarna, L. (1995). Smoking behaviors of women after diagnosis with lung cancer. *Image, 27*, 35–41.

Sarna, L. (1998). Lung cancer. In J. Holland (Ed.), *Psycho-oncology* (pp. 340–348). New York: Oxford University Press.

Sarna, L. (1999). Prevention: Tobacco control and cancer nursing. *Cancer Nursing, 22*, 21–28.

Sarna, L., Lindsey, A.M., Dean, H., Brecht, M.L., & McCorkle, R. (1994). Weight change and lung cancer: Relationships with symptom distress, functional status, and smoking. *Research in Nursing and Health, 17*, 371–379.

Sasagawa, T., Dong, Y., Saijoh, K., Satake, S., Tateno, M., & Inoue, M. (1997). Human papillomavirus infection and risk determinants for squamous intraepithelial lesion and cervical cancer in Japan. *Japanese Journal of Cancer Research, 88*, 376–384.

Sasson, M., Halley, N., & Hoffman, D. (1985). Cigarette smoking and neoplasia of the uterine cervix: Smoke constituents in cervical mucous. *New England Journal of Medicine, 312*, 315–319.

Schilling, A., Conaway, M.R., Wingate, P.J., Atkins, J.N., Berkowitz, I.M., Clamon, G.H., DiFino, S.M., & Vinciguerra, V. (1997). Recruiting cancer patients to participate in motivating their relatives to quit smoking. *Cancer, 79*, 152–160.

Schneider, N.G. (1995). Efficacy of a nicotine nasal spray in smoking cessation: A placebo-controlled, double-blind trial. *Addiction, 90*, 1671–1682.

Schwartz, A.G., & Swanson, G.M. (1997). Lung carcinoma in African Americans and whites: A population-based study in metropolitan Detroit, Michigan. *Cancer, 79*, 45–52.

Schwartz, J.S. (1987). *Review and evaluation of smoking cessation methods: The United States and Canada, 1978–1985.* Washington, DC: U.S. Government Printing Office.

Scribner, R., & Dwyer, J.M.. (1989). Acculturation and low birth weight among Latinos in the Hispanic HHANES. *American Journal of Public Health, 79*, 1263–1267.

Senore, C., Battista, R.N., Ponti, A., Segnan, N., Shapiro, S.H., Rosso, S., & Aimar, D. (1999). Comparing participants and nonparticipants in a smoking cessation trial: Selection factors associated with general practitioner recruitment activity. *Journal of Clinical Epidemiology, 2*(1), 83–89.

Shelton, D.M., Alciati, M.H., Chang, M.M., Fishman, J.A., Fues, L.A., Michaels, J., Bazile, R.J., Bridges, J.C., Rosenthal, J.L., & Kutty, L. (1995). State laws on tobacco control—United States, 1995. *Morbidity and Mortality Weekly Report, 44*, 1–28.

Shibata, A., Mack, T.M., Paganini-Hill, A., Ross, R.K., & Henderson, B.E. (1994). A prospective study of pancreatic cancer in the elderly. *International Journal of Cancer, 58*, 46–49.

Shiffman, S. (1982). Relapse following smoking cessation: A situational analysis. *Journal of Consulting and Clinical Psychology, 52*, 261–267.

Shopland, D.R., Eyre, H.J., & Pechacek, T.F. (1991). Smoking attributable cancer mortality in 1991: Is lung cancer now the leading cause of death among smokers in the United States? *Journal of the National Cancer Institute, 83*, 1142–1148.

Skjoldebrand, J., & Gahnberg, L. (1997). Tobacco preventive measures by dental care staff. An attempt to reduce the use of tobacco among adolescents. *Swedish Dental Journal, 21*, 49–54.

Solomon, L.J., & Flynn, B.S. (1993). Women who smoke. In C.T. Orleans & J. Slade (Eds.), *Nicotine addiction: Principles and management* (pp. 339–349). New York: Oxford University Press.

Sorensen, G., & Pechacek, T. (1987). Attitudes toward smoking cessation among men and women. *Journal of Behavioral Medicine, 10*, 129–137.

Sorlie, M.P., Garcia-Palmieri, M., Costas, R., Cruz-Vidal, M., & Havlik, R. (1982). Cigarette smoking and coronary heart disease in Puerto Rico. *Preventative Medicine, 11*, 304–316.

Sridhar, K.S., & Raub, W.A. (1992). Present and past smoking history and other predisposing factors in 100 lung cancer patients. *Chest, 101*, 19–25.

Stallings, M.C., Hewitt, J.K., Beresford, T., Heath, A.C., & Eaves, L.J. (1999). A twin study of drinking and smoking onset and latencies from first use to regular use. *Behavior Genetics, 29*, 409–421.

Stanton, W.R. (1995). DSM-III-R tobacco dependence and quitting during late adolescence. *Addictive Behaviors, 20*, 595–603.

Stanton, W.R., & Silva, P.A. (1992). A longitudinal study of the influence of parents and friends on children's initiation of smoking. *Journal of Applied Developmental Psychology, 13*, 423–432.

Stapleton, J.A., Russell, M.A., Feyerabend, C., Wiseman, S.M., Gustavsson, G., Sawe, U., & Wiseman, D. (1995). Dose effects and predictors of outcome in a randomized trial of transdermal nicotine patches in general practice. *Addiction, 90*, 31–42.

Steenland, K., Thun, M., Lally, C., & Heath, C. (1996). Environmental tobacco smoke and coronary heart disease in the American Cancer Society CPS-II cohort. *Circulation, 94*, 622–628.

Stewart, M.J., Brosky, G., Gillis, A., Jackson, S., Johnston, G., Kirkland, S., Leigh, G., Pawliw-Fry, B.A., Persaud, V., & Rootman, I. (1996). Disadvantaged women and smoking. *Canadian Journal of Public Health, 87*, 257–260.

Sussman, S., Parker, V.C., Lopes, C., Crippens, D.L., Elder, P., & Scholl, D. (1995). Empirical development of brief smoking prevention videotapes which target African-American adolescents. *International Journal of the Addictions, 30*, 1141–1164.

Taylor, J.A., Umbach, D.M., Stephens, E., Castranio, T., Paulson, D., Robertson, C., Mohler, J.L., & Bell, D.A. (1998). The role of N-acetylation polymorphisms in smoking-associated bladder cancer: Evidence of a gene-gene-exposure three-way interaction. *Cancer Research, 58*, 3603–3610.

Taylor, K.L., Kerner, J.F., Gold, K.F., & Mandelblatt, J.S. (1997). Ever vs. never smoking among an urban, multiethnic sample of Haitian, Caribbean, and U.S. born blacks. *Preventive Medicine, 26*, 855–865.

Terashima, T., Wiggs, B., & English, D. (1997). The effect of cigarette smoking on the bone marrow. *American Journal of Respiratory Critical Care Medicine, 155*, 1021–1026.

Thorndike, A.N., Rigotti, N.A., Stafford, R.S., & Singer, D.E. (1998). National patterns in the treatment of smokers by physicians. *JAMA, 279*, 604–608.

Tobacco Control Resource Center. (1999). *An action plan to protect the health of Massachusetts citizens and their children.* Retrieved December 1, 1999 from the World Wide Web: http://www.tobacco.neu.edu/MTCERL/blueprint.htm

Tobacco Talks. (1999). *Tobacco industry marketing to kids.* Retrieved September 21, 1999 from the World Wide Web: http://www.tobaccofreekids.org/html/tobacco_talks.html

Tominaga, S., & Kuroishi, T. (1998). Epidemiology of pancreatic cancer. *Seminars in Surgical Oncology, 15*(1), 3–7.

Tong, L., Spitz, M.R., Fueger, J.J., & Amos, C.A. (1996). Lung cancer in former smokers. *Cancer, 78*, 1004–1010.

Township of Lawrence. (1998). *An ordinance prohibiting the purchase, or within any public place, use of tobacco products by minors within the Township of Lawrence and assessing of penalties for violation thereof.* Ordinance No. 1510–97. Lawrence Township, Mercer County, New Jersey.

U.S. Department of Health Education and Welfare. (1964). *Smoking and health. Report of the Advisory Committee to the Surgeon General of the Public Health Service.* Washington, DC: Author.

U.S. Department of Health and Human Services. (1988). *The health consequences of smoking: Nicotine addiction: A report of the Surgeon General.* Rockville, MD: U.S. Office on Smoking and Health.

U.S. Department of Health and Human Services. (1990). *The health benefits of smoking cessation: A report of the Surgeon General.* Rockville, MD: Public Health Service, Centers for Disease Control.

U.S. Department of Health and Human Services. (1994). *Tobacco use among young people: A report of the Surgeon General.* Rockville, MD: Author.

U.S. Department of Health and Human Services. (1998). *Tobacco use among U.S. racial/ethnic minority groups: A report of the Surgeon General.* Washington, DC: Author, Centers for Disease Control, National Center for Chronic Disease Prevention and Health Promotion, Office on Smoking and Health.

U.S. Environmental Protection Agency. (1993). *Respiratory health effects of passive smoking: Lung cancer and other disorders.* Washington, DC: Author.

van Reek, J., Knibbe, R., & van Iwaarden, T. (1993). Policy elements as predictors of smoking and drinking behavior: The Dutch cohort study of secondary school children. *Health Policy, 26*, 5–18.

Voorhees, C.C., Stillman, F.A., Swank, R.T., Heagerty, P.J., Levine, D.M., & Becker, D.M. (1996). Heart, body, and soul: Impact of church based smoking cessation interventions on readiness to quit. *Preventive Medicine, 25,* 277–285.

Wagenknecht, L., Cutter, G., Haley, N., Sidney, S., Manolio, T., Hughes, G., & Jacobs, D. (1990). Racial differences in serum cotinine levels among smokers in the coronary artery risk development in adults study. *American Journal of Public Health, 80,* 1053–1056.

Waldron, I., & Lye, D. (1989). Employment, unemployment, occupation, and smoking. *American Journal of Preventative Medicine, 5,* 142–149.

Weibel, F.J. (1997). Health effects of passive smoking. In C.T. Bolliger & K.O. Fagerstrom (Eds.), *The tobacco epidemic* (pp. 107–121). New York: Karger.

Wewers, M.E., Jenkins, L., & Mignery, T. (1997). A nurse-managed smoking cessation intervention during diagnostic testing for lung cancer. *Oncology Nursing Forum, 24,* 1419–1423.

Whiteman, M.C., Fowkes, F.G., Deary, L.J., & Lee, A.J. (1997). Hostility, cigarette smoking and alcohol consumption in the general population. *Social Science and Medicine, 44,* 1089–1096.

Willett, W.C., Green, A., & Stampfer, M.J. (1987). Relative and absolute excess risks of coronary heart disease among women who smoke cigarettes. *New England Journal of Medicine, 317,* 1303–1309.

Wills, T.A., & Cleary, D.S. (1997). The validity of self reports of smoking: Analysis by race/ethnicity in a school sample of urban adolescents. *American Journal of Public Health, 87,* 56–61.

Wills, T.A., Schreibman, S., Benson, G., & Vaccaro, D. (1994). Impact of parental substance use on adolescents: A test of a mediational model. *Journal of Pediatric Psychology, 19,* 537–555.

Wilson, D.M., Killen, J.D., Hayward, D., Robinson, T.N., Hammer, I.K., Draemer, H.C., Varady, A., & Taylor, C. (1994). Timing and rate of sexual maturation and the onset of cigarette and alcohol use among teenage girls. *Archives of Pediatric Adolescent Medicine, 148,* 789–795.

Wingo, P.A., Ries, L.A., Giovino, G.A., Miller, D.S., Rosenberg, H.M., Shopland, D.R., Thun, M.J., & Edwards, B.K. (1999). Annual report to the nation on the status of cancer, 1973–1996. With a special section on lung cancer and tobacco smoking. *Journal of the National Cancer Institute, 91,* 675–690.

Winnail, S.D., Valois, R.F., McKeown, R.E., Sanders, R.P., & Pate, R.R. (1995). Relationship between physical activity level and cigarette, smokeless tobacco, and marijuana use among public high school adolescents. *Journal of School Health, 65,* 438–442.

Woolf, A.D. (1997). Smoking and nicotine addiction: A pediatric epidemic with sequelae in adulthood. *Current Opinions in Pediatrics, 9,* 470–477.

Worden, J.K., Flynn, B.S., Solomon, L.J., Secker-Walker, R.H., Badger, G.J., & Carpenter, J.H. (1996). Using mass media to prevent cigarette smoking among adolescent girls. *Health Education Quarterly, 23,* 453–468.

World Bank. (1999). *Curbing the epidemic: Governments and the economics of tobacco control.* Washington, DC: Author.

World Health Organization. (1999). *Combating the tobacco epidemic, WHO Report 1999: Making a difference* (pp. 65–79). Geneva Switzerland: Author.

Wynder, E.L., & Hoffman, D. (1994). Smoking and lung cancer: Scientific challenges and opportunities. *Cancer Research, 54*, 5284–5295.

Wynder, E.L., Mabuchi, K.L., & Whitmore, W.F. (1971). Epidemiology of cancer of the prostate. *Cancer, 28*, 344–360.

Wyser, C., & Bolliger, C.T. (1997). Smoking-related disorders. In C.T. Bolliger & K.O. Fagerstrom (Eds.), *The tobacco epidemic* (pp. 78–106). New York: Kargert.

Yesner, R. (1993). Pathogenesis and pathology of lung cancer. *Clinical Chest Medicine, 14*, 17–30.

Zhu, B., Liu, M., Shelton, D., Liu, S., & Giovino, G. (1996). Cigarette smoking and its risk factors among elementary school students in Beijing. *American Journal of Public Health, 86*, 368–375.

Zhu, B., Liu, M., Wang, S., He, G., Chen, D., Shi, J., & Shang, J. (1992). Cigarette smoking among junior high school students in Beijing, China, 1988. *International Journal of Epidemiology, 21*, 854–861.

Ziedonis, D.M., Wyatt, S.A., & George, T.P. (1998). Current issues in nicotine dependence and treatment. In E.F. McCance-Katz & T. Kosten (Eds.), *New treatments for chemical addictions* (pp. 1–34). Washington, DC: American Psychiatric Association.

Ziv, A., Boulet, J.R., & Slap, G.B. (1999). Utilization of physician offices by adolescents in the United States. *Pediatrics, 104*, 35–42.

CHAPTER 10

Environmental Health and Cancer Control

Barbara Sattler, RN, DrPH, and Jane A. Lipscomb, RN, PhD, FAAN

"Environmental health comprises those aspects of human health, including quality of life, that are determined by physical, chemical, biological, and social and psychological problems in the environment. It also refers to the theory and practice of assessing, correcting, controlling, and preventing those factors in the environment that can potentially affect adversely the health of present and future generations."

—World Health Organization (1993)

Introduction

The environment has radically changed over the last century. Tens of thousands of man-made chemicals have been introduced—chemical compounds that did not exist before the 1940s. These synthetic chemicals can be found in food, air, soil, and water—in workplaces, schools, homes, and communities. Many can be found in human bodies, including breast milk, in measurable amounts. Unfortunately, virtually no information exists regarding the human health effects associated with much of this steady, unnatural stream of chemicals. Of the 3,000 high-production industrial chemicals, publicly accessible toxicity data are available for only 29% of them (Goldman, 1998). For a factor with such potential for harm, a disturbing paucity of information exists about the contaminants in the environment and the health effects associated with environmental exposures (see Figures 10-1 and 10-2).

Exposure to environmental chemicals is one factor that, combined with people's dietary and smoking habits and exposure to sunlight, radiation, viruses, and other factors, can lead to the development of cancer. Simply stated, carcinogens cause cancer. Therefore, the carcinogen load in the environment (food, water, air, and soil) will affect cancer incidence. In a recent epidemiologic study of twins, in which researchers set out to identify the "gene versus environment" determinants

Figure 10-1. Information Regarding Chemical Exposures

• Of the top 20 environmental pollutants that were reported to the Environmental Protection Agency (EPA) in 1997, nearly three-quarters were known or suspected neurotoxics. This accounted for more than a billion pounds of neurotoxics being released into the air, water, and land.
• 1.2 billion pounds of pesticide products are intentionally and legally released each year in the United States.
• More than 50% of Americans live in an area that exceeds current national ambient air quality standards for ozone, NO_2, SO_2, and particulates.
• Forty states have issued one or more health advisories for mercury in their waterways. Ten states have issued advisories for every lake and river within the state's borders.
• More than 50 million U.S. homes contain some lead-based paint.
• Mobile sources (traffic) are the number-one cause of air pollution in the United States.
• Antibiotics, 17b-estradiol, caffeine, and acetaminophen have been found in measurable quantities in national streams.
• *Consumer Reports* measured dioxin in leading-brand beef baby food that exceeded the EPA allowable quantity by 100 times.
• Thirty million Americans drink water that exceeds one or more of the EPA's safe drinking water standards. Contaminants include lead, other heavy metals, nitrites, dioxin, hydrocarbons, pesticides, radon, and cyanide. (Some of the contaminants are naturally occurring.)
• Ten million U.S. children live within four miles of a toxic waste dump.

Note. Based on information from Goldman, 1998; Schettler et al., 2000; U.S. Environmental Protection Agency, 1998a.

Figure 10-2. Human Health Concerns Associated With Environmental Exposures

• The environment has a primary role in causing cancer.
• One million children in the United States have levels of lead in their blood that exceed acceptable standards. This may be associated with a range of health effects, including behavioral (e.g., violent behavior) and cognitive effects.
• Combinations of commonly used agricultural chemicals, in levels typically found in groundwater, can significantly influence immune and endocrine systems and neurological function in lab animals.
• Thirty-seven pesticides registered for use on food are neurotoxic organophosphates.
• Environmental tobacco smoke is responsible for seven million lost school days by children.
• Radon exposure is the second leading cause of lung cancer.
• Epidemiologic studies suggest a relationship between nitrates in drinking water and juvenile diabetes.
• Twenty percent of children in Arkansas who live near a herbicide manufacturing plant have herbicide residues in their urine.
• Several pesticides and herbicides have been linked to leukemia.
• Endocrine disruptors are a diverse group of compounds that include plasticizers, polychlorinated biphenyls, many pesticides, and dioxin. These compounds are so pervasive that studies have shown them to appear in 95% of the population. The concern is that when exposure to these chemicals occurs very early in life, these compounds have the potential to disrupt critical endocrine pathways, with a potential to disrupt effects on reproductive, neurologic, and immunologic systems.
• Dioxin mimics estrogen.
• The environment plays a role in asthma. Poor indoor and outdoor air quality increases asthma's severity. Asthma is the number-one reason that children miss school and the number-one reason why they are hospitalized in the United States.

Note. Based on information from Schettler et al., 1999; U.S. Environmental Protection Agency, 1997, 1998a, 2001a.

of cancer, the environment was found to have the "principal" role in causing cancer (Lichtenstein et al., 2000).

In 1958, Congress passed the Delaney Clause, a statute that set a zero tolerance for carcinogenic additives in processed foods. This was the last time a zero-tolerance statute was passed for carcinogens in the environment. All subsequent environmental protection standards, including those for the quality of the air people breathe and the water they drink, allow for an "acceptable" amount of carcinogens based on a risk assessment. The risk assessments are based on the carcinogenic potential to affect a population of otherwise healthy, middle-aged, 154-pound, White males (Browner, 1998). Additionally, almost all risk assessments are made by extrapolating data from animal studies and animal models to predict the effects on humans. A budding body of scientific knowledge is developing regarding the vulnerability of embryos, fetuses, and children to carcinogenic and other toxic exposures. Yet, current standards do not take these vulnerabilities into account. The exception to this rule is the Food Quality Protection Act (FQPA) of 1996, which specifically calls for attention to the susceptibility of growing children to suffer bodily harm as a result of exposure to toxic pesticides in food. Several pesticides currently found on foods are known or suspected carcinogens.

The purpose of this chapter is to alert nurses to the importance of environmental health to public health and to provide an overview of environmental health principles, information, and resources essential to the successful integration of environmental health into professional nursing practice. Unfortunately, the body of nursing knowledge concerned with how environmental factors contribute to health problems is not well developed. In modern nursing, healthcare professionals must begin to integrate the new knowledge of the environment's effect on human health to develop prevention strategies, plan early detection activities, and promote policies to reduce the carcinogen load in food, water, and air.

The chapter begins by describing those concepts or basic principles that allow nurses to contribute to the risk assessment of environmental health threats and hazards. Next is a discussion of various risk-management options available to address these risks. Specific examples of sentinel occupational causes of cancer are detailed in the third section, followed by a presentation of environmental health policies. The domains of home, school, community, and work are presented as a framework for assessing risk, and examples of environmental hazards found in each of these settings are discussed. Finally, nursing implications for the integration of environmental health are presented.

As nurses are concerned with the prevention of cancer, understanding environmental health principles and, specifically, how they can reduce the carcinogen load in the environment is extremely important. The environment is one of the primary determinants of individual and community health. Nurses must understand the basic mechanisms and pathways of exposure to environmental health hazards, basic prevention and control strategies, the interdisciplinary nature of effective interventions, and the role of research, advocacy, and policy.

Healthcare professionals need to remember that environmental health is not new to nursing. Florence Nightingale was a pioneer in the field of environmental health, identifying the role of cleanliness and fresh air in healing and eloquently writing about the need and value of assessing and controlling environmental causes of disease. In the midst of unprecedented technological advances in medicine, professional nursing is just now rediscovering its strong environmental health roots. In 1997, the American Nurses Association House of Delegates passed a resolution to reduce the production of toxic pollution within the healthcare sector, thereby contributing to the reduction of the carcinogen load as well as other non-cancer-causing toxins in the environment. In this resolution, nurses are committed to educating their colleagues about medical waste issues, exploring alternatives to polyvinylchloride (PVC) plastics (which cause carcinogenic air pollutants when incinerated), creating mercury-free healthcare delivery settings, reducing dioxin emissions from hospital waste incinerators, and developing standards for by-products from the use of laser and electrosurgery units. Nurses have the potential to be environmental health pioneers within the modern healthcare industry. The goal of this chapter is to provide nurses with the background knowledge that, to date, has not been part of the traditional nursing education, enabling them to expand their practice into the critical area of environmental health.

Basic Principles of Environmental Health Risk Assessment

Humans may be exposed to chemical, biological, and radiological risks in all environments in which they live, work, play, and learn. These exposures can have an impact on human health. Many factors influence the relationship between environment and health; host factors such as age, sex, genetic makeup, and underlying diseases can affect disease outcomes, the level or dose of the exposure, and the length of time exposed. Chemical and radiological exposures can be cumulative. Nurses must assess a person's total exposure to environmental risks to understand and address potential health threats. Environmental health is based upon a public health model with an emphasis on prevention. Primary prevention in environmental health includes pollution prevention, product design, engineering controls, purchasing choices, and education.

The assessments of environmental health, potential environmental exposures, and the potential for environmentally related diseases are performed on an individual and community-wide basis. Individual environmental health assessments should take into account all of the potential exposures that a person may have in the home, workplace, school, or community. Several environmental health assessment tools have been developed that can be adapted to a variety of settings. For example, the Agency for Toxic Substances and Disease Registry (ATSDR) created a general assessment tool, as well as a tool for assessing pesticide exposures in agricultural settings. ATSDR is an agency of the U.S. Public Health Service that is responsible for investigating health effects related to hazardous wastes. The Children's Environmental Health Network, a national nonprofit organization, developed an environmental health assessment tool to identify in-home hazards to children (see Figure 10-3). A national resource guide on children's environmental health can be found on its Web site at www.cehn.org.

Figure 10-3. Environmental Hazards Checklist for Home Assessments

Family name: _____

Address: _____

Housing

Type of housing? _____ Ownership?
How old? _____ ___Rental
Condition? _____ ___Owner occupied
_____ ___Public housing

Renovation/repairs occurring? __Yes __No Describe: _____
Existence of rodents/insects? __Yes __No Describe: _____
Existence of molds/fungi? __Yes __No Describe: _____
What is source of drinking water? Describe: _____

Heating sources

Uses gas stoves/ovens for heating? __Yes __No Adequate ventilation? __Yes __No
Uses fireplaces/woodburning stoves? __Yes __No What is burned?_____
Wood smell indoors? __Yes __No
Evidence of smoke/soot? __Yes __No
Uses kerosene heaters? __Yes __No

Environmental tobacco smoke

Household members smoke? __Yes __No Regular visitors smoke? __Yes __No
Smoking allowed in the car? __Yes __No
Indoor air pollution—Formaldehyde and asbestos
Sources of formaldehyde? __Yes __No Describe: _____
(particle board, urea in foam insulation, other)
Potential asbestos hazards? __Yes __No Describe: _____
*(friable pipe/boiler insulation, old vinyl linoleum,
wall board repair, home renovation/repairs)*

Air pollution—Toxic organic hydrocarbons

Uses cleaners/polishes/air fresheners/disinfectants? __Yes __No
Uses glue solvents/varnishes/building materials? __Yes __No
Where are these materials stored? _____

Pest/mold/fungi control

Home garden? __Yes __No Use of pesticides outdoors? __Yes __No
Evidence of rodents/insects? __Yes __No Use of pesticides in home? __Yes __No
Use of pesticides on children? __Yes __No What type? _____
Is re-entry after pesticide use according to instructions? __Yes __No
Evidence of molds/fungi? __Yes __No

Pets

Are there pets in the home? __Yes __No Are the pets ill? Describe: _____

Lead

Paint in poor repair? __Yes __No
Uses leaded pottery/dishes? __Yes __No
Crafts/other activities with lead? __Yes __No
Drinking H_2O tested for lead? __Yes __No
Housemembers exposed to lead at work? __Yes __No

(Continued on next page)

Figure 10-3. Environmental Hazards Checklist for Home Assessments *(Continued)*

Playground hazards
Where do children play? _____
Any hazardous play equipment or toys? _____

Home/paraoccupational activities
Housemembers work with heavy metal solvents/dust? __Yes __No
What materials are used? _____

Medications
Housemembers use home remedies? __Yes __No   Which ones? _____
Where are medications stored? _____

Household members' occupations and activities
Housemembers' occupation and potential
exposures: Housemembers' activities and hobbies:

_____   _____
_____   _____
_____   _____
_____   _____

Surrounding neighborhood
Is home or school close to highways? __Yes __No   Near to industries? __Yes __No
Are any of the neighboring businesses
Dry cleaning? __Yes __No   Radiator/auto repair? __Yes __No
Photoprocessing? __Yes __No
Where do children spend most of their time? _____
_____

Notes _____
_____
_____

Assessment completed by: _____   Date: _____

Community environmental health assessments should include the identification of potential exposures in water (e.g., drinking water), air (e.g., indoor air), dust (e.g., lead-based paint), soil (e.g., exposures from current and previous land use), and radiation (e.g., ionizing and nonionizing). No single source is available for this information, and community-specific information often is not available. Assessments may depend on information that is extrapolated from aggregate national, statewide, county, or metropolitan exposure data. The use of Geographic Information Systems (GIS), computerized mapping of graphically related data that can be specific to environmental exposures and health outcomes, is providing an emerging method for assessing community risks to environmental exposures and potential health problems. More information on GIS may be obtained from ATSDR or geography departments in universities.

Risk is defined as the probability of an undesirable health outcome arising from exposure to a hazard (National Library of Medicine, 2001). Risk assessment, in the context of environmental health, has several different meanings. Risk assessment, in regulatory terms, refers to the use of available scientific information, usually a combination of epidemiologic, animal toxicologic, and in vitro data, to evaluate and estimate exposure to a substance and the resulting adverse health effects (National Library of Medicine). Mathematical models then are used to convert these biologic data into regulatory action.

Risk assessment includes four steps. First, hazard identification relies on toxicologic and epidemiologic studies of the potential of a substance to cause harm. Next, a dose-response evaluation measures whether the harm increased with increasing doses of the substance. Third, exposure assessment involves the measurement of the amount of the chemical or other harmful substance to which a population is exposed, with a goal of estimating the dose. Fourth, risk characterization involves estimating the public health or environmental impact of the problem based on knowledge of characteristics of the population at risk (National Research Council, 1983).

Risk assessment, in public health terms, has a much broader definition and includes individual- and community-level assessments, which were described earlier in this section. In addition to determining the nature and magnitude of the risk associated with a community's exposure to an environmental hazard, an assessment of a community's resources, including its cohesiveness and leadership, should be part of a more comprehensive risk assessment.

Environmental Epidemiology

Epidemiology plays a crucial role in the risk assessment of most environmental exposures. Epidemiologic methods developed for use in the study of chronic disease, in general, are applicable to the field of environmental epidemiology. Study designs range from experimental, the most conclusive design, to case series and cluster investigation, the least conclusive design. An experimental study design rarely is applied to environmental exposure because of the ethicalities of intentionally exposing individuals or communities to environmental hazards. Analytic designs, using cohort and case control, frequently are the design of choice to study the human health effects in relation to environmental exposures (Checkoway, Crawford-Brown, & Pearce, 1989).

Cluster investigations, a technique applied less frequently to the study of other etiologic agents thought to be associated with cancer, often are used in the field of environmental epidemiology. Cluster investigations refer to the evaluation of a reported excess of disease clustering in space or time. These investigations often are conducted in response to community concerns about an excess of cancer or birth defects (Brown, 1999; Caldwell, 1990). The highly documented investigation of childhood leukemia associated with contaminated well water in Woburn, MA, in the late 1970s, which was featured in the best-selling novel and motion picture *A Civil Action*, is an example of such an investigation (Harr, 1995). Historically, cluster investigations concerning environmental exposures have rendered mostly negative or equivocal results. In the cases where the investigations have been most convincing, the disease in question has been rare and specific for the putative etiologic exposure, such as asbestos causing mesothelioma (Brown).

Environmental epidemiology is limited by many of the same challenges inherent in the study of all chronic diseases. First, environmental exposures often are

345

poorly defined and measured, leading to the potential for misclassification of cohort members on exposure status. Second, a very limited understanding of the health effects of mixed chemical exposures makes studying the most common type of environmental exposure situations particularly challenging. Third, often a relatively small number of individuals (e.g., a community) constitute the study populations, yielding limited statistical power to detect an association between the exposure(s) of concern and health effects. Fourth, a lack of understanding of the variability in the susceptibility of segments of the populations (e.g., the poor, children, elderly) is a challenge to any epidemiologic study of a heterogeneous population and limits the ability to compare findings across studies. Finally, the long latency between many environmental exposures and the evidence of chronic disease (e.g., cancer) creates additional challenges to exposure assessment (Checkoway et al., 1989). In spite of these limitations, epidemiologic studies of environmental causes of disease have contributed greatly to the field of environmental health during the past century. With improved methods of exposure assessment, namely the increased availability of biomarkers of exposure, epidemiology will contribute even more significantly to environmental risk assessment in the future (Checkoway et al.).

Toxicology

The traditional definition of toxicology is "the science of poisons." As the understanding of how various agents can cause harm to humans and other organisms has increased, a more descriptive definition of toxicology is "the study of the adverse effects of chemicals or physical agents on living organisms." These adverse effects may occur in many forms, ranging from immediate death to subtle changes that are not realized until months or years later. They may occur at various levels within the body, such as an organ, a type of cell, or a specific biochemical process. Terminology and definitions for materials that cause toxic effects are not always used consistently in the literature. The most commonly used terms are "toxicant," "toxin," "poison," "toxic agent," "toxic substance," and "toxic chemical."

"Toxicant," "toxin," and "poison" often are used interchangeably in the literature; however, subtle differences exist. A toxic agent is anything that can produce an adverse biological effect. It may be chemical (e.g., cyanide), physical (e.g., radiation), or biological (e.g., snake venom) in form. A toxic substance is simply a material that has toxic properties. It may be a discrete toxic chemical or a mixture of toxic chemicals. For example, lead chromate, asbestos, and gasoline are all toxic substances. Lead chromate is a discrete toxic chemical. Asbestos is a toxic material that does not consist of an exact chemical composition but rather a variety of fibers and minerals. Gasoline also is a toxic substance rather than a toxic chemical in that it contains a mixture of many chemicals. Toxic substances may not always have a constant composition.

The dose-response relationship is a fundamental and essential concept in toxicology. It correlates exposures and the spectrum of induced effects. Generally, the higher the dose, the more severe the response. The dose-response relationship is based on observed data from experimental animal, human clinical, or cell studies. Knowledge of the dose-response relationship establishes causality that the chemical has induced the observed effects, establishes the lowest dose where an induced effect occurs (the threshold effect), and determines the rate at which injury builds up (the slope for the dose response).

Basic nursing education typically does not include toxicology. However, all nurses learn basic pharmacology. Toxicology is profoundly similar to pharmacology. The distinction is that pharmacology is the study of the effects of a subset of chemicals called drugs. In pharmacology, the beneficial effects as well as the unintentional side effects and toxic effects of the drugs are studied. Side effects include nonpathological reactions such as nausea and diarrhea, and toxic effects include reactions such as liver or kidney damage. Toxicologists only study the negative effects of exposures to chemicals, radiation, or biological toxicants. To assist nurses in understanding the basic principles of toxicology, a side-by-side comparison of pharmacology and toxicology terms and concepts is presented (see Figure 10-4).

Figure 10-4. Side-By-Side Comparison of Basic Concepts in Toxicology and Pharmacology

Pharmacology	Toxicology
Pharmacology is the scientific study of the origin, nature, chemistry, effects, and use of drugs.	Toxicology is the science that investigates the adverse effects of chemicals on health.
Dose refers to the amount of a drug absorbed from an administration.	Dose refers to the amount of a chemical absorbed into the body from a chemical exposure.
A drug can be administered one time, short term, or long term.	Exposure is the actual contact that a person has with a chemical. Exposure can be one time, short term, or long term.
A dose-response curve graphically represents the relationship between the dose of a drug and the response elicited.	A dose-response curve describes the relationship of the body's response to different amounts of an agent such as a drug or toxin.
Routes of administration: oral, internal, IV, dermal, or topical	Routes of entry: ingestion, inhalation, or dermal absorption
With drugs, therapeutic responses (desirable) and side effects (undesirable) occur. Beyond the therapeutic dose, a drug may become toxic.	In toxicology, only the toxic effects are of concern. Toxicity is the ability of a chemical to damage an organ system, to disrupt a biochemical process, or to disturb an enzyme system.
Potency refers to the relative amount of drug required to produce the desired response.	The potency of a toxic chemical refers to the relative amount it takes to elicit a toxic effect compared with other chemicals.
Biological monitoring is performed for some drugs—clotting time is monitored in patients on anticoagulants like warfarin. Actual drug levels are measures for some drugs like digoxin.	Biological monitoring is performed for some toxic exposures, such as blood lead levels, or metabolites of chemicals, such as cotines, for environmental tobacco smoke exposures.

Note. Based on information from Sattler, 1998.

The effects of both drugs and hazardous chemicals can be immediate (acute) or long-term or can present after a latency period often associated with cancer outcomes. Host factors must be considered when looking at therapeutic drugs or hazardous chemicals. Factors such as age, sex, genetics, weight, drugs that the person may be taking, pregnancy status, and other factors may affect the therapeutic or toxic effect of a drug or a chemical. Drugs are taken voluntarily and may be taken under the supervision of a licensed healthcare provider, whereas hazardous chemical exposures almost always are involuntary. The regulatory process by which a drug comes to the market includes several stages of testing, starting with animal testing and moving slowly and carefully on to human testing. The regulatory process for hazardous chemicals that are not food, drug, cosmetic, or pesticide in nature does not require any original toxicologic testing. As such, many household products, school art supplies, and commercial products have had little or no testing.

Resources for information regarding drugs include the *Physician's Drug Reference*, Poison Control Centers, and the National Library of Medicine. For hazardous chemicals, Poison Control Centers and the Occupational Safety and Health Administration (OSHA) manual are good sources of information, and the National Library of Medicine has a substantial holding of information that is accessible via the Internet at www.toxnet.nlm.nih.gov.

Carcinogenicity is a common toxic endpoint that scientists study. The International Agency for Research on Cancer (IARC), an agency of the World Health Organization, serves as a clearinghouse for information on research about the human carcinogenicity of various agents. IARC classifications, discussed later in this chapter, are taken into account and incorporated into the risk assessments when environmental standards are promulgated.

Nurses, particularly oncology nurses, should be aware of the environmental science underpinning standards that aim to protect people from cancer-causing exposures. As advocates, nurses belong in a collaborative role with the environmentalists and scientists who set exposure limits to carcinogens in air, water, and food. Of all the disciplines involved in deciding how many cases of exposure-related cancers are "acceptable," nurses will be the ones most inclined to say "none." As such, it would be enormously helpful for oncology nurses and their representatives to become politically active and sit at the policy-making tables.

Children and Environmental Health

Any discussion of toxicology must include consideration of the unique risks that environmental hazards pose to children. The importance of addressing this aspect is underscored by the fact that, until the present time, children routinely have not been included in environmental risk assessment. Most environmental health regulations are based on studies of adult males despite the fact that children's immature organ systems are especially sensitive to environmental hazards. Of great concern is that exposure to environmental toxicants may disrupt and cause permanent damage to the developing nervous, immune, and respiratory systems of young children. In addition, the metabolic and physiological processes of children differ dramatically from those of adults, resulting in a higher rate of absorption through cutaneous, respiratory, and gastrointestinal routes. Normal childhood behavior also poses additional risks. Children's normal exploratory behavior (e.g., hand-to-mouth activity, crawling) increases opportunities to ingest toxicants, such as lead-based paint. Their dietary habits also differ both qualitatively and quantitatively from adults in their exposure to residues on foods such as fruits. Young children consume significantly greater amounts of fruits and fruit juices than older children and adults. Children today are cumulatively exposed to more toxins throughout their lifetime than previous generations. For all of these reasons, the FQPA of 1996 includes provisions for the consideration of children's special vulnerability to environmental toxicants in future chemical risk assessments. It also requires consideration of the total estimated pesticide exposure and an additional 10-fold safety factor in permissible exposure limits for toxic pesticide exposures to children (FQPA, 1996).

Risk Management of Environmental Hazards

Risk management is the process of evaluating alternative strategies for reducing risk and prioritizing or selecting among them. Risk-management strategies often involve policy development. This policy development may include regulatory, legislative, or voluntary options and may be targeted at the local, state, national, or international level.

Environmental engineering is a critical tool in risk management. Engineering strategies to control exposure to environmental hazards is similar to what is referred to as the "hierarchy of controls" in industrial settings. The industrial hygiene model for controlling hazards follows a hierarchy beginning with changes to the work process or environment that do not rely on individual behavior change and proceeding to less effective "quick fixes" until more effective controls become available (see Figure 10-5). According to this model, the substitution of a hazardous substance with one that is less hazardous should be considered the first approach to hazard reduction (Smith & Schneider, 2000). When substitution is infeasible, isolating the worker from the hazard is considered a second line of control, followed by engineering controls such as local exhaust ventilation of hazard-

---

Figure 10-5. Industrial Hygiene Hierarchy of Control of Hazards

1. Eliminate hazard or substitute with less-hazardous chemicals.
2. Isolate the hazardous chemicals.
3. Create engineering controls such as ventilation systems to dilute the hazard.
4. Create administrative controls to reduce the amount of time a person is exposed.
5. Use personal protective equipment such as gloves, goggles, or respirators to prevent exposure.
6. Additionally, ensure that anyone working with potentially hazardous substances is trained appropriately.

Note. Based on information from Smith & Schneider, 2000.

ous fumes or dust from the breathing zone of a worker. Next in the hierarchy are administrative controls, which include policies and procedures for limiting exposure to hazards and training of workers. Finally, personal protective equipment, such as respirators, can be used when higher-level controls are unavailable, but they should be viewed as a temporary measure (Smith & Schneider).

The theory behind the "hierarchy of controls" is that it is much more effective to change the environment than to rely on changing personal behavior to reduce exposure, especially involuntary exposures found in the workplace. A relevant example of the application of hierarchy of controls can be found in the healthcare setting related to the problem of needlestick injuries. To date, 17 states and the District of Columbia have passed legislation requiring the use of safer needle devices to prevent the transmission of higher virulent infectious diseases from the nearly one million needlestick injuries incurred by U.S. healthcare workers annually (International Health Care Worker Safety Center at the University of Virginia Health System, 2001). Despite the availability of this technology for more than a decade, healthcare workers have been forced to rely on a much lower level of protection, namely universal precautions—a combination of administrative controls and personal protective equipment. This legislation mandating the use of engineering controls is a direct result of decades of advocacy on the part of labor unions representing healthcare workers.

Within the context of community exposures to environmental hazards, a similar hierarchy can be described. Source reduction clearly should be the goal of any environmental risk-management strategy. Waste minimization should be viewed as a second line of defense against environmental degradation. Reuse and recycling, although important and laudable risk-management strategies, are further down the list of desirable measures, along with emissions control and waste cleanup. Any successful risk-management program will include controlling the hazard at a number of these levels, with the goal being to apply the highest level of control whenever possible, even when such a program forces technology (i.e., the industry is pushed to develop new technology). Any risk-management strategy should include education of all involved parties regarding the nature of the risk and the costs and benefits of proposed risk-management strategies.

Coalition building and community action often are critical to successful risk management. Community members always should be "at the table" in decision making involving risk management. In addition, legal remedies, such as recent class-action lawsuits against the lead pigment industry for the public health costs associated with lead poisoning and lead abatement, may be used to manage risk in combination with the aforementioned strategies.

Finally, society as a whole debates the issue of what is "acceptable risk" relative to environmental hazards. In general, recent environmental regulations have set a level of acceptable risk at anywhere from one death in a population of one hundred thousand to one in one million. Unfortunately, workplace standards issued during the past decade have not been nearly as protective of human health. In 1998, OSHA promulgated a permissible exposure limit (PEL) for workplace exposures to 1,3-butadiene, a chemical used in the production of rubber for the tire industry. Butadiene has been associated with an increased risk of leukemia among exposed workers. The PEL for butadiene was based on a risk of more than approximately eight cancer deaths in one thousand workers (OSHA).

An important concept in the management of environmental risks is that of the Precautionary Principle, which assumes that where there are possible threats of serious or irreversible damage, lack of scientific certainty shall not be used as a reason for postponing cost-effective measures to prevent environmental degradation.

Advocacy

Advocacy, at the class or policy level, is inherent in the practice of environmental health and nursing. In an environmental health context, it involves advocating for risk-management options on the part of a community. Case advocacy is well known to professional nursing in the role of advocating for individual patients and families to solve problems or secure needed services related to their care. Class advocacy, on the other hand, is less inherent to professional nursing. Class advocacy is overtly more political and focuses on changing the system of opportunities to further the interests of a group or community. Advocacy of this type is aimed at changing policy, institutional systems, and norms, laws, or patterns of resource allocation to improve the health of the group or community.

Advocacy aimed at social change can be examined from a typology formulated by Warren (1963). He described a three-level approach to class advocacy, in which nurses must play an active role at each level.

First are collaborative approaches, such as membership on planning or advisory committees, in which citizens and authorities (or professionals) work together toward a common goal. Second, campaigning approaches (e.g., lobbying) require that citizens (in this case, nurses) work singly or collectively to persuade authorities that new problem definitions and solutions are needed. The third level is contest strategies, such as protest marches, which involve citizens organizing to force attention to community problems that they feel are being ignored or mishandled by authorities. Because nurses often are the primary healthcare providers in poor and disenfranchised communities, nurse advocacy on behalf of these communities is critical to improving their health.

Environmental justice refers to the disproportionate environmental risks that are borne by poor and minority communities. The environmental health status in poor communities is subject to a multiplying effect from poor housing stock, poor nutrition, poor access to health care, unemployment, underemployment, and employment in the most hazardous jobs. The environmental risk burden generally is greater for minorities and those who are economically disadvantaged because they are exposed to a greater number and intensity of environmental pollutants in food, air, water, homes, and workplaces.

Information sharing may be inadequate or less effective in economically disadvantaged communities because of language and literacy issues as well as the challenge of understanding technical language in warning signs and other "right to know" materials. Indicators of increased risk are measured by residents' proximity to hazardous waste sites, polluting industries, and incinerators. Poor people also are more likely to live in substandard housing with friable asbestos, deteriorating lead paint, and yards with contaminated soil. In 1993, the Environmental Justice Act was passed; this was followed in 1994 by the signing of Executive Order 12898, "Federal Actions to Address Environmental Justice in Minority Populations." These efforts created policies to more comprehensively reduce the incidence of environmental inequity by mandating that every federal agency act in a manner to address and prevent illnesses and injuries. Nurses, in their role as advocates, should be aware of the potentiating effect that racism and poverty can play on risks from environmental health exposures.

Risk Communication

Risk communication, in the context of environmental health, is the art of communicating about the potential health risks associated with environmental exposures. Four elements should be considered in risk communication: the message, the messenger, the audience, and the context.

Message: Environmental health risks often are hard to define. The exposures may be difficult to characterize; the exposed population may be very diverse in age and other important variables; exposures always will include multiple chemicals because it is the nature of the environment (whereas most scientific investigation examines individual chemicals and rarely chemical mixtures); and sometimes the science is inconclusive or nonexistent.

Messenger: For risk communication to succeed, the audience must perceive the source (messenger) of the information as trusted and credible. A variety of elements that affect trust are outlined in the risk-communication literature. Nurses are considered highly credible and trustworthy sources of information within the community.

Audience: Audiences bring their own individual biases to any forum in which environmental health risks might be discussed. Their distrust of the messenger may be based on their feelings about someone from the government, industry, or an environmental organization. An audience may trust or distrust a messenger based on his or her age, race, or gender. An excellent body of literature is available on risk perception.

Context: Risk communication does not occur in a vacuum. It usually happens when an environmental health threat has been perceived—be it a potentially contaminated water supply, an accidental release of a hazardous chemical, or a newly identified hazardous waste site adjacent to a daycare center. The conditions and context will influence the audience's ability to listen and trust. Additionally, the media can play an important part in a community's understanding and bias regarding environmental risks.

Substantial attention has been paid to understanding people's perception of risks. Sandman (1987) has compared and contrasted variables that may affect the perception of risks from exposures within the environment. Figure 10-6 indicates which characteristics usually are associated with a perception of less risk and which are associated with more risk.

The U.S. Environmental Protection Agency (EPA) proposed a code of conduct that will enhance the success of a risk-communication initiative. It is a list of basic principles that honor all of the players within a community (see Figure 10-7). Risk

Figure 10-6. Perception of Risks Based on Attributes

Less Risky	More Risky
Voluntary	Involuntary
Familiar	Unfamiliar
Controllable	Uncontrollable
Controlled by self	Controlled by others
Fair, not memorable	Memorable
Not dreaded	Dreaded
Chronic	Acute
Diffuse in time and space	Focused in time and space
Not fatal	Fatal
Immediate	Delayed
Natural	Artificial
Individual mitigation possible	Individual mitigation impossible
Detectable	Undetectable

Figure 10-7. Seven Cardinal Rules of Risk Communication

1. Accept and involve public as a legitimate partner.
2. Plan carefully and evaluate your efforts.
3. Listen to your audience.
4. Be honest, frank, and open.
5. Coordinate and collaborate with other credible sources.
6. Meet the needs of the press.
7. Speak clearly and with compassion.

Note. From Seven Cardinal Rules of Risk Communication, by V.T. Covello and F.H. Allen, 1988, Washington, DC: U.S. Environmental Protection Agency.

communication often is the responsibility of the community or public health nurse, who is called upon to bridge the communication gap between the general public and the scientific or technical community. Nurses in clinical settings may be called upon to deliver risk communication, particularly if a patient's family believes that their family member's illness is associated with an environmental exposure.

Accessing Information and the "Right to Know"

Access to information about environmental risks in food, water, and soil is provided via an array of federal and state statutes and through a variety of agencies. A range of environmental right-to-know statutes and regulations exist. Store-bought foods are labeled, an example of a consumer's right-to-know requirement. Access to information about food is provided by a number of regulations and implemented by the Department of Agriculture and the U.S. Food and Drug Administration (FDA). The food packaging company must include a list of ingredients and nutritional content, along with any health-related designations, such as "organic."

Access to information about water is provided under two statutes: the Clean Water Act and the Safe Drinking Water Act. The Clean Water Act was created to protect the nation's waterways, and the Safe Drinking Water Act protects drinking water from source water to tap. Through the Safe Drinking Water Act, those who purchase water from a water provider have the right to know what is in their drinking water. Annually, as part of the drinking water right-to-know regulations, the water utility must provide a consumer confidence report or right-to-know report listing the contaminants (chemical, biological, and radiological) that have exceeded EPA standards within the last year and their probable sources. The EPA requires testing of drinking water and the public water supply for approximately 80 chemicals and agents.

Industrial contaminants that are released into the air or water are reportable, based on the chemical and its quantity, under the right-to-know component of the Superfund Amendments and the Reauthorization Act (SARA, 1986). SARA requires polluters to report certain effluents and emissions. This information is available on the EPA Web site at www.epa.gov. These data provide the basis for information on the Web site www.scorecard.org, an excellent source for community environmental assessments.

Environmental and Occupational Causes of Cancer

Environmental (i.e., nongenetic) causes of cancer have been recognized for centuries. In 1761, John Hill, MD, of London published the first modern clinical report of environmental carcinogenesis—a description of cancer of the nasal passages among tobacco snuff users (Frumkin & Thun, 2000). In 1775, Sir Percival Pott, MD, first recognized an occupational cancer, scrotal skin cancer, among chimney sweeps who were heavily exposed to soot (Frumkin & Thun). Since then, many chemicals or other substances found in the industrial setting have been recognized as human carcinogens. The identification of environmental carcinogens is critical because most occupational cancers are completely preventable via workplace controls. Because industry sources contribute significantly to overall community exposure, the reduction of exposure to carcinogens in the industrial sector subsequently will have an impact on the health of the larger community.

Current knowledge about environmental carcinogens is derived from a combination of human, animal, and in vitro studies. Epidemiology has contributed to the understanding of the association between most industrial exposures and human carcinogens. However, epidemiologic studies of environmental causes of cancer face a number of methodological challenges, including a limited study cohort, especially in the case of workplace exposures, historically poor exposure assessment, and the problem of a long latency between exposure and the expression of disease (Checkoway et al., 1989). Moreover, epidemiologic studies are relatively expensive and may take many years to complete. Most importantly, they provide evidence of carcinogenicity after the fact. These limitations to epidemiology are extremely important considerations given the number of chemicals for which carcinogenicity testing is needed. An estimated 72,000 chemicals currently are used in commerce (excluding food additives, drugs, cosmetics, and pesticides), the majority of which have had limited testing for their effects on human health and the environment (INFORM, 1995). In fact, the EPA found that of the approximately 3,000 chemicals ever produced in the United States at an annual volume of at least one million pounds, only 7% have been fully evaluated for toxicity, and a much smaller percentage have been examined for carcinogenicity (EPA, 1998). For these reasons, animal studies and in vitro testing increasingly have played a critical role in determining the carcinogenic potential of environmental agents. In addition, the technique of analyzing structure relations for chemical configurations that are similar to known carcinogens allows for the early identification of potential carcinogens that can be tested further (Rugo & Fishman, 1997). For example, after the discovery of an association between beta-naphthylamine and bladder cancer, all benzidine-derived dyes became suspect and were recognized as potential human carcinogens (Rugo & Fishman).

In 1969, IARC initiated a program to evaluate the carcinogenic risk of chemicals to humans and to produce monographs on individual chemicals. IARC established standardized criteria for the classification of chemical carcinogens based on human, animal, and in vitro data. IARC designates chemicals and processes as human carcinogens (Group 1), probable human carcinogens (Group 2A), and possible human carcinogens (Group 2B). Group 2A chemicals reflect limited evidence in humans and sufficient evidence in animals, whereas Group 2B chemicals reflect limited evidence in humans without sufficient evidence in animals or sufficient evidence in animals without any human data. Of the 750 chemicals, industrial processes, and personal habits that IARC has evaluated to date, Group 1 contains 50 and Group 2 contains almost 250 (IARC, 2000). Several other systems for classifying carcinogens exist, including the National Toxicology Program (NTP). NTP, an organization within the National Institute of Environmental Health Sciences, develops and maintains the U.S. government's official list of known or "anticipated" human carcinogens, as of this writing, it contains 198 substances (IARC, 2000).

Reviews of the IARC lists (see Tables 10-1 and 10-2) demonstrate that the majority of human carcinogens identified to date have been associated with industrial work processes. The IARC list does not address the workplace contribution or attributable risk—the fraction of a disease that can be attributed to a specific etiology—to the overall burden of cancer. This question has been the subject of tremendous debate, but it generally is accepted that 2%–8% of all cancers can be attributed to workplace exposures (Doll & Peto, 1981). This proportion is distributed unequally across various segments of the population, with males historically experiencing a higher risk than women and, similarly, workers in the manufacturing section experiencing a disproportionate share of the burden. Less is known about cancer caused by chemical exposures outside of the workplace, where people are exposed to complex mixtures of ambient environmental carcinogens, usually at much lower levels. For environmental cancers (other than occupational), estimating an attributable fraction is much more difficult. Therefore, risk estimates for community-based exposures usually are based on extrapolated risks from occupational studies and animal testing.

Table 10-1. Established Human Occupational and Environmental Carcinogens (Internal Agency for Research on Cancer Group 1*)

Exposure	Sources of Exposure	Cancer Site
Aflatoxins	Grains, peanuts (farm workers)	Liver
4-Aminobiophenyl	Rubber industry	Bladder
Arsenic and its compounds	Insecticides	Lung, skin, hemangiosarcoma
Asbestos	Insulation, friction products, auto repair	Lung, mesothelioma, respiratory tract, gastrointestinal system
Benzene	Chemical industry	Leukemia
Benzidine	Rubber and dye industries	Bladder
Beryllium and its compounds	Aerospace, nuclear, electric, and electronics industries	Lung
Bis-Chlormethyl ether and chlormethyl methyl ether	Chemical industry	Lung
Cadmium and its compounds	Metalworking industry, batteries, soldering, coatings	Prostate
Chromium (VI) compounds	Metal plating, pigments	Lung
Coal tar pitches	Coal distillation	Skin, scrotum, lung, bladder
Coal tars	Coal distillation	Skin, lung
Dioxin (2, 3, 7, 8-Tetrachlorodibenzo-p-dioxin)	Herbicide production and application	All sites combined, lung
Erionite	Environmental (Turkey)	Mesothelioma
Ethylene oxide	Sterilant in healthcare settings	Lymphoma, leukemia
Hepatitis B and C virus	Healthcare settings	Liver
Human immunodeficiency virus	Healthcare settings	Sarcoma
Mineral oils	Machining, jute processing	Skin
Mustard gas	War gas production	Lung
2-Napthylamine	Rubber and dye industries	Bladder
Nickel compounds	Nickel refining and smelting	Lung, nasal sinus
Radon and its decay products	Indoor environments, mining	Lung
Schistosoma hematobium infection	Farming and other outdoor work in endemic areas	Bladder
Shale oils	Energy production	Skin

(Continued on next page)

Table 10-1. Established Human Occupational and Environmental Carcinogens (Internal Agency for Research on Cancer Group 1*) *(Continued)*

Exposure	Sources of Exposure	Cancer Site
Silica, crystalline	Hard rock mining, sandblasting, glass and porcelain manufacturing	Lung
Solar radiation	Outdoor work	Skin
Soot	Chimneys, furnaces	Skin, lung
Sulfuric acid containing strong inorganic acid mists	Metal, fertilizer, battery, and petrochemical industries	Larynx, lung
Talc (with asbestiform fibers)	Talc mining, pottery manufacturing	Lung
Vinyl chloride	Plastic industry	Hemangiosarcoma
Wood dust	Wood and furniture industries	Nose, sinuses

*Group 1 also includes foods, tobacco, and viruses not listed here.

Note. Based on information from IARC, 2000.

Prevention and Control of Environmental Cancer

Primary prevention of environmentally related cancer is accomplished through risk-management strategies. Progressive regulatory and voluntary actions that employ a "hierarchy of control" model of environmental hazard control hold the promise for the primary prevention of many environmentally related cancers. Primary prevention also can be achieved by increasing the awareness and environmental history-taking skills of all healthcare professionals. Often, the astute clinician is in the best position to identify a link between an environmental exposure and a health complaint. In the case of occupational exposure, the identification of an illness within an individual worker can contribute to the primary prevention of a similar illness among other exposed workers (Rosenstock & Cullen, 1994).

Secondary prevention, namely early detection through screening, also requires the enhanced recognition of the environmental-relatedness of cancers on the part of primary care and other healthcare professionals. Without training and recognition of the importance of taking an occupational and environmental health history, many opportunities for the secondary prevention of environmentally caused cancers will be missed, or workers will return to a hazardous environment where their illness may worsen. Even with an enhanced awareness of the need for appropriate history taking, the long latency period between exposure to environmental carcinogens and the expression of disease will result in many linkages left unexplored. Fortunately, the increasing availability of biomarkers of exposure (e.g., blood lead that historically has been available for assessing recent lead exposure) is likely to play a major role in both clinical practice and epidemiologic studies of environmental carcinogens over the next decade.

Table 10-2. Probable Human Occupational and Environmental Carcinogens (Internal Agency for Research on Cancer Group 2A*)

Exposure	Sources of Exposure	Cancer Site
Acrylamide	Polyacrylamide manufacturing	Thyroid, adrenal, mammary gland, skin
Benz[a]anthracene	Coal distillation	Lung
Benzidine-based dyes	Dye industry	Bladder
Benzo[a]pyrene	Coal and petroleum-derived products	Lung, skin, bladder
1, 3-Butadiene	Polymer and latex production	Skin
Captafol	Fungicide	Lung
Creosotes	Wood preservatives	Skin, scrotum
Dibenz[a, h]anthracene	Coal distillation	Lung
Diesel exhaust	Motor vehicles, mining	Lung
Diethyl sulfate	Petrochemical industry	Larynx
Dimethyl carbamoyl chloride	Chemical manufacturing	Lung
1, 2-Dimethylhydrazine	Rocket propellants and fuels, boiler water treatments, chemical reactants, medicines, cancer research	Liver
Dimethyl sulfate	Former war gas, now used in chemical industry	Lung
Epichlorhydrin	Resin manufacturing, solvent	Respiratory tract
Ethylene dibromide	Fumigant, gas additive	
Formaldehyde	Chemical manufacturing, tissue preservative	Nasopharynx
4,4'-methylene bis(2-chloraniline) (MOCA)	Resin manufacturing	Bladder
N-nitrosodiethylamine	Solvent	Bladder
N-nitrosodimethylamine	Solvent	Bladder
Polychlorinated biphenyls	Electrical equipment	Liver
Propylene oxide	Chemical industry	Liver
Styrene oxide	Chemical industry	Bladder
Tetrachlorethylene	Dry cleaning	Esophagus, lymphoma
Toluenes, a-chlorinated	Chemical manufacturing	Liver
Toluidine, para-chloro-ortho and its strong acid salts	Diazo dye manufacturing	Bladder

(Continued on next page)

Table 10-2. Probable Human Occupational and Environmental Carcinogens (Internal Agency for Research on Cancer Group 2A*) *(Continued)*

Exposure	Sources of Exposure	Cancer Site
Trichloroethylene	Metal degreasing	Liver, lymphoma
1, 2,3-Trichlopropane	Pesticide, rubber manufacturing, solvent	Oral cavity, pancreas, kidney
tris-(2, 3-Dibromopropyl) phosphate	Flame retardant, polystyrene foam manufacturing	Lung, liver, kidney
Ultraviolet radiation A, B, and C	Outdoor work	Skin
Vinyl bromide	Plastic industry	Liver
Vinyl fluoride	Chemical industry	Liver

*Group 2A also includes medications, infectious agents, and foods not listed here.

Note. Based on information from IARC, 2000.

Selected Environmental Exposures

The following occupational and environmental hazards were selected because they represent exposures with carcinogenic potential that nurses should be familiar with. They do not necessarily represent the most toxic of hazards but provide an overview of those of great importance in the field of occupational and environmental health.

Asbestos

Asbestos is a fibrous silicate mineral found around the world that generally is considered to pose the greatest carcinogenic threat in the workplace. Two classes of asbestos exist—serpentine (commercial form chrysotile) and amphiboles (commercial forms amosite and crocidolite); 90% of the asbestos in the United States is chrysotile (Rugo & Fishman, 1997). All commercial forms have been associated with an increased risk of cancer; crocidolite is thought to be the most carcinogenic mineral. Long, thin, respirable fibers are most likely to cause pulmonary disease. Asbestos causes asbestosis (a fibrosis of the lungs), lung cancer, and mesothelioma of the peritoneum and pleura. Occupations at risk for asbestos-related cancers include asbestos miners, textile manufacturers, insulation and filter-material production workers, shipyard workers, and auto mechanics (Rugo & Fishman).

Asbestos-related lung cancer first was reported in 1934 (Rugo & Fishman, 1997). Lung cancer accounts for 20% of all deaths in asbestos-exposed cohorts, and up to 4% of all lung cancer cases are attributable to asbestos exposure (Rugo & Fishman). A latency period of approximately 20 years is thought to exist with asbestos-caused lung cancer. Lung cancer risk increases after short but intense exposure to asbestos fibers. Asbestos exposure and cigarette smoking increase the risk of lung cancer exponentially. The risk of dying from lung cancer increased 5-

fold for asbestos exposure alone, 10-fold for cigarette smoking alone, and 80-fold for both asbestos and cigarette exposure (Selikoff, Hammond, & Chanrg, 1968). Therefore, workers and their families who are at potential risk of asbestos exposure should be counseled to quit or never begin smoking.

The first case reports of mesothelioma associated with asbestos were published in the 1940s, but the problem received relatively little attention until 1960 (Rugo & Fishman, 1997). Mesothelioma of the peritoneum and pleura are uncommon and are considered "signal tumors" of exposure to asbestos. Eight percent of a cohort of 17,800 asbestos insulation workers in the United States and Canada who were followed from 1967–1976 died from malignant mesothelioma (Spirtas et al., 1994). The latency period between asbestos exposure and mesothelioma is 30 years or more. Although a known dose-response relationship exists, epidemiologic data demonstrate that variable levels of exposure to asbestos can cause mesothelioma, including "take-home" fibers on workers' clothing or contact in the home environment (Stayner, Dankovic, & Lemen, 1996).

Benzene

Benzene is a cyclic hydrocarbon resulting from the distillation of petroleum and coal tar. It is widely used in the United States, and an estimated two million workers have been exposed to this substance (Rugo & Fishman, 1997). Benzene ranks in the top 20 chemicals for production volume. It has been recognized as a potent bone marrow toxicant for nearly a century (Rugo & Fishman). In 1928, the first case of acute leukemia was reported in a worker who was heavily exposed to benzene (Rugo & Fishman). Workers exposed for five years or more have a 21-fold increased risk of death from leukemia (Richardson et al., 1992). Benzene is used in the production of plastics, resins, nylon, and synthetic fibers. It also is a natural component of crude oil, gasoline, and cigarette smoke. Unleaded gasoline contains 2% benzene. Leakage from underground storage tanks is of great concern around abandoned gas stations and other waste sites because of the risk of benzene contamination of community drinking water sources. The EPA (2001b) has set a maximum permissible level of benzene in drinking water at 0.005 milligrams per liter.

Dioxin

Dioxin is a generic name used to describe a family (75 chemical congeners) of compounds known as chlorinated dibenzo-p-dioxins. The most studied and toxic chemical in the family is 2,3,7,8-tetrachlorodibenzo-p-dioxin (2,3,7,8-TCDD). 2,3,7,8-TCDD first was discovered as a by-product of chlorinated phenols in the 1950s (Harrison, 1997). Dioxin does not occur naturally nor is it intentionally manufactured. Dioxin occurs as a contaminant in the manufacturing of certain chlorinated organic compounds. Combustion of many chlorine-containing materials, such as PVC, can produce dioxin. The incineration of medical waste that includes large quantities of PVC is a significant source of environmental exposure to dioxin. Animal studies of 2,3,7,8-TCDD have shown it to be extremely toxic and the most potent carcinogen ever tested among some species of animals. Studies of cancer in workers who were exposed to dioxin reported a significant increase in soft-tissue sarcoma, cancer of the respiratory system, and all cancers combined (Fingerhut et al., 1991), supporting the classification of 2,3,7,8-TCDD as a human carcinogen. The process by which dioxin exerts its toxicity is highly complex and beyond the scope of this chapter. Dioxin is a highly persistent chemical in the environment and has a high potential for accumulation in biologic tissues. This ubiquitous chemical has been found in all media, including air, water, soil, sediments, animals, and food. Dioxin has been found in virtually all samples of adipose tissue and serum from individuals with no previous exposure. Dioxin levels in the environment have declined substantially over the past two decades, following EPA regulations to reduce dioxin emissions (EPA, 2000b). A recent EPA risk reassessment found that the risk to humans may be somewhat higher than previously believed, even though actual exposure seems to be declining among the general population.

Electric and Magnetic Fields

Electric and magnetic fields (EMFs) are invisible lines of force created whenever electricity is generated or used. Power lines, electric wiring, and electric equipment and appliances produce EMFs. People are exposed to both types of fields, but scientists are more concerned about magnetic fields. The strength of a magnetic field depends on equipment design and current flow, not equipment size, complexity, or voltage. The frequency of an EMF is measured in hertz (Hz, or cycles per second). EMFs recently have been listed by the National Toxicology Program (NTP) as possible human carcinogens (NTP, 2001). Although the epidemiologic literature is equivocal on whether EMFs cause a variety of human cancers, a number of studies have shown an increased risk of brain cancer and leukemia among electric power and line workers and childhood leukemia among children living close to power lines (National Institute for Occupational Safety and Health [NIOSH], 1996). Several preliminary studies also have associated workplace EMFs with breast cancer (NIOSH). No federal government limits for worker or community exposure to EMFs currently exist. Although etiologic research on EMFs and cancer continues, good public health and nursing practice dictate the use of simple and low-cost measures to reduce EMF exposure, along with education of workers and community members regarding the possible hazards of magnetic fields. Because magnetic fields often drop off dramatically within approximately three feet of the source, workstations should be moved out of the three-foot range of stronger EMF sources. The avoidance of close and constant exposure to small household appliances (e.g., electric bedside alarm clocks) also may reduce household exposure to EMFs.

Environmental Tobacco Smoke

Environmental tobacco smoke (ETS), or second-hand smoke, is a complex mixture of chemicals, including carbon monoxide, nitric oxide, nitrogen oxides, benzene, formaldehyde, acetaldehyde, acrolein, particulate matter, and nicotine (Children's Environmental Health Network, 1999). ETS differs from mainstream smoke because it contains more incomplete by-products of combustion. In laboratory studies of mice, it was found to be more tumorigenic than mainstream smoke (Children's Environmental Health Network). ETS causes lung cancer in nonsmokers. A recent IARC study found that exposure to passive smoking at the workplace or through a spouse resulted in a 16% increase in the risk of lung cancer

(Boffetta et al., 1998). This increased risk is modest compared with the 20-fold risk associated with active smoking (Boffetta et al.). According to 1988–1991 data from the Third National Health and Nutrition Examination Survey, approximately 9 out of 10 nonsmokers are exposed to ETS, as measured by the levels of cotinine in their blood (Pirkle et al., 1996). These data also demonstrated that 43% of children (age 2 months to 11 years) lived in a home with at least one smoker; 37% of adult nontobacco users lived in a home with a smoker or reported exposure to ETS at work. Exposure, as measured by cotinine levels, was higher among children, non-Hispanic African Americans, and men (Pirkle et al.). Given this high prevalence of exposure to second-hand smoke, ETS is estimated to cause approximately 3,000 lung cancer deaths annually in the United States (EPA, 1992). Prevention of future cases of ETS-related lung cancer depends on the dramatic limitations of passive smoking. Home ventilation systems are ineffective at filtering out ETS. Opening windows or smoking in areas of the house where nonsmokers are not present may help to reduce exposure but will not eliminate the dangers of ETS.

Polycyclic Aromatic Hydrocarbons

Polycyclic aromatic hydrocarbons (PAHs) are a group of more than 100 different chemicals that are formed during the incomplete combustion of coal, coal tar, pitch, oil and gas, and other organic substances such as tobacco or charbroiled meat (Agency for Toxic Substances and Disease Registry [ATSDR], 1996). As previously mentioned, PAHs were first implicated in the development of cancer in 1775 by Sir Percival Pott, who reported an increased risk of scrotal cancer in chimney sweeps in London (Frumkin & Thun, 2000). Exposure to PAHs has been linked to lung cancer in coke oven workers, roofers, printers, and truckers and lung, stomach, and skin cancer in experimental animals (Rugo & Fishman, 1997). PAHs present an environmental hazard when they enter the ambient outdoor air as releases from volcanoes, forest fires, burning coal, and automobile exhaust. PAHs have been found in nearly half of National Priority List (hazardous waste) sites identified by the EPA (ATSDR, 1996).

Ultraviolet Light

Ultraviolet (UV) light is a ubiquitous environmental hazard. Excessive exposure to UV rays is a recognized cause of skin cancer. Skin cancer is the most common type of cancer, with 80%–90% of cases caused by exposure to sunlight (IARC, 1992). The well-documented deterioration of the stratospheric ozone layer has resulted in increased exposure to UV rays by humans and the ecosystem over the past several decades. This deterioration has been caused, in part, by the use of chlorofluorocarbons (CFCs) and other ozone-destructive chemicals. Despite international efforts to ban the use of CFCs, they still are used worldwide.

Vinyl Chloride

Vinyl chloride is the raw material used in the production of polyvinylchloride. Vinyl chloride also results from the breakdown of substances such as trichloroethane, trichloroethylene, and tetrachloroethylene (ATSDR, 1997). Exposure to vinyl chloride occurs mainly in the workplace (ATSDR, 1997). In 1974, a clinician reported a clustering of angiosarcoma of the liver among workers exposed to vinyl chloride polymer (Rugo & Fishman, 1997). Vinyl chloride now is recognized as a potent liver carcinogen. The latency period following first exposure is 11–37 years (Laplanche, Clavel-Chapelon, Contassot, & Lanouziere, 1992). Studies have demonstrated similar hepatic lesions among highly exposed animals (Rugo & Fishman). The current permissible exposure limit set by OSHA (1998) for vinyl chloride is one part per million during an eight-hour period, which strictly limits exposure to this carcinogen. Vinyl chloride has been found in about one-third of the EPA's National Priority List sites. Vinyl chloride formed from the breakdown of other chemicals can enter the groundwater. The EPA (2001b) requires that the amount of vinyl chloride in drinking water not exceed 0.002 milligrams of vinyl chloride per liter of water.

Environmental Health Policy

An essential competency for environmental health assessments is knowledge of the federal (as well as state and local) health and environmental statutes, regulations, and practices regarding what data are collected and how to access them. Unfortunately, very little data are collected that specifically connect environmental exposures to disease outcomes. Making these connections has been left to researchers and has been investigated primarily on a case-by-case basis. For instance, in states that have registries for cancer, birth defects, or other disease outcomes, data can explore the relationship to environmental exposures where those data exist. Pollution monitoring generally is performed by governmental agencies or polluting industries and sometimes has to be reported to the government, usually the state agency designated to enforce environmental protection standards. Several environmental statutes have been promulgated to give the public the "right to know" about the hazardous chemicals in the environment.

The EPA and its state equivalent entities are the primary agencies responsible for environmental protection. Numerous federal agencies address issues related to the environment, including safety and health in the workplace. Federal agencies have become increasingly involved in examining and monitoring the impact of the environment on public health. For example, the U.S. Department of Transportation regulates the transport of hazardous materials. The FDA regulates food safety. The ATSDR is responsible for environmental health-related issues associated with hazardous waste sites that have been designated as Superfund sites by the EPA.

The Superfund designation is derived from the 1980 federal Comprehensive Environmental Response, Compensation, and Liability Act (CERCLA) created to identify and clean up industrial hazardous waste sites that pose an active threat to human health (CERCLA, 1980). Approximately 1,200 hazardous waste sites are now on the National Priority List, and approximately half of these have contaminated the groundwater. The most common contaminant found in hazardous waste sites is trichloroethylene, a known carcinogen. Human exposures from hazardous waste sites include contaminated air, groundwater/drinking water, surface water, and soil. A physical risk of fire or explosion also may exist at these sites.

Environmental statutes and regulations may be created and implemented at the state, federal, and sometimes local level. Most environmental statutes are media specific, such as air, water, soil, and food. As with occupational health statutes, states must adhere to the federal environmental statutes. States may enforce more stringent, but not less stringent, statutes and regulations.

Environmental Protection Agency

The EPA was established in 1970 to permit coordinated and effective governmental action on behalf of the environment (National Environmental Policy Act, 1970). The EPA strives to abate and control pollution systematically by proper integration of a variety of research, monitoring, standard setting, and enforcement activities. The agency coordinates and supports research and antipollution activities by state and local governments, private and public groups, individuals, and educational institutions. The EPA also reinforces efforts among other federal agencies with respect to the impact of their operations on the environment. Each state has a designated agency that is responsible for the regulatory oversight within the state of environmental regulations and standards. The EPA's Web site (www.epa.gov) is an excellent source for general information, geographically specific information, and all of the environmental acts, regulations, and standards.

Major Environmental Laws

Many of the standards for environmental laws are established to set an exposure limit based on the potential to threaten human health. Regarding cancer-causing exposures, environmental standards have been established to minimize the carcinogen load in air, water, soil, and food. Figure 10-8 lists some of the environmental laws enacted by Congress through which the EPA carries out its efforts.

Figure 10-8. Environmental Laws

National Environmental Policy Act (NEPA)
The NEPA established the U.S. Environmental Protection Agency and a national policy for the environment and provides for the establishment of a Council on Environmental Policy. All policies, regulations, and public laws shall be interpreted and administered in accordance with the policies set forth in this act.

Federal Insecticide, Fungicide, and Rodenticide Act (FIFRA)
(Summary from FIFRA 1972). FIFRA provides federal control of pesticide distribution, sale, and use. EPA was given the authority to study the consequences of pesticide usage and requires users such as farmers and utility companies to register when using pesticides. Later amendments to the law required applicators to take certification examinations, register all pesticides used in the United States, and properly label pesticides that, if in accordance with specifications, will cause no harm to the environment.

Clean Water Act (CWA)
The CWA sets basic structure for regulating pollutants to U.S. waters. The law gave the EPA the authority to set effluent standards on an industry basis and continued the requirements to set water quality standards for all contaminants in surface water. The 1977 amendments focused on toxic pollutants. In 1987, the CWA was reauthorized and again focused on toxic pollutants, authorized citizen suit provisions, and funded sewage treatment plants.

(Continued on next page)

Figure 10-8. Environmental Laws *(Continued)*

Clean Air Act
(Summary from Clean Air Act 1970). The Clean Air Act regulates air emissions from area, stationary, and mobile sources. EPA was authorized to establish National Ambient Air Quality Standards (NAAQS) to protect public health and the environment. The goal was to set and achieve the NAAQS by 1975. The law was amended in 1977 when many areas of the country failed to meet the standards. The 1990 amendments to the Clean Air Act were intended to meet unaddressed or insufficiently addressed problems such as acid rain, ground-level ozone, stratospheric ozone depletion, and air toxins. Also in the 1990 reauthoriztion, a mandate for Chemical Risk Management Plans was included. This mandate requires industry to identify "worst case scenarios" regarding the hazardous chemicals that they transport, use, or dispose of.

Occupational Safety and Health Act
The act was passed to ensure worker and workplace safety. The goal was to make sure employers provide a workplace free of hazards, such as chemicals, excessive noise, mechanical dangers, heat or cold extremes, or unsanitary conditions. To establish standards for the workplace, the act also created the National Institute for Occupational Safety and Health as the research institution for the Occupational Safety and Health Administration.

Safe Drinking Water Act (SDWA)
The SDWA was established to protect the quality of drinking water in the United States. The act authorized the EPA to establish safe standards of purity and required all owners or operators of public water systems to comply with primary (health-related) standards.

Resource Conservation and Recovery Act (RCRA)
RCRA gave EPA the authority to control the generation, transportation, treatment, storage, and disposal of hazardous waste. RCRA also set forth a framework to manage nonhazardous waste. The 1984 Federal Hazardous and Solid Waste Amendments to this act required phasing out land disposal of hazardous waste. The 1986 amendments enabled EPA to address problems from underground tanks storing petroleum and other hazardous substances.

Toxic Substances Control Act (TSCA)
TSCA gives the EPA the ability to track the 75,000 industrial chemicals currently produced or imported into the United States. EPA can require reporting or testing of chemicals that may pose environmental health risks and can ban the manufacture and import of those chemicals that pose an unreasonable risk. TCSA supplements the Clean Air Act and the Toxic Release Inventory.

Comprehensive Environmental Response, Compensation, and Liability Act (CERCLA or Superfund)
This law created a tax on the chemical and petroleum industries and provided broad federal authority to respond directly to releases or threatened releases of hazardous substances that may endanger public health or the environment.

Superfund Amendments and Reauthorization Act (SARA)
SARA amended the Comprehensive Environmental Response, Compensation, and Liability Act with several changes and additions. These changes included increased size of the trust fund; encouragement of greater citizen participation in decision making on how sites should be cleaned up; increased state involvement in every phase of the Superfund program; increased focus on human health problems related to hazardous waste sites; new enforcement authorities and settlement tools; stressing the importance of permanent remedies and innovative treatment technologies in cleanup of hazardous waste sites, and Superfund actions to consider standards in other federal and state regulations. (Under Superfund legislation, the federal Agency for Toxic Substances and Disease Registry was established.)

(Continued on next page)

Figure 10-8. Environmental Laws *(Continued)*

Emergency Planning and Community Right-to-Know Act (EPCRA)
EPCRA, also known as Title III of SARA, was enacted to help local communities protect public health safety and the environment from chemical hazards. Each state was required to appoint a State Emergency Response Commission that was required to divide their states into Emergency Planning Districts and establish a Local Emergency Planning Committee for each district.

National Environmental Education Act
This created a new and better-coordinated environmental education emphasis at the EPA. It also created the National Environmental Education and Training Foundation.

Pollution Prevention Act (PPA)
The PPA focused industry, government, and public attention on reduction of the amount of pollution through cost-effective changes in production, operation, and use of raw materials. Pollution prevention also includes other practices that increase efficient use of energy, water, and other water resources, such as recycling, source reduction, and sustainable agriculture.

Food Quality Protection Act (FQPA)
The FQPA amended the Federal Insecticide, Fungicide, and Rodenticide Act and the Federal Food, Drug, and Cosmetic Act. The act changed the way EPA regulates pesticides. The requirements included a new safety standard of reasonable certainty of no harm to be applied to all pesticides used on foods.

Chemical Safety Information, Site Security and Fuels Regulatory Act
(Amendment to Section 112 of Clean Air Act). This act removed from coverage by the Risk Management Plan (RMP) any flammable fuel when used as fuel or held for sale as fuel by a retail facility. (Flammable fuels used as a feedstock or held for sale as a fuel at a wholesale facility still are covered.) The law also limits access to off-site consequence analysis, which is reported in RMPs by covered facilities.

Note. Based on information from EPA, 2001e.

Environmental Health Risks in Home, Work, School, and Community Settings

Environmental health assessments, whether individual or community-based, should take into account all of the potential exposures that may occur in homes, workplaces, schools, or communities.

Home

Indoor environments can be affected by a variety of exposures (see Figure 10-9). Household hazardous materials often are handled, stored, and disposed of inappropriately, creating environmental health risks.

Lead dust emanating from lead-based paint poses a major threat to children. More than 50 million homes in the United States contain lead-based paint (U.S. Department of Housing and Urban Development, 1999). Lead poisoning is the most preventable of the environmentally related diseases that children suffer. A wide array of state and federal statutes and regulations exist regarding lead-based paint poisoning from both the housing inspection/remediation perspective and the health

Figure 10-9. Indoor Air Quality Exposures

- Building products (urea, formaldehyde, insulation, and asbestos—all known carcinogens)
- Lead-based paint, lead pipes, and lead solder
- Heating, ventilation, and air conditioning (carbon monoxide)
- Consumer products (aerosols for items such as hair spray, nail polish remover [acetone], air fresheners, and dry-cleaned clothes)
- Cleaning products (ammonia, chlorine)
- Arts/hobby activities (glues, paints, lead-stained glass)
- Pesticide use
- Furnishings, including carpets
- Renovation and rehab activities (paint removers, adhesives)
- Work contaminants that are taken home from workplaces

Note. Based on information from Sattler, 1998.

screening/treatment perspective. Lead-based paint was banned from indoor use in 1978 (Consumer Product Safety Commission, 1978). The symptoms of lead poisoning are varied and include neurological deficits (affecting both the peripheral nervous system and the central nervous system), renal damage, hypertension, and reproductive problems (in both males and females). Learning disabilities, hyperactivity, and mental retardation all are associated with childhood lead poisoning.

Pesticides

Pesticides are chemicals formulated to kill an undesirable organism, which may be a microbe, insect, fungus, rodent, or plant. Most pesticides have not been tested comprehensively for their effect on humans, particularly fetuses and young children. Regular indoor or outdoor use of pesticides increases the risk of leukemia in children who reside in the home. Pesticide "foggers" often have persistent active ingredients that take up residence in textiles such as stuffed animals, pillows, and other items with which children may have close contact. The FQPA addresses health risks associated with pesticides in food; however, it does not address the use of pesticides in homes and schools, on lawns, or from aerial spraying of agricultural pesticides. Pesticides that are known carcinogens are used in all of these settings (see Figure 10-10).

Asthma

Asthma rates in the United States have skyrocketed over the last decade, rising even more alarmingly in African American and Hispanic communities (American Lung Association, 2001). Many indoor air contaminants (chemical and biological) can trigger asthmatic events. Biological contaminants include bacteria, mold and mildew, mites, animal hair and dander, and pollen. Environmental tobacco smoke, another asthma trigger, is associated with a number of health problems and is attributable to as many as 10 million lost school days a year (EPA, 2001a).

Radon

Radon is the second leading cause of lung cancer in the United States (EPA, 2001c). Radon is a naturally occurring radioactive gas that is found in the soil and

---

Figure 10-10. New Provisions Related to the Protection of Infants and Children

Health-based standard: A new standard of "a reasonable certainty of no harm" that prohibits taking into account economic considerations when children are at risk.

Additional margin of safety: Requires that the EPA use an additional 10-fold margin of safety when adequate data are available to assess prenatal and postnatal development risks.

Account for children's diet: Requires the use of age-appropriate estimates of dietary consumption in establishing allowable levels of pesticides on food to account for children's unique dietary patterns.

Account for all exposures: In establishing acceptable levels of a pesticide on food, the EPA must account for exposures that may occur through other routes, such as drinking water and residential application of the pesticide.

Cumulative impact: The EPA must consider the cumulative impact of all pesticides that may share a common mechanism of action.

Tolerance reassessments: All existing pesticide food standards must be reassessed over a 10-year period to ensure that they meet the new standard to protect children.

Endocrine-disruption testing: The EPA must screen and test all pesticides and pesticide ingredients for estrogen effects and other endocrine-disrupter activity.

Registration renewal: Establishes a 15-year renewal process for all pesticides to ensure that they have up-to-date science evaluations over time.

Note. Based on information from the Food Quality Protection Act, 1996.

---

can leak into basements. All homes should be assessed for the risk of radon exposure. If high amounts are found, action should be taken to reduce radon to an acceptable level. Radon also can be found in the groundwater from which well water is drawn, which necessitates testing well water.

Drinking Water

Approximately half of the U.S. population's drinking water is derived from groundwater (i.e., wells) and the other half from surface water (i.e., reservoirs, lakes, rivers) (EPA, 1997). Drinking water obtained from private wells should be analyzed regularly to determine its fitness to drink. Drinking water that is supplied by a public water provider must be tested for approximately 80 contaminants that are regulated by the EPA. When contaminants exceed regulated standards, they must be reported to the customer either immediately, if a health threat is posed, or in summary form on an annual basis.

Food

Much of the meat and poultry produced in the United States is treated with hormones (e.g., bovine growth hormone) or antibiotics (Union of Concerned Scientists, 2000). More than 50% of the antibiotics sold in the United States are used in animal feed to improve growth. The official federal definition of "organic foods" helps consumers to choose food products that do not contain chemical and hormone additives. The U.S. Geological Survey (2001) has detected hormones and antibiotics used for veterinary purposes with livestock in national streams. (This is a function of leaching from fecal material containing hormones and antibiotics.)

School

Twenty percent of the U.S. population can be found in a school building on any given weekday (EPA, 2001d). School environments provide many of the same risks as home environments from indoor air contaminants. However, schools are more likely to use industrial-strength cleaners and pest-control measures that may create health risks for children. Integrated pest-management strategies should be implemented in all cases. This is a systematic approach to pest control that takes into account the pest's need for food, water, and nesting and uses the least toxic approaches to reduce infestations.

Carpeting, particularly in classrooms of younger children, can be a source of both chemical and biological contaminants, some of which may be asthma triggers. Readily cleanable surfaces, such as tile flooring or nonporous mats, or a rigorous cleaning program for the carpeting should be implemented to minimize unhealthy exposures.

Many schools, especially those that are expressly vocational training schools, mimic workplaces with automotive programs, art and science rooms, cosmetology programs, construction shops, and photography darkrooms. The principles of the industrial hygiene hierarchy of controls should be applied to protect the students, teachers, and staff from unhealthy exposures.

Community

Environmental health risks in the community may derive from unhealthy air, water, or soil. The Clean Air Act (1970/1990) regulates air pollution from both fixed sites (e.g., smoke stacks) and nonpoint sources (e.g., automobiles, trucks, buses). Air pollution encompasses man-made chemical emissions, including combustion products, volatile chemicals, aerosols (particulate) and their atmospheric reaction products, and heavy metals. The greatest single source of air pollution in the United States is from motor vehicles (EPA, 2000a). The burning of fossil fuel and waste incineration are two other major contributors. Health effects associated with air pollution include asthma and other respiratory diseases, cardiovascular diseases (e.g., heart disease, hypertension), cancer, immunosuppression, reproductive health problems (e.g., birth defects), and neurological problems.

Dioxins and furans are products of combustion from chlorinated compounds resulting from waste incineration and industrial processes. Because of the heavy reliance on PVC plastic in the healthcare industry and the general practice of incinerating all hospital waste, hospital incinerators are one of the leading producers of dioxin in the air in the United States (Health Care Without Harm, 2001). These carcinogens also are endocrine disrupters and considered by the EPA to be reproductive toxicants. Dioxin mimics estrogen; it "looks" like estrogen to the human body. Hospital waste should be segregated and appropriately recycled or reused. The national campaign "Health Care Without Harm" addresses the environmental health threats posed by the healthcare industry. Its

Web site (www.noharm.org) is a useful tool for learning about environmental health risks and provides information on what nurses can do about them. Another major focus of the campaign is the reduction of mercury in the healthcare industry, particularly from mercury thermometers.

Industrial sites (old and current) are sources of air, water, and soil contamination. Such sites may be designated "Brownfield" or "Superfund" sites. These designations are derived from federal environmental statutes and are given when a site is environmentally compromised and creates a health risk. Drinking water sources (both ground and surface) may be contaminated by point-source contaminants, such as industrial waste streams, or nonpoint sources, such as pesticides or fertilizer runoff. Each state must have a plan for protecting its sources of drinking water from point and nonpoint sources. Nurses can and should participate in the development of these plans. Given that 70% of the human body is water, it is vitally important that drinking water sources remain healthy and safe.

The U.S. Geological Service has detected acetaminophen, caffeine, codeine, and 17-ß estradiol in national streams. These are derived from human waste. In addition, antibiotics have been measured in aquifers near hog "factories" or concentrated animal feed organizations. Some drinking water contaminants occur naturally, such as radon and arsenic, whereas other contaminants occur cyclically with the use of agricultural chemicals, such as atrazine, which contaminates ground water during the growing season, particularly in the Midwest (Burkart, Gassman, Moorman, & Singh, 1998). Leaking chemical storage tanks (both above-ground and underground) pose hazards to the soil and groundwater and almost always are associated with human health risks.

Work

The human toll and economic burden of occupational disease and injury in the United States are staggering. Direct and indirect costs associated with occupational morbidity and mortality in 1992 were estimated at $171 billion per year for occupational illness and injury, with the greater portion of the total cost, $145 billion, attributed to injuries (Leigh, Markowitz, Fahs, Shin, & Landrigan, 1997). The comparison of these and similar data for other major chronic diseases demonstrated that the costs associated with occupational disease and injury were greater than those of AIDS ($33 billion), Alzheimer's disease ($67.3 billion), all circulatory diseases ($164.3 billion), and cancer ($170.7 billion) (Leigh et al.). Despite the huge economic burden associated with occupational injury and illness, occupational health protection for U.S. workers lags far behind that provided for workers elsewhere in the world (Ashford, 2000).

Comparable estimates for the cost of occupational injury and illness prior to the 1970 passage of occupational health legislation in the United States do not exist. However, trends in occupational injury statistics provide evidence that great strides have been made in improving worker health and safety since the passage of the OSHA Act in 1970. The act created OSHA, a regulatory agency within the U.S. Department of Labor, whose mission, a very progressive one even by current standards, is to "assure so far as possible every working man and woman in the nation safe and healthful working conditions" (National Occupational Research Agenda, 1996.) OSHA activities include promulgating health and safety standards, enforcing these standards, and providing consultation and other forms of technical assistance. The OSHA Act covers private-sector employers and civilian employees of the federal government but does not cover family farms and public-sector workers in 27 states that do not have state plans. Record keeping, a critical assessment tool for OSHA compliance, is not required in workplaces with less than 10 employees. OSHA is most readily recognized (and feared) for their compliance activity. However, in reality, OSHA's compliance activity is such that if they were to attempt to visit every workplace over which they had jurisdiction, they would make one compliance visit per workplace per 100 years.

The OSHA Act also created NIOSH, part of the Centers for Disease Control and Protection within the Department of Health and Human Services. NIOSH is the only federal agency with sole responsibility for conducting occupational health and safety research. In addition, NIOSH conducts health hazard evaluations of any sites where workers, their representatives, or management have concerns about a health hazard for which an OSHA regulation does not exist. They also make recommendations to OSHA for health and safety standards and support professional training in several occupational health disciplines, including occupational health nursing. Both OSHA and NIOSH provide innumerable high-quality resources. NIOSH has a toll-free number (800-356-4674) and Web site (www.cdc.gov/niosh); OSHA's Web site is www.osha.gov.

Occupational exposures also may be of concern to communities surrounding the work site. Industrial chemicals may be a source of environmental degradation within a community. Information regarding chemical releases from industrial sites is available via the Environmental Defense Web site at http://scorecard.org.

Nursing Implications

At the beginning of this chapter, it was noted that nurses have not developed a substantial list or protocol of nursing practices to match the emerging science about the health effects associated with environmental exposures. Rather, a small number of nurses are environmental health pioneers. The clinical expertise and leadership of nurses will be invaluable as nurses incorporate environmental health risk factors into their primary prevention work and health education, participate in policy-making activities to decrease the environmental load of carcinogens that threaten the public health, engage in nursing research in which the environmental factors associated with cancer are considered, and other ways yet to be determined by emerging pioneers.

The National Academy of Science Institute of Medicine, in preparing the report *Nursing, Health and the Environment*, gathered experts from all areas of nursing and the sciences (Institute of Medicine, 1995). The report includes recommendations for the integration of environmental health into all aspects of nursing education, practice, research, advocacy, and policy. General environmental health competencies for nurses are listed, along with a "Summary of Recommendations" (see Figures 10-11 and 10-12).

Other ways nurses can be involved in environmental health activities include generating data systems for environmental assessment and outcomes, designing "critical paths" that include environmental assessment, implementing impact studies (consumer goods and land use), and increasing nursing's visibility on environmental health issues by participating in public forums regarding environmental protection and public health. Educating citizens and legislators about health threats may be the best way to effect changes in public policy. Laws often are more effective in changing behavior than public education (e.g., bike helmet and seat belt laws). This cycle eventually must involve nurse educators who can expand the basic nursing curriculum to place more emphasis on social justice and professional role expectations in the area of environmental health.

The ways in which modern nursing practice can affect environmental health are not well defined. As nurses learn more about environmental health, opportunities for integration into their practice, education programs, research, advocacy, and policy work will become evident. Opportunities abound for those pioneering spirits within the nursing profession who are dedicated to creating healthier environments for their patients and communities.

Figure 10-11. General Environmental Health Competency for Nurses as Outlined by the Institute of Medicine

Basic knowledge and concepts
All nurses should understand the scientific principles and underpinnings of the relationship between individuals or populations and the environment (including the work environment). This understanding includes the basic mechanisms and pathways of exposure to environmental health hazards, basic prevention and control strategies, the interdisciplinary nature of effective interventions, and the role of research.

Assessment and referral
All nurses should be able to successfully complete an environmental health history, recognize potential environmental hazards and sentinel illnesses, and make appropriate referrals for conditions with probable environmental etiologies. An essential component of this is the ability to access and provide information to patients and communities and to locate referral sources.

Advocacy, ethics, and risk communication
All nurses should be able to demonstrate knowledge of the role of advocacy (case and class), ethics, and risk communication in patient care and community intervention, with respect to the potential adverse effects of the environment on health.

Legislation and regulation
All nurses should understand the policy framework and major pieces of legislation and regulations related to environmental health.

Note. Based on information from Institute of Medicine, 1995.

Figure 10-12. Summary Listing of All Recommendations in Institute of Medicine Report

Nursing practice
- Environmental health should be reemphasized in the scope of responsibilities for nursing practice.
- Resources to support environmental health content in nursing practice should be identified and made available.
- Nurses should participate as members and leaders in interdisciplinary teams that address environmental health problems.
- Communication should extend beyond counseling individual patients and families to facilitating the exchange of information on environmental hazards and community responses.
- The concept of advocacy in nursing should be expanded to include advocacy on behalf of groups and communities, in addition to advocacy on behalf of individual patients and their families.
- Nurses should conduct research regarding the ethical implications of occupational and environmental health hazards and incorporate findings into curricula and practice.

Nursing education
- Environmental health concepts should be incorporated into all levels of nursing education.
- Environmental health content should be included in nursing licensure and certification examinations.
- Expertise in various environmental health disciplines should be included in the education of nurses.
- Environmental health content should be an integral part of lifelong learning and continuing education for nurses.
- Professional associations, public agencies, and private organizations should provide more resources and educational opportunities to enhance environmental health in nursing practice.

Nursing research
- Multidisciplinary and interdisciplinary research endeavors should be developed and implemented to build the knowledge base for nursing practice in environmental health.
- The number of nurse researchers should be increased to prepare to build the knowledge base in environmental health as it relates to the practice of nursing.
- Research priorities for nursing in environmental health should be established and used by funding agencies for resource allocation decisions and to give direction to nurse researchers.
- Current efforts to disseminate research findings to nurses, other healthcare providers, and the public should be strengthened and expanded.

Nursing advocacy
- Work with community, environmental groups, and local government.
- Legislative lobbying
- Reporting community hazards
- Ideally, all nurses should be advocates for safer environments.
- Involved in implementing policy

Note. Based on information from Institute of Medicine, 1995.

References

Agency for Toxic Substances and Disease Registry. (1996). *ToxFAQs: Polycyclic aromatic hydrocarbons (PAHs)*. Retrieved June 18, 2001 from the World Wide Web: http://www.atsdr.cdc.gov/tfacts69.html

Agency for Toxic Substances and Disease Registry. (1997). *ToxFAQs: Vinyl chloride*. Retrieved June 18, 2001 from the World Wide Web: http://www.atsdr.cdc.gov/tfacts20.html

American Lung Association. (2001). *American Lung Association survey reveals startling mis-understandings about living with asthma: Race/ethnicity differences confirmed.* Retrieved June 18, 2001 from the World Wide Web: http://www.lungusa.org/asthma/merck_press1.html#race

American Nurses Association. (1997). *ANA House of Delegates resolution on reduction of health care production of toxic pollution.* Retrieved June 18, 2001 from the World Wide Web: http://www.ana.org/about/summary/vtsna1.htm

Ashford, N. (2000). Government regulations I: Occupational health and safety. In B.S. Levy & D.H. Wegman (Eds.), *Occupational health: Recognizing and preventing work-related disease and injury* (pp. 161–171). Philadelphia: Lippincott Williams & Wilkins.

Boffetta, P., Agudo, A., Ahrens, W., Benhamou, E., Benhamou, S., Darby, S.C., Ferro, G., Fortes, C., Gonzalez, C.A., Jockel, K.H., Krauss, M., Kreienbrock, L., Kreuzer, M., Mendes, A., Merletti, F., Nyberg, F., Pershagen, G., Pohlabeln, H., Riboli, E., Schmid, G., Simonato, L., Tredaniel, J., Whitley, E., Wichmann, H.E., Saracci, R., et al. (1998). Multicenter case-control study of exposure to environmental tobacco smoke and lung cancer in Europe. *Journal of the National Cancer Institute, 90,* 1440–1450.

Brown, A.M. (1999). Investigating clusters in the workplace and beyond. *Occupational Medicine, 49,* 443–447.

Browner, C.M. (1998, May 8). *Agency—Johns Hopkins School of Hygiene and Public Health—Baltimore, MD. U.S. Environmental Protection Agency speeches from the administrator.* Retrieved June 18, 2001 from the World Wide Web: http://yosemite.epa.gov/opa/admspchs.nsf/cb7284cd464285f885256457006faf39/68be89cce9c415c785256601004f1444?OpenDocument

Burkart, M.R., Gassman, P.W., Moorman, T.B., & Singh, P. (1998, December). *Estimating atrazine leaching in the Midwest.* Retrieved June 19, 2001 from the World Wide Web: http://www.nalusda.gov/ttic/tektran/data/000009/32/0000093242.html

Caldwell, G.G. (1990). Twenty-two years of cancer cluster investigations at the Centers for Disease Control. *American Journal of Epidemiology, 132*(Suppl. 1), S43–S47.

Checkoway, H., Crawford-Brown, D.J., & Pearce, N.E (1989). *Research methods in occupational epidemiology.* New York: Oxford University Press.

Children's Environmental Health Network. (1999). *Training manual on pediatric environmental health: Putting it into practice.* Berkeley, CA: Children's Environmental Health Network/Public Health Institute.

The Clean Air Act. 42 U.S.C. § 7401 (1970/1990).

Comprehensive Environmental Response, Compensation, and Liability Act, 42 U.S.C. § 9601 *et seg.* (1980).

Consumer Product Safety Commission. (1978). *Ban on lead-containing paint and certain consumer products containing lead-based paint* (Title 16 CFR Part 1303, 1977). Retrieved June 18, 2001 from the World Wide Web: http://www.access.gpo.gov/nara/cfr/waisidx_00/16cfr1303_00.html

Doll, R., & Peto, R. (1981). *The causes of cancer.* New York: Oxford University Press.

Fingerhut, M.A., Halperin, W.E., Marlow, D.A., Piacitelli, L.A., Honchar, P.A., Sweeney, M.H., Greife, A.L., Dill, P.A., Steenland, K., & Suruda, A.J. (1991). Cancer mortality in workers exposed to 2,3,7,8-tetrachlorodibenzo-p-dioxin. *New England Journal of Medicine, 324,* 212–218.

Food Quality Protection Act (PL 104-170). (1996, August 3). Title 7 United States Code at Section 1261, as amended. Retrieved June 18, 2001 from the World Wide Web: http://www.epa.gov/opppsps1/fqpa/backgrnd.htm

Frumkin, H., & Thun, M. (2000). Carcinogens. In B.S. Levy & D.H. Wegman (Eds.), *Occupational health: Recognizing and preventing work-related disease and injury* (pp. 335–354). Philadelphia: Lippincott Williams & Wilkins.

Goldman, L.R. (1998). Chemicals and children's environment: What we don't know about risks. *Environmental Health Perspectives, 106*, 875–879.

Harr, J. (1995). *A civil action*. New York: Random House.

Harrison, R. (1997). Chemicals. In J. LaDou (Ed.), *Occupational and environmental medicine* (pp. 440–482). Stamford, CT: Appleton & Lange.

Health Care Without Harm. (2001). *Incineration and HCWH.* Retrieved June 18, 2001 from the World Wide Web: http://www.noharm.org/hcwh/issues/incineration.html

International Agency for Research on Cancer. (1992). *Solar and ultraviolet radiation. IARC Monograph on Evaluating Carcinogenic Risks of Humans.* Retrieved June 18, 2001 from the World Wide Web: http://www.iarc.fr/

International Agency for Research on Cancer. (2000). *Overall evaluations of carcinogenicity to humans.* Retrieved June 18, 2001 from the World Wide Web: http://193.51.164.11/monoeval/crthall.html

INFORM, Inc. (1995). *Toxics watch 1995*. New York: Author.

Institute of Medicine. (1995). *Nursing, health and the environment: Strengthening the relationship to improve the public's health.* Washington, DC: National Academy Press.

International Health Care Worker Safety Center at the University of Virginia Health System. (2001, May 1). *State legislation on needle safety.* Retrieved June 18, 2001 from the World Wide Web: http://www.med.virginia.edu/medcntr/centers/epinet/statelist.html

Laplanche, A., Clavel-Chapelon, F., Contassot, J.C., & Lanouziere, C. (1992) Exposure to vinyl chloride monomer. Results of a cohort study after a seven-year follow-up. *British Journal of Industrial Medicine, 49*, 134–137.

Leigh, J.P., Markowitz, S.B., Fahs, M., Shin, C., & Landrigan, P.J. (1997). Occupational injury and illness in the United States. Estimates of costs, morbidity, and mortality. *Archives of Internal Medicine, 157*, 1557–1568.

Lichtenstein, P., Holm, N.V., Kerkasalo, P.K., Iliadou, A., Kaprio, J., Koskenvuo, M., Pukkala, E., Skytthe, A., & Hemminki, K. (2000). Environmental and heritable factors in the causation of cancer. *New England Journal of Medicine, 343*, 78–84.

National Environmental Policy Act, 42 U.S.C. § 4321–4327 (1970).

National Institute for Occupational Safety and Health. (1996). *NIOSH fact sheet: EMFs in the workplace* (Publication No. 96-129). Retrieved June 18, 2001 from the World Wide Web: http://www.cdc.gov/niosh/emf2.html

National Library of Medicine. (2001). *Toxicology tutor I.* Retrieved June 18, 2001 from the World Wide Web: http://newsis.nlm.nih.gov/toxtutor1/index.htm

National Occupational Research Agenda. (1996). *Foreword.* Retrieved June 18, 2001 from the World Wide Web: http://www.cdc.gov/niosh/nora.html

National Research Council. (1983). *Risk assessment in the federal government: Managing the process.* Washington, DC: National Academy Press.

National Toxicology Program. (2001). *EMF-RAPID Program: The possible effects of power-line frequency electric and magnetic fields on human health.* Retrieved June 18, 2001 from the World Wide Web: http://ntp-server.niehs.nih.gov/htdocs/liason/factsheets/EMF-Rapid.pdf

Occupational Safety and Health Administration. (1998). *OSHA regulations (Standards—29 CFR). Vinyl chloride—1910.1017.* Retrieved June 18, 2001 from the World Wide Web: http://www.osha-slc.gov/OshStd_data/1910_1017.html

Pirkle, J.L., Flegal, K.M., Bernert, J.T., Brody, D., Etzel, R.A., & Maurer, K.R. (1996). Exposure of U.S. population to environmental tobacco smoke: The third national health and nutrition examination survey, 1988 to 1991. *JAMA, 275,* 1233–1240.

Richardson, S., Zittoun, R., Bastuji-Garin, S., Lasserre, V., Guihenneuc, C., Cadious, M., Viguie, F., & Laffont-Faust, I. (1992). Occupational risk factors for acute leukaemia: A case-control study. *International Journal of Epidemiology, 24,* 1063–1073.

Rosenstock, L., & Cullen, M.R. (1994). *Textbook of clinical occupational and environmental medicine.* Philadelphia: W.B. Saunders.

Rugo, H.S., & Fishman, M.L. (1997). Occupational cancer. In J. LaDou (Ed.), *Occupational and environmental medicine* (pp. 235–271). Stamford, CT: Appleton & Lange.

Sandman, P.M. (1987). Risk communication: Facing public rage. *Environmental Protection Journal, 13*(9), 21.

Sattler, B. (1998). Curriculum materials for the Environmental Health Faculty Development Workshop, Baltimore, MD.

Schettler, T., Solomon, G., Valenti, M., & Huddle, A. (1999). *Generations at risk: Reproductive health and the environment.* Boston: Massachusetts Institute of Technology.

Schettler, T., Stein, J., Reich, F., & Valenti, M. (2000). *In harm's way: Toxic threats to development. A report by Greater Boston Physicians for Social Responsibility, prepared for a joint project with Clean Water.* Cambridge, MA: Physicians for Social Responsibility.

Selikoff, I.J., Hammond, E.C., & Chanrg, J. (1968). Asbestos exposure, smoking and neoplasia. *JAMA, 204,* 106–112.

Smith, T.J., & Schneider, T. (2000). Occupational hygiene. In B.S. Levy & D.H. Wegman (Eds.), *Occupational health: Recognizing and preventing work-related disease and injury* (pp. 161–180). Philadelphia: Lippincott Williams & Wilkins.

Spirtas, R., Heineman, E.F., Bernstein, L., Beebe, G.W., Keehn, R.J., Stark, A., Harlow, B.L., & Benichou, J. (1994). Malignant mesothelioma: Attributable risk of asbestos exposure. *Occupational and Environmental Medicine, 51,* 804–811.

Stayner, L.T., Dankovic, D.A., & Lemen, R.A. (1996). Occupational exposure to asbestos and cancer risk: A review of the amphibole hypothesis. *American Journal of Public Health, 86*(2), 179–186.

Superfund Amendments and Reauthorization Act, 42 U.S.C. § 9601 *et seg.* (1986).

Union of Concerned Scientists. (2000). *Why are antibiotics used in animal agriculture?* Retrieved June 18, 2001 from the World Wide Web: http://www.ucsusa.org/agriculture/

U.S. Department of Housing and Urban Development. (1999, April). *The Healthy Homes Initiative: A preliminary plan (Summary).* Retrieved June 18, 2001 from the World Wide Web: http://www.hud.gov/lea/HHISummary.html

U.S. Environmental Protection Agency. (1992). *Respiratory health effects of passive smoking: Lung cancer and other disorders* (Publication EPA/600/6-90/006F). Washington, DC: Environmental Protection Agency, Office of Air and Radiation.

U.S. Environmental Protection Agency. (1997). *Water on tap: A consumer's guide to the nation's drinking water.* Retrieved June 18, 2001 from the World Wide Web: http://www.epa.gov/safewater/wot/wheredoes.html

U.S. Environmental Protection Agency. (1998a). *The EPA children's environmental health yearbook.* Retrieved June 18, 2001 from the World Wide Web: http://www.epa.gov/children/whatwe/ochpyearbook.pdf

U.S. Environmental Protection Agency. (1998b). *Parent's guide to school indoor air quality.* Albany, NY: Healthy Schools Network, Inc.

U.S. Environmental Protection Agency. (2000a). *Motor vehicles and air pollution: You can make a difference.* Retrieved June 18, 2001 from the World Wide Web: http://www.epa.gov/students/motor_vehicles_and_air_pollution.htm

U.S. Environmental Protection Agency. (2000b). *Questions and answers about dioxins.* Retrieved June 18, 2001 from the World Wide Web: http://www.epa.gov/ncea/pdfs/dioxin/dioxin_questions_and_answers.pdf

U.S. Environmental Protection Agency. (2001a). *The asthma epidemic.* Retrieved June 18, 2001 from the World Wide Web: http://www.epa.gov/iaq/schools/asthma/asthma_epidemic.htm

U.S. Environmental Protection Agency. (2001b). *Current drinking water standards.* Retrieved June 18, 2001 from the World Wide Web: http://www.epa.gov/safewater/mcl.html

U.S. Environmental Protection Agency. (2001c). *Financing residential radon mitigation costs: Using the HUD 203(k) mortgage insurance program to reduce the risk of lung cancer in people.* Retrieved June 18, 2001 from the World Wide Web: http://www.epa.gov/iaq/radon/203kfact.html

U.S. Environmental Protection Agency. (2001d). *Indoor air quality tools for schools.* Retrieved June 18, 2001 from the World Wide Web: http://www.epa.gov/iaq/schools/index.html

U.S. Environmental Protection Agency. (2001e). *Major environmental laws.* Retrieved June 18, 2001 from the World Wide Web: http://www.epa.gov/epahome/laws.htm

U.S. Geological Survey. (2001, May). *Toxic substances hydrology program national reconnaissance of emerging contaminants in the nation's water resources.* Retrieved June 19, 2001 from the World Wide Web: http://toxics.usgs.gov/regional/emc.html

Wallinga, D. (1998). *Putting children first: Making pesticide levels in food safer for infants and children.* Washington, DC: Natural Resources Defense Council.

Warren, R.L. (1963). A community model. In R.L. Warren (Ed.), *The community in America* (pp. 9–20). Chicago: Rand McNally & Co.

World Health Organization. (1993). *Consultation: Sophia. Bulgaria.* Geneva, Switzerland: Author.

Appendix 10-1. Environmental Health Resources

Governmental Resources

Agency for Toxic Substances and Disease Registry (ATSDR)
Ariel Rios Building (Washington office)
1200 Pennsylvania Ave., NW
M/C 5204G
Washington, DC 20460
703-603-8729
www.atsdr.cdd.gov

ATSDR was created by the 1980 "Superfund" legislation as a part of the U.S. Department of Health and Human Services. ATSDR's mission is to prevent or mitigate adverse human health effects and diminished quality of life resulting from exposure to hazardous substances in the environment. ATSDR conducts activities in public health assessments, health investigations, exposure and disease registry, emergency response, toxicological profiles, health education, and applied research.

Centers for Disease Control and Prevention (CDC)
1600 Clifton Road
Atlanta, GA 30333
404-639-7070
www.cdc.gov

The CDC is charged with protecting the nation's public health. Within the CDC, the National Center for Environmental Health focuses on environmental health issues.

Consumer Product Safety Commission (CPSC)
4330 East-West Highway
Bethesda, MD 20814-4408
301-504-0990
www.cpsc.gov

CPSC provides information on health and safety effects related to consumer products, including chemical hazards in consumer products.

Department of Energy (DOE)
1000 Independence Ave., SW
Washington, DC 20585
800-DIAL-DOE
www.doe.gov

The DOE regulates and provides the framework for a comprehensive and balanced national energy plan. The Environment, Safety and Health Office of the DOE provides independent oversight of departmental execution of environmental, occupational safety and health, and nuclear/non-nuclear safety and environmental restoration.

Department of Health and Human Services (DHHS)
200 Independence Ave., SW
Washington, DC 20201
202-619-0257 or 877-696-6775
www.dhhs.gov

DHHS is the department of the federal executive branch most concerned with the nation's human health concerns.

Food and Drug Administration (FDA)
5600 Fishers Lane
Rockville, MD 20857-0001
888-INFO-FDA
www.fda.gov

The FDA inspects food and drug manufacturing plants and warehouses; collects and analyzes samples of foods, drugs, cosmetics, and therapeutic devices for adulteration and misbranding; and enforces the Radiation Control Act as related to consumer products. With the Department of Agriculture, the FDA assesses information about food required by a number of federal regulations.

(Continued on next page)

Appendix 10-1. Environmental Health Resources *(Continued)*

Governmental Resources

National Center for Environmental Health (NCEH)
4770 Buford Highway, NE
Atlanta, GA 30341-3724
770-488-7100
www.cdc.gov/nceh/

The mission of NCEH is to promote health and quality of life by preventing or controlling disease, injury, and disability related to the interactions between people and their environment outside of the workplace.

National Institute of Environmental Health Sciences (NIEHS)
111 Alexander Drive
Research Triangle Park, NC 27709
919-541-3345
www.niehs.nih.gov

NIEHS is the principal federal agency for biomedical research on the effects of chemical, physical, and biological environmental agents on human health and well-being. NIEHS supports research and training focused on harmful agents in the environment. Research results form the basis for preventive programs for environmentally related diseases and for action by regulatory agencies.

National Institute for Occupational Safety and Health (NIOSH)
200 Independence Ave., SW
Washington, DC 20201
202-401-6995
www.cdc.gov/niosh

NIOSH was established by the Occupational Safety and Health Act of 1970 to conduct research on occupational diseases and injuries, respond to requests for assistance by investigating problems of health and safety in the workplace, recommend standards to OSHA and the Mine Safety and Health Administration, and train professionals in occupational safety and health.

Nuclear Regulatory Commission (NRC)
11555 Rockville Pike
Rockville, MD 20852-2738
301-415-7000
www.nrc.gov

NRC licenses, inspects, and regulates civilian use of nuclear energy to protect health and safety and the environment. This is achieved by licensing individuals and companies to build and operate nuclear reactors and other facilities and to own and use nuclear materials.

Occupational Safety and Health Administration (OSHA)
200 Constitution Ave., NW
Washington, DC 20210
202-693-2000
www.osha.gov

OSHA was created within the Department of Labor under the Occupation Safety and Health Act of 1970 to promulgate and enforce national occupational health and safety standards. OSHA encourages employers and employees to reduce workplace hazards; implements new or improved safety and health programs; provides research in occupational safety and health; requires a reporting and recording system to monitor job-related illnesses and injuries; develops mandatory job safety and health standards and enforces them; and provides for the development, analysis, evaluation, and approval of state occupational safety and health programs.

U.S. Department of Agriculture (DOA)
1400 Independence Ave. SW
Washington, DC 20250
202-720-8732
www.usda.gov

DOA, as part of its food-safety administration, regulates pesticides, hormones, and antibiotics used in food supply. The USDA-Food, Nutrition and Consumer Services' (FNCS) mission is to ensure access to nutritious, healthful diets for all Americans through food assistance and nutrition education for consumers.

(Continued on next page)

Appendix 10-1. Environmental Health Resources *(Continued)*

Nongovernmental Organizations and Advocacy Organizations in Environmental Health

Alliance to End Childhood Lead Poisoning 227 Massachusetts Ave., NE, Suite 200 Washington, DC 20002 202-543-1147 www.aeclp.org	A national clearinghouse and advocacy organization focusing on lead poisoning
American Public Health Association (APHA) 1015 15th St., NW Washington, DC 20005 202-789-5600 www.APHA.org	APHA was founded in 1872 as a professional organization of physicians, nurses, educators, academicians, environmentalists, epidemiologists, new professionals, social workers, health administrators, optometrists, podiatrists, pharmacists, dentists, nutritionists, health planners, other community and mental health specialists, and interested consumers. APHA has a very active environmental health section that welcomes nursing participation. The annual conventions have a rich assortment of environmental health programs.
Association of Occupational and Environmental Clinics (AOEC) 1010 Vermont Ave., #513 Washington, DC 20005 202-347-4976 www.aoec.org	AOEC is dedicated to higher standards of patient-centered, multidisciplinary care emphasizing prevention and total health through information sharing, quality service, and collaborative research.
Association of University Environmental Health/Sciences Centers (AUESC) Mount Sinai School of Medicine One Gustave L. Levey Place New York, NY 10029 212-241-6173 www.mssm.edu/	AUESC provides a forum for all of the university-based environmental health science centers supported by the National Institute of Environmental Health.
Environmental Defense (formally the Environmental Defense Fund) 257 Park Ave. New York, NY 10010 212-505-2100 www.environmentaldefense.org	Environmental Defense is dedicated to protecting the environmental rights of all people, including future generations. Among these rights are clean air, clean water, healthy and nourishing food, and a flourishing ecosystem.
Health Care Without Harm (HCWH) HCWH c/o CHEJ PO Box 6806 Falls Church, VA 22040 703-237-2249 www.noharm.org	HCWH is a national coalition-based organization that provides education and advocacy regarding the environmental impact of the healthcare industry. (The American Nurses Association is a member organization.)

(Continued on next page)

Appendix 10-1. Environmental Health Resources (Continued)

Nongovernmental Organizations and Advocacy Organizations in Environmental Health

Healthy Schools Network 96 South Swan St. Albany, NY 12210 518-462-0632	A clearinghouse and advocacy organization for environmental health issues related to schools and school children
National Environmental Health Association (NEHA) 720 S. Colorado Blvd. Suite 970, S. Tower Denver, CO 80222 301-756-9090 www.neha.org	NEHA is a professional society of people engaged in environmental health and protection for governmental agencies, public health and environmental protection agencies, industries, colleges, and universities.
Natural Resources Defense Council 40 West 20th St. New York, NY 10011 212-727-2700 www.nrdc.org	The Natural Resources Defense Council's purpose is to safeguard the Earth: people, plants and animals, and the natural systems on which all life depends. The organization uses law and science to restore the integrity of the elements that sustain life—air, land, and water—and to defend endangered natural places.
Pesticide Education Center P.O. Box 420870 San Francisco, CA 94142-0870 415-391-8511	Founded in 1933 to educate the public about the hazards and health effects of pesticides, the Pesticide Education Center works with community groups, workers, individuals, and others harmed by or concerned about risks to their health from exposure to pesticides used in agriculture, the home and garden, and other environmental and industrial uses.
Physicians for Social Responsibility (PSR) 1101 Fourteenth St., NW, Suite 700 Washington, DC 20005 202-898-0150 www.psr.org	PSR has a major environmental health effort that includes conferences, resource materials, and advocacy.
Sierra Club 85 Second St., Second Floor San Francisco, CA 94105-3441 415-977-5500 www.sierraclub.org	The Sierra Club has eight priority campaigns: Stop Sprawl: End Runaway Growth, Protect America's Wildlands, End Commercial Logging in National Forests, Protect Water From Factory Farm Pollution, Global Warming, Human Rights, Population Stabilization, and Responsible Trade.
Society for Occupational and Environmental Health (SOEH) 6728 Old McLean Village Drive McLean, VA 22101 703-556-9222 soeh@degnon.org	SOEH includes scientists, academicians, and industry and labor representatives who seek to improve the quality of both working and living places by operating as a neutral forum for conferences involving all aspects of occupational and environmental health.

(Continued on next page)

Appendix 10-1. Environmental Health Resources *(Continued)*

Nongovernmental Organizations and Advocacy Organizations in Environmental Health

WorldWatch Institute
1776 Massachusetts Ave., NW
Washington, DC 20036
202-452-1999
www.worldwatch.org

The WorldWatch Institute is a research organization that aims to encourage a reflective and deliberate approach to global problem solving.

Other resources:

- The University of Maryland School of Nursing established a Web site on environmental health for nursing. This site includes curriculum materials, video clips from lectures and conferences, and links to Web sites of interest to nurses (EnviRN.umaryland.edu).
- The American Nurses Association created a Pollution Prevention Kit for nurses as well as excellent occupational health materials for nurses (www.nursingworld.org).
- The EPA implemented Integrated Pest Management (IPM) in schools and published a parent's guide to safe schools as one of many public health information resources. It also has a very comprehensive Web site that includes a glossary of "Terms of the Environment" (www.epa.gov).
- Information for Major Environmental Laws can be found at Web site www.epa.gov.
- The National Library of Medicine (NLM) houses the most comprehensive, Web-accessible databases and information regarding environmental health. The site includes a self-paced tutorial on toxicology. A manual for environmental health and nursing, created by Howard University, focuses on the Mississippi Delta and can be found on the NLM site (http://sis.nlm.nih.gov).
- The Children's Environmental Health Network offers an online resource guide and a training manual for healthcare providers on children's environmental health issues (http://CEHN.org).
- The Institute of Medicine report *Nursing, Health, and the Environment* provides background and recommendations for the integration of environmental health into nursing education, research, and practice, as well as policy and advocacy (www.iom.edu).
- The federal Agency for Toxic Substances and Disease Registries is an excellent source of environmental information (http://ATSDR.CDC.gov).

SECTION III

Cancer Detection

Chapter 11.

Breast Cancer Prevention and Detection: Past Progress and Future Directions

Chapter 12.

Gastrointestinal Malignancies

Chapter 13.

Gynecologic Cancers

Chapter 14.

Urologic and Male Genital Cancers

Chapter 15.

Skin Cancer Prevention and Early Detection

Chapter 16.

Prevention and Detection of Head and Neck Cancers

Chapter 17.

Tertiary Prevention: Improving the Care of Long-Term Survivors of Cancer

Chapter 18.

Genetic Counseling and Screening

OVERVIEW

Section III

Suzanne M. Mahon, RN, DNSc, AOCN®, APNG(c)

There are three levels of cancer prevention. Primary cancer prevention is true cancer prevention. Secondary prevention refers to the early detection and treatment of subclinical or early disease in people without signs or symptoms of cancer. Cancer screening is a form of secondary cancer prevention. Forms of secondary cancer prevention include the use of the Pap smear to detect atypical cervical cells or a mammogram to detect a nonpalpable breast cancer. Tertiary prevention refers to the management of an illness such as cancer to prevent progression, recurrence, or other complications. In cancer care, examples of tertiary prevention include monitoring for early signs of recurrence using tumor markers or detecting second primary malignancies or other complications such as osteoporosis early in long-term survivors. This section focuses on secondary and tertiary cancer prevention.

Secondary and tertiary cancer prevention practices are rooted in epidemiologic principles. Based on epidemiologic research, certain risk factors for specific cancers have been suggested. Cancer risk assessment is a critical component of all three levels of cancer prevention. A risk factor is a trait or characteristic that is associated with a statistically significant and increased likelihood of developing a particular disease. Helping individuals to understand their risk for developing cancer is important so that they can make the best choices possible for cancer prevention and early detection (Love, 1989; Mahon, 1998; Newell & Vogel, 1988).

The cancer risk assessment begins the educational process related to cancer prevention and early detection. Without an accurate and comprehensive risk assessment, providing individuals with appropriate and reasonable recommendations for all levels of cancer prevention is impossible. The risk factor assessment provides oncology nurses with an opportunity to teach individuals about the epidemiology, risk factors, and signs and symptoms associated with various cancers. This provides the framework individuals need to understand the importance of and rationale for cancer prevention strategies as well as information about signs and symptoms that merit further evaluation.

A cancer-screening test is the means used to detect a specific cancer. A cancer-screening test may be a single test or examination, but, more often, it is a combination of tests such as the use of a fecal occult blood test, digital rectal examination, and sigmoidoscopy to detect colorectal cancer. Tests often are combined to compensate for the limitations of one of the tests (MacLean, 1996). Specific recommendations for a screening test often vary among organizations such as the American Cancer Society (ACS), the United States Preventive Services Task Force, or the National Cancer Institute. Because each of these organizations may use variations in criteria when making recommendations, they are not universal and often are very confusing to the general public (Foltz, 2001). Nurses need to instruct patients on the strengths and limitations of various screening recommendations and help patients choose appropriate tests based on their individual cancer risk assessment.

The goal of cancer screening is to detect cancer before it is clinically apparent and when the person is without obvious signs or symptoms of disease. Screening asymptomatic individuals should result in the early detection of cancer when it is most easily treated with the least morbidity and mortality. A cancer-screening test should not be used in a symptomatic person; a symptomatic person needs a more comprehensive, diagnostic examination to rule out the possibility of cancer.

Regularly scheduled screening examinations can result in the detection of cancers of the breast, colon, rectum, cervix, prostate, testicles, oral cavity, and skin at earlier stages. These cancers account for approximately half of all new cancer cases. The combined five-year relative survival rate for these cancers is about 81%. If all Americans participated in regular screening, this rate could increase to more than 95% (ACS, 2001).

Research continues to suggest that the single most important factor in an individual ever having a screening test is a recommendation from the healthcare provider (Smith, Mettlin, Davis, & Eyre, 2000). When nurses recommend screening to an individual, the likelihood that the individual actually will undergo appropriate screening is far greater. This recommendation can come easily in the form of patient education about cancer prevention and early detection.

Section III provides a detailed discussion of each of the major tumor sites and issues related to cancer prevention and early detection. Each of these chapters includes the epidemiology and incidence of the cancer, known risk factors, possible prevention strategies, signs and symptoms, current methods for the detection of cancer, and implications for nurses.

The explosion of science in genetics and cancer is rapidly changing cancer risk assessment. It is now possible to identify individuals who are at a significantly higher risk of developing a particular cancer and develop a plan for both primary and secondary prevention. In Chapter 18, Greco provides a discussion of the role that nurses can play in providing cancer genetics services. Oncology nurses who provide secondary cancer prevention services must consider genetic principles in their assessments and recommendations for early detection. Greco also provides a framework for implementing genetics principles into the cancer risk assessment process. These principles are and will continue to become very important in the early detection of each of the major tumor sites.

Nurses who work in cancer-control activities, no matter what level of prevention, need to have a focus on wellness. This includes tertiary prevention with long-term survivors of cancer who are at risk for second primary malignancies. In the past, little attention has been given to tertiary prevention. As more individuals have cancer detected early and treated successfully, the pool of cancer survivors at risk for another malignancy will continue to grow. Chapter 17 provides an overview of what is now known about risks for second malignancies and other complications of cancer treatment and how these risks and complications are best managed. Management of these risks ultimately should improve the quality of life in cancer survivors. Nurses are challenged to implement programs to ensure that cancer survivors receive follow-up that includes screening for second cancers.

All levels of cancer prevention are aimed at healthy individuals who do not consider themselves to be ill. Cancer control requires a large amount of public education to empower individuals to take more responsibility for their health and well-being. As educators of patients and families, nurses are well suited to teach people about their cancer risk, ways to manage the risk, and how to detect cancer early, when it is most easily treated.

References

American Cancer Society. (2001). *Cancer facts and figures, 2001*. Atlanta: Author.

Foltz, A. (2001). Issues in determining cancer screening recommendations: Who, what, and when. *Oncology Nursing Forum, 27*(Suppl.), 13–17.

Love, S.M. (1989). Use of risk factors in counseling patients. *Hematology/Oncology Clinics of North America, 3*, 599–610.

MacLean, C.D. (1996). Principles of cancer screening. *Medical Clinics of North America, 80*, 1–14.

Mahon, S.M. (1998). Cancer risk assessment: Conceptual considerations for clinical practice. *Oncology Nursing Forum, 25*, 1535–1547.

Newell, G.R., & Vogel, V.G. (1988). Personal risk factors. What do they mean? *Cancer, 62*(Suppl. 8), 1695–1701.

Smith, R.A., Mettlin, C.J., Davis, K.J., & Eyre, H. (2000). American Cancer Society guidelines for the early detection of cancer. *CA: A Cancer Journal for Clinicians, 50*, 34–49.

CHAPTER 11

Breast Cancer Prevention and Detection: Past Progress and Future Directions

Janice Mitchell Phillips, PhD, RN, FAAN, and
Marva Mizell Price, DrPH, MPH, RN, CS

Introduction

The new millennium finds us witnessing many advances in breast cancer prevention and detection, particularly in the areas of genetics, primary prevention, and earlier detection. Ultimately, these advances have led to improvements in breast cancer mortality and survival rates. However, breast cancer continues to be one of the most common causes of cancer among American women. In 2001 alone, an estimated 192,200 invasive cases of breast cancer will be diagnosed, and an estimated 40,200 women will die from the disease (American Cancer Society [ACS], 2001b).

This chapter provides an overview of what currently is known about breast cancer, particularly in the areas of prevention and detection. The chapter begins with an overview of the scope of the problem and includes a discussion of current issues and trends related to breast cancer prevention and detection. Selected issues related to breast cancer and ethnic/racial minorities and the underserved are highlighted. The chapter concludes with a discussion on future directions for oncology nursing practice, education, and research.

Scope of the Problem

Incidence

Globally, breast cancer is one of the most common forms of cancer, accounting for approximately 21% of all new cancers in women (Ford, Marcus, & Lum, 1999). Excluding nonmelanoma skin cancer, breast cancer is the most common cancer among women residing in the United States, accounting for one of every

three cancers diagnosed in women (ACS, 1999). Epidemiologists estimate that during 2001 alone, 192,200 new invasive cases of breast cancer will be diagnosed in the United States. Projections also indicate that an additional 46,400 cases of in situ breast cancers will be diagnosed during this time (ACS, 2001b).

Breast cancer incidence increases with age, with 77% of new cases occurring in women age 50 and older. When all ages are considered, women ages 20–24 have the lowest age-specific incidence rate, 1.3 cases per 100,000 population, whereas women ages 75–79 have the highest incidence rate, 483.3 cases per 100,000 (Ries et al., 1999). Overall, White women have a higher incidence of breast cancer when compared to African American women. However, the reverse is true for African American women under age 50 (ACS, 2000). In fact, as shown in Figure 11-1, breast cancer incidence rates generally are lower among women of other racial and ethnic groups than among White women. An examination of the age-adjusted incidence of invasive breast cancer revealed that White, Hawaiian, and African American women have the highest breast cancer rates in Surveillance Epidemiology End Results (SEER) Program regions. The lowest rates occur among Korean, American Indian, and Vietnamese women (Ries et al.).

The age-adjusted incidence of breast cancer has changed considerably over time. For instance, trends revealed that between 1940 and 1982, the incidence of

Figure 11-1. Female Breast Cancer Incidence and Death Rates by Race and Ethnicity

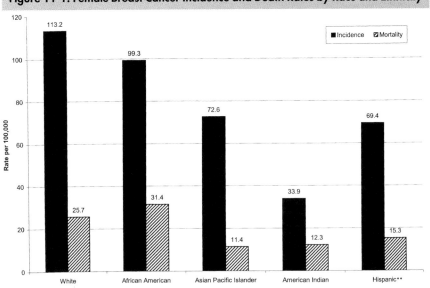

* Rates are age-adjusted to the 1970 U.S. standard population.
**Persons of Hispanic origin may be of any race.
American Cancer Society, Surveillance Research, 1999.
Data source: NCI Surveillance, Epidemiology, and End Results Program, 1999.

Note. From *Breast Cancer Facts and Figures 1999/2000* (p. 5), by the American Cancer Society, 1999, Atlanta, GA: Author. Copyright 1999 by the American Cancer Society. Reprinted with permission.

invasive breast cancer increased approximately 1% each year. The rapid increase in the number of invasive breast cancers developing during this period is attributed to the delays in childbearing and women having fewer children (ACS, 1999). This compares with the noted 4% increase in incidence between 1982 and 1988. The increase in invasive breast cancer cases during this period is attributed to increased detection through greater use of mammography. Between 1982 and 1988, the incidence of smaller tumors (< 2.0 cm) more than doubled, and the rates of larger tumors (≥ 3.0 cm) decreased approximately 27%. However, in the 1990s, breast cancer incidence rates leveled off to about 110.6 cases per 100,000 (ACS, 1999). Epidemiologists attribute this stabilization to the increased detection and earlier diagnosis noted between 1982 and 1988 (ACS, 1999).

Similarly, there have been noted increases in the number of in situ breast cancers, due in part to the increases in ductal carcinoma in situ (DCIS), a stage noted for its high curability. Between 1992 and 1996, this cancer accounted for 87% of the in situ breast cancers diagnosed among women in the SEER regions. An analysis of these trends revealed that the incidence rate of DCIS increased seven-fold faster than the incidence of invasive breast cancer, again primarily because of the increased use of mammography. Epidemiologists postulate that the increased incidence of DCIS represents a shift in the stage of diagnosis to a more curable stage rather than a true increase in breast cancer cases (ACS, 1999; Ernster, Barclay, Kerlikowske, Grady, & Henderson, 1996).

It is important to note that the increase in number of breast cancer cases diagnosed among younger women (i.e., under age 40) during the late 1980s and early 1990s has been linked to the growth and aging of the U.S. population. Breast cancer incidence among this age group began to decline in 1985 and has been declining at an average of –1.3% per year (ACS, 2000).

Mortality

In terms of mortality, breast cancer is the second leading cause of cancer death in women. Projections indicate that in the year 2001, 40,600 deaths will be attributed to breast cancer (40,200 women, 400 men [ACS, 2001b]). As shown in Figure 11-1, the highest age-adjusted mortality occurs among African American women (31.4 per 100,000), followed by White women (25.7 per 100,000) and Hispanic women (15.3 per 100,000). When compared with White women, African American women are more likely to die from breast cancer at almost every age group, except for White women age 70 and older (ACS, 2000).

Between 1990 and 1994, breast cancer mortality rates among White women declined 6.1%, representing the longest short-term decline in breast cancer in more than 40 years. However, mortality rates among African American women declined 1.0% (ACS, 1997). The racial disparities in breast cancer mortality are the result of a variety of factors, including the late stage at diagnosis for African American women and the possibility of more aggressive disease among them (ACS, 1999). The recent declines in breast cancer mortality have been attributed to the advances in breast cancer treatment and increased use of mammography screening. As more and more breast cancers are diagnosed while in situ or at earlier stages, epidemiologists predict continued reductions in breast cancer mortality (ACS, 2000).

Survival

Survival from breast cancer has increased tremendously over time because of the advances in treatment and detection. Specifically, the five-year relative survival rate for localized breast cancer has shown improvements from 72% in the 1940s to 96% today. The current five-year relative survival rate for women diagnosed with breast cancer in the localized stage is 96%, 77% for women with regional spread and 21% for women with distant metastasis (ACS, 2000). Figure 11-2 depicts the five-year relative survival rate by stage and race. As shown, the five-year survival rate is lower for women whose cancer is diagnosed at a more advanced stage. Recent data show that the relative survival rates for women diagnosed with breast cancer are 85% five years after diagnosis, 71% after 10 years, 57% after 15 years, and 52% after 20 years (ACS, 1999).

Similar to mortality rates, survival rates for African American women are less favorable when compared with their White counterparts. The five-year survival rate for all stages combined for African American women is 71.0% compared with 86% for White women. As shown in Figure 11-2, between 1989 and 1995, 51% of African American women had their breast cancers diagnosed in the localized stage compared with 62% of White women. Similarly, 35% of African American women had their breast cancers diagnosed at a regional stage compared with 29% of White women, and 9% of African American women had their breast cancers diagnosed at a distant stage compared with 6% of White women (ACS, 1999).

As with mortality rates, the differences in breast cancer survival between African Americans and Whites have been attributed to the late stage at detection and tumors that are less responsive to treatment among Africa American women. Additional factors related to this difference in survival include limited access to medical care, the presence of comorbid illnesses, as well as a variety of socioeconomic and cultural factors (ACS, 1997; Eley et al., 1994; Lannin et al., 1998).

The Science of Breast Cancer Development

Basic Anatomy and Physiology
The Normal Breast From the Embryo to the Mature Woman

This section provides an overview of the basic anatomy and physiology of breast development from the embryonic stages to the adult female breast. Review of normal growth, development, and function of the breast, also known as mammary glands, is essential to understanding the biological changes that take place in breast cancer. Breast development occurs in a cephalocaudal manner and begins early in gestation with a series of physiologic and hormonal changes taking place.

Although the breasts are mature by late adolescence, development is not fully completed until final hormonal influences occur following delivery of an infant. Early embryonic development, however, is not under the influence of hormones.

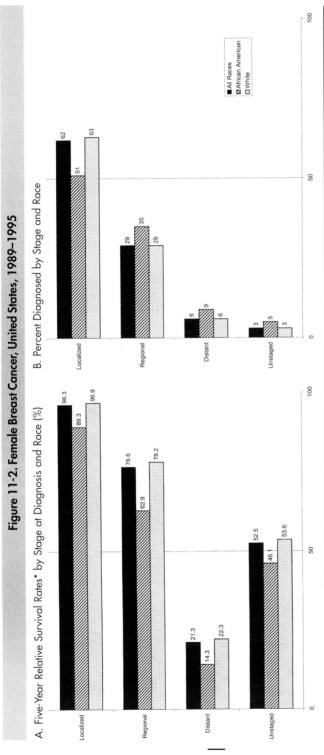

Figure 11-2. Female Breast Cancer, United States, 1989–1995

A. Five-Year Relative Survival Rates* by Stage at Diagnosis and Race (%)

B. Percent Diagnosed by Stage and Race

*Survival rates are based on follow-up of patients through 1996.
American Cancer Society, Surveillance Research, 1999.
Data source: NCI Surveillance, Epidemiology, and End Results Program, 1999.

Note. From Breast Cancer Facts and Figures 1999/2000 (p. 72), by the American Cancer Society, 1999, Atlanta, GA: Author. Copyright 1999 by the American Cancer Society. Reprinted with permission.

Fifth week of gestation: Breast development begins early in the developing embryo. During the fifth week of fetal development, a pair of milk lines develops from the axilla to the groin along the embryonic trunk. This milk line is also called the ectodermal primitive milk streak. The two ventral bands, or "galactic bands," are illustrated in Figure 11-3. Most of the band will regress, except for a small portion that develops to form a ridge on the pectoral region of the embryonic thorax, known as the mammary ridge (Harris, Lippman, Morrow, & Hellman, 1996; Tavassoli, 1999).

7th–16th week of gestation: The mammary ridge thickens and infolds into the developing chest wall during the seventh to eighth week to establish the thickened milk lines. By 10–16 weeks, the ridge flattens and cells differentiate to form the smooth muscle of the nipple and areola. At the 16th week, 15–25 epithelial strips originate from epithelial buds and branch to form the future secretory alveoli (see Figure 11-4). The Montgomery glands form around the nipple from special apocrine or sebaceous glands.

20th–32nd week of gestation: From approximately 20 weeks on into week 32 of the third trimester, placenta sex hormones (estrogen and progesterone) enter fetal circulation to produce channels or sinuses in the epithelial strips. This process evolves to join the duct and sebaceous glands. Fifteen to 25 mammary ducts are formed by the end of fetal development.

32nd–40th week of gestation: During this period, cellular differentiation takes place to develop lobular-alveoli structures and nipple-areola pigmentation. The amount of mammary gland tissue largely increases, and colostral milk (often called witch's milk) develops in the stimulated mammary tissue and ducts. The colostrum declines once placenta hormones are withdrawn, within a week after

Figure 11-3. Milk Lines

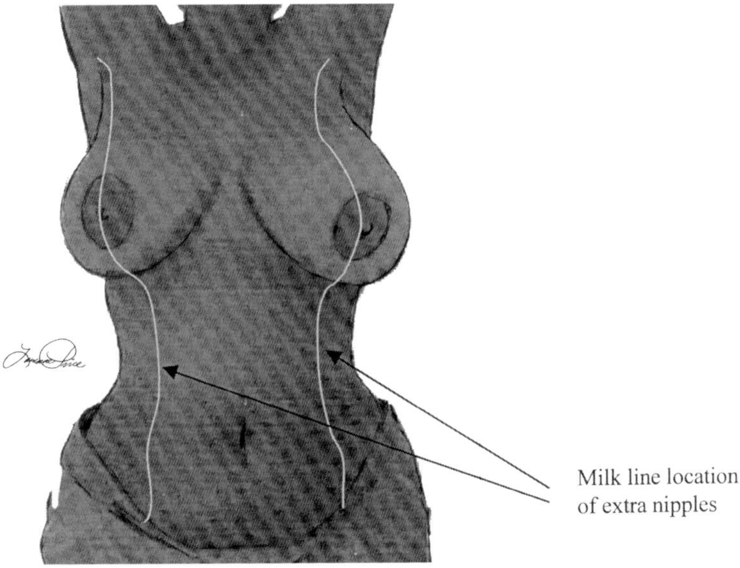

Milk line location of extra nipples

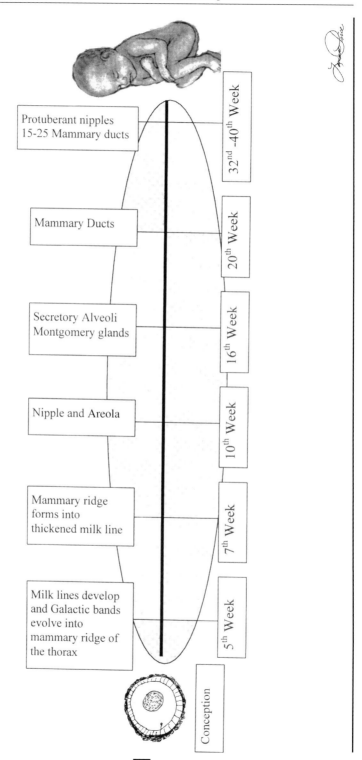

Figure 11-4. Timeline for Embryonic Development of the Breasts

Protuberant nipples 15-25 Mammary ducts — 32nd –40th Week

Mammary Ducts — 20th Week

Secretory Alveoli Montgomery glands — 16th Week

Nipple and Areola — 10th Week

Mammary ridge forms into thickened milk line — 7th Week

Milk lines develop and Galactic bands evolve into mammary ridge of the thorax — 5th Week

Conception

delivery. The mammary ducts open into shallow depressions called mammary pits. These will form the protuberant nipples.

Postnatal breast development: During the first month of postnatal development, the newborn breast can appear enlarged. As maternal placenta hormones return to normal levels, the breast tissue shrinks. Minimal changes occur from the postnatal period until puberty, with a limited number of ductal sinuses growing and branching out during childhood.

Pubertal and adolescent breast development: Most of breast growth occurs during puberty. During this phase of development, usually between ages 10–12 years, hypothalamic gonadotropin-releasing hormones are secreted into the pituitary gland. Consequently, follicle-stimulating hormone (FSH) and luteinizing hormone (LH) are released. FSH causes maturation of the ovarian follicle, and estrogen is secreted. These hormonal changes act upon the breast tissue. Estrogen is excreted from the ovarian follicle and produces further growth of the ductal system in the breast tissue. At the same time, periductal stroma proliferates.

In adolescence, estrogen is the major hormonal influence on breast growth (with progesterone in a supportive role). Estrogen acts on the ductal portion of the gland system to produce the phases of breast development that are measurable by Tanner staging. Tanner staging is classic core knowledge in the study of the development of secondary sex characteristics in pediatric and adolescent nursing. Buds develop and produce lengthening of the ductal growth. In addition, estrogen increases the volume and elasticity of periductal connective tissue. Increases in vascularity and fatty tissue further enlarge the mass of tissue beneath the areola.

Throughout adolescence and early adulthood, mammary ducts, lobules, stroma, and alveoli continue to develop from the levels of estrogen and progesterone. During these development phases, it is thought that progesterone, rather than estrogen, has the greater influence on the alveolar component of the lobules. In addition, the accumulation of fat in connective tissue continues to increase during late adolescence.

The adult female breast: Mature appearance occurs three to four years following the initial surge of estrogen and progesterone activity, with a protuberant, circular appearance to the pigmented areola and nipple. The areola diameter measures 15–60 mm. Montgomery glands are elevated ductal openings near the periphery of the areola.

The average adult breast is 10–12 cm in diameter and about 5–7 cm thick. The vertical axis of the adult breast extends from the second to the sixth vertebrae. Its horizontal axis lies between the midaxillary line and the sternal edge. The undersurface of the breast lies over the pectoral fascia, which covers the pectoralis major, the serratus anterior, and the external oblique muscles. It is attached to the overlying skin by fibrous bands known as Cooper's accessory ligaments. These connective tissue bands extend between glandular fat lobules and the skin to naturally support the breast. The axillary tail is a portion of the breast that extends into the axilla (see Figure 11-5).

The glandular portion of the breast is composed of fibrous, adipose, and epithelial tissue and is divided into 15–20 lobes, or segments, which are arranged in a radial pattern. The internal anatomy of the mature breast is shown in Figure 11-6.

Figure 11-5. Surface Anatomy of the Adult Breast

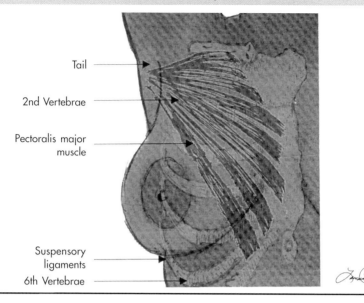

Tail

2nd Vertebrae

Pectoralis major
muscle

Suspensory
ligaments

6th Vertebrae

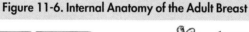

Figure 11-6. Internal Anatomy of the Adult Breast

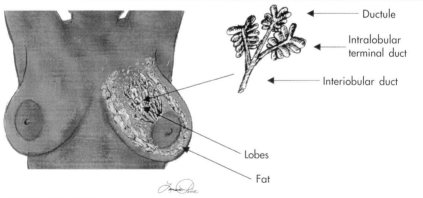

Ductule

Intralobular
terminal duct

Interiobular duct

Lobes

Fat

The functional portion of the breast is the duct system. A lobe-specific lactiferous sinus, or collecting duct, drains each of the lobules. Some of these ducts may join so that no more than 5–10 major collecting milk ducts open on the surface of the nipple. By age 13–15, the collecting ducts (see Figure 11-7) elon-

Figure 11-7. Terminal Ductal Lobular Unit

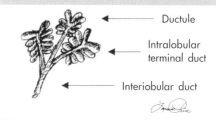

Ductule

Intralobular
terminal duct

Interiobular duct

gate from the nipple, branch out, and end in the terminal ductal lobular unit (Marchant, 1997; Tavassoli, 1999).

The terminal duct lobular unit is composed of an extralobular terminal duct, intralobular terminal duct, and ductules, which are called acinies. The ductules are the most distal structures and have a sac-like appearance. The ductules sometimes are referred to as alveolar buds when they are in a resting state, while acinies best describes the fully developed secretory unit of the breast in pregnancy and lactation (Harris et al., 1996; Marchant, 1997). The lobule is the smallest structural unit of the mammary gland and is surrounded with vascular connective tissue (Marchant). The majority of the bulk comes from the fibrous adipose tissue that surrounds the duct system.

The final stage of breast development is called lobuloalveolar differentiation and only occurs in the pregnant woman. Major changes in endocrine hormones—including placental, growth hormone levels, insulin, and glucocorticoids—produce hyperplasia of the ductal and secretory components, hypertrophy of the alveolar cells, and decrease in fat and fibrous connective tissue (Donegan & Spratt, 1995; Harris et al., 1996).

The breast at menopause: During the menopausal period, the epithelial and connective tissues of the breasts undergo progressive decrease in size while atrophy is occurring. Within the lobules, a series of intercellular changes occurs. These include thinning of the ductule cells and thickening of the cell layers that surround the epithelial cells, called basal lamina. The intercellular stroma changes into dense hyaline tissue that blends with the basal lamina. Most of the epithelium flattens and loses secretory activity. Involution of the breast tissue progresses, and there is a decrease in the ductules in the lobules. Stroma is replaced by fatty tissue. Elastic and collagen fibers change, causing sagging of the breasts. These changes in the connective tissue and support structures take place inconsistently in varying stages during the premenopausal period.

Blood and Lymph Systems of the Breast

Arterial blood supply to the breast comes from multiple sources (see Table 11-1). Lymphatic vessels arise in the periductal spaces and drain mostly into the ipsilat-

Table 11-1. Blood Supply

Location	Vessel	Portion of the Breast
Medial and central portions	Internal mammary artery	60%
Upper outer quadrant	Lateral thoracic artery	30%
Small portions of the pectoral and lateral areas	Thoracoacromial artery	10%
Outer quadrants	Third, fourth, and fifth intercostal arteries	
	Subscapular artery	
	Thoracodorsal artery	

eral axillary nodes. Both axillary and internal mammary nodes receive drainage from all four quadrants of the breast (Marchant, 1997; Tavassoli, 1999).

The breasts are drained by three groups of veins: the intercostal veins, the axillary veins, and the internal (thoracic) mammary vein perforators. Venous drainage plays a major supportive role in the spread of breast cancer to the lungs, brain, liver, bone, and other tissues.

The larger portion of the breast lymph drainage flows to the axillary nodes. Lymph can pass obstructed lymph nodes through adjoining channels. Thus, when cancer is present, lower nodes can be missed; the first metastasis may appear at a higher node. More detailed discussion of the lymphatic system in cancer progression follows in the next section on lymph flow and breast metastases (Donegan & Spratt, 1995; Harris et al., 1996; Tavassoli, 1999).

Lymph Flow and Breast Metastases

Based on a correlation of the location of carcinomas and the distribution of lymph node metastases, it appears that a preferential flow to certain pathways exists (see Figure 11-8). These routes are based on where the primary carcinoma is located in the breast (Tavassoli, 1999). Tumors located in the upper outer quadrant metastasize mainly to the axillary nodes, whereas only those located in the central or medial region of the breast may metastasize to the internal mammary chain. The major pathway for the spread of breast cancer is through the axillary nodes because these nodes receive more than 75% of the mammary lymph flow. Only tumors in the upper outer and upper central part of the breast show metastases to the interpectoral nodes (Harris et al., 1996).

The lymphatic drainage of nodes in the fifth through sixth intercostal spaces contributes to the spread of breast disease. In the presence of nodal metastases, obstruction of the physiologic routes of lymphatic flow may occur. Alternative

Figure 11-8. Breast Lymph Pathway

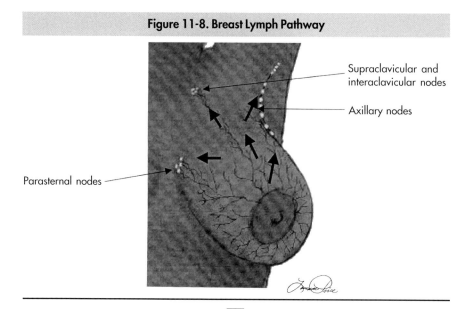

Supraclavicular and interaclavicular nodes

Axillary nodes

Parasternal nodes

pathways are thought to become important. The alternative routes include deep, substernal, and cross drainage to the contralateral internal mammary chain, superficial presternal crossover, lateral intercostal and mediastinal drainage, and spread through the rectus abdominis muscle sheath to the subdiaphragmatic and subperiotoneal plexus. The last route allows the direct spread of tumor to the liver and retroperitoneal lymph nodes. Substernal crossover has been demonstrated, using the special technique of isotope imaging of the lymph nodes, and may be of significance in early breast cancer (Tavassoli, 1999).

Common Cellular Changes for Tumor Development

During the past decade, scientists have increased investigative research in both the molecular pathogenesis of cancer and the identification of genetic predispositions. Keeping pace with the new knowledge, today's nurses are joining multidisciplinary teams to expand the role of nursing in prevention, risk analysis, and early detection of cancer. What nurses learn about cancer prevention and detection has a direct impact on the application of therapeutics for breast cancer. Considerable discussion on the biology of breast cancer is included in this chapter to further enrich the nurse's background in this area.

At least four distinct characteristics are needed for a normal cell to progress to a neoplastic cell and to give rise to an invasive cancer (Gasparini, 1999).

1. Deregulation of the cell cycle with abnormal proliferation
2. Suppression of the pathways leading to cell death
3. Assumption of altered characteristics to induce alterations of the microenvironment for growth potential
4. Tumor must avoid destruction by the immune system.

Nearly all of the breast ductal system is lined by two cell layers: the inner epithelial cell layer along the luminal side and the surrounding interrupted layer, known as myoepithelial cells. A layer of basal lamina surrounds the two cell layers. This entire structure, which is enveloped by one or more "delimiting fibroblasts" depending on the caliber of the duct, constitutes the unit structure of the breast. Any alteration in the number of these cell layers results in a pathologic change (Tavassoli, 1999).

Hormone tissue modulators and specific genetic events have been implicated in breast tumor carcinogenesis. Many breast cancers appear to develop through a series of premalignant stages. These stages are defined histologically as atypical hyperplastic proliferation of epithelial and stroma cells, and this carcinoma in situ leads to invasive cancer (Bowcock, 1999; Harris et al., 1996). This histologic progression occurs in normal cells along with numerous molecular alterations and mutations. These include changes in underlying structures of basement membrane within mammary epithelial cells that result in oncogene activation and/or tumor suppressor dysregulation or inactivation (Couch & Weber, 1998).

Oncogenes are a class of genes that cause tumor growth when activated and possess very interesting, complex behaviors. In addition, oncogenes also can prevent cell death. These genes have a strong relationship to tumor enlargement

(Roses, 1999). Their genetic changes accumulate in a complex and variable fashion: some are maintained throughout different stages of tumor development, others are specific to particular stages, whereas still others have no obvious linkage to progression. During this process, there is a general trend of the genes toward increasing mutational load. Tumor evolution is made in part by recognizable cycles of mutational diversification and clonal selection (Bowcock, 1999).

It has been suggested that mutations are causally responsible for driving mammary tumor development and that significant modifications occur in the progression of gene modeling to completely account for the complex process of gene mutation (Bowcock, 1999).

The most common molecular alterations known in breast cancer involve large-scale gains or losses of genetic material, resulting in allelic imbalances on the genetic material (Bowcock, 1999). Invasive breast cancers frequently contain multiple examples of such imbalances—most commonly losses and gains of chromosomes known to be associated with breast tumors (Bowcock). In addition, a number of genes have been indicated in breast tumorigenesis. These include the proto-oncogene products and the tumor suppressor gene products p53 (detectable in 24% of breast carcinomas), Tp53, and Rb-1 (Tavassoli, 1999).

Breast tumor evolution does not seem to follow a simple, orderly, and linear progression model; it appears to involve a more complex process characterized by periods of expansion and contraction while simultaneous evolution of multiple independent tumor regions takes place.

Over the past decade, breast cancer researchers have been identifying tumor-causing genes at a rapid pace and analyzing their relationship to pathological features of tumors. A major goal of molecular scientists and oncologists has been to be able to differentiate prognostic information as well as predictive data in relation to clinical application learned from molecular aberrations. This information could provide scientists and clinicians with the ability to tailor types of traditional and aggressive therapies. In addition, some oncologists have undertaken preliminary studies that target the more common breast cancer-related mutant gene products with novel forms of cancer treatment, including immunotherapy and gene therapy (Bowcock, 1999).

Early investigations suggested that a strong correlation may exist between genes and an increased risk for breast cancer over a woman's lifetime. Although knowledge in this area is expanding rapidly and promises to move from a laboratory environment to clinical application, recent findings caution placing too much emphasis on genetics as a cause. As many as 20% of families who are at high risk for breast cancer do not carry breast cancer genes BRCA1 and BRCA2, which has raised the possibility of a third breast cancer susceptibility gene (Tavassoli, 1999). Therefore, the development of cancer in predisposed individuals suggests that there may be a correlation of some other factors, such as environmental influences, or complex interrelation of several factors (Roses, 1999). In summary, breast cancer is characterized by progressive loss of controls of basement membrane, estrogen, and progesterone and overexpression of epidermal growth factor receptors on cell proliferation and epithelial differentiation. The epidermal growth factor is associated with genomic mutations, deletions, amplifications, and chromosomal rearrangements by causing alterations in nuclear matrix structure and function and by promoting loss of normal tissue organization and metastasis (Harris et al., 1996).

Classification of Breast Carcinoma

New findings in breast cancer research mean that there will be new approaches in how breast cancer is classified. Although it is apparent that breast cancer originates from the epithelium of mammary ducts and acini, recent pathological discoveries show that a large percentage of breast carcinomas, both ductal and lobular, take origin in the terminal duct lobular unit rather than from larger ducts. Historically and more recently, several schema have been proposed for classifying the various types of breast carcinoma. Donegan and Spratt (1995) divided cancer types into two categories—invasive and noninvasive. The following sections provide information about the most commonly occurring forms of noninvasive and invasive breast cancer.

Noninvasive Carcinoma
Ductal Carcinoma

Epithelial proliferation within the terminal ducts and lobular unit constitutes a significant site for the origination of breast cancer. In recent years, as researchers learn more about the behavior of breast cancer tumor cells, new translations of traditional classification systems have been proposed to address atypical proliferative lesions (Tavassoli, 1999). Discussion in this chapter will be based on traditional classification. Outstanding features of the major types of noninvasive and invasive breast lesions are presented in Table 11-2.

The terminal duct/lobular unit carcinoma is referred to as ductal carcinoma in situ (DCIS), or simply ductal intraepithelial neoplasia. In earlier years, this type of breast carcinoma was thought to be rare. However, widespread use of mammography has led to increased detection of this type of lesion. Usually, there is no evidence of spread to surrounding stroma tissue. The lesions in the ductal/lobular area are subdivided into two cell types, ductal and lobular. The classification depends upon the cell type, architectural pattern of cell growth and distribution, and distention of the ductules. Ductal lesions can be further divided based on atypical cell types and likelihood of becoming invasive.

DCIS noninvasive breast cancers usually can be further classified according to the architectural pattern of the lesion. These subcategories are designated as comedo, cribriform, micropapillary, papillary, solid, and combinations of patterns (Donegan & Spratt, 1995; Harris & Leininger, 1995).

Comedo carcinomas are characterized by large pleomorphic cells with abundant cytoplasm, bizarre nuclei, and frequent mitoses. Focal central necrosis is the hallmark of this variant. The necrotic material frequently becomes calcified into linear, branching, and coarse granular calcifications, which are easiest to detect mammographically. Comedo types are the largest in size and most frequently palpable lesions. It has a high rate of growth and the greatest malignant potential.

Table 11-2. Outstanding Features of Breast Carcinomas

Type	Location	Outstanding Features
Noninvasive carcinoma	Terminal ducts and lobular units	
Ductal		Frequently occurring lesion Often nonpalpable Less likely to spread to surrounding tissue
Lobular		Symptomless Found microscopically Associated with calcifications Can coexist with intraductal carcinoma Might not develop into carcinoma One-third progress to invasive cancer Marker for invasive breast cancer
Invasive carcinoma	Mammary epithelium	Single largest group and most frequently occurring of malignant mammary cancers Invades beyond basement membranes of the ducts and lobules Higher grades indicate poorer prognosis. Best prognosis with circumscribed tumors
Invasive lobular carcinoma		Second most frequently occurring form of breast cancer

Comedo type is more prone to recurrence and evolving into an invasive carcinoma (Donegan & Spratt, 1995; Harris et al., 1996). Comedo carcinomas account for up to two-thirds of DCIS (Tavassoli, 1999).

Cribriform type is typically a monomorphic population of small to medium cells with round, uniform, hyperchromatic nuclei exhibiting rare mitosis and showing a fenestrated sieve-like growth pattern. Mitosis is rarely observed, but when it is, it is limited to a single cell or small cell clusters. Necrosis is not common (Donegan & Spratt, 1995; Harris et al., 1996).

Micropapillary type consists of monomorphic, hyperchromic, proliferating tufts of small to medium-sized cells that are oriented perpendicular to the basement membrane of the involved spaces. They lack central fibrovascular cores that project into the lumen of the duct. Mitosis is infrequent. Necrosis and cellular atypia are not frequently present. Micropapillary DCIS is more frequently multifocal and multicentric than are other variants of DCIS (Donegan & Spratt, 1995; Harris et al., 1996; Tavassoli, 1999). The combination of cribriform and micropapillary patterns occurs so frequently that some authors consider them together.

The solid types of DCIS show tumor cells with well-defined margins that fill and distend the involved spaces and lack significant necrosis, fenestration, or papillations. The tumor cells may be large with atypical nuclei. There is abnormal mitosis.

Papillary, a more rare form of DCIS, constitutes only 1%–2% of breast carcinomas. DCIS lesions show projections of atypical tumor cells into the ductal lumen that, unlike the micropapillary variant, show fibrovascular cores and thus constitute true papillations (Donegan & Spratt, 1995; Harris et al., 1996).

Lobular Carcinoma

Some researchers estimate the number of cases of lobular carcinoma in situ (LCIS) to account for less than 10% of mammary cancers. LCIS is often the subject of debate. It is included here because of its high bilaterality and controversial potential for invasive malignancy. LCIS is a symptomless lesion of the breast that lacks distinguishing gross characteristics. It originates in the terminal duct lobular unit and can coexist with intraductal carcinoma (Donegan & Spratt, 1995). The diagnosis is established by microscopic examination. Most of the time, it is an incidental finding on a breast biopsy specimen that was removed for another reason, usually because of a coexisting benign or malignant lesion.

It is multicentric in about 80% of the cases and bilateral in some 15%–40% (Donegan & Spratt, 1995; Tavassoli, 1999). LCIS is found in about 1.5%–10% of biopsy specimens (Donegan & Spratt; Tavassoli). Foci of calcification in adjacent mammary lobules may be the only abnormality detected on a mammogram (Donegan & Spratt). Histologically, the calcifications can be located in normal epithelial cells adjacent to areas of lobular carcinoma in situ rather than in the involved lobules (Harris et al., 1996).

In contrast to DCIS, which is heterogeneous in its histologic appearance, the histologic features of LCIS show little variation and usually are easily recognized (Harris et al., 1996). These tumors are a solid proliferation of small cells with small, uniform nuclei. The loosely cohesive cells distort and obliterate the acini. They distend into the terminal duct/lobular units. Extension may occur to the terminal duct and produce a closely stacked or page-like appearance. Mitoses are rare and necrosis even rarer.

The differential diagnosis of LCIS includes ductal and lobular hyperplasia with various degrees of atypia. For some lesions, a definitive classification is arbitrary (Roses, 1999).

It has been observed that many of the women with LCIS will not develop breast cancer. However, LCIS is a risk factor for breast cancer development, with up to a third progressing to an invasive carcinoma (Harris et al., 1996; Tavassoli, 1999). Fifty percent of carcinomas that develop following a diagnosis of lobular neoplasia are ductal in type (Tavassoli). As a risk marker, LCIS does not specify which breast will develop invasive carcinoma; both breasts are equally at risk at about 1% per year indefinitely. LCIS is regarded as a marker that identifies a patient at increased risk of subsequent invasive breast cancer (Roses, 1999).

Invasive Carcinoma

Invasive carcinoma of the breast is a malignant neoplasm of the mammary epithelium. The neoplastic cells invade beyond the native basement membrane of the ducts and lobules in which they arise and into the surrounding stroma. Once the tumor has invaded, it has access to lymphatic and blood vessels that facilitate metastasis to both regional lymph nodes and distant sites. Although invasion beyond the basement membrane is not the sole characteristic necessary for a tumor to metastasize, it is the feature that defines the entity of invasive carcinoma and the principal one that pathologists evaluate on a morphologic basis (Roses, 1999).

Once a tumor is classified, malignant tumors are divided according to their grade and stage to further determine the degree of differentiation and prognosis. Generally, the higher the grade and stage, the poorer the prognosis. Grading includes criteria for secondary lumen formation, cellular uniformity, and mitotic count (Tavassoli, 1999). Grading schema will include a numeric designation (1,2,3, or 4) or a descriptive grade, such as moderately or poorly differentiated. The low numeric grades of well-differentiated tumors are those that cytologically and histologically deviate the least from normal, although the high-grade or poorly differentiated tumors have the least resemblance to normal cells and tissue patterns. The stage of the tumor is simply an evaluation of the extent of the tumor at the time of diagnosis and is not necessarily related to its grade. The evaluation considers size of the tumor, invasion of adjacent structures, regional lymph node involvement, and distant metastases (Tavassoli).

Carcinomas of the breast that appear to be entirely in situ rarely metastasize; in these cases, it is presumed that occult invasion exists but is not present in the histologic sections. Carcinomas may arise from other structures of the breast, notably the skin and its appendages, but these are not tumors of the mammary parenchyma (Roses, 1999).

Invasive Ductal Carcinoma

This section deals with the pathologic features of the two major forms of invasive breast carcinoma, ductal and lobular. Invasive duct carcinoma constitutes the single largest group and most frequently occurring malignant mammary tumor. The current literature gives a prevalence range of 47%–80%. The higher percentages of invasive ductal cancers have been diagnosed in the United States, whereas the lower percentages worldwide are found in Japan (Tavassoli, 1999). Invasive ductal carcinoma forms a solid tumor. However, this category of invasive carcinomas includes a wide range of histologic appearances, from those with well-formed glands to those that have little or no evidence of specific differentiation. Because of the lack of histologically evident ductal differentiation in some tumors, the terms "carcinoma, no special type" and "carcinoma, not otherwise specified" (NOS) have been proposed (Donegan & Spratt, 1995; Roses, 1999).

Cystic change is uncommon but may be a manifestation of necrosis, usually accompanied by hemorrhage in the degenerated area. The measured gross size of a mammary carcinoma is one of the most critical prognostic variables. Survival decreases with increasing tumor size; those that are irregular in shape are measured at the largest diameter. There is a coincidental rise in the rate of axillary nodal metastases in invasive carcinoma. Circumscribed tumors have a more favorable prognosis than those with irregular borders and are less likely to have axillary lymph node involvement (Harris et al., 1996).

Invasive Lobular Carcinoma

Invasive lobular carcinoma is the second most frequent form of invasive carcinoma of the breast. Invasive lobular carcinoma varies from a poorly circumscribed but defined, firm tumor to an ill-defined area of induration. The classic form of invasive lobular carcinoma is composed of small cells with uniform nuclei arranged in single file within a fibrous stroma. It is generally mildly to moderately cellular. A targetoid arrangement of tumor cells around non-neoplastic ducts often is seen (Roses, 1999).

Patterns of Anatomic Distribution, Nodal Involvement, and Disease Progression

Anatomic Distribution

Studies have described the usual sites and distribution of breast lesions. The primary site usually is described by its location by quadrant in the breast. Nearly half are located in the upper outer quadrant. This is thought to result from the increased amount of breast tissue in that quadrant (Harris et al., 1996). Figure 11-9 shows the distribution of primary sites by breast region (Donegan & Spratt, 1995).

Figure 11-9. Distribution of Primary Breast Cancer Lesions

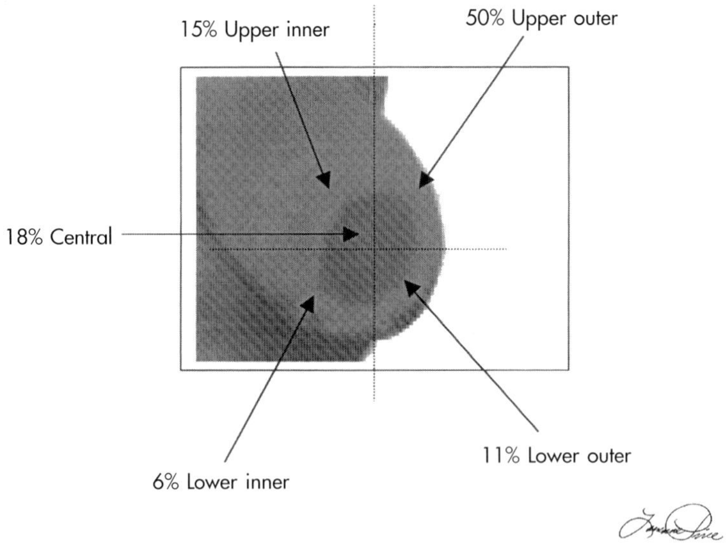

15% Upper inner

50% Upper outer

18% Central

6% Lower inner

11% Lower outer

Note. Based on information from Belcher, 1992.

Nodal Involvement

The most common sites of regional involvement of breast carcinoma are the axillary nodes. The second major nodal site of involvement is the internal mammary nodal chain that lies in intercostal spaces adjacent to the internal thoracic artery. Supraclavicular lymph node regions of involvement are associated with extensive axillary node invasion. Approximately 50% of women with breast carcinoma that is evident on clinical examination will have axillary node involvement, and another 20% will have involvement in the intramammary nodes in the intercostal spaces of the parasternal region. When supraclavicular nodes are involved, approximately one-fifth of the women also will have positive axillary nodes. Supraclavicular node involvement carries a grave prognosis because it represents a late state of axillary node involvement (Harris et al., 1996).

Disease Progression

The growth pattern of breast cancer in metastatic sites tends to be similar to that of the primary tumor. Over the past four decades, several mathematical models have been used to determine the growth rate of breast tumors. Earlier models used exponential patterns to determine tumor doubling and volume. More recent models consider many of the variables in earlier models but also observe information about the genetic and molecular biology of the disease. This includes what is known about mutation pathways and oncogenesis (Donegan & Spratt, 1995; Harris et al., 1996).

When ductal carcinoma metastasizes to the lymph nodes, it grows characteristically in cohesive nests and sheets. Lesser degrees of involvement distribute in a sinusoidal pattern. Lobular carcinoma, on the other hand, may grow in cohesive patterns, but it often has a more diffuse growth pattern, similar to growth of normal breast tissue.

Once carcinoma cells invade lymph and surrounding tissue, they may assume any of the recognized patterns of invasion, regardless of the pattern of the in situ phase. This may partly explain why almost 50% of subsequent infiltrating carcinomas observed following a diagnosis of lobular neoplasia display patterns recognized as ductal types. Occasionally, two different patterns of carcinoma may be present in different areas of the breast. Moreover, two synchronous carcinomas with identical morphologic patterns may develop in the same breast or in the opposite breast. In such cases, it is difficult to differentiate whether the lesions are different or if they represent metastases of one of the lesions. A large proportion of invasive carcinomas reflect a pure subtype, but combined patterns, with a lesion or two distinct patterns of infiltrating carcinoma within different regions of the breast, also occur. Generally, a carcinoma is designated according to the pattern dominating in 90% or more of the tumor. Infiltrating ductal carcinoma, lobular carcinoma, medullary carcinoma, and atypical medullary carcinoma have lower rates of survival, estimated to be 50% or less (Tavassoli, 1999). Diagnosis is made based on exclusion of other cellular types of breast carcinoma.

Metastatic ductal carcinoma has a higher incidence of spread to the lungs and pleura, but these are fairly common sites of spread for lobular carcinoma, as well. Lobular carcinoma more often involves the peritoneum and retroperitoneum, bone marrow, and meninges. Along with the peritoneal spread, there can be diffuse serosal involvement of abdominal and pelvic viscera, often with accompanying involvement of the walls of hollow organs of the gastrointestinal and urinary system as well as of the ovaries. Bone and liver are common sites of spread for both ductal and lobular carcinoma (Roses, 1999).

Pathologists may refer to invasive carcinoma when describing spread into lymph tissues. At other times, vascular invasion is inferred when speaking of both lymphatic and blood vessels. Some studies show a decrease in survival rates for women whose tumors have vascular invasion (Roses, 1999).

The interval to recurrence and the length of survival are the basic measurements of prognosis. Factors associated with a high frequency of recurrence correlate with reduced survival. Some treatment modalities delay, rather than reduce, the overall frequency of cancer recurrence. Survival is likely to be increased without reducing mortality of the disease in the long term (Harris et al., 1996). Overall, invasive lobular carcinoma does not have a better survival rate from invasive breast carcinoma when compared with an invasive ductal carcinoma (Roses, 1999).

Recurrence of Breast Carcinoma

Recurrence is reappearance of an original cancer in a woman after a period of clinical cure. The period between treatment and recurrence is known as the disease-free interval. This period is different from persistence, in which there is no disease-free interval. Recurrence follows primary treatment for two reasons: either the cancer was occultly disseminated before treatment, or the cancer was incompletely eliminated from local and regional tissue (Donegan & Spratt, 1995). Local-regional recurrence is recurrence in the breast or anterior chest and in its regional lymph nodes. Recurrences elsewhere are considered "distant." Local recurrence may be defined as recurrence within the soft tissues of the opposite anterior chest in the skin, breast or residual breast tissue, subcutaneous tissue, or underlying muscles. Regional recurrence refers to recurrence in unremoved regional lymph nodes in the axillary nodes, internal mammary nodes, and supraclavicular nodes (Donegan & Sprat).

Examining Breast Cancer Risk

Breast cancer is considered a heterogeneous disease resulting from a variety of factors. Risk factors associated with the development of breast cancer are multifaceted and, in some instances, not well understood. Although these factors vary from individual to individual, the presence of risk factors may or may not ensure the development of the disease. The majority of women diagnosed with breast cancer do not have any identifiable risk factors. Siedman, Stellman, and Mushinski (1982), for example, reported that 75% of women diagnosed with breast cancer have no identifiable risk factors. Their finding emerged after conducting an extensive analysis of risk factors for more than 570,000 women enrolled in one of the largest prospective studies sponsored by ACS. Since this time, many experts in the field have continued their efforts to identify and quantify risk factors related to breast cancer development and have supported the notion that all women should be considered at risk for developing breast cancer during their lifetime. When identified, risk factors often are used in determining the need for earlier and more intensive medical surveillance.

While several definitions can be used to define risk, the term "relative risk" is the one most frequently used when describing the epidemiology of breast cancer. When applied to breast cancer, this term is defined as the incidence rate of breast cancer in a population of individuals diagnosed with breast cancer with a known or suspected risk factor divided by the number of the incidence of breast cancer in a population of women without the disease. An individual with an estimated relative risk greater than 1.0 is considered to have a higher likelihood of developing breast cancer than does an individual without risk factors. In contrast, an individual estimated to have a relative risk of less than 1.0 is considered to have a lesser likelihood of developing breast cancer than an individual without risk factors. Moreover, relative risk is used to identify the strength of a relationship. For example, several factors (e.g., older age, family history, inherited genetic mutation) are associated with a relative risk greater than 4.0, placing an individual at a higher risk for developing the disease than an individual without the aforementioned risk factors (ACS, 1999, 2000; Kelsey, 1993).

Of note is that many women overestimate their personal risk for developing breast cancer. A woman residing in the United States has a 12.5%, or one in eight, lifetime risk of developing breast cancer (ACS, 1999). Women often are confused by what this statistic really means; thus, there is a continuing need to communicate to consumers that the one in eight statistic refers to the lifetime risk of developing breast cancer.

A variety of risk factors have been implicated in the development of breast cancer. Being female and age 50 or older are the two most significant risk factors for the disease. Other factors associated with the development of breast cancer include a personal or family history of breast cancer, biopsy-confirmed atypical hyperplasia, long menstrual history, history of exposure to exogenous hormones, previous breast irradiation, nulliparity, delayed childbearing (after age 30), higher socioeconomic status, and consumption of two or more alcoholic beverages a day (ACS, 2000). A history of ovarian or endometrial cancer or obesity also may increase a woman's risk of breast cancer. International variations in breast cancer incidence have shown a relationship between breast cancer and high fat intake. However, findings from studies examining the link between dietary fat consumption and breast cancer have been mixed, so continued research is under way. Additional studies are in progress to identify and examine the role of pesticides/environmental exposures, induced abortion, physical inactivity, and selective estrogen-receptor modulators (SERMs) (e.g., tamoxifen, raloxifene) in increasing or decreasing breast cancer risk (ACS, 2000).

For purposes of this discussion, breast cancer risk factors have been categorized as being either nonmodifiable or lifestyle-related. Tables 11-3 and 11-4 contain a summation of these risk factors.

The recent explosion in the amount of genetic research has marked a significant milestone in enhancing the understanding of molecular genetics and high-risk populations. Although a variety of genetic traits have been studied with regard to breast cancer, the breast cancer susceptibility genes BRCA1 and BRCA2 are the main genetic traits associated with an increased risk of breast cancer. Researchers estimate that approximately 5%–10% of breast cancer cases are related to hereditary predisposition and result from mutations or alterations in BRCA1 and BRCA2. Alterations or mutations of the gene BRCA1, located on chromosome 17, are associated with an increased risk of breast cancer, ovarian cancer, and other can-

Table 11-3. Nonmodifiable Risk Factors Associated With the Development of Breast Cancer

Nonmodifiable Risk Factors	Comments
Female gender	99% of breast cancers occur in women, 1% in men (American Cancer Society [ACS], 2001b).
Age	Aside from being female, age is the single most important risk factor (ACS, 2001b). The risk of developing breast cancer increases with age, with the majority of cases occurring after age 50 (ACS, 1999). 77% of new cases and 84% of breast cancer deaths occur in women age 50 and older (ACS, 1999).
Personal history of breast disease	The risk of developing breast cancer in the opposite breast is two to six times greater than the risk of the general population (Chen, Thompson, Somenciw, & Moa, 1999). A personal history of ductal carcinoma in situ and lobular carcinoma in situ increases the risk of developing breast cancer. A personal history of atypical hyperplasia elevates the relative risk to approximately 4%, ranging from 11%–14% over the 12–20 years post diagnosis (Ford, Marcus, & Lum, 1999).
Family history	Number of relatives affected, menopausal status, unilateral vs. bilateral breast cancer, early vs. late age at diagnosis help to identify high-risk populations. Women with a mother or sister diagnosed with breast cancer have a two to three times higher risk of developing breast cancer than women without this family history (Kelsey, 1993). Having one or more first-degree blood relatives (mother, sister, daughter) who have been diagnosed increases the risk of developing the disease (NCI, 1999). The estimated risk of breast cancer in a woman with a history of first degree relative with postmenopausal breast cancer is 1.5% and 3% if there is a history of a first-degree relative with premenopausal breast cancer; the risk increases to 8% if both mother and sister have the disease (Ford et al., 1999).
Genetic predisposition	Approximately 5%–10% of breast cancers are genetically determined, resulting from mutations or alterations in breast cancer susceptibility genes BRCA1 and BRCA2. BRCA1 and BRCA2 mutations occur in less than 1% of the general population (ACS, 2000). Genetic factors contribute to approximately 25% of breast cancers diagnosed before age 30 (Vogel, 1998b). Familial mutations are associated with a 60%–85% lifetime risk of breast cancer (Armstrong, Eisen, & Weber, 2000).
Race	Overall, White women have a higher risk of developing breast cancer; however, African American women are more likely to die of the disease (ACS, 2000; Eley et al., 1994; Ries et al., 1999).
Previous breast irradiation	Women with a previous history of high-dose ionizing radiation to the chest for medical conditions are at an increased risk of developing breast cancer (Hulka & Stark, 1995).
Menstrual history	Early onset of menarche (two to five years prior to age 16) is associated with a 10%–30% greater risk of developing breast cancer later in life (Vogel, 1998b). Delayed menopause (at age 55 or older) is associated with a 50% increased risk of developing breast cancer (Vogel, 1998b). Early menarche coupled with delayed menopause leads to a greater lifetime number of menstrual cycles, thus leading to an increased risk of developing breast cancer.

Table 11-4. Modifiable Lifestyle Risk Factors Associated With the Development of Breast Cancer

Lifestyle Factors	Comments	Recommendations
Oral contraceptives (OCPs)	Recent use of OCPs may slightly increase the risk of breast cancer; however, women who stopped using OCPs 10 years ago have the same risk as women who never used OCPs (American Cancer Society [ACS], 2000). The risk of breast cancer associated with OCPs use is small and is greatest among younger women who use OCPs for prolonged periods of time (Vogel, 1998b).	
Nulliparity	Women who have never had children or those who have their first child after age 30 have a slightly higher risk of breast cancer (ACS, 2000; Vogel, 1998b).	
Induced abortion	A large recent study has provided strong evidence that induced abortions have no overall effect on the risk of breast cancer (ACS, 2000).	
Estrogen replacement therapy (ERT)	Most studies suggest that long-term use of ERT (10 years or more) after menopause is associated with a slight increase of breast cancer (ACS, 2000). A recent study showed greater risk of breast cancer with estrogen-progestin therapy compared to estrogen alone (Schairer, Lubin, Troisi, Brinton, & Hoover, 2000). Several meta analysis studies found no positive association between ERT and breast cancer risk in women who ever used ERT compared with women who never took ERT. Still numerous findings are mixed (Vogel, 1998b).	Women should consult with their personal healthcare provider and weigh the pros and cons associated with personal use of ERT. Factors to consider include cardiovascular risk and breast cancer risk, osteoporosis, and menopausal symptoms (ACS, 2000).
Breast feeding	Studies examining the benefits of breast feeding in reducing breast cancer risk have been mixed (ACS, 2000; Kuller, 1999). Findings from the Nurses Health Study (N = 89,887) showed no important overall link between history of breast feeding and breast cancer incidence (Michels et al., 1996). Researchers recommend further studies with younger premenopausal women.	
Alcohol	Studies have established a link between alcohol intake and breast cancer development. Findings from a meta-analysis showed that two drinks a day may increase breast cancer risk by approximately 25% (ACS, 1999). A recent pooled analysis of cohort studies showed a linear increase in breast cancer incidence (Smith-Warner et al., 1998). The increased risk of breast cancer and alcohol is apparent in both pre- and postmenopausal women (Matulonis, 1999).	ACS (2000) recommends limiting the consumption of alcohol, if one drinks at all.

(Continued on next page)

Table 11-4. Modifiable Lifestyle Risk Factors Associated With the Development of Breast Cancer *(Continued)*

Lifestyle Factors	Comments	Recommendations
Smoking	Cigarettes do not appear to increase the risk of developing breast cancer; however, the link between smoking and cancers of the bladder, cervix, ureters, and pancreas is well established (Matulonis, 1999).	Do not smoke, or seek assistance to quit smoking.
Obesity	The link between obesity and breast cancer has been mixed. However, postmenopausal obesity appears to increase the risk of breast cancer (ACS, 1999). Interestingly, the reverse is true for premenopausal women (ACS, 1999; Vogel, 1998b).	It is unclear if significant weight reduction has a protective benefit on breast cancer risk (Vogel, 1998b). ACS recommends maintaining a healthy weight and becoming physically active (ACS, 2000).
Dietary fat intake	International variations in breast cancer rates suggest a link between reduced fat intake and decreased breast cancer risk; studies examining the relationship between fat intake and breast cancer risk have been mixed. Issues related to measurement and micronutrient components may account for conflicting results (Vogel, 1998b). Total fat does not appear to increase breast cancer risk in middle-aged and older women. Additional research is needed to ascertain the consequences of fat intake during the younger years and subsequent risk (Matulonis, 1999).	ACS recommends limiting the intake of high-fat foods, particularly from animal sources (ACS, 2000).
Physical activity	Eleven of the 16 recreational studies reviewed showed a 12%–60% decrease in breast cancer risk among pre- and postmenopausal women. Researchers posit that physical activity may exert its effects through changes in the menstrual cycle, reduced body size, or changes in the immune system (Gammon, John, & Britton, 1998). The protective effects may be greater in lean women who are premenopausal and have carried children to full term (ACS, 1999).	More research is needed before providers can make specific recommendations (e.g., exercise and the prevention of breast cancer) (Matulonis, 1999).

cers. Epidemiologists estimate that women with this gene have an 85% risk of developing breast cancer by age 80 and a 20% relative risk of developing breast cancer by age 40 The risk of developing breast cancer declines considerably in the seventh decade of life (Calzone, 1997; Isaacs, Peshkin, & Lerman, 2000). Alterations in the BRCA1 gene also are associated with an increased risk of prostate cancer in men and colon cancer in men and women (Calzone).

BRCA2 is more specific for breast cancer alone. Located on chromosome 13, BRCA2 is predicted to be responsible for 35% of all inherited breast cancers. Similar to BRCA1, the estimated lifetime risk of developing breast cancer by age 80 in women with BRCA2 is 85%. Alterations in BRCA2 are associated with a 15%–20% lifetime risk of developing breast cancer. Men with BRCA2 are at an increased risk of developing breast cancer. The estimated lifetime risk of developing breast cancer by age 70 in this population is 6%. Researchers caution that the actual prevalence of BRCA1 and BRCA2 is unclear and, in some instances, may be overestimated, given that prevalence rates were derived from high-risk populations (Calzone, 1997; Ford et al., 1999; Vogel, 1998a). Specific recommendations for cancer surveillance and risk reduction for individuals carrying mutations in the BRCA1 and BRCA2 genes are provided in Burke et al. (1997). Although genetic testing is now commercially available, additional research is needed before genetic testing becomes a standard of care (Ford et al.).

Clinical management of individuals who carry a BRCA1 or BRCA2 mutation is highly individualized and requires increased surveillance for breast and ovarian cancer, prophylactic surgery, and chemoprevention. Specifically, the National Human Genome Research Institute convened a special task force to identify recommendations for managing individuals who carry a BRCA1 or BRCA2 mutation. Regarding breast cancer, the task force recommended the following.

- Monthly breast self-exam (BSE) beginning at age 18–21 years
- Annual or semiannual clinical breast examination (CBE) beginning at age 25–35 years
- Yearly mammography by age 25–35 years

Regarding ovarian cancer, the task force recommended

- Transvaginal ultrasound annually or semiannually in BRCA1 mutations beginning at age 25–35
- Annual or semiannual CA-125 testing in women with BRCA1 mutation beginning at age 25–35.

These recommendations also may be applicable for women with BRCA2 mutations. Moreover, because of the increased risk of colon cancer, the task force also recommended that individuals with BRCA1 mutations undergo annual fecal occult blood testing and sigmoidoscopy every three to five years beginning at age 50. Lifestyle risk-reduction strategies include a low-fat and high-fiber diet rich in fruits and vegetables, regular exercise, and avoidance of cigarettes and excessive alcohol consumption (Myriad Genetics, Inc., 1998).

Clinical management of women who test negative for BRCA1 or BRCA2 is highly individualized and should include continued breast cancer screening (according to ACS breast cancer screening guidelines) and appropriate follow-up. Of importance, individuals who do not carry a BRCA1 or BRCA2 mutation should be reminded that such results do not infer "no risk." Rather, these individuals still carry a lifetime risk of developing breast cancer or ovarian cancer consistent with the overall population. Healthcare providers should assist these individuals in developing a personalized plan of breast health and refer them for screening and follow-up as needed.

Issues and challenges related to genetics and breast cancer are complex and include myriad psychological, social, ethical, and legal implications. As advances in molecular genetics continue, there will be an increased need for oncology nurses to become effective educators, counselors, and researchers in this area. Numerous resources are available to assist nurses in advancing their knowledge and skills with regard to breast cancer genetics, risk assessment, and counseling. A more detailed discussion of resources and implications for nursing practice can be found in the literature (Baron & Borgen, 1997; Bernhardt, Geller, Doksum, & Metz, 2000; Calzone, 1997; Oncology Nursing Society [ONS], 1998a, 1998b).

Numerous risk-assessment tools and models have been developed to assist providers and consumers in identifying a woman's risk of developing breast cancer. The Gail Model from the Breast Cancer Detection Demonstration Project is one of the most widely used models used to quantify a woman's risk of developing breast cancer. This model predicts the cumulative risk of breast cancer according to decade up to age 90 years (Armstrong, Eisen, & Weber, 2000; Gail et al., 1989). In recent years, scientists at the National Cancer Institute (NCI) and the National Surgical Adjuvant Breast and Bowel Project (NSABP) modified the Gail Model for use in the Breast Cancer Prevention Trial (BCPT). In addition to estimating breast cancer risk, the model now includes information related to tamoxifen. When estimating breast cancer risk, the modified interactive computer-based tool incorporates age, race, age at menarche, age at first live birth, number of first-degree relatives diagnosed with breast cancer, and number and histology of breast biopsies (Fisher et al., 1998; Spiegelman, Colditz, Hunter, & Hertzmark, 1994). This computerized interactive tool is available free of charge to healthcare professionals by contacting NCI at 800-4-CANCER or logging onto the NCI Web site at www.nci.nih.gov.

Another frequently used prediction model is the Claus Model, derived from data obtained from the Cancer and Steroid Hormone Study. This model incorporates the prevalence of high-penetrance genes for susceptibility of breast cancer and predicts the cumulative risk for developing breast cancer from ages 29–79. The Claus Model includes more information than the Gail Model with regard to family history, specifically first- and second-degree relatives with breast cancer and age at diagnosis. The Gail Model appears to be more appropriate for women who follow mammography screening guidelines but may underestimate the risk among young women who do not follow the guidelines. In contrast, the Claus Model seems to be more appropriate for women with a history of first- and second-degree relatives with breast cancer. Both models may yield different predictions (Armstrong et al., 2000). While no single model is appropriate for every patient, information gleaned from the use of risk-assessment models can be used to inform the decision-making process related to screening and prevention efforts targeting high-risk individuals (Isaacs et al., 2000).

While risk assessment and counseling services may be available in many medical institutions and breast cancer centers throughout the country, these services may not be readily available in many rural and underserved communities. In these instances, oncology nurses are ideally positioned and challenged to advance their personal knowledge and skill related to breast cancer risk assessment and counseling. When providing information and guidance, women must be reminded that risk assessments are highly individualized and that, in many instances, women diagnosed with breast cancer present with no identifiable risk factors. All women, regardless of risk status, should be encouraged and empowered to adopt a personal plan of breast health and be referred to additional services as needed. The National Comprehensive Cancer Network (NCCN), a composite of 17 of the leading cancer centers in the United States, has developed an extensive set of guidelines to assist healthcare providers when conducting risk assessments and providing risk reduction counseling (NCCN, 1999).

Clinical Features of Breast Cancers

Breast cancer presentation can be subtle. Any palpable finding not matched in a mirror-image location in the opposite breast is a reason for concern, including ill-defined asymmetric thickenings. The most common reason for a delay in diagnosis of breast carcinoma is failure to recognize the significance of physical findings during either BSE or CBE. Healthcare providers often reassure women that an abnormal change is merely a cyst. It is impossible to distinguish a cyst from a solid mass by palpation alone. Hormonal changes during the perimenopausal and postmenopausal period cause breast tissue abnormalities to be difficult to discern. Breast cysts become more common in women age 40 and older. The incidence of breast cancer also rises, making cysts difficult to distinguish from solid masses on breast examination alone (Harris et al., 1996).

Ductal Carcinoma

Neither BSE or CBE provides much value in detecting ductal lesions. Most cases of DCIS are nonpalpable; it is detected by mammographic calcifications. DCIS commonly is larger than indicated by mammography, involves more than a quadrant of the breast, and is unifocal in its distribution (Marchant, 1997).

Lobular Carcinoma

Neither women nor their healthcare providers are likely to detect LCIS on a breast examination. LCIS does not form a palpable mass and cannot be recognized grossly. While generally found in premenopausal women (80%–90%), it also has been recorded in postmenopausal women (Tavassoli, 1999); the true incidence varies because of a lack of clinical and mammographic signs.

Typically, women with LCIS are younger than age 55. Their average age is 10 and 15 years younger, respectively, than that of patients with infiltrating ductal and infiltrating lobular carcinoma (Donegan & Spratt, 1995). A family history of breast cancer does not seem to increase a woman's risk for LCIS (Harris et al., 1996).

Invasive Ductal Carcinoma

With rare exceptions, no clinical features are specifically associated with invasive ductal carcinoma. The lesions occur throughout the age range of breast carcinoma but are most common in women in their middle to late 50s. An exception is palpable breast carcinoma associated with Paget's disease of the nipple.

415

Women with invasive lesions present with a mass detected either by palpation or mammography; tumors generally range from 0.5 cm to 2–3 cm in size on palpation but may be massive and occupy a significant portion of the breast. Skin fixation, edema, peau d'orange, nipple retraction or discharge, Paget's disease, and even ulceration of large tumors may be seen but occur less frequently in recent years because of women's earlier detection practices (Tavassoli, 1999).

The underlying invasive carcinoma in these cases usually is of the ductal type. On the other hand, Paget's disease may originate from intraductal carcinoma limited to the lactiferous ducts. Coincidentally, there may be a palpable lesion formed by another separate carcinoma, possibly of a different histologic type, such as a rare form of mammary carcinoma with well-differentiated morphology called tubular carcinoma (Harris et al., 1996). Women with invasive duct pattern carcinoma have a worse prognosis (Tavassoli, 1999).

Invasive Lobular Carcinoma

Attention to warning signals of breast changes is important in detecting invasive breast carcinomas. Signs and symptoms such as a palpable mass, protuberances and reddening of the overlying skin, breast swelling and inflammation, skin dimpling, nipple retraction, blood-tinged nipple discharge, unexplained breast pain, and even ulcerations can be a woman's first indication of an abnormality.

Invasive lobular carcinoma occurs in women throughout the age distribution of breast carcinoma. The median age at diagnosis ranges from 45 to 56, but occurrence expands to age 86 and perhaps beyond. Women most frequently present with a tumor located in the upper outer quadrant. The lesions tend to have ill-defined margins, and occasionally the only evidence is subtle thickening or induration. Skin retraction, fixation, and other signs of advanced local disease occur with large lesions. Calcifications are not usually found in invasive lobular carcinoma. However, when found, the calcification is usually coincidentally associated with other benign lesions. Women with invasive lobular carcinoma are likely to have infiltrating disease in the opposite breast (Harris et al., 1996).

Tumor Metastasis

The spreading of breast tumor cells from the primary tumor to colonize with other sites of the body defines the metastatic process. Metastasis remains a significant contributor to patient morbidity and mortality. The metastatic process is complex, beginning with invasion at the primary site. Although the presence of lymph node metastases is the best predictor of high risk for poor prognosis, it is not known to what degree distant metastases actually result from lymphatic versus direct hematologic dissemination. After arrival at a distant organ, colonization and angiogenesis are required for the development of a metastatic focus (Bowcock, 1999).

The formation of microvessels from preexisting blood vessels is an essential step in creating an environment for tumor growth. In addition, microvesssel formation is involved in the cascade of events permitting metastasis. Most tumors appear to need angiogenesis for their growth (Bowcock, 1999).

Primary Prevention of Breast Cancer

Medical Modalities

Unlike the long history of clinical trials devoted to cancer diagnosis and treatment, breast cancer primary prevention trials represent a new and evolving area in the fight against breast cancer. Possible strategies in this area include medical and surgical modalities and lifestyle-related interventions (Ford et al., 1999). Current medical modalities include the testing of chemopreventive agents in reducing or preventing the incidence of breast cancer.

Many investigators engaged in conducting breast cancer prevention studies are focusing their efforts on testing the effectiveness of SERMs in preventing breast cancer. SERMs, noted for their estrogen-like and some antiestrogen characteristics, are being tested because of the scientific link between estrogen and breast cancer. The testing of the pharmacologic agent tamoxifen has received considerable attention during the past decade. Tamoxifen, one of the first antiestrogen drugs used in the prevention of breast cancer, was selected because of its success in reducing contralateral breast cancers and recurrence in women who have been diagnosed with breast cancer. Hence, in 1992, the BCPT was designed to evaluate tamoxifen's contribution to breast cancer prevention, cardiovascular mortality reduction, and osteoporosis prevention in women considered to be at high risk for developing breast cancer. Results from this prospective trial of 13,000 women showed that tamoxifen reduced the risk of invasive breast cancers by 49% and the risk of noninvasive breast cancers by 50% (Gail et al., 1999). The BCPT closed early in 1998 after showing a consistent benefit in preventing breast cancer.

Findings from the BCPT revealed a 45%, 39%, and 36% reduction in fractures of the hip, radius (called Colles' fracture), and spine, respectively. Because of the small number of fractures occurring in study participants, researchers cautioned that additional research is needed before definitive conclusions can be drawn (Fisher et al., 1998).

Of significance is that the rate of endometrial cancer was increased in the tamoxifen group, predominately among women age 50 and older. When endometrial cancer was diagnosed, all endometrial cancers were stage I, or localized. Similarly, the tamoxifen group experienced more cases of stroke, pulmonary embolism, and deep vein thrombosis, primarily in women age 50 and older. Tamoxifen did not alter the annual rate of ischemic disease or increase the occurrence of colon, rectal, ovarian, or other cancers. Researchers concluded that, despite the side effects associated with tamoxifen administration, tamoxifen is an appropriate preventive agent for many women who are at increased risk for breast cancer. Investigators currently are developing risk-benefit ratio tools for use with tamoxifen as a breast cancer chemopreventive agent (Fisher et al., 1998).

The side effects reported in the BCPT are similar to side effects reported in prior studies. These side effects include hot flashes, weight gain, fluid retention, vaginal discharge, nausea, and irregular menses (Aikin, 1996). Reported side effects associated with more serious consequences include endometrial cancers, other secondary cancers, thromboembolic events, and ocular toxicities (Aikin).

Similar to tamoxifen, the selective estrogen receptor modulator raloxifene has been noted to exert antiestrogen effects on breast tissue but without the estrogen-like effects on the uterus. In a study to determine if raloxifene prevents osteoporosis, researchers noted 58%–74% fewer breast cancer cases in women taking the drug versus women in the control group. These findings led researchers to initiate the current Study of Tamoxifen and Raloxifene (STAR). The STAR Trial is a large-scale randomized study comparing the effectiveness of tamoxifen and raloxifene in women at increased risk for developing breast cancer. Researchers will identify if raloxifene, like tamoxifen, is beneficial in preventing breast cancer or reducing the risk of breast cancer in women without the disease. Additional components of the study will compare the benefits and side effects of the two drugs (NCI, 2001).

Investigators with the NSABP currently are recruiting 22,000 women to participate in the STAR Trial. Women who are postmenopausal, at least 35 years of age, and deemed to have an increased risk of developing breast cancer equivalent to or greater than that of an average 60–64-year-old woman will be considered for participation. Noteworthy, all women will be randomized to receive either tamoxifen or raloxifene in the STAR Trial. Unlike tamoxifen, raloxifene is not approved by the U.S. Food and Drug Administration as a chemopreventive agent for breast cancer (ACS, 2000; Alberg, Lam, & Helzlsouer, 1999; Ford, Marcus, & Lum, 1999; NCI, 2001).

Surgical Modalities

Given the limited number of primary preventive strategies for breast cancer, researchers currently are investigating the effectiveness of prophylactic mastectomy in reducing breast cancer in extreme cases. Prophylactic mastectomy (i.e., removal of the total breast, tail of Spence, lower axillary lymph nodes, areola, and nipple) may be recommended to high-risk individuals after careful consideration of the potential risks and benefits associated with the procedure. Prophylactic mastectomy usually is followed by reconstructive procedures for cosmetic and body image concerns. High-risk populations include individuals with a strong family history of cancer or a history of the genetic susceptibility genes, DCIS, LCIS, and other premalignant lesions (Burke et al., 1997; Vogel, 1998a). Additional implications for this procedure include unreliable results on physical examination, mastodynia, and cancer phobia (Hartman et al., 1999). Prophylactic mastectomy appears to be a desirable strategy for the prevention of breast cancer because of its potential to eliminate the risk of developing breast cancer, remove occult carcinomas, and relieve the psychological distress related to the fear of developing breast cancer (Vogel, 1999b).

Despite the long history of prophylactic mastectomy, little is known about the long-term effectiveness of the procedure. To this end, Hartman et al. (1999) conducted a retrospective study of 639 women who underwent prophylactic mastectomy between 1960 and 1993: 214 at high risk and 425 at moderate risk for developing breast cancer because of family history. The control group included 403 sisters of the high-risk proband who did not undergo mastectomy. Using the Gail Model to predict the incidence of breast cancer post prophylactic mastectomy, findings showed an 89.5% reduction in the risk of breast cancer among women with a moderate risk of developing the disease and a 90%–94% reduction in the risk of breast cancer among women with a high risk of developing the disease. Similarly, the reduction in the risk of death was 100% among the moderate risk group and 81%–94% among the high-risk group. These researchers concluded that prophylactic mastectomy could significantly reduce the incidence of breast cancer (Hartman et al.).

Women who are considering prophylactic mastectomy should receive careful risk assessment and counseling regarding all possible preventive options, including the use of tamoxifen. Furthermore, women considering this option should be counseled that cancer has been documented to occur after the procedure and that there is insufficient evidence supporting the efficacy of this modality in preventing breast cancer (Burke et al., 1997).

Lifestyle Interventions

Dietary interventions, particularly those focusing on increasing fruit and vegetable intake and reducing fat consumption, currently are being evaluated as a means to protect against breast cancer. The Women's Health Initiative, established by the National Institutes of Health (NIH) in 1991, is the largest prevention study of its kind in the United States. The purposes of this longitudinal randomized clinical trial are to (a) determine whether hormone replacement therapy will prevent heart disease, (b) test whether a low-fat dietary pattern will reduce breast and colorectal cancer, and (c) examine whether calcium and vitamin D supplements will prevent osteoporotic fractures. By the close of recruitment in August 1998, 68,135 women age 50–79 enlisted for the study. Results of this study will provide valuable insights about some of the most significant health concerns affecting postmenopausal women, including breast cancer (Rossouw et al., 1995; Rossouw & Hurd, 1999).

In addition, several ongoing studies are evaluating whether a diet rich in fruits, fiber, and vegetables and low in fat is associated with a longer breast cancer-free interval in women diagnosed with breast cancer. Although the target population includes women diagnosed with breast cancer, findings from these studies may point to a means of preventing breast cancer in women with and without a history of breast cancer. More details about these and other ongoing breast cancer clinical trials can be found on NCI's CancerTrials™ Web site at http://cancertrials.nci.nih.gov/.

Early Detection of Breast Cancer

Standard Screening Tests

Cancer screening is the application of a test to detect a potential cancer in a person who is asymptomatic. There are two types of cancer screening. The first type detects cancer before it is clinically apparent, early in its natural history, and before it becomes systemic, when treatment may be more effective, less expensive, or both. In recent years, more has been learned about the issues and implications of the second type of cancer screening—that is, screening for risk factors or other markers, such as genetic or molecular, that put one at high risk for developing cancer (Reintgen & Clark, 1996).

Breast cancer is a suitable disease for which to screen because it has high prevalence and incidence. It has serious clinical consequences, measured in mortality, morbidity, and healthcare costs. The biology and natural history of the disease are amenable to screening techniques. The preclinical phase has a high prevalence in the screened population. Early-stage breast cancer is highly curable, but treatment is less effective as the disease progresses (Reintgen & Clark, 1996).

The effectiveness of breast cancer screening has been judged by several specific measures. First, comparison is made between women who are screened and their likelihood of dying from breast cancer versus those who were not screened. Second, case fatality rate measures how many women survive breast cancer for five years or longer. A third measure, case finding, is affected by lead-time and length bias. Lead-time examines two areas: time from screening diagnosis until clinical diagnosis in unscreened women and whether life is really lengthened in a screened group because the diagnosis is known only because they are screened earlier. Length bias causes screening to appear to be more effective. However, included in the screened groups will be women with slow-growing, noninvasive forms of breast carcinoma and precursor lesions. These include those carcinomas with a long preclinical phase where survival outcome appears to have been related to time of diagnosis (Harris et al., 1996; Overmoyer, 1999).

Consider that two factors that may occur in the natural history and progression of malignant breast lesions could account for the efficacy of screening and provide a biological rationale for early detection strategies: early dissemination and phenotypic progression. Should one or both of these factors occur at some stage in neoplastic development, which is dependent upon tumor size, then earlier detection and intervention may pre-empt formation of micrometastases or a more biologically aggressive primary tumor. This could lead to improved prognosis (Benson, 1998).

Over the past decade, vigilant campaigns against breast cancer took place in every region of the United States, from metropolitan areas to rural and remote communities. Nurses have been very involved in these campaigns to spread the word about the value of breast screening and early detection of breast cancer. Reintgen and Clark (1996) asserted that it makes good sense to view cancer screening as beneficial. Further, it seems most reasonable to detect cancer early, when it is small and has not spread from its primary site, rather than late, when it has metastasized to other vital organs. So, why not screen everyone to detect cancer early? Or, why screen at all when most women never get breast cancer yet many incur screening costs and some may suffer the anxiety of false-positive tests? These are questions that nurses must be prepared to address when patients and members of the community seek their advice on cancer screening. Understanding how current screening recommendations were devised will help nurses in the counseling role.

Breast Cancer Screening Decision Making:
Understanding the Evidence

Harris and Leininger (1995) advocated helping women to balance the benefits of breast screening against the harms and costs of such screening. They advised that one needs to consider the risk for dying of breast cancer, the relative reduction in that risk that will result from screening women in different age groups, and the harms and costs associated with screening. Randomized controlled trials between 1963 and 1982 weighed the risks, benefits, and costs of breast screening in various age groups (NIH, 1997). Outcomes showed that the number of lives extended increased as women grew older. Many women can weigh the evidence, costs, and benefits of screening and engage their healthcare provider in decision making about when to begin screening, whereas other women and their healthcare providers are not comfortable with such a process.

For many years, such a process led to heated discussions about the need for clear recommendations from the nation's experts in healthcare leadership. Screening at age 50 has been an artificial cutoff used as a marker for biologic changes associated with menopause, but why not consider the benefits of breast screening at age 40?

The following discussion is based on proceedings of the 1995 NIH Consensus Panel on breast cancer screening (NIH, 1997). NIH established a non-federal, nonadvocate, 12-member panel to respond to national concerns about the recommendation of a lower age limit to begin breast cancer screening. The panel represented the fields of oncology, radiology, obstetrics and gynecology, geriatrics, public health, and epidemiology. It also included patient representatives along with an additional 32 experts in oncology, surgical oncology, radiology, public health, and epidemiology.

The panel presented data regarding the effectiveness of mammography screening for women ages 40–49. The panel concluded that the data currently available do not warrant a universal recommendation for mammography for all women in their 40s. Each woman should decide for herself whether to undergo mammography. Her decision may be based not only on an objective analysis of the scientific evidence and consideration of her individual medical history, but also on how she perceives and weighs each potential risk and benefit, the value she places on each, and how she deals with uncertainty.

However, the panel concluded that it is not sufficient just to advise a woman to make her own decision about mammograms. Given both the importance and the complexity of the issues involved in assessing the evidence, a woman should have access to the best possible relevant information regarding both benefits and risks, presented in an understandable and usable form. Information should be developed and provided to women in their 40s regarding potential benefits and risks, enabling each woman to make the most appropriate decision.

The panel asserted that educational material prepared to accompany this information should lead women step-by-step through the process of using such information in the best possible way for reaching a decision. For women in their 40s who choose to have mammography performed, the costs of the mammograms should be reimbursed by third-party payors or covered by health maintenance organizations so that financial impediments will not influence a woman's decision. Additionally, a woman's healthcare provider must be equipped with sufficient information to facilitate her decision-making process.

Mammography has been shown to be effective in reducing breast cancer mortality in women ages 50–69. Currently, available evidence from randomized controlled trials indicates that for women ages 40–49, during the first 7–10 years following initiation of screening, breast cancer mortality is no lower in women who were assigned to screening than in controls. Summary data indicate a reduction of 16% in breast cancer mortality after about 10 years, with confidence intervals of two, a total of 28%. However, some studies find lower mortality from breast cancer in screened women after 10 years, while others do not. A lower mortality rate could be a result of the original screening but also could be the result of other factors, such as CBE or mammography offered to the women after age 50.

Further complicating this issue is that the charge to the panel focused on a broad age range, 40–49 years. The rationale for the charge was that evidence for recommending mammography is strong for women ages 50 and older but not as clear for 40–49-year-old women. It should be pointed out that of all the studies reviewed, only one was specifically designed originally to evaluate mammography in the 40–49-year-old age group. However, age is a continuum, and there is no abrupt biological change at age 50. Indeed, a 49-year-old woman is probably more similar to a 50-year-old woman than she is to a 40-year-old. Unfortunately, insufficient data are available at present to base recommendations for narrower age ranges. The panel concluded that presently available evidence does not warrant a universal recommendation for mammography screening of women ages 40–49. This conclusion does not preclude the possibility that older women in this age group might have a different balance of benefit and risk than younger women. Data to support this possibility are not presently available.

The effects of different ages at menopause also remain to be explored. The potential benefits of mammography for women in their 40s include earlier diagnosis and the option to choose breast-conserving therapy. These benefits must be weighed against the risks or potential risks, including those associated with false-positive tests: further diagnostic tests that may be invasive, anxiety, inconvenience, and potential risk from mammographic radiation. In addition, the impact of false reassurance given to women with false-negative screens must be considered, given the lower sensitivity of mammography in women in their 40s compared with women in their 50s.

The panel advised that professional and public education as well as disclaimers on mammography reports have increased awareness of false-negatives in women with clinical symptoms such as a palpable lump. Similarly, those recommending mammographic screening of asymptomatic women in this age group also must remind women and their physicians to continue regular CBEs and to evaluate new symptoms promptly.

Every decision to utilize or not utilize a health-related service involves weighing available scientific evidence regarding benefits and risks against personal values and prior experiences. Such decision making occurs at multiple levels, and the process differs at each level. One level is characterized by a question that nurses might pose for themselves: "Would you have this done for yourself or for someone in your immediate family?" When the available scientific evidence is equivocal and incomplete, a person's decision to act or not act will be significantly influenced by personal or family experience with the disease and by one's capacity to deal with risk and uncertainty.

Another level of decision making occurs when a healthcare clinician makes recommendations to his or her patients. Such a decision generally is based more on the strength of the scientific evidence, but the clinician's recommendations also may be colored by prior experience, personally and with other patients, as well as by assessment of the patient for whom the recommendation will be made.

Finally, there is the level of making across-the-board recommendations to a population. This decision has far-reaching implications that must be based to a much greater extent on a rigorous examination of the available scientific evidence. Of all decision levels, this level requires the strongest evidence of high benefit and low risk, particularly in the case of screening mammography, where such recommendations would be made to a healthy population. Thus, in some cases, a clinician might recommend mammography for a patient in her 40s and might do so despite a belief that the evidence is not sufficiently strong to warrant across-the-board recommendations.

The panel concluded that the data currently available do not warrant a universal recommendation for mammography for all women in their 40s. Each woman should decide for herself by considering the scientific evidence and her own medical history, also weighing each potential risk and benefit. However, advising a woman to make her own decision about mammograms is not enough. She should have access to the best possible relevant information regarding both benefits and risks, presented in an understandable and usable form. Educational material should lead women step-by-step through the process of reaching a decision.

Women will seek guidance from primary-care physicians, physicians in different specialties, and advanced practice nurses, including clinical nurse specialists and nurse practitioners. A woman's healthcare provider must be equipped with sufficient information and adequate patient-education materials to facilitate her decision-making process. Nurses are key to developing educational materials to fill this need. Another role for nursing involvement is monitoring and reviewing the latest information from research studies regarding benefits and risks of mammography for women in their 40s. This will ensure timely formulation and implementation of any new policy recommendations that may become appropriate in the future (NIH, 1997).

Over time, breast cancer has been one of the most controversial and debated diseases among those with recommended screening procedures. Questions such as at what age should screening be started, at what age should it be stopped, and how often to screen go through cycles of intense debate. Each year, scientists and sociocultural researchers learn more about breast cancer from many research perspectives. These include biologic, genetic, and epidemiological studies, and development of new modalities in screening mammography. Other important research methods include design and outcomes in clinical trials, clinical innovations, and population and cultural perspectives. National health policies have changed in the past decade to support screening for a broader population of women.

While newer technologies are being developed and are under clinical trial for detection of breast abnormality, mammography remains the single most sensitive means for early detection of breast carcinoma. Figure 11-10 shows the strengths and limitations of mammography for breast cancer screening. Other screening modalities can enhance mammography in the detection of breast cancer.

Figure 11-10. Strengths and Limitations of Breast Screening Procedures

Strengths	Weaknesses
Detects disease in its preclinical state before a woman or her healthcare provider can detect it	Fails to detect 10%–20% of carcinomas
	False reassurance
Screening is conducted efficiently and inexpensively; improved reimbursement rates.	Mammography costs vary around the country, and the cost is expensive for many women.
It is simple, inexpensive, and accessible to a large portion of the population.	Not easily accessible to remote and rural populations; approximately 50% of eligible women are screened
Acceptable sensitivity (> 80%), specificity (> 95%), and predictive values (> 20%); applied to large populations of women efficiently; quality-assurance programs vary depending on the organization and facility.	False-positive results
	Interpretation of mammographic images are difficult and remain as much an art as a science; variations exist in quality of interpretation.
It is safe and no complications are endured as a result of the screening modality.	
Improved policies by public health authorities and improved consistency on screening guidelines among healthcare organizations	Uncomfortable and occasionally painful and bruising
	May lead to additional unnecessary procedures
Randomized trials have proven its efficacy for screening women age 50 and older.	Overtreatment of some abnormalities
	Possible radiation-induced cancer

Other Screening Modalities
Ultrasound

Ultrasound is a highly useful diagnostic test to determine whether breast masses found by mammography or CBE are cystic or solid. It should not be used as a screening test. Ultrasound does not have adequate resolution to consistently visualize subtle microcalcifications that are the major mammographic signs of breast cancer. Unlike mammography, which can visualize an entire depth of breast tissue as a single image, ultrasound can depict only single planes. Visualization of an entire thickness of breast would require so many sonographic images that interpretation of a whole-breast ultrasound screening examination would be prohibitively time-consuming.

Magnetic Resonance Imaging

Magnetic resonance imaging (MRI) creates images from signals generated by the excitation of nuclear particles in a magnetic field. MRI is free of ionizing radiation as compared to conventional film/screen and digital mammography. MRI shows promise in staging cancers in dense breasts where mammography may be less effective (Roses,

1999; Shtern, Wood, & Krause, 1998). However, MRI should not be used for screening because it, too, has limited resolution. MRI usually also involves IV injection of a contrast agent and is an excessively expensive and time-consuming procedure, making it unsuitable for use in mass population screening (Roses; Shtern et al.).

Thermography

Other modalities, such as thermography, which measures variation in breast temperature; light scanning (transillumination), which records transmission of light through the breast; and radionuclide (isotope) scans, should not be used for screening because they are much less effective than mammography in detecting very small lesions (Roses, 1999; Shtern et al., 1998).

Digital Mammography and Telemammography

Digital mammography is similar to conventional film-screen mammography. It uses a dedicated electronic detector system that captures and changes the digital image into a fixed record. The transmitted image is converted into number images that are transmitted as electrical signals by telephone lines, dedicated telecommunication lines, or satellite in less than four minutes to display the x-ray information on a computer. The digital data can then be used for image analysis, review in the form of computer-enhanced images, transmission for expert consultation (telemammography), and electronic patient records for improved storage and retrieval. This will be especially advantageous for clinicians in remote areas who need expert consultation and image interpretation from breast screening centers.

Because of the advances being made in the field of telecommunications in recent years, digital mammography or telemammography will become a medium for sending mammographic images. Although digital mammography promises to overcome the limitations of conventional film/screen mammography in dense fibroglandular breast tissue, digital mammography currently is in an early stage of technical development and clinical trial (Roses, 1999; Shtern et al., 1998).

Positron-Emission Tomography and Gamma Camera Methods

Promising nuclear medicine imaging modalities that are under study include positron-emission tomography and gamma camera methods. The U.S. Food and Drug Administration recently has approved scintimammography, a gamma camera method. These methods produce images of biochemical and physiological processes in the body. Scintimammography is promising for improved imaging and screening of high-risk women. This group includes women with scars from prior biopsy or lumpectomy, women with palpable breast masses, women undergoing radiation treatment or chemotherapy to monitor treatment response, and women with positive lymph nodes but in whom conventional mammography and CBE are unable to define the primary breast tumor (Roses, 1999; Shtern et al., 1998).

Medical Free-Electron Laser

Military state-of-the-art research and development also promises improved techniques. One such method, the Medical Free-Electron Laser, uses ultrasound for computer tomography to form a breast image. The development is only in its early stages, and large clinical trials for evaluation of this technology must follow.

Industry, government, and academic partnerships are rapidly expediting many breakthrough technological products and devices for improved breast cancer screening and detection and many that offer hope for improvement in treatment, as well (Roses, 1999; Shtern et al., 1998).

Breast Cancer Screening for Women at Average Risk

Many nurses and other healthcare professionals advocate the complementary role of combining mammography with BSE and CBE. Each method should be capable of detecting cancers that are missed by one or both other modalities. Detection by CBE or BSE depends on the tactile appreciation for differences between a tumor and surrounding tissue (Foster, 1994). The sensitivity of the three complementary modalities depends on how well each is performed and also varies according to lesion size, location, shape, and composition, as well as composition of the surrounding breast tissue (Roses, 1999).

Palpable masses may not necessarily have a corresponding mammographic finding, especially in mammographically dense fibroglandular breasts. BSE may be advantageous in that it can be performed on a monthly basis and may lead to the detection of interval cancers that surface between annual mammographic and clinical screenings. Moreover, a woman who examines her breasts carefully each month may be sensitive to subtle changes occurring since her previous self-examination.

The true value of BSE probably has been underestimated in its potential effectiveness, as many women involved in such studies did not practice proper technique and did not perform BSE monthly with the recommended method and sufficient time factor. However, smaller tumors with higher survival rates are more likely to be detected by mammography than by CBE or BSE (Marchant, 1997).

Nurses are leaders in teaching and encouraging women to learn correct BSE techniques. It is rare to find a nurse who does not believe in its efficacy. ACS's (2000) BSE guidelines recommend the following.
- Ages 20–39: Monthly BSE right after the menstrual period and CBE every three years by a doctor or nurse
- Ages 40+: Monthly BSE, annual CBE close to the time of the mammogram, and first mammogram and annual mammogram thereafter.

Screening Recommendations in High-Risk Populations

In 1997, medical and healthcare organizations reached a consensus in their thinking and recommendations on the appropriate age for breast screening for low-risk women. Figure 11-11 shows which groups endorse mammography screening for women ages 40 and older on an annual basis and those who do not advise screening.

Screening is more efficient when it is targeted at individuals at high risk for breast carcinoma. Thus, identification of those at high risk is important in the design of screening strategies. Of all risk factors for breast cancer, after gender, age is the most significant. Collectively, fewer than 2% of all breast carcinomas are diagnosed before age 30.

Figure 11-11. Medical Organizations and Their Positions on Mammographic Screening of Women Ages 40–49 Years

Not Recommending	Recommending
Academy of Family Practice (begin age 50)	American Cancer Society
American College of Physicians (begin age 50)	American College of Obstetrics and Gynecology
Health Care Financing Agency (Medicare) (begin age 65)	American College of Radiology
	American College of Pathology
U.S. Preventive Services Task Force (begin age 50)	American Medical Association
	American Society of Therapeutic Radiology
	American Women's Medical Association
	National Cancer Institute
	National Comprehensive Cancer Network
	National Medical Association

Note. Based on information from Roses, 1999.

The infrequency of cancer in younger women and the density of their breasts makes screening less effective in the younger age group. Moreover, when mammography is used to screen the breasts of younger women, the theoretical risk of radiation exposure is greater (Donegan & Spratt, 1995).

About 25% of breast cancers occur in women age 30–50, and the remainder develop after age 50. Although some risk factors for breast carcinoma are known, the fact remains that more than two-thirds of all breast cancers occur in women who have no recognized risk factors. No adult woman in the United States is at such a low risk for breast cancer to merit exclusion from an effective breast cancer control program (Donegan & Spratt, 1995).

Breast Cancer Screening for Older Women

There is a lack of consensus regarding breast cancer screening recommendations for older women. Kavanagh, Singletary, Einhorn, and DePetrillo (1998) outlined ingrained beliefs that hinder development of a clear policy for women in their 70s and 80s.

- Elderly women more often have locally advanced disease at the time of initial presentation.
- Elderly women have less aggressive forms of breast cancer.
- Elderly women have a limited life expectancy from comorbid conditions other than breast cancer.
- Elderly patients cannot tolerate standard treatment.

Table 11-5 lists the proportion of women by state of residence who have never had a mammogram or CBE and who recently have had undergone a mammogram. Women older than age 65 are least likely to have had a recent mammogram.

427

Table 11-5. Mammography and Clinical Breast Exam for Women 40 Years and Older, 2000, by State

State	% Never Had a Mammogram	% Never Had a Mammogram and Clinical Breast Exam	% Recent* Mammogram 40+ Years	% Recent* Mammogram 40–64 Years	% Recent* Mammogram 65 Years and Older
Alabama	11.3	18.6	58.5	56.5	62.4
Alaska	13.8	15.5	61.7	58.6	76.8
Arizona	10.5	24.4	69.3	67.3	72.9
Arkansas	14.7	20.5	58.7	59.5	57.4
California**	N/A	N/A	63.0	60.5	68.8
Colorado	12.4	18.8	60.2	57.9	66.0
Connecticut	7.3	13.4	73.2	72.4	74.8
Delaware	7.1	13.3	75.8	74.0	79.3
District of Columbia	7.0	18.2	67.9	68.1	67.4
Florida	11.1	20.1	66.3	62.5	72.7
Georgia	12.6	19.7	60.4	59.2	63.6
Hawaii	10.5	18.6	65.8	65.9	65.6
Idaho	15.9	20.9	51.7	49.1	57.2
Illinois	12.6	19.8	63.4	64.1	69.1
Indiana	13.5	20.4	61.6	63.7	58.0
Iowa	13.1	17.8	62.8	63.4	61.9
Kansas	11.7	19.0	61.9	61.2	63.0
Kentucky	12.9	18.7	63.3	64.4	61.0
Louisiana	14.2	21.8	64.8	63.8	66.9
Maine	9.3	13.4	67.3	68.9	64.1
Maryland	9.2	15.0	69.2	67.5	73.3
Massachusetts	7.9	12.5	72.2	72.6	71.6
Michigan	8.8	15.4	69.1	68.1	71.2
Minnesota	12.7	16.6	61.3	61.2	61.6
Mississippi	16.4	22.3	51.5	54.6	45.4
Missouri	14.7	21.8	60.7	61.6	58.9
Montana	12.6	15.7	61.6	58.4	68.2
Nebraska	13.6	17.8	61.9	64.5	57.4
Nevada	10.9	19.7	61.9	58.7	69.7

(Continued on next page)

Table 11-5. Mammography and Clinical Breast Exam for Women 40 Years and Older, 2000, by State (Continued)

State	% Never Had a Mammogram	% Never Had a Mammogram and Clinical Breast Exam	% Recent* Mammogram 40+ Years	% Recent* Mammogram 40–64 Years	% Recent* Mammogram 65 Years and Older
New Hampshire	9.0	11.7	68.5	66.9	72.4
New Jersey	14.0	22.1	66.8	67.3	65.7
New Mexico	12.7	18.4	60.6	57.2	68.2
New York	9.8	17.3	68.2	69.0	66.7
North Carolina	10.9	15.5	64.8	64.2	65.9
North Dakota	12.0	15.7	62.0	60.1	65.3
Ohio	10.4	16.2	67.2	66.0	69.3
Oklahoma	17.7	22.2	55.8	54.6	58.1
Oregon	9.4	13.7	62.1	60.1	66.3
Pennsylvania	10.0	16.2	63.7	63.7	63.7
Rhode Island	8.1	13.7	71.5	71.3	72.0
South Carolina	10.0	17.5	64.8	62.7	69.3
South Dakota	13.0	16.8	62.7	61.2	65.2
Tennessee	11.9	21.7	62.6	63.2	61.5
Texas	15.1	23.0	57.2	55.0	62.2
Utah	13.6	16.5	53.0	51.5	56.7
Vermont	12.6	18.2	62.9	62.8	63.0
Virginia	11.4	19.1	61.9	58.7	69.3
Washington	10.7	14.0	58.8	57.8	61.1
West Virginia	13.6	17.7	61.6	60.3	63.9
Wisconsin	11.8	15.6	61.3	61.2	61.6
Wyoming	13.6	18.1	54.4	53.1	57.6

*Recent mammogram = within the past year
** Questions for mammogram and clinical breast exam differed and may not be comparable to other state percentages in this table.
N/A = comparable data not available.

Note. Based on information from ACS, 2001a; Behavioral Risk Factor Surveillance System, 2001.

Because women ages 70–75 and older still have a significant life expectancy, it is frequently argued that, although there are no data to demonstrate benefits of screening in this age subgroup, it is extremely likely that benefits exist and screening is worthwhile. Screening mammography is quite sensitive in this age group because of the higher fat composition of the breast tissue. It is reasonable to expect that benefits from screening women in the seventh decade and beyond will be realized well before death from another illness. Women who are in good general health have a longer-than-average life expectancy. Consensus is lacking on this issue among groups who otherwise can agree on the recommendation for women at average risk (Roses, 1999).

Follow-Up

The rationale for screening patients after treatment, or follow-up, is based on early general screening and early detection principles. The objectives of follow-up are to screen for recurrence. Recurrence of new primary lesions in the opposite breast is a frequent sequelae of treatment. The follow-up visit provides opportunity for early diagnosis and treatment. If discovered early, morbidity and mortality might be reduced by retreatment. Risk for developing another primary tumor in other organ sites also is higher in women who previously have had breast cancer.

The follow-up visit provides comprehensive management of treatment-related complications, and even evaluation of alternative treatments that the woman has heard about, considered, or tried. Psychosocial support for the individual can be assessed and coordinated through a comprehensive team approach during each subsequent visit (Donegan & Spratt, 1995).

Educating Women About Self-Examination Strategies

Although the most frequently found breast carcinomas often show no visible or palpable signs in the very early stage, the value of BSE and the importance of recommending it to women of all ages is not to be taken lightly. However, it must be stressed to women that self-examination is best accompanied by a triangular approach that includes clinical examination and age-appropriate mammography. By the time a breast carcinoma is palpable, the risk of metastatic disease increases.

The point that nurses should stress when recommending BSE is that more than 90% of breast carcinomas are found by women themselves through intuitive perception of symptoms and the incidental finding of a lump or irregularity in the breast tissue (Kavanagh et al., 1998).

All nurses play an important role in encouraging women to follow health-promotion activities, but advanced-practice nurses are in an especially good position. During a woman's clinic visit for episodic care or follow-up for chronic disease, information pertinent to breast health can be discussed. Recommendation without adequate explanation, teaching, and attention to a woman's concerns is the major reason older women may not get mammograms or perform BSE. Women rely on the healthcare professional to bring up the topic. If it is not mentioned, women may assume it is not important. Advanced-practice nurses, in particular, can address personal barriers to screening, such as a woman's unfamiliarity with breast changes and discomfort with performing BSE. Sensitivity to a woman's concerns about disrobing for exams or mammograms is important. Personal and family priorities may be barriers that need to be explored. If the costs of breast examinations and mammography are an issue, nurses may be able to provide guidance for accessing affordable care.

The amount of time the nurse clinician spends on CBE is an important variable in teaching self-care. Paying adequate attention to the CBE by performing it in an unhurried and undistracted manner indicates the importance of this component of breast care to the woman's total health. This is a good time to remind the woman that CBE is ideally performed annually, one to two weeks after the beginning of the menses (when vascular and lymph congestion from the effects of progesterone are less evident).

Demonstration and review of BSE techniques can be included with the CBE while discussing the importance of following through with screening every year. Increased knowledge among women leads to earlier diagnosis and higher cure rates for breast cancer. Public-awareness campaigns by hospitals, primary-care facilities, and local chapters of the ACS vigorously support this goal.

Widespread media campaigns tend to stress that women get mammograms. CBE and BSE often are not mentioned in public media such as television, radio, and billboard campaigns. This overshadows the importance for a woman to perform BSE and seek CBE. Large-scale clinical trials are needed to provide additional evidence about the value of BSE, and nurses can lead the way in this important endeavor.

Nursing Challenges Related to Breast Cancer Among Ethnic/Racial Minorities and the Underserved

Any discussions about breast cancer must address the concerns and issues of ethnic/racial minority and underserved women, particularly because of the disproportionate number of deaths and poor breast cancer outcomes noted among this group. Also, ethnic/racial minority and underserved women are disproportionately represented among the socioeconomically disadvantaged, a critical factor influencing the stage at diagnosis, prognosis, and survival for women diagnosed with breast cancer.

The U.S. Office of Management and Budget has established four categories for race and two categories for ethnicity. The four categories for race include American Indian or Alaska Native, African American, White, and Asian or other Pacific Islander. The two categories for ethnicity are Hispanic or Latino, and not Hispanic or Latino (NCI, 1999). These groups also are further categorized according to subgroups (i.e., native-born African Americans, Africans, Haitians, non-Spanish-speaking Caribbean Islanders of African descent).

Demographic trends predict a tremendous growth in minority populations by the year 2050. America's population today is 72% White, with a 2050 projection to 53%; 11.4% Hispanic, projected to 25%; 12.9% African American, projected to 15.4%; 4.1% Asian/Pacific Islander, projected to 8.7%; and 0.9% American Indian, projected to 1% (U.S. Bureau of the Census, 1998).

The medically underserved includes those from every ethnic and racial group. NCI (1999) defined the medically underserved as populations that have inadequate access to, or reduced utilization of, high-quality cancer prevention, screening and early detection, treatment, and rehabilitation services. Included are rural, low-literacy, and low-income populations. An effort to further define "medically underserved" currently is under way at NIH.

Ethnic and racial minorities are most likely to be disproportionately represented among the socioeconomically disadvantaged and constitute a large portion of medically underserved populations. To illustrate, recent data revealed that in 1998, 26.1% of African Americans were poor. This compares with 12.5% of Asian/Pacific Islanders, 25.6% of Hispanics, 8.2% of non-Hispanic Whites, and 10.5% of Whites (Daley, Mallett, Shapiro, Prewitt, & U.S. Bureau of the Census, 1999). Collectively, these and other factors underscore the need to examine breast cancer-related issues and trends of ethnic/racial minority and underserved women.

Reviewing the information in Table 11-1 in terms of ethnic/minority groups makes a salient point: while the incidence of female breast cancer is highest among Whites, the mortality rate is highest among African Americans (ACS, 1999). Survival data also demonstrate differences among ethnic/racial minorities and the underserved. For example, African American women are less likely than White women to survive five years, 71% versus 86%, respectively. This disparity in breast cancer outcomes has been attributed to the late stage at diagnosis and the possibility of more aggressive tumor types among African American women (ACS, 1999). Limited data are available related to the survival profiles of other ethnic/racial groups (Centers for Disease Control and Prevention [CDC], 2000).

Increasingly, poverty is being recognized as one of the most significant risk factors associated with high cancer incidence and mortality rates and poor survival. The unemployed and the "working poor" usually lack health insurance, which limits their access to screening and early detection services, state of the art treatment, and follow-up.

Breast cancer prevention and early detection for racial/ethnic minorities and the underserved was a major health objective outlined in *Healthy People 2000* (U.S. Department of Health and Human Services, 1991). The goal of this initiative was to increase the proportion of women age 50 and older (including minority and poverty-level income groups) who received a yearly CBE and mammogram to 60% by 2000 (U.S. Department of Health and Human Services, 1991). Statistics revealed that in 1994, 56% of all females age 50 and older had received a professional examination and mammogram. Specifically, the rate for African American women was 56%, compared to 50% and 38% for Hispanic and low-income women, respectively (U.S. Department of Health and Human Services, 1999).

Much of the progress toward the goals outlined in *Healthy People 2000* can be attributed to the success of the CDC's National Breast and Cervical Early Detection Program (NBCCP). The NBCCP was established in 1990 as a result of the Breast and Cervical Mortality Prevention Act. This act called for the creation of programs to increase breast and cervical cancer screening among low-income and underserved women, including older women and ethnic/racial minorities. Components of this program include (a) screening, tracking, follow-up, and case management, (b) professional education, (c) public education and outreach, (d) quality assurance and improvement, and (e) coalitions and partnerships. The NBCCP has operations in all 50 states, the District of Columbia, 6 U.S. territories, and 12 American Indian/Alaska Native organizations (Henson, Wyatt, & Lee, 1996).

Since its inception in 1990, the NBCCP has provided more than one million mammograms leading to diagnosis of more than 5,800 breast cancers. In addition, many women have received both breast and cervical cancer screening tests as a result of the NBCCP's many outreach efforts. Specifically, the distribution of screening examinations among NBCCP participants includes 53% White, non-Hispanic; 19% Hispanic; 17% Black, non-Hispanic; 6% American Indian/Alaska Native; 3% Asian; and 2% other/unknown (CDC, 2000). This national effort continues to make strides and advances in improving the breast and cervical cancer profile of ethnic/racial minority and underserved women.

Any effort to improve the breast cancer outcomes of racial/ethnic minority populations must take into account the breast cancer screening beliefs, practices, and sociocultural factors of the target populations when designing and implementing interventions. Data regarding these beliefs and practices are growing but remain limited for some racial/ethnic minorities, particularly Asian/Pacific Islanders and Native Americans. Tables 11-6–11-10 provide an overview of the cancer beliefs, barriers to screening, and implications for program planning that can be used when targeting ethnic/racial minority populations.

Individuals working with these populations must be mindful to assess for sociocultural factors that influence breast health practices. These factors are key to the design and implementation of culturally sensitive programs for ethnic/minority populations and should be incorporated accordingly. The need to avoid the "one-size fits all" approach cannot be overemphasized. Because of the diversity of racial/ethnic minority populations, a careful assessment that considers this diversity is an essential component of successful interventions.

The reader is referred to numerous authors who provide a more detailed discussion related to cancer and ethnic/racial minorities (Brant, Fallsdown, & Iverson, 1999; Burhansstipanov, 1993, 2000; Hassey-Dow, 1996; Haynes, 2000; Haynes & Smedley, 1999; Kerner, 1996; Miller et al., 1996; Olsen, 1993; ONS, 1999; Schulmeister, 1999).

Table 11-6. Breast Cancer Screening Profile: African American Women

Common Beliefs	Barriers to Screening	Implications for Program Planning
Breast cancer is a White woman's disease.	Limited education and income	Develop and disseminate educational and promotional messages depicting African American women.
Breast cancer is not a serious disease.	Distrust of the healthcare delivery system	Use African American role model intervention.
A diagnosis of breast cancer is God's will.	Limited knowledge of low/no cost screening services	Create and maintain low/no cost screening services.
	Decreased access to health care	Use lay workers to target African American women.
	Low perceived susceptibility to breast cancer	Increase perceptions related to susceptibility and perceptions related to the benefits of screening.
	Fear of finding cancer	Establish linkages with other organizations and community-based programs to promote breast cancer screening within the African American community.
	Misconceptions that without symptoms, there is no need for screening	Tailor promotional messages to meet individual needs.
	Lack of provider recommendation and support for screening	
	Fear of pain associated with mammography	

Note. Based on information from AMC Cancer Research Center, 1993; Kerner, 1996; Phillips, 1996.

Directions for Future Oncology Nursing Practice, Education, and Research

During this decade, advances in the area of breast cancer prevention and early detection will provide innumerable opportunities for ongoing involvement by oncology nurses. Promising new detection technology and treatments will no doubt have implications for oncology nursing practice, education, and research. These include, but are not limited to, the following.

Practice

• Give high priority to developing skill and expertise in conducting breast cancer risk assessments and genetic counseling services to high-risk populations.

Table 11-7. Racial/Ethnic Minority Breast Cancer Screening Profile: Hispanic Women

Common Beliefs	Barriers to Screening	Implications for Program Planning
Breast cancer cannot be detected early or cured.	Misconceptions that without symptoms, there is no need to be screened	Establish linkages with National Hispanic Leadership Initiatives in Cancer.
Cancer is a death sentence.	Lack of provider recommendation	Use client-entered and culturally relevant strategies.
Cancer is God's punishment.	Decreased access to health care	Consider level of acculturation when designing programs.
One can do little to prevent getting cancer.	Fear of finding cancer	Incorporate Spanish-language programs and approaches
	Language barriers	Emphasize caring for oneself so that one may care for her family.
	Limited education and income	Provide and disseminate bilingual educational and promotional materials
	Older age	Establish linkages with other organizations and community-based programs to promote screening within the Hispanic community such as the Hispanic Leadership Initiative on Cancer.
	Acute care orientation	
	Provider insensitivity	

Note. Based on information from AMC Cancer Research Center, 1993; Cohen & Rohally, 1993.

- Expand community outreach activities to address the needs and challenges related to the early detection of breast cancer among ethnic/minority and underserved populations.
- Incorporate ONS's *Multicultural Outcomes: Guidelines for Cultural Competence* (1999) when providing breast cancer related services to diverse populations.
- Intensify efforts to ensure and improve access to comprehensive state-of- the-art breast cancer services for all women, particularly ethnic/racial minority and underserved populations.
- Assist and empower all women to develop a personal plan for breast health.
- Work with multidisciplinary teams to facilitate professional and public awareness regarding emerging trends and issues related to breast cancer prevention and detection.
- Emphasize the benefits of screening in individuals without symptoms or identifiable risk factors.

Table 11-8. Racial/Ethnic Minority Breast Cancer Profile: Asian/Pacific Islanders

Beliefs	Barriers to Screening	Implications for Program Planning
Cancer is caused by personal lifestyle choices or external forces.	Crisis-oriented use of Westernized medicine	Create multiservice centers to reduce the need for multiple uncoordinated visits.
Illness represents an imbalance or disorder (e.g., toxic waste).	Low income/low acculturation	Develop intervention models that focus on collective rather than individual autonomy.
Illness is caused by an imbalance in morals and spirit.	Embarrassment	
	Reluctance to be examined by male providers	
	Inadequate data to design culturally acceptable and relevant screening programs	

Note. Based on information from AMC Cancer Research Center, 1993; Kagawa-Singer, 1996; Lasky, 1993.

Table 11-9. Racial/Ethnic Minority Breast Cancer Screening Profile: Native American Women

Beliefs	Barriers to Screening	Implications for Program Planning
White man's disease	Lack of access to mammography facilities	Materials should be primarily pictorial and geared toward individuals with an elementary education.
Cancer = death	Lack of provider recommendation	Present health issues as a state in which body, mind, and spirit are in harmony.
As givers of life, women may place their family's needs before their own.	Cost/lack of insurance	Consider cultural issues involving taboo and modesty must be considered when developing programs.
Fatalistic attitude regarding cancer	Misconception that without symptoms, there is no need for screening	
	Long-distance travel	
	Lack of female providers	
	Disproportionately represented among the socioeconomically disadvantaged	

Note. Based on information from AMC Cancer Research Center, 1993; Brant, 1996; Burhansstipanov & Dresser, 1993; NCI, 1996.

Table 11-10. Racial/Ethnic Minority Breast Cancer Profile: Alaska Natives

Beliefs	Barriers to Screening	Implications for Program Planning
Prolonged eye contact may be considered rude.	Preference for female providers	Listen nondefensively to village resident.
Healthcare providers are respected by Alaska Natives until they do something to destroy the respect.	Language differences	Schedule follow-up visits with written correspondences.
Unfavorable view regarding isolating physical health from mental health	Poverty and subsistence living	Establish a specific contact in the community.
	Little focus on preventive care	Do not expect to be admired for what you are being paid to do.
	Geographic factors	
	Different concept of time compared to Western culture	
	Inadequate data basic to designing culturally acceptable programs	

Note. Based on information from AMC Cancer Research Center, 1993; Burhansstipanov & Dresser, 1993; Olsen, 1993.

Education

- Integrate breast cancer prevention and detection content into nursing curricula and interdisciplinary courses.
- Incorporate issues and challenges related to reducing breast cancer mortality and improving breast cancer outcomes among diverse populations.
- Engage students in critically examining content related to breast cancer outlined in the landmark document "The Unequal Burden of Cancer."
- Give high priority to assisting students in developing beginning skills in conducting breast cancer risk assessments and counseling.

Research

- Expand outreach efforts to enhance recruitment and retention of diverse populations in breast cancer prevention clinical trials.
- Facilitate and support community participation in the design, implementation, and evaluation of breast cancer research.
- Conduct studies to evaluate the effectiveness of tailored interventions in promoting breast cancer screening and earlier detection.
- Continue to elucidate beliefs, attitudes, and practices related to breast cancer screening in diverse populations of women.

In closing, this chapter has provided an overview on breast cancer with an emphasis on prevention and detection. Breast cancer constitutes the second leading cause of cancer death among American women. As highlighted throughout the chapter, numerous advances have occurred with regard to breast cancer, particularly in the areas of genetics, prevention and detection, and the identification and management of high-risk individuals. These and other advances have led to the reductions in breast cancer mortality. The future holds much hope for conquering breast cancer, as researchers continue to unveil potential strategies that will aid in preventing breast cancer, reducing breast cancer mortality, and improving breast cancer outcomes. Oncology nurses must continue to assume their rightful place in teaching and counseling to enhance breast cancer outcomes for all women. The design and implementation of culturally sensitive interventions that target racial/ethnic minority populations should remain a high priority in any effort in the war against breast cancer.

For additional information related to breast cancer, contact these sources.

Cancer Statistics
American Cancer Society: www.cancer.org

CancerTrials™: http://cancertrials.nci.nih.gov

National Cancer Institute: www.nci.nih.gov

Surveillance, Epidemiology and End Results (SEER) Program: www.seer.ims.nci.nih.gov

Breast Cancer Resources
Breast Cancer Fund
800-487-0492
www.breastcancerfund.org

Cancer Care, Inc.
www.cancercareinc.org

The National Alliance of Breast Cancer Organizations
www.nabco.org

National Breast Cancer Coalition
www.natlbcc.org

Office of Cancer Survivorship
http://dccps.nci.nih.gov/ocs

The Susan G. Komen Cancer Foundation
www.breastcancerinfo.com

U.S. Food and Drug Administration List of Mammography Screening Facilities
www.fda.gov/cdrh/faclist.html

Y-Me National Breast Cancer Organization
www.y-me.org

Minority Health/Special Populations Resources
Celebrating Life Foundation
800-207-0992
www.celebratinglife.org

Intercultural Cancer Council (ICC)
713-798-3990
http://icc.bcm.tmc.edu

National Asian Women's Health Organization
http://nawho.org

National Library of Medicine
"Multicultural Aspects of Breast Cancer Etiology" (1999)
www.nlm.nih.gov/pubs/resources.html

Office of Minority Health Resource Center
www.omhrc.gov

Office of Special Populations Research Home Page
http://ospr.nci.nih.gov

Sisters Network
8787 Woodway Drive
Suite 4207
Houston, TX 77063
713-781-0255

This article is the result of the authors' independent work and does not reflect the views of the National Institutes of Health, the U.S. Department of Health and Human Services, or the U.S. Government.

References

Aikin, J. (1996). Tamoxifen in perspective: Benefits, side effects, and toxicities. In K.H. Dow (Ed.), *Contemporary issues in breast cancer* (pp. 59–68). Boston: Jones and Bartlett.

Alberg, A.J., Lam, A.P., & Helzlsouer, K.J. (1999). Epidemiology, prevention, and early detection of breast cancer. *Current Opinion in Oncology, 11*, 435–411.

AMC Cancer Research Center. (1993). *Breast and cervical cancer screening barriers and use among specific populations: A review of the literature prepared for public health planners* (Suppl. 2, June 1992–1993). Denver, CO: Author.

American Cancer Society. (1997). *Breast cancer facts and figures, 1997.* Atlanta: Author.

American Cancer Society. (1999). *Breast cancer facts and figures, 1999/2000.* Atlanta: Author.

American Cancer Society. (2000). *Cancer facts and figures, 2000.* Atlanta: Author.

American Cancer Society. (2001a). *Breast cancer facts and figures, 2000–2001.* Atlanta: Author.

American Cancer Society. (2001b). *Cancer facts and figures, 2001.* Atlanta: Author.

Armstrong, K., Eisen, A., & Weber, B. (2000). Assessing the risk of breast cancer. *New England Journal of Medicine, 342,* 564–571.

Baron, R.H., & Borgen, P.I. (1997). Genetic susceptibility for breast cancer: Testing and primary prevention options. *Oncology Nursing Forum, 24,* 461–468.

Behavioral Risk Factor Surveillance System. (2001). *2002 BRFSS summary prevalence report.* Atlanta: Behavioral Surveillance Branch, Division of Adult and Community Health, National Center for Chronic Disease Prevention and Health Promotion, Centers for Disease Control and Prevention.

Belcher, A.E. (1992). *Cancer Nursing.* St. Louis, MO: Mosby.

Benson, J.R. (1998). The biology of breast cancer and its relevance to screening and treatment. In M.W.E. Morgan, R. Warren, & G. Querci della Rovere (Eds.), *Early breast cancer: From screening to multidisciplinary management* (pp. 34–41). St. Leonards, Australia: Harwood Academic Publishers.

Bernhardt, B.A., Geller, G., Doksum, T., & Metz, S.A. (2000). Evaluation of nurses and genetic counselors as providers of education about breast cancer susceptibility testing. *Oncology Nursing Forum, 27,* 33–39.

Bowcock, A.M. (Ed.). (1999). *Breast cancer: Molecular genetics, pathogenesis, and therapeutics.* Totowa, NJ: Humana Press.

Brant, J.M. (1996). Breast cancer challenges in Native American women. In K.H. Dow (Ed.), *Contemporary issues in breast cancer* (pp. 243–252). Boston: Jones and Bartlett.

Brant, J.M., Fallsdown, D., & Iverson, M.L. (1999). The evolution of a breast health program for Plains Indian women. *Oncology Nursing Forum, 26,* 721–740.

Burhansstipanov, L., Dignan, M.B., Wound, D.B., Tenny, M., & Vigil, G. (2000). Native American recruitment into breast cancer screening: The NAWWA Project. *Journal of Cancer Education, 15,* 28–32.

Burhansstipanov, L., & Dresser, C.M. (1993). *Documentation of the cancer research needs of American Indians and Alaska Natives* (NIH Pub. No. 93-3603). Bethesda, MD: National Cancer Institute.

Burke, W., Daly, M., Garber, J., Botkin, J., Kahn, M.J., Lynch, P., McTiernan, A., Offit, K., Perlman, J., Petersen, G., Thomson, E., & Varricchio, C. (1997). Recommendations for follow-up care of individuals with an inherited predisposition to cancer: II. BRCA1 and BRCA2. *JAMA, 277,* 997–1003.

Calzone, K.A. (1997). Predisposition testing for breast and ovarian cancer susceptibility. *Seminars in Oncology Nursing, 13,* 82–90.

Centers for Disease Control and Prevention. (2000). *The National Breast and Cervical Cancer Early Detection Program.* Atlanta: Author

Chen, Y., Thompson, W., Semenciw, R., & Mao, Y. (1999). Epidemiology of contralateral breast cancer. *Cancer Epidemiology, Biomarkers, and Prevention, 8*, 855–861.

Cohen, R.J., & Rohally, J.A. (1993). Cancer prevention and screening among Hispanic populations. In M. Frank-Stromborg & S.J. Olsen (Eds.), *Cancer prevention in minority populations: Cultural implications for health care professionals* (pp. 203–243). St. Louis, MO: Mosby.

Couch, F.J., & Weber, B.L. (1998). Breast cancer. In B. Vogelstein & K.W. Kinzler (Eds.), *The genetic basis of human cancer* (pp. 537–563). New York: McGraw-Hill.

Daley, W., Mallett, R., Shapiro, R., Prewitt, K., & U.S. Bureau of the Census. (1999). *Current Population Report series P60-207, Poverty in the United States: 1998.* Washington, DC: U.S. Government Printing Office.

Donegan, W.L., & Spratt, J.S. (1995). *Cancer of the breast.* Philadelphia: W.B. Saunders.

Eley, J.W., Hill, H.A., Chen, V.W., Austin, D.F., Wesley, M.N., Muss, H.B., Greenberg, R.S., Coates, R.J, Correa, P., Redmond, K., Hunter, C., Herman, A.A., Kurman, R., Blacklow, R., Shapiro, S., & Edwards, B.K. (1994). Racial differences in survival from breast cancer: Results from the National Cancer Institute Black/White Survival Study. *JAMA, 272*, 947–954.

Ernster, V.L., Barclay, J., Kerilikowske, K., Grady, D., & Henderson, I.C. (1996). Incidence of and treatment for ductal carcinoma in situ of the breast. *JAMA, 275*, 913–918.

Fisher, B., Costantino, J.P., Wickerham, D.L., Redmond, C.K., Kavanah, M., Cronin, W.M., Vogel, V., Robidoux, A., Dimitrov, N., Atkins, J., Daly, M., Wieand, S., Tan-Chiu, E., Ford, L., & Wolmark, N. (1998). Tamoxifen for the prevention of breast cancer: Report of the National Surgical Adjuvant Breast and Bowel Project P-1 Study. *Journal of the National Cancer Institute, 90*, 1371–1388.

Ford, K., Marcus, E., & Lum, B. (1999). Breast cancer screening, diagnosis, and treatment. *Disease-a-Month, 45*, 340–377.

Foster, R.S. (1994). Limitations of physical examination in the early diagnosis of breast cancer. *Surgical Oncology Clinics of North America, 3*, 55–66.

Gail, M.H., Brinton, L.A., Byar, D.P., Corle, D.K., Green, S.B., Schairer, C., & Mulvihill, J.J. (1989). Projecting individualized probabilities of developing breast cancer for White females who are being examined annually. *Journal of the National Cancer Institute, 81*, 1879–1886.

Gail, M.H., Costantino, J.P., Bryant, J., Croyle, R., Freedman, L., Helzlsouer, K., & Vogel, V. (1999). Weighing the risks and benefits of tamoxifen treatment for preventing breast cancer. *Journal of the National Cancer Institute, 91*, 1829–1846.

Gammon, M.D., John, E.M., & Britton, J.A. (1998). Recreational and occupational physical activities and risk of breast cancer. *Journal of the National Cancer Institute, 90*, 100–117.

Gasparini, G. (1999). Angiogenesis in breast cancer: Role in biology, tumor progression and prognosis. In A.M. Bowcock (Ed.), *Breast cancer: Molecular genetics, pathogenesis, and therapeutics* (p. 347). Totowa, NJ: Humana Press.

Harris, J.R., Lippman, M.E., Morrow, M., & Hellman, S. (1996). *Diseases of the breast.* Philadelphia: Lippincott-Raven.

Harris, R., & Leininger, L. (1995). Clinical strategies for breast cancer screening: Weighing and using the evidence. *Annals of Internal Medicine, 122*, 539–547.

Hartman, L.C., Schaid, D.J., Woods, J.E., Crotty, T.P., Myers, J.L., Arnold, P.G., Petty, P.M., Sellers, T.A., Johnson, J.L., McDonnell, S.K., Frost, M.H., & Jenkins, R.B.

(1999). Efficacy of bilateral prophylactic mastectomy in women with a family history of breast cancer. *New England Journal of Medicine, 340,* 77–84.

Hassey-Dow, K. (1996). *Contemporary issues in breast cancer.* Boston: Jones and Bartlett.

Haynes, M.A. (2000). A conceptual framework for the planning of ethno-oncology. *Cancer, 88,* 1189–1198.

Haynes, M.A., & Smedley, B.D. (Eds.). (1999). *The unequal burden of cancer: An assessment of NIH research and programs for ethnic minorities and the medically underserved.* Washington, DC: National Academy Press.

Henson, R.M., Wyatt, S.W., & Lee, N.C. (1996). The National Breast and Cervical Cancer Early Detection Program. *Journal of Public Health Management Practice, 2*(2), 36–47.

Hulka, B.S., & Stark, A.T. (1995). Breast cancer: Cause and prevention. *Lancet, 346,* 883–887.

Issacs, C.J., Peshkin, B.N., & Lerman, C. (2000). Evaluation and management of women with a strong family history of breast cancer. In J.R. Harris, M.E. Lippman, M. Morrow, & C.K. Osborne (Eds.), *Diseases of the breast* (2nd ed.) (pp. 237–254). Philadelphia: Lippincott Williams & Wilkins.

Kagawa-Singer, M. (1996). Issues affecting Asian American and Pacific American women. In K.H. Dow (Ed.), *Contemporary issues in breast cancer* (pp. 229–241). Boston: Jones and Bartlett.

Kavanagh, J.J., Singletary, S.E., Einhorn, N., & DePetrillo, A.D. (Eds.). (1998). *Cancer in women.* Malden, MA: Blackwell Science.

Kelsey, J.L. (1993). Breast cancer epidemiology: Summary and future directions. *Epidemiologic Reviews, 15,* 256–263.

Kerner, J.F. (1996). Breast cancer in underserved minorities. In J.L. Harris, M.E. Lippman, M. Morrow, & S. Hellman (Eds.), *Diseases of the breast* (pp. 910–918). Philadelphia: J.B. Lippincott.

Kuller, L.H. (1999). Epidemiology of breast cancer. In R.B. Ness & L.H. Kuller (Eds.), *Health and disease among women: Biological and environmental influences* (pp. 201–224). New York: Oxford University Press.

Lannin, D.R., Matthews, H.F., Mitchell, J., Swanson, M.S., Swanson, F.H., & Edwards, M.S. (1998). Influence of socioeconomic and cultural factors on racial differences in late stage of presentation of breast cancer. *JAMA, 279,* 1801–1807.

Lasky, E.M. (1993). The Asian/Pacific Islander population in the United States: Cultural perspectives and their relationship to cancer prevention and early detection. In M. Frank-Stromborg & S.J. Olsen (Eds.), *Cancer prevention in minority populations: Cultural implications for health care professionals* (pp. 1–56). St. Louis, MO: Mosby.

Marchant, D.J. (1997). *Breast disease.* Philadelphia: W.B. Saunders.

Matulonis, U.A. (1999). Breast cancer: Modifiable lifestyle risk factors. In J.M. Rippe (Ed.), *Lifestyle medicine* (pp. 322–331). Malden, MA: Blackwell Science.

Michels, K.B., Willett, W.C., Rosner, B.A., Manson, J.E., Hunter, D.J., Colditz, G.A., Hankinson, S.E., & Speizer, F.E. (1996). Prospective assessment of breast feeding and breast cancer incidence among 89,887 women. *Lancet, 347,* 431–436.

Miller, B.A., Kolonel, L.N., Bernstein, L., Young, J.L., Swanson, G.M., West, D., Key, C.R., Liff, J.M., Glover, C.S., Alexander, G.A., et al. (1996). *Racial/ethnic patterns of cancer in the United States, 1988–1992* (NIH Publication No. 96-4104). Bethesda, MD: National Cancer Institute.

Myriad Genetics, Inc. (1998). *A clinical resource for health care professionals: BRCA analysis for genetic susceptibility to breast and ovarian cancer.* Salt Lake City, UT: Author.

National Cancer Institute. (1996). *Native American women: Breast cancer and mammography facts.* Bethesda, MD: Author.

National Cancer Institute. (1999). *Special populations/exceptional opportunities: Cancer control and research in minority and underserved populations* (NIH Publication No. 99-4396). Bethesda, MD: Author.

National Cancer Institute. (2001). *Study of Tamoxifen and Raloxifene (STAR) under way across North America.* Retrieved February 22, 2001 from the World Wide Web: http://cancertrials.nci.nih.gov/types/breast/prevention/star/index.html

National Comprehensive Cancer Network. (1999). NCCN Breast Cancer Risk-Reduction Guidelines. *Oncology, 13*(11a), 241–254.

National Institutes of Health. (1997). Breast cancer screening for women ages 40–49. *NIH Consensus Statement, 15*(1), 1–35.

Olsen, S.J. (1993). Cancer prevention and early detection in Native American and Alaska Native populations. In M. Frank-Stromborg & S.J. Olsen (Eds.), *Cancer prevention in minority populations: Cultural implications for health care professionals* (pp. 3–77). St. Louis, MO: Mosby.

Oncology Nursing Society. (1998a). The role of the oncology nurse in genetic counseling. *Oncology Nursing Forum, 25,* 463.

Oncology Nursing Society. (1998b). Cancer genetic testing and risk assessment counseling. *Oncology Nursing Forum, 25,* 464.

Oncology Nursing Society. (1999). *Oncology Nursing Society multicultural outcomes: Guidelines for cultural competence.* Pittsburgh: Oncology Nursing Press, Inc.

Overmoyer, B. (1999). Breast cancer screening. *Medical Clinics of North America, 83,* 1443–1466.

Phillips, J.M. (1996). Breast cancer and African American women. In K.H. Dow (Ed.), *Contemporary issues in breast cancer* (pp. 219–228). Boston: Jones and Bartlett.

Reintgen, D.S., & Clark, R.A. (1996). *Cancer screening.* St. Louis, MO: Mosby.

Ries L.A.G., Kosary, C.L., Hankey, B.F., Miller, B.A., Clegg, L.X., & Edwards, B.K. (Eds.). (1999). *SEER cancer statistics review 1973–1996* (NIH Pub. No. 99–2789). Bethesda, MD: National Cancer Institute.

Roses, D.F. (1999). *Breast cancer.* Philadelphia: Churchill Livingstone.

Rossouw, J.E., Finnegan, L.P., Harlan, W., Pinn, V.W., Clifford, C., & McGowan, J.A. (1995). The evolution of the Women's Health Initiative: Perspectives from the NIH. *Journal of the American Medical Women's Association, 50*(2), 50–58.

Rossouw, J.E., & Hurd, S. (1999). The Women's Health Initiative: Recruitment complete—Looking back and looking forward. *Journal of Women's Health, 8*(1), 3–4.

Schairer, C., Lubin, J., Troisi, S.S., Brinton, L., & Hoover, R. (2000). Menopausal estrogen and estrogen-progestin replacement therapy and breast cancer risk. *JAMA, 283,* 485–491.

Schulmeister, L.K. (1999). Cultural issues in cancer care. In C. Miaskowski & P. Buchsel (Eds.), *Oncology nursing: Assessment and clinical care* (pp. 383–401). St. Louis, MO: Mosby.

Siedman, H., Stellman, S.D., & Mushinski, M.H. (1982). A different perspective on breast cancer risk factors: Some attributable risk. *CA: A Cancer Journal for Clinicians, 32,* 301–313.

Smith-Warner, S.A., Speigelman, D., Yaun, S.S., van den Brandt, P.A., Folsom, A.R., Goldbohm, A., Graham, S., Holmberg, L., Howe, G., Marshall, J., Miller, A., Potter, J.D., Speizer, F.E., Willett, W.C., Wolk, A., & Hunter, D.J. (1998). Alcohol and breast cancer in women: A pooled analysis of cohort studies. *JAMA, 279,* 533–540.

Spiegelman, D., Colditz, G.A., Hunter, D., & Hertzmark, E. (1994). Validation of the Gail Model for predicting individual breast cancer risk. *Journal of the National Cancer Institute, 86,* 600–607.

Shtern, F., Wood, S., & Krause, C. (1998) *Image-guided diagnosis and treatment of breast cancer.* Washington, DC: U.S. Public Health Service's Office on Women's Health, U.S. Department of Health and Human Services.

Tavassoli, F.A. (1999). Normal development and anomalies. *Pathology of the breast.* Stamford, CT: Appleton & Lange.

U.S. Bureau of the Census. (1998). *Current population reports. Series P23-194, population profile of the United States 1997.* Washington, DC: U.S. Government Printing Office.

U.S. Department of Health and Human Services. (1991). *Healthy people 2000: National health promotion and disease prevention objectives* (DHHS Publication No. PHS 91–50212). Washington, DC: U.S. Government Printing Office.

U.S. Department of Health and Human Services. (1999). *Healthy people 2000 review 1998–1999: National health promotion and disease prevention objectives* (DHHS Publication No. PHS 99–1256). Hyattsville, MD: U.S. Government Printing Office.

Vogel, V.G. (1998a). Breast cancer risk factors and preventive approaches to breast cancer. In J.J. Kavanagh, S.E. Singletary, N. Einhorn, & A.D. DePetrillo (Eds.), *Cancer in women* (pp. 58–91). Malden, MA: Blackwell Science.

Vogel, V.G. (1998b). Primary prevention of breast cancer. In K.I. Bland & E.M. Copeland (Eds.), *The breast: Comprehensive management of benign and malignant diseases* (2nd ed.) (pp. 352–369). Philadelphia: W.B. Saunders.

CHAPTER 12

Gastrointestinal Malignancies

Lisa Stucky-Marshall, RN, MS, AOCN®, and
Bridget E. O'Brien, ND, RN, CS-FNP, OCN®

Introduction

Gastrointestinal (GI) malignancies comprise a significant percentage of cancers. They typically grow quietly, with minimal symptomatology, and diagnosis often is made when the disease is advanced and beyond cure. In the past decade, many new developments have occurred in the area of prevention and treatment to promote a better prognostic outcome in these diseases. The most common GI cancers have been the subject of investigation with regard to risk factors and measures for early detection.

This chapter will discuss the prevention and early detection of five GI malignancies in the order of their incidence: colorectal, gastric, hepatocellular, esophageal, and anal. Although more information currently is available about colorectal cancer (CRC) than the other four disease sites, discussions on all five will include etiology, risk factors, current trends in screening and early detection, and chemoprevention strategies for high-risk groups.

GI and oncology nurses are integral members of the healthcare team who are dedicated to caring for individuals with diseases that often are devastating. Nurses play several vital roles in their goal of improving outcomes: identifying high-risk groups for early referral, educating diverse groups on the importance of screening, early detection, and signs and symptoms of disease, and coordinating care and proper follow-up. The more nurses know about GI malignancies, the greater impact they can have on reaching their goal.

Colorectal Cancer

Introduction

CRC is the second leading cause of cancer death in the United States (Greenlee, Hill-Harmon, Murray, Bolden, & Tun, 2001). When diagnosed prior to the presentation of symptoms, the cure rate is high. Despite this fact, CRC historically has been a cancer that has received little attention in regard to early detection. Screening efforts tend to meet resistance from the general public and even from health professionals because of conflicting recommendations from various sources/schools of thought.

CRC is referred to as a "dirty cancer" because of its anatomical location. Talking about associated signs and symptoms may cause embarrassment, resulting in warning signs that go unreported. The cost of screening is another obstacle; colonoscopy easily can cost up to a few thousand dollars, including procedure room, conscious sedation, pathologist, and physician fees. Private insurance plans may reimburse for GI lab screening procedures, but Medicare did not approve coverage for CRC screening until 1998, eliminating the payment barrier for people older than 65.

Media attention is beginning to keep pace with the problem as well. In March 2000, several national organizations came together to promote "National Colorectal Cancer Awareness Month" for the first time in the United States. This effort was intended to promote awareness to both the general public and healthcare professionals regarding the need for CRC screening as part of routine health care. "Screen for Life" is another campaign created and implemented by the Centers for Disease Control (CDC) and Prevention. This campaign addresses common myths associated with CRC and educates the public on the importance of screening and early detection. Current data suggest that the majority of people in the United States do not obtain routine colorectal screening. These efforts may improve the number of people who begin CRC screening because of their own personal interest or because healthcare professionals are more informed and recommend appropriate screening.

CRC screening rates have risen slightly since 1997 but still remain at low levels (CDC, 2001). A 1999 telephone survey conducted by the Behavioral Risk Factor Surveillance System revealed that only 44% of adults age 50 and older had ever had a sigmoidoscopy or colonoscopy for screening or diagnostic purposes, and only 34% of respondents had one of those tests within the last five years. Of the respondents, 40% of adults age 50 and older reported ever having fecal occult blood testing (FOBT) using the kit at home, and only 21% reported having had the test in the previous year. Women were more likely to report having had FOBT than men, whereas more men reported having a sigmoidoscopy than women. Only 44% of adults age 50 and older had at least one of these screening tests within the recommended time interval (CDC, 2001). More current information from the same group in 1997 showed similar data with little improvement. These low numbers may relate to personal barriers, such as fear of the types of examinations performed, embarrassment, or lack of knowledge that both men and women are at risk for CRC.

Other barriers to CRC screening relate to healthcare professionals. They may lack sufficient knowledge, may not be in agreement with the recommendations, or may feel insufficient evidence is available to support CRC screening. Further, they may feel uncomfortable recommending CRC screening because it may be viewed as distasteful in the eyes of the patient.

Rationale and Appropriateness of Colorectal Cancer Screening

Guidelines exist to determine if screening is appropriate for a particular disease. Screening can be justified if it meets the following criteria: (a) it is a common disease associated with high morbidity or mortality; (b) the identified screening test used is accurate in detecting early-stage disease, is reasonable for patients, and is feasible in clinical practice; (c) treatment efforts following early detection have an impact on prognosis comparable to treatment after normal diagnosis; and (d) evidence exists that the benefits of the screening outweigh the risks and costs (Clark & Reintgen, 1996). CRC is a disease that meets all of these criteria for screening and the associated screening tests have been shown to impact mortality. Evidence shows that by removing premalignant adenomatous polyps, the incidence of CRC can be reduced. Benefits of CRC screening have been found to outweigh the risks, and cost effectiveness resembles other widely accepted screening tests (Wagner, Tunis, Brown, Ching, & Almeida, 1996; Winawer et al., 1997). Because most cancers develop from adenomatous polyps over an extended period of time, a window of opportunity is available to intercede with screening examinations to identify and remove the premalignant polyps and early-stage cancers (Winawer et al., 1997).

Incidence

CRC is the fourth most common cancer in the United States and the second leading cause of cancer death (Greenlee et al., 2001). It is a prevalent malignancy throughout the world but is found most commonly in the Western hemisphere. Approximately 135,400 new cases are estimated in 2001, with an estimated 56,700 cancer-related deaths (Greenlee et al.). Although these statistics are improving, much work still needs to be performed to increase public awareness about CRC screening. CRC can be prevented in most cases with appropriate screening (i.e., sigmoidoscopy/colonoscopy with polypectomy), and now a variety of options are available that recently have been endorsed by federal legislation. Guidelines from various national organizations also have been developed to provide more information to prescribing caregivers and offer more options to the public.

Epidemiology

CRC occurs most commonly in the Western, industrialized countries of North America, Northern Europe, and New Zealand (Parkin, Pisani, & Ferlay, 1993). Strong evidence is related to the impact of environmental factors on the incidence of colon cancer, which could influence the high rates seen in the Western world. Identifying and eliminating the causative factors from the environment or a person's diet could impact this high rate. Low-risk groups who migrate to high-risk areas have been found to take on the higher risk of the new environment. A variation from the traditional dietary practices (i.e., low fat, high in fish, low in red meat) may be responsible for recent statistical changes in Japan. The age-adjusted incidences of cancer of both the colon and rectum have risen more than threefold from 1974–1991 in Japan, approaching rates seen in the Western world (Tamura et al., 1996).

CRC incidence increases with age, with the rate of disease rising rapidly after age 50. Both genders are affected equally, and mortality figures also are equal. The lifetime risk for both men and women of developing CRC is 6% (Bedine, 1999). Males between ages 60–79 have a 3.97% chance of being diagnosed with CRC, and females in the same age range have a 3.06% chance. The incidence among African Americans is 50.4%, compared with 43.9% for Whites. Mortality rates are 23.1% for African Americans and 17.4% for Whites (Bedine).

CRC is classified into three categories based on significance: sporadic (60%), familial (30%), and hereditary (10%) (Ivanovich, Read, Ciske, Kodner, & Whelan, 1999). The American Cancer Society (ACS) has designated these three groups as average, moderate, and high risk (Byers, Levin, Rothenberger, Dodd, & Smith, 1997).

Sporadic CRC occurs without an inherited genetic mutation or extended family history of colon cancer. Familial CRC refers to familial clusters of affected members. Identifying affected members is important, as the incidence rises with more affected first-degree members (Ivanovich et al., 1999). An adenomatous polyposis coli (APC) gene mutation causes many of the familial CRCs and has been associated with an increase in CRC for people with Ashkenazi ancestry, although more study is needed in this area (Ivanovich et al.). Hereditary CRC results from the inheritance of a single gene mutation, which is a significant risk factor. Some of the common hereditary CRCs will be discussed later.

Morbidity

Diagnosed at an early stage (Dukes' A or stage I), CRC has a five-year survival rate of 90%. When metastatic disease is present, the five-year survival is 5.3% (Sandler, 1996). Unfortunately, 25% of patients present with symptoms at the time of diagnosis, indicating that the disease has metastasized and the prognosis is poor. Survival rates have improved over the last 20 years, likely related to improved surgical techniques, adjuvant chemotherapy, radiotherapy, and efforts at improving early detection (Sandler). From 1974–1976, five-year survival rates were 51% for Whites and 46% for African Americans. Rates for all stages of disease from 1986–1992 showed an increase, with Whites up to 62% and African Americans up to 53%. The survival rates for Whites are better compared with African Americans, as they typically present with an earlier stage of disease. Factors are attributed to possible healthcare access differences (Surveillance, Epidemiology, and End Results Program [SEER], 1996) (see Figure 12-1).

Pathophysiology
Anatomy/Physiology

Location of the tumor has an effect on the signs and symptoms that develop, so an understanding of the anatomy and physiology is important for nurses. The large bowel is divided into the colon and rectum, with the colon measuring four to five feet and extending from the ileocecal valve. The rectum measures six to eight inches, extending to the most distal portion, the anus. The large bowel has an important role in the absorption of water and electrolytes, fermentation of carbohydrates, and absorption of the products of this process (Kleibeuker, Nagengast, & van der Meer, 1996). This very efficient process allows a transit time of 24–72 hours, with 200 grams of stool produced per day (Kleibeuker et al.).

Anatomically, the large bowel is divided into five sections: ascending, transverse, descending, sigmoid, and rectum. The wall of the intestine has four layers: serosa, muscularis, submucosa, and mucosa. Staging of CRC is determined by the degree of tumor penetration through these layers, beyond the colon wall, and spread to distant organs.

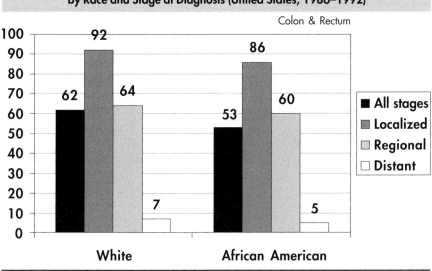

Figure 12-1. Five-Year Relative Survival Rates for Colorectal Cancer by Race and Stage at Diagnosis (United States, 1986–1992)

Note. From *SEER Cancer Statistics Review, 1973–1996,* by the Surveillance, Epidemiology, and End Results Program, 1996, Bethesda, MD: National Cancer Institute.

Common Cellular Types/Histology

Carcinogenesis in the colorectum is a multistep process resulting in malignant cell penetration and invasion into the basement membrane of the epithelium (Kleibeuker et al., 1996). The most common histological type of CRC is adenocarcinoma, with most resulting from a malignant conversion occurring in a preexisting adenomatous lesion (Boland, 1999). Some squamous cell carcinomas, adenosquamous carcinomas, lymphomas, and endocrine tumors also have been reported but are less common (Boland). Adenocarcinomas are usually of a moderate or well-differentiated grade. Approximately 20% of tumors are poorly differentiated or undifferentiated, and both are associated with a poorer prognosis. Mucin-producing tumors can occur and are associated with a worse prognosis than nonmucin-producing tumors (Boland). Multiple primary colon tumors are not uncommon and can occur simultaneously (synchronous lesions) or in different time frames (metachronous lesions) (Boland). Lesions can be in close proximity to each other or found in different locations within the colon.

Pathogenesis of Adenomatous Polyps

Most colorectal tumors develop from adenomatous polyps, which, over time, can convert to carcinoma. A polyp refers to a tissue protrusion or a mucosal mass in the colon and rectum that often is asymptomatic. Polyps can vary by the texture of the mucosal surface, size, position, color, stalk, ulceration, or bleeding (Macrae & Young, 1999). The most important characteristic of polyps is the histologic type. Polyps within the large bowel can be classified into three groups: neoplastic polyps, such as adenomatous polyps and carcinomas, non-neoplastic polyps, such as the hyperplastic polyps without malignant potential, and submucosal lesions resembling a polypoid appearance (Macrae & Young).

Hyperplastic polyps commonly are found in the colon; they are rarely larger than 4–5 mm but account for 50% or more of the small polyps of the colon (Burt & Petersen, 1996). Hyperplastic polyps are believed to have no malignant potential, although, in rare situations, adenomatous or carcinomatous changes have occurred in these types of polyps (Burt & Petersen).

Neoplastic polyps are of the most interest because of their association as precursor lesions to CRC. Their potential to become malignant is dependent on the size, histologic type, and degree of atypia. Polyps that are large (> 1 cm), with extensive villous histology or severe dysplasia, have an increased likelihood of malignancy occurring. The rate of carcinoma increases with size and changes in histology. Large villous adenomas (> 2.5 cm) may contain malignancy in up to 50% of cases, where small tubular adenomas have a malignant transformation rate of 1% (Bedine, 1999). Not all adenomatous polyps convert into carcinoma.

Direct evidence of this polyp conversion to carcinoma is limited. Several types of indirect evidence support this belief. Cancers and adenomatous polyps have the same anatomic distribution, and cancers rarely arise in the absence of adenomatous polyps. The average age of onset of adenomatous polyps precedes cancer development by several years (Winawer, Zauber, & Diaz, 1987). Patients with one or more large polyps have been found to be at increased risk of future cancer (Atkin, Morson, & Cuzick, 1992; Stryker et al., 1987), and most of these cancers develop at the site of large polyps left in place (Stryker et al.). Patients with familial adenomatous polyposis (FAP) have hundreds to thousands of polyps and a high likelihood of developing cancer. Detecting and removing adenomatous polyps in patients reduces the incidence of CRC.

The actual time to progression from an adenoma to carcinoma is not known, as no studies are available that have reported observations from small adenoma to large adenoma to cancer. An expert multidisciplinary panel estimated that the average time for an adenomatous polyp less than 1 cm in size to transform into an invasive cancer takes an average of 10 years (Winawer et al., 1993).

The progression from normal intestinal mucosa to adenomatous polyp into cancer is thought to occur after an accumulation of genetic alterations acquired after birth that promote the development of cancer (oncogenes) and the loss of tumor suppressor genes (Winawer et al., 1997) (see Figure 12-2). The order in which these mutations arise is critical and usually begins at the APC gene (Ivanovich et al., 1999). It has been hypothesized that genetic alterations cause the development of adenomatous polyps, and further genetic changes are believed to cause the polyps to progress to carcinoma (Winawer et al., 1997). People with sporadic CRC do not have an inherited genetic mutation that initiates the adenoma-to-carcinoma sequence. With the hereditary syndromes, other mutations in other genes can occur, which may accelerate the tumor initiation or tumor promotion process (Ivanovich et al.). Environmental and dietary factors may play a role in this process as well. A person's ability to form adenomatous polyps varies, and those who have polyps are likely to have a recurrence of new polyps once the others have been removed (Winawer et al., 1997).

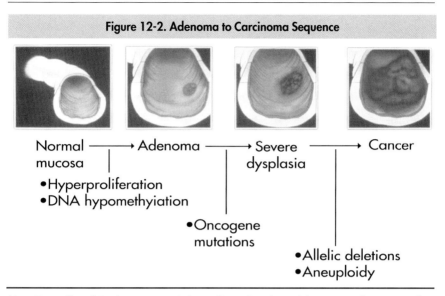

Figure 12-2. Adenoma to Carcinoma Sequence

Note. From *Clinical Teaching Project: Colorectal Neoplasia* (p. 13), by P.M. Lynch, M.I. Burrell, P.H. Green, and S. Vera, 1996, Timonium, MD: Milner-Fenwick, Inc. Copyright 1996 by Milner-Fenwick, Inc. Reprinted with permission.

Elimination of adenomatous polyps can reduce the possibility of a cancer developing. This can be achieved with endoscopic polypectomy. Surgical resection may be required for malignant polyps with poor prognostic features or those too difficult to remove by endoscopy. Colorectal screening is intended to identify the presence of adenomatous polyps, or early cancers, in people who have not developed symptoms. Polypectomy prevents the further growth and progression to CRC.

Patterns of Anatomic Site Distribution

CRC usually begins as a round lesion with a shape that may change from the sloughing and regrowth of cells. Right-sided cancers tend to grow more into the lumen and extend along one wall. Left-sided tumors grow more into the bowel wall and circumferentially, demonstrating a napkin ring or apple-core type appearance on radiologic barium enema studies (Cohen, Minsky, & Schilsky, 1997).

Tumors present different signs and symptoms, depending on the particular location in the colon. In the past, tumors more commonly were located on the left side of the colon. More recently, the distribution of cancers has shifted toward the right side of the colon. Studies have hypothesized that this increase may be related to the aging population, especially in women. Rectal cancer incidence has decreased with an increase in sigmoid and proximal colon cancers (Boland, 1999).

Patterns of Disease Progression

CRC begins as an adenoma and progresses through stages of advancing degrees of dysplasia as it grows. Growth tends to be slow at an unpredictable rate (Boland, 1999). Adenocarcinoma develops in the intestinal mucosa, usually from a polyp that has not been removed. The tumor can progress by local invasion, lymphatic extension, hematogenous spread, or implantation. Local invasion occurs as the tumor invades with direct extension and penetration through the layers of the mucosa. Once the tumor extends beyond the muscularis mucosa and infiltrates the submucosa, it is considered invasive (Hoebler, 1997). The tumor then can spread further through the lymph nodes and vascular network. The colon's lymphatic network is via the pericolic, intermediate, and principle lymph node chains (Hoebler). Spread of rectal cancer is associated with localized advancement of the tumor. Hematogenous spread most commonly results in liver metastasis, followed by lung metastasis (Cohen et al., 1997). Other sites of metastasis, such as bone or brain involvement, are uncommon without the presence of liver or lung involvement. Implantation occurs when tumor cells are released from the primary tumor and deposit onto other surfaces, such as the peritoneum. Intraluminal spread of tumor cells also can occur. Prognosis and mortality worsen during the advancing stage of disease.

Staging

No standard staging system exists for CRC, although three systems commonly are used: Dukes', Astler-Coller, and TNM. The American Joint Committee on Cancer (AJCC) and the International Union Against Cancer (UICC) codeveloped TNM staging (see Table 12-1). A combination staging of Dukes' Turnbull demonstrates carcinoma in situ and four stages of Dukes' A–D with corresponding TNM staging (see Table 12-2). All staging systems demonstrate the colorectal

Table 12-1. Comparison of Dukes' and TNM Staging Systems

Stage	Dukes'	TNM	Tumor Involvement
I	A	T1N0M0	
	B$_1$	T2N0M0	
II	B$_2$	T3N0M0	
III	C$_1$	T2N1M0	
	C$_2$	T3N1M0	
IV	D	TXNXM1	

Note. From "Alternatives in Therapy for Low Rectal Cancer," by T.D. Arnell and M.J. Stamos, 1996, Journal of Wound, Ostomy and Continence Nursing, 23, p. 152. Copyright 1996 by Mosby. Adapted with permission.

Table 12-2. TNM Classification System for Colon and Rectal Cancer

Definition of TNM

Primary Tumor (T)

TX   Primary tumor cannot be assessed.
T0   No evidence of primary tumor
Tis Carcinoma in situ: Intraepithelial or invasion of the lamina propria*
T1   Tumor invades the submucosa.
T2   Tumor invades the muscularis propria.
T3   Tumor invades through the muscularis propria into the subserosa or into nonperitonealized pericolic or perirectal tissues.
T4   Tumor directly invades other organs or structures or perforates the visceral peritoneum.**

*Note. Tis includes cells confined within the glandular basement membrane (intraepithelial) or lamina propria (intramucosal) with no extension through the muscularis into the submucosa.
**Note. Direct invasion of other organs or structures includes invasion of other segments of colorectum by way of serosa (i.e., invasion of the sigmoid colon by a carcinoma of the cecum).

Regional Lymph Nodes (N)

NX   Regional lymph nodes cannot be assessed.
N0   No regional lymph node metastasis
N1   Metastasis in one to three pericolic or perirectal lymph nodes
N2   Metastasis in four or more pericolic or perirectal lymph nodes
N3   Metastasis in any lymph node along the course of a named vascular trunk or metastasis to apical node(s) (when marked by the surgeon)

Distant Metastasis (M)

MX   Presence of distant metastasis cannot be assessed.
M0   No distant metastasis
M1   Distant metastasis

Stage Grouping

AJCC/UICC				Dukes'*
Stage 0	Tis	N0	M0	–
Stage I	T1	N0	M0	A
	T2	N0	M0	–
Stage II	T3	N0	M0	B
	T4	N0	M0	–
Stage III	Any T	N1	M0	C
	Any T	N2	M0	–
Stage IV	Any T	Any N	M1	–

*Dukes' B is a composite of better (T3, N0, M0) and worse (T4, N0, M0) prognostic groups, a Dukes' C (any T, N1, M0 and Any T, N2, M0).

Note. From AJCC Cancer Staging Manual (5th ed.) (p. 86), by American Joint Committee on Cancer, 1997, Philadelphia: Lippincott-Raven. Copyright 1997 by Lippincott-Raven. Reprinted with permission.

tumor's depth of penetration and invasion into the bowel lumen, lymphatic spread, and distant metastatic spread. Early-stage tumors (stage I–II or Dukes' A–B) are associated with a better five-year survival than late-stage tumors (stage III–IV or Dukes' C–D).

Prognostic Variables

Several variables have been identified that correlate with survival in colorectal tumors.

Age

Earlier age at onset has been thought to be associated with a worse prognosis, which has been confirmed by various studies. When stage-adjusted survival has been analyzed, no difference has been noted in relative prognosis for the younger age group in almost all reports (Umpleby & Williamson, 1984).

Gender

Women have been found to have a more favorable prognosis in several studies (Welch & Burke, 1962). Differing opinions regarding survival have been seen, with studies showing an advantage for women (Cohen et al., 1997) and others showing no difference (Bulow, 1980).

Symptoms

Five-year survival rates were different for symptomatic patients (49%) versus asymptomatic patients (71%) (Beahrs & Sanfelippo, 1971).

Obstruction/Perforation

Both obstruction and perforation have been determined to reduce survival. Obstruction is an important indicator of prognosis, independent of Dukes' stage. Perforation is important as a prognostic feature only for disease-free survival (Cohen et al., 1997).

Rectal Bleeding and Hemorrhage

Both rectal bleeding and hemorrhage have been associated with improved prognosis. This may be related to early manifestation of mucosal erosion, leading to early diagnosis, rather than being a symptom of tumor penetration (Cohen et al., 1997).

Tumor Size/Location

Tumor size itself has not been found to associate with patient outcome (Boland, 1999). Differing opinions exist on prognosis related to tumor location. However, the five-year survival tends to be lower for patients with rectosigmoid/rectal cancers compared to more proximal colon cancers (Cohen et al., 1997).

Carcinoembryonic Antigen

The value of the preoperative carcinoembryonic antigen level as an independent prognostic factor is unclear at this time (Cohen et al., 1997).

Pathologic Features

Various pathologic features are associated with worse prognosis for patients with CRC. These include adjacent organ involvement, histologic grade, colloid or mucinous cancers, vascular or perineural invasion (rectal tumors only), lymphatic invasion, and aneuploid tumors (Cohen et al., 1997).

Risk Factors

Approximately 75% of all new cases of CRC occur in people with no known predisposing risk factors (Burt, Bishop, Lynch, Rozen, & Winawer, 1990). Environmental factors, particularly those associated with diet, can affect the colonic environment and contribute to the development of CRC.

People can be stratified as average, moderate/intermediate, or high risk based on their personal and family history. Family history of colorectal carcinoma or polyps is the most important feature determining risk for CRC (Fuchs et al., 1994). Patients who are average risk have no medical condition predisposing them to CRC and only have the risk of being older than age 50. Moderate-risk individuals have a personal or family history of CRC or adenomatous polyps, with one or more parents, siblings, or children with disease but without any genetic syndrome (Winawer et al., 1997). High-risk people are those with a hereditary or medical condition such as FAP, hereditary nonpolyposis CRC (HNPCC), or a history of inflammatory bowel disease. HNPCC accounts for 5% (Rex, 1999) and FAP about 1%. Less than 1% of CRCs are associated with uncommon conditions such as inflammatory bowel diseases and some rare genetic syndromes (e.g., Peutz-Jeghers syndrome, familial juvenile polyposis) (Winawer et al., 1997). People identified as moderate or high risk need earlier screening or surveillance for CRC or its precursors to improve the duration of life.

Age

Men and women older than 40 years of age are the largest population at risk for CRC, with the risk rising sharply for those older than 50 (Hoebler, 1997). The presence of carcinogens in contact with the large intestine over the years is thought to promote this development. In addition adenomatous polyps occur in approximately 25% of people older than 50 and increase with age (Winawer et al., 1997).

Dietary/Environmental

A number of dietary components have been implicated as possible factors in the development of CRC. The major dietary factors that have been linked to CRC include fat content and fiber intake.

Fat

Diets with high fat intake (both saturated and unsaturated) may put one at greater risk for development of CRC. This diet is more common in the Western world, where people consume more red meat than poultry or fish. Fat is known to stimulate synthesis of cholesterol and bile acids in the liver that can be converted by the colonic bacteria into toxic metabolites. Efficient fat absorption takes place in the small intestine, allowing approximately 3% of the bile acids to enter the colon, with 5 grams excreted daily in the feces (Kleibeuker et al., 1996). The presence of bile acids can result in increased proliferation of the colon epithelium, resulting in other events that present inflammatory mediators and ultimately greater cell proliferation. Western diets are composed of approximately 40%–50% of calories from fat. Current ACS guidelines suggest an intake of fat of less than 65 grams per day based on a 2000-calorie diet. A multicenter trial is under way with a low-fat diet (20% of calories) that is high in fruits and vegetables to determine whether this can reduce the rate of adenoma development (Cohen et al., 1997). Recent data from a survey called the Continuing Survey of Food Intake by Individuals showed that American fat consumption decreased from 40% in the late 1970s to 33% in the mid-1990s. Only one-third of adults met the goal of 30% or less of calories from fat recommended by nutritionists (U.S. Department of Agriculture, 1999). A reduction of fat intake by 50% could lead to an estimated reduction in incidence of colon cancer of 67% and rectal cancer of 29%.

Fiber

Dietary fiber is plant material that is not easily digested by the upper GI tract (Bedine, 1999). The presence of fiber in the GI tract may be protective by increasing stool volume, decreasing the transit time, diluting the potential carcinogens, and minimizing their contact with the bowel lining.

Dietary fiber intake is controversial for impacting the risk of CRC development. Diets low in fiber are thought to put a person at greater risk for CRC development. Epidemiologic studies have revealed a correlation between high-fiber diets and low incidence of CRC, but this is dependent on the type of fiber consumed. Cellulose and bran fiber are thought to be more effective in reducing carcinogenesis than other fibers (Greenwald & Lanza, 1986). Mutagen production and bile acid concentration can depend on the type of fiber selected (Cohen et al., 1997). The Nurses Health Study (Giovannucci et al., 1995) noted an increased rate of CRC in nurses who had chronic constipation. The current fiber recommendation is 20–30 grams/day with a focus on wheat bran and cellulose. The Continuing Survey of Food Intakes by Individuals (from 1994–1996) found that a 40% increase had occurred in consumption of grain products in the diet since the 1970s, although less than one-third of adults in the United States believe that intake of grain products in the diet is important (U.S. Department of Agriculture, 1999). A recently published wheat and bran fiber research project by Alberts et al. (2000) studied 1,429 men and women with a history of polyp removal. Patients were randomized to a high wheat bran cereal supplement (13.5 grams of fiber/day) or low wheat bran fiber supplement (2 grams of fiber/day) for three years. Results indicated that although the higher dietary fiber did not impact CRC risk, as originally thought, it should continue to benefit other chronic diseases. Recurrent polyps that did develop tended to be small. Questions remain related to the short study length and the long-term follow-up needed to determine the dietary impact on these patients.

Alcohol

The association between alcohol consumption and CRC is inconsistent. Colorectal adenomas have been associated with alcohol consumption (Sandler,

1996), and beer consumption has been associated with increased risk of rectal cancers for men (Rhodes, Holmes, & Clark, 1977). The mechanism by which alcohol can contribute to CRC is its breakdown into acetaldehyde, which is a recognized carcinogen (Kroser, Bachwich, & Lichtenstein, 1997) that can result in hypomethylation, superoxide radical production, and, ultimately, carcinogenesis (Kroser et al.). Folate and methionine deficiency may play a role with alcohol in the process of carcinogenesis (Sandler).

Calcium

Calcium intake and correlation with development of CRC has been implicated, but the mechanism is not clear. The protective effect that calcium may have is likely multifactoral. Calcium intake currently is being evaluated in clinical trials to determine its effect on adenoma development and CRC.

Exercise

Physical activity appears to be protective for both men and women. The widely held hypothesis is that exercise stimulates colonic motility, decreases transit time, stimulates prostaglandins, and improves immune function (Bedine, 1999). Reducing transit time may decrease the time that bile acids and potential carcinogens remain in the colon. A sedentary occupation for an extended time is associated with a higher risk (Vena et al., 1985).

Cigarette Smoking

The risk related to cigarette smoking is conflicting. The association of smoking with CRC is a less consistent risk factor. Smoking is associated with adenoma formation, which causes an increased risk (Potter, 1996). Additional studies are needed to evaluate early onset of long-standing cigarette smoking.

Radiation

People who have received external beam pelvic irradiation may have an increased risk for CRC. Some studies have indicated a higher risk if the radiation has been low dose (Levitt, Millar, & Stewart, 1990).

Overall Risk for Colorectal Cancer

Individual risk can be categorized as average, moderate/intermediate, or high for development of CRC.

Average Risk

Average-risk individuals are those who are asymptomatic and whose major risk is being older than age 50. The average risk group comprises the majority of the population who develops CRC.

Moderate/Intermediate Risk

Moderate/intermediate-risk individuals are those with a familial CRC risk, personal history of adenomatous polyps, or CRC.

Family History of Colorectal Cancer

People without a specific genetic syndrome but with one or more first-degree relatives (e.g., parent, sibling, child) with CRC have approximately twice the risk of developing CRC as an average-risk person without a family history (Winawer et al., 1997). People with this history have what has been termed "familial colorectal cancer" (Lynch, Shaw, & Lynch, 1999). A single first-degree relative with CRC increases a person's risk significantly by age 40 (Fuchs et al., 1994); the risk is increased further if more than one first-degree relative is affected and if the cancer occurred before age 55 (St. John et al., 1993). Similar risk exists in close relatives of people having an adenomatous polyp before age 60 (Winawer et al., 1996). A second-degree relative is associated with approximately a 50% increased risk and a third-degree relative a 30% increased risk (Kroser et al., 1997). CRC in these groups is comparable to the general population in regard to the age of onset and location of tumor (Lynch et al., 1999).

Personal History of Polyps or Colorectal Cancer

People with a history of adenomatous polyps are at increased risk of CRC. One study reported that patients with a history of adenomas had a 50% risk of developing another polyp after 15 years. The risk for men was found to be 1:12 and in women 1:20 for developing cancer within that time frame (Morson & Bussey, 1985).

People with a history of CRC are at increased risk of a second (metachronous) cancer in addition to their risk of recurrence of the original cancer (Winawer et al., 1997). Information has suggested that metachronous cancers have little biological distinction from the initial cancer, except that an increased incidence may exist (Winawer et al., 1996).

High Risk

High-risk individuals are those with a genetic syndrome or medical history of inflammatory bowel disease.

Familial Adenomatous Polyposis

FAP is the most clearly detected of the inherited colon cancer syndromes and accounts for approximately 1% of new cases of CRC in the United States (Winawer et al., 1997). FAP is an autosomal dominant inherited disorder with 80%–100% penetrance. It is clinically characterized by the presence of hundreds to thousands of adenomatous polyps in the colon and rectum after the first decade of life. The syndrome results from germline mutations of the APC gene, located on the long arm of chromosome 5. Two patterns of polyp distribution have been noted, one resembling a carpet-like pattern of numerous tiny polyps that cover the surface of the colon, and the other demonstrates fewer polyps that are of slightly larger size (Burt & Jacoby, 1999). The differences in the two patterns have not been explained. Histologically, the polyps seen in FAP usually are tubular, villous, or tubulovillous adenomas. Ninety percent of polyps found are less than 5 mm, and fewer than 1% are greater than 1 cm in size (Burt & Petersen, 1996). The adenomas appear first and, over time, one or more cancers develop. Without intervention, people with

FAP have nearly a 100% likelihood of developing cancer. The average age of onset of cancer in one study was 39 years (Burt & Petersen). Patients with FAP represent the extreme end of the spectrum and serve as the prototype for the adenoma-to-carcinoma sequence (Boland, 1999). This process is terminated only after the colon is removed by prophylactic colectomy. Cancer will develop by age 21 in 7% of affected people who do not have colectomy and in 90% by age 45 (Burt & Petersen). More than 80% of people with FAP can develop small bowel adenomas, usually located near the ampulla of vater, which can develop into cancer (Terdiman, Conrad, & Sleisenger, 1999). Genetic techniques now can identify carriers of the abnormal APC gene prior to polyps developing in the offspring of the affected person (Powell et al., 1993). People with this family history should receive genetic counseling and consider genetic testing to determine if they are gene carriers. Estimates suggest that 80% of individuals in families with FAP are carriers (Winawer et al., 1997). Gene carriers should obtain flexible sigmoidoscopy surveillance annually beginning at age 10–12 to see if the gene is being expressed. If polyposis becomes evident, total proctocolectomy should be recommended and remains the only way to prevent the development of cancer. The difficulty, however, is determining when it should be performed (Winawer et al., 1997).

A newer option has been the U.S. Food and Drug Administration's (FDA) approval of celecoxib in 2000 for polyp prevention. This drug, in clinical trials, was found to reduce the number of polyps by 20 in patients with FAP. Whether this will have an impact on CRC incidence, mortality, or quality of life is unknown at this time (Steinbach et al., 2000)

Phenotypic variants of FAP can occur. Turcot's syndrome is rare and is manifested by colonic adenomatous polyposis and central nervous system tumors. Gardner's syndrome is characterized by polyposis and associated extraintestinal symptoms. The extraintestinal symptoms can include benign soft tissue tumors such as desmoid tumors, osteomas, soft-tissue tumors of the skin, supernumerary teeth, and congenital hypertrophy of the retinal pigment epithelium (Burt & Petersen, 1996). The genetic defect for both variants also occurs on chromosome 5 of the APC gene (Winawer et al., 1997).

Attenuated Familial Adenomatous Polyposis

Previously referred to as the flat adenoma syndrome, this variant of FAP is characterized by flat polyps, usually less than 1 cm in size, located in the proximal colon (Burt & Petersen, 1996). The average number of polyps in attentuated familial adenomatous polyposis (AFAP) usually is less than FAP (Burt & Petersen). Upper GI lesions can be found in the duodenum or fundus (Lynch et al., 1999). Genetic mutations occur very close to the 5' end of the APC gene. CRC will occur in most patients with AFAP, but the age of onset is late compared to FAP (age 55 versus 39) (Lynch et al., 1999).

Hereditary Nonpolyposis Colorectal Cancer

HNPCC, also known as Lynch syndrome II, accounts for approximately 5% of CRC cases (Rex, 1999). It is an autosomal dominant disorder characterized by an early onset of CRC by an average age of 45 (Lynch et al., 1993). With this syndrome, multiple synchronous and metachronous cancers are located in the colon proximal to the splenic flexure. Tumors may develop from polyps that often are multiple and flat, with more advanced pathology. The time to progression to cancer appears to be more rapid than the usual adenoma-to-carcinoma sequence (Winawer et al., 1997). HNPCC tumors tend to be mucinous and poorly differentiated but not always associated with a worse prognosis (Kroser et al., 1997). Two types of Lynch syndrome exist, based on the presence or absence of extracolonic cancers. Lynch I is not associated with a family history of other cancers. Lynch II is associated with the CRC tendency and an increased familial occurrence of extracolonic cancers. The most common extracolonic cancers are endometrial (20%–60% with HNPCC compared with 3% of general population) (Terdiman et al., 1999) but also can include ovarian, gastric, small bowel, hepatobiliary tract, and, rarely, pancreatic (Lynch et al., 1999). The presence of HNPCC traditionally has been based on the Amsterdam Criteria (see Figure 12-3), which are based on family history of CRC and the patient's age when diagnosed with cancer. These criteria include three or more relatives with CRC, one relative diagnosed at younger than age 50, one relative is a first-degree relative to the other two individuals, and the CRC involves at least two generations (Vasen, Mecklin, Kahn, & Lynch, 1991). A revised Amsterdam Criteria

Figure 12-3. Amsterdam Criteria for Hereditary Nonpolyposis Colorectal Cancer

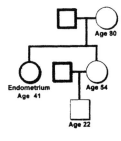

- **Three or more CRC**
- **Two or more generations**
- **One case a 1⁰ relative of the other two**
- **One affected age by 50**
- **FAP excluded**

Note. From *Clinical Teaching Project: Colorectal Neoplasia* (p. 25), by P.M. Lynch, M.I. Burrell, P.H. Green, and S. Vera, 1996, Timonium, MD: Milner-Fenwick, Inc. Copyright 1996 by Milner-Fenwick, Inc. Reprinted with permission.

was developed in 1999 by the International Collaborative Group on HNPCC. These criteria include the classical Amsterdam Criteria, but also acknowledge the presence of extracolonic cancers as part of the family history (see Figure 12-4) (Vasen, Watson, Mecklin, Lynch, & the ICG-HNPCC, 1999). Risk for CRC increases by age 21 and becomes very high by age 40. Five HNPCC genes are hMSH2, hMSH6, hMLH1, hPMS1, and hPMS2 (Boland, 1999). Together, these genes are believed to account for approximately 50%–70% of all families with HNPCC (Lynch et al., 1999). HNPCC is caused by mutations in any one of the four DNA mismatch repair genes (Winawer et al., 1997). These genes usually repair errors occurring in normal cell division. If the mismatch repair genes

---

Figure 12-4. Amsterdam Criteria II

Patient must meet ALL of the following:
• Three or more relatives with a histologically verified hereditary nonpolyposis colorectal cancer-associated cancer (colorectal cancer, small bowel cancer, endometrial cancer, ureter or renal pelvis cancer)
• One should be a first-degree relative of the other two.
• Colorectal cancer should involve at least two generations.
• One of the cases should be diagnosed before age 50.
• Familial adenomatous polyposis should be excluded in the colorectal cancer cases.

Note. Based on information from Vasen et al., 1999.

become mutated, the repair function becomes altered and instead can accelerate the buildup of genetic mutations, resulting in an accelerated adenoma-to-carcinoma progression. Patients with HNPCC express microsatellite instability (Rodriguez-Bigas et al., 1997), which, in the tumor, is a phenotypic expression of the underlying defect causing the errors in DNA replication. Currently, colorectal tumors are not tested routinely for this, although select tumors should undergo this analysis (Rodriguez-Bigas et al.).

Genetic testing should be offered to people within families of suspicion to determine the gene carriers. Genetic tests are positive in 80% of families tested, indicating the gene carriers (Winawer et al., 1997). The current recommendation for people with a family history of CRC in multiple close relatives and across generations, especially if the CRC occurs early, includes genetic counseling/early colonoscopic surveillance and testing for HNPCC. Total abdominal colectomy with ileorectal anastomosis is a consideration for patients with HNPCC because of the high incidence of metachronous cancers in patients who have undergone segmental colectomy (Ivanovich et al., 1999). Patients with multiple polyps on colonoscopy or known gene carriers could be considered for prophylactic colectomy, although the benefit of this is not known (Rodriguez-Bigas et al., 1997).

Others

Various mutations of the APC gene can occur, putting families at increased risk for colorectal adenomas and later onset of CRC. These families can be identified by analysis of the APC gene. A recent permutation in the APC gene was discovered affecting 6% of Ashkenazi Jews and has been found in 28% of the Ashkenazim who had colon cancer or a polyp and one first- or second-degree relative with CRC (Boland, 1999). This allele is rare in non-Ashkenazim groups; but the risk of cancer among people with the allele is increased but still less than with classic FAP (Laken et al., 1997).

Inflammatory Bowel Disease

The medical conditions of ulcerative colitis and Crohn's disease place people at increased risk for development of CRC, although this occurs in only 1% of all CRC cases (Winawer et al., 1997). Several factors influence the risk, including extent of disease, duration of disease, and age of onset. Ulcerative colitis tends to be more commonly associated with cancer development compared with Crohn's disease. Cancer is more likely to occur in patients with pancolitis compared with those having only left-sided disease. Dysplasia is the best marker for identifying early cancer in this group (Boland, 1999).

Signs and Symptoms

As mentioned previously, CRCs tend to grow slowly. As a tumor grows, it can give rise to several different symptoms. Symptoms depend on where the tumor is located within the colon (see Figure 12-5), but, generally, patients present with change in bowel habits, bleeding (occult or obvious), obstruction, perforation, abdominal pain, and weight loss.

Figure 12-5. Clinical Manifestations of Colorectal Cancers According to Primary Site

Right-Sided Lesions
- Dull abdominal pain
- Palpable mass in right lower quadrant
- Melena
- Anemia, malaise, indigestion, and weight loss

Left-Sided Lesions
- Change in bowel habits
- Cramps and flatulence
- Lower stool caliber
- Bright red blood in stool
- Incomplete stool evacuation

Rectal Lesions
- Bleeding
- Tenesmus

Note. From "Profiling Colorectal Cancer: Nature and Scope of the Disease," by C. Engelking, 1997, *Developments in Supportive Cancer Care, 1*(2), 38. Copyright 1997 by Meniscus Educational Institute. Reprinted with permission.

Although change in bowel habits often is considered a sign/symptom of CRC, in a retrospective case-control study, no significant differences were found in the historical frequency of bowel movements, constipation presence, or laxative use (Nakamura, Schneiderman, & Klauber, 1984).

The second symptom of bleeding is associated with tumor growth within the bowel lumen. Bleeding occurs from the trauma of the feces passing through the lumen and can occur at any location in the colon. Data from a variety of studies indicate that cancers located on the right side of the colon bleed more than those on the left (Mandel, 1996). The mean levels of blood loss were higher in patients with more advanced tumors (Offerhaus et al., 1992). Blood usually is mixed within the stool, making it difficult to identify. However, as bleeding occurs more distally, the patient often can detect it. Bleeding from tumors in the proximal colon tends to occur for longer periods of time, as the diameter of that area allows for the tumor to grow longer without obstructive symptoms. A sign of the bleeding may be iron deficiency anemia. Hematochezia or positive FOBTs may occur with tumors located in the sigmoid colon or rectum (Boland, 1999). Intermittent bleeding also can occur from large polyps.

Obstruction from the colonic lumen can produce symptoms such as abdominal distention, pain, nausea, and vomiting. Obstruction is unlikely to occur in the cecum or ascending colon because of the larger diameter and is more common in the smaller lumen of the transverse, descending, and sigmoid colon. Obstruction suggests a large tumor and poorer prognosis.

Pain occurs when tumors have penetrated the muscularis propria and invaded adjacent tissues.

Other symptoms may present that relate to the specific organ being invaded. Local invasion into the rectum can result in tenesmus.

Weight loss occurs when the tumor has metastasized. This results in loss of subcutaneous fat, appetite, weight, and strength (Boland, 1999).

Early colorectal tumors tend to produce no symptoms. People presenting with more than three of these symptoms likely have advanced disease. No correlation exists between duration of symptoms and severity of disease (Hoebler, 1997).

Overview of Screening/Early Detection

Screening currently is recommended for CRC prevention in average-, moderate-, and high-risk populations. A variety of options are available for screening for the average-risk group, with more specific guidelines for the moderate- and high-risk groups. An overview of the current tests being used will be provided, with more specific guidelines and intervals being discussed that are related to the degree of risk involved. Table 12-3 compares the sensitivity, specificity, and cost of some of the tests.

Table 12-3. Cost, Sensitivity, and Specificity of Colorectal Cancer Screening Tests

Test	Cost Per Test	Sensitivity	Specificity
Fecal occult blood testing	$10–$20	26%–92%	90%–98%
Flexibile sigmoidoscopy	$150–$500	90%	98%
Double-contrast barium enema	$300–$500	50%–80%	98%
Colonoscopy	$1,000–$1,500	75%–95%	100%

Note. From "Colorectal Cancer Screening: Making Sense of the Different Guidelines," by C.A. Burke and R. Van Stolk, 1999, Cleveland Clinic Journal of Medicine, 66, p. 307. Copyright 1999 by the Cleveland Clinic Foundation. Reprinted with permission.

Fecal Occult Blood Testing

FOBT still is the only method of screening for large populations. The procedure is inexpensive and simple and has proven to be cost effective in large studies.

If FOBT is performed every other year, mortality may be reduced; but a greater mortality reduction is noted when the procedure is performed annually (Winawer et al., 1997). The rationale of FOBT is to identify occult bleeding that may occur from larger polyps and early cancers that have not produced symptoms. Bleeding that occurs is intermittent and not evenly distributed within the stool (Mandel, 1996). Blood loss from polyps usually is less than that of cancers but is greater in larger polyps than smaller ones (Mandel et al, 1993.). The test is not designed specifically for colonic bleeding or cancer, as other areas within the GI tract can bleed and change the result of the test. The test also is not specific for blood because other substances can contain peroxidase or exhibit peroxidase activity. Red meat and certain fruits and vegetables can cause false-positive tests.

Three large randomized controlled trials have demonstrated small (15%–33%) but statistically significant reductions in CRC-associated mortality in patients older than age 45 who are undergoing annual or biannual screening with FOBT (Hardcastle et al., 1996; Kronborg, Fenger, Olsen, Jorgensen, & Sondergaard, 1996; Mandel et al., 1993). Mandel et al. (2000) followed 46,551 participants in the Minnesota Colon Cancer Control Study for 18 years who were randomly assigned to annual and biennial FOBT or usual care (control group). During the 18-year period, 417 new CRCs were identified in the annual screening group, 435 in the biennial group, and 507 in the control group. For both screening groups, the number of positive slides was associated with the positive predictive value for both adenomatous polyps of 1 cm in diameter and for CRC. This study concluded that either annual or biennial FOBT significantly reduces the incidence of CRC and may improve the cost-effectiveness of CRC screening. Unfortunately, the sensitivity of FOBT ranges from 26%–92%, making it difficult to convince physicians to promote the test to patients (Burke & van Stolk, 1999), although the newer findings from Mandel et al. (2000) do not support this. FOBT still has many criticisms in the low predictive value of a positive test for CRC. When occult blood is found in the stool, a source can be found in only 40%–50% of patients (Bedine, 1999). The significant high rates of false-positive and false-negative results that can occur with this test make people skeptical to accept its use. Many colonoscopies are performed after a positive FOBT is obtained, but they do not identify a cancer.

Patients can perform this test at home by using slides that are guaiac-based and test for peroxidase activity. Patients collect stool specimens by smearing two specimens per slide with three consecutive stool samples. For two or three days prior and throughout the collection process, patients are instructed to avoid certain medications and foods that could interfere with the sensitivity of this test (see Figure 12-6). The impact of not following specific diet and medication guidelines is not known, although with the test's low sensitivity, the directions should be adhered to closely. Alterations in the recommended process can cause false-positive tests with consumption of red meat or certain fruits and vegetables during the collection period. False-negatives can result from intake of vitamin C during the stool collection period or because the cancer or polyp did not bleed during the collection period or did not bleed enough to be detected (Winawer et al., 1997).

Figure 12-6. Recommendations for Fecal Occult Blood Testing: What to Tell Patients

In the 48–72 hours before and during testing, avoid
• Food and medications that can produce false-positive results
  – Red meat (beef, lamb), liver
  – Uncooked turnips, horseradish, broccoli, radishes
  – Aspirin in doses > 325 mg/day
• Food and medications that can produce false-negative results
  – Cantaloupe and other melons (watermelon is permitted)
  – Vitamin C supplements
Take two smears from two sites of three bowel movements (six windows).
Develop within seven days without rehydration.

Note. From "Colorectal Cancer Screening: Making Sense of the Different Guidelines," by C.A. Burke and R. Van Stolk, 1999, *Cleveland Clinic Journal of Medicine, 66,* p. 308. Copyright 1999 by the Cleveland Clinic Foundation. Adapted with permission.

Once the sampling is completed, the slides are sent to the office setting where they are developed with a hydrogen peroxide solution. A positive test results in a blue color when the developing reagent is added to the card. One positive test of one slide window is significant and requires colonoscopic evaluation. Repeating the fecal occult collection process is not necessary, and further colonic evaluation is indicated (Burke & van Stolk, 1999). Rehydration of the slides with a few drops of water before adding the developing reagent can increase the test's sensitivity, although this can decrease the specificity (Winawer et al., 1997).

Patient compliance with FOBT is variable. Obtaining stool samples is unpleasant for most, and following the dietary/medication restrictions may not always occur. Compliance tends to be higher if physicians take the time to explain the test and associated restrictions. Two studies have shown that FOBT is very underused. One study showed that only 17.3% of people age 50 and older had undergone FOBT in the previous year, and another study showed that fewer than 35% of patients had received FOBT (Anderson & May, 1995; Centers for Disease Control and Prevention, 2001). Compliance in the randomized trials ranged from 53%–75% (Mandel et al., 1993). Interventions and reminders were shown in studies to impact compliance for both patients and clinicians (Myers et al., 1991; Struewing, Pape, & Snow, 1991).

Advantages of FOBT include its ease, cost, privacy in performing, and availability in a variety of office settings. Disadvantages include its low sensitivity, the unpleasantness of stool collection by patients, and the restrictions involved during the collection process. The diagnostic examinations that could result from a positive FOBT are associated with risk, depending on the particular procedures. False-positive tests lead to anxiety for patients and false-negative tests can provide a false reassurance.

Strong direct evidence that screening reduces mortality is evident with FOBT. Most research studies used Hemoccult II® tests (SmithKline Diagnostics, Inc., Research Triangle Park, NC). Definite limitations are related to the sensitivity and false-positive results requiring additional anxiety-provoking examinations, in addition to the related costs of the further evaluations (Winawer et al., 1997).

Newer Methods of Stool Testing

Other types of FOBTs are available in addition to the guaiac-based Hemoccult II. Immunochemical tests (ELISA) can detect only hemoglobin and globin and are the most selective (Mandel, 1996). HemeSelect (Beckman Colter, Palo Alto, CA) is a hemagglutination test that is sensitive to the presence of hemoglobin. In nonrandomized trials, it was found to have a 97% sensitivity for CRC and a 76% sensitivity for adenomas larger than 1 cm. One strong advantage is that no dietary modification is necessary (Young, Macrae, & St. John, 1996). ColoCARE (Helena Laboratories, Beaumont, TX) provides a more patient-friendly way of testing stool for occult blood. Specially prepared biodegradable pads containing chemicals are sensitive to the presence of blood on the surface of stool. The pads are used to wipe after having three separate bowel movements and individually are released into the toilet bowl where they float. Within 30 seconds, if the test is positive, an area on the pad will turn blue or green. Once the testing is complete, the pad can be flushed, eliminating the direct contact with stool as compared with the Hemoccult II. Sensitivity and specificity information currently is not available for this test (Helena Laboratories, personal communication, August 2000).

Flexible Sigmoidoscopy

Flexible sigmoidoscopy is the screening procedure of choice for average-risk people. The advantage over FOBT is that it allows direct visualization of the left portion of the bowel, and lesions and polyps can be biopsied, resulting in a high sensitivity and specificity for abnormal growths in the sigmoid colon. The limitation of the examination is that 40%–60% of polyps and cancers are beyond the left side of the colon (Burke & van Stolk, 1999). The advantage is that the remaining 50% of polyps and carcinomas can be detected within the reach of the flexible sigmoidoscope (Bedine, 1999).

Several case-control studies suggest that CRC screening with flexible sigmoidoscopy may have as much as a 70% reduction in CRC-associated mortality (Newcomb, Norfleet, Storer, Surawicz, & Marcus, 1992; Selby, Friedman, Quesenberry, & Weiss, 1992).

The 60 cm fiberoptic instrument is the most common sigmoidoscope used, replacing the rigid 25 cm and flexible 35 cm scopes. The 60 cm scope should detect 40%–60% of adenomatous polyps and CRCs (Hixson, Fennarty, Sampliner, McGee, & Garewal, 1990; Selby & Friedman, 1989). The sigmoidoscope is inserted into the rectum and passed into the sigmoid and descending colon. Preparation for the examination may vary, but is usually completed one to two hours prior to the test to cleanse the distal colon. The patient lies in the left lateral position and rarely requires sedation. Lesions identified can be biopsied to determine the need for colonoscopy. The most common complication associated with flexible sigmoidoscopy is perforation of the colon. Perforation rates of 1–2/10,000 were found in large studies of sigmoidoscopies (Nelson, Abcarian, & Prasad, 1982; Winnan et al., 1980). The endoscope has the ability to transmit infection, although no infections were reported in recent large prospective series (Winawer et al., 1997). Polypectomy should not be performed in an inadequately cleansed bowel. Explosions can occur from the contact of hydrogen methane with electrocautery. Carbon dioxide is connected to the scope and introduced into the bowel before electrocautery to prevent this. If a tubular adenoma or carcinoma is found in the distal colon, the entire colon should be examined for synchronous lesions. If polyps found are small and hyperplastic, it remains controversial whether the full colon needs to be examined. A positive sigmoidoscopy is defined by the presence of any polyp larger than 1 cm in diameter or presence of a cancer (Winawer et al., 1997). Some clinicians feel the discovery of any size adenoma is cause for examination of the entire colon with colonoscopy.

Flexible sigmoidoscopy requires extensive training, but nonphysicians are performing the procedure more commonly, and it has been found to be appropriate and safe (DiSario & Sanowski, 1993; Maule, 1994; Schoenfeld et al., 1999). A large ongoing trial by the National Cancer Institute (NCI) (Prostate, Lung, Colon, and Ovary Trial) that began in 1992 is using flexible sigmoidoscopy. Study results are expected by 2008 and should provide mortality outcomes (NCI, 2000).

The advantages of flexible sigmoidoscopy is its accuracy in detecting abnormalities of the left side of the colon, need for minimal prep, and no need for conscious sedation. The disadvantages include the limited area viewed, possibly missing polyps located on the right side of the colon, and patient embarrassment and discomfort during the exam without conscious sedation.

Combination Fecal Occult Blood Testing and Flexible Sigmoidoscopy

Limited data are available addressing the combination of annual FOBT and flexible sigmoidoscopy every five years and whether the two could offer greater reductions in CRC mortality if combined. One randomized controlled trial found that two-thirds of the cancers missed by FOBT were found in the rectosigmoid area (Hardcastle et al., 1989). Sigmoidoscopy is more accurate than FOBT in detecting adenomatous polyps. When considering the benefits of each separately, it would seem a reasonable option to combine the two, although more studies are needed (Scotiniotis, Lewis, & Strom, 1999).

Colonoscopy

Colonoscopy is considered the gold standard for diagnosis of polyps and CRC. The examination has become more accepted by the public and is the most accurate and complete screening of the colon and rectum. The test usually is performed after other screening examinations, with abnormal findings, in people who are symptomatic or in high-risk groups for screening. Currently, screening colonoscopy is not covered by insurance companies in the average-risk group but is available for those with a higher risk. Although, as of July, 2000, average-risk Medicare beneficiaries were allowed a screening colonoscopy once every 10 years or at least 119 months after the previous screening colonoscopy (Health Care Financing Administration, 2001). No published studies are available that directly examine the effectiveness of colonoscopy as a screening test related to its impact on CRC mortality (Winawer et al., 1997). Indirect evidence exists showing that identifying and removing polyps reduces the incidence of CRC; detecting early CRC decreases mortality; and colonoscopy has the ability to identify both types of lesions (Winawer et al., 1996). The procedure is performed in a similar way as the flexible sigmoidoscopy but uses a longer scope to view the descending colon, transverse colon, and ascending colon to the terminal ileum. The entire colon can be viewed in 95% of patients, with the depth of penetration being dependent on the experience and skill of the endoscopist and the adequacy of the preparation (Bedine, 1999; Winawer et al., 1997). Studies suggested that colonoscopy failed to identify 25% of polyps smaller than 5 mm in size and 10% of polyps larger than 1 cm (Waye, Lewis, Frankel, & Geller, 1988). Preparation is more intense than for flexible sigmoidoscopy, requiring cleansing of the entire bowel. The most common preparation is a clear liquid diet 24 hours preceding the procedure and four liters of an isotonic nonabsorbable electrolyte solution (GoLytely® [Braintree Labs, Braintree, MA]) that patients drink the evening before during a three-to four-hour period. One gallon of fluid is unpleasant to consume but prevents the patient from becoming dehydrated with the vigorous cathartic activity that results. Two more recent preparations have been developed that may make this process easier and more palatable for patients. Oral Fleet® Phospho-soda® is a much smaller volume preparation for patients to drink. A tablet preparation new on the market called Visicol™ (InKine Pharmaceutical Co., Inc., Blue Bell, PA) has been shown to be an adequate cleansing technique for colonoscopy. The patient takes a total of 40 tablets the evening and morning before the procedure with large volumes of oral fluid intake. Improvements in the preparations given may improve compliance with this type of exam.

Colonoscopy is an outpatient procedure with IV conscious sedation to keep the patient as comfortable as possible yet able to turn from side to side, if necessary. Gastroenterologists typically perform the procedures, although some surgeons are trained in this examination. Biopsies of abnormal tissue and polyps can be obtained during the examination. Polypectomy can be performed with snare technique and electrocautery to the base of the polyp to prevent bleeding. Some polyps may need to be piecemealed to remove; surgical resection is required if the base of the polyp is too large or is located in the right colon where the colon wall is thinner. All biopsies are sent to pathology for review. Histology determines the intensity and timing of follow-up procedures (Bedine, 1999).

Complications of this procedure are not common but can include bleeding, perforation, and medication reactions. The most serious complication is perforation, occurring in 0.2% of all colonoscopies (Burke & van Stolk, 1999). Complication rates may be higher when polypectomy is performed. Older patients are not at greater risk for complications but may experience cardiac arrhythmias or respiratory depression (Winawer et al., 1997).

Advantages of colonoscopy include a view of the entire colon and the ability to remove suspicious lesions during the same examination. The conscious sedation may be viewed as an advantage for the patient by lessening the fear, embarrassment, and discomfort of the examination. The recommended interval frequency for screening is longer, from one to several years, making it easier for patients to comply. Disadvantages include the cost, potential complications, extensive preparation involved, and lack of data supporting that the benefit of this type of examination is greater than the associated risk.

Barium Enema

Barium enema radiography also has the advantage of viewing the entire colon. It can be performed with barium alone (single contrast) or with air instilled after some of the barium has been eliminated (double contrast). The latter is the better imaging method for CRC screening because the retained barium will outline abnormal lesions. A randomized study comparing double-contrast barium enema (DCBE) with flexible sigmoidoscopy to colonoscopy for symptomatic patients found that colonoscopy was more sensitive in detecting small (< 0.9 cm) polyps, but no difference was found in detecting the larger (> 0.9 cm) polyps or cancers (Rex, Lehman, Hawes, Ulbright, & Smith, 1991). A study by Rex et al. (1997) on detecting CRC compared the sensitivity of barium enema with colonoscopic examination. Results showed a sensitivity of 83% for barium enema versus 95% for colonoscopy. The insensitivity of barium enemas is related to unsatisfactory visualization of certain areas of the bowel and to interpretation errors. False-positive findings can result from stool adhering to the lining and mucosal irregularities, such as diverticular disease, that are noncancerous. Although the barium enema examines the entire intestine, its sensitivity is less than that of colonoscopy and does not allow for removal of identified polyps, requiring patients to undergo a colonoscopy if abnormalities are identified. Bowel perforation is the most common complication of DCBE but is extremely rare (Winawer et al., 1997). Any abnormalities identified with barium enema need further evaluation with colonoscopy and possible polypectomy.

Barium enema preparation begins 24 hours prior to the examination and includes diet restrictions followed by laxatives and enemas. The examination is an outpatient procedure and takes 20–30 minutes. Sedation usually is not given, although an IV antispasmodic drug can be given. A soft tube 2 cm in diameter is inserted into the rectum, and liquid barium is instilled. The patient makes position changes, facilitating the movement of barium through the bowel that is monitored by fluoroscopy. Air is instilled to provide the double contrast and aids the progression of the barium before radiographs are taken. Patients may experience some discomfort with the air instillation, especially if the procedure is performed too quickly. At completion of the examination, the patient can go home. A laxative is given to ensure that the barium is passed from the rectum, which can take one to two days (Winawer et al., 1997).

Combining DCBE with flexible sigmoidoscopy is a consideration to improve the disadvantages of both tests. In a large, ongoing Swedish study, the combination of flexible sigmoidoscopy and DCBE had a sensitivity of 98% for cancer and 99% for adenomatous polyps (Kewenter, Brevinge, Engaras, & Haglind, 1995).

Advantages to barium enema are the ability to view the entire colon with some limitations; cost, which is reasonable and covered by insurance; absence of complications associated with sedation, particularly in the elderly; and minimal risk of other complications. Disadvantages include discomfort and embarrassment associated with the examination, limited view of the rectal-sigmoid area, and limited sensitivity.

Digital Rectal Exam

Digital rectal examination has been used along with other tests, but alone it has not been shown to be an effective screening tool for CRC. Fewer than 10% of adenomas and cancers are estimated to develop within the area of the examiner's finger (Eddy, 1990). Digital rectal examination generally is included in routine gynecologic and prostate screening examinations and physicals.

Current Guidelines for Screening

In the past several years, three groups have published guidelines for screening: ACS (Byers et al., 1997), the U.S. Preventive Services Task Force (1995), and a consortium of experts from national organizations (Winawer et al., 1997). The guidelines differentiate between average-, moderate/intermediate-, and high-risk people based on their personal, family, medical, and genetic history (see Figure 12-7).

Average-Risk People

For average-risk people, screening is recommended beginning at age 50. Four options are available: FOBT, flexible sigmoidoscopy, DCBE examination, and colonoscopy. FOBT is recommended annually using three different stool samples taken from two different sites and adhering to the collection restrictions related to medications and food (see Figure 12-7). Flexible sigmoidoscopy is recommended every five years; DCBE is recommended every 5–10 years; and colonoscopy is recommended every 10 years. In 1998, Medicare began to cover the service of CRC screening with barium enema or flexible sigmoidoscopy for people older than 50. Although this decision does not guarantee other insurance carrier coverage, this service likely will be extended to all insurance holders in the near future. For average-risk people, Medicare coverage includes flexible sigmoidoscopy every four years, FOBT annually, and DCBE as an alternative procedure if a physician indicates this as the most appropriate measure (Bedine, 1999). In July 2001, Medicare began to allow screening colonoscopy for average-risk people once every 10 years (Health Care Financing Administration, 2001) and this service will likely be extended to all insured in the near future.

Moderate/Intermediate-Risk People

Guidelines for people with a family history of CRC or polyps or a personal history of polyps or cancer differ from those at average risk and will be discussed individually.

Family History of Colorectal Cancer or Adenomatous Polyps

Anyone having a sibling or child with a history of CRC should be offered the same options for screening as an average-risk person but should begin 10 years earlier (age 40). If a relative was diagnosed with CRC before age 60, had an adenomatous polyp before age 60, or if two or more first-degree relatives had CRC, a total colonic examination with DCBE or colonoscopy is recommended every five years beginning at age 40 or 10 years prior to the youngest case in the family, whichever age is younger (Burke & van Stolk, 1999).

Figure 12-7. Colorectal Screening Guidelines

Average Risk

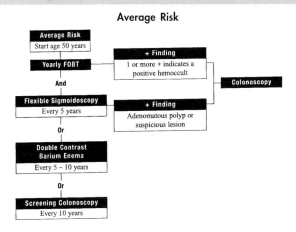

Moderate/Intermediate Risk

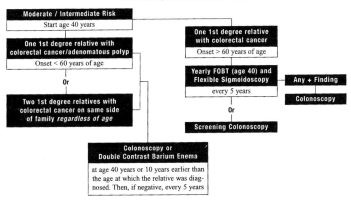

High Risk

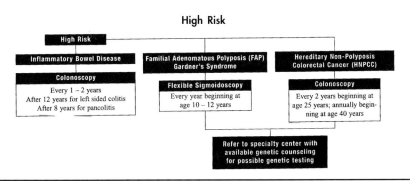

Personal History of Adenomatous Polyps

People with a history of multiple polyps or with large polyps (> 1 cm) should have them removed at colonoscopy. The colon should be examined in three years, with colonoscopy after the initial exam (Winawer et al., 1997). The interval can change for subsequent examinations, depending on the findings. A five-year interval is appropriate if subsequent examinations are negative (Burke & van Stolk, 1999; Winawer et al., 1997). Colonoscopy continues to be the preferred surveillance examination after polypectomy. A recent study by Winawer et al. (2000) compared colonoscopy with barium enema for surveillance in patients with a history of adenomatous polyps to determine whether both methods are needed for surveillance or whether DCBE could replace colonoscopy. The study confirmed that colonoscopy is the more effective method of surveillance and allows for both detection and removal of polyps during the same examination. DCBE should be reserved for those cases in which the cecum cannot be reached during colonoscopy.

Personal History of Colorectal Cancer

People with a history of CRC who have undergone a colon resection but did not undergo complete colonoscopic examination preoperatively should have a complete colon examination within one year of the surgical resection. If the preoperative examination is adequate, the next examination should be at three years after surgery and every five years thereafter (Burke & van Stolk, 1999; Winawer et al., 1997).

Family History of Familial Adenomatous Polyposis

The risk of CRC is highest in people with autosomal-dominant genetic syndromes. People with a history of FAP should receive genetic counseling with risk assessment, review of surveillance guidelines, and, if appropriate, genetic testing to determine if they are a gene carrier. A negative genetic test eliminates the possibility of FAP only if an affected family member was found to have a mutation (Winawer et al., 1997). Those with a positive test who are carriers or those with indeterminate test results should begin colorectal screening with annual flexible sigmoidoscopy at age 10–12 to determine if they are expressing the gene. If polyposis is found, prophylactic colectomy would be necessary (Winawer et al., 1997). In addition, upper endoscopy with duodenoscopy should begin once colonic adenomas appear and should be repeated at least every three years; this may need to be performed annually once lesions are found in the duodenum (Burt & Petersen, 1996). Endoscopic surveillance after ileorectal anastomosis should occur every four to six months and annually after an ileoanal anastomosis (Terdiman et al., 1999). Medicare coverage provides for a colonoscopy every two years for people in the high risk catagory (Winawer et al., 1997).

Family History of Hereditary Nonpolyposis Colorectal Cancer

For people with a family history involving multiple close relatives with CRC at an early age, genetic counseling and possible testing should be considered to determine the presence of HNPCC. Examination of the colon every one to two years should start between age 20–30 and annually beginning at age 40 (Winawer et al., 1997). Total colectomy should be performed at diagnosis of cancer, and prophylactic colectomy should be considered in known gene carriers. Annual transvaginal ultrasound or endometrial aspiration should begin at age 25–35 because of the known extracolonic spread to this area (Terdiman et al., 1999). Prophylactic hysterectomy or bilateral salpingo-oophorectomy could be considered an option for women who have been diagnosed with CRC or have been found to be a carrier through genetic testing (Burt & Petersen, 1996). Medicare coverage provides high-risk persons with a colonoscopy every two years (Winawer et al., 1997).

Personal History of Inflammatory Bowel Disease

People with a long-standing history of inflammatory bowel disease should have colonic evaluation for dysplasia as a marker for CRC risk (Burke & van Stolk, 1999; Winawer et al., 1997). People with pancolitis and left-sided disease are at greatest risk. For those with pancolitis, colonoscopic surveillance is recommended every one to two years, with biopsy beginning eight years after the onset of disease (Burke & van Stolk; Winawer et al., 1997). For those with left-sided involvement, surveillance should begin 15 years after the onset of disease. For those with dysplasia, colectomy may be encouraged. No evidence shows that this surveillance will reduce mortality in these patients. The more effective practice is colectomy, if the duration and extent of disease justifies this approach (Winawer et al., 1997).

When to Stop Screening

Screening for CRC and adenomatous polyps should continue throughout a person's life as long as an intended benefit from it exists. The decision of when to stop screening should be made by the patient and his or her physician (Burke & van Stolk, 1999).

Genetic Testing

Testing for genetic syndromes such as FAP and HNPCC is commercially available. The tests usually are performed with a blood sample, and white blood cells are extracted for analysis. Various methods are used to identify the genetic mutations. Direct gene sequencing is the most precise method but is very expensive and time-consuming. Other techniques are available, such as single-strand conformational polymorphism, denaturing gradient gel electrophoresis, and the protein truncation test (PTT). PTT is the most common test used for FAP, with a sensitivity of nearly 80% (Terdiman et al., 1999). HNPCC testing, available commercially, analyzes the mismatch repair of genes hMSH2 and hMLHI, which is where the majority of mutations occur. By limiting testing to only two mismatch repair genes, the sensitivity of HNPCC testing is restricted. Assays now are available commercially to assess microsatellite instability in tumor tissue. Because more than 90% of HNPCC-related cancers demonstrate microsatellite instability (MSI), this may be used first, followed by genetic testing in individuals with MSI-positive tumors (Rodriguez-Bigas et al., 1997). The Bethesda Guidelines were established to identify specific types of individuals who should be tested for MSI and still are being investigated (Rodriguez-Bigas et al.).

Positive and negative consequences of genetic testing need to be considered. Positive benefits occur when people can reduce the uncertainty of whether they are at risk for cancer by finding out whether a genetic mutation is present. An increased knowledge of the risk of developing cancer can aid in identifying and selecting appropriate screening. For those who test negative for a known genetic mutation, fears and anxieties may be decreased. People may have a feeling of optimism with their health and future. Detection of a mutation among one of the affected family members allows genetic testing to occur for other relatives. Those free of the mutation can be spared unnecessary extensive surveillance, and those with the mutation need counseling on the indicated surveillance.

Negative outcomes can occur because of the shortcomings of the current genetic tests. Failure to detect a mutation in an individual does not eliminate the possibility of a genetic cancer, as a mutation still may be present that the current test could not detect, or genetic variants may be identified that have an uncertain significance and outcome (Terdiman et al., 1999). Positive test results cannot predict when or if an HNPCC carrier will develop cancer. Confidentiality related to testing and costs of testing are other issues. Sequencing for hMLHI and hMSH2 can be expensive, insurers may not cover this expense, or patients may not submit the claim in fear of discrimination (Terdiman et al.). Currently, some protections are in place to prevent genetic discrimination against gene carriers. The Federal Health Insurance Portability and Accountability Act of 1996 protects gene carriers from being denied health insurance plans from employers or insurers. Several states also have passed laws to protect individuals against insurance and genetic discrimination. Updated information regarding public policy and genetic testing is available through the National Human Genome Research Institute. The screening recommendations that currently are used have not been validated for HNPCC (Terdiman et al.).

New Trends in Screening

Although several options are available for CRC screening, they are not completely acceptable to patients because of preparation difficulties, discomfort experienced during the examination, limitations with performance and safety issues, and costs. Healthcare professionals also have different opinions on the techniques available that can lead to infrequent and inconsistent prescribing by caregivers. Improved screening options are needed for patients to reduce some of these inconveniences.

Immunochemical Assays

CRCs express many nuclear antigens that can be analyzed immunohistochemically. Several antigens have been found on fecal colonocytes or in soluble feces. More research is needed in this area to develop assays, but research could result in a simple test requiring little processing time (Ahlquist & Johnson, 1999).

Exfoliated Markers/Fecal DNA

Identification of DNA mutations in stool samples has been studied. Early studies have identified K-ras, p53, and APC genes in stool of patients with CRC. In a preliminary study, identical ras mutations were identified in the stool of a patient with cancer and a patient with an adenoma (Jen, Johnson, & Levin, 1998). The challenge with this method is identifying a marker that is identical with all neoplasms and that can tolerate the environment of the colon (Ahlquist & Johnson, 1999). Alquist et al. (2000) explored the feasibility of a stool assay panel of selected DNA alterations in a blinded fashion with patients diagnosed with CRC, patients with large adenomas ($\geq$ 1 cm), and patients with normal colonoscopic exams. Analyzable DNA was obtained from all stools. Sensitivity was 91% for cancer and 82% for the adenoma group. The panel targeted point-mutations at any of the 15 mutational spots on the K-ras, APC, and p53 genes, Bat-26, and L-DNA. There were no false-positive results. This is a promising stool-screening test found to have high sensitivity and specificity for both adenomas and cancers. Larger clinical studies are needed to further evaluate this approach.

Less-Invasive Imaging

Introduced in 1994, computed tomography colonography (CTC), or virtual colonoscopy, is a technique that is minimally invasive and can be performed quickly. This exam eliminates the need to see the inside of the colon with the usual fiber-optic instruments. A bowel preparation similar to that needed for colonoscopy is required, although conscious sedation is not necessary. The entire colon can be examined with CTC within one to two minutes. The data are processed by computer software into a two- and three-dimensional view after insufflation of the colon with air or carbon dioxide. Experienced radiologists review the images when the process is complete. This technique can detect polyps and cancer, as most of these lesions protrude from the mucosa. In one study comparing CTC to colonoscopy, CTC identified 100% of polyps $\geq$ 1 cm, with a specificity of 100%; 100% of polyps $\geq$ 0.5 cm, with a specificity of 85%; and 42% of polyps , 0.5 cm (Hara et al., 1997). A more current study by Rex, Vining, and Kopecky (1999) found CTC to be inadequate as a screening test when compared with colonoscopy in identifying patients with adenomas, particularly flat adenomas. CTC needs more study within screening populations and currently is being studied in comparative trials for patients undergoing colonoscopy for symptoms or a history of polyps. Technical and diagnostic issues need to be resolved before this can become a widely used screening tool. Costs of this type of screening will need to be investigated as well. This could be an appealing screening test for patients because, unlike other tests, little discomfort is felt with the examination, and the procedure is viewed as noninvasive. In addition, there have been no reported perforations, conscious sedation is not required, and the viewing of the entire colon can take less than one minute, compared to the colonoscopy that averages 30 minutes (Dykes, 2001).

Chemoprevention Strategies

Several agents have been explored as chemopreventive agents in CRC and adenomatous polyp formation. These agents may target a particular stage in the carcinogenesis process or may interfere with multiple stages. Drugs that are being studied include nonsteroidal anti-inflammatory drugs (NSAIDs), antioxidants, folate, and calcium.

Nonsteroidal Anti-Inflammatory Agents

For over a decade, ingestion of aspirin or NSAIDs has been implicated in reducing the risk of CRC. Recent studies show that a 40%–50% reduction occurs in mortality from CRC for people using aspirin or NSAIDs on a regular basis (DuBois, 1999). Studies in humans and animal models have shown that tumors produce prostaglandins in large amounts. NSAIDs' mechanism of chemoprevention action occurs by inhibiting the formation of prostaglandin precursors. NSAIDs interrupt prostaglandin synthesis by inhibiting cyclooxygenase (COX) activity. Some examples of NSAIDs are sulindac, piroxicam, celecoxib, and aspirin. Sulindac, an NSAID related to indomethacin, has been studied in patients with FAP and was found to decrease the number of rectal polyps. Patients who stopped taking the drug were found to have a reappearance of polyps (Waddell, Ganser, Lerise, & Loughry, 1989). Two other studies revealed similar results (Giardello et al., 1993; Labayle et al., 1991) in two randomized, placebo-controlled trials in patients with FAP. Patients receiving sulindac were found to have significantly fewer polyps than the control group. Giardello et al. found a 44% reduction in total polyp number from the baseline in their study with sulindac and FAP.

Low-dose aspirin has shown to be a promising drug in reducing the rates of CRC. Giovannucci et al. (1994) performed a prospective cohort study with 51,529 U.S. healthcare professionals to investigate various potential causes of cardiovascular disease and cancer. Those who reported regular aspirin use (≥ 2 per week) had a lower risk for CRC.

Two other large studies also were performed: the Physician's Health Study and Nurse's Health Study (Giovannucci et al., 1994, 1995). The Physician's Health Study randomized 22,071 male physicians to 325 mg of aspirin on alternate days or placebo, and beta-carotene or placebo. The design was to observe the effects of aspirin on cardiovascular disease and beta-carotene on cancer. The study was terminated after five years because men in the aspirin group had a 44% reduction in the risk of myocardial infarction, and no positive effects of aspirin were found on the incidence of CRC. The Nurse's Health Study, a cohort study with registered nurses, found that nurses who took four to six low-dose aspirin tablets per week had a statistically significant reduction in CRC risk at 20 years of follow-up (Giovannucci et al., 1995).

Because of the conflicting data, more information is needed about NSAIDs and low-dose aspirin, especially the duration, dose, and associated adverse effects. A current trial through the Cancer and Leukemia Cooperative Group should bring more information about the role of aspirin in CRC chemoprevention. This study, which recently completed accrual, randomized 900 postsurgical colon resection patients with CRC to placebo or aspirin (325 mg/day) for three to four years. The study objective was to observe the effect of aspirin on recurrence of cancer and development of new adenomas.

One of the disadvantages of using NSAIDs is their adverse effects, particularly related to the kidneys and GI tract. Newer efforts to reduce the side effects have resulted in the development of COX-2 inhibitors, which have safer profiles than COX-1 inhibitors. Some investigators have reported that human CRCs have an overexpression of COX-2 compared with normal colon mucosa (Eberhart et al., 1994). COX-2 inhibitors, such as celecoxib, have been studied in preclinical models and have shown to inhibit carcinogenesis. This classification of drug is promising and, with new COX-2 inhibitors being developed, should be of interest in upcoming studies. Two NCI-sponsored trials are looking at efficacy of celecoxib for HNPCC and in sporadic polyp prevention in people who have undergone polypectomy. The FDA recently approved celecoxib as an adjunct to usual care of endoscopic surveillance and surgery to reduce the number of adenomatous colorectal polyps in patients with FAP.

Calcium

The mechanism of the chemoprevention action of calcium is through the binding of calcium to bile and fatty acids, forming insoluble complexes that can reduce the concentration of the potentially toxic bile acids that are in contact with the colonic mucosa. In addition, optimal intake of calcium may be responsible for decreased cell proliferation and increased normal cell differentiation, which may inhibit carcinogenesis (Garay & Engstrom, 1999). Studies with calcium have been inconclusive. One large randomized study followed patients with recurrent adenoma who were receiving placebo or calcium (3,000 mg daily) for four years. Patients were evaluated at one and four years with colonoscopy. Thirty-one percent of patients in the calcium group had adenomas that developed between the first and last colonoscopy compared to 38% of patients in the placebo group. This was a statistically significant reduction in risk of recurrent adenomas. In addition, polyp size was smaller in the calcium group (Baron et al., 1999). Evidence suggests that calcium has a protective effect on the colon, although the mechanism is unclear. Further studies are needed to determine the efficacy of calcium in adenoma prevention.

Antioxidants

The antioxidant vitamins of most interest are vitamins E, C, and beta-carotene. Free radicals in tissues and cells can damage DNA, proteins, carbohydrates, and lipids. Antioxidants act as free-radical scavengers and prevent tissue damage by trapping them. They also can modulate cellular differentiation and proliferation in the colorectal epithelium. Beta-carotene, a precursor to vitamin A, may have a role in deterring genetic changes by preventing DNA damage caused by free radicals (Garay & Engstrom, 1999).

In a large cohort study, the Iowa Women's Health Study observed the relationship between dietary vitamins and CRC incidence. Vitamin E was associated with a decreased cancer risk, whereas vitamins C and A were not (Bostick et al., 1993). In a Finland double-blind, placebo-controlled study, 29,133 males were randomized to receive vitamin E and beta-carotene or placebo. After a five- to eight-year follow-up, patients who had received beta-carotene showed no decrease in cancer occurrence, including CRC. Patients who received vitamin E showed a nonsignificant reduction in CRC incidence (Albanes et al., 1995). Studies also have been conducted on patients with a history of colon polyps, with most demonstrating little benefit.

Folate

Patients with CRC and adenomas may have altered DNA methylation. A study by Cravo et al. (1994) found that doses of folic acid could reverse the DNA hypomethylation present in rectal epithelium in people with adenomas or cancer. An Eastern Cooperative Oncology Group trial using folate (5 mcg/day for one year) compared with placebo for patients with a history of adenomatous polyps is ongoing (NCI, 2000). The goals of the trial are to evaluate the ability of folic acid to decrease DNA hypomethylation, determine if patients with adenomas have DNA hypomethylation of the colorectal mucosa compared to controls, and evaluate rate of adenomatous polyp recurrence.

Dithiolthiones

Oltipraz is a synthetic dithiolthione that has inhibited CRC in animals. Certain cruciferous vegetables (e.g., cabbage, Brussels sprouts, broccoli) are natural sources of this compound. Oltipraz can raise detoxification enzymes, such as glutathione, in tissue, which may have an anticancer effect (Krishnan, Ruffin, & Brenner, 1998). Further studies are needed with this agent.

Matrix Metalloproteinase Inhibitors

Matrix metalloproteinase inhibitors play a critical role in tumor invasion and metastasis. Early studies in mice and human tumors have shown that one matrix metalloproteinase inhibitor family member, matrilysin (MMP-7), frequently is expressed in adenomas. The use of these inhibitors may have a possible role in CRC prevention (Hawk & Limburg, 1999).

Nursing Challenges

The role of the nurse in the area of colorectal prevention and early detection is important and will continue to strengthen as this type of screening becomes more prevalent in the United States. Nurses have a significant role in several areas.

Patient Education/Fear Reduction

The nurse always has been instrumental in educating patients. Teaching the general public by taking part in events such as National Colorectal Awareness Cancer Month should be a focus of oncology nurses. Community education programs should explain the types of screening available, including the advantages/disadvantages of each test, interval frequency, insurance coverage, preparations for examinations, procedural differences, and the follow-up required if a positive finding exists. Other areas of teaching should include the rationale and importance of screening, signs and symptoms of CRC that should be reported, predisposing risks, and risk factor reduction in daily life. The infrequent need for screening examinations should be emphasized to patients because fear of the examination and finding cancer prevents many people from getting screened. Reinforcement of the prognostic differences in those patients diagnosed with early-stage cancers versus late-stage cancers may encourage screening.

When dealing with ethnically or culturally diverse populations, differences in cultural values and beliefs will need to be considered. Sensitivity to these differences can enhance participation and compliance with screening recommendations (Winawer et al., 1997). Access for screening should be explored to provide more options for populations that may not have the usual healthcare options available. Written materials for the general public should be available, culturally appropriate, and at a correct reading level for the intended audience.

Use of Nurse Endoscopists

Nurse endoscopists can be an asset in the area of screening with use of flexible sigmoidoscopy. Nurses have been successfully performing flexible sigmoidoscopy since the 1970s, and many studies have indicated that nurses can perform this procedure efficiently and safely. A study by Schoenfeld et al. (1999) compared patient satisfaction and technical effectiveness with flexible sigmoidoscopy performed by registered nurses, general surgeons, and gastroenterology fellows. No clinically significant differences were noted in the technical effectiveness or patient satisfaction between the groups studied. A single nonrandomized study by Maule (1994) showed similar results when comparing nurse endoscopists to gastroenterologists when reviewing depth of sigmoidoscopic insertion, identification of adenomas, and measurement of perceived discomfort with the examination.

To meet the demand for screening needs, many institutions are using nurse endoscopists or other nonphysician personnel. Ransohoff and Lang (1993) determined that if screening is performed every five years on people between the ages of 50–75, then 10 million flexible sigmoidoscopies would need to be performed, demonstrating a clear area of opportunity for nurse endoscopists. If this is the direction nurses choose to take, intensive training programs and clinical competencies are available that comply with the guidelines established by the Society for Gastroenterology Nursing and the American Society for Gastrointestinal Endoscopists. Eisemon, Stucky-Marshall, & Talamonti (2001) provided components of a competency training program and the scope of practice for a nurse endoscopist used at a large Midwestern academic center.

Ongoing evaluation of the nurse's skills should be monitored for both cognitive and technical abilities. Clinical outcomes information and patient satisfaction reports should be published for other nurses to review. Guidelines should be developed by physician organizations to assist in consistent training and defining appropriate educational levels for nurse endoscopists and nonphysicians performing flexible sigmoidoscopy (Sprout, 2000). Nonphysician endoscopists more recently have been performing colonoscopy, but little published information related to this is available.

Although Medicare does provide screening coverage for flexible sigmoidoscopy, the Health Care Financing Administration initially ruled that it would only reimburse examinations performed by physicians to ensure safe and accurate procedures (Federal Register, 1997). The Balanced Budget Act of 1998 allowed master's prepared advanced practice nurses (both NPs and CNSs) to be reimbursed for flexible sigmoidoscopy, only if they were authorized in the particular state where examinations were performed (Federal Register, 1998). This limits nonmaster's prepared nurses to performing examinations only on patients with coverage other than Medicare.

Veteran's hospitals often have delays in scheduling for flexible sigmoidoscopies. Nurse endoscopists would be an asset in this type of setting by impacting cost reduction for examinations and making screening procedures available for large groups of individuals. Creative strategies to bring this type of service to the economically challenged should be considered. Availability and access are issues for patients considering screening. When a patient has the courage to schedule an examination, if the time delay is too great, the patient may cancel and choose not to reschedule. Convenient and extended scheduling options should be provided to offset this problem. Nurse endoscopists should include patient education as part of the flexible sigmoidoscopy. Videoscoping technology allows patients to view their own examinations and can stimulate greater interest and understanding for them, improving compliance. Care, comfort measures, and reassurance provided by the nurse during the examination tempers much of the anxiety and unpleasantness patients associate with the procedure. This may determine if patients return for reexamination. A follow-up reminder should be established to ensure patients' participation and compliance with subsequent screening examinations and to determine if further evaluation is needed.

Genetic Counseling

Genetic counseling is important for patients with suspected genetic syndromes or multiple family members with cancer. Many nurses are becoming trained in genetics. For those who are not, assisting patients to find counselors who are experts in this area is important. Referring people undergoing this process who are in need of psychological support may be necessary. The nurse can assist the patient in identifying new Web site information dealing with the controversies of genetic testing and some of the discrimination issues.

Healthy Lifestyle

Nurses can promote healthy eating by suggesting low-fat foods with selections of plant sources, including fruits, vegetables, breads, and cereals. Frequent exercise, limited alcohol consumption, and cessation of smoking and tobacco use should be encouraged. Nurses also can serve as role models for these behaviors.

Chemoprevention

Nurses should promote chemoprevention trials to potentially eligible patients. Accrual strategies can be developed to identify patients who are interested in participating in these types of trials. Education about the benefits of these trials, both personal and societal, can influence one's decision to participate.

Healthcare Provider Education

The oncology nurse can assist in keeping healthcare providers up-to-date on current CRC screening guidelines. When changes occur in guidelines, dissemination of this information must occur with physicians in family practice, internal medicine, OB/GYN, and oncologists. In academic centers, education should be ongoing with medical students and residents to ensure that CRC screening becomes a normal part of a patient's health care, just as Pap smears and mammography have become in women's care. Formal education programs can be planned for physician groups focusing on guideline recommendations, possibly coinciding with CRC awareness month.

Conclusion

The nurse can serve in a variety of functions with CRC screening. As this type of screening becomes more commonplace in the general public, more nurses may be used to perform screening examinations. They should be trained properly and report their outcomes. The nurse continues to have a strong voice for patients, one that may be considered less threatening but, nonetheless, a voice that is worth listening to. Nurses should share important information with patient advocacy groups to promote colon cancer screening and early detection.

Colorectal Cancer Screening Summary

CRC remains a frequent problem in the United States and one that is likely to become easier to treat as screening efforts improve and gain more interest with the general public and healthcare providers. Nursing can serve in a variety of roles to promote awareness and eliminate some of the associated fears with CRC. Newer screening techniques are being studied, pharmacologic agents are being tested for chemoprevention, and the general public is becoming more knowledgeable about the standard of care for CRC screening. All of these efforts should impact the mortality associated with CRC by promoting more screenings and early detection.

Gastric Cancer

Epidemiology

The incidence of gastric cancer has declined progressively since 1930 by approximately 60% (McDonald, Hill, & Roberts, 1992). In the beginning of the century, gastric cancer was the leading cause of cancer deaths in the United States (Blot, Devesa, Kneller, & Fraumeni, 1991). Presently, gastric cancer is the second most common cause of cancer-related deaths in the world (Neugut, Hayek, & Howe, 1996). ACS estimated that 21,700 people in the United States will develop gastric cancer in 2001, and 12,800 individuals will die of the disease (Greenlee et al., 2001).

Even though a decrease in the incidence of gastric cancers has occurred, the number of proximal gastric and gastroesophageal adenocarcinomas continues to increase (Blot, Devesa, & Fraumeni, 1993). Other epidemic areas, including Japan, Eastern Europe, and portions of Central and South America, have not seen a decline in gastric cancer rates. The highest incidence is in Japan, where gastric cancer is the leading cause of death from malignant diseases (Nakamura et al., 1992).

In the United States, a higher incidence of gastric cancer is seen in men as compared to women, with a ratio of 2:1. The incidence is also higher in African American men as compared to White men, with a ratio of 1.5:1 (Alexander, Kelsen, & Tepper, 1997). The incidence of gastric cancer increases with age, beginning around age 40 and reaching a peak around age 70 (Lawrence & Zfuss, 1995). The mortality rates for gastric cancer have decreased during the past 60 years, but this likely represents the decrease in the incidence of the disease (Alexander et al.). The five-year survival rates have not changed significantly.

Pathophysiology

The stomach begins at the gastroesophageal junction and ends at the pyloris. It is surrounded by the structures of the diaphragm, liver, abdominal wall, transverse colon, and omentum. Structures behind the stomach include the spleen, pancreas, left adrenal, left kidney, and the splenic flexure of the colon. The area of tumor involvement directly affects the involvement of these surrounding structures.

The blood supply and the lymphatic drainage around the stomach are extensive (see Figure 12-8). Location of the tumor invasion into the arterial and venous systems greatly determines the ability to perform resection. Tumor invasion into these systems, in particular the lymphatic system, also will directly impact the spread of disease and the initial staging.

Figure 12-8. Lymphatic Drainage of the Stomach

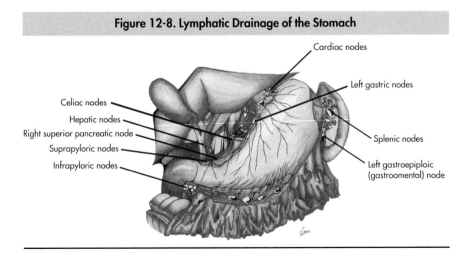

The staging of the disease is essential for planning treatment for the individual and also predicts prognosis. AJCC's TNM classification is widely accepted for staging this disease (see Table 12-4). Using this staging system, involvement of the periaortic, hepatoduodenal, retropancreatic, and mesenteric lymph nodes is considered metastatic disease.

Approximately 95% of all malignant gastric tumors are adenocarcinomas. Other malignant neoplasms of the stomach exist, but they are rare enough that when referring to gastric cancer, it typically is associated with adenocarcinoma (Blomjous et al., 1992). Other malignant tumors include squamous cell carcinoma, carcinoid tumors, leiomyosarcoma, and lymphoma.

Pattern of Disease Progression

Most gastric cancers develop in the antrum, the distal third of the stomach. More recently, a larger number of malignancies have been found in the proximal stomach and the gastroesophageal junction. The lesser curvature of the stomach is involved more frequently than the greater curvature (Alexander et al., 1997).

The individual frequently presents at a later stage of disease because the initial symptoms often are vague. This leads to presentation at a time of locally advanced disease or metastatic disease. The tumors most commonly are spread by local invasion of adjacent structures or by lymphatic spread. Tumors of the distal stomach often metastasize to infrapyloric, inferior gastric, and celiac lymph nodes. The proximal stomach metastasizes to pancreatic, pericardial, and gastric lymph nodes (McDonald et al., 1992).

Two aspects of local invasion that directly impact survival rates and prognosis include depth of invasion and involvement of the lymphatics. The five-year survival rates decrease as the depth of invasion increases (Davis, 1994) (see Figures 12-9 and 12-10). The occurrence of distant metastases also directly influences prognosis. Common sites of distant metastases include lung, adrenals, bone, liver, rectum, and the peritoneal cavity (McDonald et al., 1992). Diffuse peritoneal spread can cause obstruction in surrounding intestinal sites. A large ovarian mass, known as a Krukenburg tumor, or a large pelvic implant, known as Blumer's shelf, can produce rectal obstruction (Alexander et al., 1997).

Risk Factors

A number of risk factors exist for development of gastric adenocarcinoma (see Figure 12-11). They fall under the categories of medical conditions, genetic conditions, and environmental factors.

Medical Conditions

A wide number of studies have shown an association with the presence of Helicobacter pylori (H. pylori) infection and a risk for the development of gastric cancer. A threefold to sixfold increased risk exists, independent of the association of infection and ulcerative disease as risk factors (Faivre & Benhamiche, 1995). The specific role of H. pylori infection is unclear, but the infection is thought to be

Table 12-4. TNM Classification System for Stomach Cancer

Definition of TNM

Primary Tumor (T)

TX   Primary tumor cannot be assessed.
T0   No evidence of primary tumor
Tis Carcinoma in situ: Intraepithelial tumors without invasion of the lamina propria
T1   Tumor invades lamina propria or submucosa.
T2   Tumor invades the muscularis propria or the subserosa.*
T3   Tumor penetrates the serosa (visceral peritoneum) without invasion of adjacent structures.**
T4   Tumor invades adjacent structures.***

Note. A tumor may penetrate the muscularis propria with extension into the gastrocolic or gastro-hepatic ligaments or into the greater or lesser omentum without perforation of the visceral perito-neum covering these structures. In this case, the tumor is classified T2. If there is perforation of the visceral peritoneum covering the gastric ligaments or omenta, the tumor should be classified T3.
**Note.* The adjacent structures of the stomach are the spleen, transverse colon, liver, dia-phragm, pancreas, abdominal wall, adrenal gland, kidney, small intestine, and retroperitoneum.
***Note.* Intramural extension to the duodenum or esophagus is classified by the depth of greatest invasion in any of these sites, including the stomach.

Regional Lymph Nodes (N)

NX   Regional lymph node(s) cannot be assessed.
N0   No regional lymph node metastasis
N1   Metastasis in perigastric lymph node(s) within 3 cm of the edge of the primary tumor
N2   Metastasis in perigastric lymph node(s) more than 3 cm from the edge of the primary tumor
     or in lymph nodes along the left gastric, common hepatic, splenic, or celiac arteries

Distant Metastasis (M)

MX   Presence of distant metastasis cannot be assessed.
M0   No distant metastasis
M1   Distant metastasis

Stage Grouping

Stage 0	Tis	N0	M0
Stage IA	T1	N0	M0
Stage IB	T1	N1	M0
	T2	N0	M0
Stage II	T1	N2	M0
	T2	N1	M0
	T3	N0	M0
Stage IIIA	T2	N2	M0
	T3	N1	M0
	T4	N0	M0
Stage IIIB	T3	N2	M0
Stage IV	T4	N1	M0
	T1	N3	M0
	T2	N3	M0
	T3	N3	M0
	T4	N2	M0
	T4	N3	M0
	Any T	Any N	M1

Note. From *AJCC Cancer Staging Manual* (5th ed.) (p. 72), by American Joint Committee on Cancer, 1997, Philadelphia: Lippincott-Raven. Copyright 1997 by Lippincott-Raven. Reprinted with permission.

Figure 12-9. Depth of Penetration in Relation to T-Stage

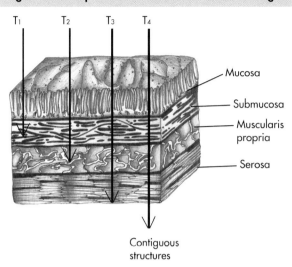

Figure 12-10. Prognosis in Relation to Depth of Invasion and Lymph Node Involvement

	Depth of Invasion	Percent With Lymph Node Involvement		Five-Year Survival	
Early Gastric Cancer	Mucosa	7%	24%	91%	78%
	Submucosa	14%		81%	
Advanced Gastric Cancer	Muscularis	45%	68%	36%	21%
	Serosa	66%		4%	

Note. From "Neoplasms of the Stomach," (p. 775) by G.R. Davis in M. Shleisenger and J. Fordtran (Eds.), *Gastrointestinal Disease* (5th ed.), 1994, Philadelphia: W.B. Saunders. Copyright 1994 by W.B. Saunders. Reprinted with permission.

associated with the development of chronic atrophic gastritis. In addition, infection with H. pylori at an early age is linked with a high gastric cancer rate in many countries (Davis, 1994). It also is believed to have a genetic or environmental component because only a small proportion of individuals with H. pylori go on to develop gastric cancer (Fuchs & Mayer, 1995). H. pylori appears to be linked with the development of gastric carcinomas in 40%–60% of cases in the world (Forman et al., 1991).

Individuals with chronic atrophic gastritis are two to three times more likely to develop gastric cancer, whether related to H. pylori infection or other causes (Fuchs & Mayer, 1995). Other causes of chronic atrophic gastritis include exposure to toxins and dietary agents, previous surgery, or chronic bile reflux into the stomach (Elder, 1995).

Figure 12-11. Risk Factors for Adenocarcinoma of the Stomach

- **Medical Conditions**
  - Helicobacter pylori infection
  - Chronic atrophic gastritis
  - Pernicious anemia
  - Gastric polyps
  - Partial gastrectomy for benign disease
- **Genetic Conditions**
  - Hereditary nonpolyposis colon cancer syndrome
  - Family history of gastric cancer
  - Blood type A
- **Dietary Factors**
  - Highly salted foods
  - Smoked foods
  - High fat
  - Low consumption of fruits and vegetables
- **Occupational Factors**
  - Coal mining
  - Processing of nickel, rubber, and timber
  - Painters
  - Fisherman
  - Printers
- **Environmental Factors**
  - Low socioeconomic status
  - Inadequate preservation of food
  - Poor nutrition
  - Poor sanitation
  - Use of well water

Another medical condition that is a risk factor for development of gastric cancer is pernicious anemia. Several studies indicate a 1%–10% incidence of gastric cancer in patients with pernicious anemia (Elder, 1995). The mechanism of action is theorized to be secondary to bacterial overgrowth, luminal pH changes, or related to chronic inflammation (Hsing et al., 1993).

Gastric polyps are another risk factor for gastric cancer. The prevalence of gastric polyps in the United States ranges from 1%–5% (Ginsberg, Al-Kawas, Fleischer, Reilly, & Benjamin, 1996). Hyperplastic polyps are the most common type of polyp and primarily occur in the gastric antrum. These polyps usually are less than 1.5 cm in diameter. If the polyps are small and multiple, they do not need to be removed (Boland & Scheiman, 1995). Fundic gland polyps account for 10%–13% of gastric polyps and have shown no evidence of malignant transformation (Ginsberg et al.). Adenomatous polyps are common in the colon yet rare in the stomach (Ginsberg et al.). The natural history of these polyps demonstrates that they are not likely to disappear and that 11% will have carcinomatous changes within four years and need to be removed. These patients need surveillance endoscopies, as new polyps develop in 25%–33% of patients after polypectomy (Ginsberg et al.).

Patients who have undergone surgery for benign disease of the stomach, in particular, peptic ulcer disease, are at increased risk for developing gastric cancer in the remaining tissue. A latent period of 15–20 years exists, and then the risk increases threefold to sixfold (Fisher et al., 1993). Interestingly, a partial surgical resection performed in Japan appeared to protect an individual from gastric cancer. This is only true for this endemic/particular area, where the incidence is so high. The protective effect theoretically results from the removal of the target organ that is susceptible to cancer (Albert, 1995).

Genetic Conditions

Genetic factors (e.g., nonpolyposis CRC) contribute to an increased risk of gastric cancer (Davis, 1994). A twofold to threefold increased risk exists in individuals who have a first-degree relative with gastric cancer (Albert, 1995). In addition, individuals with the blood type A may have an increased risk for developing the disease (Antonioli, 1990).

Environmental

Dietary factors play an important role in the risk factors for gastric disease. Diets that are high in salt, smoked or poorly preserved foods, nitrates, nitrites, and secondary amines cause a greater risk for the disease (Ramon, Serra, Cerdo, & Oromi, 1993). A large consumption of pickled foods and highly salted foods often leads to atrophic gastritis, which increases susceptibility to the development of cancer (Fuchs & Mayer, 1995). Bacteria can colonize in the stomach, leading to atrophic gastritis and the conversion of nitrates and nitrites to potentially carcinogenic compounds. Diets that are filled with raw fruits and vegetables are inversely related to gastric cancer risk (Boeing, 1991). Studies of immigrants from epidemic areas such as Japan demonstrate a decrease in the risk of gastric cancer with immigration to the West and subsequent change in their dietary patterns (Bonin, Coia, Hoff, & Schwartz, 2000). The decline in incidence of gastric cancer in the United States since 1930 has been associated with improved refrigeration (Davis, 1994).

Another environmental factor is occupational exposure to carcinogens. Coal mining and the processing of nickel, rubber, and timber all have been implicated in increasing risk. Painters, fisherman, and printers also have an associated risk in the development of gastric cancer (Fuchs & Mayer, 1995).

Low socioeconomic status also is associated with increased risk. This is likely a result of inadequate preservation of food, poor nutrition, overcrowding, and poor sanitation (Stellman & Stellman, 1996). The use of well water, which may contain high levels of nitrates or H. pylori, has been shown to be a risk factor for gastric cancer (Burstein et al., 1991).

Signs and Symptoms

Typically individuals with gastric cancer present at diagnosis with locally advanced or metastatic disease. The presenting symptoms often are vague, of variable duration, and nonspecific (Blot et al., 1991). Weight loss and abdominal pain are the most common initial signs (Davis, 1994). Other common symptoms include weakness and fatigue, nausea, anorexia, and dysphagia. Hematemesis occurs in approximately 10%–15% of patients (Bonin, Coia, Hoff, & Schwartz, 2000) (see Table 12-5).

Weight Loss

Weight loss in gastric cancer is a significant finding. In a study with 179 patients with advanced, nonmeasurable gastric cancer, more than 80% of the patients had at least a 10% weight loss. The individuals with weight loss also had a significantly shorter survival time than those who did not lose weight (DeWys, Begg, & Lavin, 1980).

Pain

Pain often suggests the specific location of the lesion. The epigastrium, back, or retrosternal areas are the most common sites for pain. In combination with pain, the individual is likely to experience symptoms of fullness, early satiety, distention, anorexia, and nausea. These vague symptoms often are self-medicated by the individual for prolonged periods of time prior to seeking treatment. Consequently, many patients present with advanced disease. Patients with more advanced cancer also may experience symptoms of cachexia, small bowel obstruction, ascites, lower extremity edema, and hepatomegaly (Boland & Scheiman, 1995).

Table 12-5. Presenting Symptoms of Gastric Cancer

Symptoms	Frequency (%)
Weight loss	61.6
Abdominal pain	51.6
Nausea	34.3
Anorexia	32.0
Dysphagia	26.1
Melena	20.2
Early satiety	17.5
Ulcer-type pain	17.1
Lower-extremity edema	5.9

Note. From "Cancer of the Stomach: A Patient Care Study by the American College of Surgeons," by H. Wanebo, B. Kennedy, J. Chimel, G. Steele, D. Winchester, and R. Osteen, 1993, Annals of Surgery, 218, p. 585. Copyright 1993 by Lippincott Williams and Wilkins. Reprinted with permission.

Prevention

Lifestyle

One of the most important areas for prevention of gastric cancer is in the alteration of nutritional factors. Nutrition has been linked directly to incidence based upon the difference in worldwide incidence and variations in diet. Nutritional counseling must include a balanced diet with fruits and vegetables, high fiber, and limited intake of salted, pickled, or smoked foods.

Other important areas of focus should include assessment and screening for high-risk groups, including individuals with genetic risk factors, low socioeconomic status, and a history of gastric polyps and pernicious anemia. Individuals should be screened as appropriate for H. pylori infection and treated with antibiotics. Screening for H. pylori should be considered in individuals of lower socioeconomic class who have other concomitant risk factors. Environmental issues, in addition to nutritional factors, may increase the transmission of H. pylori

(Schwesinger, 1996). A strong association also exists between H. pylori infection and stomach cancer in African Americans and women (Parsonnet et al., 1991). In addition, individuals with occupational exposure also should be educated on the importance of follow-up screening and the signs and symptoms of disease.

Chemoprevention

The area of chemoprevention in gastric cancer is a new and growing field. Attention to chemoprevention in this area just recently has gained importance. The main focus of study at this time is in relation to nutritional factors. Many nutrients have been suggested as having a role in chemoprevention (see Table 12-6). The specific nutrients for gastric cancer include carotenoids, vitamins A and C, and phytochemicals.

Table 12-6. Chemopreventive Agents Studied in Gastrointestinal Malignancies

Agents	Cancers
Carotenoids and vitamin A	Esophagus, gastric, colon, rectum
Vitamin C	Gastric, esophagus, colon, rectum
Vitamin D	Colon, rectum
Vitamin E	Colon, rectum
Folate	Colon, rectum
Calcium	Colon, rectum

In addition to nutrients, the role of fiber intake has been evaluated. Extensive work has been performed in the area of FAP. Studies have recognized the support for reducing bowel neoplasia by the intake of fiber supplementation (DeCosse, Miller, & Lesser, 1989). As an indirect result, this would reduce one of the risk factors for the development of gastric cancer. Similar studies on fiber intake indicated that the protective effects are not limited to the colon; case-controlled studies recognized the potential for preventing gastric cancer (Risch, Jain, & Choi, 1982).

The use of aspirin, NSAIDs, and COX-2 inhibitors primarily has been evaluated with colon and esophageal cancer, but some crossover of results applies to patients with gastric cancer. Farrow et al. (1998) observed a 50% reduced risk of noncardia gastric adenocarcinoma in patients using aspirin or NSAIDs once a week for six months or more.

Early Detection

Mass screening generally is not performed in the United States because the disease is uncommon. This type of screening can be recommended for areas of the world where a higher incidence exists, such as Japan and China (Kamschoer, Fujii, & Masuda, 1989). A variety of screening tests have been researched in Japan as a result of their mass screening programs, including double-contrast barium radiographs and upper endoscopy (Murakami et al., 1990). In some Japanese studies, screening programs yielded up to 40% of new cases of early gastric cancer (Kaneko, Nakamura, Umeda, Fujino, & Niwa, 1977).

This information is of clinical importance for screening in the United States. The principles learned from Japanese screenings should be applied to high-risk individuals. If gastric cancer is found at an early stage, it has a high cure rate; the difficulty is that it often presents at a late stage. As a result, high-risk patients should be screened in attempt to identify cases at an earlier stage. The American Society of Gastrointestinal Endoscopy recommended surveillance for individuals with a history of gastric adenoma and adenomatous polyposis, including familial polyposis (Parsonnet & Axon, 1996). Patients with adenomatous polyposis should have a gastroduodenoscopy with biopsy excision of polyps every one to two years (Kamschoer et al., 1989). Individuals with a history of a solitary adenoma should have a repeat endoscopy every one to two years (Parsonnet & Axon).

Nursing Challenges

Patient and Family Education

Patients with gastric cancer often present to the healthcare provider at a late stage of disease, which has a poor effect on prognosis. Because mass screenings are not justified for this disease in the United States, nurses must assist in the education about risk factors for gastric cancer and early signs and symptoms.

Nurses are highly skilled in educating patients and families about the importance of nutrition. They should stress the need to decrease salt intake and limit smoked or pickled foods and emphasize the importance of a diet high in fruits and vegetables and low in fats.

In addition to education regarding nutrition, nurses should identify occupational risk factors and genetic predispositions. They should assist with recommendations for genetic counseling and appropriate screening for gastric cancer in high-risk groups.

Healthcare professionals should educate the public on the symptoms of gastric cancer. Although the symptoms are notoriously vague, it is imperative to attempt to identify patients at an earlier stage of disease. The symptoms include weight loss, abdominal pain, nausea, anorexia, dysphagia, early satiety, and hematemesis. The nurse needs to convey the importance of seeking medical attention with these symptoms, rather than treating them with over-the-counter medications, thus delaying diagnosis.

Hepatocellular Cancer

Introduction

Hepatocellular carcinoma (HCC) has a wide geographic variation in incidence, with the disease being rather uncommon in the United States but extremely common in other regions of the world. Because HCC usually is diagnosed at an advanced stage, it is associated with a dismal prognosis, a median survival of less than four months (McMahon & London, 1991), and a low five-year survival rate. In the United States, HCC typically affects older populations, particularly those with a history of liver cirrhosis. Screening for this type of tumor currently is not indicated for average-risk people, but high-risk groups can benefit from screening and early detection of liver tumors. Whether screening impacts survival in high-risk groups is yet to be determined. Primary prevention of this disease is aimed at reducing risk factors, and early detection is critical in those at high risk. National practice guidelines recently have been developed to ensure consistent patient management once a suspicion of HCC is present (Benson, 1999). Efforts on identifying screening methods for those at high risk for developing HCC are being investigated, but, at present, the optimal approach still is not known.

Incidence/Epidemiology

HCC accounts for approximately 90% of adult primary liver cancer, with cholangiocarcinoma accounting for the rest (Falkson, Falkson, & Garbers, 1998). HCC usually is associated with chronic underlying liver disease, most often related to the hepatitis B or C viruses. Worldwide statistics indicate that approximately one million new cases are diagnosed annually (Carr, Flickinger, & Lotze, 1997); HCC is responsible for 250,000 deaths a year (Zhou et al., 1989); and the malignancy is the fourth most common cancer in the world (Parkin & Muir, 1992). HCC ranks first among all malignancies in Mozambique and some African countries and third in Japan and China (Okuda, 1997). In 2001, 16,200 new cases and 14,100 deaths were expected to occur from HCC in the United States (Greenlee et al., 2001). In the United States, it is the fourth most common GI malignancy and the third most lethal (Greenlee et al.). Death rates from HCC among men in low-incidence areas, such as the United States, are 1.9 per 100,000 per year compared with high incidence areas, such as Korea and China, with rates as high as 23.1–150 per 100,000 per year (Simonetti et al., 1991). HCC is an infrequent cancer in developed countries, but incidence rates are rising in the United States, Japan, United Kingdom, and France (Deuffic, Poynard, Buffat, & Valleron, 1998; El-Serag & Mason, 1999; Taylor-Robinson, Foster, Arora, Hargreaves, & Thomas, 1997). El-Serag and Mason found an increased incidence in the United States that rose from 1.4 per 100,000 between 1976 and 1980 to 2.4 per 100,000 between 1991 and 1995, likely related to hepatitis B and C viruses. With this rise, men were affected three times more than women and African Americans twice as often as Whites (El-Serag & Mason). This rising incidence is not completely understood but may relate to different etiologic agents, a larger number of patients with alcoholic cirrhosis, and better treatments that allow for longer survival from hepatitis B and C (Strauss, 1995). HCC cases may continue to rise as people infected with the hepatitis viruses remain in the latency period (El-Serag & Mason).

The incidence of HCC is higher in males than females in any geographic area, but the ratio is dependent on the region and usually is higher in those areas with higher incidence. The male to female ratio is 5:1 in areas of high incidence and 2:1 in low-incidence regions (Falkson et al., 1998).

The mean age at diagnosis worldwide is between ages 50 and 60 (Benson, 1999) but varies geographically. In sub-Saharan Africa, the peak incidence is between ages 25 and 45 and is reported to occur in the late teen years in Taiwan and Africa (Kew & Geddes, 1982). In the United States, 59.3% of patients were between ages 60 and 79, with the mean age at diagnosis being 64.6 years (Cance, Stewart, & Menck, 2000). Environmental factors may contribute to the differences in geographical distribution.

Morbidity/Mortality

HCC usually is diagnosed at an advanced stage. Prognosis is good for solitary, small (< 2 cm) lesions with negative lymph nodes and without vascular invasion, with a three-year survival of 75% (Reintgen & Albertini, 1996). Advanced tumors (stage IV) involve more than one lobe of the liver, with invasion into the hepatic vasculature or adjacent organs. The five-year survival rate for advanced disease is poor at 5%. Untreated symptomatic HCC survival rates vary from 0% at four months to 1% at two years (Okuda et al., 1985). Survival rates improve for early, small tumors where surgical resection may be an option. Unfortunately, few patients are eligible for surgical resection because of large tumor size, presence of metastatic disease, or presence of vascular invasion. Prognosis is dependent on the degree of local tumor involvement and extent of liver impairment.

Pathophysiology
Anatomy of the Liver

The liver is the largest organ in the body and is divided into two functional parts: the right and left lobes. The functions of the liver are to remove toxins from the blood, form and excrete bile into the intestines, metabolize carbohydrates, proteins, fats, and steroids, and store vitamins and minerals. Alterations in these functions can result in major metabolic problems.

Seventy percent of the liver's blood supply comes from the portal vein (Groen, 1999). The hepatic artery supplies arterial blood and venous drainage via the right and left hepatic veins, which exit the liver and enter the inferior vena cava. Liver tumors have an altered blood flow. Instead of receiving most of their blood supply from the portal vein, they receive more than 80% of their blood from the hepatic artery (Venook, 1994). Healthy livers have the ability to regenerate. Unhealthy, cirrhotic livers are unable to regenerate. Tumor can replace more than 50% of the liver without affecting the organ's function or producing symptoms (LaBrecque, 1994).

Cellular Characteristics and Natural History

Primary liver cancers usually are adenocarcinomas of two cell types: 90% are HCC that arise from liver cells and 10% are cholangiocarcinomas that arise from bile duct cells (Carr et al., 1997). A variant, known as the fibrolamellar type, is not common, usually is found in noncirrhotic livers, has a better prognosis, and often can be surgically resected (Benson, 1999). HCC tumors usually are multifocal, soft, and highly vascular and can rupture or hemorrhage. Spread of malignant cells within the liver can occur because of the vascular nature of the tumor, although 50% of patients with HCC will not have spread of their disease outside of the liver (Coleman, 1997). Metastasis is rare with HCC but can occur in the diaphragm and nearby tissues or other organs, most commonly the bone and lungs. Liver damage occurs because of malignant masses compressing on major vessels and liver tissue. Hepatic failure and GI bleeding were the leading causes of death in one study (Okuda, 1997).

Staging

Staging is important in determining the extent of disease, prognosis, and treatment options. The common staging system used for HCC is the AJCC's (1997) TNM staging system (see Table 12-7). This system evaluates tumor size, location, extent of involvement within and outside the liver, and whether metastatic disease is present. Unfavorable prognostic signs for HCC are poor performance status, tumor size occupying more than 50% of the liver, ascites, vascular invasion into the portal vein, lymph node spread, hypoalbuminemia, and hyperbilirubinemia (Carr et al., 1997).

Pathogenesis

The mechanisms in the development of HCC are unclear. The development is likely multifactoral, involving interplay of chemical, biological, and pathophysiological factors. The roles played by the various risk factors vary in different regions of the world. In experimental conditions, liver carcinogenesis requires an initiating event that impacts the cellular genome and a promoting event that impacts cell division (Strauss, 1995). Chemical carcinogens as well as chronic hepatitis B virus (HBV) infection can trigger these events (see Figure 12-12).

Liver cell regeneration is a key factor in the pathogenesis of HCC. Unlike normal livers, cell regeneration in cirrhotic livers may be oncogenic because of the abnormal hormone patterns within the environment. The liver architecture is affected, and growth factor production and oncogene expression become abnormal (Strauss, 1995).

HBV integrates the host genome and can occur near cellular proto-oncogenes. These integrations occur in random chromosomal locations in different hepatomas. Because these integrations do not always take place, it is not necessary for carcinogenesis to occur (Strauss, 1995). In addition, the tumor-suppressor gene p53 may undergo point mutations. This has been found in some HCC cases in China and South Africa in areas with HBV and aflatoxin (Bressac, Kew, Wards, & Ozturk, 1991).

Table 12-7. TNM Classification System for Liver Cancer

Definition of TNM

Primary Tumor (T)

TX   Primary tumor cannot be assessed.

T0   No evidence of primary tumor

T1   Solitary tumor 2 cm or less in greatest dimension without vascular invasion

T2   Solitary tumor 2 cm or less in greatest dimension with vascular invasion or multiple tumors limited to one lobe, none more than 2 cm in greatest dimension without vascular invasion

T3   Solitary tumor more than 2 cm in greatest dimension with vascular invasion or multiple tumors limited to one lobe, none more than 2 cm in greatest dimension, with vascular invasion or multiple tumors limited to one lobe, any more than 2 cm in greatest dimension, with or without vascular invasion

Regional Lymph Nodes (N)

NX   Regional lymph nodes cannot be assessed.

N0   No regional lymph node metastasis

N1   Regional lymph node metastasis

Distant Metastasis (M)

MX   Presence of distant metastasis cannot be assessed.

M1   No distant metastasis

M2   Distant metastasis

Stage Grouping

Stage I	T1	N0	M0
Stage II	T2	N0	M0
Stage IIIA	T3	N0	M0
Stage IIIB	T1	N1	M0
	T2	N1	M0
	T3	N1	M0
Stage IVA	T4	Any N	M0
Stage IVB	Any T	Any N	M1

Note. From *AJCC Cancer Staging Manual* (5th ed.) (p. 98), by American Joint Committee on Cancer, 1997, Philadelphia: Lippincott-Raven. Copyright 1997 by Lippincott-Raven. Reprinted with permission.

The time between exposure to the etiologic factors and tumor development can vary from a few years to several decades (Strauss, 1995). Kiyosawa et al. (1990) found that the average time between blood transfusions and the development of chronic hepatitis, cirrhosis, and HCC were 10, 21, and 29 years, respectively. The growth rate of HCC varies among patients, and these differences are not understood. In comparison to other adenocarcinomas such as breast or colon cancer, HCC tends to be slow growing. The doubling time of tumors ranges from 1–19 months, with a median of six months (Strauss). The differing double times reveal the existence of variable growth patterns in HCC. The degree of hepatic replacement by tumor and severity of liver damage can be inversely correlated with patient survival times (Okuda et al., 1985).

Figure 12-12. Pathogenesis of Hepatocellular Carcinoma

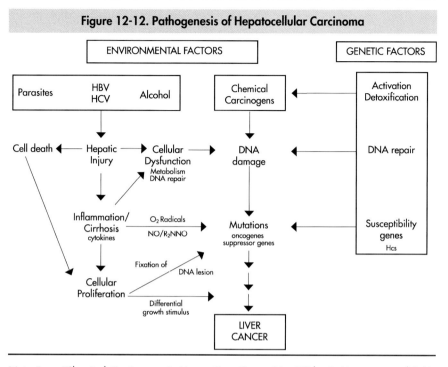

Note. From "Chemical Carcinogens in Human Liver Cancer," (p. 70) by R. Montesano and G.M. Kirby in C. Brechot (Ed.), *Primary Liver Cancer*, 1994, Boca Raton, FL: CRC Press. Copyright 1994 by CRC Press.

Etiology

HCC development occurs in stages and is related to an accumulation of risks such as infectious agents, chemicals, hormones, and genetic factors. Two viruses cause almost all of these tumors: hepatitis B and hepatitis C (Venook, 1994). The variations in these factors in the different geographic regions relate to the different incidence rates. Risk factors for the development of HCC can fall into two categories: physiologic and pathologic (see Figure 12-13).

Physiologic Factors: Age, Sex, and Race

In all geographic areas, regardless of risk, the incidence of HCC tends to increase with age. This differs in areas of high incidence, where younger groups may be affected because of HBV being acquired through birth (Colombo & Sangiovanni, 1997). People most affected worldwide are between ages 50 and 60. Males tend to develop HCC more than females, and it is unclear as to whether men have a greater susceptibility to this tumor or if they have a greater exposure to environmental risk factors. Race has no role in the development of HCC. The risk is related more to the environmental factors an ethnic group is exposed to, particularly the hepatitis viruses.

Figure 12-13. Etiologic Factors Associated With Development of Hepatocellular Carcinoma

Pathologic
• Male > Female
• Age > 50

Physiologic agents
• Viral agents
  – Hepatitis B, C
• Cirrhosis
  – Viral-related
  – Alcohol-induced
  – Hemochromatosis
• Aflatoxin exposure
• Hormones
• Thorotrast
• Increased body iron stores

Pathologic Factors
Viral Factors

The development of hepatocellular cancer almost always is related to a chronic underlying liver disease, caused by HBV and hepatitis C viruses (HCV). These viral infections can result in liver damage and cirrhosis, which eventually can lead to liver cancer.

Hepatitis B Virus

Three hundred million people are estimated to have been exposed to HBV (Maynard, 1990), and, in the United States, approximately 300,000 people acquire HBV infection each year (American Academy of Pediatrics Committee on Infectious Diseases, 1992). The worldwide distribution of chronic HBV is similar to the geographic distribution of HCC (Strauss, 1995). This correlation has been strengthened by the large amounts of HBV markers, such as HBV surface antigen (HBsAg) and anti-HBc, the antibody to the HBV core antigen (HBcAg) found in patients with HCC (Kew, Geddes, Macrab, & Bersohn, 1974). HBV DNA has been found in tissue harboring HCC as well as viral proteins, which include HBsAg and HBcAg (Strauss, 1995). HBV is of high prevalence in areas with high incidence of HCC, and the risk for HCC in carriers of HBV is much greater than for noncarriers. The relationship of the virus to the development of HCC is through chronic hepatitis and cirrhosis. Chronic hepatitis can result in hepatocyte changes resulting in nodular regeneration, dysplasia, and carcinoma (Sherlock, 1994). Nodular regeneration and cirrhosis are the most important precursor events, although HCC can develop without the presence of cirrhosis. The carcinogenesis results from a multistage process, with the end result being disorganized and rearranged hepatocyte DNA. During the course of HBV, the virus DNA integrates into the host DNA and is associated with various chromosomal deletions and translocations (Sherlock). Clinical differences appear between HBV-infected patients with HCC, depending on their geographic locations (Carr et al., 1997). African Americans with HCC do not have severe cirrhosis but have very aggressive, poorly differentiated tumors, compared with patients in the United States (Carr et al.). Routes of transmission for HBV include sexual contact, IV drug use, and blood transfusion. Fortunately, with the introduction of a hepatitis B vaccination for infants, the transmission of HBV from infected mother to offspring nearly is eliminated (Venook, 1994).

Hepatitis C Virus

HCV is known to be a risk factor for the development of cirrhosis and HCC and is the main contributor to the increased incidence of HCC around the world (Blei, 2000). Identified in the late 1980s, HCV is spread via the parenteral route or by sexual or maternal-fetal contact. Routine screening of blood for HCV began in 1992. In the United States, four million people have chronic HCV (Ince & Wands, 1999). Currently, HCV is most commonly spread through unprotected sex and infected needles with IV drug use (Heintges & Wands, 1997). With improvements in the screening of blood products, risk for HCV has been reduced. The average time between transfusion-associated infection and HCC development is 30 years (Colombo & Sangiovanni, 1997). Up to 50% of people infected with HCV cannot identify exposure to any risk factor (Ince & Wands). HCV infection causes 70% of HCC cases in Japan and approximately 30%–50% of cases in the United States (Ince & Wands). Between 15%–20% of people who are infected with HCV develop cirrhosis (Strauss, 1995).

Investigators have found that patients with HCV tend to be older than those infected with HBV, suggesting the possibility that HCV infection may take place at a later time in life. In addition, HCC in a person infected with HCV may take a much longer time to develop than in a patient with HBV (Strauss, 1995).

Some patients with cirrhosis and HCC may have both anti-HCV and HBsAg. Those who have both may be more likely to develop serious liver disease than patients infected by a single virus (Zuckerman, 1987).

The pathogenesis of HCV is unclear at this time but may be related to persistent inflammation, cellular injury, regeneration, and cirrhosis, all contributing to the carcinogenic process. Unlike HBV, HCV does not integrate into the host DNA (Khakoo, Grellier, Soni, Bhattacharya, & Dusheiko, 1996). HCV has been noted to develop into HCC without the presence of chronic hepatitis or cirrhosis (Colombo & Sangiovanni, 1997). Currently, no vaccine exists to prevent HCV.

Hepatitis Delta Virus

Hepatitis D virus (HDV) is a defective RNA virus that requires the presence of HBV to replicate and function (Dienstag & Isselbacher, 1994). HDV is uncommon in the United States, is transmitted by blood and blood products, and most commonly infects IV drug users. Conflicting data exist regarding HDV and its relationship with HCC. HDV may result in liver injury that progresses more rapidly to cirrhosis (Bonino et al., 1987). This earlier development of cirrhosis in a carrier of HDV could result in a higher risk of HCC at a younger age (Verme et al., 1991).

Alcohol

Excessive alcohol ingestion may be a risk factor for development of HCC in areas where incidence is less common. The effect of alcohol is dose dependent, and the cirrhosis that results from chronic consumption may be the basis for alcohol-related HCC cases (Colombo & Sangiovanni, 1997). In the United States, where the prevalence for HBV carriers is low, the risk for HCC was increased to 40% because of heavy alcohol consumption (Colombo & Sangiovanni). Alcohol may be a liver carcinogen only because it causes cirrhosis (Strauss, 1995).

Cirrhosis

Cirrhosis is the underlying disease in more than 80% of patients with HCC in most countries (Okuda, 1997). Fifty-six percent of patients who present with HCC have previously undiagnosed cirrhosis (Zaman, Johnson, & Williams, 1990). Cirrhosis causes progressive damage to the liver cells that results in chronic irritation, altering the body's normal control of cell growth and resulting in the development of malignant cells in the liver (Okuda). Cirrhosis can be caused by chronic alcohol use or from chronic hepatitis B or C infection. Alcoholic cirrhosis is most common as a risk factor in the United States. In a Japanese study, the three-year cumulative risk of developing HCC in people with cirrhosis was 12.5%, compared with 3.8% in people without cirrhosis (Tsukuma et al., 1993). Because HCC commonly is first seen in patients who are in their 50s–60s, cirrhosis has had time to develop, followed by HCC. Other cofactors may be involved along with cirrhosis that can increase hepatocellular proliferation, such as HBV or HCV (Khakoo et al., 1996). The annual risk of people with cirrhosis to develop HCC is 1%–6% (Ikeda et al., 1993).

A genetic disorder known as hemochromatosis can result in a rare form of cirrhosis because of deposits of iron within the liver cells. This has been associated with the development of HCC (Frogge, 1993).

Aflatoxin B

Aflatoxin B, a toxic metabolite of aspergillus flavus and related fungi, can be found in ingested foods, particularly grains and legumes in Africa and Asia where the climate and storage methods allow for higher quantities in the food (Colombo & Sangiovanni, 1997). Strong evidence is available for carcinogenic effects of aflatoxin in animals, with less conclusive evidence in humans (Peers & Dinsell, 1973). Aflatoxin B has been associated with genetic mutations, particularly the p53 gene, and allelic deletions in chromosome 17p, both of which can lead to liver cancer (Bressac et al., 1991).

Hormones

Exposure to exogenous steroidal sex hormones could increase the risk for liver adenomas and HCC. Case-control studies conducted in areas without a high incidence of HBV and HCC have shown a positive correlation between oral contraceptive use and HCC (Colombo & Sangiovanni, 1997). An association of increased risk may exist for HCC for a subset of users of oral contraceptives that contain mestranol (Kerlin et al., 1983). Current oral contraceptives do not contain mestranol; therefore, the associated risk with HCC may be eliminated (Strauss, 1995).

Thorotrast

Thorotrast, a contrast medium used in the 1950s for angiography, has been associated with the development of HCC. It is an isotope with a long half-life, and the chronic low-level internal alpha-particle radiation emitted to the liver is suspected to cause the HCC found to develop 20 years after exposure (Colombo & Sangiovanni, 1997; Strauss, 1995).

Iron

People with high body iron stores may be at risk for HCC. The persistent elevation of serum ferritin in patients with chronic liver disease may predispose them to HCC. This risk is more common in men (Strauss, 1995).

Signs and Symptoms

Early diagnosis of HCC is difficult because of the liver's ability to regenerate and mask its impaired function. The course can be silent in early stages, and symptoms may not arise until the tumor has reached an advanced stage. Patients with preexisting cirrhosis tend to have similar symptoms as patients without cirrhosis, and a sudden decline in their health may occur when a malignant process is present (Groen, 1999). Liver cancer tends to spread directly in and around the liver, and symptoms occur because of the expanding tumor in the liver. This enlargement can result in portal vein occlusion, causing ascites, esophageal varices, and edema. HCC may spread to lymph nodes, lungs, bone, adrenal glands, and the brain, causing additional symptoms. Symptoms can appear alone or in combination with others.

The most common presenting symptom is right upper quadrant pain that varies in intensity from dull and aching to very severe, requiring analgesics. This pain may radiate to the right shoulder blade and eventually may become more severe, causing sleeping difficulties. Acute onset of pain can be associated with bleeding from rupture of the tumor into the peritoneal cavity. Although this is rare, if the bleeding is not controlled, it can be life threatening (Bruix, Llovet, Bru, & Rodes, 1997). Fullness in the epigastrium or early satiety commonly are reported.

Some constitutional symptoms that may indicate advanced disease include anorexia, weight loss, malaise, and unexplained fever. These symptoms can be present in patients with cirrhotic livers, making it difficult to determine if this process is progressing or if a different etiology, such as tumor development, is creating this symptomatology.

Although not commonly a presenting complaint, jaundice can occur because of the impaired function of the noninvolved liver. Tumor or blood clots can infiltrate the biliary tree causing obstruction and jaundice in some situations (Bruix et al., 1997).

Portal hypertension results from portal vein compression and usually is a sign of advanced disease. Esophageal varices or tumor invasion into the stomach can result in hematemesis (Coleman, 1997).

Paraneoplastic syndromes can occur secondary to the tumor development and can include diarrhea, erythrocytosis, hypoglycemia, hypercalcemia, and sexual changes (Bruix et al., 1997).

Findings on physical examination can include hepatomegaly with presence of masses. Ascites is more common in patients from the West compared with Africa and Asia. It may occur from portal hypertension, cirrhosis, or tumor infiltration of the portal system and peritoneal studding by tumor (Strauss, 1995). Other findings can include peripheral edema, splenomegaly, jaundice, weight loss with muscle wasting, fever, and arterial bruit. One study showed that 14.9% of patients had a fever for an extended period of time without an obvious etiology and later was attributed to the presence of a malignant liver tumor (Ihde, Sherlock, Winawer, & Furtner, 1974).

The tumor marker known as alpha-fetoprotein (AFP) has been found to be elevated in 60%–90% of patients with HCC and varies by geographic region, with the highest of AFP-secreting tumors found in Asia (Benson, 1999). AFP is a serum protein normally synthesized by fetal liver cells, by the yolk-sac cells, and in small amounts by the fetal GI tract (Cottone & D'Antoni, 1997). AFP is not specific to HCC and can be elevated in a variety of nonmalignant conditions such as chronic hepatitis, cirrhosis, or hepatic failure. A level that has been considered specific to HCC is one above 400 ng/ml (Cottone & D'Antoni). Tumor differentiation and size have been considered important in determining the level of AFP produced (Cottone & D'Antoni). CEA is another tumor marker that may be elevated in some patients.

Prevention

Because of the poor prognosis associated with HCC and the continuing evidence linking HCC with HBV, HCV, aflatoxin exposure, and alcoholic cirrhosis, preventive measures to avoid these factors should help decrease the risk of HCC from developing.

Vaccinations

In efforts to prevent perinatal transmission of hepatitis B, the United States developed an immunization strategy for HBsAg. The likelihood of chronic HBV infection is reduced to 5%–15% when newborns are provided with this combined passive and active immunization (Katkov, 1996).

In the 1980s, the United States developed a hepatitis B immunization strategy intended to vaccinate those adults at high risk for HBV infection. The groups identified included homosexual men, heterosexual people with multiple partners, IV drug users, healthcare workers, hemodialysis patients, hemophiliacs, and people in close contact with acute or chronic HBV ("Update," 1989). After years of targeting this group, the incidence of hepatitis B increased (Centers for Disease Control and Prevention, 1989). Reasons cited for this were individual concerns about vaccine safety and difficulties in identifying high-risk individuals (Hoofnagel, 1989).

After 10 years of experience with the vaccine, it was determined that targeting specific populations could not achieve the goal of reducing HBV incidence in the United States (Katkov, 1996). In 1991, the Public Health Service recommended a universal childhood immunization strategy to eradicate the transmission of HBV (Immunization Practices Advisory Committee, 1991). This targets immunization to all infants in the United States. In 1995, the vaccine was recommended for 11–12 year old children who were not previously vaccinated. The HBV vaccination includes a three-dose series given over several months. At present 58% of all U.S. babies born receive an immunization by age 19-24 months (Folcarelli, 1999). The duration of protection offered by the HBV vaccine is unknown, although 80%–90% of people vaccinated retained protective levels of antibodies for at least five years (Dienstag & Isselbacher, 1994).

Currently, no hepatitis C vaccine is available, although efforts have been and continue to be focused on this endeavor. Current efforts to decrease the risk of this infection include screening of hepatitis C antibodies, reducing transfusion-associated hepatitis, screening for HIV risks, and using alanine aminotransferase and antibody to hepatitis B core antigen testing of donor blood (Katkov, 1996). A newer approach being studied is the chemical treatment of blood products with the goal of decreasing the virus' infective ability (Dienstag & Isselbacher, 1994). The FDA has an approved home test for HCV. This test provides an over-the-counter blood collection kit that evaluates the patient for antibodies to the HCV. The sample of blood is collected at home and mailed to a designated laboratory. The results are available in 4-10 business days (FDA, 1999).

No specific vaccine exists for hepatitis D. The hepatitis B vaccine can be used to prevent hepatitis D, and efforts focus on avoidance of blood-borne transmission of the virus (Dienstag & Isselbacher, 1994).

Avoidance of Exposure

Eliminating the risk for exposure to hepatitis B, C, and D viruses can be achieved by avoiding behaviors that lead to blood-borne transmission. Food contamination with aflatoxin easily can be reduced with better storage and agricultural methods. Reduction of alcohol consumption should be encouraged.

Chemoprevention

Few clinical trials have been conducted for HCC in the area of chemoprevention. An NCI trial performed in the People's Republic of China by Kensler et al. (1998) used oltipraz, a synthetic dithiolthione structurally related to dithiolthiones found in cruciferous vegetables. In this area of China, residents are at high risk for HCC because of aflatoxin-contaminated food ingestion. The three-arm study was double blind, randomized, and placebo controlled. The objective was to assess the ability of oltipraz to modulate levels of a biomarker of aflatoxin exposure by determining levels of aflatoxin-albumin combinations in the serum and urine. The results showed that oltipraz did not appear to affect either baseline levels or rates of decline in the biomarker of aflatoxin. A follow-up study is needed with oltipraz given over a longer duration to determine if an impact occurs on the aflatoxin burden.

Muto et al. (1996) performed a study on 89 patients with primary HCC who were deemed disease-free after having undergone surgical resection or percutaneous ethanol administration for small, solitary lesions. Because a high rate of second primary and recurrent tumors exists, this randomized, controlled study was designed to test an acyclic retinoid (polyprenoic acid) to determine whether it could impact the development of second primary tumors after curative treatment. In animal models, this agent was known to inhibit hepatic carcinogenesis and could suppress tumor growth in human cell lines. Study results suggested that oral polyprenoic acid prevented second primary tumors for those patients who were disease-free after surgical or percutaneous intervention. Further research to develop analogues of polyprenoic acid is under way with hopes that new compounds may prevent primary liver tumors (Muto et al.).

Biologic and Antiviral Therapy

Interferon, a biologic response modifier, has been widely used to treat chronic HCV infection. A series of clinical trials has shown that patients with HCV who received interferon had a sustained normalization of serum aminotransferase levels and an elimination of serum HCV RNA during treatment (Shindo et al., 1991). In a study by Imai et al. (1998), efforts were made to determine if interferon therapy had an effect on the incidence of HCC in patients with chronic hepatitis C. Results of this retrospective cohort study revealed a lower incidence of HCC in patients with a sustained response to interferon therapy compared with historical controls and nonresponders. The conclusion was that interferon therapy might decrease the risk for HCC in patients with chronic HCV. Chronic HCV infection has been eliminated with a combination treatment of interferon and ribavirin. Ribavirin, an antiviral oral nucleoside analogue, has activity against several RNA viruses and has shown lowered serum aminotransferase levels in chronic HCV. The combination of interferon and ribavirin has greater efficacy than use of interferon alone for chronic HCV (Schalm et al., 1996). However, many questions need to be answered related to optimal dose and duration of therapy, whether combination therapy should be given as first-line treatment, and the patient's tolerance to combination therapy. Large prospective studies are being conducted to answer some of these questions.

Interferon therapy may be of moderate benefit for patients with HBV-related chronic hepatitis. One study using interferon found decreased serum HBV DNA levels and undetectable hepatitis B surface antigen levels on follow-up examination (Wong et al., 1993). Interferon alpha is usually given as a subcutaneous injection dosed at 5-10 million units three times a week. In addition to lowering the concentration of the active virus, it can also decrease degenerative changes in the liver and help to prevent renal complications or human immunodeficiency virus infection (Folcarelli, 1999).

Early Detection

General screening for HCC currently does not exist in the United States for average-risk people. The most important measure of the success of a screening program for HCC is to observe a reduced mortality for this type of tumor. No reported prospective, randomized trials are available that compare mortality rates in an unscreened control population with a screened population (Haydon & Hayes, 1996). Conflicting data exist about the impact of screening on surgical cure rates. Ultrasound studies of patients with cirrhosis have identified three phases in the natural history of HCC: the nondetectable preclinical phase, the detectable preclinical phase, and the symptomatic phase (Haydon & Hayes). Successful screening programs should target the second phase prior to the onset of symptoms. Tumor diameter during the second phase is 2.5 cm compared with 10 cm during phase 3. Patients may remain asymptomatic for two or more years, and detection during this time or possible surgical resection could lead to prolonged survival (Ebara et al., 1986). The five-year survival rate for people with HCC is poor, at 5% for those with advanced disease. The model does not take into account the variations in tumor growth rates and presumes that all tumors are single and encapsulated. Survival times actually are predicted more accurately by the severity of liver impairment rather than tumor diameter at time of diagnosis (Ebara et al.).

High-Risk Groups

For the population as a whole, no randomized trials have assessed the benefit of screening for HCC; therefore, no current evidence shows that screening impacts survival. The Western world still has a low incidence of HCC, and controlled trials would require large numbers of patients followed over an extensive period of time to show a benefit for screening in the general population. A workshop sponsored by NCI has suggested screening for specific high-risk groups (McMahon & London, 1991). The groups identified included HBsAg-positive carriers and HBsAg-positive carriers with cirrhosis or a family history of HCC. At this time, HBsAg-negative patients with cirrhosis or chronic liver disease could benefit from screening, but more data are needed for specific guidelines to be provided.

Current screening tools include AFP and ultrasound. AFP is the most widely available screening blood test. As discussed earlier, it is a marker for tumor differentiation but is not specific to HCC and can be elevated in other conditions. The AFP level is elevated in 60%–90% of patients, varying with geographic distribution. The highest percentage of AFP-producing tumors is in Asia (Benson, 1999). Many analyses have shown that patients with HCC have elevated AFP levels in wide ranges because of the differing definitions of elevated level (McMahon & London, 1991). Using a high cut-off level of AFP increases the specificity but decreases the sensitivity. The level that has been considered specific to HCC is above 400 ng/ml (Cottone & D'Antoni, 1997). False-positive elevations in AFP levels can be found in patients with a flare-up of their viral hepatitis, resulting in unnecessary evaluation (Khakoo et al., 1996). At times, AFP levels may be normal or mildly elevated even in the presence of HCC. Patients with an initial, persistent AFP level of > 20 ng/ml should have close follow-up with ultrasound monitoring every three months (Cottone & D'Antoni).

The role of AFP in screening programs alone is not clear. More useful and reliable tumor markers need to be identified that can detect HCC at an early, more treatable stage. The role of AFP is limited in identifying patients with a higher risk of developing HCC from values between 20–400 ng/ml and to a diagnostic level for HCC at a value > 400 ng/ml (Cottone & D'Antoni, 1997).

Other Tumor Markers

Other tumor markers are being studied that may have greater sensitivity and specificity for the diagnosis of HCC than the current AFP test. A plasma marker, Des-gamma-carboxyprothrombin, is a prothrombin induced by the absence of vitamin K. This marker was first reported by Liebman et al. (1984) to be elevated in 67% of patients with HCC. However, other medical conditions, such as chronic hepatitis, can cause an elevation in this marker (Reintgen & Albertini, 1996). Other markers that are being studied include AFP lectin, serum alpha-L-fucosidase, tissue polypeptide antigen, and antinuclear antibodies (Cottone & D'Antoni, 1997).

Ultrasonography

Ultrasonography (US) is an inexpensive, widely accessible, easy to perform, safe, and sensitive technique that fits well with the definition of a good screening tool. Studies from Japan and Taiwan have demonstrated that ultrasound can detect small hepatocellular carcinomas (McMahon & London, 1991). No large prospective studies using ultrasound examinations have been performed in high-risk groups. It has been suggested that ultrasound is a better screening tool than AFP in HBsAg/HCV-negative populations who are less likely to have elevated AFP levels (Ebara et al., 1986). In these populations, up to 50% of tumors less than 3 cm in diameter are missed when AFP is used alone (McMahon & London). One technical problem with the use of US for screening of cirrhotic livers is the occurrence of false-positive results that require further evaluation (Haydon & Hayes, 1996).

US used in the diagnosis of small HCC had a sensitivity range from 78%–100% and a specificity range from 93%–100% (Colombo et al., 1991; Cottone et al., 1994). Other radiologic techniques, such as CT, magnetic resonance imaging, and angiography are as sensitive as US but are more expensive and expose patients to more radiation, making them not as suitable for large screening programs (Haydon & Hayes, 1996).

Difficulties with any screening involve false-negative results that provide false reassurance to patients and false-positive results that provide patients with incorrect information that they have HCC (Haydon & Hayes, 1996).

Screening Recommendations for High-Risk Groups

Currently no standard exists for the screening of high-risk groups, and limited information is available regarding particular groups to monitor and recommended screening intervals. Reported surveillance intervals vary from 3–12 months, with limited reporting on the rationale for how these intervals were chosen (Collier & Sherman, 1998). A six-month interval may be based on rationale that tumor-doubling time for HCC is estimated to be six months (range 1–19 months) (Ebara et al., 1986).

The NCI workshop developed recommendations for high-risk groups (McMahon & London, 1991) (see Table 12-8). HBsAg-positive carriers should be screened with AFP at least annually but twice annually is preferred. In populations where HCC grows more rapidly, AFP is recommended more than once annually. HBsAg-positive carriers with other risk factors (e.g., cirrhosis, family history of HCC) should have periodic US examinations and AFP. HBsAg-negative patients with chronic liver disease or cirrhosis would benefit from periodic US or AFP, but specific recommendations cannot be made with the current data that are available. Patients with elevated AFP levels should have close monitoring with US every three to six months (Cottone & D'Antoni, 1997; Zoli et al., 1996). The panel suggested a need for large prospective studies of patients with liver disease at risk for HCC. This could determine the incidence in groups with differing etiologies and the efficacy of the current screening tools that are used (McMahon & London).

Until screening standards are developed for high-risk groups, follow-up of abnormal screening tests and monitoring of these patients are left to the individual physician's clinical judgment.

Table 12-8. Suggested Screening for Individuals at High Risk for Hepatocellular Carcinoma

Risk Factor	Screening Method
Hepatitis B surface antigen *positive* carrier	Alpha-fetoprotein (AFP) preferred every six months but at least on an annual basis Populations with higher incidence of hepatocellular carcinoma should be screened every six months.
Hepatitis B surface antigen *positive* carrier with cirrhosis or family history of hepatocellular carcinoma	As above, AFP plus periodic ultrasounds
Hepatitis B surface antigen *negative* carrier with chronic liver disease or cirrhosis	Probably benefit with periodic ultrasound or AFP, although more data are needed

Note. Based on information from McMahon & London, 1991.

Future Directions

Although screening and surveillance for HCC is practiced by hepatologists worldwide, particularly for patients with cirrhosis, insufficient evidence still is available related to the impact of screening on mortality reduction (Collier & Sherman, 1998). Much more information is needed in the area of HCC to determine the efficacy and benefit of screening, appropriate interval frequency, and cost effectiveness in high-risk populations. More information is needed through prospective studies in regard to HBsAg-positive carriers and the relationship with AFP and US. Because these types of studies will require an extensive number of patients, the NCI workshop panel suggests combining study data from many institutions (McMahon & London, 1991). Because of the many differences in the growth characteristics and incidence rates of HCC, studies should be conducted among several populations. Population studies also should evaluate alcohol-related liver disease, hepatitis C, chronic liver disease, cirrhosis, and the relationships of these diseases with HCC. Evaluation of AFP and US imaging also should be included in these studies.

Current clinical trials for patients with chronic hepatitis C are investigating standard interferon therapy using different doses and schedules and in combination with other investigational agents.

Future controlled trials should focus on assessing the effectiveness of cancer therapies on the small tumors detected with screening to determine the benefit of this practice (Collier & Sherman, 1998).

Nursing Challenges

Patient/Family Education

The need for health information about HCC is significant. Ongoing health education for the general public, provided by nurses, is an important component in the prevention of the risk factors associated with HCC development. Education efforts should target risk reduction related to virus transmission, alcohol consumption, and hepatitis B vaccination for newborns and high-risk groups. High-risk patients should be encouraged to obtain screening at periodic intervals to detect early disease conducive to surgical resection. Nurses should promote participation in chemoprevention and antiviral clinical trials to high-risk patients. Patients being treated with biologic or antiviral therapies should be educated on administration technique and side-effect management. Compliance may be an issue, and the nurse should monitor this and reinforce the importance of the designated therapy. High-risk groups should be aware of signs and symptoms of HCC to ensure early reporting.

Public education should be provided to all age levels but especially younger groups. Education efforts should focus on reducing HBV and HCV transmission by encouraging people to use disposable syringes and needles, avoid tattooing and piercing, use condoms during sex, and avoid sharing razors, toothbrushes, and pierced earrings. Education should call special attention to alcohol abuse and the association with cirrhosis and HCC, particularly in younger groups.

Conclusion

Although identified risks exist for the development of HCC and efforts focus on screening and early detection, the prognosis of this disease remains poor. Identifying the high-risk groups and ensuring that they are obtaining appropriate screening for their particular risk is important. Additional study is needed among the various populations to ensure that the screening techniques used are the most efficacious. Newer, more beneficial therapies should be developed both in the areas of prevention and treatment of HCC. Guidelines for the diagnosis and treatment of HCC are available to ensure consistent and quality management of this disease once a diagnosis is confirmed.

Esophageal Cancer

Epidemiology

Esophageal cancer is fairly uncommon in the United States in relation to other areas of the world. In the United States, it represents approximately 1% of all forms of cancer (Greenlee et al., 2001). An estimated 12,300 new cases will be diagnosed in 2001, and approximately 12,100 individuals will die of this disease (Greenlee et al.). This is one of the poorest survival rates of any malignancy, second only to pancreatic cancer. The incidence in the United States is most common in elderly males. The incidence increases with age, with a median age of 67 years. The mortality rate among African Americans is three times the rate of Whites (American Cancer Society, 2000). In addition, the male-to-female ratio of prevalence rates is approximately 3:1 (Ellis, Huberman, & Busse, 1995).

Esophageal cancer has the greatest variation of any malignancy based upon geography (Roth, Putnam, Rich, & Forastiere, 1997). The World Health Organization statistics demonstrate that the mortality rates are highest in China, Puerto Rico, and Singapore. Esophageal cancer rates in China are 20–30 times that of the United States (Douglas, 1991). No specific explanation is available for these geographical variations, although nutritional and environmental factors are likely sources.

Pathophysiology

The anatomy of the esophagus originates at the level of the cricopharyngeus muscle at the level of the sixth cervical vertebrae. The length of the esophagus to the esophageal junction is approximately 25 cm. AJCC (1997) divided the esophagus into four regions for staging purposes: the cervical esophagus, extending from the cricopharyngeus to the thoracic inlet; the upper thoracic esophagus, extending from the thoracic inlet to the level of the tracheal bifurcation; the midthoracic esophagus, extending from the tracheal bifurcation to the esophagogastric junction with a lower level at 32 cm for the incisors; and the lower thoracic esophagus, the distal half of the esophagus from the tracheal bifurcation to the gastroesophageal junction. This designation is based upon strict anatomical landmarks (see Figure 12-14).

A more practical application and designation often is used, dividing the esophagus into three parts: the upper third, from the cricopharyngeus to the superior portion of the aortic arch; the middle third, from the superior portion of the aortic arch to the inferior pulmonary vein; and the lower third, from the inferior pulmonary vein to the gastroesophageal junction. This classification is useful for

Figure 12-14. Landmarks of Esophageal Anatomy

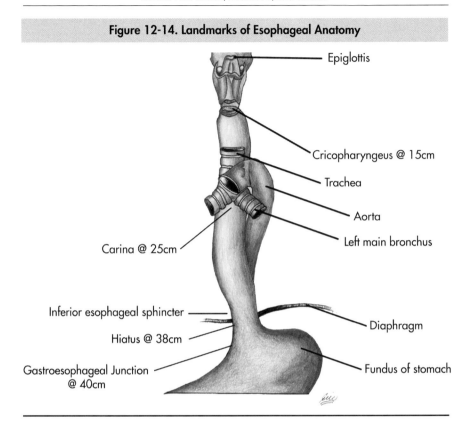

Epiglottis

Cricopharyngeus @ 15cm

Trachea

Aorta

Left main bronchus

Carina @ 25cm

Inferior esophageal sphincter

Hiatus @ 38cm

Diaphragm

Gastroesophageal Junction @ 40cm

Fundus of stomach

the distribution for the site of occurrence of disease. Approximately 15% of tumors are found in the upper third, 50% in the middle third, and 35% in the lower third (Roth et al., 1997). An extensive lymphatic supply is in the esophagus, allowing for fluids to travel to any other portion of the esophagus (see Figure 12-15). Tumors in any portion of the esophagus may drain into the cervical or supraclavicular nodes. Even though the pattern of drainage in the esophagus is unpredictable, it usually spreads longitudinally. The typical pattern of distribution is the upper third drains into the internal jugular, cervical, and supraclavicular regions; the middle third drains into the peritracheal, hilar, subcarinal, paraesophageal, periaortic, and pericardial regions; and the lower third drains into the lesser curvature, the left gastric, and celiac axis (Roth et al.).

Cellular Characteristics

Squamous cell carcinoma (> 85%) and adenocarcinoma (10%) are the two most common histological types of esophageal cancer. A rising incidence of adenocarcinoma is occurring in the United States at a rate of up to 20% (Blot et al., 1993). Because the majority of the esophagus is lined with squamous epithelium, most of

Figure 12-15. Lymphatic Drainage of the Esophagus

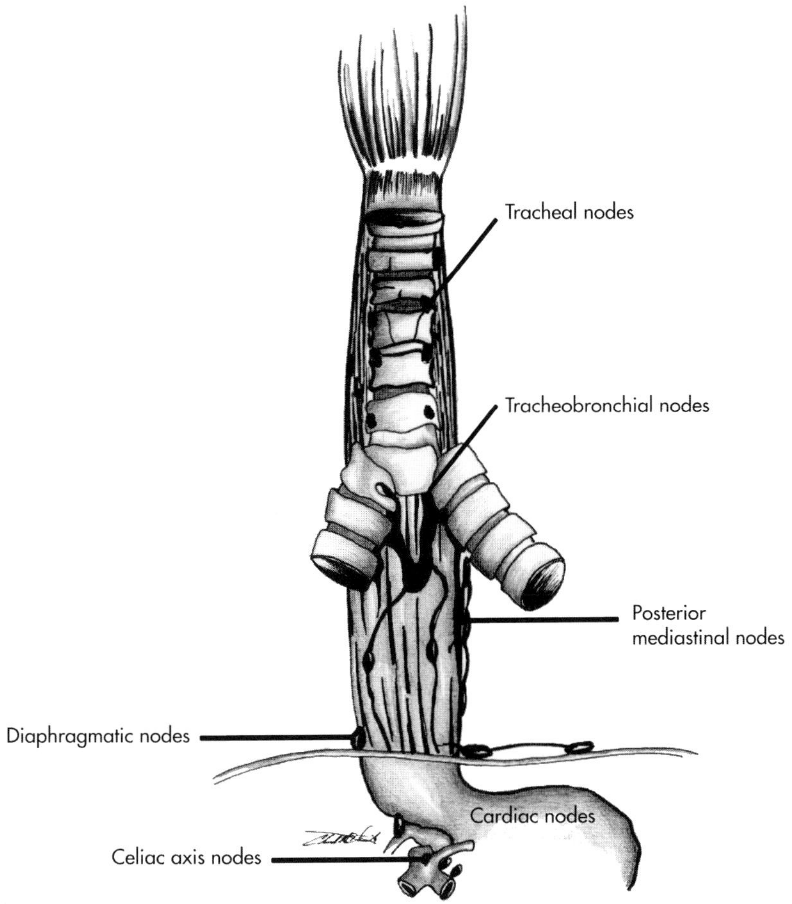

Tracheal nodes

Tracheobronchial nodes

Posterior mediastinal nodes

Diaphragmatic nodes

Cardiac nodes

Celiac axis nodes

these malignancies would be squamous cell in origin (Blot et al., 1993). Yet in the distal esophagus, an equal distribution is present of squamous cell and adenocarcinoma. These tumors often are in the esophagogastric area, and if the cellular type is adenocarcinoma, it often is a primary gastric tumor that has extended from the stomach into the esophagus.

Pattern of Disease Progression

The staging of esophageal cancer is pertinent to determine the treatment approach. The TNM staging system is outlined in Table 12-9. Esophageal tumors rarely are detected early, when they are most easily treated. Patients often

Table 12-9. TNM Classificatioin System for Esophageal Cancer

Definition of TNM

Primary Tumor (T)
TX   Primary tumor cannot be assessed.
T0   No evidence of primary tumor
Tis   Carcinoma in situ
T1   Tumor invades lamina propria or submucosa
T2   Tumor invades muscularis propria
T3   Tumor invades adventitia
T4   Tumor invades adjacent structures

Regional Lymph Nodes (N)
NX   Regional lymph nodes cannot be assessed.
N0   No regional lmph node metastasis
N1   Regional lymph node metastasis

Distant Metastasis (M)
MX   Presence of distant metastasis cannot be assessed.
N0   No distant metastasis
M1   Distant metastasis

Stage Grouping			
Stage 0	Tis	N0	M0
Stage I	T1	N0	M0
Stage IIA	T2	N0	M0
	T3	N0	M0
Stage IIB	T1	N1	M0
	T2	N1	M0
Stage III	T3	N1	M0
	T4	Any N	M0
Stage IV	Any T	Any N	M1
Stage IVA	Any T	Any N	M1a
Stage IVB	Any T	Any N	M1b

Note. From *AJCC Cancer Staging Manual* (5th ed.) (p. 66), by American Joint Committee on Cancer, 1997, Philadelphia: Lippincott-Raven. Copyright 1997 by Lippincott-Raven. Reprinted with permission.

are asymptomatic because the esophagus is rather distensible. Patients most often present to their healthcare providers with large tumors and obstructive symptoms. The five-year survival rates are directly related to the stage of disease at diagnosis. For stage 0, the five-year survival rate is more than 90%; stage I, 50%–80%; stage IIA, 15%–30%; stage IIB, 10%–30%; stage III, less than 10%; and with stage IV five-year survival is very rare (Bonin, Coia, Hoff, & Paz, 2000).

Tumors are able to spread to the adjacent tissues early in the disease as a result of the lack of serosal covering in the esophagus. In squamous cell tumors, the extent to which the tumor extends beyond the lumen wall into the adjacent structures is as high as 60% of cases (Anderson & Lad, 1982). This tumor invasion often prevents surgical resection. Tumors of the upper esophagus may invade the tissues of the carotid arteries, pleurae, laryngeal nerves, trachea, left main stem bronchus, or aortic arch. Tumors of the lower esophagus may invade the tissues of the pericardium, pleurae, descending aorta, and diaphragm. Tumor invasion of these types may make a surgical option obsolete.

The metastatic pattern for these tumors is typically via the lymphatic system. Lesions of the upper esophagus typically metastasize upward to the jugular and supraclavicular nodes. The middle esophagus tumors metastasize to the subdiaphragm and mediastinal nodes. The tumors of the lower esophagus often follow the pattern of metastasis to the lymph nodes of the abdomen.

Cancer of the esophagus can spread to almost any area of the body. Distant metastases often are not present at the time of first diagnosis. The most common sites of metastasis are the liver, lung, stomach, peritoneum, kidney, adrenal gland, brain, and bone (Roth et al., 1997).

Risk Factors

Dietary Factors

Environmental factors such as nutrition seem to play an important role in the development of esophageal tumors (see Figure 12-16). Environmental factors may be more significant than hereditary factors in this disease (Sammon, 1992). Diets that are deficient of essential vitamins (e.g., A, E, C, riboflavin, niacin, zinc) appear to increase the risk of developing esophageal cancer (Krevsky, 1995). In addition to these vitamin deficiencies, diets that have an accumulation of nitrates and potentially carcinogenic nitrosamines also are of concern. In areas of the world where the population is exposed to tannin, asbestos fiber, and water contamination by petroleum oils, the prevalence of esophageal cancer is higher. A prolonged ingestion of hot beverages also has been implied in the incidence of esophageal cancer (Stellman & Stellman, 1996). Fungal contamination of food products may be another important factor (Kirby & Rice, 1994).

Age

An age-associated increase exists in the risk of developing both squamous cell and adenocarcinoma of the esophagus. In both cases, the disease is rare for people who are younger than age 40 but increases in incidence with each decade of life (Krevsky, 1995).

Gender

Men are two to three times more likely to develop squamous cell carcinoma of the esophagus than women. In addition, they also have increased mortality rates (Kirby & Rice, 1994). Men are at 7–10 times the risk of developing adenocarcinoma of the esophagus than women (Wingo et al., 1996).

Figure 12-16. Risk Factors for Squamous Cell Carcinoma of the Esophagus

Environmental
- Geographic location
- Low soil molybdenum level
- Soil salinity
- Thermal
- Vulcanization process exposure in factory
- Water pollution by petroleum products

Dietary
- Aflatoxin
- Asbestos
- Bush tea
- Fungi (e.g., fusarium, alternaria)
- Maize consumption
- Nutritional deficiencies: Vitamins A, E, and C, riboflavin, niacin, and zinc
- Nitrosamines

Chronic irritation
- Achalasia
- Injection sclerotherapy

Reflux esophagitis
- Lye ingestion

Habits
- Alcoholic beverage consumption
- Smoking

Cultural
- Low socioeconomic status
- Race

Miscellaneous
- Hiatal hernia
- Ionizing radiation
- Papillomavirus
- Pharyngoesophageal diverticulum
- Plummer-Vinson syndrome
- Sprue
- Tylosis

Note. From "Tumors of the Esophagus" (p. 538), by B. Krevsky in W.S. Haubrich, F. Schaffner, and J.E. Berk (Eds.), *Bockus Gastroenterology*, 1995, Philadelphia: W.B. Saunders. Copyright 1995 by W.B. Saunders. Reprinted with permission.

Alcohol and Tobacco

Smoking and alcohol in combination potentiate the risk of developing squamous cell carcinoma. Individuals who smoke more than 30 grams of tobacco a day and ingest 120 grams of alcohol daily have a 44-fold increased risk of developing carcinoma of the esophagus (Franceschi et al., 1990). The role of tobacco and alcohol as a risk factor for development of adenocarcinoma is not as defined. The risk is not as significant as in squamous cell carcinoma, unless the use of tobacco and alcohol are combined in the presence of Barrett's esophagus (Kabat, Ng, & Wynder, 1993).

Barrett's Esophagus

Barrett's esophagus is defined as a progressive metaplasia of the distal esophagus as a result of prolonged reflux esophagitis and gastroesophageal reflux (Streitz, 1994). The premalignant condition is the most important risk factor for developing adenocarcinoma of the esophagus. The disorder predominantly affects White men in their 50s (Kruse, Boesby, Bernstein, & Andersen, 1993). The prevalence data of development of adenocarcinoma in the presence of Barrett's esophagus may be over exaggerated, because individuals often may not seek medical advice until they have developed complications of ulcerations, strictures, or cancer (Paraf, Flejou, Pignon, Fekete, & Potet, 1995). In addition, a case-control study demonstrated a causal relationship between esophageal adenocarcinoma and gastroesophageal reflux (Lagergren, Bergstrom, Lindgren, & Nyren, 1999).

Tylosis

Tylosis is an autosomal disorder that is characterized by hyperkeratosis of the palms and soles. Squamous cell carcinoma and tylosis are genetically linked. The dominant form is associated with a high risk for cancer development. Approximately 50% of these individuals will develop cancer by age 45, although that number increases to 95% by age 65 (Maruyama, 1992). Periodic screening is recommended for family members. Prophylactic esophagectomies have been suggested in individuals with tylosis because of the strong statistical support that they likely will develop carcinoma.

Achalasia

This disorder is an abnormal condition in which the muscle has an inability to relax. Achalasia is considered a premalignant condition (Krevsky, 1995). Patients with more than a 20-year history of achalasia have a 2%–8% prevalence rate of esophageal cancer (Meijssen, Tilanus, van Blankenstein, Hop, & Ong, 1992). These squamous cell carcinomas often will present in a later stage as a result of the symptoms mimicking the chronic esophageal complaints. These patients will have esophagitis secondary to chronic stasis and retained food, dilation, and obstruction. Annual endoscopic or radiologic screening is encouraged for patients with achalasia in an attempt to detect these malignancies at an early stage (Levine & Halorsen, 1994).

Lye Ingestion

Individuals with a history of lye ingestion have a risk of developing squamous cell cancer of the esophagus that is 1,000-fold greater than the general population (Isolauri & Markkula, 1989). Scarring and chronic inflammation are predisposing risk factors. The interval between ingestion and development of cancer is typically 40–45 years. These individuals often have an improved prognosis secondary to the fact that they usually seek medical attention early, soon after ingesting the lye. Routine screening also is recommended in these individuals (Isolauri & Markkula).

Signs and Symptoms

Dysphagia

The most common presenting sign of esophageal cancer is dysphagia or difficulty swallowing. It indicates that one-half to three-quarters of the lumen is narrowed. As a result of this narrowing, extensive involvement often occurs of the esophagus and surrounding structures. This is a negative prognostic sign. Individuals often are symptomatic for two to four months prior to seeking medical treatment (Ferguson & Skinner, 1995). The dysphagia is progressive. Initially, individuals have difficulty swallowing solids until they are unable to tolerate solid food at all. Eventually, they develop difficulty with liquids until they are unable to swallow their own saliva.

Weight Loss

Weight loss is the second most common symptom at presentation. This weight loss is often significant, usually more than 10% of total body weight. Anorexia, anemia, and dehydration are common complications to this aggressive weight loss (Coleman, 1997).

Odynophagia

Odynophagia is a severe sensation of burning or squeezing pain that occurs when swallowing. Approximately 50% of patients have odynophagia at presentation (Roth et al., 1997). It is commonly a dull pain that radiates to the back. Individuals also may have persistent substernal chest pain or episodes of hiccups. These are more ominous signs that often indicate metastatic involvement. In these cases, supraclavicular and cervical nodal metastases may be palpated (see Figure 12-17).

Prevention

Lifestyle

Important lifestyle changes have an impact on prevention of esophageal carcinomas. The intention of these lifestyle changes is to reduce an individual's risk factors for the development of this disease. Alterations in diet, including attention to keeping it low in fat and rich in vitamins and minerals, are essential changes. Cessation of smoking and limited alcohol consumption also will decrease the risk for development of esophageal cancers.

In addition to alterations in diet, decreasing obesity may influence esophageal cancer risk. The stage at which diet may attribute to this risk is unknown. Weight reduction also decreases risk for gastroesophageal reflux disease (GERD). Decreases in obesity will improve the symptoms of GERD, which is a risk factor for Barrett's esophagus.

Recent clinical trials in the area of chemoprevention demonstrated that the risk of adenocarcinoma is greatest among those with the greatest body mass and least

Figure 12-17. Signs and Symptoms of Squamous Cell Carcinoma of the Esophagus in Order of Occurrence

Dysphagia
Weight loss
Odynophagia
Vomiting
Hoarseness
Cough
Regurgitation
Hematemesis or melena
Iron-deficiency anemia
Pain
Pharyngeal discomfort
Hiccups
Horner's syndrome
Superior vena cava syndrome
Malignant pleural effusion
Malignant ascites
Bone pain
Palpable supraclavicular or cervical adenopathy

Note. From "Tumors of the Esophagus" (p. 536) by B. Krevsky in W.S. Haubrich, F. Schaffner, and J.E. Berk (Eds.), *Bockus Gastroenterology,* 1995, Philadelphia: W.B. Saunders. Copyright 1995 by W.B. Saunders. Reprinted with permission.

among those with the lowest body mass. The risk also was greatest in people who consumed the least amount of vegetables (Brown et al., 1995).

Chemoprevention

The role of chemoprevention in this disease is important because of the poor prognosis. Multiple chemoprevention trials are being developed in an attempt to improve mortality rates.

One interesting area of chemoprevention in this disease evaluates the level of cell proliferation. Because of the high level of proliferation in Barrett's esophagus, inhibitors of cell proliferation were addressed. For example, one important inhibitor called difluoromethylornithine (DFMO) was administered to eight patients with Barrett's for 12 weeks. Cell proliferation was reduced with DFMO and returned to control values when discontinued (Gerner, Garewal, Emerson, & Sampliner, 1994). Presently, multi-institutional phase II clinical trials are furthering this research base.

Another area of chemoprevention is the attempt to induce protective mechanisms, especially in the instance of Barrett's esophagus. In research trials, glutathione-S-transferase enzyme activity has a protective effect to the exposure of carcinogens (Hayes & Pulford, 1995). Glutathione was measured in patients with Barrett's metaplasia, and the enzyme activity was significantly less than in the gastric and duodenal mucosa of the same patients. This would imply that a lower level of protection exists from the development of cellular and genetic damage in the patients with Barrett's metaplasia (Peters, Roelofs, Hectors,

Nagengast, & Jansen, 1993). Further studies are continuing in this area of research to expand the knowledge base.

A third popular area of research in chemoprevention is the use of aspirin and NSAIDs. In a large population-based, case-control study, an association existed between a reduced risk of esophageal adenocarcinoma, squamous cell carcinoma, and noncardia gastric adenocarcinoma with the use of aspirin and NSAIDs (Farrow et al., 1998). Approximately a 50% reduced risk of these cancers was observed in patients who used aspirin or NSAIDs once a week for six months or more. The mechanism for this decreased risk is by reducing the prostaglandin synthesis; tumor cell growth, metastasis, and host immune function are affected (Subbaramaiah, Zakim, Weksler, & Dannenberg, 1997).

Aspirin and NSAIDs also may inhibit esophageal carcinoma by decreasing the cell proliferation in Barrett's esophagus via cyclo-oxygenase inhibition. Two isoforms of cyclo-oxygenase are COX-1 and COX-2 (DuBois, Awad, Morrow, Roberts, & Bishop, 1994). Inflammation increases prostaglandin synthesis, likely secondary to upregulation of COX-2. Inflammation is a known risk factor for epithelial carcinogenesis (Weitzman & Gordon, 1990). More recently, studies are investigating the selective COX-2 inhibitors in the area of chemoprevention because they appear to have fewer GI side effects than aspirin and NSAIDs. Because patients are able to tolerate selective COX-2 inhibitors, they are more attractive to design studies for chemoprevention.

In addition, the selective COX-2 inhibitors are being evaluated for their effect on apoptosis or programmed cell death. These agents are thought to induce apoptosis by reducing the resistance caused by COX-2 overexpression. These agents presently are being investigated to induce apoptosis in esophageal adenocarcinomas (Hughes et al., 1997).

Early Detection

Routine screening typically is not performed in the United States because of the low incidence rates. A formal screening program with recommendations is more appropriate for endemic areas such as China and Japan. In these areas, techniques of esophageal balloon cytology and flow cytometry have been evaluated for their effectiveness in mass screenings. The results of these studies have shown that these techniques are useful in identifying high-risk populations that should maintain close follow-up for malignancies (Liu et al., 1994).

High-Risk Patients

High-risk patients outside the area of endemic populations include those with Barrett's esophagus, squamous cell carcinoma in another site in the upper aerodigestive tract, tylosis, achalasia, history of lye ingestion, and prolonged and habitual alcohol and tobacco use. In addition, patients with significant risk factors, including a combination of age and gender, should be monitored closely.

Screening should include endoscopy or barium swallow and is likely to be justified in patients who are high risk or symptomatic. These procedures also should be considered in immigrants from high-risk regions (Bonin, Coia, Hoff, & Paz, 2000). Patients with achalasia or a history of lye ingestion should be screened annually with endoscopic or radiologic techniques to detect carcinomas at an early stage. As a result of variations in incidence per population, presently no specific guidelines for screening these individuals are available. The screening guidelines are to be determined by the practitioner through a prudent understanding of these high-risk groups.

Nursing Challenges

Patient and Family Education

Esophageal cancers have a poor prognosis because these tumors are identified at a late stage in the disease. Nurses must educate patients and the public about risk factors for this disease. Nurses can play a pivotal role in education about smoking cessation, decreased alcohol consumption, and the importance of dietary factors. Interactions with all patient groups, from the healthy to those undergoing therapy, should target the importance of a diet that includes essential vitamins and leads to achieving a healthy body weight.

The nurse's role in the education about signs and symptoms of esophageal cancers, especially dysphagia, odynophagia, and weight loss, also is important. The nurse should advocate for the individual who is experiencing these symptoms and assist in obtaining the appropriate level of care.

Education for the families of these individuals includes ideas for support of the patient from diagnosis to treatment. In addition, if the patient has a hereditary risk factor such as tylosis, education for screening and genetic counseling should be given to the family members. Referral to community support groups may help family members with care issues, decision making, and coping.

Anal Cancer

Epidemiology

Anal cancer includes lesions of the anus, anal canal, and anorectum. An improved survival rate of approximately 80% exists with a combined modality treatment with chemotherapy and radiation (Cummings, 1990). An estimated 3,500 new cases will be diagnosed in 2001, and approximately 500 individuals will die of the disease (Greenlee et al., 2001). Most of these tumors are epidermoid carcinoma (Shank, Cunningham, & Kelsen, 1997).

Epidermoid carcinoma of the anal region has an increasing incidence rate mainly among women, unmarried men, and people living in or near large cities (Melbye, Rabkin, Frisch, & Biggar, 1994). The incidence rate for single men is six times that for married men. In individuals younger than 35 years old, anal cancer is more common in men than women (Coia, Ellenhorn, & Ayoub, 2000).

A number of case-control studies have linked the incidence of anal cancer to sexually transmitted diseases or homosexual contact (Daling et al., 1987). In addition, a strong link exists between anal cancer and cervical cancer because of the presence of human papillomavirus (HPV) (Frisch et al., 1997). A strong association exists between the development of anal cancer and individuals with a history of male homosexual contact or genital warts (condylomata acuminata) (Daling et al.).

Pathophysiology

To understand the natural history of this disease, a distinction must be made between the anal canal and the anal margin. The upper limit of the anal canal is the anorectal ring. The anorectal ring is the muscle formed by the junction of the upper portion of the internal sphincter, the distal portion of the longitudinal muscle, the puborectalis, and the deep portion of the external sphincter (Shank et al., 1997) (see Figure 12-18). This can be palpated with a digital rectal examination. AJCC and UICC have agreed that the anal canal is measured from the anorectal ring to the anal verge (AJCC, 1997). This is an important distinction for staging and to determine appropriate margins for surgery (see Table 12-10).

Cellular Characteristics

Many different histological types of tumor cells exist, but the most common are the epidermoid (squamous) tumors. Rare histological tumors include small cell carcinomas, anorectal melanoma, or primary adenocarcinoma (Shank et al., 1997).

Pattern of Disease Progression

Cancers of the anal canal often spread by local extension, involving other organs of the pelvis. Local extension often is common at presentation. Other structures that are less likely but can be involved are the prostate, urethra, bladder, and

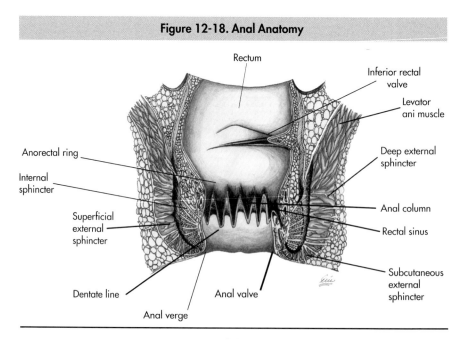

Figure 12-18. Anal Anatomy

Rectum

Inferior rectal valve

Levator ani muscle

Anorectal ring

Internal sphincter

Deep external sphincter

Superficial external sphincter

Anal column

Rectal sinus

Subcutaneous external sphincter

Dentate line

Anal valve

Anal verge

Table 12-10. TNM Classification System for Anal Cancer

Definition of TNM

Primary Tumor (T)

TX   Primary tumor cannot be assessed.
T0   No evidence of primary tumor
Tis Carcinoma in situ
T1   Tumor 2 cm or less in greatest dimension
T2   Tumor more than 2 cm but not more than 5 cm in greatest dimension
T3   Tumor more than 5 cm in greatest dimension
T4   Tumor of any size invades adjacent organ(s) (e.g., vagina, urethra, bladder). (Involvement of sphincter muscle(s) alone is not classified as T4.)

Regional Lymph Nodes (N)

NX   Regional lymph nodes cannot be assessed.
N0   No regional lymph node metastasis
N1   Metastasis in perirectal lymph node(s)
N2   Metastasis in unilateral internal iliac or inguinal lymph node(s)
N3   Metastasis in perirectal and inguinal lymph nodes or bilateral internal iliac or inguinal lymph nodes

Distant Metastasis (M)

MX   Presence of distant metastasis cannot be assessed.
M0   No distant metastasis
M1   Distant metastasis

Stage Grouping

Stage 0	Tis	N0	M0
Stage I	T1	N0	M0
Stage II	T2	N0	M0
	T3	N0	M0
Stage IIIA	T1	N1	M0
	T2	N1	M0
	T3	N1	M0
	T4	N0	M0
Stage IIIB	T4	N1	M0
	Any T	N2	M0
	Any T	N3	M0
Stage IV	Any T	Any N	M1

Note. From *AJCC Cancer Staging Manual* (5th ed.) (p. 92) by American Joint Committee on Cancer, 1997, Philadelphia: Lippincott-Raven. Copyright 1997 by Lipincott-Raven. Reprinted with permission.

seminal vesicles (Stearns, Urmacher, Sternberg, Woodruff, & Attiyeh, 1980). Disease progression also occurs through the blood supply. This pattern allows cells into the portal system for the development of liver metastases. It also permits travel to the lung and bone (Stearns et al.). Lymphatic spread also occurs. In 15%–63% of anal cancers, the inguinal lymph nodes are involved (Clark, Petrelli, Herrera, & Mittelman, 1986). Pelvic nodes and mesenteric nodes also are involved but much less frequently (Stearns et al.).

Risk Factors

The risk factors for development of anal carcinoma are primarily lifestyle behaviors, such as male homosexual practices, anal receptive intercourse in men but not women, and a history of condylomata acuminata. As a result of these lifestyle factors, a greater risk exists for viral exposure. Viral exposure to HPV and condylomata acuminata increases one's risk for disease. Anal carcinoma has been linked to condylomata acuminata in the general population even without the specific lifestyle factors (Prasad & Abcarian, 1980).

Another significant risk factor for anal cancer is human immunodeficiency virus (HIV). Increasing numbers of men with anal abnormalities are HIV-infected. Often these individuals have a concurrent HIV and HPV infection (Abrams, 1991).

Anal intraepithelial neoplasia (AIN) may develop into a malignant process. AIN is more common in HIV-positive men and is found in 15%–30% of cases. Anal cancer often develops from AIN, although it may take many years to occur. The risk of developing anal cancer from AIN increases with advanced immunosuppression (Palefsky, 1994).

Anal carcinomas also have been associated with other benign anorectal diseases and anal fistulas. A high risk of anal cancer exists after the first year of diagnosis of a benign condition, and it rapidly decreases in time (Frisch, Olsen, Bautz, & Melbye, 1995).

Cigarette smoking also is a risk factor for the development of anal cancer. In a case-control study, it was demonstrated that cigarette smoking was a major risk factor for both sexes, with a relative risk of 7.4 in women and 9.4 in men (Daling et al., 1987).

Signs and Symptoms

The symptoms of anal cancer often are confused with benign conditions of hemorrhoids and anal fissures. The most common presenting symptom is bleeding, which occurs in half of patients (Clark et al., 1986). Other common symptoms include pain, pruritis, change in bowel habits, abnormal discharge, and tenesmus or spasms of the rectum. Less frequently, the individual will present with inguinal lymphadenopathy (Greenall, Quan, & DeCosse, 1985).

The difficulty that occurs with these signs and symptoms is that they are similar to the benign conditions that people have in combination with the diagnosis of anal cancer. It is not uncommon for individuals to experience a delay in diagnosis while they are being treated for the benign condition. These individuals usually will not begin an evaluation for cancer until the benign condition is ruled out. This delay or inappropriate diagnosis occurs in one-third of patients (Pyper & Parks, 1985).

Prevention

The greatest factor that could influence the incidence of anal carcinoma is education. A variety of risk factors should be made known to the public. By increasing the awareness of the link between sexually transmitted diseases and anal cancer, lifestyle changes could occur. A successful campaign for "safe sex" practices has been linked to preventing the transmission of HIV. This should be expanded to include the risk of developing anal carcinoma.

In addition, smoking cessation programs and assistance should continue to develop for patients. Together, with a long list of diseases that one has an increased risk of developing with smoking, anal cancer should be added as a concern.

Early Detection

Along with the need for education regarding the prevention of this disease, education about the signs and symptoms should be a priority. To accomplish improvements in early detection, individuals need to be aware of the symptoms and the cross over between these symptoms with benign disease. High-risk individuals, especially male homosexuals and individuals who are immunosuppressed, need aggressive education; patients diagnosed with HPV or condylomata acuminata also should be included in this group.

In addition to education, high-risk individuals should have regular digital rectal examinations. Practitioners must follow these individuals closely for evaluation of health status and signs and symptoms of disease. Anal Pap tests or anoscopy also have been suggested for high-risk patients (Brogdon, 1997). Screening guidelines at this time do not exist, but these evaluations should be considered and discussed with those at high risk.

Chemoprevention

Currently, only one study is looking at chemoprevention of anal cancer. Clinical studies have suggested that synthetic retinoids inhibit the progression of epithelial preneoplastic conditions and some neoplastic states (Palefsky, Northfelt, Kaplan, & Critchlow, 2000). The phase I trial first is evaluating the dose of this synthetic retinoid. Second, the trial is analyzing the efficacy of isotretinoin alone or in combination with IFN alfa-2a to prevent progression or recurrence of anal intraepithelial neoplasia.

Nursing Challenges

Patient and Family Education

Nurses can provide a tremendous amount of education regarding the prevention and early detection of anal cancer. Nurses must educate the patient and the public about the risk factors and the signs and symptoms of disease. In addition, education regarding "safe sex" practices and smoking cessation are keys to improving outcomes.

Continuity of Care for Gastrointestinal Malignancies

Nurses can be of great assistance navigating patients through the healthcare system. Nurses enter the patients' experiences at all levels of the disease. During routine health examinations, the patients should be assessed for risk factors and educated on screening. If the individual is experiencing symptoms, the nurse needs to advocate for the patient regarding access to practitioners who will perform appropriate interventions for diagnosis. Nurses may follow these patients through the continuum of therapy, and, through education and advocacy, they become essential links to assisting patients with these diseases.

Nurses are able to obtain information for patients and families to assist with the explanation of a variety of diagnostic tests and treatment modalities. This assistance can provide the opportunity to make informed decisions regarding their care. Further, nurses are experts in assessing for complications or side effects of treatment and are in a position to make recommendations for management of these symptoms.

Nurses are highly skilled at providing education and support for the patient and family in a time of stress and emotional crisis. GI cancers often cannot be cured because of the late stage of disease at presentation, and the individual and family will need help in coping with emotions related to that reality. The nurse is an excellent source of emotional support, which is enhanced by directing the patient and family to formal support groups and resources, as appropriate.

Nurses are dedicated to advocating for the patient at all levels of care. Patient advocacy also includes improving access for underserved populations, especially those in high-risk groups.

Nursing can have a strong impact on early detection in these particular disease sites through the use of education that focuses on screening and chemoprevention.

Presenting patient education information on a basic, comprehensive level gives patients the knowledge they need to obtain care in a timely manner, as opposed to diminishing the importance and significance of symptoms. Starting at diagnosis, through treatment, and into follow-up care, nurses are the consistent, caring presence that is integral to the access and quality of health care.

Conclusion

Nothing is more important in the area of GI malignancies than focusing attention to early diagnosis and treatment. In this population, it is common to see patients diagnosed with advanced disease associated with a negative prognostic outcome. Areas of research are expanding regarding screening and chemoprevention, and this area of study will continue to grow.

The majority of the current research base in early detection and screening is in CRC, with the other GI malignancies slow to follow. The model of growing research interest in CRC should be duplicated to improve the research in other GI malignancies. Standards of care for screening should be provided in all areas of GI malignancies.

With the model of CRC, specific standards are available for screening and early detection. Other disease sites discussed in this chapter hopefully will follow with standards of their own. Nurses are an excellent resource to disseminate this information to the public and healthcare providers. In addition to traditional roles such as health teaching, nurses are beginning to expand to diagnostic positions as nurse endoscopists. This offers great potential to develop improved models for training in endoscopy, increase knowledge through research studies, and increase the number of screening examinations that lead to improved outcomes.

This is an exciting time of opportunity for growth regarding prevention and early detection in all areas of GI malignancies, including rich prospects for future nursing research. The improvement of patients' understanding is essential to the importance of early detection and screening, and nurses should assist with access to care. In addition, nurses should work closely with patient advocacy groups to promote screening. Concentrated efforts are needed to reduce the number of lives that are lost to these prevalent GI malignancies.

Gastrointestinal Malignancies Resources

American Cancer Society
www.cancer.org
800-ACS-2345

American Institute for Cancer Research
www.aicr.org
800-843-8114

American Liver Foundation
www.liverfoundation.org
800-223-0179

Cancer Care, Inc.
www.cancercare.org
800-813-HOPE

Colon Cancer Alliance
www.ccalliance.org
212-439-1101

Colorectal Cancer Network
www.onelist.com/subscribe/
301-879-1500

Gene Clinics
www.geneclinics.org

Genetics of Cancer
www.cancergenetics.org/

Hereditary Cancer Institute
www.medicine.creighton.edu/meschool/prevmed/hc.html
800-648-8133

National Cancer Institute's CancerNet, Physician's Data Query
www.cancernet.nci.nih.gov
800-4-CANCER

References

Abrams, D.I. (1991). Acquired immunodeficiency syndrome and related malignancies: A topical overview. *Seminars in Oncology, 18*(Suppl. 7), 41–45.

Ahlquist, D.A., & Johnson, C.D. (1999). Innovative techniques for colorectal cancer screening. *Primary Care and Cancer, 19*, 10–21.

Ahlquist, D.A., Skoletsky, J.E., Boynton, K.A., Harrington, J.J., Mahoney, D.W., Pierceall, W.E., Thibodeau, S.N., & Shuber, A.P. (2000). Colorectal cancer screening by detection of altered human DNA in stool: Feasibility of a multitarget assay panel. *Gastroenterology, 119*, 1219–1227.

Albanes, D., Heinonen, O.P., Huttunen, J.K., Taylor, P.R., Virtamo, J., Edwards, B.K., Haapakoski, J., Rautalahti, M., Hartman, A.M., & Palmgren, J. (1995). Effects of alphatocopherol and beta-carotene supplements on cancer incidence in the Alpha-Tocopherol Beta-Carotene Cancer Prevention Study. *American Journal of Clinical Nutrition, 62*(Suppl. 6), 1427S–1430S.

Albert, C. (1995). Clinical aspects of gastric cancer. In A.K. Rustgi (Ed.), *Gastrointestinal cancers: Biology, diagnosis, and therapy* (pp. 197–216). Philadelphia: Lippincott-Raven.

Alberts, D.S., Martinez, M.E., Roe, D.J., Guillen-Rodriguez, J.M., Marshall, J.R., Van Leeuwen, B., Reid, M.E., Ritenbaugh, C., & Vargas, P.A. (2000). Lack of effect of a high fiber cereal supplement on the recurrence of colorectal adenomas. *New England Journal of Medicine, 342*, 1156–1162.

Alexander, H.R., Kelsen, D.G., & Tepper, J.C. (1997). Cancer of the stomach. In V.T. DeVita, Jr., S. Hellman, & S.A. Rosenberg (Eds.), *Cancer: Principles and practice of oncology* (5th ed.) (pp. 1021–1054). Philadelphia: Lippincott-Raven.

American Academy of Pediatrics Committee on Infectious Diseases. (1992). Universal hepatitis B immunization. *Pediatrics, 89*, 795–800.

American Cancer Society. (2000). *Cancer facts and figures, 2000.* Atlanta: Author.

American Joint Committee on Cancer. (1997). *AJCC cancer staging manual* (5th ed.). Philadelphia: Lippincott-Raven.

Anderson, L.L., & Lad, T.E. (1982). Autopsy findings in squamous cell carcinoma of the esophagus. *Cancer, 50*, 1587–1590.

Anderson, L.M., & May, D.S. (1995). Has the use of cervical, breast, and colorectal cancer screening increased in the United States? *American Journal of Public Health, 85*, 840–842.

Antonioli, D.A. (1990). Gastric carcinoma and its precursors. *Monographs in Pathology, 31*, 144–180.

Atkin, W.S., Morson, B.C., & Cuzick, J. (1992). Long-term risk of colorectal cancer after excision of rectosigmoid adenomas. *New England Journal of Medicine, 326*, 658–662.

Baron, J.A., Beach, M., Mandel, J.S., van Stolk, R.U., Haile, R.W., Sandler, R.S., Rothstein, R., Summers, R.W., Shover, D.C., Beck, G.J., Bond, J.H., & Greenberg, E.R. for the Calcium Polyp Prevention Study Group. (1999). Calcium supplements for the prevention of colorectal adenomas. *New England Journal of Medicine, 340*, 101–108.

Beahrs, O.H., & Sanfelippo, P.M. (1971). Factors in the prognosis of colon and rectal cancer. *Cancer, 28*, 213–218.

Bedine, M.S. (1999). Colorectal carcinoma: Etiology, diagnosis, and screening. *Comprehensive Therapy, 25*(3), 163–168.

Benson, A. (1999). NCCN practice guidelines for hepatobiliary cancers. *Oncology, 13,* 265–292.

Blei, A. (2000, April). Hepatocellular carcinoma—A clinical overview. In M. Talamonti (Chair), *Liver-directed therapy and primary hepatocellular cancer and secondary liver tumors.* Symposium conducted at the Robert H. Lurie Comprehensive Cancer Center of Northwestern University, Chicago, IL.

Blomjous, J.G., Hop, W.C., Langenhorst, B.L., ten Kate, F.J., Eykenboom, W.M., & Tilanus, H.W. (1992). Adenocarcinoma of the gastric cardia. Recurrence and survival after resection. *Cancer, 70,* 569–574.

Blot, W.J., Devesa, S.S., & Fraumeni, J.F. (1993). Continuing climb in rates of esophageal adenocarcinoma: An update. *JAMA, 270,* 1320.

Blot, W.J., Devesa, S.S., Kneller, R.W., & Fraumeni, J.F. (1991). Rising incidence of adenocarcinoma of the esophagus and gastric cardia. *JAMA, 265,* 1287–1298.

Boeing, H. (1991). Epidemiological research in stomach cancer: Progress over the last ten years. *Journal of Cancer Research in Clinical Oncology, 117,* 133–143.

Boland, C.R. (1999). Malignant tumors of the colon. In T. Yamada (Ed.), *Textbook of gastroenterology* (3rd ed.) (pp. 2023–2082). Philadelphia: Lippincott-Raven.

Boland, C.R., & Scheiman, J.M. (1995). Tumors of the stomach. In T. Yamada (Ed.), *Textbook of gastroenterology* (2nd ed.) (pp. 1494–1522). Philadelphia: Lippincott-Raven.

Bonin, S.R., Coia, L.R., Hoff, P.M., & Paz, I.B. (2000). Esophageal cancer. In R. Pazdur, L.R. Coia, W.J. Hoskins, & L.D. Wagman (Eds.), *Cancer management: A multidisciplinary approach* (4th ed.) (pp. 201–214). Melville, NY: PRR, Inc.

Bonin, S.R., Coia, L.R., Hoff, P.M., & Schwartz, R.E. (2000). Gastric cancer. In R. Pazdur, L.R. Coia, W.J. Hoskins, & L.D. Wagman (Eds.), *Cancer management: A multidisciplinary approach* (4th ed.) (pp. 215–225). Melville, NY: PRR, Inc.

Bonino, F., Negro, F., Baldi, M., Brunetto, M.R., Chiaberge, E., Capalbo, M. Maran, E., Lavarini, C., Rocca, N., & Rocca, G. (1987). The natural history of chronic delta hepatitis. In M. Rizetto, J.L.B. Erin, & R.M. Purcell (Eds.), *Progress in clinical and biological research* (Vol. 234) (pp. 145–152). New York: Alan R. Liss.

Bostick, R.M., Potter, J.D., McKenzie, D.R., Sellers, T.A., Kushi, L.H., Steinmetz, K.A., & Folsom, A.R. (1993). Reduced risk of colon cancer with high intake of vitamin E: The Iowa Women's Health Study. *Cancer Research, 53,* 4230–4237.

Bressac, B., Kew, M., Wards, J., & Ozturk, M. (1991). Selective GTOT mutations of p53 gene into hepatocellular carcinomas from Southern Africa. *Nature, 350,* 429–431.

Brogdon, C.F. (1997). Human immunodeficiency virus (HIV) and related cancers. In S.E. Otto (Ed.), *Oncology nursing* (3rd ed.) (pp. 268–283). St. Louis, MO: Mosby.

Brown, L.M., Swanson, C.A., Gridley, G., Swanson, G.M., Schoenberg, J.B., Greenberg, R.S., Silverman, D.T., Pottern, L.M., Hayes, R.B., & Schwartz, A.G. (1995). Adenocarcinoma of the esophagus: Role of obesity and diet. *Journal of the National Cancer Institute, 87,* 104–109.

Bruix, J., Llovet, J.M., Bru, C., & Rodes, J. (1997). Clinical presentation. In T.L. Livraghi, M. Makuuchi, & L. Buscarini (Eds.), *Diagnosis and treatment of hepatocellular carcinoma* (pp. 53–66). London: Greenwich Medical Media.

Bulow, S. (1980). Colorectal cancer in patients less than 40 years of age in Denmark. *Diseases of the Colon and Rectum, 23,* 327–336.

Burke, C.A., & van Stolk, R. (1999). Colorectal cancer screening: Making sense of the different guidelines. *Cleveland Clinic Journal of Medicine, 66,* 303–311.

Burstein, M., Monge, E., Leon-Barua, R., Lozano, R., Berendson, R., Gilman, R.H., Legua, H., & Rodriguez, C. (1991). Low peptic ulcer and high gastric cancer prevalence in a developing country with a high prevalence of infection by *Helicobacter pylori. Journal of Clinical Gastroenterology, 13,* 154.

Burt, R.W., Bishop, D.T., Lynch, H.T., Rozen, P., & Winawer, S.J. (1990). Risk and surveillance of individuals with heritable factors for colorectal cancer. *Bulletin of the World Health Organization, 68,* 655–665.

Burt, R.W., & Jacoby, R.F. (1999). Polyposis syndromes. In T. Yamada (Ed.), *Textbook of gastroenterology* (3rd ed.) (pp. 1995–2022). Philadelphia: Lippincott-Raven.

Burt, R.W., & Petersen, G.M. (1996). Familial colorectal cancer: Diagnosis and management. In G.P. Young, P. Rozen, & B. Levin (Eds.), *Prevention and early detection of colorectal cancer* (pp. 171–194). Philadelphia: W.B. Saunders.

Byers, T., Levin, B., Rothenberger, D., Dodd, G.D., & Smith, R.A. (1997). American Cancer Society guidelines for screening and surveillance for early detection of colorectal polyps and cancer: Update 1997. *CA: A Cancer Journal for Clinicians, 47,* 154–160.

Cance, W.G., Stewart, A.K., & Menck, H.R. (2000). The National Cancer Data Base Report on Treatment Patterns for Hepatocellular Carcinomas. *Cancer, 88,* 912–920.

Carr, B.I., Flickinger, J.C., & Lotze, M.T. (1997). Hepatobiliary cancers. In V.T. DeVita, S. Hellman, & S.A. Rosenberg (Eds.), *Cancer: Principles and practice of oncology* (5th ed.) (pp. 1987–1113). Philadelphia: Lippincott-Raven.

Centers for Disease Control and Prevention. (1989). *Hepatitis surveillance: Report no. 52.* Atlanta: U.S. Public Health Service.

Centers for Disease Control and Prevention. (2001). *Colorectal cancer prevention and control initiatives.* Retrieved August 9, 2001 from the World Wide Web: http://www.cdc.gov/cancer/colorctl

Clark, J., Petrelli, N., Herrera, L., & Mittelman, A. (1986). Epidermoid carcinoma of the anal canal. *Cancer, 57,* 400–406.

Clark, R.A., & Reintgen, D.S. (1996). Principles of cancer screening. In D.S. Reintgen & R.A. Clark (Eds.), *Cancer screening* (pp. 1–20). St. Louis, MO: Mosby.

Cohen, A.M., Minsky, B.D., & Schilsky, R.L. (1997). Cancers of the gastrointestinal tract. In V.T. DeVita, S. Hellman, & S.A. Rosenberg (Eds.), *Cancer: Principles and practice of oncology* (5th ed.) (pp. 1144–1188). Philadelphia: Lippincott-Raven.

Coia, L.R., Ellenhorn, J.D.I., & Ayoub, J.P. (2000). Colorectal and anal cancers. In R. Pazdur, L.R. Coia, W.J. Hoskins, & L.D. Wagman (Eds.), *Cancer management: A multidisciplinary approach* (4th ed.) (273–299). Melville, NY: PRR, Inc.

Coleman, J. (1997). Esophageal, stomach, liver, gallbladder, and pancreatic cancers. In S.L. Groenwald, M. Goodman, M.H. Frogge, & C.H. Yarbro (Eds.), *Cancer nursing: Principles and practice* (4th ed.) (1082–1144). Boston: Jones and Bartlett.

Collier, J., & Sherman, M. (1998). Screening for hepatocellular carcinoma. *Hepatology, 27,* 273–278.

Colombo, M., de Franchi, R., Del Ninno, E., Sangiovanni, A., DeFazio, C., Tommasini, M., Donato, M.F., Piva, A., DiCarlo, V., & Dioguardi, N. (1991). Hepatocellular carcinoma in Italian patients with cirrhosis. *New England Journal of Medicine, 325,* 675–680.

Colombo, M., & Sangiovanni, A. (1997). Etiology. In T.I. Livraghi, M. Makuuchi, & L. Buscarini (Eds.), *Diagnosis and treatment of hepatocellular carcinoma* (pp. 17–24). London: Greenwich Medical Media.

Cottone, M., & D'Antoni, A. (1997). Early detection and serum markers. In T.I. Livraghi, M. Makuuchi, & L. Buscarini (Eds.), *Diagnosis and treatment of hepatocellular carcinoma* (pp. 67–78). London: Greenwich Medical Media.

Cottone, M., Turri, M., Caltagirone, M., Parisi, P., Orlando, A., Fiorentino, G., Virdone, R., Fusco, G., Grasso, R., & Simonetti, R.G. (1994). Screening for hepatocellular carcinoma in patients with child's A cirrhosis: An 8-year prospective study by ultrasound and alpha-fetoprotein. *Journal of Hepatology, 21,* 1029–1034.

Cravo, M., Fidalgo, P., Pereira, A., Gouveia-Olivera, A., Chaves, P., Selhub, J., Mason, J.B., Mira, F.C., & Leitao, C.N. (1994). DNA methylation as an intermediate biomarker in colorectal cancer: Modulation by folic acid supplementation. *European Journal of Cancer Prevention, 3,* 473–479.

Cummings, B.J. (1990). Anal cancer. *International Journal of Radiation Oncology, Biology, and Physics, 19,* 1309–1315.

Daling, J.R., Weiss, N.S., Hislop, T.G., Maden, C., Coates, R.J., Sherman, K.J., Ashley, R.L., Beagrie, M., Ryan, J.A., & Corey, L. (1987). Sexual practices, sexually transmitted diseases, and the incidence of anal cancer. *New England Journal of Medicine, 317,* 973–977.

Davis, G.R. (1994). Neoplasms of the stomach. In M. Shleisenger & J. Fordtran (Eds.), *Gastrointestinal disease* (5th ed.) (pp. 763–848). Philadelphia: W.B. Saunders.

DeCosse, J.J., Miller, H.M., & Lesser, M.L. (1989). Effect of wheat fiber and vitamins C and E on rectal patients with familial adenomatous polyposis. *Journal of the National Cancer Institute, 81,* 1290.

Deuffic, S., Poynard, T., Buffat, L., & Valleron, A.J. (1998). Trends in primary liver cancer. *Lancet, 351,* 214–215.

DeWys, W.D., Begg, D., & Lavin, P.T. (1980). Prognostic effect of weight loss prior to chemotherapy in cancer patients. *American Journal of Medicine, 69,* 491.

Dienstag, J.L., & Isselbacher, K.J. (1994). Acute hepatitis. In K.J. Isselbacher, E. Braunwald, J.D. Wilson, J.B. Martin, A.S. Fauci, & D.L Kasper (Eds.), *Harrison's principles of internal medicine* (13th ed.) (pp. 1458–1478). New York: McGraw-Hill.

DiSario, J.A., & Sanowski, R.A. (1993). Sigmoidoscopy training for nurses and resident physicians. *Gastrointestinal Endoscopy, 39,* 29–32.

Douglas, H.O. (1991). Overview of gastrointestinal cancer: Two decades of progress. In A.R. Moossa, S.C. Schimpff, & M.C. Robson (Eds.), *Comprehensive textbook of oncology* (2nd ed.) (847–853). Baltimore: Williams & Wilkins.

Dubois, R.N. (1999). Cyclooxygenase and colorectal cancer prevention. In M.C. Perry (Ed.), *1999 educational book* (pp. 189–192). Alexandria, VA: American Society of Clinical Oncology.

DuBois, R.N., Awad, J., Morrow, J., Roberts, L.J., & Bishop, P.R. (1994). Regulation of eicosanoid production mitogenesis in rat intestinal epithelial cells by transforming growth factor and phorbolester. *Journal of Clinical Investigation, 93,* 493–498.

Dykes, C.M. (2001). Virtual colonoscopy: A new approach for colorectal cancer screening. *Gastroenterology Nursing, 24*(1), 5–11.

Ebara, M., Ohto, M., Shinagawa, T., Sugiura, N., Kimura, K., Matsutani, S., Morita, M., Saisho, H., Tsuchiya, Y., & Okuda, K. (1986). Natural history of minute hepatocellular carcinoma smaller than three centimeters complicating cirrhosis: A study in 22 patients. *Gastroenterology, 90,* 289–298.

Eberhart, C.E., Coffey, R.J., Radhika, A., Giardiello, F.M., Ferrenbach, S., & DuBois, R.N. (1994). Up-regulation of cyclooxygenase 2 gene expression in human colorectal adenomas and adenocarcinomas. *Gastroenterology, 107,* 1183–1188.

Eddy, D.M. (1990). Screening for colorectal cancer. *Annals of Internal Medicine, 113,* 373–384.

Eisemon, N., Stucky-Marshall, L., & Talamonti, M.S. (2001). Screening for colorectal cancer: Developing a preventive healthcare program utilizing nurse endoscopists. *Gastroenterology Nursing, 24*(1), 12–19.

El-Serag, H.B., & Mason, A.C. (1999). Rising incidence of hepatocellular carcinoma in the United States. *New England Journal of Medicine, 340,* 745–750.

Elder, J.B. (1995). Carcinoma of the stomach. In W.S. Haubrich & F. Schaffner (Eds.), *Bockus gastroenterology* (5th ed.) (pp. 854–874). Philadelphia: W.B. Saunders.

Ellis, F.H., Huberman, M., & Busse, P. (1995). Cancer of the esophagus. In G.P. Murphy, W. Lawrence, & R.E. Lenhard (Eds.), *American Cancer Society textbook of clinical oncology* (pp. 293–303). Atlanta: American Cancer Society.

Faivre, J., & Benhamiche, A.M. (1995). Gastric carcinoma: New developments in the field. *Gastroenterology, 90,* 2213–2216.

Falkson, G., Falkson, C.I., & Garbers, L.M. (1998). Hepatocellular carcinoma. In A.B. Benson (Ed.), *Gastrointestinal oncology* (pp. 83–101). Boston: Kluwer Academic Publishers.

Farrow, D.C., Vaughan, T.L., Hansten, P.D., Stanford, J.L., Risch, H.A., Gammon, M.D., Chow, W.H., Dubrow, R., Ahsan, H., Mayne, S.T., Schoenberg, J.B., West, A.B., Rotterdam, H., Fraumeni, J.F., & Blot, W.J. (1998). Use of aspirin and other nonsteroidal anti-inflammatory drugs and risk of esophageal and gastric cancer. *Cancer Epidemiological Biomarkers Prevalence, 7,* 97–102.

Federal Register. (1997, October 31). *Rules and regulations* (No. 62, 211). Washington, DC.

Federal Register. (1998, November 2). *Rules and regulations* (No. 63, 211). Washington, DC.

Ferguson, M.K., & Skinner, D.B. (1995). Carcinoma of the esophagus and cardia. In G.A. Zuidema (Ed.), *Shackelford's surgery of the alimentary tract* (4th ed.) (305–332). Philadelphia: W.B. Saunders.

Fisher, S.G., Davis, F., Nelson, R., Weber, L., Goldberg, J., & Haenszel, W. (1993). A cohort study of stomach cancer risk in men after gastric surgery for benign disease. *Journal of the National Cancer Institute, 85,* 1303–1310.

Folcarelli, P.H. (1999). Problems of the liver, gallbladder, and pancreas. In G.A. Harkness and J.R. Dincher (Eds.), *Medical-surgical nursing: Total patient care* (10th ed.) (pp. 1099 – 1120). St. Louis: Mosby.

Forman, D., Newell, D.G., Fullerton, F., Yarnell, J.W., Stacey, A.R., Wald, N., & Sitas, F. (1991). Association between infection with Helicobacter pylori and risk of gastric cancer: Evidence from a prospective investigation. *BMJ, 302,* 1302–1305.

Franceschi, S., Talamini, R., Barra, S., Baron, A.E., Negri, E., Bidoli, E., Serraino, D., & La Vecchia, C. (1990). Smoking and drinking in relation to cancers of the oral cavity, pharynx, larynx, and esophagus in northern Italy. *Cancer Research, 50,* 6502–6507.

Frisch, M., Glimelius, B., van den Brule, A.J.C., Wohlfahrt, J., Meijer, C.J.L., Walboomers, J.M.M., Goldman, S., Svensson, C., Adami, H.O., & Melbye, M. (1997). Sexually transmitted infection as a cause of anal cancer. *New England Journal of Medicine, 337,* 1350–1358.

Frisch, M., Olsen, J.H., Bautz, A., & Melbye, M. (1995). Benign anal lesions and the risk of cancer. *New England Journal of Medicine, 331,* 300–302.

Frogge, M.H. (1993). Gastrointestinal cancers: Esophogus, stomach, liver, and pancreas. In S.L. Groenwald, M.H. Frogge, M. Goodman, & C.H. Yarbro (Eds.), *Cancer nursing: Principles and practice* (3rd ed.) (pp. 1022–1029). Boston: Jones and Bartlett.

Fuchs, C.S., Giovannucci, E.L., Colditz, G.A., Hunter, D.J., Speizer, F.E., & Willet, W.C. (1994). A prospective study of family history and risk of colorectal cancer. *New England Journal of Medicine, 331,* 1669–1674.

Fuchs, C.S., & Mayer, R.J. (1995). Gastric carcinoma. *New England Journal of Medicine, 333,* 32–41.

Garay, C.A., & Engstrom, P.F. (1999). Chemoprevention of colorectal cancer: Dietary and pharmacologic approaches. *Oncology, 13,* 89–97.

Gerner, E.W., Garewal, H.S., Emerson, S.S., & Sampliner, R.E. (1994). Gastrointestinal tissue polyamine contents of patients with Barrett's esophagus treated with alpha-difluoromethylornithine. *Cancer Epidemiology, Biomarkers, and Prevention, 3,* 325–330.

Giardello, F.M., Hamilton, S.R., Krush, A.J., Piantadosi, S., Hylind, L.M., Celano, P., Booker, S.V., Robinson, C.R., & Offerhaus, G.J. (1993). Treatment of colonic and rectal adenomas with sulindac in familial adenomatous polyposis. *New England Journal of Medicine, 328,* 1313–1316.

Ginsberg, G.C., Al-Kawas, F.H., Fleischer, D.E., Reilly, H.F., & Benjamin, S.B. (1996). Gastric polyps: Relationship of size and histology to cancer risk. *American Journal of Gastroenterology, 91,* 714–717.

Giovannucci, E., Egan, K.M., Hunter, D.J., Stampfer, M.J., Golditz, G.A., & Willet, W.C. (1995). Aspirin and the risk of colorectal cancer in women. *New England Journal of Medicine, 333,* 609–614.

Giovannucci, E., Rimm, E.B., Stampfer, M.J., Colditz, G.A., Ascherio, A., & Willet, W.C. (1994). Aspirin use and the risk for colorectal cancer and adenoma in male health professionals. *Annals of Internal Medicine, 121,* 241–246.

Greenall, M.J., Quan, S.H., & DeCosse, J. (1985). Epidermoid cancer of the anus. *British Journal of Surgery, 72*(Suppl. 1), S97–S103.

Greenlee, R.T., Hill-Harmon, M.O. Murray, T., Bolden, S., & Thun, I.M. (2001). Cancer statistics, 2001. *CA: A Cancer Journal for Clinicians, 51,* 15–36.

Greenwald, P., & Lanza, E. (1986). Role of dietary fiber in the prevention of cancer. In V.T. DeVita, S. Hellman, & S.A. Rosenberg (Eds.), *Important advances in oncology* (p. 37). Philadelphia: Lippincott.

Groen, K.A. (1999). Primary and metastatic liver cancer. *Seminars in Oncology Nursing, 15*(1), 48–57.

Hara, A.K., Johnson, C.D., Reed, J.E., Ahlquist, D.A., Nelson, H., MacCarty, R.L., Harmsen, W.S., & Ilstrup, D.M. (1997). Detection of colorectal polyps with CT colography: initial assessment of sensitivity and specificity. *Radiology, 205,* 59–65.

Hardcastle, J.D., Chamberlain, J.O., Robinson, M.H., Moss, S.M., Amar, S.S., Barfour, T.W., James, P.D., & Mangham, C.M. (1996). Randomised controlled trial of fecal-occult blood screening for colorectal cancer. *Lancet, 348,* 1472–1477.

Hardcastle, J.D., Thomas, W.M., Chamberlain, J., Pye, G., Sheffield, J., James, P.D., Balfour, T.W., Amar, S.S., Armitage, N.C., & Moss, S.M. (1989). Randomised, controlled trial of fecal-occult blood screening for colorectal cancer. Results for the first 107,349 subjects. *Lancet, 1*, 1160–1164.

Hawk, E.T., & Limburg, P.J. (1999). Agent development in colorectal cancer chemoprevention: Current status and future trends. In M.C. Perry (Ed.), *1999 educational book* (pp. 193–199). Alexandria, VA: American Society of Clinical Oncology.

Haydon, G.H., & Hayes, P.C. (1996). Screening for hepatocellular cancer. *European Journal of Gastroenterology and Hepatology, 8*, 856–860.

Hayes, J.D., & Pulford, D.J. (1995). The glutathione S-transferase supergene family: Regulation of GST and the contribution of the isoenzymes to cancer chemoprotection and drug resistance. *Critical Review of Biochemical Molecular Biology, 30*, 445.

Health Care Financing Administration. (2001). *HCFA targets the number two cancer killer.* Retrieved July 23, 2001 from the World Wide Web: http://www.hcfa.gov/news/pr2001/pr010314.htm

Heintges, T., & Wands, J.R. (1997). Hepatitis C virus: Epidemiology and transmission. *Hepatology, 26*, 521–526.

Hixson, L.J., Fennarty, M.B., Sampliner, R.E., McGee, D., & Garewal, H. (1990). Prospective study of the frequency and size distribution of polyps missed by colonoscopy. *Journal of the National Cancer Institute, 82*, 1769–1772.

Hoebler, L. (1997). Colon and rectal cancer. In S.L. Groenwald, M.H. Frogge, M. Goodman, & C.H. Yarbro (Eds.), *Cancer nursing: Principles and practice* (4th ed.) (pp. 1036–1054). Boston: Jones and Bartlett.

Hoofnagel, J.H. (1989). Toward universal vaccination against hepatitis B virus. *New England Journal of Medicine, 321*, 1333–1334.

Hsing, A.W., Hansson, L.E., McLaughlin, J.K., Nyren, O., Blot, W.J., Ekbom, A., & Fraumeni, J.F. (1993). Pernicious anemia and subsequent cancer: A population-based cohort study. *Cancer, 71*, 745–750.

Hughes, S.J., Nambu, Y., Soldes, O.S., Hamstra, D., Rehemtulla, A., Iannettoni, M.D., Orringer, M.B., & Beer, D.G. (1997). Fas/APO-1 (CD95) is not translocated to the cell membrane in esophageal adenocarcinoma. *Cancer Research, 57*, 5571–5578.

Ihde, D.C., Sherlock, P., Winawer, S.J., & Furtner, J.G. (1974). Clinical manifestations of hepatoma. *American Journal of Medicine, 56*, 83–91.

Ikeda, K., Saitoh, S., Koida, I., Arase, Y., Tsubota, A., Chayama, K., Kumada, H., & Kawanishi, M. (1993). A multivariate analysis of risk factors for hepatocellular carcinogenesis: A prospective observation of 795 patients with viral and alcoholic cirrhosis. *Hepatology, 18*, 47–53.

Imai, Y., Kawata, S., Tamura, S., Yabuuchi, I., Noda, S., Inada, M., Maeda, Y., Shirai, Y., Fukuzaki, T., Kaji, I., Ishikawa, H., Matsuda, Y., Nishikawa, M., Seki, K., & Matsuzawa, Y. (1998). Relation of interferon therapy and hepatocellular carcinoma in patients with chronic hepatitis C. *Annals of Internal Medicine, 129*, 94–99.

Immunization Practices Advisory Committee. (1991). Hepatitis B virus: A comprehensive strategy for eliminating transmission in the United States through universal childhood vaccination. *Morbidity and Mortality Weekly Report, 40*, 1–25.

Ince, N., & Wands, J.R. (1999). The increasing incidence of hepatocellular carcinoma. *New England Journal of Medicine, 340*, 798–799.

Isolauri, J., & Markkula, H. (1989). Lye ingestion and carcinoma of the esophagus. *Acta Chirurgica Scandinavica*, *155*, 269–271.

Ivanovich, J.L., Read, T.E., Ciske, D.J., Kodner, I.J., & Whelan, A.J. (1999). A practical approach to familial and hereditary colorectal cancer. *American Journal of Medicine*, *107*, 68–77.

Jen, J., Johnson, C., & Levin, B. (1998). Molecular approaches for colorectal cancer screening. *European Journal of Gastroenterology and Hepatology*, *10*, 213–217.

Kabat, G.C., Ng, S.K.C., & Wynder, E.L. (1993). Tobacco, alcohol intake, and diet in relation to adenocarcinoma of the esophagus and gastric cardia. *Cancer Causes and Control*, *4*, 123–132.

Kamschoer, G.H.M., Fujii, A., & Masuda, Y. (1989). Gastric cancer detected by mass survey: A comparison between mass survey and outpatient detection. *Scandanavian Journal of Gastroenterology*, *24*, 813–817.

Kaneko, E., Nakamura, T., Umeda, N., Fujino, M., & Niwa, H. (1977). Outcome of gastric carcinoma detected by gastric mass survey in Japan. *Gut*, *18*, 626.

Katkov, W.N. (1996). Hepatitis vaccines. *Medical Clinics of North America*, *80*, 1189–1200.

Kensler, T.W., He, X., Otieno, M., Egner, P.A., Jacobson, L.P., Chen, B., Wang, J.S., Zhu, Y.R., Zhang, B.C., Wang, J.B., Wu, Y., Zhang, Q.N., Quian, G.S., Kuang, S.Y., Fang, X., Li, Y.F., Yu, L.Y., Prochaska, H.J., Davidson, N.E., Gordon, G.B., Gorman, M.B., Zarba, A., Enger, C., Munoz, A., Helzlsouer, K.J., & Groopman, J.D. (1998). Olitpraz chemoprevention trial in Quidong, People's Republic of China: Modulation of serum aflatoxin albumin adduct biomarkers. *Cancer Epidemiology, Biomarkers, and Prevention*, *7*, 127–134.

Kerlin, P., Davis, G.L., McGill, D.B., Weiland, L.M., Adson, M.A., & Sheed, P.F. (1983). Hepatic adenoma and focal nodular hyperplasia: Clinical, pathologic, and radiologic features. *Gastroenterology*, *84*, 994–1002.

Kew, M.C., & Geddes, E.W. (1982). Hepatocellular carcinoma in rural southern African blacks. *Medicine*, *61*, 98–108.

Kew, M.C., Geddes, E.W., Macrab, G.M., & Bersohn, I. (1974). Hepatitis B antigen and cirrhosis in Bantu patients with primary liver cancer. *Cancer*, *34*, 538–541.

Kewenter, J., Brevinge, G., Engaras, B., & Haglind, E. (1995). The yield of flexible sigmoidoscopy and double-contrast barium enema in the diagnosis of neoplasms in large bowel in patients with a positive Hemoccult test. *Endoscopy*, *27*, 159–163.

Khakoo, S.I., Grellier, L., Soni, P.N., Bhattacharya, S., & Dusheiko, G.M. (1996). Etiology, screening, and treatment of hepatocellular carcinoma. *Medical Clinics of North America*, *80*, 1121–1145.

Kirby, T.J., & Rice, T.W. (1994). The epidemiology of esophageal cancer: The changing face of a disease. *Chest Surgery Clinics of North America*, *4*, 217–225.

Kiyosawa, K., Sodeyama, T., Tanaka, E., Gibo, Y., Yoshizawa, K., Nakano, Y., Furuta, S., Akahane, Y., Nishioka, K., & Purcell, R.H. (1990). Interrelationship of blood transfusion, non-A, non-B hepatitis and hepatocellular carcinoma: Analysis by detection of antibody to hepatitis C virus. *Hepatology*, *12*, 671–675.

Kleibeuker, J.H., Nagengast, F.M., & van der Meer, R. (1996). Carcinogenesis in the colon. In G.P. Young, P. Rozen, & B. Levin (Eds.), *Prevention and early detection of colorectal cancer* (pp. 45–62). Philadelphia: W.B. Saunders.

Krevsky, B. (1995). Tumors of the esophagus. In W.S. Haubrich, F. Schaffner, & J.E. Berk (Eds.), *Bockus gastroenterology* (pp. 534–558). Philadelphia: W.B. Saunders.

Krishnan, K., Ruffin, M.T., & Brenner, D.E. (1998). Clinical models of chemoprevention for colon cancer. *Hematology/Oncology Clinics of North America, 12*, 1079–1114.

Kronborg, O., Fenger, C., Olsen, J., Jorgensen, O.D., & Sondergaard, O. (1996). Randomised study of screening for colorectal cancer with fecal-occult blood test. *Lancet, 348*, 1467–1471.

Kroser, J.A., Bachwich, D.R., & Lichtenstein, G.R. (1997). Risk factors for the development of colorectal carcinoma and their modification. *Hematology/Oncology Clinics of North America, 11*, 547–578.

Kruse, P., Boesby, S., Bernstein, I.T., & Andersen, I.B. (1993). Barrett's esophagus and esophageal adenocarcinoma. Endoscopic and histologic surveillance. *Scandanavian Journal of Gastroenterology, 28*, 193–196.

Labayle, D., Fischer, D., Vielh, P., Drouhin, F., Pariente, A., Bories, C., Duhamel, O., Trousset, M., & Attali, P. (1991). Sulindac causes regression of rectal polyps in familial adenomatous polyposis. *Gastroenterology, 101*, 635–639.

LaBrecque, D. (1994). Liver regeneration: A picture emerges from the puzzle. *American Journal of Gastroenterology, 89*, 86–96.

Lagergren, J., Bergstrom, R., Lindgren, A., & Nyren, O. (1999). Symptomatic gastroesophageal reflux as a risk factor for esophageal adenocarcinoma. *New England Journal of Medicine, 340*, 825–831.

Laken, S.J., Petersen, G.M., Gruber, S.B., Oddoux, C., Ostrer, H.L., Giardiello, F.M., Hamilton, S.R., Hampel, H., Markowitz, A., Klimstra, D., Jhanwar, S., Winawer, S., Offit, K., Luce, M.C., Kinzler, K.W., & Vogelstein, B. (1997). Familial colorectal cancer in Ashkenasim due to a hypermutable tract in APC. *Nature Genetics, 17*, 79–83.

Lawrence, W., & Zfuss, A. (1995). Gastric neoplasms. In G.P. Murphy, W. Lawrence, & R.E. Lenhard (Eds.), *American Cancer Society textbook of clinical oncology* (pp. 281–292). Atlanta: American Cancer Society.

Levine, M.S., & Halorsen, R.A. (1994). Esophageal carcinoma. In R.M. Gore, M.S. Levine, & I. Laufer (Eds.), *Textbook of gastrointestinal radiology* (pp. 447–478). Philadelphia: W.B. Saunders.

Levitt, M.D., Millar, D.M., & Stewart, J.O. (1990). Rectal cancer after pelvic irradiation. *Journal of the Royal Society of Medicine, 83*, 152–154.

Liebman, H.A., Furie, B.C., Tong, M., Blanchard, R.A., Lo, J.K., Lee, S.D., & Coleman, M.S. (1984). Des-gamma-carboxyl (abnormal) prothrombin as a serum marker of primary hepatocellular carcinoma. *New England Journal of Medicine, 310*, 1427–1431.

Liu, S.F., Shen, Q., Dawsey, S.M., Wang, G.Q., Nieberg, R.K., Wang, Z.Y., Weiner, M., Zhou, B., Cao, J., & Yu, Y. (1994). Esophageal balloon cytology and subsequent risk of esophageal and gastric cardia in the high risk Chinese population. *International Journal of Cancer, 57*, 775–780.

Lynch, H.T., Shaw, T.G., & Lynch, J. (1999). The genetics of colorectal cancer. *Primary Care and Cancer, 19*(6), 27–31.

Lynch, H.T., Smyrk, T.C., Watson, P., Lanspa, S.J., Synch, J.F., Lynch, P.M., Cavalieri, R.J., & Boland, C.R. (1993). Genetics, natural history, tumor spectrum and pathology of hereditary nonpolyposis colorectal cancer: An updated review. *Gastroenterology, 104*, 1535–1549.

Macrae, F.A., & Young, G.P. (1999). Neoplastic and non-neoplastic polyps of the colon and rectum. In T. Yamada (Ed.), *Textbook of gastroenterology* (3rd ed.) (pp. 2023–2082). Philadelphia: Lippincott.

Mandel, J.S. (1996). Colon and rectal cancer. In D.S. Reintgen & R.A. Clark (Eds.), *Cancer screening* (pp. 55–91). St. Louis, MO: Mosby.

Mandel, J.S., Bond, J.H., Church, T.R., Snover, D.C., Bradley, G.M., Schuman, L.M., & Ederer, F. (1993). Reducing mortality from colorectal cancer by screening for fecal occult blood. Minnesota Colon Cancer Control Study. *New England Journal of Medicine, 328,* 1365–1371.

Mandel, J.S., Church, T.R., Bond, J.H., Ederer, F., Geisser, M.S., Mongin, S.J., Snover, D.C., & Schuman, L.M. (2000). The effect of fecal occult-blood screening on the incidence of colorectal cancer. *New England Journal of Medicine, 343,* 1603–1607.

Maruyama, M. (1992). Early diagnosis of gastrointestinal cancer. In I. Laufer & M.S. Levine (Eds.), *Double contrast gastrointestinal radiology* (2nd ed.) (pp. 495–532). Philadelphia: W.B. Saunders.

Maule, W.F. (1994). Screening for colorectal cancer by nurse endoscopists. *New England Journal of Medicine, 330,* 183–187.

Maynard, J.E. (1990). Hepatitis B: Global importance and need for control. *Vaccine, 8*(Suppl. 1), S18–S20.

McDonald, J.S., Hill, M.C., & Roberts, J.M. (1992). Gastric cancer: Epidemiology, pathology, detection, and staging. In J.D. Ahlgren & J.S. McDonald (Eds.), *Gastrointestinal oncology* (pp. 151–158). Philadelphia: Lippincott.

McMahon, B.J., & London, T. (1991). Workshop on screening for hepatocellular carcinoma. *Journal of the National Cancer Institute, 83,* 916–919.

Meijssen, M.A., Tilanus, H.W., van Blankenstein, M., Hop, W.C., & Ong, G.L. (1992). Achalasia complicated by esophageal squamous cell carcinoma: A prospective study in 195 patients. *Gut, 33,* 155–158.

Melbye, M., Rabkin, C.S., Frisch, M., & Biggar, R.J. (1994). Changing patterns of anal cancer incidence in the United States, 1940–1989. *American Journal of Epidemiology, 139,* 772–780.

Morson, B.C., & Bussey, H.J.R. (1985). Magnitude of risk for cancer in patients with colorectal adenomas. *British Journal of Surgery, 72*(Suppl.), S23–S25.

Murakami, R., Tsukuma, H., Ubukata, T., Nakanishi, K., Fujimoto, I., Kawashima, T.,Yamazaki, H., & Oshima, A. (1990). Estimation of validity of mass screening program for gastric cancer in Osaka, Japan. *Cancer, 65,* 1255–1260.

Muto, Y., Moriwaki, H., Ninomiya, M., Adachi, S., Saito, A., Takasaki, K.T., Tanaka, T., Tsurumi, K., Okuno, M., Tomita, E., Nakamura, T., & Kojima, T. (1996). Prevention of second primary tumors by an acyclic retinoid, polyprenoic acid, in patients with hepatocellular carcinoma. *New England Journal of Medicine, 334,* 1561–1565.

Myers, R.E., Ross, E.A., Wolf, T.A., Balshem, A., Jepson, C., & Millner, L. (1991). Behavioral interventions to increase adherence in colorectal cancer screening. *Medical Care, 29,* 1039–1050.

Nakamura, G.J., Schneiderman, L.J., & Klauber, M.R. (1984). Colorectal cancer and bowel habits. *Cancer, 54,* 1475–1477.

Nakamura, K., Ueyama, T., Yao, T., Xuan, Z.X., Ambe, K., Adachi, Y., Yakeishi, Y., Matsukuma, A., & Enjoji, M. (1992). Pathology and prognosis of gastric carcinoma. Findings in 10,000 patients who underwent primary gastrectomy. *Cancer, 70,* 1030–1037.

National Cancer Institute. (2000, October 17). *Questions and answers about the Prostate, Lung, Colorectal, and Ovarian Cancer Screening Trial.* Retrieved August 2, 2001 from the World Wide Web: http://cis.nci.nih.gov/fact/5_12.htm

Nelson, R.L., Abcarian, H., & Prasad, M.L. (1982). Iatrogenic perforation of the colon and rectum. *Diseases of the Colon and Rectum, 25,* 305–308.

Neugut, A.I., Hayek, M., & Howe, G. (1996). Epidemiology of gastric cancer. *Seminars in Oncology, 23,* 281–291.

Newcomb, P.A., Norfleet, R.G., Storer, B.E., Surawicz, T., & Marcus, P.M. (1992). Screening sigmoidoscopy and colorectal cancer mortality. *Journal of the National Cancer Institute, 84,* 1572–1575.

Offerhaus, G.J., Giardiello, F.M., Krush, A.J., Booker, S.V., Tersmette, A.C., Kelley, N.C., & Hamilton, S.R. (1992). The risk of upper gastrointestinal cancer in familial adenomatous polyposis. *Gastroenterology, 102,* 1980–1982.

Okuda, K. (1997). Epidemiology. In T.I. Livraghi, M. Makuuchi, & L. Buscarini (Eds.), *Diagnosis and treatment of hepatocellular carcinoma* (pp. 3–17). London: Greenwich Medical Media.

Okuda, K., Ohtsuki, T., Obata, H., Tomimatsu, M., Okazaki, N., Hasegawa, H., Nakajima, Y., & Ohnishi, K. (1985). Natural history of hepatocellular carcinoma and prognosis in relation to treatment. *Cancer, 56,* 918–928.

Palefsky, J.M. (1994). Anal human papillomavirus infection and anal cancer in HIV-positive individuals. *AIDS, 8*(3), 283–295.

Palefsky, J.M., Northfelt, D.W., Kaplan, L.D., & Critchlow, C. (2000). *Chemoprevention of anal neoplasia arising secondary to anogenital human papillomavirus infection in people with HIV infection.* Clinical trial sponsored by theNational Institute of Allergy and Infectious Diseases and Hoffman-LaRoche. Retrieved July 23, 2001 from the World Wide Web: http://www.clinicaltrials.gov/ct/gui/

Paraf, F., Flejou, J.F., Pignon, J.P., Fekete, F., & Potet, F. (1995). Surgical pathology of adenocarcinoma arising in Barrett's esophagus. *American Journal of Surgical Pathology, 19,* 183–191.

Parkin, D.M., & Muir, C.S. (1992). Cancer incidence in five continents. *IARC Scientific Publications, 120,* 145–173.

Parkin, D.M., Pisani, P., & Ferlay, J. (1993). Estimates of the worldwide incidence of eighteen major cancers in 1985. *International Journal of Cancer, 54,* 594–606.

Parsonnet, J., & Axon, A.J.R. (1996). Principles of screening and surveillance. *American Journal of Gastroenterology, 91,* 847–852.

Parsonnet, J., Friedman, G.D., Vandersteen, D.P., Chang, Y., Vogelman, J.H., Orentreich, N., & Sibley, R.K. (1991). Helicobacter pylori infection and the risk of gastric carcinoma. *New England Journal of Medicine, 325,* 1127.

Peers, F.G., & Dinsell, C.A. (1973). Dietary alfatoxins and liver cancer: A population-based study in Kenya. *British Journal of Cancer, 27,* 473–484.

Peters, W.H., Roelofs, H.M., Hectors, M.P., Nagengast, F.M., & Jansen, J.B. (1993). Glutathione and glutatione S-transferases in Barrett's epithelium. *British Journal of Cancer, 67,* 1413–1417.

Potter, J.D. (1996). Epidemiologic, environmental, and lifestyle issues in colorectal cancer. In G.P. Young, P. Rozen, & B. Levin (Eds.), *Prevention and early of detection of colorectal cancer* (pp. 23–44). Philadephia: W.B. Saunders.

Powell, S.M., Petersen, G.M., Krush, A.J., Booker, S., Jen, J., Giardiello, F.M., Hamilton, S.R., Vogelstein, B., & Kinzler, K.W. (1993). Molecular diagnosis of familial adenomatous polyposis. *New England Journal of Medicine, 329,* 1982–1987.

Prasad, M.L., & Abcarian, H. (1980). Malignant potential of perianal condyloma acuminatum. *Diseases of the Colon and Rectum, 23,* 191–197.

Pyper, P.C., & Parks, T.G. (1985). The results of surgery for epidermoid carcinoma of the anus. *British Journal of Surgery, 72,* 712–714.

Ramon, J.M., Serra, L., Cerdo, C., & Oromi, J. (1993). Dietary factors and gastric cancer risk. A case-control study in Spain. *Cancer, 71,* 1731–1735.

Ransohoff, D.F., & Lang, C.A. (1993). Sigmoidoscopic screening in the 1990s. *JAMA, 26,* 1278–1281.

Reintgen, D.S., & Albertini, J. (1996). Miscellaneous tumors. In D.S. Reintgen & R.A. Clark (Eds.), *Cancer screening* (pp. 196–218). St. Louis, MO: Mosby.

Rex, D.K. (1999). Current recommendations for colorectal cancer screening. *Primary Care and Cancer, 19*(6), 1–5.

Rex, D.K., Lehman, G.A., Hawes, R.H., Ulbright, T.M., & Smith, J.J. (1991). Screening colonoscopy in asymptomatic average-risk people with negative fecal occult blood tests. *Gastroenterology, 100,* 64–67.

Rex, D.K., Rahmani, E.Y., Haseman, J.H., Lemmel, G.T., Kaster, S., & Buckley, J.S. (1997). Relative sensitivity of colonoscopy and barium enema for detection of colorectal cancer in clinical practice. *Gastroenterology, 112,* 17–23.

Rex, D.K., Vining, D., & Kopecky, K.K. (1999). An initial experience with screening for colon polyps using spiral CT with and without CT colography (virtual colonoscopy). *Gastrointestinal Endoscopy, 50,* 309–313.

Rhodes, J.B., Holmes, F.F., & Clark, G.M. (1977). Changing distribution of primary cancer in the large bowel. *JAMA, 235,* 1641–1643.

Risch, H.A., Jain, M., & Choi, N.W. (1982). Dietary factors and the incidence of cancer of the stomach. *American Journal of Epidemiology, 122,* 947.

Rodriguez-Bigas, M.A., Boland, C.R., Hamilton, S.R., Henson, D.E., Jass, J.R., Khan, P.M., Lynch, H., Perucho, M., Smyrk, T., Sobin, L., & Srivastava, S. (1997). A National Cancer Institute workshop on hereditary nonpolyposis colorectal cancer syndrome: Meeting highlights and Bethesda guidelines. *Journal of the National Cancer Institute, 89,* 1758–1762.

Roth, J.A., Putnam, J.B. Jr., Rich, T.A., & Forastiere, A.A. (1997). Cancer of the esophagus. In V.T. DeVita, Jr., S. Hellman, & S.A. Rosenberg (Eds.), *Cancer principles and practice of oncology* (5th ed.) (pp. 980–1019). Philadelphia: Lippincott-Raven.

St. John, D.J., McDermott, F.T., Hopper, J.L., Debney, E.A., Johnson, W.R., & Hughes, E.S. (1993). Cancer risk in relatives of patients with common colorectal cancer. *Annals of Internal Medicine, 118,* 785–790.

Sammon, A.M. (1992). A case-control study of diet and social factors in cancer of the esophagus in Transkei. *Cancer, 69,* 860–865.

Sandler, R.S. (1996). Epidemiology and risk factors for colorectal cancer. *Gastroenterology Clinics of North America, 25,* 717–731.

Schalm, S.W., Brouwer, J.T., Chemello, L., Alberti, A., Bellobuono, A., Ideo, G., Schwartz, R., & Weiland, O. (1996). Interferon-ribavirin combination therapy for chronic hepatitis C. *Digestive Diseases and Sciences, 41*(Suppl. 12), 131S–134S.

Schoenfeld, P.S., Cash, B., Kita, J., Piorkowski, M., Cruess, D., & Ransohoff, D. (1999). Effectiveness and patient satisfaction with screening flexible sigmoidoscopy performed by registered nurses. *Gastrointestinal Endoscopy, 49*, 158–162.

Schwesinger, W.H. (1996). Is Helicobacter pylori a myth or the missing link? *American Journal of Surgery, 172*, 411–417.

Scotiniotis, I., Lewis, J.D., & Strom, B.L. (1999). Screening for colorectal cancer and other GI cancers. *Current Opinion in Oncology, 11*(4), 305–311.

Selby, J.V., & Friedman, G.D. (1989). U.S. Preventive Services Task Force. Sigmoidoscopy in the periodic health examination of asymptomatic adults. *JAMA, 261*, 594–601.

Selby, J.V., Friedman, G.D., Quesenberry, C.P., & Weiss, N.S. (1992). A case-control study of screening sigmoidoscopy and mortality from colorectal cancer. *New England Journal of Medicine, 326*, 653–657.

Shank, B., Cunningham, J.D., & Kelsen, D.P. (1997). Cancer of the anal region. In V.T. DeVita, Jr., S. Hellman, & S.A. Rosenberg (Eds.), *Cancer principles and practice of oncology* (5th ed.) (pp.1234–1251). Philadelphia: Lippincott-Raven.

Sherlock, S. (1994). Viruses and hepatocellular carcinoma. *Gut, 35*, 828–832.

Shindo, M., DiBisceglie, A.M., Cheung, L., Shih, J.W., Feinstone, C.K., & Hoofnagle, J.H. (1991). Decrease in serum hepatitis C viral RNA during alpha-interferon therapy for chronic hepatitis C. *Annals of Internal Medicine, 115*, 700–704.

Simonetti, R.G., Camma, C., Fiorella, F., Politi, F., d'Amico, G., & Pagloiar, O.L. (1991). Hepatocellular carcinoma. *Digestive Disease Science, 36*, 962–972.

Sprout, J. (2000). Nurse endoscopist training: The next step. *Gastroenterology Nursing, 23*, 111–115.

Stearns, M.W., Urmacher, C., Sternberg, S.S., Woodruff, J., & Attiyeh, F. (1980). Cancer of the anal canal. *Current Problems in Cancer, 4*(12), 1–44.

Stellman, J.M., & Stellman, S.D. (1996). Cancer and the workplace. *CA: A Cancer Journal for Clinicians, 46*, 70–92.

Strauss, R.M. (1995). Hepatocellular carcinoma: Clinical, diagnostic, and therapeutic aspects. In A.K. Rustgi (Ed.), *Gastrointestinal cancers: Biology, diagnosis, and therapy* (pp. 479–496). Philadelphia: Lippincott-Raven.

Steinbach, G., Lynch, P.M., Phillips, R.K., Wallace, M.H., Hawk, E., Gordon, G.B., Wakabayashi, N., Saunders, B., Shen, Y., Fujimura, T., Li-Kuo, S., & Levin, B. (2000). The effect of celecoxib, a cyclooxygenase-2 inhibitor, in familial adenomatous polyposis. *New England Journal of Medicine, 342*, 1946–1952.

Streitz, J.M. (1994). Barrett's esophagus and esophageal cancer. *Chest Surgery Clinics of North America, 4*, 227–240.

Struewing, J.P., Pape, D.M., & Snow, D.A. (1991). Improving colorectal cancer screening in a medical residents' primary care clinic. *American Journal of Preventive Medicine, 7*(2), 75–81.

Stryker, S.J., Wolff, B.G., Culp, C.E., Libbe, S.D., Ilstrup, D.M., & MacCarty, R.L. (1987). Natural history of untreated colonic polyps. *Gastroenterology, 93*, 1009–1013.

Subbaramaiah, K., Zakim, D., Weksler, B., & Dannenberg, A.J. (1997). Inhibition of cyclooxygenase: A novel approach to cancer prevention. *Proceedings of the Society for Experimental Biology and Medicine, 216*, 201–210.

Surveillance, Epidemiology, and End Results Program. (1996). *SEER cancer statistics review, 1973–1996*. Bethesda, MD: National Cancer Institute.

Tamura, K., Ishiguro, S., Munakata, A., Yoshida, Y., Nakaji, S., & Sugawara, K. (1996). Annual changes in colorectal carcinoma incidence in Japan. *Cancer, 78*, 1187–1194.

Taylor-Robinson, S.D., Foster, G.R., Arora, S., Hargreaves, S., & Thomas, H.C. (1997). Increase in primary liver cancer in the U.K., 1979–94. *Lancet, 350*, 1142–1143.

Terdiman, J.P., Conrad, P.G., & Sleisenger, M.H. (1999). Genetic testing in hereditary colorectal cancer: Indications and procedures. *American Journal of Gastroenterology, 94*, 2344–2356.

Tsukuma, H., Hiyamam, T., Tanaka, S., Nakao, M., Yabuuchi, T., Kitamura, T., Nakanishi, K., Fujimoto, I., Inoue, A., Yamazaki, H., & Kawashima, T. (1993). Risk factors for hepatocellular carcinoma among patients with chronic liver disease. *New England Journal of Medicine, 328*, 1797–1801.

Umpleby, H.C., & Williamson, R.C.N. (1984). Carcinoma of the large bowel in the first four decades. *British Journal of Surgery, 71*, 272–277.

Update on hepatitis B prevention. (1989). *Morbidity & Mortality Weekly Report, 36*, 353–360.

U.S. Department of Agriculture. (1999). *Results from the 1994–96 continuing survey of food intakes by individuals.* Washington, DC: Author.

U.S. Food and Drug Administration. (1999, April 29). *FDA talk paper: FDA approves first home test for hepatitis C virus.* Rockville, MD: U.S. Food and Drug Administration, U.S. Department of Health and Human Services, Public Health Service. Retrieved October 29, 2001 from the World Wide Web: http://www.fda.gov/bbs/topics/ANSWERS/ANS00952.html

U.S. Preventive Services Task Force. (1995). *A guide to clinical preventative services* (2nd ed.). Washington, DC: Department of Health and Human Services.

Vasen, H.F., Mecklin, J.P., Kahn, P.M., & Lynch, H.T. (1991). The International Collaborative Group on hereditary non-polyposis colon cancer (ICG-HNPCC). *Diseases of the Colon and Rectum, 34*, 424–425.

Vasen, H.F., Watson, P., Mecklin, J.P., & Lynch, H.T. (1999). New clinical criteria for hereditary nonpolyposis colorectal cancer (HNPCC, Lynch syndrome) proposed by the International Collaborative group on HNPCC. *Gastroenterology, 116*, 1453–1456.

Vena, J.E., Graham, S., Zielezny, M., Swanson, M.K., Barnes, R.E., & Nolan, J. (1985). Lifetime occupational exercise and colonic cancer. *American Journal of Epidemiology, 122*, 357–365.

Venook, A.P. (1994). Treatment of hepatocellular carcinoma: Too many options? *Journal of Clinical Oncology, 12*, 1323–1334.

Verme, G., Brunetto, M.R., Oliveri, F., Baldi, M., Forzani, B., Piantino, P., Ponzetto, A., & Bonino, F. (1991). Role of hepatitis delta virus infection in hepatocellular carcinoma. *Digestive Diseases Science, 36*, 1134–1136.

Waddell, W.R., Ganser, G.F., Lerise, E.J., & Loughry, R.W. (1989). Sulindac for polyposis of the colon. *American Journal of Surgery, 157*, 175–179.

Wagner, J.L., Tunis, S., Brown, M., Ching, A., & Almeida, R. (1996). Cost-effectiveness of colorectal cancer screening in average-risk adults. In G. Young & B. Levin (Eds.), *Prevention ad early detection of colorectal cancer* (pp. 321–356). Philadelphia: W.B. Saunders.

Waye, J.D., Lewis, B.S., Frankel, A., & Geller, S.A. (1988). Small colon polyps. *American Journal of Gastroenterology, 83*, 120–122.

Weitzman, S.A., & Gordon, L.I. (1990). Inflammation and cancer: Role of phagocyte-generated oxidants in carcinogenesis. *Blood, 76,* 655–663.

Welch, C.E., & Burke, J.F. (1962). Carcinoma of the colon and rectum. *New England Journal of Medicine, 266,* 211.

Winawer, S.J., Fletcher, R.H., Miller, L., Godlee, F., Stolar, M.H., Mulrow, C.D., Woolf, S.H., Glick, S.N., Ganiats, T.G., Bond, J.H., Rosen, L., Zapka, J.G., Olsen, S.J., Giardiello, F.M., Sisk, J.E., Van Antwerp, R., Brown-Davis, C., Marciniak, D.A., & Mayer, R.J. (1997). Colorectal cancer screening: Clinical guidelines and rationale. *Gastroenterology, 112,* 594–642.

Winawer, S.J., Stewart, E.T., Zauber, A.G., Bond, J.H., Ansel, H., Waye, J.D., Hall, D., Hamlin, A.A., Schapiro, M., O'Brien, M.J., Sternberg, S., & Gottlieb, L.S. (2000). A comparison of colonoscopy and double-contrast barium enema for surveillance after polypectomy. *New England Journal of Medicine, 342,* 1766–1772.

Winawer, S.J., Zauber, A.G., & Diaz, B. (1987). The national polyp study: Temporal sequence of evolving colorectal cancer from the normal colon [Abstract]. *Gastrointestinal Endoscopy, 33,* A167.

Winawer, S.J., Zauber, A.G., Gerdes, H., O'Brien, M.J., Gottlieb, L.S., Sternberg, S.S., Bond, J.H., Waye, J.D., Schapiro, M., Panish, J.F., Kurtz, R.C., Shike, M., Ackroyd, F.W., Stewart, E.T., Skolnick, M., & Bishop, D.T. (1996). Risk of colorectal cancer in the families of patients with adenomatous polyps. *New England Journal of Medicine, 334,* 82–87.

Winawer, S.J., Zauber, A.G., Ho, M.N., O'Brien, M.J., Gottlieb, L.S., Sternberg, S.S., Waye, J.D., Schapiro, M., Bond, J.H., & Panish, J.F. (1993). Prevention of colorectal cancer by colonoscopic polypectomy. The National Polyp Study Workgroup. *New England Journal of Medicine, 329,* 1977–1981.

Wingo, P.A., Bolden, S., Tong, T., Parker, S.L., Martin, L.M., & Heath, C.W. Jr. (1996). Cancer statistics for African Americans. *CA: Cancer Journal for Clinicians, 46,* 113–125.

Winnan, G., Berci, G., Panish, J., Talbot, T.M., Overholt, B.F., & McCallum, R.W. (1980). Superiority of the flexible to the rigid sigmoidoscopy in routine proctosigmoidoscopy. *New England Journal of Medicine, 302,* 1011–1012.

Wong, D.K., Cheung, A.M., O'Rourke, K., Naylor, C.D., Detsky, A.S., & Heathcote, J. (1993). Effect of alpha-interferon treatment in patients with hepatitis B antigen-positive chronic hepatitis B: A meta-analysis. *Annals of Internal Medicine, 119,* 312–323.

Young, G.P., Macrae, F.A., & St. John, D.J.B. (1996). Clinical methods for early detection: Basis, use, and evaluation. In G.P. Young, P. Rozen, & B. Levin (Eds.), *Prevention and early detection of colorectal cancer* (pp. 241–270). Philadelphia: W.B. Saunders.

Zaman, S.N., Johnson, P.J., & Williams, R. (1990). Silent cirrhosis in patients with hepatic carcinoma: Implications for screening in high incidence and low incidence areas. *Cancer, 65,* 1607–1610.

Zhou, X.D., Tang, Z.Y., Yu, Y.Q., Yang, B.H., Lin, Z.Y., Lu, J.Z., Ma, Z.C., & Tang, C.L. (1989). Long-term survivors after resection for primary liver cancer. Clinical analysis of 19 patients surviving more than ten years. *Cancer, 63,* 2201–2206.

Zoli, M., Magalotti, D., Bianchi, G., Gueli, C., Marchesini, G., & Pisi, E. (1996). Efficacy of a surveillance program for early detection of hepatocellular carcinoma. *Cancer, 78,* 977–985.

Zuckerman, A.J. (1987). Viral superinfection. *Hepatology, 7,* 184–185.

CHAPTER 13

Gynecologic Cancers

Kathleen Farley Omerod, RN, MS, AOCN®

Introduction

The American Cancer Society (ACS) estimated that in 2000, 77,500 women in the United States would be diagnosed with gynecologic cancer and 26,500 women would die of these diseases (ACS, 2000). The fear and uncertainty that accompany the diagnosis of gynecologic cancer present many challenges to a woman. The news of a gynecologic pathology causes a severe, all-encompassing threat to her physical, spiritual, psychological, and social well-being, as well as that of her family. Nurses are in a unique position to provide holistic care for women undergoing evaluation for gynecologic cancer. Nurses must also care for women at risk for gynecologic cancer, providing valuable information about the cause and prevention of these diseases.

Cervical Cancer

Epidemiology

ACS estimated that in 2000, 12,800 women would be diagnosed with cervical cancer and 4,600 women would die from this disease (ACS, 2000). Cervical cancer is considered a preventable cancer because it has a long premalignant phase. Since 1940, the age-adjusted death rate from cervical cancer has decreased 70%. This primarily can be attributed to the use of the Papanicolaou (Pap) smear. However, cervical cancer is the leading cause of cancer-related deaths of women in developing countries, where the incidence is 75% higher than the ideal set by the World Health Organization (WHO) (Lovejoy, 1999). Additionally, the incidence of precancerous lesions, or cervical intraepithelial neoplasia (CIN), has risen dramatically, in part because of improved technology for CIN screening. The median age of occurrence of cervical cancer is 45–50 years; the mean age for CIN is in a woman's third decade. Most (85%–90%) cervical cancers are of squamous cell origin histologically. The rest are adenocarcinomas (Branda, 1994). Most of the definitive epidemiologic information relates to squamous cell carcinoma of the cervix.

Cervical cancers typically occur in women ages 35–55 years. The cause of a large percentage of squamous cell cancers of the cervix appears to be a sexually transmitted factor or cofactor. Risk factors for these squamous cell tumors are similar to those for other sexually transmitted diseases and include early age at first coitus, multiple sex partners, low socioeconomic status, cigarette smoking, and a history of sexually transmitted disease.

Risk factors for adenocarcinomas are not so obvious (Branda, 1994). Sexual transmission does not appear to play a major role in the pathogenesis of such tumors. Oral contraceptive use has been associated with a slightly increased risk but is not an established risk factor. The proportion of adenocarcinomas to squamous cell carcinomas has increased over the past two decades, probably because of the decreasing incidence of squamous cell carcinomas (DiSaia & Creasman, 1997).

Adenocarcinoma of the cervix arises from the endocervical canal. As a result, Pap smear screening may miss these cancers. Adenocarcinomas tend to produce fewer early symptoms and are more likely to be diagnosed at a later stage than squamous cell carcinomas. The lesions are typically bulky and expand the cervical canal to create the so-called barrel-shaped lesions of the cervix (DiSaia & Creasman, 1997). The spread pattern of these lesions is similar to that of squamous cell cancer, with direct extension accompanied by metastasis to regional pelvic lymph nodes. Local recurrence of adenocarcinoma is more common than local recurrence of squamous cell carcinoma, resulting in the commonly held belief that adenocarcinoma lesions are more radioresistant than are squamous cell lesions. Hence, many oncologists recommend combined radiotherapy and surgery for treatment. Survival statistics relative to adenocarcinoma are comparable to those of squamous cell carcinoma, stage for stage (DiSaia & Creasman).

Clear-cell adenocarcinoma of the cervix and vagina has been associated with first-trimester exposure to a nonsteroidal synthetic estrogen. The most common synthetic estrogen associated with the occurrence of clear-cell carcinoma is diethylstilbestrol (DES). Because DES is no longer prescribed for women experiencing high-risk pregnancies, the incidence of this rare disease has decreased steadily since its peak in 1975. The age range of young women diagnosed with clear-cell adenocarcinoma of the cervix or vagina is 7–34 years. Women younger than age 15 have more aggressive tumors than do women over age 19 (DiSaia & Creasman, 1997).

Pathogenesis

Figure 13-1 shows the female reproductive organs. The cervix is one of the two major parts of the uterus. The corpus of the uterus is immediately above and adjacent to the cervix. The narrowest part of the corpus is the lower portion, or isthmus, of the uterus. The isthmus is immediately above the cervix. The cervix, extending from the isthmus to the vagina, is the narrow, cylindrical segment of the uterus that lies, in most instances, at 90 degrees to the anterior vaginal wall. In

Figure 13.1. Female Reproductive Organs

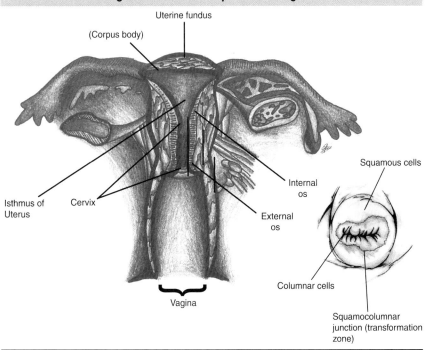

Uterine fundus

(Corpus body)

Squamous cells

Internal
os

Isthmus of
Uterus

Cervix

External
os

Columnar cells

Vagina

Squamocolumnar
junction (transformation
zone)

most women, the cervix measures 2–4 cm in length. Anteriorly, the cervix is separated from the bladder by fatty tissue and is connected laterally by broad ligaments and parametrium. The cervix receives its blood supply through the parametrium. The lowest portion of the cervix projects into the vault of the vagina and is covered by a mucous membrane.

The endocervical canal is the passageway between the external os and the internal os (McCance & Huether, 1998). It is lined with columnar epithelial cells. The ectocervix and the vagina are lined with squamous epithelial cells. The point at which these two types of epithelial cells meet is called the squamocolumnar junction, or transformation zone. The transformation zone is the usual site of carcinoma of the cervix.

The majority of squamous cell carcinomas are thought to arise from a precancerous cervical condition in the transformation zone (McCance & Huether, 1998). Such lesions are termed CIN or cervical dysplasia. CIN is graded according to the degree of involvement of the epithelium, or as CIN I, II, or III. CIN III represents full-thickness neoplasia of the epithelium. The likelihood of progression to invasive cancer is much greater at CIN III than at CIN I (Richart, 1993).

Cytologic and histologic abnormalities of CIN include nuclear pleomorphism, increased nucleus-to-cytoplasm ratio, nuclear alteration, hyperchromaticity, abnormal chromatin distribution, and increased mitotic figures. The degree of dysplasia is based on the proportion of squamous epithelium replaced by atypical cells and the severity of cytologic abnormality.

In CIN I, neoplasia extends to less than one-third the thickness of the epithelium. CIN II describes one-third to two-thirds involvement. CIN III describes a situation in which neoplasia extends from two-thirds to the full thickness of the epithelium, without invading the underlying stroma (Richart, 1993).

CIN, regardless of severity, generally is asymptomatic and not grossly visible on inspection of the cervix. Risk factors for the development of CIN are essentially the same as those for invasive squamous cell carcinoma of the cervix (Parazzini et al., 1992).

Much has been written about adenocarcinoma in situ arising from the endocervical epithelium. This lesion is much less common than CIN, and much less is known about its natural history (Andersen & Arffman, 1989; Muntz et al., 1992). Evidence definitely suggests, however, that adenocarcinoma in situ develops into invasive adenocarcinoma.

Invasive squamous cell carcinoma of the cervix spreads through direct invasion into adjacent tissues and metastasizes through lymphatic and vascular dissemination. The route of proliferation is from the cervix to the vaginal mucosa, extending microscopically to the myometrium of the lower uterine segment, to the paracervical lymph nodes, to regional and distant lymphatics, and then by direct extension to adjacent structures or parametria. Extension to involve the bladder or rectum may occur with or without the presence of a vesicovaginal or rectovaginal fistula.

The presence of lymph node involvement correlates with the stage and grade of the malignancy (DiSaia & Creasman, 1997). Lymph node involvement in stage I disease is 15%–20% and involvement in stage II is 25%–40%; in stage III disease, it is assumed that at least 50% of women have positive lymph nodes.

Risk Factors

Lack of screening or infrequent screening is the most significant risk factor in the development of cervical neoplasia. A number of epidemiologic studies have identified a positive association between squamous cervical cancer and multiple social and physical characteristics (see Figure 13-2).

The association of cervical cancer risk and sexual behavior is the most consistent epidemiologic finding. The two most important sexual determinants of risk include early age at first intercourse and lifetime number of sex partners. The sexual behavior of the male partner also has been found to affect a woman's risk of cervical cancer (Zunzunegui, Kink, Coria, & Charlet, 1986). Husbands of women with cervical cancer had

Figure 13-2. Risk Factors for Cervical Cancer

Intercourse at an early age
Multiple sexual partners
Male risk factors
Human papilloma virus
Cigarette smoking
Oral contraceptive use
Immunocompromise
Low socioeconomic status

Note. From "Screening and Prevention of Gynecologic Malignancies" (p. 18) by S.A. Nolte and J.R. Walczak in G.J. Moore-Higgs, L.A. Almadrones, B. Colvin-Huff, L.M. Gossfeld, and J.H Eriksson (Eds.), *Women and Cancer: A Gynecologic Nursing Perspective* (2nd ed.), 2000, Boston: Jones and Bartlett. Copyright 2000 by Jones and Bartlett. Reprinted with permission.

more sex partners, had intercourse at an earlier age, and had a greater history of venereal disease than did husbands of women without cervical cancer (Duncan et al., 1990). Women married to men who previously had wives with cervical cancer also are at greater risk for developing cervical cancer (Graham et al., 1979). Wives of men with penile cancer also are at increased risk (Maden et al., 1993).

A variety of agents, such as herpes simplex virus type-2 (HSV-2), have been implicated as sexually transmitted factors or cofactors in the development of squamous cervical neoplasia. However, the sexually transmitted factor currently considered most serious is human papilloma virus (HPV). Over the past few decades, an enormous amount of data have accumulated regarding HPV. Although strong evidence supports the etiologic role of certain HPV types, it appears that other factors or circumstances must also be at work for cervical neoplasia to occur (Dillner, 2000; Koss, 1987; Syrjanen & Syrjanen, 1985; Walker et al., 1989). A large percentage of women test positive for HPV, but only a small percentage of women develop cervical neoplasia.

Cigarette smoking has been implicated as a risk factor for cervical cancer, especially squamous cell carcinoma (Sook, 1991). Cotinine and nicotine have been shown to exert mutagenic activity in the cervical mucus of smokers. Cigarette smoking produces local immunosuppression in cervix epithelium, which may increase the likelihood of developing HPV-related neoplasia (Winkelstein, 1990). Women who report ever smoking cigarettes regularly have a risk of HPV-related neoplasia that is 50% higher than that of women who have always been nonsmokers. Women who smoke 40 or more cigarettes per day and women who have smoked for 40 years or longer have a significant twofold risk (Coker, Rosenberg, McCaan, & Hulka, 1992).

The relationship of oral contraceptives to cervical neoplasia has been studied extensively. Oral contraceptives are related to invasive cervical cancer, as the WHO Collaborative Study of Neoplasia and Steroid Contraceptives (1985) reported. According to this study, increased risk of cervical neoplasia was noted with any use of oral contraceptives, with the greatest increase in women who used them for five years or more. The mechanism of action of oral contraceptives on the cervical epithelium is unclear. Evidence suggests that cervical epithelium is subject to a variety of proliferative changes resulting from oral contraceptive use; however, further research is needed to study these changes and their causes. Several studies have demonstrated that women who use barrier methods, such as a diaphragm or condoms, have a lower cervical cancer risk than do women who use hormonal contraceptives (Hannaford, 1991).

DiSaia and Creasman (1997) noted that women exposed to DES in utero have an increased incidence of clear-cell adenocarcinoma of the vagina and cervix. The cause of this increased risk is unknown.

Some epidemiologic reports suggest that immunosuppression may be a risk factor for developing cervical cancer. Women who are iatrogenically immunosuppressed because of medical conditions or organ transplantation have a greater incidence of cervical cancer as well as other malignancies of the reproductive tract and anus. Women who undergo renal transplantation have an incidence of cervical cancer five times higher than that of age-matched controls (Penn, 1986). The progressive immunosuppression associated with human immunodeficiency virus (HIV) infection has prompted concern regarding its impact on the potential for cervical neoplasia in HIV-positive women (Feingold et al., 1990). The progression from HPV infection to the development of cervical neoplasia in HIV-positive women has been correlated to the degree of immunosuppression (Schafer, Friedmann, Meilke, Schwartlander, & Koch, 1991). One in five HIV-positive women with no evidence of cervical disease developed biopsy-confirmed squamous intraepithelial lesions (SILs) within three years, highlighting the importance of cervical screening programs for these women (Maiman et al., 1990). Women at high risk for HIV infection should undergo a yearly screening, including a Pap smear and gynecologic examination. Women with symptomatic HIV infection or CD-4 cell counts greater than $200/mm^3$ should have a screening every six months.

Studies show that cervical cancer predominantly affects women in lower socioeconomic classes. The risk among women in the lowest social class is approximately five times that of women in the highest class. The role that social class exerts is unclear but may be related to poor diet, inadequate education, rural location, inadequate access to health care, or being underinsured or a member of a racial minority (Brinton & Fraumeni, 1986).

Signs and Symptoms

Early symptoms are subtle, making it difficult for a woman to recognize that she may have cervical cancer. The initial symptom is a painless, thin, watery or blood-tinged vaginal discharge and irregular or postcoital bleeding (DiSaia & Creasman, 1997). A premenopausal woman may describe what seems to be an increase in menstrual periods. The bleeding may become continuous, with resulting anemia. In postmenopausal women, bleeding is more likely to prompt early medical attention.

All these symptoms are associated with a tumor mass. Lesions are friable and bleed easily with trauma, so sexual activity or douching causes sloughing and bleeding of the lesion. Progressive bleeding and a foul discharge are associated with large, bulky, necrotic tumors. These advanced lesions often bleed spontaneously and shed necrotic debris.

Late symptoms indicate more advanced or recurrent disease and include referred pain to the flank or leg. This is secondary to involvement of the uterus, pelvic wall, or sciatic nerve. Dysuria, hematuria, rectal bleeding, or constipation may herald bladder or rectal invasion. Persistent edema of one or both lower extremities results from extensive pelvic wall disease that blocks lymphatic and venous flow. Uremia may result from ureteral obstruction associated with advanced lateral pelvic disease (Hopkins & Morely, 1993).

Primary Prevention

Squamous cancer of the cervix appears to be a "venereal" disease in the sense that its association with sexual behavior has been the most consistent epidemiologic finding. The primary means of preventing cervical cancer is delaying sexual activity until age 20 and restricting sexual activity to monogamous relationships.

Smoking cessation should be encouraged to decrease the risk of developing CIN and cancer. Information regarding the purpose, need, and frequency of Pap smear screening may promote better compliance with screening efforts (Franco, 1991).

Figure 13-3 summarizes risk-reducing behaviors of which all adolescents, especially women, should be aware. Adolescents should know that women with multiple sex partners and women who begin intercourse before age 18, when the columnar cells of the cervix are most susceptible to squamous metaplasia, are at increased risk for cervical cancer. Adolescents should understand that risk increases progressively with the number of partners and each partner's number of partners. Because sexual abstinence is ideal but difficult to achieve, most health education programs advocate use of a barrier contraceptive—specifically, condom use. Safe-sex guidelines and HIV-prevention strategies have been compiled and may be useful in educating young women about prevention of cervical neoplasia (Nolte, Sohm, & Koons, 1993).

Figure 13-3. Risk-Reducing Behaviors

Limit sexual activity in the teen years.
Limit the number of sexual partners.
Develop safe sexual practices by using barrier contraception: diaphragm and condoms.
Health education before girls become sexually active regarding risks of sexual contact: safe sexual practices and disease prevention methods; the purpose, need, and frequency of Pap smear and pelvic examinations.
Stop smoking: obtain referral to smoking cessation programs, prescription for medical treatment.
Seek prompt medical treatment of cervical intraepithelial neoplasia.

Note. From "Screening and Prevention of Gynecologic Malignancies" (p. 18) by S.A. Nolte and J.R. Walczak in G.J. Moore-Higgs, L.A. Almadrones, B. Colvin-Huff, L.M. Gossfeld, and J.H Eriksson (Eds.), *Women and Cancer: A Gynecologic Nursing Perspective* (2nd ed.), 2000, Boston: Jones and Bartlett. Copyright 2000 by Jones and Bartlett. Reprinted with permission.

Women should be advised of the health risks of cigarette smoking, including the fact that it increases the risk of cervical cancer. Nursing strategies to help women stop smoking could include the use of educational materials; counseling; referral to smoking-cessation programs; and, when appropriate, medical treatment that includes pharmacologic interventions and nicotine replacement.

Twenty-five percent of women with cervical cancer and 40% of women who die of cervical cancer are age 50 or older (Mandelblatt, Andrews, Kerner, Zauber, & Burnett, 1991). A disproportionate number of these women present with locally advanced invasive cervical cancer, which may explain their relatively poor survival rate. Women older than 65 with early-stage disease experience longer disease-free intervals than younger women experience. Screening may have a significant impact on morbidity and mortality among older women. Education regarding the importance of regular screening is paramount for older women.

Secondary Prevention: Early Detection

The Pap smear, originally intended to detect cervical cancer, has evolved into a technique to screen for cervical precancerous conditions. If lesions are histologically confirmed as being precancerous, treatment may prevent them from progressing to invasive cancer. In the United States and other countries where cervical cytologic screening programs are widespread, the incidence of and mortality from invasive cancer have decreased.

ACS, the National Cancer Institute (NCI), and the American College of Obstetricians and Gynecologists published a widely accepted consensus statement in 1988 recommending that women who are, or have been, sexually active or have reached the age of 18 have a Pap smear and pelvic examination annually. After a woman has had three consecutive annual examinations with normal findings, the Pap smear may be performed less frequently, at the physician's discretion. The Pap smear has been established as an inexpensive, reliable test for secondary prevention of cervical cancer. The greater the number of negative smears a woman has had, the lower her risk of developing invasive cervical cancer. False-negative rates are estimated at 10%–20% (van der Graaf, Vooijs, Gaillard, & Go, 1987). In the presence of invasive cancer, the false-negative rate actually appears to be much higher and is attributed to obscuring inflammation, resulting in a delay in diagnosis and a reduced chance of survival.

Several factors have led most healthcare professionals in the United States to recommend annual screening. These factors include the relatively high false-negative rate of the Pap smear; the frequent difficulty in determining the risk status of an individual woman; recent evidence that the transit time from CIN to invasive cancer in some women is quite short; and the opportunity to screen for other medical conditions, including other malignancies. The false-positive rate of the Pap smear is unknown but may be substantial. This leads to a different set of problems for women: anxiety; expense associated with establishing a differential diagnosis; and, in some cases, unnecessary treatment. Despite these limitations, a properly retrieved sample that is used to produce a well-fixed, well-stained, and correctly interpreted Pap smear is the best means of screening for cervical cancer.

A woman scheduled for a Pap smear should not be menstruating. She should not douche, have intercourse, use tampons, or use intravaginal medication for at least 24 hours before the examination.

To collect the cells needed to make a Pap smear, the clinician begins by inserting a speculum in the vagina (see Figure 13-4). The speculum, lubricated only with water or a specialized lubricant, is carefully placed to expose the cervix. The clinician rotates an Ayre spatula 360 degrees to gently scrape the entire circumference of the external cervical area (see Figure 13-5) to harvest cells from the area of the transformation zone. Meticulous technique in obtaining a Pap smear is essential in reducing false-negative results. To avoid contamination of the cell sample with foreign material, the clinician should use a dry, cotton-tipped applicator to gently remove excess cervical mucus; the use of general-purpose lubricants must be avoided. The specimen is quickly, but gently and evenly, spread on a glass slide. An additional sample may be taken from the vaginal pool or the posterior vaginal fornix; it is important to obtain an adequate sample from the endocervical canal. This is best done with a cytobrush or endocervical brush (see Figure 13-6). Also important is rapid fixation of the specimen with a cytofixative to avoid air-drying artifact.

Figure 13-4. Inserting a Speculum Into the Vagina

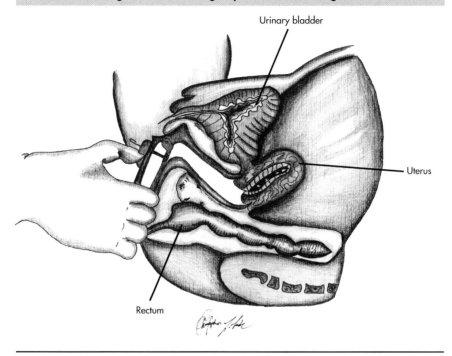

Urinary bladder

Uterus

Rectum

Figure 13-5. Using a Spatula to Scrape Cells From the External Cervical Area for a Pap Smear

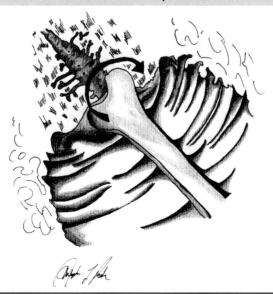

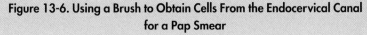

Figure 13-6. Using a Brush to Obtain Cells From the Endocervical Canal for a Pap Smear

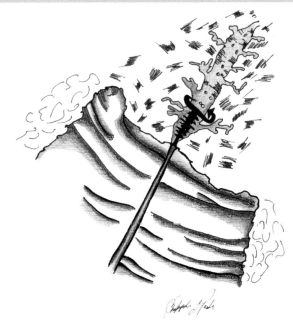

An adequate patient history must accompany the smear, including the date of the patient's last menstrual period and information about hormonal medications and prior genital tract neoplasia and treatment.

In certain populations, such as postmenopausal women, obtaining an adequate endocervical sample is especially important. Getting endocervical cells can be challenging because estrogen loss causes the transformation zone to migrate up the cervix. The healthcare professional may need to take extra time to position the patient in a way that allows him or her to obtain the sample. A variety of specula should be available in the event of a stenotic os. Stenosis may occur as a part of the aging process. It may also occur after radiation therapy to the vagina, cervix, or uterus. The Pap smear is useful for detecting extracervical gynecologic cancers and should not be discontinued after hysterectomy. One-third of women still have an intact cervix after hysterectomy (DiSaia & Creasman, 1997).

Controversy exists regarding the need for Pap smear screening in elderly women, though cervical cancer remains an important health problem into old age. To promote decreased morbidity and mortality associated with cervical cancer, Medicare coverage was extended in 1990 to include triennial Pap smear screening for all women.

The Bethesda System of reporting Pap smear results designates and promotes precise communication regarding cytologic results (see Figure 13-7). This system includes three main categories: a statement of specimen adequacy, a general cat-

Figure 13-7. Bethesda System for Reporting Cervical Cytologic Diagnoses

Squamous Cell
- Atypical squamous cells
  - of undetermined significance (ASC-US)
  - cannot exclude HSIL (ASC-H)
- Low grade squamous intraepithelial lesion (LSIL) encompassing: HPV/mild dysplasia/CIN 1
- High grade squamous intraepithelial lesion (HSIL) encompassing: moderate and severe dysplasia, CIS/CIN 2 and CIN 3
  - with features suspicious for invasion (if invasion is suspected)
- Squamous cell carcinoma

Glandular Cell
- Atypical
  - endocervical cells (NOS or specify in comments)
  - endometrial cells (NOS or specify in comments)
  - glandular cells (NOS or specify in comments)
- Atypical
  - endocervical cells, favor neoplastic
  - glandular cells, favor neoplastic
- Endocervical adenocarcinoma in situ
- Adenocarcinoma
  - endocervical
  - endometrial
  - extrauterine
  - not otherwise specified (NOS)

Note. From *NCI Bethesda System 2001 Terminology,* by the National Cancer Institute, 2001, retrieved February 22, 2002 from the World Wide Web: http://bethesda2001.cancer.gov/terminology.html

egorization of normal or abnormal, and a descriptive diagnosis. Epithelial cell abnormalities are divided into low- and high-grade groups. Low-grade SIL includes mild dysplasia (CIN I) and HPV lesions; high-grade SIL includes moderate dysplasia (CIN II) and severe dysplasia, or carcinoma in situ (CIN III). The Bethesda System also includes an evaluation of hormonal state, infection, reactive and reparative changes, and glandular cell components.

Recognizing the inherent false-negative rate of the Pap smear, researchers have developed a few alternative or adjunctive methods of cervical screening. These include ThinPrep® (Cytyc Corp., Boxborough, MA) Pap smear cytopathology, colposcopy, the acetic acid test, cervicography, and Schiller's test.

ThinPrep Pap Smear Cytopathology

This technology allows the health professional to collect the sample as a cell suspension in a liquid medium and prepare from it a monolayer of cells on a glass slide. The collecting device, either a cytobrush or a spatula, delivers the cellular sample into a solution that is then processed as a cell suspension. In the process, blood, mucus, and inflammatory debris are eliminated, rendering the epithelial component easy to evaluate under a microscope. ThinPrep technology is credited with considerably decreasing the number of smears that are unsatisfactory because of obscuring artifacts. Thus, ThinPrep smears have reduced the need for repeated exams. In contrast to the traditional Pap smear method, the ThinPrep method ensures a greater number of diagnostic cells per slide; this contributes to accurate diagnosis. Clinical trials have demonstrated that the ThinPrep method is more sensitive regarding the detection of cervical abnormalities than the traditional method. ThinPrep technology offers increased diagnostic accuracy with the potential to reduce false-negative cervical cytology (Linder & Zahniser, 1997).

Colposcopy

Colposcopy consists of examining the vagina and cervix with a colposcope, a specialized endoscope. Colposcopy is the usual method of evaluating a cervix following the report of an abnormal Pap smear. Prior studies have demonstrated some improvement in screening sensitivity by combining the Pap smear and colposcopy (Nolte & Hanjani, 1990). Cost and the need for expertise in colposcopy make using colposcopy for routine screening impractical, however.

For satisfactory colposcopy, the entire transformation zone (squamocolumnar junction) must be examined because most cervical cancers begin in this area. The colposcope magnifies the cervix 10–20 times. The healthcare professional may apply 3%–5% acetic acid to the transformation zone to remove mucus, dehydrate cells, and accentuate abnormalities, such as mosaicism, punctation, and white epithelium. A green filter helps the healthcare professional to see the vascular pattern. All abnormal areas are biopsied. In nonpregnant woman, endocervical curettage is performed.

Depending on the results of this evaluation, the plan of management for CIN lesions varies widely, from observation only to hysterectomy. A large percentage of women with a significant CIN lesion (CIN II or III) are treated with a locally ablative method (laser or cryotherapy), large-loop excision of the transformation zone, or cone biopsy. Evaluating women long-term has revealed that some go on to develop invasive cancer. Hysterectomy is offered to healthy women with CIN III who do not intend to have any more children.

Acetic Acid Test

Van Le, Broekhuizen, Janzer-Steele, Behar, and Samter (1993) reported the results of three studies that investigated whether acetic acid application and visual examination, by themselves, could detect CIN that was missed during evaluation of a Pap smear. The acetic acid test did appear to detect CIN in a few women who had a normal Pap smear, but false-positive and false-negative rates were high.

Cervicography

Cervicography consists of taking a picture of what is seen through the colposcope after applying acetic acid to the cervix (Boselli et al., 2000). The picture is sent to an expert for interpretation. Some studies of this technique as a screening method report high false-positive and false-negative rates. The technique is significantly more expensive than a Pap smear.

Schiller's Test

Schiller's test consists of applying Lugol's iodine solution to the cervix and evaluating the resulting color. Normal ectocervical tissue contains glycogen, so it turns mahogany brown. Pale areas should be biopsied. False positives are too frequent to make this test useful for screening.

Nursing Challenges

Nurses have a critical role in promoting Pap smear screening among healthcare professionals and the public and preparing a woman for the test. Nurses should ensure that women know what the Pap smear procedure is, when they should have a Pap test, and what the results mean. Such education, if it led to universal screening of women, could largely eliminate invasive cervical cancer.

In addition, nurse practitioners (NPs) have a substantial impact on the overall accuracy of Pap smear screening. The quality of smears collected by NPs does not differ from that of smears obtained by medical practitioners (Mitchell, 1993). In a two-year study examining the relationship between various levels of experience and the ability to obtain adequate Pap smears, the NPs had the second highest rating the first year. In addition, when compared to first- through fourth-year residents and attending staff, NPs had the highest percentage of successful smears in the second year.

Ovarian Cancer

Introduction

In the past decade, the outlook for women with advanced ovarian cancer has improved with early detection, the use of advanced surgical procedures, and adjuvant therapy. Early detection and screening include the use of genetic information so women at highest risk can be offered treatment earlier. New surgical procedures have resulted in more precise diagnoses and therapeutic interventions that cause less morbidity. Platinum-based chemotherapy regimens combined with paclitaxel have improved the disease-free survival rate. Most important, ovarian cancer recently has received much-needed national attention that has resulted in increased support for resources and research.

The remarkable work of the Ovarian Cancer National Alliance and the National Ovarian Cancer Coalition has increased the involvement of ovarian cancer survivors in public education and in securing support for research and resources for women with ovarian cancer. The diligent efforts of these survivors have paid off. Since 1998, September has been designated as National Ovarian Cancer Month.

Early detection of ovarian cancer drastically improves survival rates. To effect change in the morbidity and mortality associated with ovarian cancer, it is necessary to identify those women at increased risk, ensure prompt treatment, and improve treatment to prevent invasion and metastasis.

Epidemiology

In the United States, a woman's lifetime risk of ovarian cancer from birth to age 70 is approximately 1.8% (ACS, 2000). Ovarian cancer incidence appears to be the highest in North America and northern Europe and lowest in Japan; it occurs more commonly in White women than other ethnic groups, but this difference may be narrowing. The mean age at diagnosis is 59 years, and the incidence increases with age, peaking in the eighth decade (ACS).

Stage, age, lymph node status, grade, histology, presence of ascites, and race are all predictors of survival. However, the overall survival rate for all stages—that is, 35%—has remained constant for the past 30 years (Creasman, 1997b).

Pathophysiology

The more than 30 types of ovarian cancer differ in regard to cell type of origin. The three main types of cells within the ovary are epithelial, germ, and sex-cord stromal cells. Each develops from a different source.

Epithelial cells cover the surface of the ovary and develop from the peritoneum, endometrium, endocervix, and endosalpinx. Epithelial cancers are derived from epithelial cells and constitute approximately 90% of all ovarian cancers. The main histologic subtypes of epithelial ovarian cancer are serous (the most common), endometrioid, mucinous, clear cell, and poorly differentiated adenocarcinomas (Ozols, Schwartz, & Eifel, 1997).

Germ cells are precursors of ova. Cancers derived from germ cells are more common in younger women. The most common type of germ-cell cancer is dysgerminoma.

Sex-cord stromal cells secrete hormones and connect the different components of the ovary. Cancers derived from these cells are called sex-cord stromal tumors and have the capacity to secrete estrogen or testosterone. The most common of these tumors are granulosa cell tumors.

Although the precise mechanism of ovarian carcinogenesis is unknown, the natural history of ovarian cancer is thought to begin with malignant transformation of the epithelial lining of inclusion cysts within the ovarian stroma. The cells replicate, the tumor penetrates the ovarian capsule, and malignant cells spread throughout the peritoneal lining of the pelvis and abdomen. At this point, the cells may attach directly to the adjacent organs of the pelvis or the small or large intestines, or they may circulate, in clockwise fashion with the peritoneal fluid, to the pericolic gutters and diaphragmatic surfaces or omenta, where implants may grow (Ozols, Rubin, Dembo, & Robboy, 1997).

Only 25% of women with newly diagnosed ovarian cancer present with stage I disease; 75% present with malignant cells outside the ovaries at the time of diagnosis (Ozols, Rubin, et al., 1997). Therefore, strategies must be developed for prevention or early detection to control this disease process.

Risk Factors

The specific causes of ovarian cancer are still unknown. All women are at risk. Age; heredity; diet; and environmental, reproductive, and chemical factors have been identified as potentially causative (Narod et al., 1995). Like breast cancer, ovarian cancer risk increases at age 40, and the incidence peaks in the eighth decade.

In general, ovarian cancer is believed to occur as a sporadic genetic mutation rather than a hereditary cancer syndrome. Only 3%–9% of ovarian cancers are thought to be caused by a hereditary cancer syndrome (Ford et al., 1998). Family history of ovarian cancer is among the strongest risk factors for the disease. Women who have two or more first-degree relatives (mother, sister, daughter) or second-degree relatives (grandmother, aunt) who have had ovarian cancer have a greater risk of developing the disease than women who do not.

Familial clusters of ovarian cancer suggest a genetic component. Researchers have conducted several case-controlled studies in an attempt to estimate the magnitude of the genetic contribution, with the largest of these studies showing relative risks of 3.6% and 2.9% associated with ovarian cancer in first- and second-degree relatives, respectively (Ford et al., 1998). Women with a positive family history of ovarian cancer are diagnosed in their early 40s or younger. The risk also increases if other family members have developed ovarian cancer before menopause or if there is a family history of breast, endometrial, colon, rectal, or pancreatic cancer in either female or male relatives.

A predisposing cancer gene, such as BRCA1 and BRCA2, accounts for approximately 5% of all ovarian cancers. More than 50% of women with BRCA1 mutations who develop ovarian cancer are younger than 50 years old. The lifetime risk of ovarian cancer conferred by a BRCA1 mutation has been estimated to be 60%, and the risk for carriers of a BRCA2 mutation has been estimated to be 27% (Breast Cancer Linkage Consortium, 1999). These risks greatly exceed the population risk of 1.8% by age 70. However, these cumulative risk estimates are made on the basis of studies of families with multiple instances of early-onset breast or ovarian cancer; a risk estimate made on the basis of a sample of (mostly) unaffected Jewish individuals was much lower. The risks conferred by BRCA1 or BRCA2 mutations, ascertained through women with cancer but unselected for family history, may be different. The cancer risks for carriers also may vary by specific mutation and among ethnic groups (Weber, 1996).

In North America, the incidence of ovarian cancer is higher among Ashkenazi Jewish women than non-Jewish women. Three common mutations are reported in this population: two in BRCA1 (18delAG and 5382insC) and one in BRCA2 (6174delT). The combined frequency of these three mutations in the Ashkenazic population is approximately 2%. These mutations may account for 30%–60% of all early-onset breast or ovarian cancer in this ethnic population (Moslehi et al., 2000; Struewing et al., 1997).

Three hereditary cancer syndromes have been identified: site-specific familial ovarian cancer, in which two or more first-degree relatives or a first- and second-degree relative have or had ovarian cancer; breast-ovarian cancer syndrome, in which breast and ovarian cancers occur among first- and second-degree relatives; and family cancer syndrome, or Lynch syndrome II, in which a family history of colorectal, endometrial, ovarian, pancreatic, or other type of cancer exists in male or female relatives (Lynch, Lynch, & Conway, 1993).

The highest incidence of ovarian cancer occurs in industrialized countries, particularly those countries of Europe and North America, implicating environmental factors as risk factors. Ovarian cancer is more common in women from industrialized Western countries than in women from other parts of the world, with the exception of Japan. The Japanese rate is lower than the U.S. rate but higher than the rate elsewhere. However, Japanese women who immigrate to the United States develop an increased risk of ovarian cancer that approaches, but does not reach, the rate of White American women (Piver, Baker, Piedmonte, & Sandecki, 1991).

Meat and animal fat characterize the diet of people in industrialized nations. Do diets high in meat and animal fat—as well as high in alcohol, cigarette, and coffee consumption—contribute to ovarian cancer? The results of studies conflict (Cramer, Welch, Hutchinson, Willett, & Scully, 1984; Mettlin & Piver, 1990). Obesity is associated with a slight increase in risk, but studies did not demonstrate that cigarette and coffee consumption increased risk (Kuper, Titus-Ernstoff, Harlow, & Cramer, 2000).

Exposure of the ovaries to industrial by-products, triazine herbicides, and radiation have not been proven to be risk factors (Polychronopoulou et al., 1993). Migration of chemicals to the peritoneal cavity via the vagina and reproductive organs may account for exposure to carcinogens. Tests of talc and asbestos exposure as causes of ovarian cancer lack statistical significance (Tzonou et al., 1993).

Exogenous use of estrogens alone has not been associated with an increased risk of ovarian cancer. No evidence suggests that menopausal hormone replacement therapy increases the risk of developing ovarian cancer (Whittemore et al., 1988).

Signs and Symptoms

The initial spread of ovarian cancer is clinically "silent." Approximately 75%–85% of women have advanced disease at the time of diagnosis. A significant number of women with disease seemingly confined to the ovaries have microscopic spread at the time of diagnosis (Ozols, Rubin, et al., 1997).

Ovarian cancer is difficult to detect because its symptoms and potential signs are vague. The symptoms women often describe include distention, dyspepsia, bloating, gastrointestinal disturbances, and vague pelvic discomfort. These symptoms typically occur in advanced stages, when tumor growth creates pressure on the bladder and rectum, and ascites begins to form. Approximately 10% of ovarian cancers are found in the early stages (Ozols, Rubin, et al., 1997). A woman may experience vague symptoms for many months before the tumor becomes apparent.

Primary Prevention

Even though the exact etiology of ovarian cancer is unknown, current epidemiologic and genetic data suggest several prevention strategies. These include oral contraceptive use, diet modification, and prophylactic oophorectomy.

The risk of ovarian cancer correlates with the length of time a woman has ovulated. As uninterrupted ovulation cycles continue, the probability of developing ovarian cancer increases. Pregnancy, lactation, tubal ligation, oral contraceptive use, and early menopause suppress ovulating cycles and seem to decrease risk. The cascade of epithelial events prompted by ovulation include minor trauma; a bathing of the surrounding tissue with estrogen-rich follicular fluid; and increased proliferation of epithelium, particularly near the point of ovulation, with resulting inclusions into the ovarian parenchyma. Whittemore (1994) suggested that some of or all these events may lie in the causal path of ovarian cancer. This theory is consistent with most of the endocrine-related risk factors, except for the risks associated with infertility.

For a decade researchers have known that oral contraceptives decrease the risk of ovarian cancer in young women. The longer a woman takes oral contraceptives, the greater the protection, and the protection persists for many years after stopping. Subsequent multiple studies have substantiated the initial studies (Fathalla, 1971; Hankinson et al., 1992; WHO Collaborative Study of Neoplasia and Steroid Contraceptives, 1989). A woman who uses oral contraceptives for a total of five years can significantly decrease her risk of ovarian cancer by up to 60%. Even women with a BRCA mutation who have used oral contraceptives for a total of five years may decrease their risk of developing ovarian cancer (Creasman, 1997b).

Epidemiologic studies to evaluate risk factors for epithelial ovarian cancer indicate a higher incidence in nulliparous or low-parity women. Women who have been pregnant and have breast-fed for at least three months have a smaller chance of developing ovarian cancer than do nulliparous women and women without a history of contraceptive use (Whittemore et al., 1988).

All women should be counseled regarding the beneficial effects of a low-fat diet that is high in vitamin A. The benefits of such a diet in regard to the prevention of ovarian cancer and other cancers are well established. Nurses can help women make lifestyle modifications so their diets include low-fat, high-fiber foods and an adequate number of vegetables and fruits. Nurses can support women in their attempts to exercise regularly; limit alcohol intake; and avoid carcinogens, such as cigarettes.

Tubal ligation or hysterectomy also may decrease the risk of developing ovarian cancer but not to the extent that oral contraceptives do (Whittemore et al., 1988).

Women older than age 40 who are about to undergo a hysterectomy for a noncancerous condition involving the uterus, such as uterine fibroids, may decide to have an oophorectomy during the procedure to eliminate the risk of ovarian cancer (Creasman, 1997b). A woman considering an elective oophorectomy at the time of hysterectomy for benign disease should be counseled based on age, parity, risk factors, menstrual status, family and personal history, likelihood of postoperative follow-up, and cultural factors. Nurses are in a key position to assist women with this highly individual decision by providing information and counseling regarding the potential benefits and consequences of oophorectomy.

Prophylactic oophorectomy for women with family risk factors is controversial because it may not offer total protection from intra-abdominal carcinoma. Numerous reports have provided evidence that intra-abdominal carcinomatosis can arise from celomic epithelium after prophylactic oophorectomy (Chen, Schooley, & Flam, 1985; Narod et al., 1998; Tobacman et al., 1982). For women with an inherited familial hereditary cancer syndrome, the National Institutes of Health (NIH) Consensus Development Conference on Ovarian Cancer (NIH, 1994) recommended use of oral contraceptives before childbearing and prophylactic oophorectomy after childbearing, preferably by age 35. Those women with unequivocally high genetic risk for ovarian cancer (i.e., women who have two or more first-degree relatives with ovarian cancer) should be counseled and considered for prophylactic oophorectomy when childbearing is not an interest. Such a woman must consider the long-term physiologic and psychologic effects of oophorectomy, which may necessitate hormone replacement therapy, and management of menopausal symptoms. Prevention and screening for osteoporosis also are considerations.

Secondary Prevention: Early Detection

Currently, no procedure can reliably detect ovarian cancer in its early stage. Available screening techniques include pelvic examination (ovarian palpation), ultrasound examinations, evaluation of CA 125 and other tumor markers, and combined-modality approaches. The objective of cancer screening is to find the disease in a precancerous stage, prior to malignant transformation, or at an early, highly curable stage. Unfortunately, little is understood about the natural history of ovarian cancer. Experts cannot even confirm whether all ovarian cancers begin as precancerous lesions.

Ovarian cancers may not progress in an orderly fashion from stage I to IV. If they do, the length of time the cancer spends in each stage is unknown. Reports exist of women developing peritoneal carcinomatosis following oophorectomy. These reports suggest that the peritoneum, like the ovarian epithelium, is of embryologic origin and undergoes malignant transformation at the same time as either the ovary or the primary cancer.

A screening test must meet several criteria before it can be considered feasible and cost-effective. It should be simple to perform, inexpensive, acceptable to the patient and to the people performing it, safe, relatively painless, and valid. Sensitivity, specificity, and predictive values measure the validity of the test. Ideally, a test should have both a high sensitivity and specificity, but an increase in one usually leads to a decrease in the other.

In addition, a positive predictive value is dependent on the prevalence of the disease in the study population. If, for example, only women with a positive family history of ovarian cancer were screened, a much less specific test could be performed to keep the positive predictive value at 10%. The vast majority of women destined to develop ovarian cancer have a negative family history and probably would not benefit from a screening program.

In the United States , 43 million women are older than age 45. Screening all U.S. women by using pelvic ultrasound and CA 125 assessment would cost 14 billion dollars per year. No evidence to date suggests that such screening would significantly increase early diagnosis or improve survival rates for women with ovarian cancer. A screening test for ovarian cancer must have a specificity of 99.6% to make a true impact on the disease. Assuming 100% sensitivity, a test for women older than age 45 must have a specificity of 99.6% to achieve a 10% positive predictive value; a test for women older than age 45 and women with a BRCA1 mutation must have a specificity of 90% to achieve a 10% positive predictive value (Creasman, 1997b).

Pelvic Examinations

Detecting an asymptomatic pelvic mass through routine pelvic examination may identify an ovarian carcinoma before abdominal dissemination (see Figure 13-8). No data report the frequency with which annual rectopelvic examination detects ovarian cancer in asymptomatic women, however. Furthermore, no evidence suggests that detecting ovarian cancer by such means alters morbidity or mortality. Thus, although the healthcare establishment continues to recommend yearly pelvic examinations for women past the age of 40, the benefit of these examinations as screenings for ovarian cancer has not been established (Ozols, Rubin et al., 1997).

Figure 13-8. The Pelvic Examination

A pelvic examination consists of (a) a digital exam, (b) palpation of the rectum and uterus, and (c) bimanual palpation.

(a) a digital exam

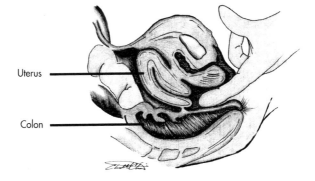

Uterus

Colon

(b) palpation of the rectum and uterus

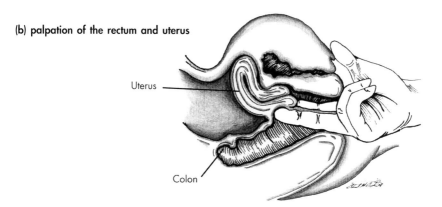

Uterus

Colon

(c) bimanual palpation

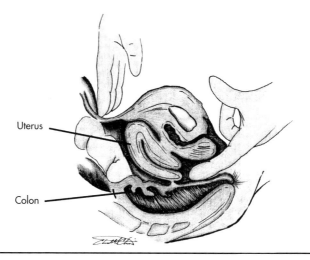

Uterus

Colon

Ultrasonography

Abdominal ultrasonography is a screening procedure that is easy to perform, acceptable by most women, and essentially free of complications. However, abdominal ultrasonography is not sufficiently specific to be useful as a routine screening procedure. In a prospective study of more than 5,000 self-referred asymptomatic women undergoing annual transabdominal ultrasonography at King's College Hospital, London, five women with primary ovarian cancer (three with borderline tumors) were identified from a total of 15,977 scans. To diagnose the five cases, 338 laparotomies were performed. The laparotomies revealed that an additional four women had metastatic ovarian cancer. Although the apparent detection rate was 100%, the false-positive rate was 2.3% and the specificity was 97.7%; therefore, the odds that an abnormal transabdominal ultrasound indicated the presence of a primary ovarian cancer were 1 in 67 (Campbell, Bhan, Roysten, Whitehead, & Collins, 1989).

Recently, transvaginal ultrasonography with color Doppler flow has been proposed as a more specific alternative to abdominal ultrasonography as a screening test. Transvaginal ultrasonography with color Doppler flow offers increased resolution capable of detecting slight morphologic changes in the ovary (Van Nagell et al., 1991), and it can detect intraovarian vascular changes. The ability to track ovarian neovascularization, which the Doppler component reveals by detecting impeded blood flow, may help healthcare professionals to distinguish benign from malignant ovarian tumors. Initial results are promising; however, studies are needed to determine the actual accuracy of this new technique.

CA 125

Overall, more than 80% of women with advanced ovarian cancer have an elevated CA 125 level (a level greater than 35 u/ml) (Bast et al., 1983). CA 125, a protein associated with the surface of ovarian cancer cells, is expressed in 80% of nonmucinous epithelial ovarian cancers. Nevertheless, the CA 125 test is not useful in detecting early-stage disease because it is accurate only 50% of the time, particularly in premenopausal women. Noncancerous conditions may decrease the accuracy of the CA 125 test; conditions such as pregnancy, endometriosis, uterine fibroids, liver disease, and benign ovarian cysts may elevate CA 125 levels. Tracking the CA 125 level is one way of measuring a woman's response to ovarian cancer therapy (Gard & Houghton, 1994).

Multimodal Screening

Preliminary studies using serum CA 125 levels, pelvic examinations, and ultrasonography have demonstrated that ovarian cancer can be detected in asymptomatic women. However, these procedures are associated with a significant false-positive rate such that an unacceptably large number of negative laparotomies would result if each "positive" screening test resulted in surgical exploration aimed at diagnosing early ovarian cancer. A recent review of uncontrolled trials of ovarian cancer screenings of 36,000 women showed that 29 cases of ovarian cancer were identified, but only 12 (41%) were stage I (Cronin, Weed, Connor, & Prorok, 1998). Survival is unlikely to be significantly affected by an earlier diagnosis of advanced-stage disease. Based on these considerations, the NIH Consensus Conference on Ovarian Cancer (NIH, 1994) did not recommend ovarian cancer screening for women without risk factors.

Compared to women with a BRCA mutation who undergo prophylactic surgery, women with a BRCA mutation who do not undergo surgery may be at significantly increased risk for the development of ovarian cancer (40%) as well as breast cancer (60%) by age 70. Therefore, women who do not have prophylactic surgery require more intensive clinical surveillance (Burke et al., 1997). Women with family histories consistent with a genetic predisposition to hereditary cancers require more intensive evaluations when presenting with abdominal or pelvic symptoms, even if the symptoms are vague.

The NIH consensus statement concluded that women at increased risk should have, at least annually, a comprehensive gynecologic examination (a pelvic exam that includes a rectovaginal exam), a test for serum marker CA 125, and a transvaginal or transabdominal ultrasonography screening. The NIH made this recommendation despite the lack of data supporting the use of these measures for ovarian cancer screening (NIH, 1994).

Research Initiatives

To effect change in the morbidity and mortality associated with ovarian cancer, it is necessary to identify those individuals at increased risk and clinically apply the understanding of the biochemical and molecular biology of ovarian carcinogenesis, improve available treatment, and prevent invasion and metastasis. Ovarian carcinogenesis, invasion, and metastasis require a complex cascade of interrelated genetic, molecular, and biochemical events that regulate aberrations affecting cell-cycle control, apoptosis, adhesion, angiogenesis, transmembrane-signaling DNA repair, and genomic stability (Plagxe, Deligdisch, Dotting, & Chen, 1995). Specific genetic aberrations found in ovarian cancer include amplification or over-expression of ErbB2 and PIK3CA (Katso et al., 1997). These regions of recurrent abnormality may encode genes that contribute to ovarian cancer progression as a result of abnormal copy number or mutation.

The metastatic processes of cellular adhesion, migration, extracellular matrix degradation, invasion into host parenchyma, proliferation, and neovascularization are influenced by numerous regulatory molecules. These include epidermal growth factor (EGF) and receptors (EGFR/ErbB); urinary-type plasminogen (uPA) and receptor (uPAR); telomerase; and lysophospholipids, such as lysophosphatidic acid (LPA) (Ellerbrock, Fishman, Kearns, Bafetti, & Stack, 1999; Fishman, Kearns, Bafetti, & Stack, 1998). Preliminary data indicate that LPA upregulates proteinase uPA and matrix metalloproteinase (MMP) expression and enhances invasion. Telomerase is expressed in malignant, abnormal ovarian epithelium. The detection of proteinase and active MMPs, uPA and uPAR, EGFR/ErbB1, and lyso-phospholipids may be detected in serum (Ellerbrock et al.). These biomarkers may be useful in the detection of early-stage ovarian cancer in women deemed at increased risk. The effectiveness of these biomarkers in cancer screening must be compared to the effectiveness of the established marker, CA 125.

Ovarian epithelial dysplasia had been characterized by morphometric methods, revealing specific changes in the architecture and cytologic characteristics of the ovarian surface. Retrospective analysis of women with stage I ovarian carcinoma assessed the presence of cellular and nuclear atypia in noncancerous tissue adjacent to the primary tumor. Atypia was more common in the women with cancer and was defined as the presence of nuclear pleomorphism or irregular chromatin distribution. Cellular atypia was defined as presence of stratification or loss of polarity. The presence of nuclear atypia was used to define ovarian intraepithelial neoplasia, which is believed to precede the development of ovarian cancer (Plagxe et al., 1995).

Ovarian surface epithelium (OSE) sampling via the ovarian Pap test currently is being evaluated. This newly developed minimally invasive office laparoscopic procedure allows a direct view of the ovaries and permits the healthcare professional to take samples from the ovaries and peritoneum for detailed cytologic evaluation. Direct sampling of tissue from the ovaries and peritoneum is required to screen for premalignant or early malignant changes of the ovary and peritoneal epithelium (Runowicz, 1995).

The development of novel biomarkers and evaluation of the OSE is a project of the National Ovarian Cancer Early Detection Program (NOCEDP). NOCEDP is sponsored by NCI and represents the largest integrated program of clinicians, scientists, and institutions with complementary expertise focusing on asymptomatic women at increased risk. The clinical research program includes ovarian cancer risk assessment and the evaluation of the molecular and biochemical interactions regulating ovarian carcinogenesis. This work may translate into screening tests and new tumor markers for the early detection of ovarian cancer.

Little is known about the etiology of ovarian cancer at the molecular and genetic levels. Use of the ovarian Pap test affords the ability to compare ovarian epithelium from asymptomatic women at increased risk for the development of ovarian cancer to samples showing the changes associated with ovarian cancer. By comparing these samples, it may be possible to develop molecular profiles of the changes relevant to the tumor progression of sporadic ovarian cancer. This work may reveal early genomic or biologic changes that will allow detection of early-stage epithelial ovarian cancer and identify markers of premalignant changes.

Nursing Challenges

The issues of genetic counseling and cancer risk for women who are at increased risk for ovarian cancer are of great importance (Daly & Lerman, 1993; Runowicz, 1995). Specifically trained oncology nurses can provide cancer genetic counseling and calculate risk information while providing education and emotional support (Calzone, 1997; Loescher, 1998). These nurses are uniquely positioned to promote the health of women at risk for ovarian cancer and tailor assessment plans to their social, educational, and economic status. This is particularly true in regard to women considering prophylactic surgery. In addition, nurses can mobilize strategies from other aspects of oncology nursing care—such as support groups, educational seminars, and peer or individual counseling—that may be beneficial in reducing the stress of receiving genetic information or cancer risk assessment. Nurses are in a unique position to help women at risk for ovarian cancer to understand the information they receive and the consequences of it (Mahon, 1998).

Conclusion

The reality of early detection of ovarian cancer is on the horizon. The benefits of a centralized program for early detection will be manifest at several levels. First, and perhaps most important, promotion of a "national program" funded by NCI and supported by the Ovarian Cancer National Alliance and National Ovarian Cancer Coalition will enhance women's awareness of and improve access to early-detection clinics throughout the United States. Second, the cost-benefit ratio gained through a coordinated effort will be profound. Third, the potential for scientists to benefit by expanding their access to preliminary-result data is enormous. Last, the ability of researchers to measure the impact of participating in a clinical research program for the early detection of ovarian cancer will improve. This may result in increased cost-effectiveness of screening and a better quality of life for women with ovarian cancer.

Endometrial Cancer

Cancer of the endometrium is the most common invasive gynecologic cancer and the fourth most frequently diagnosed cancer among American women today. Currently, endometrial cancer is predominantly a disease of postmenopausal women, with an average age at diagnosis of 61 years. However, 25% of cases occur in premenopausal women, and 5% occur in women younger than 40 years of age. Survival rates for endometrial cancer are 76% for women with stage I, 50% for those with stage II, 30% for those with stage III, and 9% for those with stage IV disease (ACS, 2000).

Epidemiology

Endometrial cancer rates are highest in North America and northern Europe; intermediate in Israel, southern Europe, and Latin America; and low in Asia and Africa (Muir, Waterhouse, Mack, Powell, & Whelan, 1987). The disease is rare before the age of 45, but the risk rises sharply among women in their late 40s to middle 60s. The age-adjusted incidence for Whites is approximately twice as high as for non-Whites, with reasons for discrepancy remaining largely undefined. Within the last several decades in the United States, a dramatic change in the incidence pattern for endometrial cancer has occurred, characterized by a marked increase that peaked around 1975. Considerable evidence has linked this rise and fall with the widespread use of estrogen replacement therapy in the late '60s and early '70s (White, 1993).

Temporal changes in endometrial cancer rates may be affected by several factors: the use of exogenous estrogens; hysterectomy rates (i.e., decreased numbers of women with uteri); the proportion of older women in the population (75% of women are diagnosed after age 50); and changes in the prevalence of specific risk factors (e.g., obesity, nulliparity) (White, 1993).

Pathophysiology

The uterus occupies the space between the bladder and the rectum and is divided structurally and functionally into two parts—the corpus (or body) and the cervix—which are separated by a slight narrowing of the uterus known as the isthmus. This is the location of the internal os of the cervix. The cervix is divided into the supravaginal portion (which is close to the bladder) and the vaginal portion (which projects into the cavity of the vagina). The walls of the uterus are composed of muscular tissue called the myometrium. The epithelial membrane that lines the uterine corpus is called the endometrium. The principal ligaments that support the uterus are the broad ligaments, the round ligaments, the uterosacral ligaments, and the cardinal ligaments. Blood is supplied to the uterus by the uterine artery, which is a branch of the hypogastric, or internal iliac, artery. The uterine artery enters the wall of the uterus at the isthmus. The lymphatics of the myometrium drain into the subserosal network of lymphatics, which coalesce into larger channels before leaving the uterus. Lymph flows from the fundus toward the adnexa and the infundibulopelvic ligaments. Lymph flow from the lower and middle thirds of the uterus tends to spread in the base of the broad ligaments toward the lateral pelvic sidewall (Barkat, Park, Grigsby, Muss, & Norris, 1997).

Cancer of the endometrium arises from the glandular component of the endometrial mucosa. The disease may be locally confined to a polyp, or it may spread diffusely throughout the endometrial lining. The disease commonly involves the upper portion of the uterine cavity (Huang, Berek, & Fu, 1992). Endometrial tumor growth tends to be slow, invading the myometrium and advancing toward the isthmus and cervix. Extrauterine spread occurs by direct extension of tumor cells through the fallopian tubes, resulting in peritoneal implants. Lymphatic invasion of the tumor results in metastasis to the pelvic, aortic, and inguinal lymph nodes. Hematogenous metastasis to distant sites frequently involves the pulmonary system (Morrow, Curtin, & Townsend, 1993).

The initial pathologic evaluation of endometrial tissue determines the cell type and histologic grade. Following surgery, depth of myometrial invasion and lymph node involvement are defined by pathologic diagnosis. The evaluation also must include a thorough microscopic evaluation of the cervix for evidence of tumor extension (Barkat et al., 1997). These factors determine prognosis and assist in developing an individualized treatment plan.

Grade 1 endometrial cancers are well differentiated and generally associated with a good prognosis. Grade 2 cancers are moderately differentiated and suggest an intermediate prognosis, and grade 3 cancers are poorly differentiated lesions, which suggest a poor prognosis. As the cancer becomes less differentiated, the risk of deep myometrial invasion and lymph node metastases increases (DiSaia & Creasman, 1997; Piver, Lele, Barlow, & Blumenson, 1982).

Endometrioid adenocarcinoma is the most common histologic cell type found in endometrial cancer, accounting for 75%–85% of all cases (Wilson et al., 1990). There are four main variants of adenocarcinoma. Adenocanthoma is composed of benign squamous metaplasia and adenocarcinoma. Adenocanthoma lesions tend to be well differentiated. Adenosquamous carcinoma contains a malignant squamous component, which is poorly differentiated and associated with extrauterine spread (Barkat et al., 1997). Papillary adenocarcinoma tends toward myometrial invasion and peritoneal surface involvement. This cell subtype is common in African American women and older women (DiSaia & Creasman, 1997). Secretory adenocarcinoma is an uncommon cell subtype that usually is well differentiated and suggests a favorable prognosis.

Mucinous carcinoma is a rare cell type and common in the endocervix. Serous carcinoma is a poor prognostic and an aggressive tumor type associated with early lymphatic and myometrial spread (Barkat et al., 1997). Clear-cell carcinoma often occurs in older women and tends to be aggressive, suggesting a poor prognosis.

Figure 13-9 lists histologic cell types relating to endometrial cancer. Overall prognosis is dependent on both uterine and extrauterine factors. Uterine factors include histologic cell type, tumor grade, depth of myometrial invasion, occult extension to the cervix, and vascular space invasion. Extrauterine factors include intraperitoneal and adnexal spread, positive peritoneal cytology, pelvic lymph node metastases, and aortic lymph node involvement (Sutton, 1990). The uterus may or may not be enlarged; therefore, enlargement is not a reliable indicator. To adequately evaluate prognostic factors and extent of disease, a surgical staging procedure is necessary. In 1988, the International Federation of Gynecology and Obstetrics defined surgical-stage criteria based on degree of myometrial invasion, endocervical involvement, nodal spread, and metastatic disease.

Figure 13-9. Classification of Histologic Cell Types

Endometrioid adenocarcinoma	Serous carcinoma
Adenocanthoma	Clear-cell carcinoma
Adenosquamous carcinoma	Squamous carcinoma
Papillary carcinoma	Undifferentiated carcinoma
Secretory carcinoma	Mixed types
Mucinous carcinoma	Metastatic carcinoma

Note. From "Cancer of the Endometrium" (p. 169) by B.M. Paniscotti in G.J. Moore-Higgs, L.A. Almadrones, B. Colvin-Huff, L.M. Gossfeld, and J.H. Eriksson (Eds.), *Women and Cancer: A Gynecologic Nursing Perspective* (2nd ed.), 2000, Boston: Jones and Bartlett. Copyright 2000 by Jones and Bartlett. Reprinted with permission.

Risk Factors

Risk factors for endometrial cancer have been well defined and include age, obesity, polycystic ovarian syndrome, parity, infertility, diabetes mellitus, hypertension, use of unopposed estrogen therapy or tamoxifen, adenomatous hyperplasia, and Lynch syndrome II (see Table 13-1) (Parazzini, La Vecchia, Bocciolone, & Franceschi, 1991; White, 1993).

Postmenopausal women are at the greatest risk for endometrial cancer; the average age at diagnosis is 61 years (White, 1993). Most studies have indicated that the age at menopause is directly related to the risk of developing endometrial cancer. About 70% of all women diagnosed with endometrial cancer are postmenopausal (Morrow et al., 1993). Most studies support the assertion that there is nearly a twofold risk associated with natural menopause after age 52 than before age 49 (Barkat et al., 1997). The effect of late age at menopause on risk may reflect prolonged exposure of the uterus to estrogen stimulation in the presence of anovulatory (progesterone-deficient) cycles. The interrelationships among menstrual factors, age, and weight are complex, and the biologic mechanisms of these variables operating in the pathogenesis of endometrial cancer are subject to substantial speculation.

Several studies found that, among younger women, the effects of age at menarche were stronger than among older women, although this trend was not consistently demonstrated (Parazzini et al., 1991; Schottenfeld, 1995). The extent to which these relationships reflect increased exposure to ovarian hormones or other correlates of early menarche (e.g., increased body weight) is unresolved. However, approximately 25% of the cases occur in premenopausal women, and 5% are diagnosed before age 40.

Obesity is a well-recognized risk factor for endometrial cancer. Obesity may account for as many as 25% of the cases (Hill & Austin, 1996). Very heavy women appear to have a disproportionately high risk. Women weighing 200 pounds or more have a risk that is seven times greater than that of women weighing less than 125 pounds (Brinton et al., 1992). Obesity appears to affect both premenopausal and postmenopausal endometrial cancer. Abnormalities in endogenous estrogen production or metabolism and lack of progesterone effect on the endometrial lining associated with obesity may account for this increased risk.

Epidemiologic studies also have evaluated the etiologic role of dietary factors. Geographic differences in disease rates (i.e., high rates in Western societies and low rates in Eastern societies) suggest that diet, especially the high content of animal fat in Western diets, plays a role (Barbone, Austin, & Partridge, 1993). A correlation may exist between total fat intake and endometrial cancer incidence. Higher levels of plasma estrone, estradiol, and prolactin are found among women consuming a high-fat or omnivorous diet rather than a low-fat or vegetarian diet.

Hormonal and reproductive factors play an important role in the development of endometrial cancer. Endogenous estrogen production associated with polycystic ovary syndrome has been identified as a risk factor. Endometrial proliferation associated with this syndrome may be reversed by treatment with clomiphene citrate or progesterone or by wedge resection of the ovary (DiSaia & Creasman, 1997; Fu, Gambone, & Berek, 1990).

Nulliparity is a recognized risk factor for endometrial cancer (Brinton et al., 1992). The risk of endometrial cancer decreases with increasing parity; evidence from the Iowa Women's Health Study (McPherson, Sellers, Potter, Bostick, &

Table 13-1. Risks for Endometrial Cancer

Characteristic	Increased Risk
Obesity	
> 30 lb.	3x
> 50 lb.	10x
Nulliparous	2x
Late menopause	2.4x
"Bloody" menopause	4x
Diabetes mellitus	2.8x
Hypertension	1.5x
Unopposed estrogen	9.5x
Complex atypical hyperplasia	29x

Note. From "Corpus: Epithelial Tumors" (p. 860) by R.R. Barkul, R.C. Park, P.W. Grigcby, H.D. Muss, and H.J. Norris in W.J. Hoskins, C.A. Perez, and R.C. Young (Eds.), *Principles and Practice of Gynecologic Oncology*, 1996, Philadelphia: J.B. Lippincott. Copyright 1996 by J.B. Lippincott. Reprinted with permission.

Folsom, 1996) supports the association of endometrial cancer with early age at menarche, late age at natural menopause, and total length of ovulation span. However, infertility and ages at first and last pregnancy may be unrelated to risk after adjustment for gravity. Results suggest that a miscarriage late in reproductive life, followed by lack of a subsequent full-term pregnancy, may be a marker for progesterone deficiency and supports the "unopposed" estrogen hypothesis for the etiology of endometrial cancer.

The relationship between exogenous hormones and risk of endometrial cancer has received considerable attention. Many studies found that any use of estrogen replacement therapy is associated with a 2- to 12-fold elevation in risk of endometrial cancer (Brinton & Hoover, 1993; Hulka, 1994; Kelsey & Whitmore, 1994). In most investigations, the increased risk was not observed unless the drugs were used for at least two to three years, and longer use of estrogen generally was associated with higher risk (Brinton & Hoover; Hulka; Kelsey & Whitmore).

The associations of risk with estrogen replacement therapy are strongest among women who are thin, nondiabetic, and normotensive (Brinton et al., 1992; Hulka, 1994; Kelsey & Whitmore, 1994). These findings suggest that estrogen metabolism differs in these groups of women or that risk is already so high for obese, hypertensive, or diabetic women that exposure to exogenous estrogens has only a small additional effect.

Further evidence of the role of exogenous hormones in the pathogenesis of endometrial cancer derives from studies that evaluated the effects of oral contraceptives. These studies demonstrated that users of sequential oral contraceptives (i.e., contraceptives containing a high dose of estrogen and a weak dose of progestin) had a significantly higher risk of endometrial cancer than did women using estrogen-progestin combination pills (Rosenblatt & Thomas, 1991).

A number of clinical trials and population-based case-control studies indicated an increased risk of endometrial cancer among tamoxifen-treated women with breast cancer. This is consistent with the estrogenic effects of tamoxifen on the endometrium (Fornander, Hellstrom, & Morberger, 1993; Peters-Engl et al., 1999; van Leeuwen et al., 1994). The report of the National Surgical Adjuvant Breast and Bowel Project (NSABP) B-14 trial revealed data regarding the rates of endometrial and other cancers (Fisher et al., 1994). Women with breast cancer who had node-negative, estrogen receptor–positive, invasive breast cancer were randomly assigned to receive placebo or tamoxifen (20 mg/day). Data regarding rates of endometrial and other cancers were analyzed on 2,843 women enrolled in this study and 1,220 tamoxifen-treated women registered in NSABP B-14. Two of the 1,424 women assigned to receive placebo developed endometrial cancer; however, both subsequently received tamoxifen for treatment of breast cancer recurrence. Fifteen women randomized to tamoxifen treatment developed endometrial cancer. Eight additional cases of uterine cancer occurred in the 1,220 tamoxifen-treated women. Seventy-six percent of the endometrial cancers occurred in women age 60 or older. The mean duration of tamoxifen therapy was 35 months, with 36% of the endometrial cancers developing within two years of therapy and six occurring less than nine months after treatment started. This suggests that some of the cancers may have been present prior to the start of tamoxifen therapy. The average annual hazard rate for endometrial cancer in the placebo group was 0.2/1,000 and 1.6/ 1,000 for the randomized tamoxifen-treated group. The relative risk of an endometrial cancer occurring in the randomized tamoxifen-treated group was 7.5%. Similar results were seen in the 1,220 women who received tamoxifen. The risks of tamoxifen treatment in inducing endometrial cancer must be weighed against the benefits of tamoxifen in reducing breast cancer recurrence and new contralateral breast cancers. Taking into account the increased cumulative rate of endometrial cancer, there was a 38% reduction in the five-year cumulative hazard rate in the tamoxifen-treated group. Thus, the benefit of tamoxifen therapy for breast cancer outweighs the reported potential increase of endometrial cancer.

Progesterone has been shown to produce regressive changes in endometrial hyperplasia, a presumed precursor of endometrial cancer. The idea of combining estrogen therapy with progestins to combat carcinogenic effect recently has evoked widespread enthusiasm. Women receiving combined therapy have had lower rates of endometrial hyperplasia than have women receiving estrogens alone. The effect of combined therapy on the occurrence of endometrial cancer remains less clear.

A hereditary pattern, Lynch syndrome II, is associated with endometrial cancer. Lynch syndrome II is characterized by a significant genetic association between hereditary nonpolyposis colorectal cancer and the development of endometrial carcinoma. Other cancers noted in the same families include carcinoma of the ovary, urologic system, stomach, small bowel, pancreas, and breast. Healthcare professionals caring for women with endometrial cancer must obtain a complete family history to determine the possibility of Lynch syndrome II (Lynch, Bardawil, & Harris, 1978; Lynch, Ens, & Lynch, 1990; Whitehead, Hillard, & Crook, 1990).

Signs and Symptoms

The cardinal symptom of both endometrial hyperplasia and endometrial cancer is abnormal vaginal bleeding. In women younger than age 45, the development of endometrial cancer may be associated with obesity and a history of anovulation. Endometrial cancer sometimes is diagnosed during an evaluation for infertility, when symptoms include spotting or unusually heavy menstrual bleeding (menometrorrhagia) or scant menstruation (oligomenorrhea). In postmenopausal women, vaginal bleeding is an indicator of malignancy and should be investigated to rule out atrophic vaginitis or medicinal withdrawal bleeding. Any bleeding that occurs 12 months after menses have stopped is considered abnormal. A purulent, sometimes blood-tinged vaginal discharge also may be a presenting symptom of endometrial cancer. Pelvic pressure, pain, ascites, and hemorrhage may indicate advanced disease (Barkat et al., 1997).

Primary Prevention

Hormonal imbalance is the single most significant causative factor relating to endometrial cancer (Kelsey & Whitmore, 1994). The endometrial lining is controlled in a cyclic fashion by estrogen and progesterone. The actual etiology of the progression of normal cells to cancer is unknown. Therefore, it is vital to consider the risk factors in the disease process. Factors that reduce the risk of developing endometrial cancer are the use of combination oral contraceptives, which reduces menstrual proliferation, and weight loss, which reduces estrone production from adipose tissue (Morrow et al., 1993).

Endometrial hyperplasia is an overgrowth of the endometrial lining of the uterus as a result of prolonged estrogenic stimulation of the endometrium. Endometrial hyperplasia may clinically present as abnormal bleeding with excessive blood loss, may indicate anovulation and infertility, or may result from unopposed estrogen use.

In addition, endometrial hyperplasia may precede endometrial cancer; endometrial hyperplasia is considered a precursor to endometrial cancer, and it may occur with endometrial cancer. The term *endometrial hyperplasia* refers to the histopathologic state of the endometrial glands and stroma. The histopathologic classification accepted by the International Society of Gynecologic Pathologists consists of three categories: simple (cystic without atypia), complex (adenomatous without atypia), and atypical (simple cystic with atypia or complex adenomatous with atypia).

Endometrial hyperplasia with cellular atypia is considered premalignant. Endometrial hyperplasia without atypia is benign. However, the endometrium continues to be predisposed to the development of cancer in the absence of cytologic atypia based on the underlying pathophysiologic state (Morrow et al., 1993). Hyperplasia progresses to cancer in 1% of women with simple hyperplasia. The progression rate for women with complex hyperplasia is 3%. When atypia accompanies hyperplasia, the progression rate to cancer is much higher. The rate rises to 8% for women with simple atypical hyperplasia and 29% in cases of complex atypical hyperplasia (Barkat et al., 1997).

Women with atypical hyperplasia may be treated by periodic use of progestins or hysterectomy, depending on age and reproductive desires. Hysterectomy is the preferred treatment for women with complex atypical hyperplasia. This approach not only cures the usual presenting symptoms of abnormal bleeding but also confers prophylaxis against the almost 30% risk of later developing endometrial cancer (DiSaia & Creasman, 1997). Those women treated with progestins should have a dilatation and curettage (D&C) performed before treatment to rule out the occasional occult carcinoma not detected by biopsy. A progestin should be administered at least 10–14 days each month and endometrial biopsies performed at three- to four-month intervals to assess treatment results. The addition of progestins to the regimens of women treated with exogenous estrogens may prevent endometrial hyperplasia and the subsequent development of cancer (Barkat et al., 1997; Persson et al., 1989).

Another preventive measure for perimenopausal women with fluctuating levels of estrogen who are amenorrheic or hypermenorrheic or for any woman with a suspected condition of unopposed endogenous estrogen production is periodic treatment with a progestin. This creates scheduled withdrawal bleeding and prevents hyperplasia. A progesterone challenge may be helpful in defining this group of women. This test involves challenging a nonpregnant amenorrheic woman with progesterone to see if withdrawal bleeding occurs. If bleeding does occur, endometrial sampling may be performed to confirm a diagnosis. Appropriate treatment and follow-up then can be established (Barkat et al., 1997).

Secondary Prevention: Early Detection

No effective screening test exists for endometrial cancer. The pelvic exam enables the clinician to detect only whether the uterus is of abnormal size. Even though Pap smear screening is effective for cervical cancer, it detects only an occasional endometrial cancer if the vaginal pool is sampled. Currently, the American College of Obstetricians and Gynecologists (ACOG) and ACS recommend an annual pelvic exam and Pap smear screening (ACOG, 1997; ACS, 2000). Sampling of the endometrium is neither cost-effective nor indicated for the general population and, for asymptomatic women, is not required before or during hormone replacement therapy (ACOG).

The standard method of assessing uterine bleeding and diagnosing endometrial cancer is the formal fractional D&C. Before dilating the cervix, the endocervix should be curetted. Careful sounding of the uterus is then accomplished; dilatation of the cervix is performed, followed by systematic curetting of the entire endometrial cavity. Cervical and endometrial specimens should be kept separate and forwarded for pathologic diagnosis. Fractional D&C provides the maximum amount of tissue from the endometrial cavity and the opportunity for examination while the woman is relaxed under anesthesia (DiSaia & Creasman, 1997). Outpatient procedures, such as endometrial biopsy or aspiration curettage coupled with endocervical sampling, are definitive if positive for cancer. However, if sampling techniques fail to provide sufficient diagnostic information, a fractional D&C is mandatory.

Results of endometrial biopsies correlate well with endometrial curettings (Creasman, 1997b). However, the methods individually or combined may miss an existing endometrial carcinoma because the sampling is random and does not include the entire endometrium. If a biopsy or curettage obtains the endometrium, 15%–25% of women with a diagnosis of atypical hyperplasia may have a uterine cancer (Creasman, 1997a). In cases of women with atypical hyperplasia, treatment that does not include hysterectomy should be actively followed with endometrial sampling and D&C if results are unclear.

Nursing Challenges

Nurses can play an important role in the prevention of endometrial cancer by promoting risk-reduction strategies. These include annual pelvic examination, sequencing progesterone with estrogen replacement therapy, use of oral contraceptives for birth control, regular medical check-ups for control of medical conditions (e.g., diabetes, hypertension), and diet modifications for weight control or weight loss. Any woman with abnormal uterine bleeding should be encouraged to seek timely medical evaluation. By educating women about endometrial cancer, nurses give them the information women need to take responsibility for their health and well-being. Education is vitally important in reducing the morbidity and mortality associated with the disease.

Summary

Nurses will continue to play an important role in the prevention and early detection of gynecologic cancers. NPs can provide screening examinations and refer patients for diagnostic evaluations when appropriate. Nurses can teach patients about primary prevention strategies. As more is learned about genetic predisposition for gynecologic cancers, new roles for nurse geneticists will emerge. Nurses can help to meet the psychosocial needs of women being evaluated for gynecologic cancer and help to promote adjustment. Perhaps the most important role nurses have in caring for women being evaluated for gynecologic cancer is as the patients' advocate and educator. By teaching women about their risk-factor profile, primary prevention strategies, signs and symptoms of disease, and the strengths and limitations of screening examinations, nurses help patients to become more actively involved in their care. This should ultimately improve patients' quality of life and decrease the mortality associated with gynecologic cancers.

References

American Cancer Society. (2000). *Cancer facts and figures, 2000.* Atlanta: Author.

American College of Obstetricians and Gynecologists. (1997). *Routine cancer screening* (ACOG Committee Opinion #185). Washington, DC: Author.

Andersen, E.S., & Arffmann, E. (1989). Adenocarcinoma in situ of the uterine cervix: A clinco-pathologic study of 36 cases. *Gynecologic Oncology, 35,* 1–7.

Barbone, F., Austin, H., & Partridge, E.E. (1993). Diet and endometrial cancer: A case control study. *American Journal of Epidemiology, 137,* 393–403.

Barkat, R.R., Park, R.C., Grigsby, P.W., Muss, H.B., & Norris, H.J. (1997). Corpus: Epithelial tumors. In W.J. Hoskins, C.A. Perez, & R.C. Young (Eds.), *Principles and practice of gynecologic oncology* (2nd ed.) (pp. 859–896). Philadelphia: Lippincott.

Bast, R.C., Klug, T.L., St. John, E., Jenison, E., Niloff, J.M., Lazarus, H., Berkowitz, R.S., Leavitt, T., Griffiths, C.T., Parker, L., Zurawski, V.R., & Knapp, R.C. (1983). A radio-immunoassay using a monoclonal antibody to monitor the course of epithelial ovarian cancer. *New England Journal of Medicine, 309,* 883–887.

Boseli, F., DeMartis, S., Rivasi, F., Toni, A., Abbiati, R., & Chiossi, G. (2000). The Italian experience of a Pap test and speculoscopy based screening programme. *Journal of Medical Screening, 7,* 160–162.

Branda, J.A. (1994). Pathology of cervical carcinoma and its prognostic implications. *Seminars in Oncology, 21,* 3–8.

Breast Cancer Linkage Consortium. (1999). Cancer risks in *BRCA2* mutation carriers. *Journal of the National Cancer Institute, 91,* 1310–1316.

Brinton, L.A., Berman, M.L., Mortel, R., Twiggs, L.B., Barrett, R.J., Wilbanks, G.D., Lannom, L., & Hoover, R.N. (1992). Reproductive, menstrual and medical risk factors for endometrial cancer: Results from a case-control study. *American Journal of Obstetrics and Gynecology, 167,* 1317–1325.

Brinton, L.A., & Fraumeni, J.F. (1986). Epidemiology of uterine cervical cancer. *Journal of Chronic Disease, 39,* 1051–1065.

Brinton, L.A., Hoover, R.N., & The Endometrial Cancer Collaborative Group. (1993). Estrogen replacement therapy and endometrial cancer risk: Unresolved issues. *Obstetrics and Gynecology, 81,* 265–271.

Burke, W., Daly, M., Garber, J., Botkin, J., Kahn, M.J., Lynch, P., McTiernan, A., Offit, K., Perlman, J., Petersen, G., Thomason, E., & Varricchio, C. (1997). Recommendations for follow-up care of individuals with an inherited predisposition to cancer. *JAMA*, 277, 997–1003.

Calzone, K. (1997). Genetic predisposition testing: Clinical implications for oncology nurses. *Oncology Nursing Forum, 24*, 712–718.

Campbell, S., Bhan, V., Roysten, P., Whitehead, M.I., & Collins, W.P. (1989). Transabdominal ultrasound screening for early ovarian cancer. *BMJ, 299*, 1363–1367.

Chen, K.T.K., Schooley, J.L., & Flam, M.S. (1985). Peritoneal carcinomatosis after prophylactic oophorectomy. *Gynecologic Oncology, 47*, 395–397.

Coker, A.L., Rosenberg, A.J., McCann, M.F., & Hulka, B.S. (1992). Active and passive cigarette smoke exposure and cervical intraepithelial neoplasia. *Cancer Epidemiology, Biomarkers, and Prevention, 1*, 349–356.

Cramer, D.W., Welch, W.R., Hutchinson, G.B., Willett, W., & Scully, R. (1984). Dietary animal fat in relation to ovarian cancer risk. *Obstetrics and Gynecology, 63*, 833–838.

Creasman, W.T. (1997a). Endometrial cancer: Incidence, prognostic factors, diagnosis, and treatment. *Seminars in Oncology, 24*, S1–140–50.

Creasman, W.T. (1997b). Ovarian cancer screening. *American College of Obstetricians and Gynecologists, 2*, 1–2, 14.

Cronin, K.A., Weed, D.L., Connor, R.J., & Prorok, P.C. (1998). Case-controlled studies of cancer screening: Theory and practice. *Journal of the National Cancer Institute, 90*, 498–504.

Daly, M.B., & Lerman, C. (1993). Ovarian cancer risk counseling: A guide for the practitioner. *Oncology, 7*(11), 27–34.

Dillner, J. (2000). Trends over time in the incidence of cervical neoplasia in comparison to trends over time in human papilloma infection. *Journal of Clinical Virology, 19*, 7–23.

DiSaia, P.J., & Creasman, W.T. (1997). *Clinical gynecologic oncology* (4th ed.). St. Louis, MO: Mosby.

Duncan, M.E., Tibaux, G., Pelzer, A., Reimann, K., Peutherer, J.F., Simmonds, P., Young, H., Jamil, Y., & Daroughar, S. (1990). First coitus before menarche and risk of sexually transmitted disease. *Lancet, 335*, 338–340.

Ellerbrock, S.M., Fishman, D.A., Kearns, A.S., Bafetti, L.M., & Stack M.S. (1999). Ovarian carcinoma regulation of matrix metalloproteinase-2 and membrane type 1 matrix metalloproteinase through beta1 integrin. *Cancer Research, 59*, 1635–1641.

Fathalla, M.F. (1971). Incessant ovulation: A factor in ovarian neoplasia. *Lancet, 2*, 163.

Feingold, A.R., Vermund, S.H., Burk, R.D., Kelley, K.F., Schrager, L.K., Schreiber, K., Munk, G., Friedland, G.H., & Klein, R.S. (1990). Cervical cytologic abnormalities and papillomavirus in women infected with human immunodeficiency virus. *Journal of Acquired Immune Deficiency Syndrome, 3*, 896–903.

Fisher, B., Costantino, J.P., Redmond, C.K., Fisher, E.R., Wickerham, D.L., & Cronin, W.M. (1994). Endometrial cancer in tamoxifen-treated breast cancer patients: Findings from the National Surgical Adjuvant Breast and Bowel Project (NSABP) B-14. *Journal of the National Cancer Institute, 86*, 527–537.

Fishman, D.A., Kearns, A.M., Bafetti, L.M., & Stack, M.S. (1998). Regulation of ovarian cancer metastasis: Tumor cell adhesion upregulates proteinase activity. *Gynecologic Oncology, 68*, 78.

Ford, D., Easton, D.F., Stratton, M., Narod, S., Godgar, D., Ford, D., Easton, D.F., Stratton, M., Narod, S., Goldgar, D., Devilee, P., Bishop, D.T., Weber, B., Lenoir, G., Chang-Claude, J., Sobol, H., Teare, M.D., Struewing, J., Arason, A., Scherneck, S., Peto, J., Rebbeck, T.R., Tonin, P., Neuhausen, S., Barkardottir, R., Eyfjord, J., Lynch, H., Ponder, B.A., Gayther, S.A., Zelada-Hedman, M., et al. (1998). Genetic heterogeneity and penetrance analysis of the BRCA1 and BRCA2 genes in breast cancer families. *American Journal of Human Genetics, 62,* 676–689.

Fornander, T., Hellstrom, A.C., & Moberger, B. (1993). Descriptive clinicopathologic study of 17 patients with endometrial cancer during or after adjuvant tamoxifen in early breast cancer. *Journal of the National Cancer Institute, 85,* 1850–1855.

Franco, E.L. (1991). Viral etiology of cervical cancer: A critique of the evidence. *Review of Infectious Disease, 13,* 1195–1206.

Fu, Y.S., Gambone, J.C., & Berek, J.S. (1990). Pathophysiology and management of endometrial hyperplasia and carcinoma. *Western Journal of Medicine, 153,* 50–61.

Gard, G.B., & Houghton, R.S. (1994). An assessment of the value of serum CA-125 measurements in the management of epithelial ovarian carcinoma. *Gynecologic Oncology, 53,* 283–289.

Graham, S., Priore, R., Graham, M., Browne, R., Burnett, W., & West, D. (1979). Genital cancer in wives of penile cancer patients. *Cancer, 44,* 1870–1874.

Hankinson, S.E., Colditz, G.A., Hunter, D.J., Spencer, T.L., Rosner, B., & Stampfer, M.J. (1992). A quantitative assessment of oral contraceptive use and risk of ovarian cancer. *Obstetrics and Gynecology, 80,* 708–714.

Hannaford, P.C. (1991). Cervical cancer and methods of contraception. *Advances in Contraception, 7,* 317–324.

Hill, H., & Austin, H. (1996). Nutrition and endometrial cancer. *Cancer Causes and Control, 7,* 19–32.

Hopkins, M.P., & Morley, G.W. (1993). Prognostic factors in advanced stage squamous cell cancer of the cervix. *Cancer, 72,* 2389–2393.

Huang, S.F., Berek, F.S., & Fu, Y.S. (1992). Pathology of endometrial carcinoma. In M. Coppleson (Ed.), *Gynecologic oncology: Fundamental principles and clinical practice* (2nd ed.) (pp. 753–773). New York: Churchill Livingstone.

Hulka, B.S. (1994). Links between hormone replacement therapy and neoplasia. *Fertility and Sterility, 62,* 1685–1755.

Katso, R.M.T., Manek, S., O'Bryne, K., Playford, M.P., LeMeuth, V., & Ganesan, T.S. (1997). Molecular approaches to diagnosis and management of ovarian cancer. *Cancer and Metastasis Reviews, 16,* 81–107.

Kelsey, J.L., & Whitmore, A.S. (1994). Epidemiology and primary prevention of cancers of the breast, endometrium and ovary. A brief overview. *Annals of Epidemiology, 4,* 89–95.

Koss, L.G. (1987). Cytologic and histologic manifestations of human papillomavirus infection of the female genital tract and their clinical significance. *Cancer, 60,* 1942–1950.

Kuper, H., Titus-Ernstoff, L., Harlow, B.L., & Cramer, D.W. (2000). Population-based study of coffee, alcohol and tobacco use and risk of ovarian cancer. *International Journal of Cancer, 88,* 313–318.

La Vecchia, C., Franceschi, S., Decarli, A., Gallus, G., & Tognoni, G. (1984). Risk factors for endometrial cancer at different ages. *Journal of the National Cancer Institute, 73,* 667–671.

Linder, J., & Zahniser, D. (1997). The ThinPrep Pap test. A clinical review of studies. *Acta Cytologica, 41,* 30–38.

Loescher, L.J. (1998). DNA testing for cancer predisposition. *Oncology Nursing Forum, 25,* 1317–1327.

Lovejoy, N.C. (1999). Multinational approaches to cervical screening: A review. *Cancer Nursing, 19,* 126–134.

Lynch, H.T., Bardawil, W.A., & Harris, R.E. (1978). Multiple primary cancers and prolonged survival: Familial colonic and endometrial cancers. *Diseases of the Colon and Rectum, 21,* 165.

Lynch, H.T., Ens, J.A., & Lynch, J.F. (1990). The Lynch syndrome II and urological malignancies. *Journal of Urology, 143,* 24–28.

Lynch, H.T., Lynch, J.F., & Conway, T.A. (1993). Hereditary ovarian cancer. In S.C. Rubin & G. Sutton (Eds.), *Ovarian cancer* (pp. 189–217). New York: McGraw-Hill.

Maden, C., Sherman, K.J., Beckmann, A.M., Hislop, X.G., The, C.Z., Ashley, R.L., & Daling, J.R. (1993). History of circumcision, medical conditions and sexual activity and risk of penile cancer. *Journal of the National Cancer Institute, 85,* 19–24.

Mahon, S.M. (1998). Cancer risk assessment: Conceptual considerations for clinical practice. *Oncology Nursing Forum, 25,* 1535–1547.

Maiman, M., Fruchter, R.G., Serur, E., Remy, J.C., Feuer, G., & Boyce, J. (1990). Human immunodeficiency virus infection and cervical neoplasia. *Gynecologic Oncology, 38,* 377–382.

Mandelblatt, J., Andrews, H., Kerner, J., Zauber, A., & Burnett, W. (1991). Determinants of late stage diagnosis of breast cancer and cervical cancer: The impact of age, race, social class, and hospital type. *American Journal of Public Health, 81,* 646–649.

McCance, K.L., & Huether, S.E. (1998). *Pathophysiology: The biological basis for disease in adults and children* (3rd ed.). St. Louis, MO: Mosby.

McPherson, C.P., Sellers, T.A., Potter, J.D., Bostick, R.M., & Folsom, A.R. (1996). Reproductive factors and risk of endometrial cancer. The Iowa Women's Health Study. *American Journal of Epidemiology, 143,* 1195–1202.

Mettlin, C.J., & Piver, S.M. (1990). A case-control study of milk drinking and ovarian cancer risk. *American Journal of Epidemiology, 132,* 871–876.

Mitchell, H. (1993). Pap smears collected by nurse practitioners: A comparison with smears collected by medical practitioners. *Oncology Nursing Forum, 20,* 807–810.

Morrow, P.C., Curtin, J.P., & Townsend, D.E. (1993). Reproductive, menstrual and medical risk factors for endometrial cancer: Results from a case-control study. *American Journal of Obstetrics and Gynecology, 167,* 1317–1325.

Moslehi, R., Chu, W., Karlan, B., Fishman, D., Risch, H., Fields, A., Smotkin, D., Ben-David, Y., Rosenblatt, J., Russo, D., Schwartz, P., Tung, N., Warner, E., Rosen, B., Friedman, J., Brunet, J.S., & Narod, S.A. (2000). BRCA1 and BRCA2 mutation analysis of 208 Ashkenazi Jewish women with ovarian cancer. *American Journal of Human Genetics, 66,* 1259–1272.

Muir, C., Waterhouse, J., Mack, T., Powell, J., & Whelan, S. (Eds.). (1987). *Cancer incidence in five continents* (Vol. 5). Lyon, France: IARC Scientific Publications.

Muntz, H.G., Bell, D.A., Lage, J.M., Goff, B.A., Feldman, S., & Rice, L.W. (1992). Adenocarcinoma in situ of the uterine cervix. *Obstetrics and Gynecology, 80,* 935–939.

Narod, S.A., Ford, D., Devilee, P., Barkadottir, R.B., Eyfjord, J., Lenoir, G., Serova, O., Easton, D., & Goldgar, D. (1995). Genetic heterogeneity of breast-ovarian cancer revisited. *American Journal of Human Genetics, 57*, 957–958.

Narod, S.A., Risch, H., Moslehi, R., Dorum, A., Neuhausen, S., Olsson, H., Provencher, D., Radice, P., Evans, G., Bishop, S., Brunet, J.S., & Ponder, B.A., for the Heredity Ovarian Clinical Study Group. (1998). Oral contraceptives and the risk of hereditary ovarian cancer. *New England Journal of Medicine, 339*, 424–428.

National Institutes of Health. (1994). Ovarian cancer: Screening, treatment, and follow-up. *National Institutes of Health Consensus Statement, 12*, 1–30.

Nolte, S., & Hanjani, P. (1990). Intraepithelial neoplasia of the lower genital tract. *Seminars in Oncology Nursing, 6*, 181–189.

Nolte, S., Sohm, M.A., & Koons, B. (1993). Prevention of HIV infection in women. *Journal of Obstetric, Gynecologic, and Neonatal Nursing, 22*, 884–885.

Ozols, R.F., Rubin, S.C., Dembo, A.L., & Robboy, S.J. (1997). Epithelial ovarian cancer. In W.J. Hoskins, C.A. Perez, & R.C. Young (Eds.), *Principles and practice of gynecologic oncology* (pp. 731–782). Philadelphia: J.B. Lippincott.

Ozols, R.F., Schwartz, P.E., & Eifel, P.J. (1997). Ovarian cancer, fallopian tube carcinoma and peritoneal carcinoma. In V.T. De Vita, Jr., S. Hellman, & S.A. Rosenberg (Eds.), *Cancer: Principles and practice of oncology* (5th ed.) (pp. 1502–1539). Philadelphia: Lippincott-Raven.

Parazzini, F., La Vecchia, C., Bocciolone, L., & Franceschi, S. (1991). The epidemiology of endometrial cancer. *Gynecologic Oncology, 41*, 1–16.

Parazzini, F., La Vecchia, C., Negri, E., Fedele, L., Franceschi, S., & Gallotta, L. (1992). Risk factors for cervical intraepithelial neoplasia. *Cancer, 69*, 2276–2282.

Penn, I. (1986). Cancers of the anogenital region in renal transplant recipients: Analysis of sixty-five cases. *Cancer, 58*, 611–616.

Persson, I., Adami, H.O., Bergkvist, L., Lindgren, A., Pettersson, B., Hoover, R., & Schairer, C. (1989). Risk of endometrial cancer after treatment with oestrogens alone or in conjunction with progestogens: Results of a prospective study. *BMJ, 298*, 147–151.

Peters-Engel, C., Frank, W., Danmayr, E., Friedl, H.P., Leodolter, S., & Medl, M. (1999). Association between endometrial cancer and tamoxifen treatment of breast cancer. *Breast Cancer Research and Treatment, 54*, 255–260.

Piver, M.S., Baker, T.R., Piedmonte, M., & Sandecki, A.M. (1991). Epidemiology of ovarian neoplasia. *Proceedings of the American-European Conference on the Ovary* (pp. 364–366). Montreaux, Switzerland: Excerpta Media International Congress Series.

Piver, M.S., Lele, S.B., Barlow, J.J., & Blumenson, L. (1982). Paraortic lymph node evaluation in stage I endometrial carcinoma. *Obstetrics and Gynecology, 59*, 97–100.

Plagxe, S.C., Deligdisch, L., Dotting, P.R., & Chen, C.J. (1995). Ovarian intraepithelial neoplasia demonstrated in patients with stage I ovarian carcinoma. *Gynecologic Oncology, 38*, 367–372.

Polychronopoulou, A., Tzonou, A., Hsieh, C.C., Kaprinis, G., Rebelakos, A., Toupadaki, N., & Trichopoulos, D. (1993). Reproductive variables, tobacco, ethanol, coffee and somatometry as risk factors for ovarian cancer. *International Journal of Cancer, 55*, 402–407.

Richart, R.M. (1993). Controversies in the management of low-grade cervical intraepithelial neoplasia. *Cancer, 71*, 1413–1421.

Rosenblatt, K.A., & Thomas, D.B. (1991). Hormonal content of combined oral contraceptives in relation to the reduced risk of endometrial carcinoma. The WHO Collaborative Study of Neoplasia and Steroid Contraceptives. *International Journal of Cancer, 49,* 870–874.

Runowicz, C. (1995). Office laparoscopy as a screening tool for early detection of ovarian cancer. *Journal of Cellular Biochemistry, 23,* 238–242.

Schafer, A., Friedmann, W., Meilke, M., Schwartlander, B., & Koch, M.A. (1991). The increased frequency of cervical dysplasia-neoplasia in women infected with the human immunodeficiency virus as related to the degree of immunosuppression. *American Journal of Obstetrics and Gynecology, 164,* 593–599.

Schottenfeld, D. (1995). Epidemiology of endometrial neoplasia. *Journal of Cellular Biochemistry, 23,* 151–159.

Sook, A.K. (1991). Cigarette smoking and cervical cancer: Meta-analysis and critical review of recent studies. *American Journal of Preventive Medicine, 7,* 208–213.

Struewing, J., Hartge, P., Wacholder, S., Baker, S.M., Berlin, M., McAdams, M., Timmerman, N.M., Brody, L.C., & Tucker, M.A. (1997). The risk of cancer associated with specific mutations of BRCA1 and BRCA2 among Ashkenazi Jews. *New England Journal of Medicine, 336,* 1401–1408.

Sutton, G.P. (1990). The significance of positive peritoneal cytology in endometrial cancer. *Oncology, 4,* 21–26.

Syrjanen, K.J., & Syrjanen, S.M. (1985). Human papilloma virus (HPV) infections related to cervical intraepithelial neoplasia (CIN) and squamous cell carcinoma of the uterine cervix. *Annals of Clinical Research, 17,* 45–56.

Tobacman, J.K., Greene, M.H., Tucker, M.A., Costa, J., Kase, R., & Fraumeni, J.F. (1982). Intra-abdominal carcinomatosis after prophylactic oophorectomy in ovarian-cancer-prone families. *Lancet, 2,* 795–797.

Tzonou, A., Polychronopoulou, A., Hsieh, C.C., Rebelakos, A., Karakatsani, A., & Trichopoulos, D. (1993). Hair dyes, analgesics, tranquilizers and perineal talc application as risk factors for ovarian cancer. *International Journal of Cancer, 55,* 408–410.

van der Graaf, Y., Vooijs, G.P., Gaillard, H.L., & Go, D.M. (1987). Screening errors in cervical cytology screening. *Acta Cytologica, 31,* 434–438.

Van Le, L., Broekhuizen, F.F., Janzer-Steele, R., Behar, M., & Samter, T. (1993). Acetic acid visualization of the cervix to detect cervical dysplasia. *Obstetrics and Gynecology, 8,* 293–295.

van Leeuwen, F.E., Benraadt, J., Coeberg, J.W., Kiemeny, L.A., Gimbrere, C.H., Otter, R., Schouten, L.J., Damhuis, R.A., Bontenbal, M., Diepenhorse, F.W., et al. (1994). Risk of endometrial cancer after tamoxifen treatment of breast cancer. *Lancet, 343,* 448–452.

Van Nagell, J.R., DePriest, P.D., Puls, L.E, Donaldson, E.S., Gallion, H.H., Pavlik, E.J., Powell, D.E., & Kryscio, R.J. (1991). Ovarian cancer screening in postmenopausal women by transvaginal sonography. *Cancer, 68,* 458–462.

Walker, J., Bloss, J.D., Liao, S.Y., Berman, M., Bergen, S., & Wilczynski, S.P. (1989). Human papillomavirus genotype as a prognostic indicator in carcinoma of the uterine cervix. *Obstetrics and Gynecology, 74,* 781–785.

Weber, B.L. (1996). Genetic testing for breast cancer. *Scientific American Society of Medicine, 3,* 12–21.

White, L.N. (1993). An overview of screening and early detection of gynecologic malignancies. *Cancer, 71*(Suppl. 4), 1400–1405.

Whitehead, M.I., Hillard, T.C., & Crook, D. (1990). The role and use of progestogens. *Obstetrics and Gynecology, 7*(Suppl. 4), 59–76.

Whittemore, A.S. (1994). Characteristics relating to ovarian cancer risk: Implications for prevention and detection. *Gynecologic Oncology, 55*(3 Part 2), S15–S19.

Whittemore, A.S., Wu, M.L., Paffenbarger, R.S., Sarles, D.L., Kampert, J.B., Grosser, S., Jung, D.L., Ballon, S., & Hendrickson, M. (1988). Personal and environmental characteristics related to epithelial ovarian cancer II. Exposures to talcum powder, tobacco, alcohol, and coffee. *American Journal of Epidemiology, 128*, 1228–1240.

WHO Collaborative Study of Neoplasia and Steroid Contraceptives. (1985). Invasive cervical cancer and combined oral contraceptives. *BMJ, 290*, 961–965.

WHO Collaborative Study of Neoplasia and Steroid Contraceptives. (1989). Epithelial ovarian cancer and combined oral contraceptives. *International Journal of Epidemiology, 18*, 538–545.

Wilson, T.O., Podratz, K.C., Gaffey, T.A., Malkasian, G.D., O'Brien, P.C., & Naessens, J.M. (1990). Evaluation of unfavorable histologic subtypes in endometrial adenocarcinoma. *American Journal of Obstetrics and Gynecology, 162*, 418–423.

Winkelstein, W. (1990). Smoking and cervical cancer—Current status: A review. *American Journal of Epidemiology, 131*, 945–957.

Zunzunegui, M.V., Kink, M.C., Coria, C.F., & Charlet, J. (1986). Male influence on cervical cancer risks. *American Journal of Epidemiology, 123*, 302–307.

CHAPTER 14

Urologic and Male Genital Cancers

Mary Magee Gullatte, RN, MN, ANP, AOCN®, FAAMA,
James K. Bennett, MD, and Corlis L. Archer, MD

Introduction

Cancers of the male genitalia include prostate, testes, and penis; female genital cancers include the cervix, uterus, ovary, vulva, and vagina. The urinary system cancers include urethra, bladder, kidney, and ureters. This chapter will provide specific information about prevention, detection, and control of cancers that affect the bladder, kidney, testis, penis and urethra, and prostate.

Table 14-1 shows trends in the five-year relative cancer risk by race for cancers of the kidney, prostate, testis, and bladder. Table 14-2 shows estimates from the American Cancer Society (ACS) regarding the number of new cases of urologic and male genital cancer in 2001, and Table 14-3 shows the number of deaths expected from these cancers in the same year (ACS, 2001).

Bladder Cancer

Incidence and Epidemiology

Although the overall rate of new cancer cases is declining, the incidence of bladder cancer in the United States is slowly increasing, concurrent with the increase in the number of older people in the U.S. population (Montie, Smith, & Sandler, 2000). ACS estimated that a total of 54,300 new cases of bladder cancer would be diagnosed in the United States in 2001 (ACS, 2001). The incidence of bladder cancer is associated with age, environmental carcinogens (including cigarette smoke), male gender, and race.

Bladder cancer seems strongly linked to age. Wingo, Ries, Rosenberg, Miller, and Edwards (1998) reported that 70% of the cases of bladder cancer in men and

Table 14-1. Percentages Representing Five-Year U.S. Cancer Survival Rates 1974–1995

Cancer Site	White			African American			All Races		
	1974–1976	1980–1982	1989–1995	1974–1976	1980–1982	1989–1995	1974–1976	1980–1982	1989–1995
Bladder	74	79	82	48	58	62	73	78	81
Colon	51	56	62	46	49	52	50	55	62
Prostate	68	75	93	58	65	84	67	73	92
Rectum	49	53	60	42	38	51	49	52	60
Testis	79	92	96	76	90	88	79	92	95

Note. Based on information from Ries et al., 1998.

Table 14-2. Estimated New Cancer Cases by Site and Sex: United States, 2001

System	Male	Female
Urinary		
Bladder	39,200	15,100
Kidney and renal pelvis	18,700	12,100
Ureters and other urinary organs	1,500	900
Genital		
Prostate	198,100	NA
Testis	7,200	NA
Penis and other genitalia	1,200	NA

NA = not applicable
Note. Based on information from ACS, 2000.

Table 14-3. Estimated Cancer Deaths by Site and Sex: United States, 2001

System	Male	Female
Urinary		
Bladder	8,300	4,100
Kidney and renal pelvis	7,500	4,600
Ureters and other urinary organs	300	200
Genital		
Prostate	31,500	NA
Testis	400	NA
Penis and other genitalia	300	NA

NA = not applicable
Note. Based on information from ACS, 2001.

74% of cases in women occurred in people older than age 65. The mean age at the time of diagnosis is 68 years for men and 69 years for women (Kantoff, Shipley, Gallagher, Loughlin, & Soto, 1996).

Known environmental carcinogens initiate or promote malignant growth. In the case of bladder carcinoma, carcinogens in cigarette smoke have emerged as significant risk factors in the development of this malignancy. The male-to-female ratio in regard to bladder cancer incidence has historically been 3:1; however, the gender-related discrepancy seems to be narrowing with the increase in smoking among females. In fact, if the number of women smokers continues to increase at the present rate, the male-to-female bladder cancer ratio may soon be 1:1. The bladder cancer rate for women even may surpass that of men (Parker, Tong, & Bolden, 1997).

The role gender plays in bladder cancer incidence is believed to be related to the cause and effect of men being heavier smokers than women. With female smoking patterns increasing, the numbers are equalizing and the reverse may soon be true.

From the perspective of race in the United States, Whites have an incidence of bladder cancer that is twice that of African Americans and Hispanics (ACS, 2001). The lowest reported U.S. rates refer to U.S. Asian populations (ACS, 2001).

Mortality

ACS estimated that the number of bladder cancer deaths in 2001 would be 12,400 (ACS, 2001). Mortality rates reflect the age factor, with 83% of men and 87% of women bladder cancer deaths to occur to those age 65 and older (Montie, Smith, & Sandler, 2000).

Most bladder cancers are minimally invasive to noninvasive at the time of diagnosis; however, women present with more advanced stages than do men (Fleshner et al., 1996). Although the incidence is higher in Whites than in African Americans, the reverse is true in regard to mortality. Stage for stage, the survival rate of African Americans is less than that of Whites (Parker et al., 1997).

Etiology and Risk Factors

A number of factors determine the initiation and progression of bladder cancer: activation and inactivation mechanisms, efficiency of the DNA-repair process, and the ability of the immune system to eradicate abnormal cells (Madajewicz, 1995). The etiology of bladder cancer is unknown; however, studies indicate the following associated risk factors: age, gender, and race; long-term exposure to aniline dyes, textiles, and paint; long-term ingestion of food additives; smoking; and chronic infection or irritation of the bladder. Table 14-4 lists the risk factors related to bladder cancer and their effects.

Cigarette Smoking

In the United States, cigarette smoking accounts for approximately 50% of bladder cancer cases (Vineis, Martone, & Randone, 1995). Smoking may be responsible for as many as 40% of the bladder cancer cases in men and 26% of the cases in women (Lind, 1997). Vineis et al. reported that smoking cessation is

Table 14-4. Risk Factors Associated With Bladder Cancer

Possible Risks	Etiology
Occupational High bladder cancer risk is associated with these industries: • Textile • Rubber • Leather • Printing • Dye (including hair dyes) • Aluminum	Arylamines, O-toludine, and benzidines are chemical by-products associated with the cited industries. Long-term exposure to these and other substances can initiate or promote bladder cancer.
Environmental • Automobile exhaust	
Lifestyle • Cigarette smoke	Cigarette smoke contains polycyclic aromatic hydrocarbons and aromatic amines, which are carcinogens (Madajewicz, 1995). Risk increases with amount of smoking as well as the type of tobacco leaf smoked. Black-leaf tobacco, which is air-cured, causes a higher risk than does blond (flue-cured) tobacco. Black-leaf tobacco contains a higher concentration of arylamine carcinogens. These carcinogens are metabolized in the liver by N-acetylation. "Slow" acetylators are homozygous for the slow acetylator gene and increase the risk of bladder carcinoma. Slow acetylation makes the liver less effective; hence, greater concentrations of the aromatic amine compounds reach the bladder mucosa and cells (Vineis, Martone, & Randone, 1995).
• Chronic bladder infection or irritation	S. haematobium infection leads to production and urinary excretion of tryptophan metabolites, which are carcinogenic (Richie, Shipley, & Yagoda, 1989).
• Schistosomiasis haematobium	Reports suggest that patients who, as a result of chronic infection, have had an in-dwelling Foley catheter for 10 years or more have a risk of bladder cancer that is 16–20 times higher than risk in the general population (Navon, Soliman, & Khonsari, 1997).
Medications • Cyclophosphamide • Phenacetin	Metabolites from cyclophosphamide and phenacetin come in constant contact with the bladder mucosa, increasing risk. Phenacetin-containing drugs have been removed from the market because of their carcinogenic risk.

Note. Based on information from Gullatte, 2001; Madajewicz, 1995; Montie et al., 2000; Navon et al., 1997; Richie et al., 1989; Vineis et al., 1995.

associated with a dramatic drop in bladder cancer risk; however, Montie et al. (2000) reported an associated risk at the age of starting to smoke and an increased risk 10–15 years after quitting. Risk does not appear to vary with use of filtered verses unfiltered cigarettes.

Occupational Exposures

Occupational exposures may account for up to 25% of all bladder cancers (Miller, 1996). Workers in rubber, coal, coke, textile, paint, and machinery industries are at greater than average risk for bladder cancer. Silverman, Levin, and Hoover (1989) reported that bladder cancer risk becomes unusually high in groups that had been employed in these industries for more than 10 years. Improved exposure-reduction practices in the workplace are decreasing bladder cancer risk in the leather and rubber industries.

Medications and Food Additives

Research shows that long-term exposure to certain medications or food additives increases the risk of bladder cancer. These include cyclophosphamide, phenacetin, and some artificial sweeteners (cyclamates and saccharin). Long-term use of phenacetin reportedly increases the risk of transitional cell carcinoma (TCC) of the bladder and the renal pelvis (Talar-Williams, Hijazi, & Walther, 1996). Over time, oral cyclophosphamide use can cause as much as a 30-fold increase in bladder cancer (Talar-Williams et al.). In a study reported by Fernandes, Manivel, Reddy, and Ercole (1996), patients who were treated with cyclophosphamide and developed bladder cancer had highly aggressive tumors. Patients receiving cyclophosphamide therapy need close cytologic surveillance to detect bladder cancer at an early stage, should it occur.

Researchers have conducted studies to determine if coffee, alcohol, or artificial sweeteners are risk factors for bladder cancer; however, associations, if present, are weak at best, with no dose-response relationships confirmed (Madajewicz, 1995; Miller, 1996).

Infection and Irritation

An association between infection of the bladder by the flatworm Schistosomiasis haematobium and bladder cancer was postulated over 100 years ago (Madajewicz, 1995). Infection with schistosomiasis ova is rare in the United States. It is prevalent on the African continent, however, especially in Egypt, where it is endemic. Chronic bladder irritation by schistosomiasis or other long-term bladder infectors is typically associated with squamous cell carcinoma (SCC) of the bladder (Montie et al., 2000). A study by La Vecchia, Negri, D'Avanzo, Savoldelli, and Franceschi (1991) demonstrated a quantitative relationship between chronic urinary tract infection and bladder cancer.

Pathophysiology

The bladder is a reservoir for urine. It consists of smooth muscle fibers arranged in spiral, longitudinal, and circular bundles. The muscles lining the bladder are predominantly transitional and squamous epithelial in origin. TCC accounts for 90% of bladder malignancies; SCC and adenocarcinoma account for 8% and 2%, respectively (Kantoff et al., 1996; Lind, 1998; Parzuchowski & Wallace, 1997).

The pathologic grade and stage of bladder cancer cells are based on the American Joint Committee on Cancer (AJCC) tumor-node-metastasis (TNM) classification. The grade and stage of the cancer determine treatment and prognosis. Most bladder cancers are low grade and noninvasive at the time of diagnosis. TCC can appear grossly exophytic or nodular. The majority of lesions are exophytic or papillary in appearance.

Molecular Genetics

Molecular assays and genetic coding are making it possible to pinpoint and decode genetic markers that may indicate malignant transformation before it occurs (Cairns & Sidransky, 1999). The science and technology of genetic alteration and transformation are heralding a new era in cancer prevention, detection, and control.

The p53 tumor-suppressor gene plays a vital role in apoptosis and the binding of tumor-transforming proteins (e.g., SV40 large T antigen) and in induction of the cell-cycle regulator p21 gene, the protein inhibitor of the cyclin-dependent kinases (Offit, 2000). Mutations of the p53 gene are among the most common genetic alterations found in malignancies (Chang, Syrjanen, & Syrjanen, 1995). A p53 tumor-suppressor gene alteration has been identified in a number of cancers, including cancer of the bladder. The presence of the p53 gene mutation or overexpression is associated with decreased patient survival and aggressive features of bladder tumors (Offit, 1998). Loss of alleles near the p53 locus on chromosome 17 has recently been implicated as a final phase in the carcinogenesis of bladder cancer (Isaacs, Carter, & Ewing, 1991). The ability to recognize and map these molecular genetic signals will significantly advance cancer research, prevention, early detection, and treatment.

Signs and Symptoms

Hematuria is the most common presenting sign and symptom of bladder cancer. Others include irritative voiding symptoms (e.g., urinary urgency, frequency, and hesitancy; dysuria) and recurrent bladder infections (Gullatte, 2001; Lind, 1997; Parzuchowski & Wallace, 1997). Weight loss, decrease in appetite, a feeling of pelvic fullness, abdominal pain, and flank pain may be present in patients who present at an advanced stage. Often these malignancies originate at the base of the bladder and involve the ureters (Kantoff et al., 1996; Lind, 1997; Parzuchowski & Wallace). Be alert for bladder cancer when patients present with intermittent hematuria, which is characteristic of the disease. Because hematuria may resolve with time or antimicrobial therapy for urinary tract infection, the clinician may not immediately test for bladder cancer, thus delaying diagnosis (Murphy, Morris, & Lange, 1997).

Prevention

The precise etiology of bladder cancer is unknown; however, cigarette smoking is a known, highly associated risk factor. For this reason, public awareness of the importance of smoking cessation is crucial to bladder cancer prevention. Increased public and professional education to heighten individuals' awareness of bladder cancer, its signs and symptoms, and the associated risk factors is also vital.

Because bladder cancer risk increases with exposure to infections associated with specific geographic regions, travelers can lower their risk by taking preventive measures. The Centers for Disease Control and Prevention maintains a Web site page (www.cdc.gov/travel/) that provides information about diseases and infections endemic to certain areas. By checking the site, a traveler can learn how to minimize health risks associated with his or her destination.

Chemoprevention is the use of chemical and dietary interventions to retard, block, reverse, or alter human susceptibility to carcinogens (Morse & Stoner, 1993). The use of botanicals in chemoprevention is gaining momentum as an alternative and complementary therapy in the treatment of bladder cancer. Table 14-5 describes clinical trials related to urologic and male cancers; the trials are sponsored by the National Cancer Institute (NCI). Among the trials the table describes is a phase III clinical trial to determine whether high-dose multivitamins have a chemopreventive efficacy beyond that of standard therapy in reducing the risk of bladder cancer recurrence in patients with resected TCC at stage 0 or stage I. To date, no preliminary data have been released.

Early Detection

In about three-fourths of the patients diagnosed with bladder cancer, gross hematuria is the most common clinical finding and the symptom that most frequently brings them to a healthcare provider (Murphy et al., 1997; Parzuchowski & Wallace, 1997). Any patient presenting with microscopic or gross hematuria should undergo a diagnostic workup and evaluation.

The most common and easily accessible screening measure is urinalysis, which can be performed in most office settings. If urinalysis indicates infection, the patient should be appropriately treated and a follow-up urinalysis should be performed. In the absence of infection, the patient should be referred to a urologist for further evaluation. The recommended workup for hematuria includes a urine test to evaluate cytology, an intravenous pyelogram (IVP), and cystoscopy. A bladder biopsy is performed when a suspicious lesion is noted during cystoscopy. Further diagnostic workup is done to determine the stage of invasive bladder tumors. Figure 14-1 is an illustration of bladder cancer and surrounding structures.

Grégoire et al. (1997) reported that urine cytology can play a major role in the detection and monitoring of urinary bladder cancer. However, cytology has limitations. For the detection of bladder cancer, cytologic evaluation is not a standalone diagnostic tool. The sensitivity of cytology is 60%, with a specificity of 70%–80% in detecting bladder cancer (Grossman, 1998). Urine cytology is not objective; it involves human variability in interpreting results. Furthermore, cytology will not yield valid results unless the clinician collects an adequate number of cells. Urine cytology is invaluable in the detection and follow-up of high-grade cancers with abnormal morphology; however, in tests of low-grade tumors that closely resemble normal cells, the sensitivity can be as low as 10%–40%

Table 14-5. National Cancer Institute Trials Related to Urologic and Male Genital Cancers

Site	Type	Phase	Status	Objective
Bladder	Prevention	III	Active	• Determine whether high-dose multivitamins have chemopreventive efficacy beyond that of standard therapy in reducing the risk of recurrence in patients with resected stage 0 and I (T1 and Tis). • Determine the effect of the regimen on development of transitional cell carcinoma of the bladder.
Kidney (renal cell)	Genetic	NA	Active	• Correlate specific mutations and their associated protein domains with the disease severity score in patients with inherited urologic malignant disorders. • Determine improved diagnostic indicators for genetic disorders by using linked markers, mutation screening, or other techniques. • Determine the genetic etiology of hereditary urologic malignancies. • Characterize urologic malignant disorders as genetic disease; evaluate candidate genes. • Detect disease manifestations in individuals at risk for von Hippel-Lindau (VHL) and characterize the genetic events associated with hereditary renal cell carcinoma. • Detect occult disease manifestations in individuals known to have VHL. • Identify chromosome VHL gene mutations and make genotype and phenotype correlation.
Prostate	Prevention and treatment	I	Active	• Determine the pharmacokinetic parameters of two preparations of genistein in patients with no history or asymptomatic patients with early prostate cancer or other malignancy. • Determine the toxic effects of each preparation when administered to these patients as a single dose.
Prostate	Prevention and treatment	III	Active	• Determine the effects of two dietary regimens on levels of prostate-specific antigen (PSA) in patients with prostate cancer. • Determine the compliance of these patients with the dietary regimen. • Evaluate the effects of the dietary regimen on participants' quality of life. • Evaluate the effects of the diet on participants' PSA and anxiety. • Evaluate the effects of the dietary regimen on participants' obesity, high blood pressure, and serum cholesterol.

(Continued on next page)

584

Table 14-5. National Cancer Institute Trials Related to Urologic and Male Genital Cancers *(Continued)*

Site	Type	Phase	Status	Objective
Prostate	Screening	NA	Active	• Determine whether screening with digital rectal exam plus a serum PSA test can reduce mortality from prostate cancer in men ages 55–74. • Assess other screening variables for the above, including sensitivity, specificity, and positive predictive value. • Assess the mortality and predictive value of biologic and prognostic characterization of tumor tissue as intermediate end points.
Prostate	Genetic	NA	Active	• Determine the location of the prostate cancer disease

NA = not applicable
Note. Based on information from NCI, 2000.

Figure 14-1. Bladder Cancer and Surrounding Structures in the Male and the Female

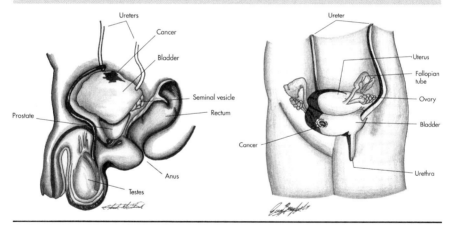

(Montie et al., 2000). A urine sample for cytologic evaluation may be a sterile specimen obtained through catheterization or during cystoscopy. Bladder washing yields a larger cellular component than does collecting a sample through catheterization; therefore, using bladder washing rather than catheterization improves cytologic sensitivity (Raitanen et al., 2000; van der Poel et al., 1997).

The U.S. Food and Drug Administration (FDA) approved the use of urinary nuclear matrix protein (NMP22) for the detection of occult or rapidly recurring bladder cancer after transureteral resection. Stampfer et al. (1998) concluded that NMP22 may perform better than urine cytology as a diagnostic tool. NMP22 is not a first-line diagnostic assay.

Screening for bladder cancer has not been widely advocated in the United States because of the relatively low prevalence of the disease in America (Montie et al., 2000). Patients with a history of bladder cancer may be at risk of recurrence. Smokers and workers in the rubber, coal, coke, textile, paint, and machinery industries are at greater risk than the general population. Educating the public about bladder cancer risk factors and the importance of regular health assessments is key to reducing bladder cancer morbidity and mortality.

Renal Cell Cancer

Incidence and Epidemiology

Cancer of the kidney accounts for approximately 3% of all cancers in adults (ACS, 2001). ACS estimated that cancers of the kidney and renal pelvis (see Table 14-6) would account for an estimated 30,800 new cancer cases in males and females in 2001 (ACS, 2001). The renal pelvis encompasses the lower part of the kidney, where urine collects before entering the ureter and continuing to the bladder. The most common cancer of the kidney is renal cell carcinoma (RCC), accounting for 95% of kidney tumors (Kassabian & Graham, 1995). RCC is more prevalent in urban U.S. populations than in other kinds of U.S. populations. It affects twice as many men as women, and the median age range of people affected is 57–60 years (McLaughlin & Lipworth, 2000; Simons & Marshall, 2000).

Hereditary factors have been strongly linked to RCC. Reportedly, up to 35% of patients with von Hippel-Lindau (VHL) syndrome develop RCC (Malek, Omesa, & Benson, 1987). VHL syndrome is an autosomal dominant trait produced by the VHL tumor-suppressor gene located on chromosome 3p 25–26 (Wittebol-Post, Hes, & Lips, 1998).

The VHL suppressor-gene mutation can affect up to 14 target organs, resulting in a loss of gene function. Patients with RCC should be assessed for the presence of VHL. This assessment should include taking a family history and mapping a pedigree. The patient should have a clinical and radiologic workup to determine the presence of subclinical manifestations of VHL gene mutation. The information gained should be used to assess the patient for tumor development in other areas, such as the retina (Lliopoulos & Eng, 2000). Evidence suggests an increased incidence of RCC in individuals with autosomal dominant polycystic kidney (Gnarra et al., 1993; Grégoire, Torres, & Halley, 1987). Based on Surveillance, Epidemiology and End Results (SEER) data, 70% of cancers of the kidney are RCC: 15% arise in the renal pelvis, 8% in the ureter, 4% in the urethra, and 3% in other sites within the kidney (Devesa et al., 1990).

Racial and ethnic patterns of this disease are changing. Since the 1970s, incidence rates appear to be rising in the United States among the four

Table 14-6. Cancer of the Kidney and Renal Pelvis, Incidence and Mortality by Sex: United States 2001

	Incidence	Mortality
Male	18,700	7,500
Female	12,100	4,600
Combined	30,800	12,100

Note. Based on information from ACS, 2000.

major race and gender groups (McLaughlin & Lipworth, 2000). Chow, Devesa, and Warren (1999) reported that rates are increasing for African American men by 3.9% per year and 4.3% per year for African American females. The annual rate for White men is 2.3% and for White women is 3.1%.

Mortality

RCC causes a relatively high mortality rate in all racial and ethnic populations, with men's mortality rates about twice as high as women's, regardless of age (Miller, 1996). ACS estimated 12,100 deaths in 2001 from cancer of the kidney and renal pelvis (ACS, 2001). Mortality rates for African Americans are comparable to those of Whites.

Etiology and Risk Factors

Multiple factors have been implicated in the pathogenesis of RCC. The most prevalent is the use of tobacco (e.g., cigars, cigarettes, smokeless tobacco). More than 3,000 chemicals are present in tobacco smoke, including 60 known carcinogens (e.g., nitrosamines, polycyclic aromatic hydrocarbons). The activated compounds of tobacco trigger activation of DNA enzymes. Researchers believe these enzymes interfere with the normal growth of cells. Tobacco can be both a promoter and an initiator of human cancers. Compared to nonsmokers, smokers have about twice the risk of RCC and about four times the risk of renal pelvis cancer than do nonsmokers (Miller, 1996). Other strongly associated risk factors include obesity, chronic analgesic use, familial risks, and workplace exposures. Table 14-7 cites the exposure risks and the suspected etiology of risk factors associated with RCC. Coffee and alcohol have been studied relative to RCC risk. Investigators have found no definitive link between either substance and RCC.

Pathophysiology

The kidneys are between the peritoneum and the muscles of the back, at the level of the last two ribs. The main function of the kidneys is to purify the blood, enabling reabsorption of essential nutrients into the bloodstream. The body contains two kidneys; one kidney can do the needed work. The kidney is a bean-shaped organ with an intricate system of nephrons and tubules. During the blood-filtering process, urine is formed and travels via the ureters to the bladder. Urine is eliminated through the urethra.

RCC develops in the proximal tubules and accounts for 85% of all renal parenchymal tumors. TCC develops in the renal pelvis. In children, the most common renal malignancy is Wilms' tumor.

The four basic histologic RCC types are clear cell (associated with VHL), granular cell, papillary, and sarcomatoid (Fromowitz & Bard, 1990). RCC metastasizes through the blood system, from the renal vein or inferior vena cava, with direct extension via the lymph channels. Because RCC develops in the retroperitoneum, it often grows undetected until it has spread. Therefore, in most cases, RCC is not diagnosed until it has reached a late stage. Direct invasion of RCC, via the abdominal lymph nodes, accounts for about 45% of cases at the time of diagnosis. Invasion via the inferior vena cava accounts for 10%–15% of cases;

Table 14-7. Risk Factors Associated With Renal Cell Carcinoma

Possible Risks	Etiology
Occupational The following sites are associated with a high risk of renal cell carcinoma (RCC). • Workplaces that use or produce cadmium, asbestos, rubber, leather, fluoroacetamide, dimethyl nitrosamines • Coke ovens • Oil refineries • Gas stations	Data conflict regarding the carcinogenic effect of the items listed at left. A large-scale international study found a moderate association of asbestos exposure and RCC (Mandel, McLaughlin, & Schlehofer, 1995). Asbestos fibers can be deposited in the kidney. Wong and Raabe (1989) found no definitive link between RCC risk and work in an oil refinery or gas station; Pukkala (1995) reported high risk.
Lifestyle • Cigarette smoke • Obesity	The effect of obesity on RCC risk is unclear. Some studies indicate that a history of cyclic weight swings, which are accompanied by hormonal changes, may be a risk factor (Newsom & Vurgin, 1987).
Genetic • von Hippel–Lindau (VHL) • Polycystic kidney disease	The VHL gene, on the short arm of chromosome 3, is believed to be the early target of mutation or chromosomal loss in pathogenesis.
Medications • Phenacetin • Acetaminophen • Diuretics • Estrogens	Data conflict regarding the carcinogenic effect of the items listed at left. Phenacetin-containing drugs have been removed from the market because of their carcinogenic risk. Acetaminophen is a metabolite of phenacetin; however, McCredie, Pommer, and McLaughlin (1995) reported little evidence to suggest that it is an RCC risk. McLaughlin, Blot, and Fraumeni (1988) reported a strong association between antihypertensive medications, such as diuretics, and RCC; more recent studies disprove an association (McLaughlin, Chow, & Mandel, 1995). All the medication associations cited here were based on chronic use and exposure to the specific metabolites of the drugs, contact with renal tissue, and exposure over time.

Note. Based on information from Mandel et al., 1995; McCredie et al., 1995; McLaughlin et al., 1988, 1990, 1995; Newsom & Vurgin, 1987; Pukkala, 1995; Wong & Raabe, 1989.

lymph node invasion accounts for 10%–13%. The most common sites of metastasis are lungs, bones, liver, and brain (Murphy et al., 1997; Richie, Stolbach, & Atkins, 1996). RCC usually progresses and metastasizes rapidly after diagnosis. RCC spawns paraneoplastic syndromes, anemia, abnormal liver function, fever, weight loss, and erythrocytosis.

Signs and Symptoms

In RCC, the "classic triad" of abdominal cancer signs and symptoms—a mass in the abdomen or flank, pain, and hematuria—usually denote advanced disease. Hematuria is the most common presenting sign of RCC. Pain is also usually present. The paraneoplastic syndromes associated with RCC and the fact that the kidney performs a major endocrine function often account for the incidental diagnosis of RCC. The endocrine-related signs and symptoms of RCC make it elusive and a challenge to diagnose (Motzer, 2000; Simons & Marshall, 2000).

Prevention

RCC risk factors suggest that the key to RCC prevention is behavior and lifestyle modification. Because cigarette smoking is the number-one risk factor associated with this disease, a tobacco-free lifestyle is the first priority for prevention. Other preventive strategies include dietary modifications (eating a low-fat diet rich in fruits and vegetables) and physical conditioning to maintain ideal body weight (obesity is a risk factor for RCC). No chemoprevention trials are currently under way in regard to RCC.

Early Detection

As many as 50% of RCC cases are initially detected when patients are being evaluated for other medical or surgical conditions (Konnak & Grossman, 1990; Smith et al., 1989). Aso and Homma (1992) and Tsukamoto et al. (1991) reported that 75% of incidentally detected RCCs are confined to the renal capsule and lend themselves to surgical resection. Most of these patients report gross hematuria.

TCC of the renal pelvis and ureter account for approximately 500 cases of cancer per year. As with RCC, cigarette smoking is a significant risk factor for this cancer (Jensen, Knudsen, McLaughlin, & Sorenson, 1988). Other associated risk factors include obesity, dietary fat intake, phenacetin, and occupational exposure to asbestos and petroleum (O'Rourke, 2001).

Simons & Marshall (2000) reported that 75% of TCC patients present with microscopic or gross hematuria. In the primary care setting, these patients should be referred to a urologist for further evaluation or diagnostic testing. An evaluative workup should include an IVP or intravenous urogram (IVU), urine cytology, and cystoscopy.

An IVU that shows parenchymal calcification is highly suggestive of RCC; therefore, an IVU should be the first imaging study to evaluate the urinary tract of patients with RCC symptoms (Hilton, 2000).

Testicular Cancer

Incidence and Epidemiology

ACS (2001) estimated that 7,200 new cases of testicular cancer would be diagnosed in the United States in 2001. Cancer of the testis accounts for approximately 1% of male cancers. In the United States, testicular cancer occurs most frequently in young White males, with the average age at onset being 35. The age-adjusted incidence of cancer of the testis is 4.5 times higher in Whites than in African Americans; the rates for Asians, Native Americans, and Hispanics are between those of Whites and those of African Americans (Moul, Schanne, & Thompson, 1994).

Overall, testicular cancer is an uncommon malignancy. In the United States, cancer of the testis most frequently occurs in White males ages 20–34. The next highest incidence for White males is in men ages 35–39, and the lowest rate for White males relates to men ages 15–19 (Ries, Kosary, & Hankey, 1998). The incidence of testicular cancer may be higher in men with a family history of the disease.

Mortality

ACS estimated that testicular cancer would cause 400 deaths in the United States in 2001 (ACS, 2001). Advances in detection and treatment over the past two decades are associated with a 60% decrease in mortality (Ries et al., 1998).

Etiology and Risk Factors

Risk factors for the development of cancer of the testis are unknown; however, failure of the testis to descend (cryptorchidism) increases the risk of testicular cancer by 3–14 times (Garnick, Krane, Scully, & Weber, 1996; Small & Torti, 2000). Significant structural and functional abnormalities result in males with cryptorchidism, including testicular hypoplasia (Madajewicz, 1995). Androgenic hormones are essential for normal testicular embryonogenesis. Through the 1940s and 1960s, prenatal estrogen was administered when spontaneous abortion was a threat. Male offspring of mothers who received prenatal estrogen were at an increased risk for testicular cancer. Use of prenatal estrogen has been shown to increase the risk of cryptorchidism in association with testicular hypoplasia (Dupree, Pike, & Henderson, 1983). A 40-fold increase in testicular cancer is associated with testicular feminization syndrome and cases in which the testes remained in the abdomen. In cases of genotypically male but phenotypically female patients, this syndrome may be misdiagnosed as ovarian cancer rather than testicular cancer (Rutgers & Scully, 1991).

Researchers continue to explore the genetic basis of testicular cancer. Murty and Changanti (1998) and Nicholson and Harland (1995) reported that genetic predisposition accounts for one-third of germ-cell tumors, with one or more predisposing genes mapping to 4qcen-13 and 12q regions (Leahy et al., 1995). In 1982, chromosomal studies to map a susceptibility gene for testicular cancer identified an isochromosome on the short arm of chromosome 12 (Atkin & Baker, 1982). Subsequent studies revealed the i(12p) chromosome in 80% of all subsets of germ-cell tumors, including carcinoma in situ (Chaganti, Rodriguez, & Bosl, 1993; Mosteret, van de Pol, & Olde-Weghuis, 1996).

Pathophysiology

The testes originate as intra-abdominal organs. During development of the fetus, the testes descend gradually into the scrotum. These oval-shaped structures have a twofold function: they are the sites where sperm are made, and they produce the male sex hormone, testosterone. Each testis is suspended in the scrotum by the spermatic cord. The spermatic cord contains the vas deferens, which transports sperm away from the testis, testicular artery, and vein. Sperm are stored in the epididymis before traveling along the vas deferens during ejaculation.

Testicular cancers are categorized into two types: germ cell and non-germ cell. More than 90% of testicular tumors are of the germ-cell type. Histologically, testicular cancers are classified as seminomas or nonseminomas. Nonseminoma malignancies account for 60% of all germ-cell tumors (Small & Torti, 2000) (see Table 14-8). The specific cell types are important because the histology determines the rate of metastasis, treatment, and prognosis. At diagnosis, approximately 60% of testicular cancers are localized, 24% are regional, and 14% are distant stage (Ries et al., 1998). Early in its development, testicular cancer spreads via the lymph nodes; later, it spreads via the hematic system.

Table 14-8. Types of Testicular Cancer

Type	Percentage of Testicular Tumors	Notes
Seminomas	40	
Classic	93	Usually occur in men 40–50 years old
Spermatocytic	7	Usually occur in men with a median age of 65
Nonseminomas	60	
Embryonal tumors	20–24	Usually occur in men ages 15–35
Teratomas	25–30	Aggressive tumors with a highly malignant potential; usually occur in men 20–30 years old
Choriocarcinomas (yolk-sac tumors)	≤ 1	Aggressive tumors; usually occur in men 20–30 years old
Stromal-cell tumors	3–4	Rare but most aggressive of germ-cell tumors

Note. Based on information from Garnick et al., 1996; Murphy et al., 1997; Nichols et al., 2000; Small & Torti, 2000.

Signs and Symptoms

The most common presenting sign of testicular cancer is a painless, pea-sized lump or swelling in the scrotum. Many believe that painless masses are not cancerous and so do not need to be evaluated. This is a misconception; painless lumps can be cancerous. When detected early, cancer of the testis is a highly curable cancer.

Other signs and symptoms of testicular cancer are indistinguishable from those of acute epididymitis, and they have been observed in 25% of patients with malignancies of the testes (Small & Torti, 2000). Choriocarcinoma, accounting for 10% of testicular malignancies, produces human chorionic gonadotropin hormone. Hence, gynecomastia may be a concomitant sign of testicular cancer. Figure 14-2 lists other signs and symptoms.

Prevention

No definitive cause of testicular cancer has been identified; hence, no targeted prevention strategies have been identified. However, the known strong association

---

Figure 14-2. Signs and Symptoms Associated With Testicular Cancer

- Dragging sensation in the scrotum
- Dull aching or pain in the scrotum
- Gynecomastia
- Chronic cough, dyspnea, hemoptysis (usually from lung metastasis)
- Ureteral obstruction
- Low back pain
- Abdominal pain (late symptom)

Note. Based on information from Garnick et al., 1996; Murphy et al., 1997.

---

between cryptorchid testes and testicular cancer does warrant attention. Surgical correction of an undescended testis when a boy is 2–5 years old has been shown to decrease testicular cancer risk. Madajewicz (1995) suggested that immunization against mumps could significantly decrease the incidence of mumps-induced testis atrophy, thereby lowering the risk of testicular cancer associated with mumps.

Early Detection

ACS recommends regular testicular self-examination (TSE) for men from puberty through their 40s. A man should examine each testicle monthly, supporting the testicle with one hand and, with the other, gently rotating the testicle between the thumb and four fingers. TSE is easily performed in the shower while using warm water and lather as lubricants. Masses of the testicle are hard and firm. Male teens should be educated regarding the risk of testicular cancer and taught the TSE technique. Healthcare providers may contact a local ACS chapter to get teaching aids (pictoral "shower cards," videos, and models) and instruction on how to teach patients about TSE.

Diagnosis of testicular cancer often is delayed because the man is hesitant to report symptoms to a healthcare provider. Clinicians also may delay diagnosis of a scrotal mass, believing it to be an infectious or inflammatory process (Garnick et al., 1996). A lump in the scrotum could represent epididymitis, hydrocele, or result from testicular trauma.

Testicular ultrasonography is a sensitive and specific test that can discriminate between a malignant and nonmalignant condition; nonmalignant conditions include hydrocele, varicocele, spermatocele, testicular torsion, and epididymitis (Small & Torti, 2000). Patients with a suspicious mass should be referred to a urologist for further evaluation and diagnostic workup.

Testicular tumors account for only 1% of all male cancers; therefore, mass screening for testicular cancer is not recommended.

Penile and Urethral Cancer

Incidence and Epidemiology

ACS (2001) estimated 1,200 new cases of penile and urethral cancer in the United States in 2001. Penile and urethral carcinomas are rare in the United

States; their incidence is 10%–20% higher in Asia, Africa, and South America (Pettaway, Balbay, & Grossman, 2000). The reported incidence of urethral cancer is less than 0.1% of that of genitourinary cancers in general (Grabstald, 1973). Pettaway et al. reported that cancer of the urethra is the only urologic cancer with a higher incidence in women than men. In men, cancer of the urethra usually occurs after age 50; cancer of the penis usually is diagnosed in men in their 60s (Fair & Yang, 1992; Walton & Olsson, 1992).

Mortality

ACS (2001) estimated that, in 2001, 300 men would die from cancer of the penis or urethra. Like mortality rates regarding many other types of cancer, the incidence of death from penile and urethral cancer is directly related to the stage of the disease at the time of diagnosis.

Etiology and Risk Factors
Penile Cancer

The preponderant risk factor for cancer of the penis is the presence of foreskin. The religious practice of male circumcision among the Jewish population is believed to be associated with the lower incidence of penile cancer among Jews. Among males whose foreskin is removed in early infancy, the incidence of cancer of the penis is rare. The male's age at circumcision seems to be significant. Bissada, Morcos, and el-Senoussi (1986) and Brinton et al. (1991) reported that the protective effect of circumcision diminishes if the male is circumcised in late childhood or adulthood. The presence of inflammation in a closed preputial environment predisposes a man to the development of penile cancer (Pettaway et al., 2000). A correlation between phimosis and penile cancer has been reported in up to 50% of patients with penile carcinoma (Bissada et al.; Maden et al., 1993; Pettaway et al.).

Urethral Cancer

The etiology of cancer of the urethra remains unknown. Kaplan, Bulkey, and Grayhack (1967) and Ray, Canto, and Whitmore (1977), reported that 25%–75% of men with cancer of the urethra reported a history of urethral strictures. Of those men, 33%–50% reported venereal disease. In women, polyps, coitus, fibrosis, and caruncles all have been reported as associated risk factors for urethral carcinoma; however, scientific evidence to support the reports is lacking (Marshall, Uson, & Melicow, 1960; Mevorach, Cos, & di Sant'Agnese, 1990). No conclusive evidence exists to explain the increased risk of cancer of the urethra in women.

Pathophysiology
Penile Cancer

The unstimulated penis is a flaccid structure. Attached to the anterior and lateral walls of the pelvic arch, in front of the scrotum, it is composed of three longitudinal columns of erectile tissue connected by fibrous bands and covered with skin (Jacob & Francone, 1974).

The penis transports urine from the bladder via the urethra. It is the male reproductive organ, through which sperm-containing semen passes. The head of the penis, called the glans, is protected by a loose fold of skin called the prepuce, or foreskin. The glans and prepuce make a substance called smegma. Smegma serves as a lubricant, allowing easy movement (retraction) of the foreskin. As discussed, the most significant risk factor for penile cancer is presence of foreskin.

Penile cancer usually appears as a mass, a persistent sore, or an ulcer on the glans or prepuce (Gullatte, 2001; Kassabian & Graham, 1995) (see Figure 14-3). Penile cancer usually grows slowly. It can be cured if detected early. Some clinical lesions are precancerous, including benign condylomata acuminatum and carcinoma in situ (seen with erythroplasia of Queyrat or Bowen's disease) (Pettaway et al., 2000). Unfortunately, after finding an abnormality on the penis, most men wait for more than one year before seeking medical care (Fair, Fuks, & Scher, 1993; Gullatte, 2001). When the cancer extends beyond the penis, it usually involves the groin and pelvic lymph nodes. Metastasis also may occur, via the lymphatics, in the lungs and bones (Kassabian & Graham).

Figure 14-3. Malignancies of the Glans and Prepuce

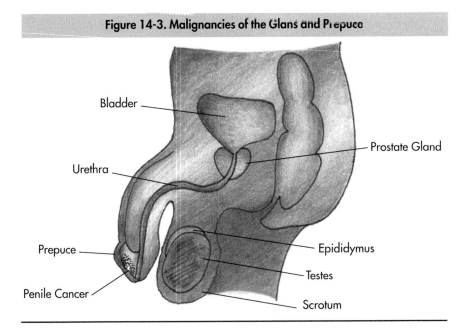

Urethral Cancer

Male: The urethra of an adult male is approximately 21 cm long and divided into five sections: fossa navicularis urethra, penile (pendulous) urethra, bulbous urethra, membraneous urethra, and prostatic urethra. The types of cells lining the urethra change as it traverses from the meatus to the prostate. Pathologically, male urethral cancers are classified into three groups based on the location of the lesion. Ascending from the glans to the prostate, they are penile cancer, bulbomembranous cancer, and prostatic cancer. The majority (59%) of male urethral cancers occur posteriorly, involving the bulbomembranous urethra. Thirty-three percent of male urethral cancers are penile cancers and 7% are prostatic cancers (Srinivas & Khan, 1988).

Female: The urethra of an adult female is approximately 4 cm long. The cells lining the urethra are mixed stratified squamous epithelium and transitional cell epithelium. Fifty percent of urethral cancers in women occur in the distal urethra and are squamous cell cancers. Squamous cell and distal urethral cancers make up 70% of all female genitourinary cancer cases (Grabstald, 1973; Srinivas & Khan, 1988).

Signs and Symptoms
Penile Cancer

The most common sign of penile cancer is a painless ulcer or growth on the penis. This lesion may go undetected if the glans is covered by the prepuce. Other signs include a foul-smelling discharge, from beneath the foreskin, that looks like soft cheese. Inguinal adenopathy may occur in a late stage of the disease (see Figure 14-4).

Figure 14-4. Signs and Symptoms Associated With Penile Cancer

- Swollen inguinal nodes
- Reddish rash (small, crusty bumps) or blue-brown flat growths
- Painless ulcer or nodule
- Phimosis
- Pain, bleeding (late signs)

Note. Based on information from Fair et al., 1993; Kassabian & Graham, 1995; Nettina, 1997.

Urethral Cancer

Patients may present with symptoms that mimic the symptoms of several benign disorders: urethritis, prostatitis (in men), strictures, and cystitis (Pettaway et al., 2000). Patients are often treated for benign conditions until the condition persists or worsens, prompting further medical evaluation.

Prevention
Penile Cancer

Poor hygiene by uncircumcised males is the primary risk factor for penile cancer. Prevention of penile cancer is associated with effective personal hygiene and circumcision. Safe-sex practices should include the use of condoms to prevent transmission of genital herpes and condyloma. Education of males regarding the signs and symptoms of penile cancer is key to early detection and prompt medical intervention.

Urethral Cancer

In as much as sexually transmitted diseases are risk factors for urethral cancer, employing safe-sex practices is prudent. To date, no chemoprevention trials related to penile or urethral carcinomas are under way.

Early Detection
Penile Cancer
Each man must take responsibility for early detection of penile cancer, through personal examination, because no laboratory or radiologic test screens for penile cancer specifically. Physical examination by a clinician should include inspection of the glans and, for uncircumcised men, the foreskin. Biopsy of a suspicious lesion is a diagnostic measure.

Urethral Cancer
Distal urethral tumors in women are usually visible as a protruding growth from the meatus (Pettaway et al., 2000). When women present for cervical screening examination, inspection of the external genitalia and perineum are part of the routine examination. Nurses should instruct male and female patients to inspect their external genitourinary anatomy on a monthly basis and to alert a healthcare provider to any abnormalities. Because cancers of the male and female genitourinary anatomy are relatively rare in the United States, mass U.S. screenings are not recommended.

Prostate Cancer
Incidence and Epidemiology
Prostate cancer is a leading cause of death in men in the United States. ACS estimated 198,100 new prostate cancer cases in the United States in 2001 (ACS, 2001). The incidence rate of prostate cancer is disproportionately high for African Americans. For African American men in 2001, prostate cancer is expected to account for 37% of all male cancers, or 25,300 cases (ACS, 2000, 2001). Incidence is also high among Blacks of the Caribbean and Blacks in the northeastern region of Brazil (Madajewicz, 1995; Roach, 1998).

Age plays a significant role in prostate cancer incidence. The median age at diagnosis is 70 years, and risk increases with each decade after age 50 (Kassabian & Graham, 1995).

Mortality
Prostate cancer is second only to lung cancer as the leading cause of cancer death in men in the United States (ACS, 2001). Prostate cancer mortality of African American men is higher than that of any other U.S. racial or ethnic group (ACS, 2000, 2001). ACS estimated that 6,100 African American men would die of prostate cancer in 2001, a number that accounts for 19% of cancer deaths among African American men. During 1990–1995, twice as many African American men were expected to die of prostate cancer than were U.S. Whites. The prostate cancer mortality estimate for African American men was five times that of Asians and Pacific Islanders (ACS, 2000, 2001). Prostate cancer mortality rates are declining for Whites and African Americans, probably because prostate-specific antigen (PSA) screening has increased early detection. In the United States, the mortality rate is highest for African American men and lowest for Jewish men (ACS, 2000,

2001; Gullatte, 2001; Zinner, 1991). The five-year survival rate for prostate cancer significantly increases when the cancer is diagnosed at a localized stage. The survival rate drops to 30% when diagnosis is at a late stage (ACS, 2000, 2001).

Etiology and Risk Factors

Table 14-9 lists factors that have been suggested as risks for prostate cancer development. The high incidence of prostate cancer in Western society seems to correlate with a high-fat diet. Circulating testosterone levels decrease by as much as 30% in men who stop eating a high-fat diet in favor of a vegetarian, low-fat diet (Dennis & Resnick, 2000; Hill & Wynder, 1979; Kolonel, 1996).

Other factors associated with an increased risk of prostate cancer are age and smoking. Men older than age 50 are more likely to get prostate cancer than are men younger than age 50. However, it is important to note that, for African American men, the median age of diagnosis for prostate cancer is 45. Laboratory studies involving rats have led to evidence of an increased rate of prostate cancer growth among those exposed to the chemicals produced by smoking (Johansson, Landstrom, Bjermer, & Henriksson, 2000).

Some studies and anecdotal reports have suggested a link between sexual activity and prostate cancer and a link between vasectomy and prostate cancer (Heshmat, Kovi, Herson, Jones, & Jackson, 1975; Kirby, Christmas, & Brawner, 1996). The data conflict regarding the influence of sexual activity on the development of prostate cancer; more research is needed. The same is true for conflicting studies suggesting a relationship between vasectomy and prostate cancer (Giovannucci, Ascherio, & Rimm, 1993; Giovannucci, Tosteson, & Speizer, 1993).

Table 14-9. Risk Factors for Prostate Cancer[a]

Risk Factor	Correlations
Age	Greater age, greater risk
Diet	Higher animal-fat intake, higher risk Lower intake of yellow vegetables and green vegetables, higher risk
Genetic proclivity	Dominance of specific autosomal gene, higher risk
Hormone level	Higher dihydrotestosterone and testosterone levels, higher risk
Infection[b]	Infection with gonococcus, herpes simplex II, or RNA virus; higher risk
Pollution	Higher cadmium exposure, higher risk
Race	African American, Scandinavian, U.S. White, or Western European; higher risk
Radioactivity	Higher exposure to Cr^{51}, Fe^{59}, Co^{60}, Zn^{65}, or tritium; higher risk
Sexual history	In men, early sexual experience and multiple sex partners; higher risk
Urban living	Living in an urban area, higher risk

[a] Some studies indicate a correlation between vasectomy and prostate cancer risk; others do not.
[b] Studies do not uniformly support a correlation between infection and prostate cancer risk.

Workers exposed to chemicals in the rubber, textile, chemical, drug, cadmium, oxide dust, fertilizer, and atomic energy industries have an increased risk of developing prostate cancer (Gullatte, 2001; Kolonel, 1996).

Epidemiologic studies indicate a familial clustering of prostate cancer and show that first-degree relatives of patients with prostate cancer have a risk of developing the disease that is two to three times higher than that of men without a similar family history (Ornstein, Dahut, Liotta, & Emmert-Buck, 1999). Researchers estimate that 10% of prostate cancers are inherited and that more than 43% of patients with prostate cancer who are younger than 55 have an inheritable form of the disease (Gronberg et al., 1997; Walsh, 1998). In 1997, Cooney et al. reported the first susceptibility locus (1q24-25)/AKA HPC1. Since that time, other researchers have suggested that another chromosome, at locus 1p36, is the prostate cancer susceptibility gene. With continued research, a definitive breakthrough in the search for the prostate cancer susceptibility gene soon should be forthcoming (Morton & Isaacs, 1998; Ornstein et al.).

Pathophyslology

As Figure 14-5 shows, the prostate is a walnut-shaped gland that is an integral part of the male reproductive system. At the base of the bladder, the prostate surrounds the urethra. The gland produces the fluid that mixes with semen to form seminal fluid. The seminal vesicles are accessory sex glands. The seminal vesicles join the vas deferens and drain into the prostatic urethra via the ejaculatory ducts (Bostwick, MacLennan, & Larson, 1999).

The prostate has three zones: the peripheral, central, and transitional zones. The peripheral zone is the largest and contains about 70% of the glandular tissue

Figure 14-5. Cancer of the Prostate

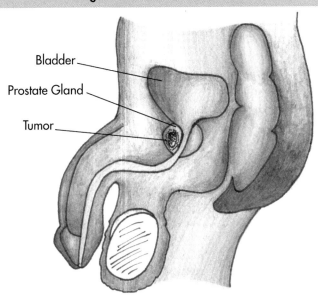

Bladder

Prostate Gland

Tumor

of the prostate. Most cancers develop in the peripheral zone. The central and transitional zones compose the remaining 30% of the prostate. The transition zone is the smallest and accounts for most cases of benign prostatic hyperplasia (BPH), a noncanerous enlargement of the prostate.

The prostate consists of epithelial and stromal cells as well as basal and neuroendocrine cells, macrophages, and lymphocytes (Scher, Issacs, Zelefsky, & Scardino, 2000). The epithelial cells, which predominate, are the sites of PSA and prostate-specific acid phosphatase (PAP) production and secretion. PSA and PAP constitute the prostatic fluid of the ejaculate (Scher et al.).

Prostate growth depends on hormones. One of these hormones, testosterone, stimulates prostate growth as well as the growth of prostate cancer cells. The progression of prostate cancer is usually slow and steady. Growth signals for prostate cancer result from a combination of genetic (induced by DNA damage) and epigenetic (not induced by DNA damage) events controlled by the difference in cell growth and cell death (Scher et al., 2000).

Ninety-five percent of all prostate cancer develops in glandular cells (Kantoff et al., 1996). Prostate cancer spreads via the lymphatic system and by direct extension. It commonly metastasizes to bone but also can locally invade surrounding organs in the pelvis, such as the bladder and seminal vesicles.

Signs and Symptoms

In the early stages, prostate cancer is asymptomatic but can present in combination with an enlarged prostate, causing urine-outflow problems. In later stages, symptoms and signs of prostate cancer usually are associated with metastatic involvement or local spread and may include hematuria, bone pain, and weight loss. Table 14-10 cites other signs and symptoms of local and locally invasive prostate cancer.

Mettlin (1997) reported that 58% of patients present with localized cancer. This high percentage is believed to be a direct result of efforts to promote digital rectal examination (DRE) and the PSA test. (As mentioned in the discussion of mortality, however, African American men tend to be diagnosed when the disease is at an advanced stage.)

Table 14-10. Signs and Symptoms of Localized Prostate Cancer

Stage	Signs	Symptoms
Local	Low-volume urine stream	Urinary urgency Urinary frequency Urinary hesitancy Sensation of incomplete emptying
Locally invasive	Blood in the urine Persistent incontinence Impotence Bleeding from the rectum Blood in the seminal fluid	Voiding pain Pain in the lower abdomen

Prevention and Screening

The exact etiology of prostate cancer is unknown. Prostate cancer continues to be a major health problem despite the success of screening and early-detection initiatives. Routine screening for prostate cancer continues to be employed despite the lack of prospective, randomized, controlled trials that prove its effectiveness, because prostate cancer rarely causes symptoms until it is in an advanced stage (Goolsby, 1998; Scher et al., 2000).

Maintaining a low-fat diet and avoiding known environmental risk factors are potential preventive measures. Certain nutrients, which may be contained in the human diet, may interfere with the development of cancer. These include beta-carotene; vitamins A, C, E, and B_{12}; and the trace elements selenium and zinc (Madajewicz, 1995). Chemoprevention researchers have evaluated these dietary nutrients to determine their effect on preventing cancer cell growth or increasing apoptosis. Some researchers suggest that diets high in fruits, vegetables, and soy proteins may offer some protection from prostate cancer development (Bylund et al., 2000; Lichtenstein, Ornish, Rippe, & Willett, 1999; Miller, 1996).

In 1997, NCI announced the completion of recruitment for the first large-scale trial to study prostate cancer prevention. The Prostate Cancer Prevention Trial (PCPT), including a total of 18,000 participants at 22 sites across the United States, is designed to determine if the drug finasteride prevents prostate cancer. Finasteride is an FDA-approved drug for the treatment of BPH. Men enrolled in PCPT are randomized to take either finasteride or a placebo every day for seven years. Finasteride blocks the growth of the prostate by decreasing the levels of dihydrotestosterone, one of the hormones that affect prostate growth. To determine if finasteride prevents prostate cancer, PCPT researchers will compare the disease prevalence in the control (placebo-taking) group with that in the experimental (finasteride-taking) group at the end of seven years.

Other studies are under way to determine if chemoprevention can inhibit or reverse the carcinogenic effect of prostatic intraepithelial neoplasm (PIN). These studies are evaluating the effects of synthetic retinoids, polyamine synthesis inhibitors, and antiandrogens, compounds shown to have preventive effects, in vitro and in vivo, on prostate carcinogenesis (Nelson, Gleason, & Brawer, 1996).

Early Detection

DRE (see Figure 14-6) has been the gold standard of prostate cancer screening because of the location of most prostatic lesions. Seventy percent of prostate cancers develop in the peripheral zone, where a DRE can detect them (Murphy et al., 1997; von Eschenbach, 1997; Waldman, 2000; Zinner, 1991). In the past decade, the serum level of PSA has been used successfully as a screening measure along with the DRE. Men age 50 and older, as well as African American men in their 40s, should have a DRE and PSA test as part of their annual physical examination (Moul, 1998; Murphy et al.).

In evaluating specific tests, three indices should be considered: sensitivity, the percentage of positive tests that result because patients actually have the disease; specificity, the percentage of negative tests that result because patients do not have the disease; and cost. PSA is a blood-specific antigen whose level is elevated in the

Figure 14-6. Digital Rectal Examination

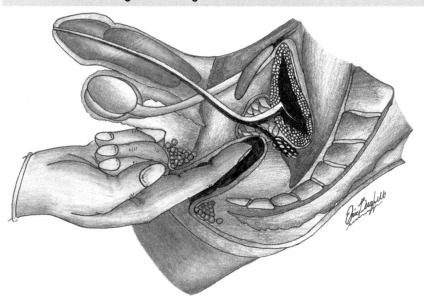

presence of several diseases of the prostate (e.g., infection, BPH, cancer). The principal strengths of the PSA test are its superior sensitivity, reasonable cost, and patient acceptance (ACS, 2001).

In combination with the DRE, PSA testing is the best screening measure for prostate cancer. Nevertheless, the test is surrounded by controversy. First, some researchers and clinicians believe that PSA values have different significance according to race. Some researchers believe that, in men who have no clinical or histologic evidence of cancer, total PSA tends to be higher in African Americans than in White Americans (Catalona, Partin, & Slaw, 2000). If that is true, a single or age-adjusted PSA reference range established for White men may not be applicable to African American men (Henderson et al., 1997; Morgan et al., 1996). Clinicians typically use a free PSA level less than 25% as the level that prompts them to recommend prostate biopsy. Reports have suggested that using this percentage could lead to underdiagnosis of early-stage prostate cancer in African American men (Fowler, Bigler, Kilambi, & Landi, 1999; Fowler et al., 2000; Schroder et al., 2000).

The second point of controversy relates to the three PSA measures: total PSA, a measure of serum PSA bound to protease inhibitor; free PSA, a measure of serum PSA unbound to protease inhibitor; and complexed PSA, a measure of PSA complexed with various protease inhibitors, including %-1-antichymotrypsin and %-1-antitrypsin, to the exclusion of free PSA (Brawer et al., 2000). A test of free PSA is necessary when total PSA is 4.0–10.0 ng/ml (Vashi, Wojno, & Hendricks, 1997). In such cases, Brawer et al. reported a 85%–95% sensitivity, revealing that the specificity of complexed PSA testing was higher than that of total PSA testing and equivalent to that of testing the ratio of free PSA to total PSA. This research indicated that complexed PSA can be used as a single assay measure to screen and detect prostate cancer, eliminating the need to test total PSA.

Other researchers have pointed out the significant number of false positives that PSA testing produces. False positives lead to unnecessary workups and invasive prostate biopsies for men who do not have the disease. For example, the natural history of PIN, believed to be a precursor of prostate cancer, is variable; no reliable predictive screening marker has been identified (Keefe & Meyskens, 2000). In cases of PIN, the false-positive rate produced by a PSA test for prostate cancer is as high as 25%–50%. Overall, the positive predictive value of PSA screening is approximately 30% (Keefe and Meyskens). PSA testing also results in a number of false negatives. In these cases, prostate cancer goes undetected. Studies have demonstrated that as many as 25% of men with a normal PSA level (a level less than 4 ng/ml) have disease beyond the prostate (Lu-Yao & Yao, 1997).

Although controversy remains, ACS and the American Urologic Association currently recommend that PSA screening, in combination with DRE, begin at age 40 years in African American men and men who have first-degree relatives with prostate cancer; all other men should begin screening at age 50 (Powell et al., 2000).

Other diagnostic tests for prostate cancer include transrectal ultrasound (TRUS) screening. TRUS is used to evaluate prostate size, as a follow-up evaluation after a DRE or a PSA test produces abnormal results, and to guide an automatic needle that takes a prostate sample for biopsy (see Figure 14-7).

Figure 14-7. Transrectal Prostate Sampling for Biopsy

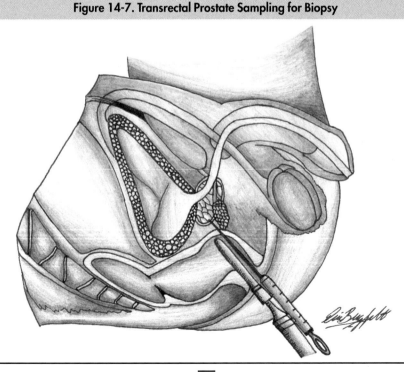

Education of men at high risk for developing prostate cancer is crucial to reducing prostate cancer mortality rates.

ACS's National Prostate Cancer Detection Project showed that—after five years of annual testing by means of PSA screening, the DRE, and TRUS—91.7% of cancers were detected while still localized (Mettlin, 1997). PSA tests can result in false positives if the serum antigen is sampled after the patient has had a DRE (Dew et al., 1999). A DRE can increase PSA by approximately two times the normal level (Wallach, 1996). Therefore, DRE should be performed after serum PSA is collected.

In 1993, NCI launched a longitudinal screening trial to study the effect of screening procedures in reducing morbidity and mortality from prostate, lung, colorectal, and ovarian cancer (PLCO). The randomized and controlled PLCO trial, known as the PLCO Cancer Screening Trial, includes 74,000 men and 74,000 women ages 55–74 at 10 cancer centers throughout the United States. The prostate arm of the trial has a design power of 90% to determine a 20% reduction of prostate cancer mortality from a baseline and three subsequent annual screenings consisting of PSA testing and the DRE (Gohagan, Prorok, Kramer, & Cornett, 1994). Current data indicate that the median age of African American men with prostate cancer is 45 (ACS, 2001). Therefore, some experts are concerned that the PLCO trial, because of the age range of enrollees, will produce few results relevant to African American men. Keefe and Meyskens (2000) predicted that, in the future, genetic testing will be able to identify men whose prostate cancer will be highly aggressive and those whose cancer will progress slowly.

Table 14-5 lists several active chemotherapy prevention, screening, and genetic trials currently under way through NCI. To find out more about these trials, visit CancerTrials™ (http://cancertrials.nci.nih.gov), a Web site produced by NCI that lists clinical trials being conducted across the United States.

Recruiting minorities into clinical trials remains a challenge. Researchers (Harris, Gorelick, Samuels, & Bempong, 1996; Mouton, Harris, Rovi, Solorzano, & Johnson, 1997) have tried to explain why minority participation in clinical trials tends to be less than nonminority participation. The reasons they present include

- Lack of trust in an institution or medical staff to provide safe and effective care in the best interest of the study subject
- Lack of minority researchers approaching the subjects
- Concern about being the subject of experimentation and feeling like a "guinea pig"
- Lack of knowledge related to the benefits of clinical trials and the ability to withdraw without harm
- Fear of changing from a treatment or medication that seems to be working to an unknown treatment or medication
- Costs of care
- The influence of family and friends who do not support participation because of reasons listed previously
- Barriers relating to language and culture.

For many African Americans, the realities of the Tuskegee Syphilis Study, 1932–1972 still come to mind when asked to participate in a clinical trial. In the Tuskegee study, the U.S. Public Health Service withheld treatment to known syphilis patients without their knowledge or consent (Brooks, 1997–1998; Savitt, 1982). To many, the Tuskegee trials confirm suspicions of racism in clinical testing—a suspicion that will take science decades of hard work to overcome (Gavaghan, 1995; Gorelick, Harris, Burnett, & Bonecutter, 1998).

Despite these seemingly insurmountable barriers, researchers must find a way to increase minority participation in clinical trials (Svensson, 1989; Swanson & Ward, 1995). This is particularly important in regard to trials relating to breast cancer and prostate cancer, diseases that seem to have ethnic-specific components. Increasing minority participation has the potential to equalize early-detection rates in minority and nonminority populations (Roberson, 1994).

Nursing Challenges and Opportunities

Weinstein (1991) reported that 50%–80% of human cancers have exogenous causes and are, therefore, preventable. This fact suggests that nursing opportunities associated with urinary and male genital cancers include patient and community education related to prevention, screening, and early detection and access to preventive and follow-up care. Table 14-11 lists resources that may be helpful to nurses in their educational efforts. Each person must be encouraged and taught to be an advocate for his or her own health. This advocacy must take the form of behavior and lifestyle changes when appropriate—changes such as smoking cessation, achieving a healthful diet, and reaching a weight appropriate to height and age. The evidence suggests that about one-third of the 500,000 cancer deaths in the United States are related to dietary factors and another third are related to cigarette smoking (ACS, 2001; Tariq et al., 2000).

Nursing and Bladder Cancer

Educating patients about the early signs and symptoms of bladder cancer is important because no specific screening test for bladder cancer exists. Bladder cancer is the fourth most common cancer in men and the eighth most common cancer in women (Lamm, 1998; Murphy et al., 1997). About 80% of patients experience micro- or macroscopic hematuria as a presenting sign. Patients should be instructed to seek medical care when experiencing unusual or abnormal urinary symptoms. These symptoms include urinary frequency or hesitancy or a burning sensation. Adults 60–80 years old should have regular annual physicals, including a urine screening for microscopic hematuria. Individuals of any age who have been treated with cyclophosphamide and pelvic radiation are at greater than average risk for bladder cancer and also should be assessed annually. The Occupational Safety and Health Administration (OSHA) requires all employers to have a workplace hazard and safety program to protect employees from hazardous work conditions, including exposure to environmental and chemical toxins. Nurses participating in public and community education programs can increase public awareness of OSHA requirements as well as knowledge and awareness of cancer risks and early-detection strategies.

Table 14-11. Genitourinary Cancer Resources for Healthcare Professionals and the Public

Organization	Functions	Internet Address
American Cancer Society 1599 Clifton Road NE Atlanta, GA 30329 800-ACS-2345	Offers services to patients, families, and professionals. Supports cancer research and offers service and educational programs. Local divisions and units at the community level.	www.cancer.org
American Foundation for Urologic Disease 1128 N. Charles St. Baltimore, MD 21201 800-242-2383	Educates patients, the public, and healthcare professionals about urologic diseases and dysfunction, including prostate cancer, bladder health, and sexual function. Supports research.	www.afud.org
American Institute for Cancer Research 1759 R St. NW Washington, DC 20009 800-843-8114	Provides information about cancer prevention through diet and nutrition.	www.aicr.org
Cancer Research Foundation of America 1600 Duke St., Suite 110 Alexandria, VA 22314 800-227-2732	Funds research and provides educational materials about early detection and nutrition.	www.preventcancer.org
CaP CURE (Association for the Cure of Cancer of the Prostate) 1250 Fourth St., Suite 360 Santa Monica, CA 90401 800-757-2873	Provides funding for research designed to improve diagnosis and treatment of prostate cancer.	www.capcure.org
Kidney Cancer Association 1234 Sherman Ave., Suite 203 Evanston, IL 60202 800-850-9132	Supports research. Provides information about diagnosis and treatment of kidney cancer. Sponsors support groups and provides physician referral information.	www.nkca.org
US TOO International 5003 Fairview Ave. Downers Grove, IL 60515 800-80USTOO	Prostate cancer support group organization. Increases awareness of prostate cancer in the community. Provides latest information about treatment.	www.ustoo.org
National Cancer Institute 31 Center Dr. Building 31, Room 10A16 MSC 2580 Bethesda, MD 20892 800-4-CANCER	Provides cancer information to patients, families, and healthcare professionals.	www.nih.nci.gov

Nursing and Kidney Cancer

To date, no screening test exists for cancer of the kidney. Public and community education initiatives aimed at risk reduction and early detection, as well as timely access to medical care, are the cornerstones of reducing mortality from this disease.

Nursing and Testicular Cancer

The most consistent occupational risk associated with testicular cancer among professional and white-collar workers is sedentary lifestyle (Murphy et al., 1997). Nurses should make the public aware of this risk and help give patients the information they need to choose prudent exercise programs.

Nurses should ensure that men know that TSE is the best screening plan for early detection of testicular cancer. Every male older than 15 years of age should know how to perform TSE. Nurses can make educational materials—videos, booklets, and TSE cards (i.e., cards produced by ACS or NCI)—readily available. Nurse practitioners or physicians should perform testicular examinations during athletes' annual physical examinations. These encounters lend themselves to teaching as the clinician demonstrates testicular examination. Healthcare providers should be sensitive to patients' sexuality issues related to self-image and some patients' hesitancy to perform TSE. Nurses can educate parents about the need for early surgical correction of cryptorchidism.

Nursing and Penile and Urethral Cancer

Young parents should be educated about circumcision and the importance of hygiene practices for uncircumcised males. Young adults should be educated about safe-sex practices that help prevent the transmission of sexually transmitted diseases. Men should be instructed to seek prompt medical attention regarding abnormal genital findings. Nurses can heighten adult males' awareness of risk factors associated with penile and urethral cancers, the symptoms of these diseases, and when to seek medical advice. Both men and women should be educated about the risk factors associated with urethral cancer as well as the symptoms to report to their healthcare provider.

Nursing and Prostate Cancer

Although prostate cancer incidence rates are declining, prostate cancer remains the leading cause of cancer death in American men. Nurses must educate men regarding controllable risk factors and promote screening. Table 14-12 lists Web sites that may be helpful to nurses who are designing educational programs. Prostate cancer screening programs should be offered in the community to increase public awareness of cancer prevention, screening, and early detection.

Future Directions

Breakthroughs in genetics will affect disease prevention, early detection, and treatment strategies relating to genitourinary cancers. The Human Genome Project

Table 14-12. Prostate Cancer Web Sites

Site	Internet Address
Prostate Cancer Home Page Sponsored by TAP Pharmaceuticals. Provides information about prostate cancer diagnosis and treatment.	http://prostate.com
Astra Zeneca Sponsored by pharmaceutical company. Provides general information about prostate cancer.	www.prostateinfo.com
Centerwatch Lists, by state, clinical trials relating to prostate cancer.	www.centerwatch.com
Uromed Corporation Sponsored by supplier of brachytherapy products. Provides general information about prostate cancer.	www.uromed.com
Web MD Provides information about prostate cancer and other cancers.	http://webmd.com
Cancer Prevention and Control Produced by the Centers for Disease Control. Provides information about prostate cancer.	www.cdc.gov/cancer
Office of Disease Prevention and Health Promotion Sponsored by the U.S. government. Provides statistical and research information about health issues and disease.	http://odphp.osophs.dhhs.gov
Prostate Cancer Research and Education Foundation Conducts research to increase public awareness about prostate cancer.	www.prostatecancer.com
CancerNet Sponsored by the National Cancer Institute. Provides information about clinical trials and other information about prostate cancer and resources for patients.	http://cancernet.nci.nih.gov

holds great promise for researchers. It promises not only to unlock the mystery of chromosomal and cellular mutation, but also to teach clinicians the right time to interfere to arrest the mutation process.

The findings of large-scale clinical trials, like the PLCO Cancer Screening Trial, will significantly reduce cancer incidence and mortality in the next millennium. Researchers must strategize to overcome the factors that deter many minorities, women, and the elderly from participating in clinical trials. Equal participation will help minimize the disparities between the morbidity and mortality rates of minority populations and those of nonminority populations.

Researchers should launch a greater number of controlled chemoprevention studies to evaluate the safety and effectiveness of herbal therapies in cancer prevention and control. One recent study investigated the effect of epigallocatechin gallate (EGCG), the main constituent of Japanese green tea, and green-tea polyphenols on tumor necrosis factor-alpha (TNF-α). The researchers, working in a phase I trial in Japan, found strong evidence that EGCG inhibits the release of TNF-α from cells (Fujiki et al., 2000). The study demonstrated that green tea is a cancer preventive. Two U.S. studies, one at the M.D. Anderson Cancer Center, in Houston, TX, and another at Memorial Sloan-Kettering Cancer Center, in New York, NY, currently are investigating the preventive effects of green tea.

Other studies of chemoprevention suggest that daily intake of saw palmetto, beta-carotene, vitamin E, and selenium may help prevent prostate cancer (Gerber, 2000; Janson, 1999; Marshall, 2000; "Prostate Cancer Prevention Trial," 1997). Trials such as these may help broaden the knowledge base of cancer prevention.

References

American Cancer Society. (2000). *Cancer facts and figures for African Americans 2000–2001* (pp. 2–3). Atlanta: Author.

American Cancer Society. (2001). *Cancer facts and figures, 2001*. Atlanta: Author.

Aso, Y., & Homma, Y. (1992). A survey on incidental renal cell carcinoma in Japan. *Journal of Urology, 147*, 340–343.

Atkin, N.B., & Baker, M.C. (1982). Specific chromosome change, i(12p), in testicular tumors? *Lancet, 2*, 1349.

Bissada, N.K., Morcos, R.R., & el-Senoussi, M. (1986). Post-circumcision carcinoma of the penis: Clinical aspects. *Journal of Urology, 135*, 283–285.

Bostwick, D.G., MacLennan, G.T., & Larson, T.R. (1999). *Prostate cancer*. Atlanta: American Cancer Society.

Brawer, M.K., Cheli, C.D., Neaman, I.E., Goldblatt, J., Smith, C., Schwartz, M.K., Bruzek, D.J., Morris, D.L., Sokoll, L.J., Chan, D.W., Yeung, K.K., Partin, A.W., & Allard, W.J. (2000). Complexed prostate-specific antigen provides significant enhancement of specificity compared with total prostate-specific antigen for detecting prostate cancer. *Journal of Urology, 163*, 1476–1480.

Brinton, L.A., Li, J.Y., Rong, S.D., Huang, S., Xiao, B.S., Shi, B.G., Zhu, Z.J., Schiffman, M.H., & Dawsey, S. (1991). Risk factors for penile cancer: Results from a case-control study in China. *International Journal of Cancer, 47*, 504–509.

Brooks, J. (1997, December–1998, January). Minority participation in clinical trials: The impact of the Tuskegee Syphilis Study. *Closing the Gap: A Newsletter of the Office of Minority Health*, pp. 1–5.

Bylund, A., Zhang, J.X., Bergh, A., Damber, J.E., Widmark, A., Johansson, A., Adlercreutz, H., Aman, P., Shepherd, M.J., & Hallmans, G. (2000). Rye bran and soy protein delay growth increase apoptosis of human LNCaP prostate adenocarcinoma in nude mice. *Prostate, 42*, 304–314.

Cairns, P., & Sidransky, D. (1999). Molecular methods for the diagnosis of cancer. *Biochimica et Biophysica Acta, 1423*, C11–C18.

Catalona, W.J., Partin, A.W., & Slawin, K.M. (2000). Percentage of free PSA in black versus white men for detection and staging of prostate cancer: A prospective multicenter clinical trial. *Urology, 55*, 372–376.

Chaganti, R.S., Rodriguez, E., & Bosl, G.J. (1993). Cytogenetics of male germ-cell tumors. *Urology Clinics of North America, 20*, 55–56.

Chang, F., Syrjanen, S., & Syrjanen, K. (1995). Implications of the p53 tumor-suppressor gene in clinical oncology. *Journal of Clinical Oncology, 13*, 1009–1022.

Chow, W.H., Devesa, S.S., & Warren, J.L. (1999). The rising incidence of renal cell cancer in the United States. *JAMA, 281*, 1628–1631.

Cooney, K.A., McCarthy, J.D., Lange, E., Huang, L., Miesfeldt, S., Montie, J.E., Oesterling, J.E., Sandler, H.M., & Lange, K. (1997). Prostate cancer susceptibility locus on chromosome 1q: A confirmatory study. *Journal of the National Cancer Institute, 89*, 955–959.

Dennis, L.K., & Resnik, M.I. (2000). Analysis of recent trends in prostate cancer incidence and mortality. *Prostate, 42*, 247–252.

Devesa, S.S., Silverman, D.T., McLaughlin, J.K., Brown, C.C., Connelly, R.R., & Fraumeni, J.F. (1990). Comparison of the descriptive epidemiology of urinary tract cancers. *Cancer Causes and Control, 1*(2), 133–141.

Dew, T., Coker, S., Saadeh, F., Mulvin, D., Copcoat, M.J., & Sherwood, R.A. (1999). Influence of investigative and operative procedures on serum prostate-specific antigen concentration. *Annals of Clinical Biochemistry, 36*, 340–346.

Dupree, R.H., Pike, M.C., & Henderson, B.E. (1983). Estrogen exposure during gestation and risk of testicular cancer. *Journal of the National Cancer Institute, 71*, 1151–1155.

Fair, R.W., Fuks, Z.Y., & Scher, H.I. (1993). Cancer of the urethra and penis. In V.T. DeVita, S. Hellman, & S.A. Rosenberg (Eds.), *Cancer: Principles and practice of oncology* (pp. 1114–1125). Philadelphia: Lippincott.

Fair, W.R., & Yang, C.R. (1992). Urethral carcinoma in males. In M.I. Resnick & E.D. Kursh (Eds.), *Current therapy in genitourinary surgery* (p. 157). St. Louis, MO: Mosby.

Fernandes, E.T., Manivel, J.C., Reddy, P.K., & Ercole, C.J. (1996). Cyclophosphamide associated bladder cancer: A highly aggressive disease—Analysis of 12 cases. *Journal of Urology, 156*, 1931–1933.

Fleshner, N.E., Herr, H.W., Stewart, A.K., Murphy, G.P., Mettlin, C., & Menck, H.R. (1996). The National Cancer Data Base report on bladder carcinoma. *Cancer, 78*, 1505–1515.

Fowler, J.E., Bigler, S.A., Kilambi, N.K., & Landi, S.A. (1999). Relationships between prostate-specific antigen and prostate volume in black and white men with benign prostate biopsies. *Urology, 53*, 1175–1178.

Fowler, J.E., Sanders, J., Bigler, S.A., Rigdon, J., Kilambi, N.K., & Land, S.A. (2000). Percent free prostate-specific antigen and cancer detection in black and white men with total prostate-specific antigen 2.5 to 9.9 ng/ml. *Journal of Urology, 163*, 1467–1470.

Fromowitz, F.B., & Bard, R.H. (1990). Clinical implications of pathologic subtypes of renal cell carcinoma. *Seminars in Urology, 8*, 31–50.

Fujiki, H., Suganuma, M., Okabe, S., Sueoka, E., Suga, K., Imai, K., & Nakachi, K. (2000). A new concept of tumor promotion by tumor necrosis factor-alpha, and cancer prevention agents (-)-epigallocatechin in gallate and green tea—A review. *Cancer Detection and Prevention, 24*, 91–99.

Garnick, M.B., Krane, R.J., Scully, R.E., & Weber, E.T. (1996). Cancer of the testis. In R.T. Osteen (Ed.), *Cancer manual* (9th ed.) (pp. 471–481). Boston: American Cancer Society, Massachusetts Division.

Gavaghan, H. (1995). Clinical trials face lack of minority group volunteers. *Nature, 373,* 178.

Gerber, G.S. (2000). Saw palmetto for the treatment of men with lower urinary tract symptoms. *Journal of Urology, 163,* 1408–1412.

Giovannucci, E., Ascherio, A., & Rimm, E.B. (1993). A prospective cohort study of vasectomy and prostate cancer in U.S. men. *JAMA, 269,* 873–877.

Giovannucci, E., Tosteson, D., & Speizer, F.E. (1993). A retrospective cohort study of vasectomy and prostate cancer in U.S. men. *JAMA, 269,* 878–914.

Gnarra, J.R., Glenn, G.M., Latif, F., Anglard, P., Lerman, M.I., Zbar, B., & Linehan, W.M. (1993). Molecular genetic studies in sporadic and familial renal cell carcinoma. *Urologic Clinics of North America, 2,* 207–216.

Gohagan, J.K., Prorok, P.C., Kramer, B.S., & Cornett, J.E. (1994). Prostate cancer screening in the Prostate, Lung, Colorectal and Ovarian Cancer Screening Trial of the National Cancer Institute. *Journal of Urology, 152,* 1905–1909.

Goolsby, M.J. (1998). Screening, diagnosis, and management of prostate cancer: Improving primary care outcomes. *Nurse Practitioner, 23,* 11–41.

Gorelick, P.B., Harris, Y., Burnett, B., & Bonecutter, F.J. (1998). The recruitment triangle: Reasons why African Americans enroll, refuse to enroll, or voluntarily withdraw from a clinical trial. *Journal of the National Medical Association, 90,* 141–145.

Grabstald, H. (1973). Proceedings: Tumors of the urethra in men and women. *Cancer, 32,* 1236–1255.

Grégoire, J.R., Torres, V.E., & Halley, K.E. (1987). Renal epithelial hyperplastic and neoplastic proliferation in autosomal dominant polycystic kidney disease. *American Journal of Kidney Diseases, 9,* 27–38.

Grégoire, M., Fradet, Y., Meyer, F., Têtu, B., Bois, R., Bédard, G., Charrois, R., & Naud, A. (1997). Diagnostic accuracy of urinary cytology, and deoxyribonucleic acid flow cytometry and cytology on bladder washings during follow-up for bladder tumors. *Journal of Urology, 157,* 1660.

Gronberg, H., Isaacs, S.D., Smith, J.R., Carpten, J.D., Bova, G.S., Freije, D., Xu, J., Meyers, D.A., Collins, F.S., Trent, J.M., Walsh, P.C., & Isaacs, W.B. (1997). Characteristics of prostate cancer in families potentially linked to the hereditary prostate cancer 1 (HPC1) locus. *JAMA, 278,* 1251–1255.

Grossman, H.B. (1998). New methods for detection of bladder cancer. *Seminars in Urologic Oncology, 16,* 17–22.

Gullatte, M.M. (2001). Cancer prevention, screening, and early detection. In S. Otto (Ed.), *Oncology nursing* (4th ed.) (pp. 30–48). St. Louis, MO: Mosby.

Harris, Y., Gorelick, P.B., Samuels, P., & Bempong, I. (1996). Why African Americans may not be participating in clinical trials. *Journal of the National Medical Association, 88,* 630–634.

Henderson, R.J., Eastham, J.A., Culkin, D.J., Kattan, M.W., Whatley, T., Matai, J., Venable, D., & Sartor, O. (1997). Prostate-specific antigen (PSA) and PSA density: Racial differences in men without prostate cancer. *Journal of the National Cancer Institute, 89,* 134–138.

Heshmat, M.Y., Kovi, J., Herson, J., Jones, G.W., & Jackson, M.A. (1975). Epidemiologic association between gonorrhea and prostatic carcinoma. *Urology, 6,* 457–460.

Hill, P.B., & Wynder, E.L. (1979). Effect of a vegetarian diet and dexamethasone on plasma prolactin, testosterone and dehydroepiandrosterone in men and women. *Cancer Letters, 7,* 273–282.

Hilton, S. (2000). Imaging of renal call carcinoma. *Seminars in Oncology, 27*, 150–159.

Isaacs, W.B., Carter, B.S., & Ewing, C.M. (1991). Wild-type p53 suppresses growth of human prostate cancer containing mutant p53 alleles. *Cancer Research, 51*, 4716–4720.

Jacob, S.W., & Francone, C.A. (1974). *Structure and function in man* (pp. 541–542). Philadelphia: W.B. Saunders.

Janson, M. (1999). *All about saw palmetto and prostate health.* Garden City Park, NY: Avery Publishing Group.

Jensen, O.M., Knudsen, J.B., McLaughlin, J.K., & Sorensen, B.L. (1988). The Copenhagen case-control study of renal pelvis and ureter cancer: Role of smoking and occupational exposures. *International Journal of Cancer, 41*, 557–561.

Johansson, S., Landstrom, M., Bjermer, L., & Henriksson, R. (2000). Effects of tobacco smoke on the growth and radiation response of Dunning R3327 prostate adenocarcinoma in rats. *Prostate, 42*, 253–259.

Kantoff, P.W., Shipley, W.U., Gallagher, J., Loughlin, K.R., & Soto, E.A. (1996). Cancer of the bladder. In R.T. Osteen (Ed.), *Cancer manual* (9th ed.) (pp. 462–470). Boston: American Cancer Society, Massachusetts Division.

Kaplan, G.W., Bulkey, G.J., & Grayhack, J.T. (1967). Carcinoma of the male urethra. *Journal of Urology, 98*, 365–371.

Kassabian, V.S., & Graham, S. (1995). Urologic and male genital cancers. In G.P. Murphy, W. Lawrence, & R.E. Lenhard (Eds.), *American Cancer Society textbook of clinical oncology* (pp. 309–329). Atlanta: American Cancer Society.

Keefe, K.A., & Meyskens, F.L. (2000). Cancer prevention. In M.D. Abeloff, J.O. Armitage, A.S. Lichter, & J.E. Niederhuber (Eds.), *Clinical oncology* (pp. 318–365). New York: Churchill Livingstone.

Kirby, R.S., Christmas, T.J., & Brawner, M. (1996). *Prostate cancer* (pp. 23–29). Wilmington, DE: Times Mirror International.

Kolonel, L.N. (1996). Nutrition and prostate cancer. *Cancer Causes and Control, 7*, 83–94.

Konnak, J.W., & Grossman, H.B. (1990). Renal cell carcinoma as an incidental finding. *Journal of Urology, 134*, 1094–1096.

La Vecchia, C., Negri, E., D'Avanzo, B., Savoldelli, R., & Franceschi, S. (1991). Genital and urinary tract diseases and bladder cancer. *Cancer Research, 51*, 629–631.

Lamm, D.L. (1998). Bladder cancer: Twenty years of progress and the challenges that remain. *CA: A Cancer Journal for Clinicians, 48*, 263–268.

Leahy, M.G., Tonks, S., Moses, J.H., Brett, A.R., Huddart, R., Forman, D., Oliver, R.T., Bishop, D.T., & Bodmer, J.G. (1995). Candidate regions for a testicular cancer susceptibility gene. *Human Molecular Genetics, 4*, 1551–1555.

Lichtenstein, A., Ornish, D., Rippe, J., & Willett, W.C. (1999). The best diet for healthy adults. *Patient Care for Nurse Practitioners, 2*(11), 30–52.

Lind, J. (1997). Urinary tract cancers. In C. Varricchio (Ed.), *A cancer source book for nurses* (7th ed.) (pp. 316–326). Atlanta: American Cancer Society.

Lind, J. (1998). Nursing care of the client with cancer of the urinary system. In J.K. Itano & K.N. Taoka (Eds.), *Core curriculum for oncology nursing* (pp. 421–447). Philadelphia: W.B. Saunders.

Lliopoulos, O., & Eng, C. (2000). Genetic and clinical aspects of familial renal neoplasms. *Seminars in Oncology, 27*, 138–149.

Lu-Yao, G.L., & Yao, S.L. (1997). Population-based study of long-term survival in patients with clinically localised prostate cancer. *Lancet, 349*, 906–910.

Madajewicz, S. (1995). Genitourinary cancer. In P. Greenwald, B.S. Kramer, & D.L. Weed (Eds.), *Cancer prevention and control* (pp. 659–671). New York: Marcel Dekker.

Maden, C., Sherman, K.J., Beckmann, A.M., Hislop, T.G., Teh, C.Z., Ashley, R.L., & Daling, J.R. (1993). History of circumcision, medical condition, and sexual activity and risk of penile cancer. *Journal of the National Cancer Institute, 85*, 19–24.

Malek, R.S., Omesa, P.J., & Benson, R.C. (1987). Renal cell carcinoma in von Hippel-Lindau syndrome. *American Journal of Medicine, 82*, 236–238.

Mandel, J.S., McLaughlin, J.K., & Schlehofer, B. (1995). International renal-cell cancer study. IV occupation. *International Journal of Cancer, 61*, 601–605.

Marshall, F.C., Uson, A.C., & Melicow, M.M. (1960). Neoplasms and caruncles of the female urethra. *Surgery, Gynecology and Obstetrics, 110*, 723.

Marshall, J.R. (2000). Chemoprevention of prostate cancer in a high-risk population. *Oncology Economics, 1*, 40–44.

McCredie, M., Pommer, W., & McLaughlin, J.K. (1995). International renal-cell cancer study. II. Analgesics. *International Journal of Cancer, 60*, 345–349.

McLaughlin, J.K., Blot, W.J., & Fraumeni, J.F. (1988). Diuretics and renal cell cancer. *Journal of the National Cancer Institute, 80*, 378.

McLaughlin, J.K., Chow, W.H., & Mandel, J.S. (1995). International renal-cell cancer study. VIII. Role of diuretics, other anti-hypertensive medications and hypertension. *International Journal of Cancer, 63*, 216–221.

McLaughlin, J.K., Hrubec, Z., Heineman, E.F., Blot, W.J., & Fraumeni, J.F. (1990). Renal cancer and cigarette smoking: 26-year follow-up of U.S. veterans. *Public Health Reports, 105*, 535–537.

McLaughlin, J.K., & Lipworth, L. (2000). Epidemiologic aspects of renal cell cancer. *Seminars in Oncology, 27*, 115–123.

Merrill, R.M., & Stephenson, R.A. (2000). Trends in mortality rates in patients with prostate cancer during the era of prostate-specific antigen screening. *Journal of Urology, 163*, 503–510.

Mettlin, C.J. (1997). Observations on the early detection of prostate cancer from the American Cancer Society National Prostate Cancer Detection Project. *Cancer, 80*, 1814–1817.

Mevorach, R.A., Cos, L.R., & di Sant'Agnese, P.A. (1990). Human papilloma virus type 6 in grade I transitional cell carcinoma of the urethra. *Journal of Urology, 143*, 126–128.

Miller, B.A. (Ed.). (1996). *Racial/ethnic patterns of cancer in the United States 1988–1992* (NIH Publication No. 96-4104). Bethesda, MD: National Cancer Institute.

Montie, J.E., Smith, D.C., & Sandler, H.M. (2000). Carcinoma of the bladder. In M.D. Abeloff, J.O. Armitage, A.S. Lichter, & J.E. Niederhuber (Eds.), *Clinical oncology* (pp. 1800–1822). New York: Churchill Livingstone.

Morgan, T.O., Jacobson, S.J., McCarthy, W.F., Jacobson, D.J., McLeod, D.G., & Moul, J.W. (1996). Age-specific reference ranges for serum prostate-specific antigen in black men. *New England Journal of Medicine, 335*, 304–310.

Morse, M.A., & Stoner, G.D. (1993). Cancer chemoprevention: Principles and prospects. *Carcinogenesis, 14*, 1737–1746.

Morton, R.A., & Isaacs, W.B. (1998). Molecular genetics of prostate cancer: Clinical applications. *JAMA, 90*(Suppl. 11), 728–731.

Mosteret, M.M.C., van de Pol, M., & Olde-Weghuis, D. (1996). Comparative genomic hybridization of germ-cell tumors of the adult testis: Conformation of karyotypic findings and identification of a 12p-amplicon. *Cancer Genetics and Cytogenetics, 89,* 146–152.

Motzer, R.J. (2000). Renal cell carcinoma: Progress against an elusive tumor. *Seminars in Oncology, 27,* 113–114.

Moul, J.W. (1998). Use of prostate-specific antigen in black men: Age-adjusted reference ranges for maximal cancer detection. *Journal of the National Medical Association, 90*(Suppl. 11), 710–712.

Moul, J.W., Schanne, F.J., & Thompson, I.M. (1994). Testicular cancer in blacks: A multicenter experience. *Cancer, 73,* 388–393.

Mouton, C.P., Harris, S., Rovi, S., Solorzano, P., & Johnson, M.S. (1997). Barriers to black women's participation in cancer clinical trials. *Journal of the National Medical Association, 89,* 721–727.

Murphy, G.P., Morris, L.B., & Lange, D. (1997). *Informed decisions: The complete book of cancer diagnosis, treatment, and recovery* (pp. 643–647). Atlanta: American Cancer Society.

Murty, V.V., & Changanti, R.S. (1998). A genetic perspective of male germ cell tumors. *Seminars in Oncology, 25,* 133–144.

National Cancer Institute. (2000). *Trials related to urologic and male genital cancers.* Retrieved June 20, 2000 from the World Wide Web: http://www.clinicaltrials.nci.nih.gov

Navon, J.D., Soliman, H., & Khonsari, F. (1997). Screening cystoscopy and survival of spinal cord injured patients with squamous cell cancer of the bladder. *Journal of Urology, 157,* 2109–2111.

Nelson, P.S., Gleason, T.P., & Brawer, M.K. (1996). Chemoprevention for prostate intraepithelial neoplasia. *European Urology, 30,* 269–278.

Nettina, S. (1997). *Lippincott's pocket manual of nursing practice* (pp. 142–154). Philadelphia: J.B. Lippincott.

Newsom, G.D., & Vurgin, D. (1987). Etiologic factors in renal cell adenocarcinoma. *Seminars in Nephrology, 7,* 109–116.

Nichols, C.R., Timmerman, R., Foster, R.S., Roth, B.J., & Einhorn, L.H. (2000). Neoplasms of the testis. In J.F. Holland & E. Frei (Eds.), *Cancer medicine* (pp. 1596–1601). Hamilton, Ontario: Decker.

Nicholson, P.W., & Harland, S.J. (1995). Inheritance and testicular cancer. *British Journal of Cancer, 71,* 421–426.

Offit, K. (1998). *Clinical cancer genetics: Risk counseling and management.* New York: John Wiley.

Offit, K. (2000). Genetics in clinical oncology. In M.D. Abcloff, J.O. Armitage, A.S. Lichter, & J.E. Niederhuber (Eds.), *Clinical oncology* (pp. 138–157). New York: Churchill Livingstone.

Ornstein, D.K., Dahut, W.L., Liotta, L.A., & Emmert-Buck, M.R. (1999). Review of AACR [American Association for Cancer Research] meeting: New research approaches in the prevention and cure of prostate cancer. *Biochimica et Biophysica Acta, 1424*(1), R11–R19.

O'Rourke, M.E. (2001). Genitourinary cancers. In S. Otto (Ed.), *Oncology nursing* (4th ed.) (p. 238). St. Louis, MO: Mosby.

Parker, S.L., Tong, T., & Bolden, S. (1997). Cancer statistics, 1997. *CA: A Cancer Journal for Clinicians, 47*, 5–27.

Parzuchowski, J., & Wallace, M. (1997). Genitourinary cancers. In S. Otto (Ed.), *Oncology nursing* (4th ed.) (pp. 164–195). St. Louis, MO: Mosby.

Pettaway, C.A., Balbay, M.D., & Grossman, H.B. (2000). Penis and urethra. In M.D. Abeloff, J.O. Armitage, A.S. Lichter, and J.E. Niederhuber (Eds.), *Clinical oncology* (pp. 1885–1905). New York: Churchill Livingstone.

Powell, I.J., Banerjee, M., Novallo, M., Sakr, W., Grignon, D., Wood, D.P., & Pontes, J.E. (2000). Should the age-specific prostate-specific antigen cutoff for prostate biopsy be higher for black than white men older than 50 years? *Journal of Urology, 163*, 146–149.

Prostate cancer prevention trial recruitment of 18,000 men completed. (1997). Retrieved June 6, 2000 from the World Wide Web: http://cancernet.nci.nih.gov

Pukkala, E. (1995). Cancer incidence among Finnish oil refinery workers, 1971–1994. *Journal of Occupational Environmental Medicine, 40*, 675–679.

Raitanen, M.P., Marttila, T., Kaasinen, E., Rintala, E., Aine, R., Tammela, T.L.J., & Finnbladder Group. (2000). Sensitivity of human complement factor H related protein (BTA STAT) test and voided urine cytology in the diagnosis of bladder cancer. *Journal of Urology, 163*, 1689–1692.

Ray, B., Canto, A.R., & Whitmore, W.F. (1977). Experience with primary carcinoma of the urethra. *Journal of Urology, 117*, 591–594.

Richie, J.P., Shipley, W.U., & Yagoda, A. (1989). Cancer of the bladder. In V.T. DeVita, S. Hellman, & J. Rosenberg (Eds.), *Cancer principles and practice of oncology* (pp. 1008–1022). Philadelphia: Lippincott.

Richie, J.P., Stolbach, L., & Atkins, M. (1996). Cancer of the kidney. In R.T. Osteen (Ed.), *Cancer manual* (9th ed.) (pp. 434–445). Boston: American Cancer Society, Massachusetts Division.

Ries, L.A.G., Kosary, C.L., & Hankey, B.F. (1998). *SEER cancer statistics review 1973–1995.* Bethesda, MD: National Cancer Institute.

Roach III, M. (1998). Is race an independent prognostic factor for survival from prostate cancer? *Journal of the National Medical Association, 90*(Suppl. 11), 713–719.

Roberson, N. (1994). Clinical trials participation: Viewpoint from racial/ethnic groups. *Cancer, 74*(Suppl. 9), 2687–2691.

Rutgers, J.L., & Scully, R.E. (1991). The androgen insensitivity syndrome (testicular feminization): A clinicopathologic study of 43 cases. *International Journal of Gynecological Pathology, 10*, 126.

Savitt, T. (1982). The use of blacks for medical experimentation and demonstration in the Old South. *Journal of Southern History, 28*, 331–348.

Scher, H.I., Issacs, J.T., Zelefsky, M.J., & Scardino, P.T. (2000). Prostate cancer. In M.D. Abeloff, J.O. Armitage, A.S. Lichter, & J.E. Niederhuber (Eds.), *Clinical oncology* (pp. 1823–1884). New York: Churchill Livingstone.

Schroder, F.H., van der Cruijsen-Koeter, I., De Koning, H.J., Vis, A.N., Hoedemaecker, R.F., & Kranse, R. (2000). Prostate cancer detection at low prostate-specific antigen. *Journal of Urology, 163*, 806–812.

Silverman, D.T., Levin, L.I., & Hoover, R.N. (1989). Occupational risks of bladder cancer in the United States: White men. *Journal of the National Cancer Institute, 81,* 1472–1480.

Simons, J.W., & Marshall, F.F. (2000). Kidney and ureter. In M.D. Abeloff, J.O. Armitage, A.S. Lichter, & J.E. Niederhuber (Eds.), *Clinical oncology* (pp. 1784–1799). New York: Churchill Livingstone.

Small, E.J., & Torti, F.M. (2000). Testes. In M.D. Abeloff, J.O. Armitage, A.S. Lichter, & J.E. Niederhuber (Eds.), *Clinical oncology* (pp. 1906–1945). New York: Churchill Livingstone.

Smith, S.J., Bosniak, M.A., Megibow, A.J., Hulnick, D.H., Horii, S.C., & Raghavendra, B.N. (1989). Renal cell carcinoma. Earlier discovery and increased detection. *Radiology, 170,* 699–703.

Srinivas, V., & Khan, S.A. (1988). Male urethral cancer: A review. *International Urology and Nephrology, 20,* 61.

Stampfer, D.S., Carpinito, G.A., Rodriguez-Villanueva, J., Willsey, L.W., Dinney, C.P., Grossman, H.B., Fritsche, H.A., & McDougal, W.S. (1998). Evaluation of NMP22 in the detection of transitional cell carcinoma of the bladder. *Journal of Urology, 159,* 394–398.

Svensson, C. (1989). Representation of American blacks in clinical trials of new drugs. *JAMA, 261,* 263–265.

Swanson, G.M., & Ward, A.J. (1995). Recruiting minorities into clinical trials: Towards a participant-friendly system. *Journal of the National Cancer Institute, 87,* 1747–1759.

Talar-Williams, C., Hijazi, Y., & Walther, M. (1996). Cyclophosphamide-induced cystitis and bladder cancer in patients with Wegener granulomatosis. *Annals of Internal Medicine, 124,* 477.

Tariq, N., Jenkins, D.J.A., Vidgen, E., Fleshner, N., Kendall, W.C., Story, J.A., Singer, W., D'Costa, M., & Struthers, N. (2000). Effect of soluble and insoluble fiber diets on serum prostate-specific antigen in men. *Journal of Urology, 163,* 114–118.

Tsukamoto, T., Kumamoto, Y., Yamazaki, K., Miyao, N., Takahashi, A., Masumori, N., & Satoh, M. (1991). Clinical analysis of incidentally found renal carcinoma. *European Urology, 19,* 109–113.

van der Poel, H.G., Boon, M.E., van Stratum, P., Ooms, E.C., Wiener, H., Debruyne, F.M., Witjes, J.A., Schalken, J.A., & Murphy, W.M. (1997). Conventional bladder wash cytology performed by four experts versus quantitative image analysis. *Modern Pathology, 10,* 976–982.

Vashi, A.R., Wojno, K.J., & Hendricks, W. (1997). Determination of the "reflex range" and appropriate cut points for percent free prostate-specific antigen in 413 men referred for prostatic evaluation using the AxSYM system. *Urology, 49,* 19.

Vineis, P., Martone, T., & Randone, D. (1995). Molecular epidemiology of bladder cancer: Known chemical causes of bladder cancer—Occupation and smoking. *Urology Oncology, 1,* 137.

von Eschenbach, A. (1997). American Cancer Society guidelines for the early detection of prostate cancer: Update. *CA: A Cancer Journal for Clinicians, 47,* 261–264.

Waldman, A.R. (2000). Screening and early detection. In J. Held-Warmkessel (Ed.), *Contemporary issues in prostate cancer: A nursing perspective* (pp. 24–35). Boston: Jones and Bartlett.

Wallach, J. (1996). *Interpretation of diagnostic tests.* Boston: Little, Brown & Co.

Walsh, P.C. (1998). Early age at diagnosis in families providing evidence of linkage to the hereditary prostate cancer locus (HPC1) on chromosome 1. *Journal of Urology, 160,* 265–266.

Walton, G.R., & Olsson, C.A. (1992). Localized squamous cell carcinoma of the penis. In M.I. Resnick & E.D. Kursh (Eds.), *Current therapy in genitourinary surgery* (p. 138). St. Louis, MO: Mosby.

Weinstein, I.B. (1991). Cancer prevention: Recent progress and future opportunities. *Cancer Research, 51*(Suppl. 18), 5080–5085.

Wingo, P.A., Ries, L.A., Rosenberg, H.M., Miller, D.S., & Edwards, B.K. (1998). Cancer incidence and mortality 1973–1995: A report card for the U.S. *Cancer, 82,* 1197–1207.

Wittebol-Post, D., Hes, F.J., & Lips, C.J.M. (1998). The eye in von Hippel-Lindau disease: Long term follow-up of screening and treatment—Recommendations. *Journal of Internal Medicine, 243,* 555–561.

Wong, O., & Raabe, G.K. (1989). Critical review of cancer epidemiology in petroleum industry employees, with a quantitative meta-analysis by cancer site. *American Journal of Medicine, 15,* 283–310.

Zinner, N.R. (1991). Prostate cancer. In M. Dollinger, E.H. Rosenbaum, & G. Cable (Eds.), *Everyone's guide to cancer therapy* (pp. 485–495). Kansas City, MO: Andres & McMeel.

CHAPTER 15

Skin Cancer Prevention and Early Detection

Catherine C. Burke, APRN, BC

Introduction

Skin cancer is the most common form of cancer in the United States. The National Cancer Institute's analysis of the Surveillance, Epidemiology, and End Results (SEER) program data found an annual rise in the incidence of melanoma approaching 4% from 1973–1996 (Gloeckler et al., 1999). Malignant melanoma accounts for 75% of all skin cancer deaths. An estimated 51,400 people will be diagnosed with malignant melanoma in the year 2001, and approximately 7,800 will die from the disease (Greenlee, Hill-Harmon, Murray, & Thun, 2001). Frequent and early metastasis, late detection, and inadequate primary treatment are factors contributing to this high mortality rate. More than one million cases of nonmelanoma skin cancers (NMSCs), which include basal cell carcinoma (BCC) and squamous cell carcinoma (SCC), also occur each year. Although the mortality caused by NMSC is low, the rising incidences of BCC and SCC place an economic burden on society and cause significant patient morbidity in terms of disfigurement and functional impairment.

Although most nurses would agree that skin cancer prevention and early detection is important, screening activities usually are not a part of routine clinical practice. Primary care providers usually do not perform skin assessments for the early diagnosis of melanoma, and they typically are a low priority during acute care visits. Heywood, Sanson, Ring, and Mudge (1994) reported that in Australia, where skin cancer incidence is highest, most men and women did not receive recommended skin cancer screening from their general practitioners. Another survey of 216 people with malignant melanoma found that in the year prior to diagnosis, only 20% received a total skin examination by a physician, and only 24% had performed a skin self-examination (Geller et al., 1992).

Commonly cited barriers to skin screening include inadequate educational preparation, lack of time, and inadequate reimbursement for preventive care (Wender, 1995). Lack of expertise is perhaps the greatest barrier. Most primary healthcare providers never were taught how to examine the skin and are not confident in their ability to accurately recognize cutaneous melanoma. In addition, most patients in nondermatology settings do not have significant problems/conditions during skin examination, making it difficult for physicians to develop and maintain clinical skills (Kirsner, Muhkerjee, & Federman, 1999; Wender).

Reductions in mortality, morbidity, and treatment costs that are associated with early diagnosis underscore the value of skin cancer screening. Incorporating skin examinations into routine clinical assessments may improve early detection rates. Early diagnosis of thin lesions significantly reduces the morbidity and mortality associated with melanoma, and more than 90% of patients present with a primary lesion visible on the skin (Reintgen, Ross, Bland, Seigler, & Balch, 1993). A recent study reported that tumor thickness was significantly less for physician-detected melanomas as compared to self-detected melanomas (Epstein, Lange, Gruber, Mofid, & Koch, 1999). Another study found that patients who received periodic skin examinations tended to have thinner and less invasive cutaneous melanomas than did patients whose tumors were diagnosed during the first examination (Richert, D'Amico, & Rhodes, 1998).

Educating the public about skin cancer prevention and promoting monthly skin self-examinations are other approaches that easily can be incorporated into clinical practice. Most skin cancers are linked to ultraviolet radiation (UVR) exposure. Preventive practices such as use of sunscreens, protective clothing, and avoidance of sun exposure during peak intensity may reduce the current rising incidence trends. Skin self-examinations may lead to early diagnosis and treatment. Miller et al. (1996) found that lack of awareness and knowledge of skin self-examination were the most common reasons for not practicing it. Individuals who are taught to examine their skin regularly are the ones most likely to recognize an abnormal or changing lesion.

The inclusion of skin cancer prevention and detection information, both during training programs and through continuing-education courses, enables nurses to provide these services to their patients. This chapter discusses skin cancer risk factors and risk assessment, the components of a comprehensive skin assessment, how to recognize suspicious skin lesions and make appropriate referrals, and how to educate the public about skin cancer.

Risk Factors

Table 15-1 outlines the major risk factors for skin cancer. Analyses of major risk factors for melanoma also are available in the literature to help clinicians to identify high-risk individuals (MacKie, Freudenberger, & Aitchison, 1989; Rhodes, Weinstock, Fitzpatrick, Mihm, & Sober, 1987; Robinson, 1997).

Table 15-1. Major Skin Cancer Risk Factors

Nonmelanoma Skin Cancer	Melanoma
Exposure to ultraviolet radiation (UVR) • Squamous cell carcinoma (SCC): Chronic, cumulative • Basal cell carcinoma (BCC): Intense, intermittent	Exposure to UVR • Intense, intermittent • History of three or more painful or blistering sunburns prior to age 20 • Use of tanning beds/sunlamps
Influential factors • Residence close to equator • Residence at high altitude • Ozone depletion	Influential factors • Residence close to equator • Residence at high altitude • Ozone depletion
Genetic predisposition • Burns easily, freckles, tans poorly • Fair skin (type I or II) • Blue or green eyes • Red or blond hair	Genetic predisposition • Burns easily, freckles, tans poorly • Fair skin (type I or II) • Blue or green eyes • Red or blond hair
Prior history skin cancer/precancer	Prior history skin cancer/precancer Dysplastic nevi Numerous acquired nevi Giant congenital nevi (> 20 cm)
Family history • Runs in families, related to similar skin types and UVR exposure	Family history • First-degree relative with melanoma • Melanoma-prone family
Genetic syndromes • Xeroderma pigmentosum • Basal cell nevus syndrome • Albinism	Genetic syndromes • Xeroderma pigmentosum • Albinism
Immunosuppression • SCC	Immunosuppression
Occupational exposures • Arsenic (BCC and SCC) • Products derived from petroleum and coal (SCC)	Occupational exposures
Other risk factors • Scars, burns, ulcerations (SCC) • Psoralen and ultraviolet A (PUVA) therapy (SCC) • Tobacco/alcohol abuse (SCC) • Exposure to ionizing radiation (SCC > BCC)	Other risk factors • PUVA therapy

Ultraviolet Radiation

Exposure to UVR is responsible for more than 90% of all skin cancers. The three spectral ranges of UVR (UVA—long wavelength, UVB—midline wavelength, and UVC—shortest wavelength) are outlined in Table 15-2. *The Ninth Report on Carcinogens 2000* (National Institute of Environmental Health Service, 2000) lists solar radiation as a known human carcinogen, citing a causal relation-

Table 15-2. Ultraviolet Radiation

Type	Wavelength	Effect
UVA	Long wavelength (320 nm–400 nm) Deep penetration to dermis and subcutaneous tissue	• Damages connective tissue (photoaging of skin). Characterized by deep wrinkles, leathery coarseness, and lentigines • Damages blood vessels • May burn corneas, resulting in retinal damage and cataracts • Interacts with topical and systemic chemicals and medications • May cause erythema (sunburn); immediate and delayed tanning
UVB	Midline wavelength (280 nm–320 nm) Superficial penetration to stratum corneum and epidermis	• Associated with sunburn, tanning, and skin cancers
UVC	Shortest wavelength (250 nm–280 nm) Absorbed by earth's atmosphere	• None

ship between UVR exposure and the development of melanoma and NMSC. Sun exposures can be chronic and episodic. NMSCs are associated with chronic, cumulative exposure involved with regular outdoor occupations and leisure activities. The majority of lesions occur on the head, neck, forearms, and back of the hands. Some studies suggest that acute exposures may be more important in determining BCC risk (Gallagher et al., 1995; Rosso et al., 1996; Zanetti et al., 1996). In a population-based case-control study of 226 patients with BCC and 406 randomly matched controls, Gallagher et al. (1995) found no association between cumulative sunlight exposure and BCC. Significant risk factors for BCC include having fair skin, freckles, increased recreational sun exposure during childhood and adolescence, and a history of severe childhood sunburn (Gallagher et al., 1995). A multicenter case-control study (Rosso et al.; Zanetti et al.) evaluated risk for SCC and BCC according to sun exposures and skin type. The study population included 1,549 patients with BCC, 228 patients with SCC, and 1,795 randomly selected controls. The investigators found that a history of sunburns, young age at first sunburn, and recreational exposures were associated with an increased risk of BCC.

Cutaneous melanoma is associated with episodic, intense exposures. Individuals who spend the majority of their time indoors may experience acute sun exposures during outdoor recreational activities on weekends and vacations. Intense exposures occurring during childhood, adolescence, and young adulthood, in particular, are associated with increased melanoma risk. Individuals who experience three or more blistering sunburns prior to age 20 are at increased risk for melanoma later in life (Rigel & Carucci, 2000).

UVA exposure also may come from artificial sources, such as tanning beds and sunlamps. Indoor tanning is associated with both acute and chronic adverse effects. Acute effects may range from mild erythema (sunburn), pruritus, and skin dryness to a severe burn. Photosensitive and phototoxic reactions also may occur. Chronic effects of UVA exposure include photoaging of the skin, ocular damage, and skin cancer (Spencer & Amonette, 1995; Spencer & Amonette, 1998).

A history of chronic tanning with UVA light has been associated with melanoma, and exposure to sun lamps or sun beds is listed as a known human carcinogen (National Institute of Environmental Health Service, 2000). Westerdahl et al. (1994) found an overall risk increase in people who reported more than 10 exposures per year and a significant risk in users younger than 30. These findings were supported in a recent case-control study, in which regular sun bed use was associated with a significantly increased risk for melanoma (Westerdahl, Ingvar, Masback, Jonsson, & Olsson, 2000). The magnitude of risk correlated with the number of sun bed uses per year, the total number of exposures, and the number of years of regular use. Autier et al. (1994) also reported an increased risk for melanoma in sun bed users, especially in those who experienced intense exposure or skin burn. However, no increase in melanoma risk was associated with sun bed use that started after 1980. Two possible explanations were offered: the long latency period that usually exists between exposure and malignancy and the change in tanning equipment from emitting UVA and UVB to emitting UVA alone.

Skin cancer risk varies according to race and ethnicity. Hair, eye, and skin color and freckling in response to sun exposure are independent characteristics for risk. Melanin in the skin provides natural photoprotection, and individuals with dark complexions are the least susceptible. Skin cancers are most common in people who have type I or II skin, blue or green eyes, blond or red hair, and a fair complexion and who burn easily and tan poorly (see Table 15-3).

UVR exposure is influenced by geographic area of residence and atmospheric conditions (ozone). UVR is most intense in sunny climates near the equator and increases 4% in intensity for every 1,000 feet of elevation (Wentzell, 1996). Proximity to the equator is especially worrisome when combined with a fair-skinned population. Because the earth's ozone layer is very efficient in absorbing UV rays from the sun, only UVA radiation and a small amount of UVB radiation reach the earth's surface. The amount of UV radiation present in natural sunlight is dependent on the ozone, and UVB radiation is especially sensitive to ozone changes.

Table 15-3. Cutaneous Phenotype and Skin Cancer Risk

Skin Cancer Risk	Skin Type	Sunburn or Tanning History
Highest	I	Always burns, never tans
	II	Always burns, tans minimally
	III	Burns often, tans gradually
	IV	Burns minimally, tans well
	V	Burns rarely, tans profusely
Lowest	VI	Never burns, deeply pigmented skin

Man-made chlorofluorocarbons are responsible for ozone depletion, with the major effect being an increase in UVB radiation exposure (Kripke, 1988). A 1% reduction in the ozone level is estimated to cause a 2% increase in skin cancer incidence (Henriksen, Dahlback, Larsen, & Moan, 1990).

Genetic Factors

A personal or family history of skin cancer is a significant risk factor. Anyone with a prior history of skin cancer or precancerous lesions has sun-damaged skin and therefore is at risk for another skin cancer. A personal history of NMSC also places an individual at increased risk for melanoma (Marghoob et al., 1995). NMSCs are not inherited but tend to run in families based on similar skin types and UVR exposure.

Melanoma risk is increased in individuals who have one or more first-degree relatives with melanoma. Most melanomas are nonfamilial, but approximately 10% of cases develop in individuals with a familial predisposition (Fraser, Goldstein, & Tucker, 1997). A melanoma-prone family is a family in which melanoma has occurred in two or more first-degree relatives (e.g., parents, siblings, offspring). Two melanoma predisposition genes have been identified. CDKN2A has been mapped to the short arm of chromosome 9, and CDK4 has been mapped to the long arm of chromosome 12 (Fraser et al.). Most melanomas (60%–80%) that occur in melanoma-prone family members are not associated with an identified gene mutation, and the penetrance of known mutations is not understood. Routine genetic testing within melanoma-prone families, therefore, is not currently recommended (Kefford, Newton, Bergman, & Tucker, 1999).

Members of melanoma-prone families tend to develop numerous cutaneous melanomas, with the first occurring at a young age. Tucker et al. (1993) found that among 23 melanoma-prone families, 10% of individuals developed melanoma before age 20. Identification of at-risk children is important so that routine skin screening can begin by age 10 (Fraser et al., 1997). Increased surveillance has proven to be of value in this high-risk population. Members of melanoma-prone families tend to have thinner lesions at diagnosis as compared to individuals who develop nonfamilial melanomas (Robinson, 1997; Tucker et al., 1993).

Dysplastic nevi are the single best markers of melanoma risk. In the United States, dysplastic nevi, or atypical moles, occur in approximately 10% of Whites (Seykora & Elder, 1996). They easily are confused with melanoma because they have one or more of the characteristic features (diameter ≥ 6 mm, asymmetry, irregular or indistinct border, and variegated color [e.g., tan, brown, pink, black]) of cutaneous melanoma. One or more lesions may be present anywhere on the body. Covered or unusual areas, such as the back, scalp, buttocks, and breasts, may be involved. The incidence of dysplastic nevi has been correlated to UVR and especially to intense sun exposure.

Dysplastic or atypical nevi both are potential precursors of malignant melanoma and significant markers of increased melanoma risk. Melanoma risk associated with dysplastic nevi is variable between patients and is independent of the risk associated with multiple benign nevi. The presence or absence of a personal or family history of malignant melanoma is the most important criteria to determine a patient's magnitude of risk. In the United States, the average White person's lifetime risk for developing melanoma is approximately 1%. Those who have dysplastic nevi in the absence of personal and family history have a moderate increase (approximately 6%) in lifetime risk. Individuals at greatest risk are those who have one or more dysplastic nevi and either a personal or family history of melanoma (Conrad et al., 1999; Seykora & Elder, 1996; Skender-Kalnenas, English, & Heenan, 1995; Slade et al., 1995; Tucker et al., 1997). In a prospective study of 23 melanoma-prone families, Tucker et al. (1993) found that melanoma risk was increased 85 times among family members who had dysplastic nevi alone and 229 times in family members who had both dysplastic nevi and a prior melanoma.

The total number of dysplastic nevi present and their degree of atypia also help to determine an individual's overall melanoma risk. Tucker et al. (1997) reported a twofold increase in risk associated with the presence of one dysplastic nevus and a 12-fold increase in risk associated with 10 or more dysplastic nevi. Other factors, including skin type, immune status, and prior sun exposure, also should be considered.

Patients with dysplastic nevi should receive full-body examinations by a dermatologist at regular intervals. The frequency of examinations should be determined by the patient's estimated risk. Careful surveillance has been shown to increase the likelihood that subsequent melanomas will be diagnosed at an early, curable stage (Carey et al., 1994; Kang, Barnhill, Mihm, Fitzpatrick, & Sober, 1994). Regular ophthalmologic examinations should be encouraged because patients may have an increased risk of ocular nevi and ocular malignant melanoma. Dysplastic nevi and risk for melanoma also are increased in family members, so they should be encouraged to receive routine skin screening.

Nevi should be monitored carefully for change (e.g., asymmetry, border irregularity, variegated color, increased size), and any suspicious mole should be excised. The addition of baseline cutaneous photographs may help the examiner identify subtle changes. Rivers et al. (1990) found that change in a clinical feature, best demonstrated through comparison to a baseline photograph, was the best indicator of malignancy. Clinically normal skin should be inspected carefully because the patient's risk is increased whether or not the dysplastic lesions are removed.

Numerous acquired melanocytic nevi (nondysplastic) are an independent risk factor for melanoma, with risk increasing in proportion to the total number of nevi (≥ 2 mm in diameter) present (Holly, Kelly, Shpall, & Chiu, 1987; MacKie et al., 1989; Swerdlow et al., 1986). Tucker et al. (1997) found that in the absence of dysplastic nevi, patients with numerous small melanocytic nevi had approximately a twofold increase in risk, and those with both small and large nondysplastic nevi had a fourfold increase. Because these moles are considered markers of risk and not precursor lesions, surgical excision is not indicated.

Acquired nevi generally develop beginning in early childhood and continue to occur until about age 40. New moles after the age of 40 are uncommon. The number of melanocytic nevi an individual has by age 20 is linked to cumulative sun exposure, number of severe sunburns, and fairness of skin (Gallagher et al., 1990; Williams & Pennella, 1994).

Individuals with large congenital melanocytic nevi (LCMN), defined as nevi that are either ≥ 20 cm in diameter or are predicted to be that size in adulthood, are at a significantly increased risk for melanoma. LCMN is a rare condition occurring in fewer than 1 in 20,000 infants (Sober & Burstein, 1995). Marghoob et al. (1996) estimated a five-year cumulative risk of 4.5%. Melanomas in these individuals often develop at a young age and are associated with a poor prognosis. A review of 289 patients with LCMN found that 67 patients (23%) developed melanoma, with half of the cases occurring prior to age five (DeDavid et al., 1997). Full-thickness excision of the nevi, when surgically feasible, often is recommended to reduce risk. However, surgical removal is not completely preventive because melanoma may occur elsewhere. In the DeDavid et al. study, approximately half of the patients developed cutaneous melanoma within the nevus. The other cases included primary central nervous system melanoma (31%), metastatic melanoma with an occult primary (15%), and cutaneous melanoma outside of the nevus (3%). Life-long periodic examinations, including total skin assessment and neurological evaluation, are recommended. The degree of risk associated with small (< 1 cm in diameter) and intermediate-sized nevi (1– < 20 cm) is unknown, but some investigators estimated the risk to be small (Marghoob et al., 1996; Swerdlow, English, & Qiao, 1995).

Patients with certain genetic disorders are at increased risk for skin cancers. Xeroderma pigmentosa is a rare autosomal recessive disorder in which patients' bodies are not able to repair cellular DNA damage caused by UVR exposure. Approximately 5% of these patients develop melanoma (Ruiz & Orozco, 1997). Albinism and basal cell nevus syndrome also are associated with an increased skin cancer risk.

Immunosuppression

Numerous acquired melanocytic nevi and dysplastic nevi are identified risk factors for melanoma. For those with a history of immunosuppression, such as survivors of childhood cancer, the increased risk for melanoma is associated with the effect immunosuppression has on nevi. In children, studies indicated that immunosuppression caused by cancer chemotherapy and organ transplantation increases total nevus counts and induces atypical nevi (Baird, McHenry, & MacKie, 1992; Green et al., 1993; Hughes, Cunliffe, & Bailey, 1989; Smith et al., 1993). These individuals should be encouraged to avoid excessive UVR exposure, employ sun protection measures, and receive total skin screening as part of their routine long-term surveillance (Green et al.).

Immunosuppression occurring in adults also is associated with increased numbers of both benign and atypical nevi, and these individuals are considered to be at risk for melanoma. Grob et al. (1996) found that immunosuppression itself, regardless of the cause, was responsible.

Individuals who are chronically immunosuppressed, such as organ transplant recipients, patients with lymphoproliferative disorders, and those taking immunosuppressive medications, also are at a significantly increased risk for NMSC, especially SCC. The development of SCC among renal transplant recipients is a significant problem. As compared to the general population, the ratio of BCC to SCC is reversed, with SCC being three times more common and also occurring in younger individuals. Bavinck et al. (1996) suggested that immunosuppression, regardless of the cause, was responsible for the increased incidence of SCC among these patients.

Prolonged immunosuppression and UVR exposure are associated with an increased incidence of SCC. Hartevelt, Bavinck, Kootte, Vermeer, and Vandenbroucke (1990) observed a cumulative skin cancer incidence that rose from 10% after 10 years to 40% after 20 years post-transplant and an overall incidence of SCC that was 253 times higher than that of the general population. An even higher incidence of SCC was observed in a group of 1,158 renal transplant recipients (Bavinck et al., 1996). UVR exposure is another important risk factor. Multiple lesions are common, with most occurring on skin surfaces that are chronically exposed to the sun (Barksdale, O'Conner, & Barnhill, 1997; Bavinck et al., 1993; Gupta, Cardella, & Haberman, 1986).

Occupational Risks

Occupational exposures have been associated with skin cancer risk. Products derived from petroleum and coal (e.g., tar, pitch, heavy tar oil, carbon black, crude paraffin, asphalt, mineral oil) are associated with SCC. Arsenic exposure is associated with NMSC. Arsenic previously was used in medicines to treat psoriasis. In industry, it is used in the manufacture of ceramics, fireworks, herbicides, insecticides, paints, and semiconductors and is a by-product of copper smelting operations, textile printing, and silver refining. People who are exposed tend to develop multiple tumors that may occur on unusual sites, such as the palms, soles, and sun-protected skin.

Although no occupational exposures are associated with melanoma, high socioeconomic status has been implicated as a risk factor. Recreational activities may explain this finding. Wealthy individuals are more likely than others to expose themselves to intense, intermittent sun exposure during leisure time and vacations in sunny climates (Pion, Rigel, Garfinkel, Silverman, & Kopf, 1995).

Other Risk Factors

Other risk factors for SCC have been reported. Individuals may develop a lesion in an area of trauma, such as a scar, burn, chronic ulceration, or sinus tract. In deeply pigmented people, scarring processes are the most common predisposing factor for SCC (Barksdale et al., 1997).

PUVA therapy, which combines psoralens with UVA for the treatment of severe psoriasis, is an established risk factor for SCC (Morison et al., 1998). In a prospective multicenter study, Stern and Laird (1994) observed a strong dose-dependent relationship between exposure to PUVA and SCC. Increased risk was associated with long-term exposure and total cumulative dose. They also noted that many patients developed tumors on non-sun-exposed skin, which is unusual for SCC among the general population. PUVA therapy also has been linked to melanoma. Stern, Nichols, and Vakeva (1997) prospectively followed 1,380 patients with psoriasis who were treated with PUVA and noted a modest increase in the incidence of melanoma beginning 15 years after initial treatment; this was associated mostly with high dosages of PUVA.

SCCs of the lip and oral mucosa are associated with tobacco use, chronic UVR exposure, intake of alcoholic beverages, and chronic irritation. SCC and BCC may occur in a radiation therapy field following treatment for cancer (e.g., Hodgkin's disease, lymphoma, breast cancer). Radiation therapy also was used in the past to treat benign conditions such as acne vulgaris. Skin areas that were exposed to such treatments also are at risk for NMSC.

Anatomy and Function of the Skin

This section reviews the normal anatomy and physiology of the skin. Prior to performing skin assessments, a basic understanding of skin anatomy is needed to recognize the origin of NMSC and cutaneous melanoma. In addition, once a malignancy is established, a description of the depth of invasion as it relates to subepithelial layers is important.

Epidermis

The skin is composed of three layers: epidermis, dermis, and subcutaneous tissue (see Figure 15-1). The epidermis is the most superficial and is approximately 0.1 mm thick, depending on the site (see Figure 15-2). It has five layers predominantly composed of two types of cells, the keratinocytes and dendritic cells. Keratinocytes are flat, scale-like stratified squamous epithelial cells that make up 90% of the epidermis. The dendritic cells include the Langerhans' cells and melanocytes. Langerhans' cells are a type of macrophage that make up 4% of the epidermis and serve as the initial receptors for the body's cutaneous response to external antigens. Melanocytes are found in the stratum germinativum between

Figure 15-1. Three Layers of the Skin

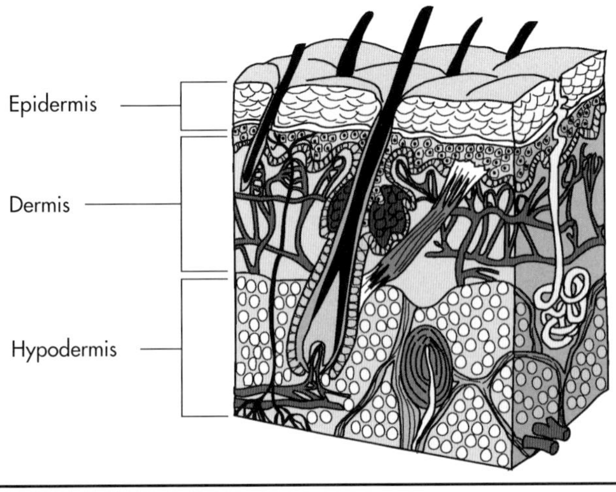

Note. LifeArt image copyright 2002 by Lippincott Williams & Wilkins. All rights reserved.

Figure 15-2. Zones of the Epidermis

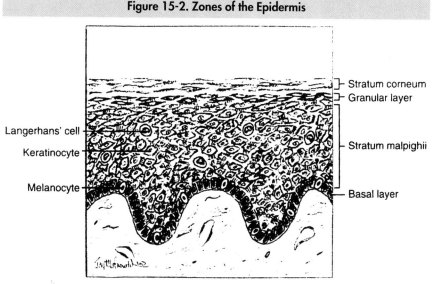

Note. From *Andrew's Diseases of the Skin: Clinical Dermatology* (9th ed.) (p.3), by R.B. Odom, W.B. James, and T.G. Berger (Eds.), 2000, Philadelphia: W.B. Saunders. Copyright 2000 by W.B. Saunders. Reprinted with permission.

basal cells. Melanocytes produce the pigment melanin, which is responsible for shielding the skin from UVR by absorbing radiant energy.

The epidermis rejuvenates itself through keratinization, the process of morphological and biochemical differentiation of the keratinocyte from basal cell in the stratum germinativum to a cornified cell in the stratum corneum. The end product is keratin, a highly resilient, insoluble fibrous protein that enables the skin to serve as a major physical barrier that is relatively impermeable to water and electrolytes.

The epidermis is avascular and derives nutritional support from the dermis. The basement membrane is the junction between the two layers, providing a semipermeable filter that permits the exchange of cells and fluid. It also provides structural support for the epidermis and helps to hold the epidermis and dermis together.

Dermis

The dermis is the support layer of the skin, providing strength, resiliency, stability, and flexibility. It functions to prevent mechanical trauma and to maintain homeostasis. The dermis binds large amounts of water and thereby represents a water-storage organ. The dermis is 1–4 mm thick and consists of the upper papillary layer and the lower reticular layer. The reticular layer makes up the bulk of the dermis, absorbing most of the skin's physical stress. The dermis is composed of connective tissue, water, and an interstitial component (ground substance). The connective tissue contains collagen, elastic fibers, and reticulum. The major component of connective tissue is collagen, a fibrous protein produced by fibroblasts. It is the most important stress-resistant material of the skin, providing tensile strength and the ability to resist stretching. Elastic fibers are responsible for the skin's resiliency; together with ground substance, they are believed to be responsible for preventing overstretching. The reticulum are immature collagen fibers found in the papillary dermis. Ground substance is a gel-like, amorphous material accounting for much of the volume of the dermis. It molds to irregular objects and has a great capacity to bind water.

The cells found in the dermis include fibroblasts, mast cells, macrophages, and histiocytes. In addition to collagen, fibroblasts produce elastic fibers, reticular fibers, and ground substance. In the upper dermis, the fibroblast is called the dermal dendrocyte and has immunologic and reparative functions. Histiocytes and mast cells serve in the body's line of defense against pathogens. Histiocytes, normally present in small numbers around blood vessels, are known as macrophages when they phagocytize bacteria and travel through the dermis as tissue monocytes during pathologic conditions.

The dermis also is responsible for thermoregulation and sensory innervation. It houses and supports vasculature; sensory (afferent) nerve fibers for pain, touch, and temperature; autonomic motor nerves (innervating blood vessels, glands, and arrectores pilorum muscles), lymphatic vessels; muscle fibers; hair follicles; sebaceous glands; apocrine glands; and eccrine glands. The sebaceous glands and shorter hair follicles originate in the dermis.

Subcutaneous Tissue

The subcutaneous tissue is the innermost layer of skin. Its main functions are to insulate underlying tissue from extreme temperatures, absorb mechanical shock, and store energy (calories) as fat. The deeper hair follicles and sweat glands originate in this layer.

Skin Appendages

The skin appendages include both the cornified appendages (nails and hair) and the glandular appendages (sebaceous glands, apocrine sweat glands, and eccrine sweat glands). The nails are epidermal cells converted to hard plates of keratin. The nail includes the nail plate and the tissue around it. The nail plate lies in a nail groove, an invagination of the epidermis. The nail bed lies directly underneath, providing support and adherence for the nail plate. The vascularity of the nail bed gives the nail its characteristic pink color.

Hairs are derived from the hair follicles of the epidermis. The hair follicle is an invagination of the epidermis with layers of cells that make up the matrix of the hair follicle and produce the keratin in mature hair. Melanocytes present in the hair shaft provide hair color. The two types of adult hair are vellus and terminal. Vellus hairs are fine, short, nonpigmented hairs of the body. Terminal hairs are found primarily on the scalp, brows, and extremities; they are coarse, thick, and pigmented. The sebaceous glands, present everywhere on the skin except the palms and soles, secrete the complex lipid substance sebum. Sebum is thought to waterproof and lubricate the hair and skin, control epidermal water loss, and inhibit the growth of fungi and bacteria. Apocrine sweat glands are found primarily in the axillae and genital region and do not develop until puberty. Although they have no proven function, these glands secrete an odorless milky substance that becomes malodorous when mixed with the bacteria found in the hair follicles and on the skin surface. The eccrine sweat glands are located everywhere on the skin surface, with the highest concentration found on the forehead, palms, and soles. Although eccrine sweat glands respond to thermal, emotional, and gustatory stimuli, heat is their primary stimulus. By responding to thermal stimuli, the eccrine glands help to regulate body temperature through water secretion (Du Vivier, 1991; Sauer & Hall, 1996; Seidel, Ball, Dains, & Benedict, 1991).

Nonmelanoma Skin Cancer

NMSC is the most common malignancy in the United States, with approximately 1.3 million cases occurring annually (American Cancer Society, 2000). It accounts for approximately 90% of all skin cancers. The exact incidence is difficult to determine, however, because many NMSCs are treated in outpatient settings and are not registered (Marks, 1995). The annual mortality rate is 1,200–2,000 people (Barksdale et al., 1997), and the annual cost of treatment exceeds $500 million (Preston & Stern, 1992). More than 90% of NMSCs occur on skin surfaces receiving chronic sun exposure (e.g., head, neck, forearms, dorsa of the hands). Precursor lesions for SCC include actinic keratosis (AK) and Bowen's disease. No known precursor lesion exists for BCC (Preston & Stern).

Precursor Lesions

AKs, or solar keratoses, are rough, scaly macules or papules caused by cumulative exposure to UVR. They are the most common precancerous skin lesions and typically occur on chronically sun-exposed areas of the body. These include the face (e.g., forehead, cheeks, nose, temples, vermilion border of the lower lip), neck, and dorsa of the hands and forearms. In males, bald scalps and helices of the ears may be affected. Although single lesions may occur, multiple lesions in groups or clusters are more common. Risk factors for AKs are the same as those for SCC.

AKs are more easily diagnosed by palpation than by inspection because they are elevated, irregular, discrete, and have a rough (sandpaper-like) texture. They may appear pink or erythematous and become yellow-brown or brown with the development of an adherent scale. Most patients are asymptomatic; however, tenderness, burning, or pruritus may occur. Marks, Rennie, and Selwood (1988a) reported that the rate of conversion of any individual AK to SCC was low. In their study, the risk of malignant transformation of an AK to SCC was less than one per thousand per year. Ablative treatment generally is recommended, and treatment options include cryotherapy, surgical removal, retinoic acid, topical 5-fluorouracil cream, and acid peels. The regular use of broad-spectrum sunscreens prevents actinic damage and also may induce remissions in those who apply them and reduce their sun exposure (Naylor & Farmer, 1997; Thompson, Jolley, & Marks, 1993).

AKs are sensitive indicators of sunlight exposure and skin cancer risk (Marks, Rennie, & Selwood, 1988b; Sober & Burstein, 1995). Any person diagnosed with AKs has sun-damaged skin and therefore is at increased risk for subsequent premalignant disease and NMSCs, especially SCC. Such individuals should be examined at regular intervals, with the treated area carefully inspected for local recurrence.

Bowen's disease, an intraepidermal or in situ SCC, also is caused by chronic sun exposure. Lesions occur predominantly on sun-exposed sites such as the scalp and ears in men and on the lower extremities in women (Kossard & Rosen, 1992). Lesions on non-sun-exposed skin may result from arsenic exposure, radiation therapy, and human papilloma virus infections. Usually presenting as solitary lesions, they have distinctive features: sharply demarcated borders, elevated erythematous plaques, and areas of scales and crusts. A biopsy may be required to differentiate Bowen's disease from eczema, psoriasis, superficial BCC, invasive SCC, or Paget's disease. The rate of malignant transformation to Bowenoid SCC is 5%–11% and typically takes years to occur because the lesions grow slowly by lateral extension (Vargo, 1991). Lesion invasion into the dermis often is signaled by ulceration. Treatment measures include electrodissection and curettage, cryosurgery, excisional surgery, and topical 5-fluorouracil cream. As with individuals with AKs, follow-up skin examinations and sun-protection education is required.

Basal Cell Carcinoma

BCC is the most common skin cancer, accounting for approximately 75% of all NMSCs (Gloster & Brodland, 1996). It originates in the basal layer of epidermal cells, and its incidence is rising not only in older adults (> 60 years of age) but also in those younger than age 35. It occurs primarily on skin surfaces that receive chronic sun exposure, such as the head (e.g., nose, cheek, forehead, ears), neck, and forearms. However, the incidence of BCC does not correlate with cumulative sun exposure as closely as the incidence of SCC does. Tanning bed use was implicated as a risk factor for development of BCC in women younger than 30 (Dinehart, Dodge, Stanley, Franks, & Pollack, 1992). BCC also occurs on non-sun-exposed skin, implicating other causes for its development such as genetic factors and exposure to chemicals and ionizing radiation. Zanetti et al. (1996) found that the trunk was the second most common site for BCC in both men and women. BCCs are rare in African Americans, but, when seen, usually develop on the head and neck and most often are pigmented. This often leads to a delayed or missed diagnosis.

BCC is a slow-growing tumor that spreads by direct extension and rarely metastasizes. Although it is the least aggressive skin cancer, BCC should not be disregarded. Significant local tissue destruction, invasion of vital structures, and disfigurement can occur if it is left untreated. The cure rate approaches 100% if lesions are treated early and completely (Preston & Stern, 1992).

Clinical Characteristics

Four types of BCC exist. The most common is the nodular type. The typical initial presentation is a small, firm, well-demarcated, dome-shaped papule that is pearly white, pink, or skin colored. As the tumor grows, the epidermis thins but remains intact, giving a waxy or shiny (translucent) appearance. An ulceration with crusting may occur centrally or peripherally. Other classic features of nodular

BCC are raised, rolled, well-circumscribed borders and the presence of telangiectasias over the border and surface. Patients usually are asymptomatic but may experience pruritus or bleeding at the site. Nodular BCCs usually occur on the face (especially the nose) and rarely metastasize.

The superficial type of BCC usually originates on the trunk or extremities, often in actinic-damaged skin. The lesions vary in size and may appear as flat, erythematous or pink, scaling plaques or papules. Shallow erosions or crusts may be present, encircled by well-demarcated threadlike borders that are raised and pearly. Single or multiple lesions may occur. Superficial BCC may be associated with arsenic ingestion. It also may be mistaken for a benign inflammatory condition such as psoriasis or eczema.

A third type of BCC, the pigmented form, may be mistaken for melanoma until histologically confirmed, because the melanin pigmentation may cause the lesion to appear blue, brown, or black. Lesions may have shiny, papillary borders and telangiectasias. This type of BCC is most common in dark-skinned patients. It also may be associated with arsenic ingestion.

Morpheaform is the rarest and most aggressive histologic subtype of BCC. It is a firm, scar-like lesion that is flat or depressed, appears white or pale yellow, and has ill-defined margins. Morpheaform lesions lack the translucent appearance typical of other types of BCC. Although telangiectasias are common, ulceration usually is absent. Because subclinical spread usually is present and recurrence frequently occurs after treatment, this tumor is best treated by surgical excision or Moh's micrographic surgery.

Squamous Cell Cancer

SCC, a tumor of the keratinizing cells of the epidermis, is the second most common skin cancer, accounting for 20% of NMSCs (Gloster & Brodland, 1996). Although lesions occur anywhere on the skin and mucous membranes, they usually arise on areas chronically exposed to UVR. Typical primary sites include the top of the nose, forehead, helices of the ears, lower lip, and dorsa of the hands. SCC also may occur in traumatized or chronically inflamed skin, such as scars, sinus tracts, and stasis ulcers (this is the most frequent site of SCC in African Americans).

Most SCCs (95%) occur in males who are older than 40. The aggressiveness of SCC varies, and the overall five-year cure rate for cutaneous tumors ranges from 75%–90% (Bernstein, Lim, Brodland, & Heidelberg, 1996). Compared with BCCs, SCCs have a faster growth rate, less well-defined margins, and a greater metastatic potential. Regional lymph node and distant metastasis occur in less than 5% of cases (Kwa, Campana, & Moy, 1992). The mortality rate is 1%–2% (Preston & Stern, 1992). Tumors grow locally but can extensively invade subcutaneous tissue, muscle, and bone.

The frequency of metastasis is related to anatomic site, histologic features, etiology, host immunosuppression, lesion size, and prior treatment (Kwa et al., 1992). Common routes of metastases are via lymphatic channels and perineural invasion. SCCs of the lower lip are associated with a higher rate of metastasis and mortality than lesions occurring at other sites. Higher metastatic rates also are seen with lesions occurring on the oral mucosa, penis, scrotum, and anus. SCCs arising in sun-damaged skin have the lowest risk of recurrence. Poorly differentiated tumors, lesions that are deeply invasive, and those that are > 2 cm in size are more likely to metastasize and recur. Recurrent SCCs and those arising in scars, wound sites, and areas of prior irradiation also have a greater incidence of metastases. Late diagnosis may contribute to the aggressive nature of SCCs arising in scars. Other risk factors for metastasis include immunosuppression and lesions that occur on sun-protected skin in the absence of a predisposing cause.

Clinical Characteristics

Because the presentation of SCC varies, all persistent ulcers or lesions should be considered for biopsy. Most SCCs appear as firm, erythematous or flesh-colored nodules or plaque-like lesions. They are round to irregular in shape, with margins that tend to be elevated and indistinct. Ulceration, crust, or scales may be present. Characteristic findings in BCCs—rolled, pearly borders and telangiectasias—usually are absent. Hyperkeratotic SCCs and those occurring on a mucocutaneous surface may appear white. Patients may report sensations of "crawling" or tenderness that are not typically associated with BCCs. When occurring on the lip, SCC usually develops on the lower lip in an area of chronic actinic cheilitis and is associated with tobacco usage. It typically begins as a scaling, rough papule or ulceration and progresses into a large, fungating lesion. SCC occurring on the nail bed, nail folds, and nail matrix is associated most frequently with immunosuppression.

Treatment of Nonmelanoma Skin Cancer

The key to effective treatment of NMSC is early detection and adequate initial treatment. When detected early, virtually all NMSCs are small, superficial lesions with little risk for recurrence or metastasis. Additionally, localized ablation or surgery is unlikely to result in a functional or cosmetic impairment for the patient. An invasive procedure associated with significant morbidity and cost may be required to eradicate a large lesion. The total removal or destruction of a tumor is the foremost treatment goal. If this goal is not achieved, all other treatment objectives will be compromised. Other important treatment goals are maximal preservation of normal tissue structure and function, minimal morbidity, and an optimal cosmetic result. Major treatments include electrosurgery (curettage and electrodessication), surgical excision, cryosurgery, radiation therapy, Moh's micrographic surgery, and laser therapy (Fleming, Amonette, Monaghan, & Fleming, 1995).

Post-Treatment Surveillance

Individualized follow-up is important to detect recurrent and subsequent disease. Most NMSCs are cured by primary treatment. Local recurrence is uncommon (Preston & Stern, 1992). Recurrences usually are caused by either an aggressive tumor or inadequate treatment. Careful follow-up allows for the early diagnosis and prompt treatment of recurrent tumors. Most lesions that recur are cured by additional local therapy.

In contrast, patients are at high risk of developing additional NMSCs. Frankel, Hanusa, and Zitelli (1992) reported that of 101 patients with SCC who were followed during a five-year period, 52% developed new lesions. The greatest incidence of new lesions was observed during the first year of follow-up. Two studies evaluating the risk of developing a second BCC within five years of initial treatment found one or more BCCs in 53% and 36% of patients (Marghoob et al., 1993; Robinson, 1987); therefore, patients should be examined carefully at regular intervals. In addition, monthly skin self-examination and sun protection methods should be taught to the patient and family members. Skin type and environmental exposures are significant risk factors for NMSC, and lesions tend to occur within families (Kibarian & Hruza, 1995).

Melanoma

A dramatic rise in incidence of melanoma has occurred during the past 60 years. In 1935, the lifetime melanoma risk for Whites living in the United States was 1:1,500. Lifetime risk is currently 1:74 (Rigel & Carucci, 2000). Melanoma also is a disease of the relatively young. Approximately half of all people diagnosed with melanoma are younger than 55 years of age, and approximately 30% are younger than 45 (Gloster & Brodland, 1996). It rarely occurs in children (0–12 years of age), and people younger than 20 represent only 1%–4% of all cases of malignant melanomas (Ruiz & Orozco, 1997).

Early detection and prompt treatment of cutaneous melanoma is essential. Surgery is the treatment of choice and is curative if the tumor is completely excised before metastasis occurs. Conversely, treatment of metastatic melanoma is rarely curative. Tumor thickness, measured as Breslow's thickness, is used to predict prognosis. Breslow's thickness is measured in millimeters from the top of the granular cell layer to the deepest point of tumor extension. The odds of survival are linked closely to the thickness of the primary tumor at the time of removal. Patients presenting with thin melanomas (< 1 mm) usually have localized disease and cure rates exceed 95%. Patients presenting with thick melanomas (> 4 mm) are at high risk for both nodal and distant metastases and have poor survival rates (Reintgen, Balch, Kirkwood, & Ross, 1997).

Cutaneous melanomas grow in two ways: radially (horizontal growth) within the epidermis and vertically into the dermis and subcutaneous tissues. Radial growth within the epidermis is considered an in situ growth phase. Lesions usually are flat or have a slightly papular surface. A clinically detectable papule, nodule, or plaque may occur with vertical growth. The radial growth phase may last from months to years, and the lesion may measure several centimeters in diameter. Lesion diameter may not correlate with vertical growth. These early, thin lesions have little risk of metastasis, and cure rates approach 100% with simple excision.

Four histologic subtypes of cutaneous melanoma exist: superficial spreading melanoma, nodular melanoma, lentigo maligna melanoma, and acral lentiginous melanoma. With the exception of nodular melanomas, all subtypes exhibit an in situ growth phase, making early detection possible. Any lesion exhibiting change should be considered for biopsy.

An excisional biopsy, removing the entire lesion along with a margin of normal tissue, is the preferred method because the entire tissue specimen can be histologically evaluated. Alternatively, an incisional (removing a small part of the lesion) or punch biopsy may be used to establish the diagnosis when excision is not feasible because of anatomic constraints or cosmetic concerns. The most suspicious area of the lesion, such as the most raised or irregular, should be selected. Shave biopsy should not be performed because it can interfere with accurate evaluation of lesion thickness (Langley & Sober, 1998; National Institutes of Health [NIH] Consensus Development Panel, 1992).

Not all melanomas are easily recognized. Change is the watchword during the clinical skin examination and the most important characteristic that should be observed in a lesion. The ABCD acronym, developed by the American Cancer Society, offers a guideline to help the lay public and primary healthcare clinicians to recognize a suspicious pigmented lesion (see Figure 15-3). Key observation points include asymmetry, irregular border, varied pigmentation pattern, and size larger than 6 mm. Increased size and change in color are the most common characteristics associated with early melanoma. Small size should not reduce the level of suspicion, however, because early melanomas may be detected when less than 6 mm in diameter. Later signs of melanoma include elevation (i.e., change in lesion height from flat or slightly raised), the presence of sensation (e.g., itching, tenderness, pain), bleeding, and ulceration.

The Glasgow Seven-Point Checklist is another tool that was established to improve the early recognition of melanoma by patients and general practitioners. The checklist, revised in 1989, consists of three major features and four minor features (see Figure 15-3). The major features include change in lesion size, shape, and color of a new or preexisting cutaneous lesion; the minor features are presence of inflammation, crusting or bleeding, sensory change, and a diameter $\geq$ 7 mm.

Figure 15-3. Warning Signs of Melanoma

American Cancer Society's ABCD System		Glasgow Seven-Point Checklist
Asymmetry	One half is unlike the other. Lesion cannot be folded evenly onto itself.	**Major signs** Change in size Change in shape Change in color
Border	Irregular, notched, hazy, and poorly defined	**Minor signs** Inflammation
Color	Varied color from one area to another Shades of brown, black, gray, red, and white may be present.	Crusting or bleeding Sensory change Diameter $\geq$ 7 mm
Diameter	Larger than 6 mm (size of a pencil eraser)	

Referral to a dermatologist is indicated for all pigmented lesions containing at least one major feature, and the additional presence of any minor feature is further indication that the lesion should be suspected for melanoma (MacKie, 1990). Although use of the seven-point checklist has been effective in improving the detection of early melanomas, some investigators have criticized the system for a lack of specificity, allowing many unnecessary referrals for patients with benign lesions. Others contend that the system's high-sensitivity is critical, and general healthcare providers will improve their ability to recognize benign lesions with education and experience (Healsmith, Bourke, Osborne, & Graham, 1994; Higgins, Hall, Todd, Murthi, & du Vivier, 1992).

Clinical Characteristics

Superficial spreading melanomas are the most common, accounting for 70% of all melanomas (Langley & Sober, 1998). Although most commonly seen on the trunk and back (males) or lower legs (females), they may occur on any skin surface. They often arise in a preexisting nevus. Variegation in color, including dark brown, black, blue-gray, pink, or gray-white, is a characteristic feature. Hypopigmented areas of regression also may be present. Lesions may present initially as an asymmetric pigmented macule or plaque, and lesion borders may become irregular with growth. Radial tumor growth may last from months to years before vertical growth occurs.

Nodular melanomas make up 15%–30% of all melanomas (Langley & Sober, 1998). Like the superficial spreading subtype, they may occur anywhere on the skin but are most common on the head, neck, and trunk. They may arise in nevi or on previously normal skin. Identification of nodular melanomas may be difficult because they lack many of the classic features associated with melanoma. Nodular melanomas are the most aggressive subtype because of their rapid clinical onset. Vertical growth begins from the start. Early diagnosis is difficult because no identifiable radial growth phase exists. Lesions often are uniform in color (e.g., blue-black, bluish red, amelanotic) and may present as a raised, shiny, dome-shaped nodule. Conversely, lesions may present as a papule or as a pedunculated lesion. Lesions may be symmetric with regular borders. Ulceration and bleeding also may occur.

Lentigo maligna melanoma accounts for 4%–15% of all melanomas (Langley & Sober, 1998). In contrast to the other subtypes, incidence is linked to cumulative rather than intermittent sun exposure. It is most common in fair-skinned adults who are older than 60 and occurs equally in men and women. The lesions arise from premalignant lentigo maligna in chronically sun-exposed skin such as the head and neck. Lentigo maligna presents as a slow-growing, ill-defined, pigmented patch with various shades of color. Lentigo malignas may resemble other skin lesions such as seborrheic keratoses, dysplastic nevi, or lentigines, making clinical recognition difficult. The premalignant radial growth phase may last for many years before invasion occurs. The clinical indication of invasive lentigo maligna melanoma is a raised papular or nodular area within the lesion. Although the risk of progression from lentigo maligna to lentigo maligna melanoma has been reported to be low, careful follow-up or excision is indicated once a diagnosis of lentigo maligna has been made (Weinstock & Sober, 1987).

Acral lentiginous melanoma, the rarest subtype, accounts for 2%–8% of all melanomas (Langley & Sober, 1998). It occurs with similar incidence across nationalities, but it is the most common form of melanoma among dark-skinned people. It is most common in adults older than 60. Acral lentiginous melanomas may occur on the palms and soles, on mucosal surfaces, and beneath the nail plate (subungual lesions). The plantar surface of the foot is the most common site. Although early diagnosis is possible because radial growth precedes vertical growth, the diagnosis usually is delayed. Acral lentiginous melanoma presents clinically as a macular lesion with variegated colors and irregular borders.

Subungual lesions are uncommon and usually occur in the great toe and thumb. Lesions may present with the rapid onset of diffuse nail plate discoloration or as a longitudinal pigmented band within the nail plate. Concomitant pigmentation in the proximal or lateral nail folds (Hutchinson's sign) is considered diagnostic and is associated with a poorer prognosis (Cockerell, Howell, & Balch, 1993; Lang, 1998; Langley & Sober, 1998; Rose, 1998; Swetter, 1996). A uniform screening system for subungual melanoma recently was proposed (Levit, Kagen, Scher, Grossman, & Altman, 2000).

Post-Treatment Surveillance

Patients who have had a cutaneous melanoma are at increased risk for developing another primary lesion because their underlying personal risk profile remains unchanged. Up to 10% of patients will develop a second primary melanoma (Gloster & Brodland, 1996). Melanoma survivors also are at risk for tumor recurrence, which usually occurs within 10 years. Late recurrences beyond 10 years are uncommon but have been reported (McEwan, Smith, & Matthews, 1990; Tsao, Cosimi, & Sober, 1997). Lifetime surveillance is recommended, with frequency determined by risk for recurrence (e.g., tumor thickness, stage of disease). Patients may be examined as often as every three or six months for the first two to five years and then annually thereafter (Lang, 1998; Poo et al., 1999; Ross, 1996).

The benefit of close surveillance is well established. Patients who develop subsequent melanomas are more likely to have thinner lesions at diagnosis. Ariyan, Poo, Bolognia, Buzaid, and Ariyan (1995) observed that patient prognosis was determined by the original (thickest) melanoma and was unchanged among those who developed subsequent, thinner lesions. In addition, close follow-up enables the examiner to evaluate treatment outcomes, assess patient rehabilitation, and detect the presence of early tumor recurrences. The examination should include total-body skin examination and palpation of the excision site and regional lymph nodes. Patient education, stressing the importance of monthly skin self-examination and sun-protection methods, should complement the surveillance program (NIH Consensus Development Panel, 1992; Poo et al., 1999).

First-degree relatives of patients with melanoma also are at increased risk. Familial tendency for melanoma partly is related to inherited factors such as skin type, presence of dysplastic or numerous acquired nevi, and sun sensitivity. Family members should be encouraged to have their skin examined annually, perform skin self-examination on a monthly basis, and limit their exposure to UVR.

Primary Skin Cancer Prevention

"There is no such thing as a healthy tan" is the most important message that should be communicated to the public. UV-induced DNA damage to the skin occurs first, and the increase in skin pigmentation (tanning) is the response of the injured skin. Many people believe that sunscreens can be used to increase the amount of time they spend in the sun. However, effective sun protection requires sunscreen use in combination with sun avoidance and protective clothing (see Table 15-4).

Table 15-4. Skin Cancer Prevention

Protective Activity	Examples
Avoid sun-seeking behavior.	• Limit sun exposure between 10 am–3 pm ("Short shadow, seek shade"). • Do not work on a tan. • Avoid tanning salons and sunlamps. • Pay attention to the ultraviolet index. • Use extra precautions when at higher altitudes or when near the equator.
Exercise caution on cloudy days.	• Approximately 80% of UVR (ultraviolet radiation) penetrates thick cloud cover.
Exercise caution around reflective surfaces.	• Reflective surfaces may increase UVR exposure by as much as 90%.
Wear protective attire.	• Tightly woven, dark fabrics that are loose fitting offer the most protection. • Wear wide-brimmed hats and labeled sunglasses.
Use sunscreens and lip balm.	• Use sunscreens daily. • Use a broad-spectrum sunscreen with an SPF of 15 or higher. • Chose a sunscreen based on skin type, physical activity, and environmental conditions. • Apply sunscreen at least 15–30 minutes before going outdoors. • Apply a thick coat of sunscreen to exposed skin. • Reapply sunscreens frequently based on environmental conditions and physical activity. • Use lip balm with an SPF of at least 15.
Use sun-protective measures with children.	• Use broad-spectrum sunscreens specially formulated for children. • Provide supervision to ensure that sunscreens are used and applied correctly.
Use special care with infants (0–6 months).	• Primary protection is sun avoidance and use of protective clothing. • Sunscreens may be used sparingly when physical protection is inadequate (American Academy of Pediatrics, 1999).

Note. Based on information from Goldsmith et al., 1996; Naylor & Farmer, 1997; Wentzell, 1996.

Avoid Sun-Seeking Behavior

Individuals should limit their sun exposure between 10 am and 3 pm. UVB radiation is the strongest during this time, with approximately 60% of these damaging rays occurring in the four hours around midday (Wentzell, 1996). The simple slogan "short shadow, seek shade" can help people remember that they should avoid the midday sun. Objects cast less shadow when the sun is directly overhead and most intense. Therefore, when one's shadow is less than his or her actual height, safety measures should be taken. Taking shelter beneath a canopy, umbrella, or tree are simple strategies that may significantly reduce exposure.

Deliberate tanning using artificial light (e.g., tanning salons, sunlamps) also should be avoided. Many people have reported the use of tanning devices to protect themselves from sunburn prior to vacationing in a sunny climate. However, UVA-induced tans are not completely protective, and this practice should be discouraged.

Another service that assists the public in implementing sun-protection measures is the UV index, which predicts the amount of UVR that will reach the earth's surface at noon the following day. This information alerts the public about the potential risks of exposure and helps them to plan outdoor activities accordingly on days when UVR intensity is expected to be high.

Individuals should take special precautions when around reflective surfaces, on cloudy days, and according to geographic location. UVR exposure may be increased by as much as 90% around reflective surfaces such as sand, water, concrete, and snow. Similarly, clouds and fog scatter UVR but absorb very little. Approximately 80% of UVR penetrates thick cloud cover. Increased UVR exposures also occur to those living at or near the equator and at high altitudes. Overexposure to the sun also can occur through a closed window, such as while riding in a car. Window glass blocks UVB radiation; however, it does not block UVA.

Wear Protective Attire

Long-sleeve shirts and long pants offer the most protection against UVR. All garments should cast a shadow when held up to the sunlight to be considered protective. Some general rules exist about clothing and sun protection. The weave of a fabric is more important than its thickness or weight, with tightly woven garments offering the most protection (Welsh & Diffey, 1981). Loose-fitting clothing tends to be more protective because stretching a fabric relaxes the weave. For the same reason, fabrics with the ability to stretch, such as Lycra® (du Pont, Wilmington, DE), tend to be less protective. Darker fabrics offer greater protection than do lighter ones. Dry clothing also is more protective; most wet garments become transparent and the air space between the clothing and the skin is eliminated. Cotton fabrics offer the least protection when wet because they absorb the most water. Special sun-protective clothing is available. One example is Solumbra™ (Sun Precautions, Everett, WA), a fabric of woven nylon with a sun protection factor (SPF) of more than 70 when dry and more than 65 when wet.

A broad-brimmed hat should be worn to protect the top of the head (especially bald spots), face, neck, and ears. The hat should be tightly woven with a brim of at least three to four inches. UVB radiation can be reduced by 70% to the head and neck if a four-inch-wide brim hat is worn (Gloster & Brodland, 1996). New legionnaire-type hats with flaps that protect the ears and back of the neck also are available. Other styles of hats do not provide satisfactory protection. Peaked baseball-style caps, for example, protect the nose but do not shade the neck or other areas of the face (Diffey & Cheeseman, 1992).

Sunglasses that provide UVA and UVB protection should be worn to protect the eyes from retinal damage and cataracts. Protection is provided by an invisible chemical applied to the lenses to absorb UV radiation, not the darkness of the lenses. Protective sunglasses block 99%–100% of the full UV spectrum, and they should be labeled accordingly. Sunglasses that either are unlabeled or have a nonspecific label should not be worn. The size, shape, and wearing position of the sunglasses are other factors that should be considered. Large, close-fitting lenses that shade the eyes from all sides offer the most protection (American Academy of Pediatrics, 1999).

Wear Sunscreen

Regular use of sunscreens with an SPF of 15 during the first 18 years of life may reduce the lifetime incidence of NMSC by as much as 78% (Stern, Weinstein, & Baker, 1986). Chemical sunscreens contain agents that absorb or filter UVR, thereby decreasing the quantity of radiation penetrating the epidermis. They include aminobenzoic acid esters (ABA, formerly PABA), cinnamates, salicylates, benzophenones, dibenzomethanes, and anthranilates.

Physical sunscreens are opaque or pigmented formulations that form a protective barrier to scatter, reflect, or physically block UVR. They generally provide a broader spectrum of coverage and protect against UVA and UVB. Examples include those containing titanium dioxide, zinc oxide, kaolin, talc, iron oxide, and colored clays.

Commercial sunscreens are made up of a mixture of organic chemicals that absorb various wavelengths of UV light. Some products combine chemical agents with physical ones. The term "sunblock" often is misunderstood. Sunblock, by definition, is any sunscreen with an SPF of 15 or greater.

One goal of sunscreen use is to prevent erythema (sunburn). The SPF rating relates to UVB exposures and sunburn. Sunburn is delayed UVB-induced erythema. It is caused by an increase in blood flow to affected skin. It begins about four hours after exposure and peaks in 8–24 hours. In addition to erythema, DNA damage and the activation of inflammatory pathways also occur (Naylor, 1997). No standard measurement of UVA protection is available. Parsol 1789 (avobenzene) and micronized zinc are the most effective UVA blockers.

The calculation of an individual's minimal erythematous dose (MED) can be used to estimate the amount of sun protection he or she will receive from a sunscreen. MED is the minimum time of sunlight exposure necessary to induce a barely perceptible redness in the skin within 24 hours of exposure to noontime sun. SPF is the ratio of time required to produce minimal erythema on skin covered with sunscreen to the time required to produce the same degree of erythema without sunscreen. MED multiplied by SPF approximates the length of time an individual may spend in the sun using a specific sunscreen without getting sunburned.

This calculation strictly is an estimate and does not take time of day, environmental conditions, or physical activities into consideration. Wind, heat, humidity, and high altitudes decrease the efficacy of sunscreens. Swimming and heavy perspiration also reduce their effectiveness.

An estimated 80% of a person's total lifetime sun exposures are incidental. These are multiple, brief exposures that are not intended to produce tanning. Incremental damage occurs with each exposure to UVR, as evidenced by photoaging, wrinkling, and blotchy skin pigmentation. Skin damage is cumulative over a person's lifetime and is dependent on time spent in the sun and the magnitude of sun exposures. Sunscreens can prevent DNA damage associated with these suberythemal exposures and should be used regularly when one plans to be outdoors for more than 20 minutes (Farmer & Naylor, 1996; Naylor, 1997). Everyone should use a broad-spectrum agent with an SPF of at least 15. No chemical sunscreen blocks UVR completely. Broad-spectrum products filter UVA II (range of 320 nm–340 nm) and UVB radiation. SPF 15 sunscreens block approximately 93% of UVR (American Academy of Pediatrics, 1999). Individuals with fair skin, a history of skin cancer, or those with photosensitivity disorders (e.g., lupus, polymorphous light eruption, taking photosensitizing medications) should use a sunscreen with a higher SPF. Wind, heat, humidity, light reflection, altitude, and nearness to the equator also must be considered. SPF 30 sunscreens block approximately 97% of UVR (American Academy of Pediatrics). Sunscreens with a higher SPF are not associated with an increase in skin irritation. In addition, sunscreens can be selected based on physical activity to achieve the most protection. Sweat-resistant products should be selected during strenuous outdoor exercise because they provide protection for up to 30 minutes of heavy perspiration. Water-resistant or waterproof preparations should be used while engaged in swimming, as they offer about 40 minutes and 80 minutes of protection, respectively. All times are approximate (Farmer & Naylor).

Possible adverse effects of chemical sunscreens are contact dermatitis and drug-induced photosensitivities. Contact dermatitis reactions include skin irritation, which is most common, and allergic contact dermatitis, a hypersensitivity reaction. These may be caused by the high concentration of chemicals contained in a sunscreen. Preservatives, fragrances, or other additives also may be responsible. A patch test, the application of sunscreen to a small area of skin prior to whole body use, can be used to measure an individual's sensitivity to a particular sunscreen. Two types of drug-induced photosensitivities are caused by UVR absorption by the skin in combination with a photosensitizing chemical. The sensitizing chemical can be a medication or part of an ordinary topical preparation (e.g., cosmetics, lotions, shampoo, hair dye, soap). Phototoxicity is more common. This reaction is characterized by the rapid onset of an exaggerated or intense sunburn that usually resolves in one week. The response is dose dependent but not immune related and may occur with the first sun exposure. In contrast, photoallergic photosensitivity is an immune-mediated reaction that is not dose dependent. In this reaction, the causative agent is antigenic. It is characterized by a delayed and slowly resolving inflammatory response that occurs after prior or prolonged sun exposure (Funk, Dromgoole, & Maibach, 1995; Gonzalez & Gonzalez, 1996).

Basic education about sunscreen use and application should be emphasized. Everyone should use sunscreens regularly, including those who have dark skin or tan easily. Artificial tanning lotions may be recommended to individuals who want a tan. They do not protect the skin from UVR, however, and sunscreens should be used. Sunscreen should be applied at least 15–30 minutes before going outdoors to allow absorption into the skin. All areas of exposed skin should be covered, with special attention paid to often-neglected areas such as the earlobes, lips, nose, bald spots, and the back of the neck. A thick coat is required to achieve the product's stated SPF. As a general rule, about one ounce should be used for total skin coverage. Most people do not apply sunscreens thickly enough, and a thin application results in decreased protection. Such individuals might benefit from a product with a higher SPF.

Sunscreens also should be reapplied liberally and frequently about every one to two hours, based on outdoor activity. Those who are exposed to strong winds, heavy perspiration, or swimming should consider more frequent applications. Reapplication does not increase the amount of protection but maintains the product's intended SPF. Many additional products such as body lotions, make-up, and moisturizers contain sunscreens. Regular use of these products should be encouraged. Exposure to UVR is a major risk factor for SCC of the lips. Like sunscreens, lip protection should be reapplied frequently and after eating, drinking, and swimming.

Physical sunscreens are very effective and spread easily on the skin but wash off easily and may stain clothing. In the past, they have been unsightly, messy, and impractical for covering large areas of the skin. However, the newer micronized formulations (e.g., ultramicronized zinc oxide) are broken down into minute particles that blend into the skin and are not noticeable. Physical sunscreens offer some advantages over chemical sunscreens. They provide broad-spectrum protection from UVA and UVB and are less dependent on the technique of application. In addition, they are not antigenic and therefore are not associated with sensitivity reactions. They are an excellent choice for those who cannot tolerate chemical sunscreens and for those who experience photosensitivity. The major disadvantage to physical sunscreens is that they are occlusive, blocking sweat glands and skin pores. Regular use may promote skin conditions such as folliculitis and acne. They do offer excellent protection and especially are useful on skin areas that burn easily, such as the nose and tops of the ears.

Sun Precautions and Children

Severe sunburns during childhood and the development of numerous melanocytic nevi are known risk factors for melanoma. Sun avoidance and sunburn prevention are critical to reduce lifetime risk. It is essential to protect young skin, establish good skin-care habits, and supervise protection practices. Children should use broad-spectrum sunscreens that are specially formulated for them. A patch test should be performed to determine skin sensitivity. Sunscreens with an alcohol base are not recommended for children younger than age 12 because these products may cause stinging, burning, and eye irritation. Products containing lanolin, the preservative paraben, and fragrances also should be avoided to prevent a future contact allergy. Children should be supervised to ensure that sunscreens are used and applied correctly. Parents can further promote sunscreen use by sending sunscreen to a child's school or daycare facility and requesting that personnel assist the child prior to going outdoors. The ultimate goal should be that regular sunscreen use becomes a lifelong habit.

Sun avoidance, protective clothing, and use of shade are the primary preventive measures that should be used for infants under six months of age. Sunscreens may be applied to small areas, such as the back of the hands and face, in situations where physical protection is not adequate. Sunscreens were not recommended for infants in the past for fear that they lacked the ability to metabolize topical agents absorbed through the skin. Harmful effects from sunscreen use never have been reported (American Academy of Pediatrics, 1999).

Secondary Cancer Prevention: Comprehensive Skin Examination

Total skin evaluation is a comprehensive visual inspection that is brief, noninvasive, inexpensive, and easy to perform. In addition to detecting suspicious lesions, patients with obvious signs of sun-induced skin damage, such as photoaged skin, wrinkling, and solar lentigines, can be identified during the examination and counseled about prevention. The examination also provides an opportunity for teaching the patient skin self-examinations, which can be performed using mirrors to visualize hard-to-see areas or with the help of a partner.

Risk Assessment

The American Academy of Dermatology recommends an annual total skin evaluation and regular skin self-examinations for all adults. Total skin evaluation begins with risk assessment. To expedite the screening process, the patient should be asked to complete a short risk assessment tool that the clinician reviews before and during the examination (see Figure 15-4). The risk assessment provides essential information that allows the clinician to individualize recommendations for routine screening and prevention. It allows the clinician to evaluate the patient's current sun protection practices so that "bad habits" can be corrected and appropriate suggestions made. The risk assessment also helps the clinician to identify high-risk individuals for referral to a dermatologist.

Referral of high-risk patients often is recommended because dermatologists are more proficient at recognizing subtle skin changes that could indicate malignancy (Robinson, 1997). High-risk patients also benefit from increased surveillance, with the frequency of examinations determined by the patient's estimated risk. Referral should be considered for members of melanoma-prone families, those with a prior history of skin cancer, patients who are immunosuppressed, and those with multiple or atypical moles.

Specific concerns the patient has regarding his or her skin also should be elicited at this time. Although skin cancers often are diagnosed in asymptomatic indi-

Figure 15-4. Skin Cancer Screening—Questionnaire

	Yes	No
Family History		
1. Do you have any relatives who have had precancerous lesions?		
2. Do you have any relatives who have had precancerous moles?		
3. Do you have any relatives who have had skin cancer? If yes, what type?		
Personal History		
1. Have you ever had precancerous lesions?		
2. Have you ever had precancerous moles?		
3. Have you ever had skin cancer? If yes, what type? When were you diagnosed?		
4. Have you ever had chronic exposure to arsenic, coal tar, petroleum products, or creosate?		
5. Have you ever had radiation treatment to your skin?		
6. Have you worked outdoors extensively? If yes, for how many years?		
7. Have you regularly participated in outdoor activities? If yes, for how many years?		
8. What is your skin's response to sun exposure? Burn easily Burn after three to four hours Never burn		
9. Did you ever get a painful or blistering sunburn before you were 20 years old? If yes, how many times?		
10. How many times a year do you get sunburned?		
11. Have you ever used sunlamps or tanning salons?		
12. Do you use sunscreen regularly? If yes, what SPF?		
13. Do you have a sore that has not healed in three weeks?		
14. Do you have a mole that has changed in size, color, shape, or has been bleeding?		
15. Do you have a mole in an area that is rubbed easily or irritated?		
16. Do you have any other concerns regarding your skin? If yes, please describe.		

Note. Figure courtesy of The University of Texas M.D. Anderson Cancer Center. Used with permission.

viduals who were not aware of them, many patients seek skin screening for a specific complaint. Patients should be questioned about any skin changes they have observed, including new moles and lesions or changes in existing ones (e.g., size, shape, color) and symptomatic lesions (e.g., sores that have not healed, lesions that itch or bleed). All areas of patient concern warrant special attention during the screening examination.

Equipment

Proper lighting, a magnification lens (5x–10x, and a measuring device in centimeters facilitate the screening examination. Adequate lighting enables the examiner to evaluate subtle color changes in an identified lesion. Natural sunlight provides the best illumination, but it is impractical in most clinical settings. Direct light from a 60-watt examination bulb is a satisfactory substitute. A magnification lens is essential when close or detailed visualization is required. For example, magnification is effective in detecting translucency and telangiectasias, which are common findings in BCCs, and irregular pigmentation patterns, which may be indicative of malignant melanoma. A centimeter ruler should be used to provide the exact measurements of any skin lesion. Imprecise measurements (e.g., "quarter-sized") and subjective estimates should be avoided. Irregular lesions may require more than one measurement of length and width. In this instance, a sketch of the lesion on a body chart may help to clearly illustrate the lesion's dimensions and location.

Photography is another tool that can be incorporated into the skin examination and enhances the close follow-up of high-risk patients (Shriner, Wagner, & Glowczwski, 1992). Baseline total-body photographs provide a visual record of the patient's skin. In one setting, patients had a total of 36 color photographs taken of all anatomic sites (with the exception of the hairy scalp and perineum) in overview and full-frame close-up (Rhodes, 1998). In another setting, a series of 14 baseline photographs was used to provide full coverage of the skin surface (Kelly, Yeatman, Regalia, Mason, & Henham, 1997).

Photographs of atypical moles and skin surfaces with numerous moles are useful tools in the recognition of new moles and subtle skin changes over time. Melanocytic nevi can be photographed individually to record pigmentation patterns, and a ruler usually is included next to the nevus for measurement. Several studies have found that combining baseline photography with serial examination facilitates the early diagnosis of melanoma in patients with dysplastic nevi (Kelly et al., 1997; MacKie, McHenry, & Hole, 1993; Tiersten et al., 1991).

Baseline photographs also help to limit the cost and morbidity associated with frequent surveillance. In addition to improving the clinician's ability to recognize suspicious skin changes, they also document the stability of a given mole, indicating when excision may not be required (Rhodes, 1998). Comparing serial photographs to baseline pictures may help the examiner recognize new or changing moles. In place of standard photography, some centers use computer-assisted, high-resolution digital video photography. This technique allows for easy storage and retrieval, and images collected over time can be analyzed for change.

The use of full-body photography may assist high-risk individuals with monthly skin self-examinations. Self-detection of early melanomas requires the individual to recognize any changes during monthly self-examinations. An inability to remember the skin's previous appearance is a major problem associated with self-detection. Hanrahan, Hersey, Menzies, Watson, and D'Este (1997) found that study volunteers viewing computer-generated pictures over long intervals had difficulty recognizing change in a lesion and the development of a new lesion on previously normal skin. Initial skin photographs may improve an individual's ability to self-detect skin cancer because a baseline is provided to monitor for change.

Patient Preparation

Total skin evaluation requires that the patient be completely undressed so that all body surfaces can be inspected. An examination gown should be worn, with areas of skin exposed as they are examined. For a thorough examination, small areas of skin should be concentrated on one at a time. It is a disservice to the patient to limit the examination in any way. Studies have shown that total skin examination needs to be performed to detect most malignant melanomas (Friedman, Rigel, Silverman, Kopf, & Vossaert, 1991). Rigel et al. (1986) found that patients receiving total skin examination were 6.4 times more likely to have a melanoma detected than were patients receiving a partial examination. Limiting the skin assessment to an area of patient complaint (e.g., "spot check") should be avoided because an asymptomatic skin malignancy may be missed. Bandages, prosthetic devices (e.g., hearing aids, eyeglasses, dentures), and cosmetics should be removed so that lesions are not hidden or obscured.

Procedure for Inspection and Palpation

A full-body assessment includes inspection and palpation of the head (scalp, face, and mucous membranes), neck, trunk, upper extremities (including fingernails and palms of the hands), external genitalia, and lower extremities (including toenails and soles of the feet). The skin can be assessed systematically from scalp to feet or incorporated into the routine physical examination and assessed as the various anatomic areas are inspected and palpated. The examiner should give special attention to areas of the body that are difficult for the patient to see, such as the scalp, back, buttocks, soles of the feet, behind the ears, and backs of the legs (Kopf, Salopek, Slade, Marghoob, & Bart, 1995).

Total skin examination begins with the head and neck. The scalp is inspected and palpated, using fingers to part the hair. A blow-dryer may be used to facilitate scalp assessment.

Next, the skin surfaces and skin folds over the face should be inspected carefully. The examination should include the temples, forehead, nose, cheeks, and lips. The creases around the nose should be evaluated. Skin beneath facial hair (e.g., beards, mustaches) also should be assessed. The preauricular and postauricular areas and both sides of the pinna should be examined. Neck assessment should include inspection and palpation of the anterior, posterior, and lateral sides.

The mucous membranes of the mouth should be assessed for erythroplakia (red patches) and leukoplakia (white patches). Erythroplakias are superficial, red velvety patches occurring in the oral cavity and pharynx. Identified lesions should be biopsied because this condition commonly is associated with underlying dysplasia, carcinoma in situ, or invasive cancer. Leukoplakia, a flat, sharply defined, grayish-white plaque, is an AK localized to the mucous membranes. The lesion may feel rough or leathery on palpation and cannot be rubbed off. Common areas of occurrence include the lips (primarily the lower lip) and oral cavity, where single or multiple lesions may be present. Lesions should be biopsied to determine the presence of dysplasia or an invasive cancer. When underlying dysplasia is not present, the condition rarely advances to malignancy. However, when dysplasia is present, approximately 20%–30% of cases progress to SCC if left untreated. Smoking (cigarette, cigar, and pipe), smokeless tobacco, sunlight, alcohol, and chronic irritation are known etiologic factors for development of leukoplakia.

Total skin examination continues with evaluation of the trunk. Assessment should include the anterior and posterior surfaces, including the axillae, breasts, abdomen, umbilicus, and surfaces beneath any hair. A simple way to recognize sun-induced skin changes (sun-damaged skin) is to compare the skin from the patient's underarms (skin that receives little sun exposure) to the skin of the outer arms (skin that receives chronic sun exposure). Examination of the upper and lower extremities includes the anterior, posterior, medial, and lateral surfaces. In addition, the dorsal and palmar or plantar surfaces of the hands and feet, web spaces between the fingers and toes, the fingernails and toenails, and surfaces beneath hair should be examined. Examination of the external genitalia and buttocks completes the assessment. In women, a thorough examination of the external genitalia, including vulvar inspection and speculum examination of the vaginal mucosa, generally is not performed during routine skin screening. Women therefore should be encouraged to obtain annual pelvic examinations.

Recognizing Suspicious Lesions

The presence of lesions, scars, and nevi should be noted and evaluated for subtle changes that may indicate malignancy. The most important characteristic to note is change from the previous examination or change by patient report. Any preexisting lesion that exhibits a change in color, size, shape, or appearance that is unusual or different as compared to other moles should be considered for biopsy. Late signs and symptoms include bleeding, tenderness, and surface elevation. If a malignant lesion is suspected, the patient should be questioned about its duration, rate of growth, and the effects of previous treatment. Likewise, a new lesion that is irregular in shape or color, continues to grow, or bleeds should be considered for biopsy. Any pigmented lesion that the examiner considers worrisome or unusual also should be biopsied. Danger signs in moles or nevi are presented in Figure 15-3 (Lang, 1998; Robinson, 1997).

Patient Education

At the conclusion of the examination, the patient should have learned about his or her skin cancer risk factors, preventive strategies, and self-examination. Preventive practices such as use of sunscreens, protective clothing, and avoidance of sun exposure during peak intensity may reduce the current rising incidence trends.

Preventive strategies for children should be taught to parents because intense sun exposure during childhood and adolescence is a known risk factor for future skin cancer. Family history is a significant risk factor for both cutaneous melanoma and NMSC. Therefore, family members of patients with skin cancer should be recruited for regular skin screening and targeted for preventive education.

Patients should be taught to examine their skin regularly and seek medical attention for changes in skin growths or the appearance of new lesions. Lack of knowledge is probably the most important reason for patients failing to seek medical care for early cutaneous melanomas (Rhodes, 1995). One case-control study found that skin self-examinations significantly reduced the mortality associated with melanoma (Berwick, Begg, Fine, Roush, & Barnhill, 1996). Having a partner check areas that are difficult to see also will facilitate the examination.

Informational pamphlets from organizations such as the Skin Cancer Foundation, American Academy of Dermatology, and American Cancer Society should supplement verbal instructions. Booklets that provide instructions on skin self-examination and illustrate both melanoma and nonmelanoma skin cancers help to teach patients how to examine their skin accurately and recognize abnormalities.

Nursing Challenges

The analysis of SEER cancer data (1973–1996) showed that the increase in melanoma mortality is less than the rate of increase in the incidence of disease (Gloeckler et al., 1999). Prompt recognition of cutaneous melanomas may be attributed to the efforts made in public and professional education, leading to more tumors being diagnosed at an early stage.

Public-education programs focusing on primary prevention and early detection have been associated with a reduction in melanoma mortality rates. Exposure to sunlight is the major environmental risk factor for skin cancer. Optimal sun safety incorporates sun avoidance, physical protection, and use of sunscreens with an SPF of 15 or greater. Mass media and educational campaigns focusing on sensible exposure have been effective in changing attitudes and beliefs. For example, primary prevention programs in Australia have led to substantial changes in behavior, with people avoiding the midday sun, wearing protective clothing and wide-brim hats, and using sunscreens.

Attitudes, knowledge, and beliefs about suntans and exposure to sunlight need to be changed. Despite the known dangers associated with excessive UVR exposure, having a tan continues to be socially desirable. Most people know that they need be sun safe but often do not translate their knowledge into personal practice. Studies indicate that more work needs to be done to motivate people to change their sun-related behaviors. In a nationwide telephone survey, most White adults (59%) reported that they had sunbathed over the past year, and a quarter admitted to frequent sunbathing. Only 25% of sunbathers routinely used a sunscreen with an SPF of 15 or higher. Individuals in the youngest age group (16–25 years of age) sunbathed frequently and were least likely to use the recommended sunscreen (Koh et al., 1997).

Another national telephone survey measured the American Academy of Dermatology's progress over 10 years in increasing public knowledge about skin cancer and promoting risk-reduction behaviors (Robinson, Rigel, & Amonette, 1997). The study found that although knowledge was increased significantly, a rise in sunburns (30%–39%) and tanning bed use (2%–6%) occurred among Whites. Sunscreen use increased (35%–53%), but not all respondents used a product with an SPF ≥ 15 or applied the sunscreen correctly.

Public-awareness programs are most effective when used to target high-risk groups based on factors such as geographic location, occupation, and age. Children and teenagers are a particularly important high-risk group. Robinson, Rademaker, Sylvester, and Cook (1997) interviewed teenagers to determine their knowledge and attitudes about sun exposure and use of sun-protection measures. Although most teens were knowledgeable about the dangers associated with sun exposure, they reported extensive outdoor exposures and sunburning. Consequently, teaching sun safety to young people and encouraging them to practice these behaviors regularly is important. The use of artificial tanning devices, which are easily accessible and popular with teenagers and young adults, should be discouraged. One strategy to reach the young is to enlist the support of adults as educators and role models in promoting sun safety; therefore, programs targeted to parents, teachers, daycare workers, camp counselors, and coaches may be very effective.

Teaching individuals how to examine their skin and encouraging self-examination on a regular basis is the final component of public education. Older men who develop melanoma have the highest mortality rates. This may be explained by the fact that most lesions arise on the torso where they cannot be seen easily. Having a partner to assist in self-examination may improve early detection. A survey by Koh et al. (1992) found that of 216 incident cases of cutaneous melanoma, either the patient, a family member, or a friend discovered the majority of tumors (74%). Medical personnel initially detected 26% of the cases. In addition to patients and family members, professional groups such as hairdressers, barbers, and massage therapists also should be targeted for education, as they may be able to detect suspicious lesions while working with their clients.

In addition to educating the public about sun safety, nurses should support local and national early-detection initiatives. The American Academy of Dermatology has sponsored free annual screenings since 1985. Although such programs have detected many skin cancers, provided professional education, and raised public awareness, mass screening of the entire population is impractical by logistical and financial barriers. Some have suggested that targeting high-risk populations for screening may be the most cost-effective method to increase the proportion of cancers found (Koh et al., 1990).

Ultimately, the ability to detect skin cancers early will depend on a combination of patient and professional awareness (Weinstock, 1998). Innovative teaching strategies that combine verbal instructions with written "how-to" information and graphic illustrations of early cancers can help individuals to learn how to perform a skin self-examination and recognize the warning signs of skin cancer (e.g., ABC's of melanoma). Likewise, nondermatologists can be educated to recognize and evaluate suspicious skin lesions. Skin examinations usually are omitted in primary healthcare settings, often because the examiner does not feel confident in his or her ability to perform them. McCormick, Masse, Cummings, and Burke (1999) found that nurses who participated in a skin cancer education program were more knowledgeable, better able to perform skin screening, and better able to educate their patients about prevention. Oncology nurses should take a lead role in fostering professional education for themselves and others so that all nurses can serve as better advocates for their patients.

Conclusion

Routine skin assessments and patient education related to skin cancer prevention and early detection are strategies that may reduce the morbidity and mortality associated with skin cancer. This chapter reviewed how to examine the skin, major risk factors for skin cancer, signs and symptoms, and preventive strategies. To be most effective, the skin examination should be a comprehensive head-to-toe visual inspection that includes an assessment of skin cancer risk. Symptomatic or changing lesions should be evaluated carefully during the examination, and any questionable lesion should be referred for biopsy. In addition to the benefit of early detection, the inclusion of total skin examination into routine patient care also provides an opportunity to discuss with patients and family members the importance of skin self-examinations, sun protection methods, and the need to obtain regular skin screenings (Chiarello, 1997).

References

American Academy of Pediatrics. Committee on Environmental Health. (1999). Ultraviolet light: A hazard to children. *Pediatrics, 104,* 328–333.

American Cancer Society. (2000). *Cancer facts and figures, 2000.* Atlanta: Author.

Ariyan, S., Poo, W.J., Bolognia, J., Buzaid, A., & Ariyan, T. (1995). Multiple primary melanomas: Data and significance. *Plastic and Reconstructive Surgery, 96,* 1384–1389.

Autier, P., Dore, J.F., Lejeune, F., Koelmel, K.F., Geffeler, O., Hille, P., Cesarini, J.P., Lienard, D., Liabeuf, A., Joarlette, M., Chemaly, P., Hakim, K., Koeln, A., & Kleeberg, U.R. (1994). Cutaneous malignant melanoma and exposure to sunlamps or sunbeds: An EORTC multicenter case-control study in Belgium, France and Germany. *International Journal of Cancer, 58,* 809–813.

Baird, E.A., McHenry, P.M., & MacKie, R.M. (1992). Effect of maintenance chemotherapy in childhood on numbers of melanocytic naevi. *BMJ, 305,* 799–801.

Barksdale, S.K., O'Conner, N., & Barnhill, R. (1997). Prognostic factors for cutaneous squamous cell and basal cell carcinoma: Determinants of risk of recurrence, metastasis, and development of subsequent skin cancers. *Surgical Oncology Clinics of North America, 6,* 625–638.

Bavinck, J.N., De Boer, A., Vermeer, B.J., Hartevelt, M.M., Van Der Woude, F.J., Claas, F.H.J., Wolterbeek, R., & Vandenbroucke, J.P. (1993). Sunlight, keratotic skin lesions and skin cancer in renal transplant patients. *British Journal of Dermatology, 129*, 242–249.

Bavinck, J.N., Hardie, D.R., Green, A., Cutmore, S., MacNaught, A., O'Sullivan, B., Siskind, V., Van Der Woude, F.J., & Hardie, I.R. (1996). The risk of skin cancer in renal transplant recipients in Queensland, Australia. *Transplantation, 61*, 715–721.

Bernstein, S.C., Lim, K.K., Brodland, D.G., & Heidelberg, K.A. (1996). The many faces of squamous cell cancer. *Dermatologic Surgery, 22*, 243–254.

Berwick, M., Begg, C.B., Fine, J.A., Roush, G.C., & Barnhill, R.L. (1996). Screening for cutaneous melanoma by skin self-examination. *Journal of the National Cancer Institute, 88*, 17–23.

Carey, W.P., Jr., Thompson, C.J., Synnestvedt, M., Guerry, D., Halpern, A., Schultz, D., & Elder, D.E. (1994). Dysplastic nevi as a melanoma risk factor in patients with familial melanoma. *Cancer, 74*, 3118–3125.

Chiarello, S.E. (1997). Should everyday be melanoma Monday? *Archives of Dermatology, 133*, 569–571.

Cockerell, C.J., Howell, J.B., & Balch, C.M. (1993). Think melanoma. *Southern Medical Journal, 86*, 1325–1333.

Conrad, N., Leis, P., Orengo, I., Medrano, E.E., Hayes, T.G., Baer, S., & Rosen, T. (1999). Multiple primary melanoma. *Dermatologic Surgery, 25*, 576–581.

DeDavid, M., Orlow, S.J., Provost, N., Marghoob, A.A., Rao, B.K., Huang, C.L., Wasti, Q., Kopf, A.W., & Bart, R.S. (1997). A study of large congenital melanocytic nevi and associated malignant melanomas: Review of cases in the New York University Registry and the world literature. *Journal of the American Academy of Dermatology, 36*, 409–416.

Diffey, B.L., & Cheeseman, J. (1992). Sun protection with hats. *British Journal of Dermatology, 127*, 10–12.

Dinehart, S.M., Dodge, R., Stanley, W.E., Franks, H.H., & Pollack, S.V. (1992). Basal cell carcinoma treated with Moh's surgery. *Journal of Dermatologic Surgery and Oncology, 18*, 560–566.

Du Vivier, A. (1991). *Atlas of skin cancer*. Philadelphia: Lippincott.

Epstein, D.S., Lange, J.R., Gruber, S.B., Mofid, M., & Koch, S.E. (1999). Is physician detection associated with thinner melanomas? *JAMA, 281*, 640–643.

Farmer, K.C., & Naylor, M.F. (1996). Sun exposure, sunscreens, and skin cancer prevention: A year-round concern. *Annals of Pharmacotherapy, 30*, 662–672.

Fleming, I.D., Amonette, R., Monaghan, T., & Fleming, M.D. (1995). Principles of management of basal and squamous cell carcinoma of the skin. *Cancer, 75*, 699–703.

Frankel, D.H., Hanusa, B.H., & Zitelli, J.A. (1992). New primary nonmelanoma skin cancer in patients with a history of squamous cell carcinoma of the skin: Implications and recommendations for follow-up. *Journal of the American Academy of Dermatology, 26*, 720–726.

Fraser, M.C., Goldstein, A.M., & Tucker, M.A. (1997). The genetics of melanoma. *Seminars in Oncology Nursing, 13*, 108–114.

Friedman, R.J., Rigel, D.S., Silverman, M.K., Kopf, A.W., & Vossaert, K.S. (1991). Malignant melanoma in the 1990s: The continued importance of early detection and the role of physician examination and self-examination of the skin. *CA: A Cancer Journal for Clinicians, 41*, 201–226.

Funk, J.O., Dromgoole, S.H., & Maibach, H.I. (1995). Sunscreen intolerance. *Dermatologic Clinics, 13*, 473–481.

Gallagher, R.P., Hill, G.B., Bajdik, C.D., Fincham, S., Coldman, A.J., McLean, D.I., & Threlfall, W.J. (1995). Sunlight exposure, pigmentary factors, and risk of nonmelanocytic skin cancer: I. Basal cell carcinoma. *Archives of Dermatology, 131*, 157–163.

Gallagher, R.P., McLean, D.I., Yang, P., Coldman, A.J., Silver, H.K.B., Spinelli, J.J., & Beagrie, M. (1990). Suntan, sunburn, and pigmentation factors and the frequency of acquired melanocytic nevi in children. *Archives of Dermatology, 126*, 770–776.

Geller, A.C., Koh, H.K., Miller, D.R., Clapp, R.W., Mercer, M.B., & Lew, R.A. (1992). Use of health services before the diagnosis of melanoma: Implications for early detection and screening. *Journal of General Internal Medicine, 7*(2), 154–157.

Gloeckler, L.A., Kosary, C.L., Hankey, B.F., Miller, B.A., Clegg, L.X., & Edwards, B.K. (Eds.). (1999). *SEER cancer statistics review 1973–1996*. Bethesda, MD: National Cancer Institute.

Gloster, H.M., Jr., & Brodland, D.G. (1996). The epidemiology of skin cancer. *Dermatologic Surgery, 22*, 217–226.

Goldsmith, L., Koh, H.K., Bewerse, B., Reilly, B., Wyatt, S., Bergfeld, W., Geller, A.C., & Walters, P.F. (1996). Proceedings from the national conference to develop a national skin cancer agenda. *Journal of the American Academy of Dermatology, 34*, 822–823.

Gonzalez, E., & Gonzalez, S. (1996). Drug photosensitivity, idiopathic photodermatoses, and sunscreens. *Journal of the American Academy of Dermatology, 35*, 871–885.

Green, A., Smith, P., McWhirter, W., O'Regan, P., Battistutta, D., Yarker, M.E., & Lape, K. (1993). Melanocytic naevi and melanoma in survivors of childhood cancer. *British Journal of Cancer, 67*, 1053–1057.

Greenlee, R.T., Hill-Harmon, M.B., Murray, T., & Thun, M. (2001). *Cancer statistics 2000. CA: A Cancer Journal for Clinicians, 51*, 15–36.

Grob, J.J., Bastuji-Garin, S., Vaillant, L., Roujeau, J.C., Bernard, P., Sassolas, B., & Guillaume, J.C. (1996). Excess of nevi related to immunodeficiency: A study in HIV-infected patients and renal transplant recipients. *Journal of Investigative Dermatology, 107*, 694–697.

Gupta, A.K., Cardella, C.J., & Haberman, H.F. (1986). Cutaneous malignant neoplasms in patients with renal transplants. *Archives of Dermatology, 122*, 1288–1293.

Hanrahan, P.F., Hersey, P., Menzies, S.W., Watson, A.B., & D'Este, C.A. (1997). Examination of the ability of people to identify early changes of melanoma in computer-altered pigmented skin lesions. *Archives of Dermatology, 133*, 301–311.

Hartevelt, M.M., Bavinck, J.N., Kootte, A.M.M., Vermeer, B.J., & Vandenbroucke, J.P. (1990). Incidence of skin cancer after renal transplantation in the Netherlands. *Transplantation, 49*, 506–509.

Healsmith, M.F., Bourke, J.F., Osborne, J.E., & Graham, R.B. (1994). An evaluation of the revised seven-point checklist for the early diagnosis of cutaneous malignant melanoma. *British Journal of Dermatology, 130*, 48–50.

Henriksen, T., Dahlback, A., Larsen, S.H.H., & Moan, J. (1990). Ultraviolet-radiation and skin cancer. Effect of an ozone layer depletion. *Photochemistry and Photobiology, 51*, 579–582.

Heywood, A., Sanson, R.F., Ring, I., & Mudge, P. (1994). Risk prevalence and screening for cancer by general practitioners. *Preventive Medicine, 23*, 152–159.

Higgins, F.M., Hall, P., Todd, P., Murthi, R., & du Vivier, A.W.P. (1992). The application of the seven-point check-list in the assessment of benign pigmented lesions. *Clinical and Experimental Dermatology, 17*, 313–315.

Holly, E.A., Kelly, J.W., Shpall, S.N., & Chiu, S. (1987). Number of melanocytic nevi as a major risk factor for malignant melanoma. *Journal of the American Academy of Dermatology, 17*, 459–468.

Hughes, B.R., Cunliffe, W.J., & Bailey, C.C. (1989). Excess benign melanocytic naevi after chemotherapy for malignancy in childhood. *BMJ, 299*, 88–91.

Kang, S., Barnhill, R.L., Mihm, M.C., Jr., Fitzpatrick, T.B., & Sober, A.J. (1994). Melanoma risk in individuals with atypical nevi. *Archives of Dermatology, 130*, 999–1001.

Kefford, R.F., Newton, J.A., Bergman, M.A., & Tucker, M.A. (1999). Counseling and DNA testing for individuals perceived to be genetically predisposed to melanoma: A consensus statement of the Melanoma Genetics Consortium. *Journal of Clinical Oncology, 17*, 3245–3251.

Kelly, J.W., Yeatman, J.M., Regalia, C., Mason, G., & Henham, A.P. (1997). A high incidence of melanoma found in patients with dysplastic naevi by photographic surveillance. *Medical Journal of Australia, 167*, 191–194.

Kibarian, M.A., & Hruza, G.J. (1995). Nonmelanoma skin cancer: Risks, treatment options, and tips on prevention. *Postgraduate Medicine, 98*, 39–58.

Kirsner, R.S., Muhkerjee, S., & Federman, D.G. (1999). Skin cancer screening in primary care: Prevalence and barriers. *Journal of the American Academy of Dermatology, 41*, 564–566.

Koh, H.K., Bak, S.M., Geller, A.C., Mangione, T.W., Hingson, R.W., Levenson, S.M., Miller, D.R., Lew, R.A., & Howland, J. (1997). Sunbathing habits and sunscreen use among white adults: Results of a national survey. *American Journal of Public Health, 87*, 1214–1217.

Koh, H.K., Caruso, A., Gage, I., Geller, A.C., Prout, M.N., White, H., O'Conner, K., Balash, E.M., Blumental, G., Rex, I.H., Jr., Wax, F.D., Rosenfeld, T.L., Gladstone, G.C., Shama, S.K., Koumans, J.A, Baler, G.R., & Lew, R.A. (1990). Evaluation of melanoma/skin cancer screening in Massachusetts. *Cancer, 65*, 375–379.

Koh, H.K., Miller, D.R., Geller, A.C., Clapp, R.W., Mercer, M.B., & Lew, R.A. (1992). Who discovers melanoma? Patterns from a population-based survey. *Journal of the American Academy of Dermatology, 26*, 914–919.

Kopf, A.W., Salopek, T.G., Slade, J., Marghoob, A.A., & Bart, R.S. (1995). Techniques of cutaneous examination for the detection of skin cancer. *Cancer, 75*, 684–690.

Kossard, S., & Rosen, R. (1992). Cutaneous Bowen's disease: An analysis of 1001 cases according to age, sex, and site. *Journal of the American Academy of Dermatology, 27*, 406–410.

Kripke, M.L. (1988). Impact of ozone depletion on skin cancers. *Journal of Dermatologic Surgery and Oncology, 14*, 853–857.

Kwa, R.E., Campana, K., & Moy, R.L. (1992). Biology of cutaneous squamous cell carcinoma. *Journal of the American Academy of Dermatology, 26*, 1–26.

Lang, P.J., Jr. (1998). Malignant melanoma. *Medical Clinics of North America, 82*, 1325–1358.

Langley, R.G.B., & Sober A.J. (1998). Clinical recognition of melanoma and its precursors. *Hematology Oncology Clinics of North America, 12*, 699–715.

Levit, E.K., Kagen, M.H., Scher, R.K., Grossman, M., & Altman, E. (2000). The ABC rule for clinical detection of subungual melanoma. *Journal of the American Academy of Dermatology, 42*, 269–274.

MacKie, R.M. (1990). Clinical recognition of early invasive malignant melanoma: Looking for changes in size, shape and colour is successful. *BMJ, 301*, 1005–1006.

MacKie, R.M., Freudenberger, T., & Aitchison, T.C. (1989). Personal risk factor chart for cutaneous melanoma. *Lancet, 2*, 487–490.

MacKie, R.M., McHenry, P., & Hole, D. (1993). Accelerated detection with prospective surveillance for cutaneous malignant melanoma in high-risk groups. *Lancet, 341*, 1618–1620.

Marghoob, A., Kopf, A.W., Bart, R.S., Sanfilippo, L., Silverman, M.K., Lee, P., Levy, E., Vossaert, K.A., Yadav, S., & Abadir, M. (1993). Risk of another basal cell carcinoma developing after treatment of a basal cell carcinoma. *Journal of the American Academy of Dermatology, 28*, 22–28.

Marghoob, A.A., Schoenbach, S.P., Kopf, A.W., Orlow, S.J., Nossa, R., & Bart, R.S. (1996). Large congenital melanocytic nevi and the risk for the development of malignant melanoma. *Archives of Dermatology, 132*, 170–173.

Marghoob, A.A., Slade, J., Salopek, T.G., Kopf, A.W., Bart, R.S., & Rigel, D.S. (1995). Basal cell and squamous cell carcinomas are important risk factors for cutaneous malignant melanoma. *Cancer, 75*, 707–714.

Marks, R. (1995). An overview of skin cancers: Incidence and causation. *Cancer, 75*, 607–612.

Marks, R., Rennie, G., & Selwood, T.S. (1988a). Malignant transformation of solar keratoses to squamous cell carcinoma. *Lancet, 1*, 795–797.

Marks, R., Rennie, G., & Selwood, T.S. (1988b). The relationship of basal cell carcinomas and squamous cell carcinomas to solar keratoses. *Archives of Dermatology, 124*, 1039–1042.

McCormick, L.K., Masse, L.C., Cummings, S.C., & Burke, C. (1999). Evaluation of a skin cancer prevention module for nurses: Change in knowledge, self-efficacy, and attitudes. *American Journal of Health Promotion, 13*, 282–289.

McEwan, L., Smith, J.G., & Matthews, J.P. (1990). Late recurrence of localized cutaneous melanoma: Its influence on follow-up policy. *Plastic and Reconstructive Surgery, 86*, 527–534.

Miller, D.R., Geller, A.C., Wyatt, S.W., Halpern, A., Howell, J.B., Cockerell, C., Reilly, B.A., Bewerse, B.A., Rigel, D., Rosenthal, L., Amonette, R., Sun, T., Grossbart, T., Lew, R.A., & Koh, H.K. (1996). Melanoma awareness and self-examination practices: Results of a United States survey. *Journal of the American Academy of Dermatology, 34*, 962–970.

Morison, W.L., Baughman, R.D., Day, R.M., Forbes, P.D., Hoenigsmann, H., Krueger, G.G., Lebwohl, M., Lew, R., Naldi, L., Parrish, J.A., Piepkorn, M., Stern, R.S., Weinstein, G.D., & Whitmore, S.E. (1998). Consensus workshop on the toxic effects of long-term PUVA therapy. *Archives of Dermatology, 134*, 595–598.

National Institute of Environmental Health Service. (2000). *Ninth report on carcinogens 2000.* Research Triangle Park, NC: Author.

National Institutes of Health Consensus Development Panel. (1992). Diagnosis and treatment of early melanoma. *JAMA, 268*, 1314–1319.

Naylor, M.F. (1997). Erythema, skin cancer risk, and sunscreens. *Archives of Dermatology, 133*, 373–375.

Naylor, M.F., & Farmer, K.C. (1997). The case for sunscreens: A review of their use in preventing actinic damage and neoplasia. *Archives of Dermatology, 133,* 1146–1154.

Pion, I.A., Rigel, D.S., Garfinkel, L., Silverman, M.K., & Kopf, A.W. (1995). Occupation and the risk of malignant melanoma. *Cancer, 75*(Suppl. 2), 637–644.

Poo, W.J., Ariyan, S., Lamb, L., Papac, R., Zelterman, D., Hu, G.L., Brown, J., Fischer, D., Bolognia, J., & Buzaid, A.C. (1999). Follow-up recommendations for patients with American Joint Committee on Cancer stages I–III malignant melanoma. *Cancer, 86,* 2252–2258.

Preston, D.S., & Stern, R.S. (1992). Nonmelanoma cancers of the skin. *New England Journal of Medicine, 327,* 1649–1662.

Reintgen, D., Balch, C.M., Kirkwood, J., & Ross, M.I. (1997). Recent advances in the care of the patient with malignant melanoma. *Annals of Surgery, 225,* 1–14.

Reintgen, D., Ross, M., Bland, K., Seigler, H.F., & Balch, C. (1993). Prevention and early detection of melanoma: A surgeon's perspective. *Seminars in Surgical Oncology, 9,* 174–187.

Rhodes, A.R. (1995). Public education and cancer of the skin. What do people need to know about melanoma and nonmelanoma skin cancer? *Cancer, 75,* 613–636.

Rhodes, A.R. (1998). Intervention strategy to prevent lethal cutaneous melanoma: Use of dermatologic photography to aid surveillance of high-risk groups. *Journal of the American Academy of Dermatology, 39,* 262–267.

Rhodes, A.R., Weinstock, M.A., Fitzpatrick, T.B., Mihm, M.C., Jr., & Sober, A.J. (1987). Risk factors for cutaneous melanoma: A practical method of recognizing predisposed individuals. *JAMA, 258,* 3146–3154.

Richert, S.M., D'Amico, F., & Rhodes, A.R. (1998). Cutaneous melanoma: Patient surveillance and tumor progression. *Journal of the American Academy of Dermatology, 39,* 571–577.

Rigel, D.S., & Carucci, J.A. (2000). Malignant melanoma: Prevention, early detection, and treatment in the 21st century. *CA: A Cancer Journal for Clinicians, 50,* 215–236.

Rigel, D.S., Friedman, R.J., Kopf, A.W., Weltman, R., Prioleau, P.G., Safai, B., Lebwohl, M.G., Eliezri, Y., Torre, D.P., Binford, R.T., Cipollaro, V.A., Biro, L., Charbonneau, D., & Mosettis, A. (1986). Importance of complete cutaneous examination for the detection of malignant melanoma. *Journal of the American Academy of Dermatology, 14,* 857–860.

Rivers, J.K., Kopf, A.W., Vinokur, A.F., Rigel, D.S., Friedman, R.J., Heilman, E.R., & Levenstein, M. (1990). Clinical characteristics of malignant melanoma developing in persons with dysplastic nevi. *Cancer, 65,* 1232–1236.

Robinson, J.K. (1987). Risk of developing another basal cell carcinoma: A 5-year prospective study. *Cancer, 60,* 118–120.

Robinson, J.K. (1997). A 28-year-old fair-skinned woman with multiple moles: Clinical crossroads. *JAMA, 278,* 1693–1699.

Robinson, J.K., Rademaker, A.W., Sylvester, J.A., & Cook, B. (1997). Summer sun exposure: Knowledge, attitudes, and behaviors of Midwest adolescents. *Preventive Medicine, 26,* 364–372.

Robinson, J.K., Rigel, D.S., & Amonette, R.A. (1997). Trends in sun exposure knowledge, attitudes, and behaviors: 1986 to 1996. *Journal of the American Academy of Dermatology, 37,* 179–186.

Rose, L.C. (1998). Recognizing neoplastic skin lesions. *American Family Physician, 58*, 873–884.

Ross, M.I. (1996). Staging evaluation and surveillance for melanoma patients in a fiscally restrictive medical environment. *Surgical Clinics of North America, 76*, 1423–1432.

Rosso, S., Zanetti, R., Martinez, C., Tormo, M.J., Schraub, S., Sancho-Garnier, H., Franceschi, S., Gafa, L., Perea, E., Navarro, C., Laurent, R., Schrameck, C., Talamini, R., Tumino, R., & Wechsler, J. (1996). The multicenter south European study 'Helios' 1I: Different sun exposure patterns in the aetiology of basal cell and squamous cell carcinomas of the skin. *British Journal of Cancer, 73*, 1447–1454.

Ruiz, R.M., & Orozco, M.C. (1997). Malignant melanoma in children. *Archives of Dermatology, 133*, 363–371.

Sauer, G.C., & Hall, J.C. (1996). *Manual of skin diseases* (7th ed.) (pp. 1–8). Philadelphia: Lippincott-Raven.

Seidel, H.M., Ball, J.W., Dains, J.E., & Benedict, G.W. (1991). *Mosby's guide to physical examination* (2nd ed.). St. Louis, MO: Mosby.

Seykora, J., & Elder, D. (1996). Dysplastic nevi and other risk markers for melanoma. *Seminars in Oncology, 23*, 682–687.

Shriner, D.L., Wagner, R.F., & Glowczwski, J.R. (1992). Photography for the early diagnosis of malignant melanoma in patients with atypical moles. *Cutis, 50*, 358–362.

Skender-Kalnenas, T.M., English, D.R., & Heenan, P.J. (1995). Benign melanocytic lesions: Risk markers or precursors of cutaneous melanoma? *Journal of the American Academy of Dermatology, 33*, 1000–1007.

Slade, J., Marghoob, A.A., Salopek, T.G., Rigel, D.S., Kopf, A.W., & Bart, R.S. (1995). Atypical mole syndrome: Risk factor for cutaneous malignant melanoma and implications for management. *Journal of the American Academy of Dermatology, 32*, 479–494.

Smith, C.H., McGregor, J.M., Barker, J.N.W., Morris, R.W., Rigden, S.P.A., & MacDonald, D.M. (1993). Excess melanocytic nevi in children with renal allografts. *Journal of the American Academy of Dermatology, 28*, 51–55.

Sober, A.J., & Burstein, J.M. (1995). Precursors to skin cancer. *Cancer, 75*(Suppl. 4), 645–650.

Spencer, J.M., & Amonette, R.A. (1995). Indoor tanning: Risks, benefits, and future trends. *Journal of the American Academy of Dermatology, 33*, 288–298.

Spencer, J.M., & Amonette, R.A. (1998). Tanning beds and skin cancer: Artificial sun + old sol = real risk. *Clinics in Dermatology, 16*, 487–501.

Stern, R.S., & Laird, N. (1994). The carcinogenic risk of treatments for severe psoriasis. *Cancer, 73*, 2759–2764.

Stern, R.S., Nichols, K.T., & Vakeva, L.H. (1997). Malignant melanoma in patients treated for psoriasis with methoxsalen (psoralen) and ultraviolet radiation (PUVA). *New England Journal of Medicine, 336*, 1041–1045.

Stern, R.S., Weinstein, M.C., & Baker, S.G. (1986). Risk reduction for nonmelanoma skin cancer with childhood sunscreen use. *Archives of Dermatology, 122*, 537–545.

Swerdlow, A.J., English, J., MacKie, R.M., O'Doherty, C.J., Hunter, J.A.A., Clark, J., & Hole, D.J. (1986). Benign melanocytic naevi as a risk factor for malignant melanoma. *BMJ, 292*, 1555–1559.

Swerdlow, A.J., English, J.S.C., & Qiao, Z. (1995). The risk of melanoma in patients with congenital nevi: A cohort study. *Journal of the American Academy of Dermatology, 32*, 595–599.

Swetter, S.M. (1996). Malignant melanoma from the dermatologic perspective. *Surgical Clinics of North America, 76,* 1287–1298.

Thompson, S.C., Jolley, D., & Marks, R. (1993). Reduction of solar keratoses by regular sunscreen use. *New England Journal of Medicine, 329,* 1147–1151.

Tiersten, A.D., Grin, C.M., Kopf, A.W., Gottlieb, G.J., Bart, R.S., Rigel, D.S., Friedman, R.J., & Levenstein, M.J. (1991). Prospective follow-up for malignant melanoma in patients with atypical-mole (dysplastic-nevus) syndrome. *Journal of Dermatologic Surgery and Oncology, 17,* 44–48.

Tsao, H., Cosimi, A.B., & Sober, A.J. (1997). Ultra-late recurrence (15 years or longer) of cutaneous melanoma. *Cancer, 79,* 2361–2370.

Tucker, M.A., Fraser, M.C., Goldstein, A.M., Elder, D., Guerry, D., & Organic, S.M. (1993). Risk of melanoma and other cancers in melanoma-prone families. *Journal of Investigative Dermatology, 100*(Suppl. 3), 350S–355S.

Tucker, M.A., Halpern, A., Holly, E.A., Hartge, P., Elder, D.E., Sagebiel, R.W., Guerry, D., & Clark, W.H., Jr. (1997). Clinically recognized dysplastic nevi: A central risk factor for cutaneous melanoma. *JAMA, 277,* 1439–1444.

Vargo, N.L. (1991). Basal and squamous cell carcinomas. An overview. *Seminars in Oncology Nursing, 7,* 13–25.

Weinstock, M.A. (1998). Issues in the epidemiology of melanoma. *Hematology Oncology Clinics of North America, 12,* 681–698.

Weinstock, M.A., & Sober, A.J. (1987). The risk of progression of lentigo maligna to lentigo maligna melanoma. *British Journal of Dermatology, 116,* 303–310.

Welsh, C., & Diffey, B. (1981). The protection against solar actinic radiation afforded by common clothing fabrics. *Clinical and Experimental Dermatology, 6,* 577–581.

Wender, R.C. (1995). Barriers to effective skin cancer detection. *Cancer, 75,* 691–698.

Wentzell, J.M. (1996). Sunscreens. The ounce of prevention. *American Family Physician, 53,* 1713–1719.

Westerdahl, J., Ingvar, C., Masback, A., Jonsson, N., & Olsson, H. (2000). Risk of cutaneous malignant melanoma in relation to use of sunbeds: Further evidence for UVA carcinogenicity. *British Journal of Cancer, 82,* 1593–1599.

Westerdahl, J., Olsson, H., Masback, A., Ingvar, C., Jonsson, N., Brandt, L., Jonsson, P., & Moller, T. (1994). Use of sunbeds or sunlamps and malignant melanoma in southern Sweden. *American Journal of Epidemiology, 140,* 691–699.

Williams, M.L., & Pennella, R. (1994). Melanoma, melanocytic nevi, and other melanoma risk factors in children. *Journal of Pediatrics, 124,* 833–845.

Zanetti, R., Rosso, S., Martinez, C., Navarro, C., Schraub, S., Sancho-Garnier, H., Franceschi, S., Gafa, L., Perea, E., Tormo, M.J., Laurent, R., Schrameck, C., Cristofolini, M., Tumino, R., & Wechsler, J. (1996). The multicenter south European study 'Helios' 1: Skin characteristics and sunburns in basal cell and squamous cell carcinomas of the skin. *British Journal of Cancer, 73,* 1440–1446.

CHAPTER 16

Prevention and Detection of Head and Neck Cancers

Robin L. Coyne, MS, RN, CS-FNP

Introduction

Cancer of the head or neck is a devastating diagnosis. The patient may face disfigurement and some degree of loss in very basic functions, such as eating, speaking, and even breathing. Empathetic family members and healthcare providers are affected by what they see the patient going through. Although head and neck cancers are relatively rare in relation to lung, breast, or prostate cancer, the morbidity is extreme, and the five-year survival rate for the various disease sites is approximately 64% (Hoffman, Karnell, Funk, Robinson, & Menck, 1998). When detected early, however, head and neck cancers are curable. Stage I or II disease is considered curable at 80% and 60%, respectively (Vokes, Weichselbaum, Lippman, & Hong, 1993). Unfortunately, 60% of head and neck cancers occurring in the United States are not detected until advanced stages (Clayman, Lippman, Laramore, & Hong, 1997).

The surgical interventions and radiation therapy necessary to achieve local control of head or neck cancer can cause functional, structural, and cosmetic deficits. Many of those afflicted experience changes in mastication and speech as well as altered visual, auditory, and olfactory function. Quality of life may suffer significantly. Changes in function and appearance may contribute to diminished self-esteem, depression, and social isolation.

The purpose of this chapter is to review disease progression and the risk factors, genetic predispositions, and signs and symptoms associated with malignancies of the head and neck. The chapter will discuss prevention of head and neck cancers and early-detection strategies, and it will highlight research considerations and nursing challenges.

Epidemiology and Etiology

According to Hoffman et al. (1998), cancers of the head and neck accounted for 6.6% of all malignancies reported to the National Cancer Data Base from 1985–1994. Figure 16-1 shows the prevalence of different types of head and neck cancer categorized by site. The overall five-year survival rate associated with the types described in the National Cancer Data Base was 64%. Patients with lip cancer had the best prognosis, with a five-year survival rate of 91.1%. Patients with cancer of the hypopharynx had the worst survival rate (31.4%).

The American Cancer Society (ACS) estimated that 58,700 Americans would be diagnosed with cancer involving structures of the head or neck in 2000. Of that number, 12,900 were expected to die of their malignancies. Cancer of the oral cavity will account for 22,000 cases. Cancer of the thyroid will contribute 18,400 cases, and malignancies of the larynx and pharynx will account for 10,100 and 8,200 new diagnoses, respectively.

Cancers of the oral cavity, larynx, and pharynx predominantly affect men in their fifth or sixth decade of life, despite a gradual rise of disease occurrence among women. This trend is reflective of the increased use of tobacco products by the female population (Shugars & Patton, 1997). Prevalence is greater among African Americans than Whites. Early detection of head and neck cancer in the African American population is the exception and not the rule.

Tobacco use is the primary risk factor associated with head and neck malignancies. Excessive alcohol use in conjunction with tobacco potentiates the development of cancer, especially in the oral cavity. Shaha and Strong (1995) estimated that 80%–85% of all head and neck malignancies can be attributed to tobacco use in conjunction with alcohol. Poor dietary habits associated with alcohol abuse may

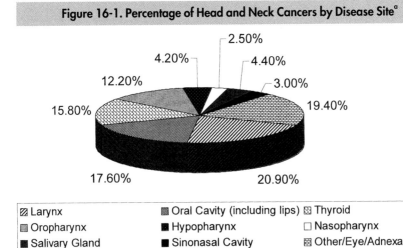

Figure 16-1. Percentage of Head and Neck Cancers by Disease Site[a]

2.50%
4.20%
4.40%
12.20%
3.00%
15.80%
19.40%
17.60%
20.90%

▨ Larynx	▨ Oral Cavity (including lips)	▨ Thyroid
▨ Oropharynx	■ Hypopharynx	☐ Nasopharynx
■ Salivary Gland	■ Sinonasal Cavity	▨ Other/Eye/Adnexa

[a] Based on 295,022 U.S. cases, 1985–1994

further increase the risk of cancer. Ultraviolet radiation is responsible for the majority of lip cancers, although chronic irritation from tobacco use also may be a factor (Pogoda & Preston-Martin, 1996).

Genetic abnormalities, such as Bloom's syndrome and Li-Fraumeni syndrome, are closely associated with head and neck cancers (Shaha & Strong, 1995). The human papilloma virus and the Epstein-Barr virus (EBV) have been implicated in malignancies of the larynx and the nasopharynx, respectively (Trizna & Schantz, 1992). Environmental and occupational hazards also have been identified.

Malignancies of the major and minor salivary glands typically present in the fourth to sixth decade of life. It is not uncommon for those afflicted to have undergone radiation treatment for acne or tonsillar or thymic enlargement at a young age (Ward & Levine, 1998). Cancers of the major and minor salivary glands, nasal cavity, and paranasal sinus are less common. Thyroid cancer is the most common endocrine gland malignancy.

Thyroid cancer is a disease that affects the young and old. The disease is most lethal in the elderly. Thyroid malignancies most commonly occur in females. In the overall population, the age at diagnosis is 25–65 (Horsley & Fratkin, 1995).

As with salivary gland cancer, therapeutic radiation has been linked to thyroid cancer. The latency period for disease development following treatment with ionizing radiation is 5–35 years (Stanford & Evans, 1999). Thyroiditis has not been correlated with the development of thyroid malignancies; however, severe Hashimoto's thyroiditis has been associated with lymphoma (Horsley & Fratkin, 1995).

Nasopharyngeal malignancies occur in a younger population than is typical of other head and neck cancer sites. The disease is two to three times more prevalent in men than women. The disease is 20 times more common in Asia than in North America (Clayman et al., 1997).

Pathophysiology

The majority of head and neck cancers develop in the mucous membranes of the upper aerodigestive tract. The upper aerodigestive tract begins at the commissure of the lips; extends to the cervical esophagus; and encompasses the oral cavity, pharynx, and larynx. Malignancies may occur at any juncture along the upper aerodigestive tract. The hidden vestibule extending from the skull base to the sixth cervical vertebra is commonly known as the pharynx. The pharynx is further divided into the nasopharynx, the oropharynx, and the hypopharynx.

Lips and Oral Cavity

Figure 16-2 shows the structures of the oral cavity. The oral cavity begins at the lips and contains the anterior two-thirds of the tongue, the floor of the mouth, the hard palate, the buccal mucosa, and the gingivae (Clayman et al., 1997). The posterior aspect of the oral cavity is contiguous with the oropharynx. Together, the oral cavity and the oropharynx support the activities of mastication, swallowing,

Figure 16-2. The Oral Cavity: Anatomic Subsites

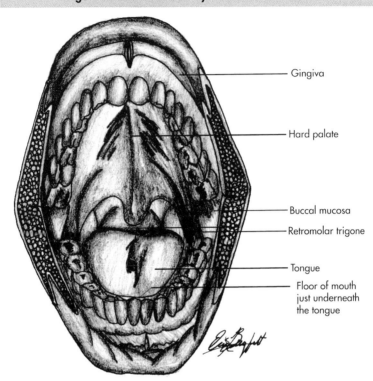

Gingiva

Hard palate

Buccal mucosa

Retromolar trigone

Tongue

Floor of mouth just underneath the tongue

and articulation. The floor of the mouth, the ventrolateral tongue, and the soft palate are especially high-risk sites for tumor development because of the pooling of alcohol inferiorly and the distribution of tobacco carcinogens superiorly (Mashberg & Barsa, 1984). A salivary gland tumor is a unique entity that will be discussed later in this chapter.

Larynx

The larynx is a cartilaginous framework covered by mucosa. The cricoid cartilage, the thyroid cartilage, and the arytenoid cartilages form the foundation of the structure and are supported by ligaments and fibrous membranes. Surrounding muscle creates the movement of the larynx that results in speech.

Cancer of the larynx typically is classified as supraglottic, glottic, or subglottic. Supraglottic malignancies account for 30% of laryngeal malignancies; glottic, 65%; and subglottic, 5% (Clayman et al., 1997). The supraglottic larynx encompasses the epiglottis, false cords, ventricles, aryepiglottic folds, and arytenoids. The glottis is the plane in which the true vocal cords lie. The subglottic larynx is just inferior to the true vocal cords, extending to the cricoid cartilage. The supraglottic larynx is rich in lymphatics; the glottic area is devoid of lymphatic drainage. Consequently, supraglottic cancers are much more likely to develop nodal metastases than are glottic malignancies. Primary subglottic cancer is extremely rare, although carcinoma from adjoining laryngeal structures may extend locally into this area (Spaulding, Hahn, & Constable, 1987).

Oropharynx and Hypopharynx

The oropharynx extends from the soft palate to the epiglottis. The oral cavity is anterior to the oropharynx, the nasopharynx is superior to it, and the larynx and hypopharynx are inferior to it. The tongue base, tonsils, and soft palate are within the oropharynx. Malignancies of the oropharynx are most likely to develop in the base of the tongue or in the tonsils (Vokes et al., 1993).

The hypopharyngeal portion of the pharynx begins at the epiglottis and ends at the inferior aspect of the cricoid cartilage. At the juncture with the cartilage, it meets the esophagus. Within the hypopharynx are two cul-de-sacs known as the pyriform sinuses, the posterior cricoid area, and the posterior and lateral pharyngeal walls. The pyriform sinus is the most common site for hypopharyngeal malignancies (Haggood, 1997). The hypopharynx is difficult to see and assess without specialized training. Generally, hypopharyngeal cancers grow extensively before symptoms appear and the condition is diagnosed. The majority of patients present with advanced nodal disease, and more than 20% have progressed to distant metastasis at the time of diagnosis (Wolf, Lippman, Laramore, & Hong, 1992).

Tobacco and alcohol promote cancer of the oropharynx and hypopharynx. Iron deficiency anemia (Plummer-Vinson syndrome) has been linked to cancers of the pyriform sinus. Typically, malignancies of the pharynx occur in male patients ages 50–80 (Gleich & Gluckman, 1998).

Nasopharynx

In terms of location, the nasopharynx is superior to the soft palate and posterior to the nares (see Figure 16-3). The nasal and oral portions of the pharynx connect via the pharyngeal isthmus. The isthmus closes off the nasopharynx during swallowing. The nasopharynx consists of a roof, a posterior wall, a floor, and two lateral walls. The lateral walls contain the openings of the eustachian tubes.

Malignancies of the nasopharynx generally develop before the age of 50. The disease is two to three times more prevalent in men than women. Much like salivary gland malignancy, nasopharyngeal carcinoma is not strongly connected to tobacco or alcohol use. Instead, nasopharyngeal carcinoma has been linked to Asian ancestry, frequent consumption of salted fish, and EBV (Vokes et al., 1993). Salted fish consumption poses a risk because the fish contain a high concentration of nitrosamines, a known carcinogen (Fee, 1998).

Nose and Paranasal Sinuses

The nose consists of a framework of bone, hyaline, and cartilage that is covered by skin. Paired nares are separated by the nasal septum. The nares open to the face and meet the nasopharynx posteriorly. Each naris is composed of a roof, a floor, and a lateral and medial wall and is divided into three regions: the nasal vestibule, the respiratory region, and the olfactory region. Opening into the lateral walls of the nasal cavity are four paired sinuses. The maxillary, frontal, ethmoid, and sphe-

Figure 16-3. Regions of the Head and Neck

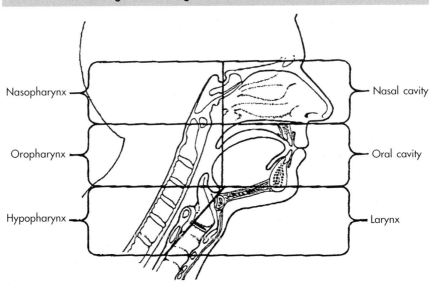

Note. From "Head and Neck Cancers" (p. 230) by A.S. Haggood in S.E. Otto (Ed.), *Oncology Nursing* (3rd ed.), 1997, St. Louis, MO: Mosby. Copyright 1997 by Mosby. Reprinted with permission.

noid sinuses collectively warm and humidify air while filtering some particles. Each sinus is connected to the nasal cavity by apertures that allow air flow and movement of mucus. Because the nasal cavity and sinuses are contiguous, tumors developing in one site often spread locally and encroach on adjacent structures—the orbits, oral cavity, oropharynx, and, in advanced cases, the skull base (Clayman et al., 1997; Rassekh, 1998).

Major and Minor Salivary Glands

The major and minor salivary glands work together to produce 500–1,500 cc of saliva each day (Ward & Levine, 1998). The three major salivary glands occur in pairs. The paired parotid glands are the largest salivary glands (see Figure 16-4). They are wedge-shaped structures situated just anterior to the external auditory canal. The sublingual glands are contained in the mucosa of the floor of the mouth and are accompanied by the submandibular glands in the submandibular triangle, which is formed by the mandible and surrounding muscles.

Eighty percent of tumors developing in the salivary glands are benign (Clayman et al., 1997). Malignant tumors of the salivary glands are different from other head and neck cancers because of their weak association to tobacco products.

Of the salivary glands, cancer growth has the greatest affinity for the parotid gland. Malignancies in this location account for 85% of salivary gland cancers. Cancers of the submandibular and the sublingual glands are much less common, accounting for 8%–15% and 1%, respectively (Ward & Levine, 1998).

The minor salivary glands number in the thousands and are scattered through-

Figure 16-4. Major and Minor Salivary Glands

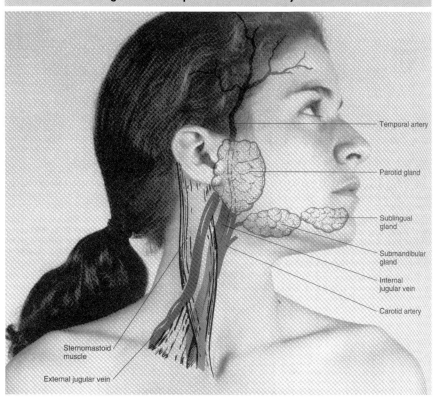

Note. From "Head and Neck, Including Lymphatics" (p. 278) by M.M. Andrews and J. Keithly in C. Jarvis (Ed.), *Physical Examination and Health Assessment,* 1992, Philadelphia: W.B. Saunders. Copyright 1992 by W.B. Saunders. Reprinted with permission.

out the oral cavity and soft palate. Only 5%–6% of all salivary gland tumors are minor salivary gland malignancies.

Salivary gland cancer usually occurs in the fourth to sixth decades of life. Often, those who develop the disease underwent therapeutic radiation as children. Unlike the majority of head and neck cancers, salivary gland malignancies are not strongly linked to tobacco or alcohol consumption.

Thyroid

The thyroid gland is the largest endocrine gland in the body. The thyroid is composed of two lateral lobes connected by an isthmus. It is affixed to the trachea and ascends with swallowing. The gland plays a major role in maintaining metabolism by producing thyroxine and triiodothyronine.

Thyroid cancer is a disease that strikes both young and old. Women are more likely to be afflicted than men. Individuals with a history of receiving therapeutic radiation are at increased risk. Exposure to mantle radiation as a treatment for

Hodgkin's disease increases the risk of thyroid cancer 16 times (Norton, Levin, & Jensen, 1993). Conversely, treatment of the thyroid with radioactive iodine is not associated with an increased risk of carcinoma. Papillary and follicular cancer have been linked to iodine deficiencies and autoimmune thyroid disease (Stanford & Evans, 1999).

Histology

Of all head and neck cancers, 85%–90% are squamous cell carcinomas (SCCs). SCC is most prevalent in the oral cavity, larynx, oropharynx, hypopharynx, nasopharynx, nasal cavity, and paranasalsinus. Other cancer types typical in these areas include sarcoma, malignant melanoma, lymphoma, and verrucous carcinoma.

Mucoepidermoid cancers account for 34% of all salivary gland malignancies. Development of mucoepidermoid malignancies occurs most often in the parotid gland. Adenoid cystic carcinoma ordinarily affects the submandibular gland and minor salivary glands. Adenocarcinoma, acinic cell carcinoma, and SCC are less common variants of salivary gland carcinomas (Ward & Levine, 1998).

Papillary and follicular carcinomas account for 75% and 10% of primary thyroid malignancies, respectively. A mixed type, papillary-follicular carcinoma occurs less frequently and behaves like papillary cancer. Medullary cancer of the thyroid is associated with an autosomal dominant trait. The types of medullary carcinoma that are inherited include familial medullary thyroid carcinoma and multiple endocrine neoplasia types 2a and 2b (Horsley & Fratkin, 1995).

Other primary malignancies of the thyroid include lymphoma, sarcoma, SCC, and anaplasia. Anaplastic thyroid cancer has the worst prognosis, with a two-year survival rate of zero. Disease that metastasizes to the thyroid from breast, lung, and kidney cancers and from melanoma have been described (Shaha, 1998; Stanford & Evans, 1999).

Patterns of Disease Progression

Cancers of the oral cavity, pharynx, and larynx first spread locally, with extension into surrounding structures. The lymph system gradually filters cancer cells, with resultant cervical lymphadenopathy. An enlarged lymph node is often the first identifying characteristic of head and neck cancer. The pattern of lymph node involvement may predict the anatomic location of an occult tumor.

Oral cavity malignancies metastasize most readily to the submandibular, submental, or upper cervical lymph nodes, whereas laryngeal and hypopharyngeal cancers metastasize to deep cervical lymph nodes along the midjugular, lower jugular, and peritracheal lymphatic chains (see Table 16-1). Perineural spread may occur along associated cranial nerves.

Disease of the nasal cavity and paranasalsinus often spreads to neighboring structures. Depending on the location of tumor development, the skull base, the orbits, the oral cavity, and the oropharynx may be invaded by tumor (Clayman et al., 1997).

Table 16-1. Distribution of Lymphatics and Cranial Nerve Involvement

Site	Lymph Nodes	Cranial Nerves	Notes About Metastasis
Oral cavity	Submandibular Submental Upper cervical	V, trigeminal XII, hypoglossal	Infrequent lymph node metastasis in lips, alveolar ridge, and hard palate. Aggressive, often bilateral lymph node involvement in floor of mouth, buccal mucosa, retromolar trigone, and oral tongue.
Oropharynx	Upper jugular Jugulodigastric Retropharyngeal	IX, glossopharyngeal X, vagus	
Nasopharynx	Bilateral cervical Posterior triangle Supraclavicular	II, optic III, oculomotor IV, trochlear VI, abducens IX, glossopharyngeal X, vagus XI, spinal accessory XII, hypoglossal	
Hypopharynx	Lower jugular Upper and middle jugular chain	IX, glossopharyngeal X, vagus	Rich lymphatics; cancer of the lower hypopharynx may metastasize to lower cervical chain, posterior cervical triangle.
Larynx	Prelaryngeal Pretracheal Jugulo-omohyoid Jugulodigastric	X, vagus Recurrent laryngeal nerve	Supraglottic: rich lymphatics, bilateral metastasis Glottic: scant lymphatic drainage, ipsilateral metastasis Subglottic: primary tumor rare
Nasal cavity Paranasal sinus	Submandibular Submaxillary Retropharyngeal Jugular	I, olfactory	
Salivary glands	Intraglandular Paraglandular Deep jugular	VII, facial (mandibular division) XII, hypoglossal	
Thyroid	Lymphatics accompanying arterial circulation	Recurrent laryngeal nerve	

Note. Based on information from Haggood, 1997; Schleper, 1989.

Involvement of the second division of the trigeminal nerve may be detected, and the patient may report sensation changes in the skin of the upper lip (Rassekh, 1998). Malignancies that are primary to the nasal cavity will metastasize to the submandibular lymph nodes. Tumors of the paranasal sinuses spread via lymphatic drainage to the submaxillary, retropharyngeal, and jugular lymph nodes (Haggood, 1997).

Patients with thyroid cancer usually present with a single, asymptomatic nodule that is noted during a routine clinical examination. Carcinoma of the thyroid may spread locally to surrounding cervical lymph nodes. A hard, fixed thyroid nodule associated with cervical lymphadenopathy is highly suggestive of a malignancy (Horsley & Fratkin, 1995).

A painless mass or swelling may be the first indication of salivary gland cancer. Nodal metastasis follows the intraglandular and paraglandular lymphatics to the deep jugular nodes (Haggood, 1997). Ward and Levine (1998) reported that facial weakness or palsy may occur if malignancy from the parotid gland invades the facial nerve (the facial nerve divides the parotid gland).

Distant metastasis of head and neck cancer most frequently involves the lungs. Other sites of metastasis may include mediastinal lymph nodes, the liver, or the brain (Shaha & Strong, 1995). Development of second primary tumors occurs at an annual rate of 3%–7% in individuals treated for cancers of the head and neck. Second primary tumor occurrence supports the concept of field cancerization. *Field cancerization* refers to chronic insult to the mucosal lining of the upper aerodigestive tract, with resultant cellular changes attributed to repeated carcinogenic exposure (Clayman et al., 1997).

Risk Factors

Personal Factors

Most head and neck cancers involving the upper aerodigestive tract occur in men in their fifth or sixth decade. The average age at diagnosis is 60–69 (Hoffman et al., 1998). Currently, men are twice as likely to develop malignancies of the upper aerodigestive tract than are women. In the 1950s, men were six times more likely to develop head and neck cancer than were women. The increase in the number of women smokers accounts for the difference. African Americans have a higher rate of cancer of the oral cavity and pharynx than do Whites, and African Americans' prognosis is typically poorer (Hoffman et al.). Individuals of Asian ancestry may be at increased risk for nasopharyngeal cancer because of genetic abnormalities and consumption of salted fish (Fee, 1998; Shaha & Strong, 1995).

Women are twice as likely to develop thyroid cancer as are men. Thyroid malignancies are known to affect individuals of all ages but generally are diagnosed in patients ages 25–65.

Individuals in lower socioeconomic levels are more likely to be afflicted with head and neck cancers than are their upper-class counterparts. A great majority of patients from lower socioeconomic groups present with advanced (stage III and stage IV) head and neck cancers. Men of divorced, widowed, or single status are more greatly affected by the disease than are married men.

Use of Tobacco, Marijuana, Alcohol, or Betel Nut

Tobacco in any form is the primary risk factor for cancers of the upper aerodigestive tract. Habitual use of cigarette, pipe, cigar, or smokeless tobacco has been proven to increase an individual's overall risk of cancer development. Tar from tobacco is a component of a number of cancer initiators, promoters, and co-carcinogens. Marijuana should be considered extremely carcinogenic because it contains four times more tar than cigarettes (Clayman et al., 1997). The risk of a cigarette smoker developing head and neck cancer is 2–18 times that of a person who never smoked. The risk of individuals who habitually smoke a pipe or cigars is 12 times higher than that of someone who never smoked. According to Nelson (1998), cigar use has increased 250% since 1993.

In the 1970s, smokeless tobacco was touted as the safe alternative to cigarettes, and its use increased. This increase may account for the increased incidence of oral cavity malignancies in individuals younger than 40. The National Cancer Advisory Board of the National Cancer Institute (NCI), which had recognized this risk in 1985, subsequently issued a resolution to control smokeless tobacco use. The surgeon general issued a report in 1986 concluding that the use of smokeless tobacco posed a significant health risk and should not be considered a safe alternative to cigarette smoking (U.S. Department of Health and Human Services, 1986). Reports by the U.S. Department of Health and Human Services (1990) supported allegations of a causal relationship between smokeless tobacco use and cancer development, specifically in the oral cavity.

Most people know that the risk of cancer decreases with each year after smoking cessation; however, ex-smokers will probably never be able to reduce their risk to the level of people who never smoked (Haggood, 1997).

The habit of reverse smoking (i.e., placing the lighted end of the cigarette in the mouth) is a common practice in developing countries and significantly increases the risk of cancer of the hard palate (Baden, 1987).

Excessive alcohol use is strongly correlated with cancers of the upper aerodigestive tract. Alcohol exposure damages the epithelial cells of the upper aerodigestive tract both independently and in combination with tobacco. A number of alcohol metabolites—specifically, acetaldehyde—have been proven to be carcinogenic in animal studies (Blot, 1992). Alcohol may act as a solvent, increasing the potency of other carcinogens. Alcohol also may be responsible for interrupting the delivery of necessary nutrients at a cellular level. Some researchers hypothesize that excessive abuse of alcohol may suppress immune function and block the breakdown of tobacco metabolites and other carcinogens in the liver. Of all the carcinogens studied, alcohol has the strongest association with oral cancer. In combination with tobacco, alcohol is responsible for 75% of all oral and pharyngeal cancers (Blot et al., 1988).

Betel nut chewing, popular in India, also is associated with an increased risk of oral cancer (Shaha & Strong, 1995).

Poor Nutrition

Poor dietary habits resulting in deficiencies of vitamins A, C, and E have been linked to cancer of the upper aerodigestive tract. Poor nutrition and alcoholism, both risk factors for head and neck malignancies, usually occur concurrently. Epidemiology and laboratory studies have led to the discovery that, on epithelial cells, vitamin A acts much like a hormone by promoting normal growth and cellular differentiation (Whelan, 1999). Foods rich in nitrosamines, such as salted fish, cured meats, and pickled vegetables, may promote tumor development in tissues of the nasopharynx (Xu, Shen, Jin, & Xu, 1991). High-fat diets that lack fruits and vegetables generally are thought to be a factor in cancer development (ACS, 2000).

Poor Oral Hygiene

Poor oral hygiene, ill-fitting dentures and dental prostheses, and sharp teeth have been suggested as risk factors for cancer of the oral cavity, but actual risk factors are unknown. Gorsky and Silverman (1984) found no correlation between denture use and oral cancer in 400 patients who were evaluated. Although some researchers have speculated that mouthwashes containing high concentrations of alcohol increase the risk of oral cancer, the evidence to date is inconclusive (Elmore & Horwitz, 1995).

Environmental and Occupational Factors

Exposure to asbestos, hydrocarbons, and radiochemicals may pose some risk in the development of head and neck cancer. Nasal and paranasal sinus cancers have been associated with exposure to chemicals, wood, leather, chromium, and radium (Rassekh, 1998). Wood dust has been associated with nasopharyngeal cancer. Some researchers have suggested that asbestos exposure promotes cancer of the larynx; however, this assertion remains controversial (Vokes et al., 1993).

Ionizing and ultraviolet radiation also are factors in malignancy promotion. Studies of atomic bomb survivors and patients receiving therapeutic radiation for cancer or other diseases have identified high-dose radiation as carcinogenic. The thyroid gland is one of the sites most commonly affected by ionizing radiation exposure (ACS, 2000). Chronic, unprotected exposure to sunlight is almost solely responsible for the development of lip cancer (Pogoda & Preston-Martin, 1996).

The concept that viruses play a role in malignancy development is becoming widely accepted. In patients with nasopharyngeal cancer, the immunoglobulin G (IgG) and IgA antibody titers for EBV reveal levels of IgG and IgA that are higher than those found in the general population. Antibody titers have been used as tumor markers to determine high-risk individuals in Asia. Disease recurrence following definitive treatment also may be predicted according to titer levels (Shaha & Strong, 1995; Vokes et al., 1993). Identifying the DNA of EBV in an occult neck mass serves as confirmation of a nasopharyngeal primary tumor (Feinmesser et al., 1992). The DNA of the human papilloma virus (HPV) has been isolated in tumors throughout the upper aerodigestive tract. HPV most commonly is found in tumors of the tonsils. Well known as precursors to cervical cancer, the high-risk strains—16, 18, 33, and 31—are associated with cancers of the head and neck. Interestingly, women with a history of carcinoma in situ or invasive cervical cancer have a risk of head and neck cancer that is two to four times as high as that of women without a history of cervical cancer (Gillison, Koch, & Shah, 1999). Some researchers hypothesize that the herpes simplex virus may have a mutagenic effect on epithelial cells. Elevated herpes antibody titers have been identified in patients with cancers of the head or neck (Trizna & Schantz, 1992).

Genetic Predisposition

Bloom's syndrome, an autosomal recessive growth disorder, is associated with a high rate of malignant neoplasms that appear in young people. The average age of a patient at malignancy diagnosis is 25 (Wong & Hashisaki, 1996). Growth retardation, short stature, facial erythema, skin sensitivities, and infertility characterize Bloom's syndrome (Berkower & Biller, 1988).

Li-Fraumeni syndrome is an autosomal dominant disorder associated with a mutation of the p53 tumor suppressor gene. The result is the early onset of sarcomas and breast, laryngeal, and lung carcinomas (Trizna & Schantz, 1992).

In the absence of autosomal recessive or dominant traits that stimulate cancer development, genetic instability, independently or in combination with tobacco or alcohol, is probably a force that drives head and neck cancers. Mutagen-induced chromosomal fragility has been identified as an independent risk factor for head and neck malignancies (Schantz, Hsu, Ainslie, & Moser, 1989). Cytogenic alterations, resulting in chromosomal loss or gain, have been identified in head and neck tumors. Allelic loss involving the p53 tumor suppressor gene, with resultant loss of protective activity, may spur the growth of abnormal cells. Such mutations have been suggested as an explanation for the development of head and neck malignancies in nonsmokers and nondrinkers (Schantz & Ostroff, 1997).

Interpretation of Risk Data

When instituting prevention and early-detection strategies directed at head and neck malignancies, healthcare providers should direct their efforts to populations at greatest risk. Those who habitually use tobacco and alcohol are at greatest risk of head and neck cancers. Reducing tobacco and alcohol use undoubtedly would significantly reduce morbidity and mortality from these cancers.

A comprehensive patient history may direct healthcare providers' attention to other, less obvious, factors posing risk. Healthcare professionals should be alert to a history that includes chronic environmental or occupational exposure to chemicals, therapeutic ionizing radiation, actinic radiation, or a family history of cancer. Ancestry and immigrant status should prompt healthcare professionals to find out if the patient practices culture-linked activities that are potentially harmful—such as reverse smoking, betel-nut chewing, or frequent consumption of salted fish—and provide information that could help the patient to abandon unhealthful practices.

Signs and Symptoms

ACS has identified seven warning signs of cancer. Four of these, alone or in combination, may indicate cancer of the head and neck: dysphagia, chronic ulceration, persistent hoarseness, or a lump in the neck (Shaha & Strong, 1995). Figure 16-5 lists other symptoms, which often are site specific.

Late signs relative to all sites include unexplained weight loss, pain relating to referred otalgia, headache or facial discomfort, and cranial nerve paralysis per-

Figure 16-5. Common Signs and Symptoms of Head and Neck Cancer by Site

Nasal Cavity/Para-nasal sinus
- Symptoms of chronic sinusitis
- Epistaxis
- Nasal obstruction
- Numbness or tingling, upper lip
- Toothache
- Increased lacrimation
- Rhinorrhea
- Diplopia
- Proptosis

Salivary Gland
- Painless swelling
- Rapidly growing, painless mass
- Facial asymmetry
- Otalgia

Thyroid Gland
- Asymptomatic nodule
- Cystic nodules
- Cervical lymphadenopathy
- Neck pain
- Hoarseness
- Dysphagia
- Dyspnea

Oral Cavity
- Painful ulceration
- Slurred speech
- Bleeding in oral cavity
- Exophytic mass
- Difficulty chewing
- Painful swelling in jaw or mouth
- Trismus[a]

Oropharynx
- Dysphagia
- Change in voice
- Airway obstruction[a]
- Stridor

Nasopharynx
- Unilateral otitis media
- Nasal obstruction
- Epistaxis
- Double vision
- Change in visual acuity
- Hearing loss
- Tinnitus
- Loss of smell

Larynx
- Hoarseness
- Change in voice
- Dysphagia
- Airway obstruction[a]
- Stridor

Hypopharynx
- Odynophagia
- Dysphagia
- Referred otalgia
- Globus sensation
- Hoarseness[a]

[a] Symptom of head and neck cancer in a late stage.
Note. Based on information from Haggood, 1997.

taining to the site of cancer involvement (Shaha & Strong, 1995). In regard to salivary gland cancer, pain at the time of diagnosis usually signifies a poor prognosis. Facial weakness or palsy indicates facial nerve involvement that is common with parotid gland malignancies (Ward & Levine, 1998).

Precursor Lesions

Oral leukoplakia and erythroplasia are known premalignancies of the oral cavity and oropharynx. Leukoplakia is a white or gray plaque or thickened, irregular lesion found in the mucosa that does not scrape off. Erythroplasia is a velvety red lesion. Erythroleukoplakia of the oropharynx consists of lesions with a characteristic speckled pattern. This type of lesion usually is white, with areas of bright-red velvety plaques within an irregular border (NCI, 1994).

Oral leukoplakia is six times more prevalent in smokers than nonsmokers. The lesions often are multifocal, supporting the theory of field cancerization as described by Sporn and Lippman (1997). Leukoplakia transforms into malignancy at a rate of 5%. Cancer develops in 17.5%–36% of people with erythroplakia. The rate of spontaneous regression of leukoplakia and erythroplakia is 30%–40% and 5%, respectively. Cessation of tobacco use, within one year, results in regression or complete resolution in 75% of leukoplasia cases (Lippman, 1997).

Primary Prevention

Lifestyle Modification

The majority of cancers involving the upper aerodigestive tract are avoidable. Primary prevention strategies can significantly affect morbidity and mortality associated with the disease. Tobacco avoidance is the best defense. Healthcare professionals should implement interventions about tobacco early and often. Children, teenagers, and young adults must recognize the risk of tobacco use. The goal in this age group is tobacco avoidance. In addition, the public must recognize smokeless tobacco, cigars, and pipe smoking as hazards rather than safe alternatives to cigarettes. Healthcare professionals must learn to identify high-risk individuals and develop ways to educate them about their risk of developing head and neck cancer, the signs and symptoms of the disease, risk-reducing behaviors, and the importance of early detection.

ACS recommends that a patient's history of tobacco use be assessed and documented at each healthcare visit. ACS reminds physicians, nurse practitioners, and staff nurses to *ask* about tobacco use, *advise* patients to quit, *assist* patients in quitting, and *arrange* follow-up (Shaha & Strong, 1995). Nicotine replacement therapy combined with behavioral therapy may result in successful tobacco cessation. No compelling evidence supports the efficacy of nicotine replacement in the absence of professional support and guidance, however (Hughes & Miller, 1984).

Healthcare providers also should assess patients' alcohol consumption. A number of screening questionnaires are available to help healthcare providers to identify individuals at high risk for substance abuse: the Alcohol Use Disorders Identification Test, the Michigan Alcoholism Screening Test, the Drug Abuse Screening Test, and the CAGE questionnaire (U.S. Department of Health and Human Services, 1998). Referral to a chemical dependency program is warranted in all cases of suspected alcohol addiction or chronic abuse.

Nutrition counseling is of the utmost importance for high-risk individuals because chronic alcohol use has been associated with malnutrition. Research has shown that deficiencies of vitamins A, C, and E contribute to malignancy formation. ACS (2000) recommends a diet low in fat and nitrosamines that includes five fruits and vegetables a day. According to Winn et al. (1984), adequate fruit and vegetable intake may decrease the risk of oral and pharyngeal cancer by 30%–50%.

Chemopreventive Strategies

Chemoprevention is the use of pharmaceutical agents to reverse, suppress, or prevent premalignant transformation and cancer development in high-risk individuals. The belief that chemical agents may prevent cancer involves the concept of field cancerization or "multistep" carcinogenesis (Sporn & Lippman, 1997). Cancer progression in the upper aerodigestive tract serves as an excellent model of both concepts because the mucosa in the tract are continually exposed to carcinogens.

Researchers are studying numerous agents to determine their efficacy in preventing the transformation of oral leukoplakia into cancer and the occurrence of second primary tumors. Retinoids, natural and synthetic derivatives of vitamin A, are the most frequently studied class of chemopreventives in regard to head and neck cancer. 9-*cis*-retinoic acid (9-cRA) and 13-*cis*-retinoic acid (13-cRA) are natural compounds, and researchers are evaluating their effect on the upper aerodigestive tract. Hong et al. (1986) established that 13-cRA in high doses resulted in a clinical regression of oral leukoplakia in 67% of patients (16 of 24) versus 10% of patients (2 of 20) on placebo. The study, however, was limited because of substantial 13-cRA toxicity and the relapse of more than 50% of participants within the second or third month after therapy. A second clinical trial tested 13-cRA at lower doses. Patients were randomized to retinoid therapy, and those who received 13-cRA received a high dose for three months. Nine months of maintenance therapy with low-dose 13-cRA or beta-carotene followed. The results were positive in that only 8% of patients (2 of 24) on 13-cRA experienced a relapse. Fifty-five percent of patients (16 of 29) who received beta-carotene relapsed (Lippman et al., 1993). Similar studies have revealed that retinoids given to patients following definitive treatment for aerodigestive tract cancer were effective in decreasing the occurrence of second primary tumors (Lippman, 1997).

Currently, the U.S. Food and Drug Administration approves no single chemopreventive agent for the prevention of head and neck cancer. A number of promising agents are on the horizon, however, and clinical research regarding chemoprevention continues to escalate. Although chemopreventive agents will not be "magic pills" for preventing and curing cancer, healthcare providers and the lay public will need to recognize them as complements to current and future prevention strategies.

Secondary Prevention and Early Detection
Efficacy of Screening

Unfortunately, studies show that screening for head and neck cancer does not have a significant impact on survival. Population-based community screenings identify only a small number of premalignancies or malignancies (Clayman, Chamberlain, Lee, Lippman, & Hong, 1995; Prout, Sidari, Witzburg, Grillone, & Vaughan, 1997). Even screening in high-risk populations produces a low yield of suspicious lesions. Despite these facts, experts in the field do encourage healthcare providers to conduct routine screening, especially in high-risk patients (Bonner, 1998; Schantz & Ostroff, 1997). The location of the oral cavity makes the mouth amenable to screening. ACS endorses a comprehensive physical examination that includes a thorough oral examination every three years for individuals older than age 20 and annually for individuals older than age 40 (Shaha & Strong, 1995).

The U.S. Preventive Services Task Force neither supports nor opposes routine oral examinations for the detection of cancer or premalignancies. Healthcare providers, however, are encouraged to incorporate the oral examination into practice when assessing patients with a history of tobacco use. The task force does support annual dental examinations, especially in individuals older than age 65 (U.S. Department of Health and Human Services, 1998).

Screening Techniques

No nationally recognized screening recommendations relative to head and neck sites exist. This chapter will suggest techniques for taking a history and conducting a physical examination designed to detect head and neck cancers.

Taking a History

Before each head and neck examination, ask the patient about current and past tobacco and alcohol use. It is important to document the type of tobacco used and the duration of exposure. If the patient is currently a smoker, learn about the patient's attempts at smoking cessation and identify the variables that negatively affected the attempts (Campbell, 1998). Record the individual's occupation. A history suggesting exposure to potentially carcinogenic chemicals may increase the risk of head and neck cancer. Ask if the patient has a history of therapeutic radiation and document the patient's family history of cancer, paying particular attention to multiple cancer occurrence in the maternal or paternal line. Early onset of multiple cancers within a family may suggest a genetic predisposition to malignancy development (Muirhead, 2000). If genetic susceptibility is suspected, genetic counseling may be considered.

A crucial element of the history is the review of head and neck symptomatology (White & Spitz, 1993). As Figure 16-5 shows, the symptoms associated with head and neck cancer may include, but are not limited to, diplopia, blurred vision, ptosis, proptosis, change in visual acuity, otalgia, tinnitus, dysphagia, odynophagia, hoarseness, globus sensation, numbness or tingling of the face, or enlarged lymph or salivary glands.

Conducting an Examination

Face, scalp, and neck: Thorough inspection of the skin of the scalp, face, and neck is the starting point of head and neck evaluation. Most nonmelanoma skin cancers develop above the neck. Palpate the facial skin and parotid glands, with the purpose of identifying masses or lesions. Assess the cranium for normalcy of shape and size. Inspect the face for symmetry.

Ears: Otoscopic examination of the ears may reveal lesions of the external auditory canal or bulging of the tympanic membrane. Abnormalities of the middle ear may signify involvement of the eustachian tubes.

Nose: To allow examination of the nasal cavities, ask the patient to sit upright, raise the chin, and flare the nostrils, as if he or she were sniffing. Insert the nasal speculum in each naris and study the mucosa of the anterior nasal cavity and septum (Foreman & Callender, 1998). Look for and document ulcerative areas and polyps.

Oral cavity: Begin with a general survey of the lips. Note skin changes, the presence of lesions, and cracking.

Prior to inspecting the oral cavity, ask the patient to remove dentures or other dental appliances. Use adequate lighting while looking inside the mouth. Develop a systematic method of performing the mouth exam and repeat it for each patient to minimize the chance of missing abnormalities. Use a tongue blade to hold the cheek away from the gums and retract the lips.

Begin by observing the condition of the teeth. Inspect the gingivae for bleeding, discoloration, swelling, or nodular areas. Ask the patient to "open wide" so that all surfaces of the buccal mucosa can be examined. Normal buccal mucosa is pink, moist, and without evidence of lesions. White, plaquelike lesions may represent oral leukoplakia. SCC may appear as an indurated lesion that is erythemic. Inspect the palate, the tongue, and the floor of the mouth for suspicious lesions, swellings, nodules, induration, or ulcerations. The U-shaped area involving the floor of the mouth is particularly susceptible to tumor formation (Schleper, 1989). To fully evaluate the tongue, ask the patient to position the tip of the tongue on the roof of the mouth and to move it to the right or left lateral buccal mucosa. Finally, depress the tongue with a tongue blade to inspect the posterior pharynx for signs of asymmetry or masses.

Following visual inspection of the oral cavity and posterior pharynx, don gloves to perform bimanual palpation of the floor of the mouth. Place one finger under the tongue while placing the other hand under the jaw for stabilization. Palpate the floor of the mouth. This allows assessment of the submandibular, sublingual, and minor salivary glands. To palpate the tongue, ask the patient to extend the tongue beyond the lips, then hold the tip of the tongue with a piece of gauze and palpate the tongue with the free hand (U.S. Department of Health and Human Services, 1998). Thickened areas and masses identified during the bimanual examination should be further evaluated.

Examining each component of the pharynx and larynx means using a dental mirror to get an indirect view of the areas or conducting an endoscopic evaluation. Both techniques require special training, and the extent of the head and neck assessment may be limited by the training and resources available. If the screening reveals suspicious symptoms or unexplained abnormalities, the patient should be referred to an otolaryngologist or head and neck surgeon. Panendoscopy (laryngoscopy, bronchoscopy, and esophagoscopy) is used routinely to assess abnormalities and obtain tissue biopsies of suspicious areas along the upper aerodigestive tract.

Neck: Inspect the neck for symmetry and tracheal deviation. Using the fingers, explore the anterior, posterior, and supraclavicular areas to assess the lymph nodes. Figure 16-6 shows the node locations. To palpate the anterior deep cervical chain, place both hands on either side of the trachea. Using circular motions, apply gentle pressure to find and assess prominent nodes or masses. Palpate the submental lymph nodes with the fingertips of one hand. Using similar circular motions and pressure, survey the posterior, cervical, and supraclavicular lymph nodes. Document enlarged lymph nodes or neck masses, citing the size, consistency, mobility, and location of the node. Ask the patient how long the enlargement or mass has existed.

To palpate the thyroid gland, stand behind the patient. Ask the patient to sit upright and flex the head forward slightly, relaxing the neck muscles. Place the fingertips of the right hand on the right lobe of the thyroid while the left hand gently displaces the trachea slightly to the right. Press gently on the right lobe, ask the patient to swallow, and assess the lobe as it ascends in the neck. Repeat on the left side. Document enlargement or nodularity of the thyroid gland.

Figure 16-6. Lymph Nodes of the Head and Neck

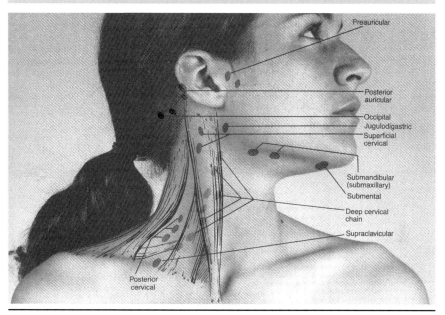

Note. From "Head and Neck, Including Lymphatics" (p. 281) by M.M. Andrews and J. Keithly in C. Jarvis (Ed.), *Physical Examination and Health Assessment,* 1992, Philadelphia: W.B. Saunders. Copyright 1992 by W.B. Saunders. Reprinted with permission.

Cranial nerves: Assess the cranial nerves systematically throughout the head and neck examination or at the close of the assessment. Knowledge of each cranial nerve's function and associated assessment technique is required to identify abnormalities. Table 16-2 lists the cranial nerves and tells how to assess each one.

Following Up on an Examination

Address any suspicious findings in a timely manner by ensuring that the patient is referred to the appropriate specialist. Experts agree that referral to an otolaryngologist is necessary for any patient with hoarseness persisting for longer than two weeks (Dettelbach, Eibling, & Johnson, 1994; Garrett & Ossoff, 1999; Hoare, Thomson, & Proops, 1993). Studies have shown that early endoscopic examination of patients complaining of hoarseness promotes accurate diagnosis and expedites treatment in the presence or absence of malignancy.

If a premalignant lesion of the oral cavity is suspected, biopsy is indicated. McGuirt (1999) recommended that a neck mass presenting in anyone older than age 40 should be considered a malignancy until proven otherwise. Antibiotic trials for lymphadenopathy should not exceed two weeks.

At the close of any head and neck examination, tell the patient about the importance of annual screening. Reinforcing the purpose of the examination may motivate the patient to follow up on a routine basis. If histologic tests confirm the presence of oral leukoplakia or erythroplakia, the patient must follow up with

---

Table 16-2. Cranial Nerves

Cranial Nerve	Relates to	Assessment
I, olfactory	Sense of smell	Perform "sniff" test (test olfactory capabilities by assessing patient's ability to recognize common scents [e.g., peppermint extract]).
II, optic	Vision	Test visual acuity and fields of vision, check pupils.
III, oculomotor	Pupillary constriction, eye opening, extraocular movement	Check pupils for size, reactivity, accommodation. Check eye movement (six cardinal gazes). Check for ptosis.
IV, trochlear	Downward and inward motion of the eye	Check eye movement (six cardinal gazes).
V, trigeminal (three divisions: ophthalmic, maxillary, and mandibular)	*Motor functions:* temporal and masseter muscles, lateral movement of the jaw *Sensory functions:* facial sensation	*Motor functions:* Palpate temporal and masseter muscles; note strength. *Sensory functions:* Ask patient to close eyes; check sensation on each side of the forehead, cheeks, and jaw by using sharp and dull ends of a safety pin. Check perception of light touch by using a cottonball.
VI, abducens	Lateral movement of the eye	Check eye movement (six cardinal gazes).
VII, facial	*Motor functions:* facial movement *Sensory functions:* Taste on anterior two-thirds of the tongue	Inspect face for symmetry. Inspect frown, smile, eye closure, and puffed cheeks.
VIII, acoustic (cochlear division affects hearing; vestibular division affects balance)	Hearing and balance	Assess hearing.
IX, glossopharyngeal	*Motor functions:* pharynx *Sensory functions:* posterior eardrum and ear canal, pharynx, and posterior tongue	Assess voice quality. Inspect pharynx, soft-palate movement. Check gag reflex.
X, vagus	*Motor functions:* palate, pharynx, and larynx *Sensory functions:* pharynx and larynx	See IX.
XI, spinal accessory	Movement of the sternocleidomastoid muscle and superior portion of the trapezius	Inspect trapezius muscles. Use both hands to check bilateral shoulder shrug.
XII, hypoglossal	Movement of the tongue	Inspect tongue. Assess speech quality.

Note. Based on information from Bates et al., 1995.

testing every three to four months. Referral to a chemoprevention clinical trial may be appropriate. Encourage biannual dental examinations, which complement medical evaluation. Encourage tobacco cessation and the prudent use of alcohol, if any, and reinforce the encouragement frequently.

Nursing Challenges

Because nurses are clinicians, educators, advocates, and risk counselors, they play an important role in the prevention of cancer of the upper aerodigestive tract, nasal cavity and sinuses, salivary glands, and thyroid. Nurses can encourage a healthful lifestyle and serve as role models. For nurses, the primary challenge lies in catalyzing behavior modification, often the most difficult pill a patient has to swallow. Patients must realize the detrimental effects of certain behaviors before they can be self-motivated to change their lifestyle. Creative motivational strategies—such as smoking-cessation programs based in the community, hospital, or workplace—may help smokers to quit. Individuals struggling with alcohol abuse may need guidance to establish healthful coping mechanisms and develop self-esteem. Every patient interaction should be an opportunity to provide information about cancer risk reduction. Continuity of health care can be achieved by reinforcing the information at future appointments and encouraging annual cancer screening. Table 16-3 lists resources that may help nurses to develop creative motivational strategies and help to provide patients with information they need.

The National Oral Cancer Awareness Program (NOCAP) was established to help to nurses identify individuals at increased risk and provide appropriate information regarding risk reduction (Bonner, 1998). The goals of the program—which is supported by a number of groups in various disciplines with an interest in reducing the incidence of oral cancer—are to assemble a database of oral cancer programs and projects, increase public awareness of oral cancer, increase healthcare professionals' awareness of oral cancer, screen high-risk populations within the community, and develop a national support group for patients with oral cancer and their families. Educational opportunities for healthcare professionals and the lay public available through NOCAP may help in the promotion and early detection of cancer of the upper aerodigestive tract. Information about NOCAP is available on the Internet at www.oralcancer.org.

Supporting open access to health care is an ongoing challenge for nurses. Nurses should develop and promote preventive health services for all individuals, regardless of race and socioeconomic level.

Nurse-researchers can address the challenge of developing creative screening opportunities for use in communities. Although reports suggest that screening specifically for head and neck cancers may not be effective (Clayman et al., 1995; Prout et al., 1997), comprehensive cancer screening in communities may be. A worthy research goal could be to develop an effective multidisciplinary screening approach that increases early detection of all types of cancer but—because it is a "one-stop" screening effort—uses relatively few human and financial resources.

Table 16-3. Internet Resources Regarding Head and Neck Cancer

Site Name	Sponsoring Organization	Content
Support for People With Oral and Head and Neck Cancer www.spohnc.org	Support for People With Oral and Head and Neck Cancer (a patient-directed self-help organization)	Provides information and support to people with head and neck cancer
Oral Cancer Information Center www.oralcancer.org	Oral Cancer Information Center	Provides information about oral cancer, clinical trials, and research. Sells educational materials for use by healthcare professionals. May provide, to qualifying patients, free samples of nonprescription products.
Ear Nose and Throat Information www.sinuscarecenter.com	Sinus Care Center of Jackson (a private practice in Flowood, MS)	Provides general information about the ear, nose, and throat as well as specific information about smoking and cancer
OncoLink www.cancer.med.upenn.edu/ disease/headneck	University of Pennsylvania Cancer Center	Provides general information about head and neck cancers, symptom management, and psychosocial support. Presents information about clinical trials and research, financial issues, and resources. Publishes book reviews and meeting announcements.
American Academy of Otolaryngology—Head and Neck Surgery www.aaohns.org	American Academy of Otolaryngology—Head and Neck Surgery is a professional organization of physicians and other healthcare providers. (AAO-HNS)	Provides general information for patients and healthcare providers about the ears, nose, and throat and related structures of the head and neck.
Society of Otorhinolaryngology and Head-Neck Nurses www.sohnnurse.com	Society of Otorhinolaryngology and Head-Neck Nurses (SOHN) is a professional nursing organization whose members specialize in ear, nose, throat, and head and neck surgery patient care.	Provides information for professionals about ear, nose, throat and head/neck patient management.

Conclusion

Although relatively rare, cancers of the head and neck can be devastating—both physically and emotionally. A plethora of research is on the horizon with the purpose of identifying chemical compounds that will prevent head and neck cancer. The viral component of cancer development is being evaluated, and it is not unrealistic to consider a future in which a vaccine will be able to help prevent head and neck malignancies. Biomarkers may help to identify high-risk populations. While continually supporting these efforts, nurses should strive to educate patients, evaluate risk, support patients diagnosed with cancer, and create new screening opportunities.

References

American Cancer Society. (2000). *Cancer facts and figures, 2000.* Atlanta: Author.

Baden, D. (1987). Prevention of cancer of the oral cavity and pharynx. *CA: A Cancer Journal for Clinicians, 37,* 49–59.

Bates, B., Bickley, L.S., & Hoekelman, R.A. (1995). *A guide to physical examination and history taking* (6th ed.). Philadelphia: J.B. Lippincott.

Berkower, A.S., & Biller, H.F. (1988). Head and neck cancer associated with Bloom's syndrome. *Laryngoscope, 98,* 746–748.

Blot, W.J. (1992). Alcohol and cancer. *Cancer Research, 52*(Suppl. 7), 2119–2123.

Blot, W.J., McLauglin, J.K., Winn, D.M., Austin, D.F., Greenberg, R.S., Preston-Martin, S., Bernstein, L., Schoenberg, J., Stemhagen, A., & Fraumeni, J.F. (1988). Smoking and drinking in relation to oral and pharyngeal cancer. *Cancer Research, 48,* 3282–3287.

Bonner, P., (1998). The national oral cancer awareness program. *ORL-Head and Neck Nursing, 16*(2), 15–21.

Campbell, B. (1998). History, physical exam and endoscopic evaluation. In L.G. Close, D.L. Larson, & J.P. Shah (Eds.), *Essentials of head and neck oncology* (pp. 49–58). New York: Thieme.

Clayman, G.L., Chamberlain, R.M., Lee, J.J., Lippman, S.M., & Hong, W.K. (1995). Screening at a health fair to identify subjects for an oral leukoplakia chemoprevention trial. *Journal of Cancer Education, 10*(2), 88–90.

Clayman, G.L., Lippman, S.M., Laramore, G.E., & Hong, W.K. (1997). Head and neck cancer. In J.F. Holland, R.C. Bast, D.L. Morton, E. Frei, III, D.W. Kufe, & R.R. Weichselbaum (Eds.), *Cancer medicine* (pp. 1645–1710). Baltimore: Williams & Wilkins.

Dettelbach, M., Eibling, D.E., & Johnson, J.T. (1994). Hoarseness. *Postgraduate Medicine, 95,* 143–162.

Elmore, J.G., & Horwitz, R.I. (1995). Oral cancer and mouthwash use: Evaluation of the epidemiologic evidence. *Otolaryngology Head and Neck Surgery, 113,* 253–261.

Fee, W.E. (1998). Nasopharynx. In L.G. Close, D.L. Larson & J.P. Shah (Eds.), *Essentials of head and neck oncology* (pp. 205–211). New York: Thieme.

Feinmesser, R., Miyazaki, I., Cheung, R., Freeman, J.L., Noyek, A.M., & Dosh, H.M. (1992). Diagnosis of nasopharyngeal cancer by DNA amplification of tissue by fine-needle aspiration. *New England Journal of Medicine, 326,* 17–21.

Foreman, D.S., Callender, D.L. (1998). Head and neck cancer. In K.L. Boyer, M.B. Ford, A.F. Jodkins, & B. Levin (Eds.), *Primary care oncology* (pp. 41–57). Philadelphia: W.B. Saunders.

Garrett, C.G., & Ossoff, R.H. (1999). Hoarseness. *Medical Clinics of North America, 83*(1), 115–123.

Gillison, M.L., Koch, W.M., & Shah, K.V. (1999). Human papillomavirus in head and neck squamous cell carcinoma: Are some head and neck cancers a sexually transmitted disease? *Current Opinion in Oncology, 11*(3), 191–199.

Gleich, L., & Gluckman, J.L. (1998). Hypopharynx and cervical esophagus. In L.G. Close, D.L. Larson, & J. P. Shah (Eds.), *Essentials of head and neck oncology* (pp. 211–223). New York: Thieme.

Gorsky, M., & Silverman, Jr., S. (1984). Denture wearing and oral cancer. *Journal of Prosthetic Dentistry, 52*, 164–170.

Haggood, A.S. (1997). Head and neck cancers. In S.E. Otto (Ed.), *Oncology nursing* (3rd ed.) (pp. 227–267). St. Louis, MO: Mosby.

Hoare, T.J., Thomson, H.G., & Proops, D.W. (1993). Detection of laryngeal cancer—The case for early specialist assessment. *Journal of the Royal Society of Medicine, 86*, 548–549.

Hoffman, H.T., Karnell, L.H, Funk, G.F., Robinson, R.A., & Menck, H.R. (1998). The National Cancer Database report on cancer of the head and neck. *Archives of Otolaryngology—Head and Neck Surgery, 124*, 951–962.

Hong, W.K., Endicott, J., Itri, L.M., Wilhelm, D., Batsakis, J.G., Bell, R., Fofonoff, S., Byers, R., Atkinson, E.N., Vaughan, C., Toth, B.B., Kramer, A., Dimery, I.W., Skipper, P., & Strong, S. (1986). 13-*cis*-retinoic acid in the treatment of oral leukoplakia. *New England Journal of Medicine, 315*, 1501–1505.

Horsley, III, J.S., & Fratkin, M.J. (1995). Cancer of the thyroid and parathyroid glands. In G.P. Murphy, W. Lawrence, Jr., & R.E. Lenhard, Jr. (Eds.), *American Cancer Society textbook of clinical oncology* (2nd ed.) (pp. 355–377). Atlanta: American Cancer Society.

Hughes, J.R., & Miller, S.A. (1984). Nicotine gum to help stop smoking. *JAMA, 252*, 2855–2858.

Lippman, S.M. (1997). Head and neck chemoprevention: Recent advances. *Cancer Control, 4*(2), 128–135.

Lippman, S.M., Batsakis, J.G., Toth, B.B., Weber, R.S., Lee, J.J., Martin, J.W., Hays, G.L., Goepfert, H., & Hong, W.K. (1993). Comparison of low-dose isotretinoin with beta-carotene to prevent oral carcinogenesis. *New England Journal of Medicine, 328*, 15–20.

Mashberg, A., & Barsa, P. (1984). Screening for oral and oropharyngeal squamous carcinomas. *CA: A Cancer Journal for Clinicians, 34*, 262–268.

McGuirt, W.F. (1999). The neck mass. *Medical Clinics of North America, 83*, 219–234.

Muirhead, G. (2000). Genetic testing for cancer. *Patient Care for the Nurse Practitioner, 3*(2), 46–60.

National Cancer Institute. (1994). *Tobacco effects in the mouth* (Publication 94-3330). Washington, DC: U.S. Government Printing Office.

Nelson, N.J. (1998). "Big smoke" has big risks: Daily cigar use causes cancer, heart disease. *Journal of the National Cancer Institute, 90*, 562–564.

Norton, J.A., Levin, B., & Jensen, R.T. (1993). Cancer of the endocrine system. In V.T. DeVita, S. Hellman, & S.A. Rosenberg (Eds.), *Cancer: Principles and practice of oncology* (2nd ed.) (pp. 1333–1435). Philadelphia: J.B. Lippincott.

Pogoda, J.M., & Preston-Martin, S. (1996). Solar radiation, lip protection and lip cancer rise in Los Angeles County women. *Cancer Causes and Control, 7*, 458–463.

Prout, M.N., Sidari, J.N., Witzburg, R.A., Grillone, G.A., & Vaughan, C.W. (1997). Head and neck cancer screening among 4611 tobacco users older than forty years. *Otolaryngology—Head and Neck Surgery, 116*, 201–208.

Rassekh, C.H. (1998). Nose and paranasal sinus. In L.G. Close, D.L. Larson, & J.P. Shah (Eds.), *Essentials of head and neck oncology* (pp. 124–134). New York: Thieme.

Schantz, S.P., Hsu, T.C., Ainslie, N., & Moser, R.P. (1989). Young adults with head and neck cancer express increased susceptibility to mutagen-induced chromosome damage. *JAMA, 262*, 3313–3315.

Schantz, S.P., & Ostroff, J.S. (1997). Novel approaches to the prevention of head and neck cancer. *Proceedings of the Society for Experimental Biology and Medicine, 216*, 275–282.

Schleper, J.R. (1989). Prevention, detection, and diagnosis of head and neck cancers. *Seminars in Oncology Nursing, 5*, 139–149.

Shaha, A.R. (1998). Thyroid. In L.G. Close, D.L. Larson, & J.P. Shah (Eds.), *Essentials of head and neck oncology* (pp. 124–134). New York: Thieme.

Shaha, A.R., & Strong, E.W. (1995). Cancer of the head and neck. In G.P. Murphy, W. Lawrence, Jr., & R.E. Lenhard, Jr. (Eds.), *American Cancer Society textbook of clinical oncology* (2nd ed.) (pp. 355–377). Atlanta: American Cancer Society.

Shugars, D.C., & Patton, L.L. (1997). Detecting, diagnosing and preventing oral cancer. *Nurse Practitioner, 22*(6), 105–129.

Spaulding, C.A., Hahn, S.S., & Constable, W.C. (1987). The effectiveness of treatment of lymph nodes in cancer of the pyriform sinus and supraglottis. *International Journal of Radiation Oncology, Biology and Physics, 13*, 963–968.

Sporn, M.B., & Lippman, S.M. (1997). Chemoprevention of cancer. In J.F. Holland, E. Frei, R.C. Bast, Jr., D.L. Morton, E. Frei III, D.W. Kufe, & R.R. Weichselbaum (Eds.), *Cancer medicine* (pp. 1645–1710). Baltimore: Williams & Wilkins.

Stanford, P.A., & Evans, D.B. (1999). Endocrine cancer: The thyroid, parathyroid, adrenal glands, and pancreas. In K.L. Boyer, M.B. Ford, A.F. Jodkins, & B. Levin (Eds.), *Primary care oncology* (pp. 98–124). Philadelphia: W.B. Saunders.

Trizna, Z., & Schantz, S.P. (1992). Hereditary and environmental factors associated with risk and progression of head and neck cancer. *Otolaryngologic Clinics of North America, 25*, 1089–1103.

U.S. Department of Health and Human Services. (1986). *The health consequences of using smokeless tobacco: A report of the advisory committee to the surgeon general* (Publication NIH 86-2874) (pp. 33–94). Rockville, MD: Author.

U.S. Department of Health and Human Services. (1990). *The health benefits of smoking cessation* (Publication CDC 90-8416). Rockville, MD: Author.

U.S. Department of Health and Human Services. (1998). *Clinician's handbook of preventive services* (U.S. Government Printing Office Publication 1998-433-082) (2nd ed.) (pp. 201–221). Washington, DC: Author.

Vokes, E.E., Weichselbaum, R.R., Lippman, S.M., & Hong, W.K. (1993) Head and neck cancer. *New England Journal of Medicine, 328*, 184–194.

Ward, M.J., & Levine, P.A. (1998). Salivary gland tumors. In L.G. Close, D.L. Larson, & J.P. Shah (Eds.), *Essentials of head and neck oncology* (pp. 146–158). New York: Thieme.

Whelan, P. (1999). Retinoids in chemoprevention. *European Urology, 35*, 424–428.

White, L.N., & Spitz, M.R. (1993). Cancer risk and early detection assessment. *Seminars in Oncology Nursing, 9*, 188–197.

Winn, D.M., Ziegler, R.G., Pickle, L.W., Gridley, G., Blot, W.J., & Hoover, R.N. (1984). Diet in the etiology of oral and pharyngeal cancer among women from the southern United States. *Cancer Research, 44*, 1216–1222.

Wolf, G., Lippman, S.M., Laramore, G., & Hong, W.K. (1992). Head and neck cancer. In J.F. Holland, E. Frei, R.C. Bast, Jr., D.W. Kufe, D.L. Morton, & R. Weichselbaum (Eds.), *Cancer medicine* (3rd ed.) (pp. 1174–1221). Philadelphia: Lea & Febiger.

Wong, B.J.F., & Hashisaki, G.T. (1996). Treatment of Bloom syndrome patients: Guidelines and a report on a case. *Otolaryngology—Head and Neck Surgery, 114,* 295–298.

Xu, H.X., Shen, X.H., Jin, Z.L., & Xu, X.B. (1991). Analysis of volatile N-nitrosamines in beer and food in China. In I.K. O'Neill, J. Chen, & H. Bartsch (Eds.), *Relevance to human cancer of N-nitroso compounds, tobacco smoke and mycotoxins* (IARC Scientific Publications No. 105) (pp. 230–231). New York: Oxford University Press.

CHAPTER 17

Tertiary Prevention: Improving the Care of Long-Term Survivors of Cancer

*Suzanne M. Mahon, RN, DNSc, AOCN®, APNG(c)
and Melanie Williams, RN, BSN*

Introduction

Tertiary cancer prevention includes the ongoing surveillance and early detection of second primary malignancies and other treatment-related complications in cancer survivors. Tertiary prevention is an emerging role for oncology nurses. The care and rehabilitation of patients with cancer should include strategies to promote the early detection of second cancers as well as to reduce risk factors for second malignancies and other long-term complications.

An ever-growing population of cancer survivors are living longer after their initial cancer diagnosis. Current estimates suggest that more than 8.8 million people with a history of cancer are alive (American Cancer Society [ACS], 2001). More than 50% of patients diagnosed with cancer are disease-free five or more years after their initial diagnosis. This is largely because of earlier detection of malignancy and the development of more effective therapies.

Although more people are living longer after an initial diagnosis of cancer, treatment modalities and the underlying genetic basis of many cancers predispose survivors to developing second primary malignancies. Another complication that recently has become more evident is the development of osteoporosis in women with hormone-dependent malignancies.

This chapter focuses on two areas of tertiary cancer prevention: the risk for developing and the detection of second primary malignancies and the prevention and detection of osteoporosis in women with hormone-dependent malignancies. Each area includes a discussion of the epidemiology and etiology of the problem, known risk factors, appropriate nursing assessment and screening, and treatment, when appropriate.

Second Primary Cancers

Introduction

The observation of multiple primary cancers was first reported in 1889 (Neugut, Meadows, & Robinson, 1999). Initial criteria for classifying multiple primary cancers first were reported in the 1930s. Despite these published reports, little attention has been directed toward screening for second primary cancers. Only recently has attention been focused on the medical and psychosocial needs of long-term survivors of malignancy. The National Cancer Institute (NCI) recently established the Office of Cancer Survivorship. A major focus of this office is on risks for developing second primary cancers. As people with cancer live longer after the initial diagnosis and usually experience high levels of function after treatment, providing preventive therapies and screening for the late consequences of the first diagnosis is becoming increasingly important.

A second primary cancer is defined as the occurrence of a new cancer that is biologically independent of the original primary cancer. Second primary cancers may occur because of genetic predisposition to a second cancer (e.g., ovarian cancer after breast cancer in women with a BRCA1 or BRCA2 mutation) or through a common environmental exposure, such as intense ultraviolet exposure and the subsequent development of multiple skin cancers. Treatment with chemotherapeutic agents, especially alkylating agents, is another etiologic source. Treatment with radiation therapy has been associated with the development of second primary cancers. Still other second cancers probably occur as a result of random chance. Understanding the etiology, risk factors, and subsequent development of a second cancer ultimately should result in improved screening and surveillance for survivors (Hancock & Tucker, 1998).

Incidence of Second Primary Cancers

The exact incidence of second primary malignancies varies by the site. Data on the exact incidence are difficult to obtain, as many registries do not have the ability to effectively identify cases that are subsequent primary cancers (Morris, Perkins, Wright, Snipes, & Young, 1996). NCI has collected the largest set of data through the Surveillance, Epidemiology, and End Results (SEER) Program. The data are available through the SEER Program Web site (http://seer.cancer.gov). In 1973, second primary cancers accounted for 6.1% of the cancers in men and 6.3% of the cancers in women. In 1996, the number of second primary cancers registered increased to 11.4% in men and 11.8% in women. The reason for the increase in this incidence, in part, probably is because survivors are living longer after an initial diagnosis as a result of earlier detection and improved treatment (Robinson, 1999). Neugut et al. (1999) cautioned that a cancer survivor in the United States has roughly twice the chance of developing a second malignancy as an individual from the general population has of developing a first cancer. When reviewing the literature, many anecdotal reports exist on the incidence of second primary cancers, but few data are available on the value of follow-up of patients with a single cancer for the purposes of detection of a second primary tumor. Quantification of the risk factors for second cancers is important to develop appropriate guidelines for follow-up, but, to date, little work has been performed in this area (Hemminki & Vaittinen, 1999).

Etiology

The exact etiology of a second primary cancer is not always clear. Many of these cancers are thought to be treatment related. To date, most of the second primary cancers that are associated with radiotherapy for childhood cancers have been bone and soft tissue sarcomas and carcinomas of the thyroid gland, breast, and skin (Inskip, 1999). Factors that influence the development of second malignancies include the total dose and number of fractions, the source of energy, combinations with chemotherapeutic agents, and age at exposure (i.e., younger age increases risk) (Rodriguez & Ash, 1996).

Chemotherapeutic agents also have been associated with second primary cancers, especially alkylating agents, vinca alkaloids, antimetabolites, and antitumor antibiotics (Schottenfeld, 1996). Alkylating agents, in particular, have been associated with leukemias, myelodysplastic syndrome, sarcomas, and bladder cancer (Felix, 1999).

Genetic predisposition also plays an important etiologic role in the development of second malignancies. Many of the hereditary cancers are inherited in an autosomal dominant fashion. Germline mutations result in the mutated gene in all embryonic cells (the "first hit"). Further exposure to carcinogens results in loss of the second normal allele and subsequent development of cancer (the "second hit"). This germline mutation results in the first hit in all embryonic cells and subsequent increase in the risk of multiple cancers. Second breast and ovarian cancers are associated with mutations in BRCA1 and BRCA2. Table 17-1 shows other syndromes associated with multiple primary malignancies.

The impact of environmental exposure cannot be overlooked. Second cancers may develop because of prolonged exposure to an environmental carcinogen. Velie and Schatzkin (1999) noted that only a small subset of second primary cancers are diagnosed at the same time, known as synchronous lesions. Most second primary cancers occur years after the first cancer. These are known as metachronous lesions. This may be related to the fact that even with a similar carcinogen load, some anatomic sites may differ in the timing of neoplastic events or have more resistance. Rigel and Carucci (2000) noted that a previous history of nonmelanoma or melanoma skin cancer increases the risk of a second melanoma or nonmelanoma skin cancer. This often is related to long-term environmental exposure to ultraviolet light. Similarly, tobacco use is associated with multiple primary cancers in the aerodigestive tract and cervix.

Table 17-1. Genetic Predisposition to Multiple Primary Cancers

Genetic Syndrome/Mutation	Associated Primary Cancers
BRCA1/BRCA2 mutations	Breast Ovarian
Von Hippel-Landau disease	Retinal and central nervous Hemangioblastomas Renal cell carcinoma Pheochromocytoma
Neurofibromatosis type 1	Vestibular schwannoma Astrocytoma Meningioma
Nevoid basal cell carcinoma (Gorlin) syndrome	Multiple basal cell carcinomas Brain tumors
Cowden syndrome	Breast cancer Thyroid cancer Genitourinary tract tumors
Familial adenomatous polyposis	Multiple colorectal polyps/cancers
Hereditary nonpolyposis colorectal cancer (Lynch I)	Multiple site-specific colorectal cancers
Hereditary nonpolyposis colorectal cancer (Lynch II)	Multiple colonic lesions Endometrium Ovary Renal tract Small bowel
Muir-Torre syndrome	Same as Lynch II but affected family member also may develop benign and malignant skin lesions.
Dysplastic nevus/melanoma	Multiple malignant melanomas
Peutz-Jegher	Intestine Breast Uterus and ovary Testicle
Xeroderma pigmentosum	Basal and squamous cell skin cancers Melanomas Aerodigestive cancers
Ataxia-telangiectasia	Non-Hodgkin's lymphoma Leukemia Breast cancer
Bloom syndrome	Non-Hodgkin's lymphoma Leukemia Gastrointestinal cancer
Li-Fraumeni syndrome	Sarcomas Breast cancer Brain cancer Leukemia Adrenocortical carcinoma

Note. Based on information from Bishop & Kolodner, 1999; Eng & Maher, 1999; Schneider, 1995; Schottenfeld, 1996.

Risks of Second Primary Cancers Associated With Specific Cancer Types

Second Primary Cancers Associated With Breast Cancer

Breast cancer is the most frequently diagnosed cancer among women, with an estimated 192,900 new cases annually (ACS, 2001). The relative five-year survival rate for localized breast cancer is approximately 96%. This improved long-term survival rate has created an ever-growing number of people at risk for the development of other cancers.

Breast cancer: Women with breast cancer have been reported to have three to four times the risk of a second breast cancer in the unaffected breast (Schottenfeld, 1996). Contralateral breast cancer accounts for 40%–50% of all second tumors in women with breast cancer. The risk of a second primary breast cancer is increased in women when the primary breast cancer is classified as lobular carcinoma; a history of biopsy for benign breast disease exists; or a history of breast cancer, endometrial cancer, or ovarian cancer exists in a first-degree relative (Schottenfeld).

Estimates certainly vary, but the incidence of contralateral breast cancer is approximately 1% per year (Daly & Costalas, 1999). It increases to 3% per year in women with a history of breast cancer in a first-degree relative. Estimates suggest that approximately 15% of breast cancer survivors will have a second, contralateral breast cancer (Daly & Costalas). The overall relative risk is 3.0. Relative risk compares an individual's risk for developing a particular cancer. For example, if the risk of developing breast cancer in a woman with no known risk factors is 1.0, a comparison can be made to a woman who has one or more risk factors. For a woman with a relative with premenopausal breast cancer, the relative risk may be 5.1. This means she has 5.1 times the chance of developing breast cancer compared to a woman without risk factors. Risk is highest in women who are younger than age 45 years at diagnosis (Breast Cancer Linkage Consortium, 1999). This risk may be, in part, because of BRCA1 and BRCA2 gene mutations. Risk may be increased in women who have received radiotherapy because of scattered radiation exposure (Schottenfeld, 1996), although the magnitude of the risk is unknown. Obedian, Fischer, and Haffty (2000) reported that in a trial of radiation therapy after lumpectomy, as compared to mastectomy, no increased risk of second malignancies to the contralateral breast was seen in women receiving radiation therapy.

Endometrial cancer: Epidemiologic studies suggest that an increased risk of developing endometrial cancer exists in long-term survivors of breast cancer. The overall relative risk is 1.72 and increases in women who are age 70 and older (Daly & Costalas, 1999). This may be related to a shared hormonal etiology between breast and endometrial cancer, as well as aging. Genetic factors such as hereditary nonpolyposis colorectal cancer (HNPCC) also may account for some of the increased risk. More recently, treatment with tamoxifen has been identified as a risk factor for developing endometrial cancer (Assikis, Neven, Jordan, & Vergote, 1996). Because many women with breast cancer are treated with tamoxifen, this risk cannot be overlooked.

Ovarian cancer: Ovarian cancer is another common second malignancy seen in survivors of breast cancer. The disease is estimated to occur in 5%–26% of breast cancer survivors, with a relative risk of 1.2–2.4 (Daly & Costalas, 1999). The risk for developing an ovarian cancer after breast cancer probably is related to BRCA1 and BRCA2 gene mutations and, in some cases, HNPCC.

Colorectal cancer: After breast cancer, a woman also is at risk for developing colorectal cancer. The relative risk is estimated to be 2–3 (Daly & Costalas, 1999). The etiologic basis for this risk may be related to dietary factors, including consumption of a diet high in animal fat or shared genetic factors. A high-fat diet has been associated with both breast and colorectal cancers (ACS, 2000; Willett, 1999).

Other cancers: After primary treatment for breast cancer, treatment-related second primary cancers may occur. These most often include hematologic malignancies. The risk of leukemia is estimated to be 1.29% at 10 years after chemotherapy (Parikh & Advani, 1996). This risk is relatively small, considering the benefits of chemotherapy.

Second Primary Cancers Associated With Ovarian Cancer

Each year, an estimated 23,100 women are diagnosed with ovarian cancer (ACS, 2000). The overall risk of a second cancer is approximately 20% greater in women who have had ovarian cancer and survive at least five years (Travis et al., 1996). The survival rates for ovarian cancers are not as encouraging as for other gynecologic and breast cancers in women. Seventy-eight percent of patients with ovarian cancer live one year after diagnosis; the five-year relative survival rate for all stages is 50%. For those women who have localized disease, the relative survival rate is 95%; however, only 25% of ovarian cancer cases are detected at the localized stage. Travis et al. estimated that one in five women with ovarian cancer is expected to develop a new malignancy within 20 years if she survives her initial primary cancer. Risk for a second gynecologic malignancy is low because most of these women are treated initially with a primary radical hysterectomy.

Breast cancer: Treatment for ovarian cancer often results in ablation of gonadal function, but this does not necessarily mean a reduced risk for developing breast cancer. Relative risk may be as high as 4.0 (Travis et al., 1996). This elevated risk may be, in part, because of shared risk factors, including nulliparity, early menarche, and late menopause. Women younger than age 40 diagnosed with ovarian cancer may have a BRCA1 or BRCA2 mutation, which substantially increases their risk for developing breast cancer.

Colorectal cancer: An increased risk for developing colorectal cancer exists in women who have survived gynecologic cancer (Travis et al., 1996). Further, ovarian cancers have been associated with HNPCC, suggesting that genetic determinants may influence the development of both ovarian and colorectal cancers.

Second Primary Cancers Associated With Endometrial Cancer

In the United States, endometrial cancer is the most common gynecologic cancer, with an estimated 38,300 new cases annually. It also is the most curable gynecologic cancer. The five-year relative survival rate is 95% if the cancer is detected early and 64% if diagnosed at the regional stage (ACS, 2001).

Zimmerman and Westhoff (1999) noted that research on second primary cancers following endometrial cancer is very limited. Risk for developing a second primary is highest in the breast and colon.

Breast cancer: Breast cancer can occur after a diagnosis of endometrial cancer. The relative risk is estimated to be 1.3–4.1 (Zimmerman & Westhoff, 1999). The development of breast cancer after endometrial cancer may occur in both long- and short-term survivors of endometrial cancer and therefore is not thought to be related to treatment. The etiology of developing breast cancer after endometrial cancer is most likely because of their shared risk factors. These include number of years of menstrual cycles, nulliparity, and postmenopausal obesity. Shared genetic factors are another suspected etiologic cause, including HNPCC.

Colorectal cancer: Women who have been treated successfully for endometrial cancer are at risk for developing a second primary colorectal cancer. The relative risk is estimated to range from 1.19–5.92 (Zimmerman & Westhoff, 1999). The risk is thought to be related to a common shared genetic etiology, particularly HNPCC. Women with a personal or family history of colorectal cancer or endometrial cancer, in particular, should be considered at high risk.

Second Primary Cancers Associated With Colorectal Cancer

Colorectal cancers are the third most common cancers in men and women (ACS, 2001). ACS estimated that 135,400 people are diagnosed each year with colorectal cancer. Once a person is diagnosed, the risk for a second colorectal cancer is higher. The relative risk is estimated to be 3.3 for men and 3.2 for women (Neugut & Gold, 1999).

As with many of the other cancers associated with second primary cancers, hereditary predisposition is a significant risk factor, including HNPCC and familial adenomatous polyposis (FAP). A personal history of polyps places a person at risk for developing subsequent polyps and possibly colorectal cancer.

Breast cancer: The relative risk of developing breast cancer after colorectal cancer is estimated to be 1.26 (Neugut & Gold, 1999). This may be related to hormonal factors. High parity seems to reduce the risk for colon cancer. Women with a history of early menarche, a long interval between the birth of the first and second child, late parity, or nulliparity are at higher risk for developing both breast and ovarian cancers.

Ovarian cancer: The risk for developing ovarian cancer after colorectal cancer appears to be higher than the risk of developing breast cancer. Neugut and Gold (1999) estimated that the relative risk for developing a subsequent ovarian cancer is 3.0. This risk appears to be bidirectional (i.e., colorectal cancer after ovarian cancer or ovarian cancer after colorectal cancer). Like the risk for developing breast cancer after colon cancer, the risk of developing ovarian cancer may be related to the hormonal factors of early menarche, late parity, or nulliparity.

Endometrial cancer: The risk of developing endometrial cancer after colon cancer is estimated to be 1.6–2.0 (Neugut & Gold, 1999). Like the risk of developing a second breast or ovarian cancer after colon cancer, the risk of a second endometrial cancer probably is related to hormonal factors.

Other cancers: After cancer of the colon and rectum, an increased risk exists for developing cancer of the kidneys, bladder, and prostate. The relative risk for developing kidney or bladder cancer is 1.5–2.0 in both men and women (Neugut & Gold, 1999). A slightly increased risk also exists for developing prostate cancer. The estimated relative risk after colon cancer is estimated to be 1.3.

Skin Cancer

With approximately 1.4 million cases of skin cancer diagnosed annually in the United States, a large group of survivors of skin cancer are at risk for second primary malignancies. Most nonmelanoma skin cancers, which are the basal and squamous cell types, are highly curable. An estimated 1,900 deaths occur annually from these cancers (ACS, 2001). The incidence of melanoma is increasing; it is diagnosed in approximately 51,400 people a year, with an estimated 7,800 annual deaths. For those with localized melanoma, the relative five-year survival rate is 88% (ACS, 2001).

Malignant melanoma: Approximately 5% of patients with melanoma will go on to develop a second primary melanoma (Berwick, 1999). This is hypothesized to be related to genetic predisposition. In many cases, a second melanoma is thinner than the first primary melanoma. This may be because of improved follow-up and screening.

Nonmelanoma skin cancers: Multiple primary nonmelanoma skin cancers are more common in men than women. Approximately 20% of those who develop one basal cell or squamous cell skin cancer go on to develop a second primary nonmelanoma skin cancer (Berwick, 1999). This may be because of environmental exposure to ultraviolet light or immune suppression.

Prevention Strategies

Primary prevention efforts can be applied to long-term survivors of cancer. When a survivor is identified with good prognostic factors, efforts need to be made to prevent additional cancers. These efforts are similar to those identified for people who are asymptomatic.

The identification of those with a genetic predisposition for developing malignancy can be a step toward primary prevention in some high-risk families. A number of familial cancer syndromes are associated with multiple primary cancers, including retinoblastoma, FAP, HNPCC, Li-Fraumeni syndrome, von Hippel-Lindau disease, neurofibromatosis, Cowden syndrome, Peutz-Jeghers syndrome, multiple endocrine neoplasia, Gorlin's syndrome, and hereditary breast/ovarian cancer syndrome. When individuals from these families are identified, a program for prevention should be developed, when possible, as well as a program of increased surveillance. For example, a woman with a BRCA1 or BRCA2 mutation may consider a prophylactic oophorectomy to prevent ovarian cancer and tamoxifen to prevent a recurrence of the first breast cancer and to prevent a second primary breast cancer (Eisen, Rebbeck, Wood, & Weber, 2000; Smith & Hillner, 2000).

Smoking cessation could eliminate many cancers. In particular, multiple cancers of the head and neck region could be reduced with cessation of tobacco use.

Similarly, these cancers could be reduced by avoiding heavy alcohol consumption. Cancer survivors may be more receptive to teaching and actually trying to modify these lifestyle habits because they better understand the seriousness of a diagnosis of malignancy.

The implementation of a healthy diet and regular exercise could further reduce the number of cancers, especially colorectal cancers and cancers of the aerodigestive system, breast, and endometrium. ACS's *Goals for Nutrition in the Year 2000* makes the following recommendations: avoid weight gain in adulthood, perform 30 minutes of moderate exercise on most days, eat five or more servings of fruits and vegetables daily, decrease consumption of red meat, and increase consumption of cereal products (Willett, 1999). Cancer survivors should be reminded of these healthy habits. Some people may benefit from consultation with a dietician, who can make specific recommendations.

Many second cutaneous cancers could be reduced by the proper and consistent use of sunscreen, protective clothing, and hats, in addition to reducing ultraviolet exposure.

Screening Strategies

Healthcare providers who work with long-term survivors of cancer are well suited to provide the comprehensive risk assessments and education patients need about developing a second cancer. The process of selecting appropriate screening strategies begins with an individual risk assessment. Each cancer survivor should be considered individually. Risk factors should be documented and interpreted to the patient. The risk factor assessment should guide the selection of appropriate screening strategies.

Specific guidelines for screening for second primary malignancies presently are not available. Currently, screening for second cancers is similar to screening for first cancers when following the guidelines for screening in asymptomatic people, which is published by ACS (2001). These guidelines need to be tailored to the individual risks of the cancer survivor. For example, ACS recommends colorectal cancer screening in all people beginning at age 50. Average-risk people may opt to have flexible sigmoidoscopy and fecal occult blood testing. A 45-year-old woman who has been treated successfully for breast cancer probably has a higher-than-average risk of developing colorectal cancer. She may be considered moderate risk and be referred for full colonoscopy. In cases where a survivor has undergone genetic testing and is known to carry a BRCA1 or HNPCC mutation, screening may be performed more frequently or tests may be added, such as a transvaginal ultrasound, to monitor for ovarian cancers.

Cancer survivors also need to be educated about the signs and symptoms of second malignancies that should be reported. This education helps to make patients better advocates for themselves and more involved in their care.

Appropriate self-examination also should be discussed with long-term survivors of cancer. Women should be taught proper breast self-examination techniques during the course of a professional examination. This enables women to better appreciate their own anatomical landmarks. Women who have had breast surgery should be taught how to examine the affected breast and what constitutes a normal and abnormal finding. All survivors probably can benefit from knowing how to properly examine their skin. Many survivors have received photosensitizing chemotherapy and need to know how to protect their skin from further damage and how to examine for changes that might signal an early skin cancer.

Psychosocial Concerns

Anxiety and fear about cancer recurrence has been documented as a concern in long-term survivors of cancer. Little is known about how much survivors realize they are at risk for a second primary cancer and how fearful cancer survivors are of developing a second primary cancer. This problem has received little attention. Every cancer survivor has a different risk of developing a second primary cancer. Clearly, efforts need to be made to better understand patients' perceptions and anxiety related to this risk.

Information should be communicated in a nonthreatening way about a second risk for cancer. Survivors need to understand that their prognosis actually is excellent when concern shifts to screening for second cancers and that screening and prevention recommendations are being given to detect cancers early and further increase long-term survival and quality of life. Just as assessment of risk for second malignancies should occur in long-term follow-up, assessment of overall adjustment and quality of life also should take place. For patients having difficulty adjusting to long-term survival, further intervention with a healthcare professional with expertise in psychosocial management may be indicated. Holistic care also includes spiritual care to help patients to draw from their inner strength to promote healing, identify the people and things that give meaning to their lives, and find hope for the future.

Nursing Challenges

Regular follow-up appointments provide an opportunity for continuity of care and to assess for long-term adjustment to the cancer diagnosis. Resources are available to facilitate understanding of the psychosocial changes that occur in long-term survivors as well as resources for the early detection and prevention of cancers. Figure 17-1 provides some of these resources. Efforts should be made to help survivors to become active participants in their long-term follow-up. Healthcare professionals have an opportunity to teach survivors about healthy lifestyles and the importance of cancer screening and to impart this information to patients' family members. After treatment is completed, the stress levels of patients and families often are lower, and they may be more receptive to this teaching.

Healthcare providers who manage the long-term follow-up of cancer survivors need to consider not only follow-up to detect recurrence but also active screening to detect second malignancies. The selection of an appropriate screening method only can be made with the knowledge of the risk for developing a second cancer. An important aspect of this follow-up is patient education that includes information about the magnitude of the risk, strategies for primary prevention, and appropriate screening. Robinson (1999) stressed that although many case reports are

Figure 17-1. Selected Resources for Long-Term Survivors Related to Second Malignancies

National Cancer Institute (NCI)
This site contains the most recent and accurate cancer information from NCI. An entire section of publications is aimed at cancer genetics, prevention, and detection. The user may search the site by disease type and order or download publications (www.nci.nih.gov).

The NCI Office of Cancer Survivorship (OCS)
The mission of OCS is to enhance the quality and length of survival of all people diagnosed with cancer and to minimize or stabilize adverse sequelae of cancer survivorship. OCS conducts and supports research that both examines and addresses the long- and short-term physical, psychological, social, and economic effects of cancer and its treatment among pediatric and adult survivors of cancer and their families (http://dccps.nci.nih.gov/ocs/).

Facing Forward: A Guide for Cancer Survivors (NCI publication)
A concise overview of important survivor issues, including ongoing health needs, psychosocial concerns, insurance, and employment. Order publication through NCI's Web site or by calling 800-4-CANCER.

National Coalition of Cancer Survivorship
This organization has a wide range of resources for people who have been treated successfully for cancer. Many resources to facilitate psychosocial adjustment to a diagnosis of cancer are available (www.cansearch.org or 301-650-9127).

available on the incidence of multiple primary malignancies, very little data exist on the value of follow-up and screening of patients with a single cancer with the intent to detect a second primary cancer.

Although the exact incidence and etiology of all second primary cancers is not completely clear, efforts should be made to consistently identify and monitor individuals at higher risk after the completion of cancer treatment. A recent study suggested that few healthcare providers consistently assess and recommend screening to detect second cancers. Mahon, Williams, and Spies (2000) reported that in a study of 321 oncology nurses caring for long-term survivors, the screening activities performed most consistently were mammogram, clinical breast examination, and Pap smear. Screening activities that were least likely to be recommended included colorectal cancer screening, endometrial biopsy, and screening for osteoporosis. These researchers also noted that when screening is recommended, a physician most likely initiates it. Because of the time nurses spend with patients and the educational opportunity associated with these tests, nurses need to be more proactive in initiating screening and prevention strategies.

One way to ensure that screening is carried out is to develop protocols, which can be implemented at an institution. They may help to ensure that recommendations are discussed consistently, especially in the realm of prevention. Protocols may include educational information such as written materials, visual diagrams, anatomical models, and videotapes to supplement the education.

Osteoporosis

Follow-up care of long-term survivors of cancer also considers conditions that have the potential to further complicate the original problem. Osteoporosis is one of these considerations. It is important to understand the scope of the problem and the treatment measures that decrease the risk of fractures. Osteoporosis is defined as a systemic skeletal disease characterized by low bone mass and microarchitectural deterioration of bone tissue with a consequent increase in bone fragility and susceptibility to fracture (Consensus Development Conference, 1993). Figure 17-2 provides a photo of the differences between normal and osteoporotic bone. Ten million Americans have osteoporosis of the hip, and an additional 19 million have low bone mass (Melton, 1999).

Figure 17-2. Differences Between Normal and Osteoporotic Bone

Normal Bone Structure

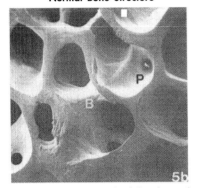

Deteriorated Bone Structure

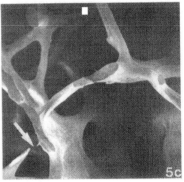

An electron micrograph of iliac bone demonstrates normal trabecular strength and architecture on the left and compromised trabecular number and connectivity on the right.

Note. From "A Simple Method for Correlative Light and Scanning Electron Microscopy of Human Iliac Crest Bone Biopsies: Qualitative Observations in Normal and Osteoporotic Subjects," by D.W. Dempster, E. Shane, W. Horbert, and R. Lindsay, 1986, *Journal of Bone and Mineral Research, 1,* 15–21. Copyright 1986 by the American Society for Bone and Mineral Research. Reprinted with permission.

At age 50, a White woman has nearly a 40% chance of developing an osteoporotic fracture during her remaining lifetime. By age 60–70, only one in nine women in the United States has "normal" bone mineral density (BMD); almost one out of three women has osteoporosis, and the rest have osteopenia (see Figure 17-3). After age 80, 70% of women have osteoporosis (Ross, 1996).

Women of all races are at risk for bone loss, osteoporosis, and fractures. Although women of different races may achieve different peak BMD, all will lose bone mass at a similar rate. For example, African American women achieve a higher peak bone mass in general but still lose bone density at the same rate as White women (Perry et al., 1996). Therefore, African American women are at risk

---

Figure 17-3. Definitions of Osteoporosis

Normal: Bone mineral density (BMD) within 1 standard deviation (SD) of the young adult reference mean (> –1 SD)

Osteopenia: BMD more than 1 SD below the young adult mean but less than 2.5 SD below this value (–1 SD to –2.5 SD)

Osteoporosis: BMD 2.5 SD or more below the young adult mean (< –2.5 SD)

Severe or Established Osteoporosis: BMD more than 2.5 SD below the young adult mean in the presence of one or more fragility fractures (< –2.5 SD + fracture)

Note. Based on information from World Health Organization, 1994.

for osteoporosis, although the effects may be seen later in life than for White women. Osteoporosis also is not gender specific. Twenty to thirty percent of osteoporotic fractures occur in men (Cooper, Campion, & Melton, 1992).

An estimated 1.3 million osteoporotic fractures occur annually in the United States. This includes more than 500,000 vertebral fractures, 250,000 distal forearm fractures, and 250,000 hip fractures (Nevitt, 1994). Demographic changes could cause the annual number of hip fractures to double from 238,000 in 1986 to 512,000 in 2040 (Melton, 1993).

Osteoporosis has significant economic consequences. The cost of fractures in the United States may be as much as $20 billion per year, with hip fractures accounting for more than one-third of the total cost (Melton, 1993). In 1995, an estimated $13.8 billion was spent on osteoporotic fractures (Ray, Chan, Thamer, & Melton, 1997). Among women age 45 years and older, hip fractures account for more than half of all osteoporosis-related hospital admissions in the United States (Ray et al.).

The social costs of osteoporosis are even higher. Sixty percent of women older than 80 have vertebral compression fractures, suggesting that these are the most common osteoporotic fractures. Vertebral compression fractures are associated with height loss, limited range of motion, muscle weakness, a protruding abdomen, and thoracic kyphosis (Lyles et al., 1993). Vertebral fractures resulting from osteoporosis can cause pain, debilitation, and impaired balance that can lead to falls. These fractures can limit an individual's ability to perform activities of daily living, restricting function in employment as well as in social and recreational activities.

Once a woman experiences two or more vertebral fractures, osteoporosis begins to have a noticeable impact on emotional functioning. High levels of anxiety result from a very real fear of falling, and future fractures and can lead to inactivity, depression, and diminished self-esteem (Gold, 1996).

Mortality associated with osteoporosis also is significant. Most mortality is related to hip fractures. Men and women are two to five times more likely to die during the first 12 months following a hip fracture compared with people of the same age and gender in the general population without hip fractures (Ross, 1996). Virtually all patients are hospitalized following a hip fracture. The average length of hospitalization is between 20 and 30 days. Almost half of all patients with hip fractures in the United States are discharged to a long-term care/rehabilitation facility, and more than one-third are rehospitalized during the year following the fracture (Magaziner, Simonsick, Kashner, Hebel, & Kenzora, 1990). At two months following hospital discharge, fewer than 40% of patients have regained their prefracture walking ability, and only about 25% have recovered their previous capacity to perform physical activities of daily living (Magaziner et al.).

Osteoporosis in Survivors of Cancer

These figures regarding osteoporosis represent a staggering health problem. Relatively little systematic data are available on the exact risk and incidence of osteoporosis in survivors of breast cancer, but there is concern that this may be an important health problem (Ganz, 2000). From a public health perspective, the number of women with a near-normal life expectancy after a diagnosis of localized breast cancer will continue to increase because of early diagnosis and improved therapy. An estimated 500,000 women are 50 years old and have survived at least five years after localized breast cancer (Vassilopoulou-Sellin & Theriault, 1994). An additional 20,000 women are estimated to be added to this figure each year. The combination of premature menopause, prolonged estrogen deficiency, and the toxic effects of chemotherapeutic agents on bone puts breast cancer survivors at especially high risk for low bone mass, osteoporosis, and fractures.

Survivors of breast cancer potentially face several decades of estrogen deficiency. Premenopausal women who have been treated successfully for breast cancer are subjected to premature menopause because of cytotoxic treatment (Goodwin, Ennis, Pritchard, Trudeau, & Hood, 1999). The risk of menopause with adjuvant chemotherapy ranges from 53%–89%. Current medical opinion generally suggests that estrogen replacement therapy (ERT) is contraindicated in this population. These figures do not consider the number of women diagnosed with postmenopausal breast cancer who have good prognostic factors and also are estrogen deficient.

Further research indicates that women with breast cancer are at increased risk for fractures. The prevalence of vertebral fractures in women with breast cancer without skeletal metastasis was nearly five times greater than that in controls. The incidence of vertebral fractures in women with soft tissue metastasis was more than 20 times greater than in controls (Kanis, 1999). Even these data may be underestimated by nearly 25%, because half of the women with breast cancer were receiving a bisphosphonate.

Patients who have been treated successfully for malignancies should not have to suffer the morbidity and mortality associated with osteoporosis just because they may not be candidates for ERT. Awareness of recent improvements in diagnostic and treatment modalities can prevent the devastating effects of osteoporosis in these cancer survivors.

Pathophysiology of Osteoporosis

An understanding of normal bone remodeling is necessary to appreciate the pathophysiology of osteoporosis and comprehend the mechanism of action of current therapies approved by the U.S. Food and Drug Administration (FDA). Bone is living tissue and undergoes constant repair, or remodeling. Bone remodeling consists of phases of resorption and formation. These events are coupled and occur in bone-remodeling units. The bone-remodeling unit consists of osteoblasts and osteoclasts. The osteoclasts are the bone cells responsible for bone resorption, and the osteoblasts are responsible for bone formation. The osteoclasts will create a cavity in the bone called the resorption pit that subsequently will be filled by osteoblasts. The rate at which this process occurs is known as bone turnover (see Figure 17-4).

Figure 17-4. Bone Turnover

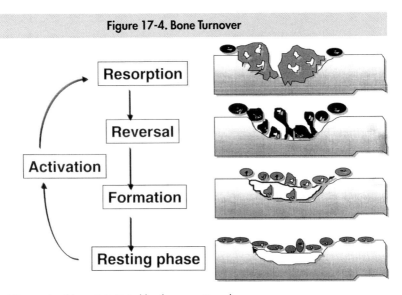

The remodeling cycle of bone is initiated by the resorption phase.

Note. From "Bone Density Measurement and the Management of Osteoporosis" (p. 142) by C.C. Johnson, C.W. Slemenda, and L.J. Melton in N.J. Favus (Ed.), *Primer on the Metabolic Bone Diseases and Disorders of Mineral Metabolism,* 1996, Philadelphia: Lippincott-Raven. Copyright 1996 by Lippincott-Raven. Reprinted with permission.

In osteoporosis, the coupling of the bone-remodeling unit is impaired. The resorption pit created by the osteoclast is not refilled completely by the osteoblast. This results in a net deficit of total bone formation. Ultimately, this deficit results in lower bone mass, damage of bone microarchitecture, increased bone fragility, and fractures (see Figure 17-2).

Peak bone mass usually is achieved between ages 30 and 35. Estrogen deficiency in the first 5–10 years immediately following menopause can result in an accelerated loss of bone mass. Without estrogen replacement, women can lose up to 30% of their bone mass during this period (Riis, 1995). After this time, a gradual but continual loss of bone occurs. This pattern of bone loss is illustrated in Figure 17-5. The loss of bone mass increases bone fragility and increases susceptibility for fractures. The sites for fracture most associated with low bone mass and osteoporosis include the distal forearm, the hip, and the vertebrae (Kanis, 1994).

In patients with malignancy, both bone formation and bone resorption may be impaired. This impairment may be because of the effects of the disease or medica-

Figure 17-5. Pattern of Bone Loss

Bone loss in women

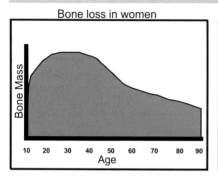

Fracture incidence in women

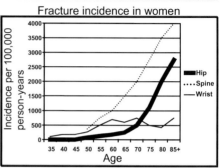

As bone mass decreases with age, there is an exponential increase in fracture risk.

Note. From *Osteoporosis: Critique and Practicum* (p. 179), by R.D. Wasnich, P.D. Ross, J.M. Vogel, and J.W. Davis, 1989, Honolulu, HI: Banyan Press. Copyright 1989 by Banyan Press. Adapted with permission; and "Epidemiology of Osteoporosis," by C. Cooper and L.J. Melton, 1992, *Trends in Endocrinology and Metabolism, 3*, p. 225, Copyright 1992 by Elsevier Science. Reprinted with permission.

tions used to treat the disease. The medications used may have a direct effect on osteoclasts or osteoblasts, or they may impair gonadal function, inducing menopause. The resulting estrogen deficiency from menopause impairs the bone remodeling cycle by increasing bone resorption beyond bone formation. The result is a net loss of bone mass.

Risk Factors for Osteoporosis

All women have some risk for losing bone mass and developing osteoporosis and sustaining a fracture. This risk increases steadily after menopause, especially if the patient remains estrogen deficient. Risk for osteoporosis and subsequent fracture is significantly higher in some groups of women. To provide a more effective management strategy, identification and early detection of women at higher risk for developing osteoporosis is critical. A number of factors contribute to low bone mass (see Figure 17-6). Risk factors for osteoporosis that increase fracture risk and are particularly significant in long-term survivors of malignancy include estrogen deficiency, exposure to certain medications used in the treatment of malignancy, history of a previous fracture, and the malignancy itself.

Estrogen deficiency: Estrogen deficiency is one of the most significant contributors to low bone mass in postmenopausal women. Estrogen deficiency is thought to affect both the osteoclasts and osteoblasts (Guise & Mundy, 1998; Kanis, 1994; Mundy, 1996). Estrogen deficiency can cause rapid loss of bone immediately following menopause. Menopause in breast cancer survivors may occur naturally, surgically following the removal of both ovaries, or medically following the administration of some medications and, in particular, chemotherapeutic agents.

Chemotherapeutic agents often used in the treatment of breast and gynecologic malignancies that are associated with gonadal dysfunction and an earlier meno-

Figure 17-6. Risk Factors for Osteoporosis

Genetic Factors
- White or Asian
- Personal or family history of osteoporosis or fracture
- Small body frame (< 127 lbs.)

Lifestyle Factors
- Smoking
- Inactivity
- Nulliparity
- Excessive exercise (causing amenorrhea)
- Estrogen deficiency
- Early natural menopause
- Late menarche

Nutritional Factors
- Milk intolerance
- Life-long low dietary intake
- Vegetarian diet
- Excessive alcohol intake
- Consistently high protein intake

Medical Disorders
- Anorexia nervosa
- Thyrotoxicosis
- Hyperparathyroidism
- Cushing's syndrome
- Type I diabetes mellitus
- Alterations in gastrointestinal and hepatobiliary function
- Occult osteogenesis imperfecta
- Mastocytosis
- Rheumatoid arthritis
- Prolactinoma
- Hemolytic anemia, hemochromatosis, and thalassemia
- Ankylosing spondylitis

Medications
- Thyroid replacement medications
- Glucocorticoids
- Anticoagulants (heparin)
- Chemotherapeutic agents
- Gonadotropin-releasing hormone agonist or antagonist therapy
- Anticonvulsants
- Extended tetracycline use
- Diuretics producing calciuria
- Phenothiazine derivatives
- Cyclosporine

Note. Based on information from Avioli, 1994; Dempster & Lindsay, 1993.

pause include cyclophosphamide, methotrexate, 5-fluorouracil, and doxorubicin (Averette, Boike, & Jarrell, 1990). Up to 89% of women receiving these agents will have a premature chemotherapy-induced menopause (Goodwin et al., 1999). Premature menopause related to the use of these agents results in estrogen deficiency at a younger age. As adjuvant chemotherapy is becoming a standard treatment for premenopausal women with both node-negative and node-positive breast cancer, chemotherapy-induced menopause will be seen more frequently.

The administration of ERT to women with malignancies that are thought to have a hormonal etiology (such as breast or endometrial cancer) is very controversial. Most of these women will not be candidates for ERT. Studies that address the use of ERT in women diagnosed with breast and endometrial cancer are scarce and preliminary (Roy, Sawka, & Pritchard, 1996). Follow-up time is short. Prospective studies are being conducted, but it will be many years before definitive results are available (Vassilopoulou-Sellin & Theriault, 1994). Presently, the decision of whether ERT should be used is made on an individual basis and only after the expected benefits and potential consequences (including an early recurrence) are discussed.

The question of whether ERT might modify a woman's risk of developing breast cancer is controversial and unclear. Women who are considered to be at higher risk for developing breast or endometrial cancer often will choose to not take ERT. The estrogen deficiency in these women also places them at significant risk for developing osteoporosis and fracture.

Medications that contribute to bone loss: Many medications are associated with bone loss (see Figure 17-6). Oncology nurses especially need to be aware of medications used in the treatment of malignancy that contribute to bone loss, osteoporosis, and fractures. Drugs that may have a negative effect on bone mass include cyclophosphamide, doxorubicin, glucocorticoids, and methotrexate. The negative effects of these drugs may be the direct toxic effect on skeletal metabolism or gonadal tissues. The toxic effect on gonadal function results in premature menopause and subsequent estrogen deficiency.

Cyclophosphamide has been shown to induce ovarian failure and premature menopause in patients with breast cancer (Kayuama, Wada, & Nishizawa, 1977). In a recent study by Headley, Theriault, LeBlanc, Vassilopoulou-Sellin, and Hortobagyi (1998), menopause was induced in more than 80% of premenopausal patients treated with 5-fluorouracil, doxorubicin, and cyclophosphamide.

In animal studies, methotrexate and doxorubicin have been shown to reduce bone formation by nearly 60% (Friedlander, Tross, Doganis, Kirkwood, & Baron, 1984). Methotrexate also has been shown to increase bone resorption (May, Mercill, McDermott, & West, 1996). Even though methotrexate has been shown to have a negative effect on bone formation and bone resorption, the effect of low-dose methotrexate on BMD and fracture risk is unclear (Carbone et al., 1999).

Glucocorticoid use is associated with significant bone loss and increased risk for fracture. It appears that fracture risk with glucocorticoids is dose and duration dependent, although doses as low as 2.5 mg of prednisone or equivalent per day have been shown to increase fracture risk (Van Staa, Leufkens, Abenhaim, Zhang, & Cooper, 2000). Glucocorticoids appear to diminish osteoblast function, increase osteoclast activity, reduce intestinal calcium absorption, and impair gonadal function. The combination of these mechanisms synergistically contributes to bone loss and an increased risk for fractures.

The American College of Rheumatology (ACR) Task Force on Osteoporosis (1996) recommended that BMD testing be performed on any patient who is or will be on long-term glucocorticoid therapy to determine fracture risk. In addition, ACR recommended that preventive bone health measures be implemented for all patients on steroid therapy. These preventive measures include adequate intake of calcium and vitamin D, exercise, fall risk prevention, and lifestyle modifications (e.g., smoking cessation, moderation of alcohol consumption) (Paget et al., 1998).

Tamoxifen, which commonly is used in the management of breast cancer, is an estrogen antagonist with weak agonist activity. Most of the studies to determine the effect of tamoxifen on BMD and fracture risk in women with breast cancer have had a small sample size or were not designed specifically to assess these endpoints. Measurement of BMD in women with breast cancer treated with tamoxifen suggested that tamoxifen exerts a neutral or estrogenic effect on bone, such that bone mass is preserved (Kalef et al., 1996; Love, 1994; Wright et al., 1994). The long-term effects of tamoxifen on bone mass and fracture risk are not known.

History of previous fracture: A history of a previous osteoporotic fracture also is a significant risk factor for future fractures. Women with a single previous vertebral fracture experienced subsequent spine fractures at a rate 2.6–3.0 times greater than women without previous fractures, independent of bone mass. Women with a low bone mass and one previous fracture at baseline have a 25-fold increased risk of subsequent spine fractures, compared to women with high bone mass and no previous fractures (Ross, 1991). Women with vertebral fractures also are at increased risk for a nonvertebral fracture, including hip fractures (Klotzbuecher, Ross, Landsman, Abbott, & Berger, 2000; Melton, Atkinson, Cooper, O'Fallon, & Riggs, 1999).

In addition to increasing fracture risk, prevalent vertebral fractures also have been shown to significantly impair quality of life. Women with an existing vertebral fracture have an increase in hospital stays and limited activity days because of back pain (Nevitt et al., 2000). Multiple vertebral fractures result in height loss, permanent disfigurement, depression, loss of self-esteem, and fear of future fractures.

Two-thirds of all vertebral fractures are asymptomatic (Cooper, Atkinson, O'Fallon, & Melton, 1992). For this reason, a comprehensive history and physical assessment are critical (see Figure 17-7). Something as benign as reaching for dishes in the cabinet, weeding the garden, or carrying a child can result in a fragility vertebral fracture. A fragility fracture is an atraumatic fracture sustained from a fall of standing height or less. It is not uncommon for long-term survivors of breast or endometrial cancer to experience a fragility fracture without prior warning or symptoms.

Malignancy: Breast cancer may have a generalized effect on the skeleton. Biological markers on bone turnover have shown an increase in the activity of osteoclast function in patients presenting with cancer. Breast cancer tumors may increase the release of parathyroid hormone-related protein, transforming growth factor (alpha or beta), and cytokines (Guise & Mundy, 1998).

Figure 17-7. Evaluation of the Patient With Osteoporosis

History
- Alcohol consumption
- Tobacco use
- Weight-bearing exercise
- Nutrition assessment
- Medication use
- Any genetic or medical conditions associated with failure of bone gain or bone loss
- Fall risk assessment, including strength testing, gait, and balance evaluation
- Any fracture after age 40
- Menstrual history
- Tallest height and current height
- Back pain
- Family history of osteoporosis
- Surgical history

Laboratories
- Primary evaluation
  - Complete blood cell count
  - Serum chemistry including calcium, phosphate, liver enzymes, total alkaline phosphatase, creatinine, and electrolytes
  - Urinalysis, including pH
  - Bone mineral density testing
- Secondary evaluation
  - Thyrotropin
  - 24-hour urinary calcium excretion
  - Erythrocyte hormone concentration
  - 25-hydroxyvitamin D concentration
  - Dexamethasone suppression and other tests for hyperadenocorticism
  - Acid-base studies
  - Serum or urine protein electrophoresis
  - Bone marrow examination or bone biopsy
  - Undecalcified iliac bone biopsy with double tetracycline labeling

Medical History
1. Height at age 30? Any loss of height noticed?
2. Medications: heparin, thyroid medications, diuretics, alendronate/etidronate, hormone replacement/birth control pills, phenytoin/phenobarbital, prednisone, calcium, calcitonin, vitamins
3. Dietary history—specifically for dairy products, lactose intolerance, vegetarian, caffeine intake
4. Fractures? How did they occur?
5. Family history of fractures, Dowager's hump, osteoporosis
6. Physical activity
7. Menstrual history
8. Pain, functional limitations, psychosocial consequences

Physical Examination
A general physical examination should be performed on each patient with focus on
1. Accurate measurement of height and weight at each visit
2. Neck examination for thyroid enlargement
3. Spine examination for kyphosis, pain over the spinous processes, and muscle spasm
4. Evaluation of men for androgen deficiency
5. Breast examinations and education on self-examination for women if estrogen replacement is being considered
6. Assessment of gait stability, visual acuity, and fall risk

Screening and Diagnostic Evaluation for Osteoporosis

Low bone mass is the single most accurate predictor of increased fracture risk (Cummings et al., 1993). BMD testing can diagnose osteoporosis before fractures occur. The identification of people at risk for developing osteoporosis is critical so that further diagnostic evaluation and prevention can be implemented when indicated. Oncology nurses should remember that women who have survived breast and endometrial cancer are at a higher risk for developing osteoporosis because of estrogen deficiency and exposure to the medications used to treat these malignancies that have a direct toxic effect on bone cells or gonadal function. For these women, a discussion of osteoporosis and bone densitometry and possibly referral for further evaluation is appropriate, especially for women who are in long-term follow-up. Ganz (2000) noted that the risk of osteoporosis is high enough in premenopausal women diagnosed with breast cancer to consider ordering a baseline evaluation.

The current definition of osteoporosis is dependent on bone mass or the presence of a fragility fracture. BMD is expressed as standard deviation (SD) from the mean. The World Health Organization (1994) suggested definitions for osteoporosis (see Figure 17-3). Normal BMD is a value within 1 SD of the young adult reference mean. Low bone mass (osteopenia) is defined as BMD values between 1.0 and 2.5 SD below the young adult mean. Osteoporosis is defined as BMD values more than 2.5 SD from the young adult mean. Severe or established osteoporosis is defined as BMD greater than 2.5 SD below the young adult mean in the presence of one or more fragility fractures. A 75-year-old woman's bone mass always will be compared to a 30-year-old woman's bone mass (young adult mean) to determine fracture risk.

Bone densitometry should be considered when the patient's bone mass or fracture risk could affect clinical decision making (Miller, Bonnick, & Rosen, 1996). The following are clinical situations in which BMD may be indicated: estrogen deficiency, suspected osteopenia on x-ray, asymptomatic primary hyperparathyroidism, long-term glucocorticoid therapy, and monitoring the efficacy of osteoporosis treatment (see Figure 17-8). As bone mass decreases, risk of fracture increases exponentially. For each SD decrease in bone mass, the risk for fracture doubles at the spine and increases 2.5 times at the hip.

Bone densitometry also can help women to make decisions regarding measures to prevent fractures (Wasnich, 1993). After densitometry, women who reported below-normal results were almost five times more likely to begin therapy than women with normal BMD (Rubin & Cummings, 1992).

The most common method of measuring bone mass and currently the "gold standard" is dual x-ray absorptiometry (DXA). DXA subjects the patient to a radiation exposure equivalent to one-tenth the exposure of a chest x-ray (Johnston, Slemenda, & Melton, 1996). Other methods to determine BMD include quantitative computerized tomography, peripheral DXA, radiographic absorptiometry, ultrasound, single x-ray absorptiometry, or dual photon-absorptiometry (see Figure 17-9).

Figure 17-8. Indications for Bone Mineral Density Measurements (Bone Mass Measurement Act)

The Health Care Financing Administration passed the Bone Mass Measurement Act July 1, 1998. It provides national coverage for reimbursement of bone mineral density (BMD) tests in qualified Medicare beneficiaries. The following individuals are eligible for coverage.
• Estrogen-deficient women at clinical risk for osteoporosis
• Patients with vertebral abnormalities
• Patients receiving long-term glucocorticoid therapy (> 7.5 mg of prednisone qd or equivalent for more than three months)
• Patients with hyperparathyroidism
• Patients being monitored for evaluation of any osteoporosis drug therapy approved by the U.S. Food and Drug Administration

The National Osteoporosis Foundation's guidelines suggest that BMD testing be performed in the following individuals.
• All women 65 years of age or older regardless of additional risk factors
• All postmenopausal women younger than 65 years of age who have at least one additional risk factor other than menopause
• All postmenopausal women who seek treatment for fractures
• All women considering osteoporosis drug therapy whose decision might be influenced by BMD testing
• All women taking hormone replacement therapy for a prolonged period

Note. Based on information from Department of Health and Human Services, 1998; Lindsay, 1996.

Figure 17-9. Dual X-Ray Absorptiometry

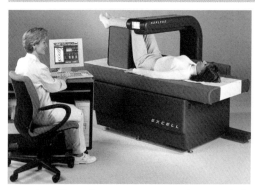 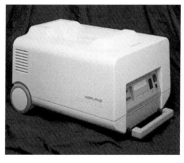

Examples of bone density measurement devices include devices that measure bone density at the hip and spine and portable devices that measure bone density at the wrist.

Note. Photos courtesy of Norland Medical Systems, Inc. Used with permission.

Because more than 30% of bone must be lost to determine osteopenia by routine x-ray, this method of detection is not used to determine bone density (Lane, Riley, & Wirganowicz, 1996). Radiographs can be used, however, to determine the presence of vertebral fractures and confirm fractures at other sites.

At the time that a fracture is confirmed, an interview should be conducted with the patient to determine the circumstances surrounding the fracture. The assessment should determine whether the fracture was a result of trauma or fragility. A fragility fracture itself can confirm the diagnosis of osteoporosis when any other underlying conditions are excluded. If the fracture is a result of a fall, risk-reduction strategies should be discussed (see Figure 17-10).

Once low bone mass has been determined, secondary causes must be ruled out. The major conditions contributing to decreased bone mass include genetic traits, lifestyle factors, nutritional factors, medical disorders, and certain medications (see Figure 17-6). Low bone mass in patients with cancer also may be related to metastatic lesions.

Clinical Implications of Risk Assessment

It is impossible to accurately predict BMD based on risk factors (Ribot, Tremollieres, & Pouilles, 1995). Consequently, most risk factors are not adequate predictors of fracture risk. Assessment and identification of risk factors can direct the clinician toward secondary causes of bone loss and osteoporosis. A risk factor assessment also can provide potential strategies for management of fracture risk, including changes in lifestyle, fall risk, or nutrition.

Another clinical assessment to incorporate into routine follow-up of women is a height measurement. This should be compared with other previous measure-

Figure 17-10. Fall Risk Reduction Strategies

Assess for factors that increase fall risk.
• The use of sedatives, hypnotics, alcohol, and psychotropic agents
• Postural hypotension
• Cognitive impairment
• Muscle strength, range of motion, gait, and ambulation
• Visual impairment
• Presence of small pets that may obstruct walkways or pathways

Minimize environmental hazards.
• Label all medications.
• Address disabilities.
• Sit on the side of the bed for a minute before rising.
• Correct vision problems.
• Adequately light stairways, hallways, and bathrooms.
• Implement gait and strength exercises.
• Discontinue the use of throw rugs.
• Arrange furniture to allow for unobstructed traffic flow.
• Maintain dry floors; address any leaks.
• Use nightlights and install handrails on stairs and in the bathroom.
• Remove hazardous electrical cords.
• Wear sturdy shoes with rubber, nonskid soles.
• Adjust hemlines.

ments, if available, or other self-reports to determine if height has been lost. Significant loss of height ($\geq$ 2 inches) may indicate the presence of one or more vertebral fractures and is suggestive of osteoporosis and the need for further diagnostic evaluation (Hunt, 1996).

Primary Prevention of Osteoporosis

Ideally, primary prevention measures to reduce the risk of developing osteoporosis are initiated in adolescence and continued through life. All women should receive information about these prevention practices, regardless of whether they have osteoporosis. The goals of prevention of osteoporosis include optimizing bone mass and preserving skeletal integrity (American Association of Clinical Endocrinologists and American College of Endocrinology, 1996). These measures include adequate calcium and vitamin D intake, regular weight-bearing exercise, smoking cessation, alcohol moderation, and pharmacologic intervention, when appropriate.

Calcium Intake

In providing advice about calcium intake, the intent is to ensure sufficient calcium to maintain calcium balance. Women who do not attain an average peak bone mass as young adults may be at higher risk for osteoporosis in the future (Dempster & Lindsay, 1993). Calcium can reduce the rate of bone loss at or after menopause. The NIH Consensus Conference (1994) recommended 1,500 mg of elemental calcium daily for women 65 years of age and older and for postmenopausal women younger than 65 who are not undergoing ERT. Postmenopausal women younger than 65 who are receiving ERT should take 1,000 mg of elemental calcium daily. Table 17-2 lists sources for dietary calcium. Calcium supplements should be taken with meals, because an acidic environment will facilitate calcium absorption (American Association of Clinical Endocrinologists and American College of Endocrinology, 1996). Patients with a history of kidney stones should take calcium supplements under medical supervision.

A vitamin D deficiency easily can be overlooked. Vitamin D helps to ensure that calcium is absorbed from the gastrointestinal (GI) tract. A vitamin D deficiency can cause a secondary hyperparathyroidism, which will increase bone turnover and increase bone loss. A vitamin D deficiency also may impair mineralization and cause osteomalacia. Vitamin D is synthesized naturally, following approximately 10 minutes of daily exposure to natural sunlight, and also is found in eggs, butter, and milk. Most multivitamins contain 400 IU, and some calcium supplements also contain vitamin D.

Exercise

The amount, duration, and intensity of exercise that is optimal for preserving bone mass in adults is unknown. Weight-bearing exercises generally are assumed to be most beneficial to bone. These exercises include such activities as tennis or walking. Swimming is not considered a weight-bearing exercise and

Table 17-2. Dietary Sources of Calcium

Source	Amount of Calcium (in mg)
Yogurt (1 cup)	400
Low-fat dry milk (¼ cup)	375
Ricotta cheese (½ cup)	350
Evaporated milk (½ cup)	350
Sardines (3 oz.)	324
Milk shake (10 oz.)	319
Milk (1 cup)	300
Swiss cheese (1 oz.)	275
Soft-serve ice milk (1 cup)	275
Cheese pizza (¼ of a 12-inch pizza)	232
Salmon (canned with bones, 3 oz.)	203
Cheddar cheese (1 oz.)	200
Spaghetti with meat balls (1 cup)	124
Dried beans (cooked, 1 cup)	100
Greens (½ cup)	100
Broccoli (½ cup)	89
Cottage cheese (½ cup)	75
Nuts (¼ cup)	75

Note. Based on information from National Dairy Council, 2001.

Population	Recommended Daily Calcium Intake
Children	800–1,200 mg
Adolescents and young adults	1,200–1,500 mg
Adults	
Postmenopausal women	
On estrogen	1,000–1,500 mg
Not on estrogen	1,500 mg
All adults older than age 65	1,500 mg

Note. Based on information from American Association of Clinical Endocrinologists & American College of Endocrinology, 1996.

therefore has a limited, if any, effect on bone mass. Even though some controversy exists regarding the effect of exercise on bone mass and fracture risk, exercise does have cardiovascular benefits and may improve agility and, therefore, the patient's ability to prevent or break a fall (American Association of Clinical Endocrinologists & American College of Endocrinology, 1996) (see Figure 17-10).

Calcium and vitamin D supplementation and an exercise regimen are insufficient to prevent the devastating consequences of osteoporosis and fractures. These strategies, however, are essential to any prevention or therapeutic regimen. All of the pharmacologic clinical trials discussed subsequently have control arms that include calcium- and vitamin D-replete subjects. Any increases in bone mass and reductions in fracture risk are in addition to those seen with calcium and vitamin D supplementation alone.

Pharmacologic Management of Osteoporosis

The primary goals of pharmacologic therapy for osteoporosis are to increase bone mass, stop or reverse bone loss, and reduce the incidence of fractures. The FDA has approved ERT, raloxifene, alendronate, and risedronate for the prevention of osteoporosis and alendronate, risedronate, raloxifene, and calcitonin for the treatment of osteoporosis.

The National Osteoporosis Foundation has suggestions for indications for treatment (Lindsay & Meunier, 1998) (see Figure 17-11), which rely primarily on bone mass and the presence of risk factors. Any patient who already has sustained a fragility fracture has osteoporosis and should be considered for treatment.

Figure 17-11. Recommendations for Treatment

American Association of Clinical Endocrinologists
• Consider preventive intervention when the T-score ranges from −1.5 to −2.5.
• Consider therapeutic intervention when the T-score is −2.5 or lower.
• Consider therapeutic intervention when preventive intervention is ineffective and bone loss continues.

National Osteoporosis Foundation
• Initiate therapy when T-score is below −2 in the absence of risk factors.
• Initiate therapy when T-score is below −1.5 when other risk factors are present.
• Initiate therapy in women older than 70 with multiple risk factors (especially those with previous nonhip, nonspine fractures) who are at high enough risk of fracture to initiate treatment without bone mineral density testing.

Note. Based on information from American Association of Clinical Endocrinologists & American College of Endocrinology, 1996; Lindsay & Meunier, 1998.

All of the therapies that will be discussed are considered antiresorptives. That is, they act to inhibit osteoclast number or function. This inhibition of the osteoclast results in a reduction of bone turnover and a net gain in bone mass. Currently, no FDA-approved anabolic therapies stimulate bone formation.

Estrogen Replacement Therapy

ERT currently is approved for the prevention of osteoporosis in postmenopausal women. In prospective trials, estrogen has been shown to slow bone loss following menopause or increase bone density by as much as 6% (Bone et al., 2000; Lufkin et al., 1992; Ravn et al., 1999; Writing Group for the PEPI Trial, 1996).

ERT is most beneficial if initiated at the onset of menopausal symptoms and continued indefinitely (Lindsay, 1996). Data suggest that once estrogen therapy is discontinued, bone loss may resume at a rate consistent with the early postmenopausal period (Greenspan et al., 1999).

Women who are on ERT and subsequently diagnosed with breast cancer usually will be advised to discontinue ERT immediately. These women need to be identified as being at increased risk for osteoporosis.

Numerous observational studies support estrogen therapy as effective in the reduction of vertebral fractures by as much as 50%–80%. The study of osteoporotic fractures suggested that current users of ERT had a reduction in fracture risk, and women who started ERT within five years of menopause and used ERT for more than 10 years had a relative risk for wrist fractures (0.25) and hip fractures (0.27) (Cauley et al., 1995).

Prospective data determining the efficacy of estrogens on fracture risk are limited. Lufkin et al. (1992) studied 75 postmenopausal women age 47–75 who had at least one vertebral fracture at baseline. Treatment with transdermal estrogen for one year reduced the incidence of vertebral fracture by 61%. Eight new fractures were found in seven women in the estrogen group (21% or 7:34). In the placebo group, 20 new fractures were found in 12 women (35% or 12:34). The group fracture rate in the estrogen group was 23 fractures per 100 people compared to 58 fractures in the placebo group. This is a different reporting method for fracture risk compared to other fracture trials.

In the Postmenopausal Estrogen/Progestin Intervention (PEPI) study, 875 women were randomized to receive either placebo or an estrogen/progestin regimen for three years (Writing Group for the PEPI Trial, 1996). No significant reduction was observed in the incidence of clinical fractures between the placebo and estrogen-treated groups. In contrast, a five-year study of 464 early postmenopausal women randomized to receive HRT alone, vitamin D alone, HRT and vitamin D, or placebo demonstrated a significant 71% reduction in symptomatic, nonvertebral fractures in the group that received HRT alone (Cauley et al., 1995).

Currently, no prospective studies are available that assess hip fracture risk reduction with ERT. Retrospective studies have shown that ERT may reduce hip fracture risk up to 50% (Reid, Torgerson, Thomas, & Campbell, 1996). Estrogen generally is considered a first-line management because of its positive effect on lipid profile and bone, potential cardiovascular benefits, and cerebrovascular benefits.

Only 30% of women continue ERT 12 months after initiating therapy (Hammond, 1994). Nonacceptance largely is because of concerns about side effects (e.g., spotting/menstrual bleeding, weight gain) and the potential increase in cancer risk (Hammond; Ravnikar, 1987). Women who have had a previous diagnosis of breast or endometrial cancer or who are considered at high risk for these malignancies may not be candidates for ERT.

Raloxifene

Raloxifene is the first selective estrogen-receptor modulator approved for the prevention and treatment of osteoporosis. When raloxifene binds to the estrogen receptor, it produces either an estrogen agonist or antagonist activity, depending on the tissue location of the receptor.

Raloxifene currently is approved by the FDA for both the prevention and treatment of osteoporosis in postmenopausal women. Raloxifene 60 mg/day is the FDA-approved dose.

The Multiple Outcomes of Raloxifene Evaluation (MORE) study evaluated the effect of raloxifene on the risk of vertebral fractures. In this study, 7,705 women with osteoporosis with low BMD and with or without a prevalent vertebral fracture received either 60 mg or 120 mg raloxifene or placebo. All participants received 500 mg supplemental calcium and 400 IU vitamin D daily. Roughly one-third of the participants had at least one vertebral fracture when the study began (Ettinger et al., 1999).

A three-year study (Ettinger et al., 1999) analyzed 6,828 women. BMD increased in the raloxifene-treated group by 2.6% at the spine and 2.1% at the femoral neck. Overall, a 40% reduction occurred in new vertebral fractures in the raloxifene-treated group. In the group treated with the FDA-approved dose of 60 mg/day, a 30% reduction (6.6%, 148:2,259) in new vertebral fractures was seen compared to placebo (10.1%, 231:2,292). Women in the 60 mg treatment group who had low bone mass on entry but no vertebral fracture had a 50% reduction in new vertebral fractures (4.5%, 68:1,522 versus 2.3%, 35:1,490). Women in the raloxifene 60 mg treatment group with low BMD and a prevalent vertebral fracture had a 30% reduction in new vertebral fractures (14.7%, 113:769) compared to placebo (21.2%, 163:770) (Ettinger et al.). Currently, no studies demonstrate hip fracture risk reduction with raloxifene treatment.

Also reported in the MORE trial was a 70% reduction in the development of invasive breast cancer in patients treated with raloxifene (Cummings et al., 1999). No effect was found on the endometrium. Raloxifene has not been studied in survivors of breast, endometrial, and ovarian cancers.

The most commonly reported side effects in women taking raloxifene are hot flashes, leg cramps, and an increase of venous thromboembolic events. Raloxifene, therefore, is contraindicated in women with an active or a past history of venous thromboembolic events. Raloxifene should be discontinued at least 72 hours before and during periods of immobility, such as prolonged bed rest, immobility because of travel, or postsurgical recovery. Therapy can be resumed once the patient is fully mobile.

Raloxifene should not be administered with cholestyramine because this drug interferes with raloxifene absorption. If administered with warfarin, the prothrombin time must be monitored carefully. It should be used with caution when administered with other highly protein-bound drugs, such as indomethacin, naproxen, diazepam, clofibrate, diazoxide, or ibuprofen. Raloxifene does not control menopausal symptoms.

Lipid changes also are seen with raloxifene therapy. Raloxifene has been shown to lower LDL cholesterol levels, although not as great as seen with estrogen, without a change in HDL cholesterol levels. Raloxifene does not cause an increase in triglycerides (Delmas et al., 1997).

Alendronate

Alendronate can be used in postmenopausal women who are at higher risk for developing osteoporosis. This includes women who are unable or unwilling to receive ERT. In a four-year clinical trial of early postmenopausal women (age 45–60) with normal bone density, alendronate 5 mg/day increased BMD at the hip and spine by 3%–4% (Ravn et al., 1999).

Alendronate also is approved by the FDA for the treatment of postmenopausal osteoporosis and for the treatment of glucocorticoid-induced osteoporosis in men and women. In various clinical trials, alendronate has been shown to improve BMD in the spine by 8%–10% and BMD in the hip by 3%–6% (Black et al., 1996; Cummings et al., 1998; Liberman et al., 1995).

The Fracture Intervention Trial (FIT) was designed to assess the efficacy of alendronate on fracture risk in postmenopausal women (Cummings et al., 1998). FIT has two treatment arms. The Clinical Fracture study was a four-year, multicenter study that looked at 4,432 postmenopausal women ages 55–80 without previous vertebral fractures. Patients received either placebo or 5 mg alendronate daily for the first two years and either placebo or 10 mg daily for the following 2.25 years (Cummings et al., 1998).

The Clinical Fracture arm found a 44% reduction in new vertebral fractures in the alendronate-treated group (2.1%, 43:2,077) versus the placebo group (3.8%, 78:2,218). A 56% reduction occurred in hip fracture risk in patients treated with alendronate who had a femoral neck T-score on entry of $\leq$ –2.5 (2.2% in the placebo group versus 1% in the alendronate group). No reduction occurred in hip fracture risk observed in patients with a femoral neck T-score at entry > –2.5 (0.4% in the placebo group versus 0.8% in the alendronate group).

The Vertebral Fracture arm of FIT studied 2,027 postmenopausal women ages 55–81 with osteoporosis who had experienced at least one vertebral fracture. In this three-year study, patients received either placebo or 5 mg alendronate daily for the first two years, and then placebo or 10 mg alendronate daily for the third year (Black et al., 1996).

In the Vertebral Fracture arm, new vertebral fractures occurred in 15% (145:965) of patients on placebo and 8.0% (78:981) of patients who received alendronate for three years. This resulted in a 47% reduction in new vertebral fractures in patients treated with alendronate. Additionally, a 90% reduction occurred in multiple vertebral fractures in the group treated with alendronate.

The Vertebral Fracture group also found a 51% reduction in hip fractures among patients who received alendronate for three years (2.2%, 22:1,005 in the placebo group versus 1.1%, 11:1,005 in the alendronate group).

In the fall of 2000, the FDA approved alendronate for once-weekly dosing (Merck & Co., Inc., 2000). Alendronate 70 mg orally per week has been approved for the treatment of osteoporosis in postmenopausal women and to increase bone density in men. Alendronate 35 mg orally per week has been approved for the prevention of osteoporosis in postmenopausal women.

Alendronate is poorly absorbed and has specific dosing instructions. It should be taken with 6–8 ounces of plain water after an overnight fast and at least 30 minutes before ingesting any other food, beverage, or medication. Patients should not lie down for at least 30 minutes after taking alendronate to prevent esophageal reflux and irritation and should remain upright until after the first meal of the day (Merck & Co., Inc., 1997). Some pharmacists and physicians interpret the directions "take on an empty stomach" to mean that it can be taken 30 minutes before lunch or dinner, provided the patient has not eaten between meals. This makes it easier for nursing home residents who often complain about being awakened at 6:30 am to take the pill and sit upright until breakfast arrives. Alendronate should be swallowed whole, and patients should not chew or suck the tablet (see Figure 17-12).

Alendronate, like other bisphosphonates, can cause upper GI irritation. Postmarketing reports indicated some incidences of esophagitis, gastric ulcers, and duodenal ulcers (Bauer et al., 2000).

Figure 17-12. Patient-Education Points Regarding Alendronate and Risedronate

1. After getting up for the day, swallow your tablet with a full glass (6–8 oz.) of plain water. Do not take alendronate or risedronate with mineral water, coffee, tea, or juice.
2. After swallowing your tablet, do not lie down—stay fully upright (sitting or standing) for at least 30 minutes and until after your first food of the day. Do not chew or suck the tablet. This will help the tablet reach your stomach quickly and help avoid irritation of your esophagus (the tube that connects your mouth with your stomach).
3. After swallowing the tablet, wait at least 30 minutes before taking your first food, beverage, or other medication of the day, including antacids, calcium supplements, and vitamins. The tablet is effective only if taken when your stomach is empty.
4. Do not take your medication at bedtime or before getting up for the day.
5. If you have difficulty or pain upon swallowing, chest pain, or new or worsening heartburn, stop taking the medication and call your doctor.
6. Take the tablet once a day, every day.
7. It is important that you continue taking it for as long as your doctor prescribes it. The medication can treat your osteoporosis or help you from getting osteoporosis only if you continue to take it.
8. If you miss a dose, do not take it later in the day. Continue your usual schedule of one tablet once a day the next morning.

Note. Based on information from Aventis Pharmaceuticals, 2000; Merck & Co. Inc., 1997.

Alendronate should not be used in patients with abnormalities of the esophagus that may delay esophageal emptying (i.e., stricture or achalasia) or esophageal abnormalities such as difficulty swallowing or gastroesophageal reflux disease. Alendronate is contraindicated in patients with an inability to stand or sit upright for at least 30 minutes and patients with hypercalcemia. Hypocalcemia must be corrected before initiating therapy.

Risedronate

Risedronate is a pyridinyl bisphosphonate approved by the FDA for the prevention and treatment of postmenopausal osteoporosis. Risedronate also is approved for the prevention and treatment of glucocorticoid-induced osteoporosis in men and women who are either initiating or continuing systemic glucocorticoid treatment for chronic diseases.

In various clinical trials, risedronate has been shown to improve BMD in the spine by 4%–6% and in the femoral neck by 1%–3% in postmenopausal women with low BMD and a prevalent vertebral fracture (Harris et al., 1999; Reginster et al., 2000).

The Vertebral Efficacy with Risedronate Trial, or VERT, was designed to assess the efficacy of risedronate in the prevention of vertebral fractures in postmenopausal women with established osteoporosis (Harris et al., 1999; Reginster et al., 2000). VERT had a North American arm and an international arm. VERT was a randomized, double-blind, multicenter, placebo-controlled study. The North American arm enrolled 2,458 postmenopausal women with at least one vertebral fracture at baseline and low BMD (Harris et al.). This study compared a control group receiving only calcium and vitamin D to groups receiving 2.5 mg or 5 mg risedronate per day for three years. The 2.5 mg/day of risedronate arm was discontinued after one year. Of the 2,458 patients enrolled, 450 subjects in the placebo arm and 489 subjects in the 5 mg/day risedronate arm completed the study.

The North American study found a 41% reduction in new vertebral fractures in the group treated with 5 mg/day of risedronate (11.3%, 61:696) versus the placebo group (16.3%, 93:678). Overall, the risedronate group demonstrated a 39% reduction in nonvertebral fractures; however, no significant reduction was found in hip fracture risk.

The international arm studied 1,226 postmenopausal women with low BMD and at least two vertebral fractures at baseline (Reginster et al., 2000). In this three-year study, patients received either 2.5 mg or 5 mg risedronate per day or placebo. The 2.5 mg/day of risedronate group was discontinued after two years. The international arm demonstrated a 49% reduction in new vertebral fractures during the three years of the study. New vertebral fractures occurred in 29% of the placebo subjects versus 18.1% in the risedronate group. The international arm of VERT demonstrated a 33% overall reduction in nonvertebral fractures; however, no significant reductions were found in hip fracture risk.

A recent study assessed the effect of risedronate on hip fracture risk. A total of 9,497 patients were enrolled into two groups of the study. All patients had to be at least 70 years old to participate. Risedronate, 2.5 mg and 5 mg, and placebo were evaluated. During the three years of the study, an overall 30% reduction in hip fracture risk was seen in the risedronate groups (McClung et al., 2001).

Like alendronate, risedronate should be taken with 6–8 ounces of plain water after an overnight fast and 30 minutes before any other food, beverage, or medication. Patients should not lie down for at least 30 minutes after taking risedronate and until after the first meal of the day. The pill should be swallowed whole, and patients should not chew or suck the tablet (Aventis Pharmaceuticals, 2000) (see Figure 17-12). Like other bisphosphonates, the most common side effects of risedronate are GI problems such as dyspepsia and nausea.

Risedronate should not be used in patients with abnormalities of the esophagus that may delay esophageal emptying (i.e., stricture or achalasia) or cause esophageal abnormalities such as difficulty swallowing or gastroesophageal reflux disease. Risedronate is contraindicated in patients with hypercalcemia and is not recommended for use in patients with renal impairment.

Calcitonin

Calcitonin is a hormone secreted by the thyroid gland that works as an antiresorptive agent by inhibiting osteoclastic function. Calcitonin is approved by the FDA for the treatment of osteoporosis in women who are at least five years postmenopausal with low bone mass (Novartis Pharmaceuticals Corp., 1995). Calcitonin has been available in the injectable form in the United States for more than 30 years.

Calcitonin has been shown to increase BMD by 2%–4% in postmenopausal women who already have experienced a vertebral fracture (Gennari, Agnusdei, & Camporeale, 1991). No conclusive data are available at this time to support that calcitonin can reduce fracture risk. Studies are ongoing at the request of the FDA.

Some studies suggested that calcitonin may be beneficial to reduce the painful effects of vertebral fractures (Gennari et al.).

The Prevent Recurrence of Osteoporotic Fractures study examined prevention of vertebral fractures in 1,255 postmenopausal women with a prevalent vertebral fracture and low BMD (Chestnut et al., 2000). Participants received either placebo or 100 IU, 200 IU, or 400 IU per day of salmon calcitonin nasal spray. All women received 1 g calcium and 400 IU vitamin D daily.

An analysis of all data found that after five years of therapy, those who received 200 IU intranasal calcitonin daily had a 36% reduction in the relative risk of new vertebral fractures (29.5%, 60:203 in the placebo group versus 19.3%, 40:207 in the 200 IU group). No statistically significant reduction was found in nonvertebral fracture risk or hip fracture risk (Blank & Bockman, 1999; Silverman et al., 1998).

The intranasal form of calcitonin has been available since October 1995. When given by the intranasal route, calcitonin has been shown to increase spinal bone mass in postmenopausal women with established osteoporosis but not in early postmenopuasal women. No evidence has shown that calcitonin will increase BMD at the hip. Figure 17-13 describes nursing considerations for calcitonin.

Figure 17-13. Nursing Considerations for Calcitonin

- Periodic nasal examinations are recommended. The development of mucosal alterations occurred in up to 9% of patients receiving intranasal calcitonin. Patients should notify their healthcare provider if they develop significant nasal irritation.
- Provide careful instruction on pump assembly. Patients should be instructed on priming of the pump and nasal introduction.
- Patients should alternate nostrils with the administration of intranasal calcitonin daily.

Note. Based on information from Novartis Pharmaceuticals Corp., 1995.

Nursing Challenges

Nurses need to include an assessment for osteoporosis for their perimenopausal and postmenopausal female patients. Particular care should be given so as to not overlook this potential problem in women whose long-term prognosis is favorable and who are not good candidates for ERT.

Assessment for and education regarding osteoporosis also should be a significant component of cancer screening and early detection programs. Women who seek cancer-screening services often have questions about the risks and benefits of ERT. This information usually is included in education about breast and endometrial cancer prevention. This discussion needs to be balanced, including comprehensive information about the strengths and limitations of ERT. In particular, women who decide not to take ERT because of a higher risk for breast or endometrial cancer should be encouraged to seek further evaluation for osteoporosis. Assessment for osteoporosis easily can be included with the cancer risk assessment and provides a foundation for education about women's health and well-being. Written materials can help to reinforce this education (see Figure 17-14).

Figure 17-14. Selected Resources for Information on Osteoporosis

Organizations	Web Sites
Older Women's League 666 Eleventh St. NW, Suite 700 Washington, DC 20001 (202-783-6686 or 800-TAKEOWL)	North American Menopause Society (NAMS) www.menopause.org Evista® (raloxifene) www.evista.com
National Osteoporosis Foundation PO Box 96616, Department ME Washington DC 20077-7456 800-464-6700 or 202-223-2226	Merck & Co., Inc. www.merck.com Fosamax® (alendronate) www.fosamax.com
North American Menopause Society c/o University Hospitals Department of OB/GYN 11100 Euclid Ave. Cleveland, OH 44106 216-844-8748	Actonel® (risedronate) www.actonel.com International Osteoporosis Foundation www.osteofound.org
Dairy Council 10255 W. Higgins Road, Suite 900 Rosemont, IL 60018-5616 847-803-2000, ext. 220 or 800-974-6455, toll-free fax	National Osteoporosis Foundation www.nof.org Dairy Council www.milk.co.uk
Merck & Co., Inc. Patient information: 800-505-WISH Pharmacist information: 800-NCS-MERCK	Older Women's League www.owl-national.org
Arthritis Foundation PO Box 19000 Atlanta, GA 30326 800-283-7800	American Cancer Society www.cancer.org CA: A Cancer Journal for Clinicians www.ca-journal.org
	American Society of Clinical Oncology www.asco.org
	American Society for Bone and Mineral Research www.asbmr.org
	International Society for Clinical Densitometry www.iscd.org
	Local Osteoporosis Education Link www.loel.net/store/default.asp?
	International Bone and Mineral Society www.bonekey-ibms.org
	Arthritis Foundation www.arthritis.org

As the issue of osteoporosis gains more public attention, patients may have more questions about their risk for developing it. Little is known about the attitudes and concerns of women with hormone-dependent malignancies and concerns related to estrogen deficiency. In one randomly selected group of 224 women with breast cancer, 27% felt they needed some treatment related to menopause, and 70% were concerned about menopause-related risk of osteoporosis (Vassilopoulou-Sellin & Theriault, 1994). This study suggested that women with breast cancer are aware of and concerned about the possible consequences of estrogen deficiency; however, 78% of the women in this study were unwilling to even consider ERT because of fears of recurrence. Clearly, oncology nurses cannot overlook this concern, whether patients verbalize it or not.

Oncology nurses can incorporate assessment of osteoporosis into routine visits for follow-up for women who have survived breast and endometrial cancer. Women who have a higher risk for development of osteoporosis should be counseled about the importance of diagnostic evaluation.

Many patients with cancer mistakenly believe that osteoporosis is the same as bone metastasis. Oncology nurses need to provide clear education that normal bone remodeling and hypercalcemia or metastatic lesions associated with malignancy are two entirely different physiologic processes that have different implications for treatment and long-term survival.

Many long-term survivors of breast and endometrial cancer may question why attention is being given to osteoporosis. In the past, little could be done to medically manage osteoporosis, so, in most cases, evaluation for osteoporosis was not viewed as relevant. With the development of nonhormonal medications, a new hope exists of preventing fractures, treating this disease, and, ultimately, improving the long-term quality of life for women with osteoporosis. Patients also may experience some hope and a sense of reassurance regarding their malignancy if the focus of the discussion is on a complication related to long-term survival.

Oncology nurses also can be key providers of education about what the patient can expect when scheduled for bone density testing. During DXA, a woman will be asked to remove any clothing with metal parts (e.g., zippers, snaps, underwire bras). The examination usually takes about 5–10 minutes per site (hip, spine, or forearm). The radiation exposure with a DXA examination is equivalent to one-tenth of a chest radiograph (Johnston et al., 1996). To image the spine, patients will be asked to lie flat on their back on the imaging table. To further stabilize the spine, patients are asked to elevate their legs on a foam wedge (see Figure 17-9). To image the hip, patients again are asked to lie flat on their back, and the hip is immobilized by using a brace on the ankle. The "gold standard" is to image one hip and the spine at the same appointment. Patients may be asked to not take their calcium supplements several days prior to imaging to decrease the probability of false-positive readings, because unabsorbed calcium in the GI tract will elevate BMD. A history of previous fractures at the hip or spine will compromise the results. A thorough history should be elicited before the examination so alternate or peripheral sites can be considered for evaluation. Peripheral sites include the wrist, calcaneus, or phalanges. No special preparation is needed before imaging these sites.

If a woman is diagnosed with osteoporosis or bone loss, options for medical management need to be discussed. Nurses can offer clarification about how to take medications correctly (see Figures 17-12 and 17-13).

Nurses also need to obtain a dietary history and provide education about dietary sources of calcium (see Figure 17-8) and vitamin D and differences in calcium supplements. Calcium supplements should be selected based on their content of elemental calcium, which can be determined by carefully reading the label. Encouraging patients to engage in weight-bearing exercise and implement strategies to reduce risk of falls also should be included in patient education.

Many women will be distressed if they are diagnosed with osteoporosis. Nurses need to emphasize that a low BMD does not mean a fracture will occur but that the risk is higher. Current therapeutic options can reduce fracture risk by 30%–90% (see Table 17-3). Patients should be reminded that they can help reduce their risk of a fracture related to osteoporosis. Providing education is the primary means of support. A number of written resources on osteoporosis are available. For further information, women may want to contact some of the organizations listed in Figure 17-14.

Table 17-3. Comparison of Therapies Available for the Prevention and Treatment of Osteoporosis

Drug/Dose	Osteoporosis Indication	Increases in Bone Mineral Density	Spine Fracture Risk Reduction	Hip Fracture Risk Reduction
Estrogen (various): Transdermal or oral	Prevention	2%–5% spine, 1%–3% hip	Prospective data: No statistically significant risk reductions; retrospective: 30%–80%	No prospective data; retrospective: 50%
Raloxifene 60 mg/qd po	Prevention and treatment	2%–3% spine, 1%–3% hip	30%	No significant reduction
Alendronate 5 or 10 mg/qd po or 70 mg/week po or 35 mg/week po	Prevention and treatment	8%–10% spine, 3%–6% hip	44%–47%	51%–56%
Risedronate 5 mg/qd po	Prevention and treatment	4%–6% spine, 1%–3% hip	41%–49%	30%
Nasal calcitonin 200 IU/qd intranasal	Treatment of women who are more than five years postmenopausal	1%–3% spine	33%	No significant reduction

Note. Based on information from Aventis Pharmaceuticals, 2000; Black et al., 1996; Blank & Bockman, 1999; Eli Lilly & Co., 1997; Ettinger et al., 1999; Harris et al., 1999; Hodgson et al., 2001; Liberman et al., 1995; Lindsay, 1996; Lufkin et al., 1992; McClung et al., 2001; Merck & Co., Inc., 2000; Meunier, 1998; Novartis Pharmaceuticals Corp., 1995; Reginster et al., 2000.

Clearly, osteoporosis is an emerging concern for long-term survivors of cancer. Nurses should not underestimate the important role they will play in helping to identify women at higher risk for developing osteoporosis. The early identification and management of osteoporosis ultimately can improve the long-term quality of life for these women.

Conclusion

Providing tertiary prevention practices is becoming an increasingly important role for nurses. The increasing number of cancer survivors puts many people at risk for developing both second malignancies and osteoporosis. The exact number of people affected is difficult to quantify but is significant in number. More research is needed to better understand the risks for developing second cancers and osteoporosis so that appropriate screening guidelines can be developed. Patients should be instructed that tertiary prevention measures are implemented when prognostic factors are good, and recommendations for screening ultimately are made to improve quality of life. This needs to be communicated to patients in a caring and hopeful manner. Healthcare providers need to increase their awareness and knowledge of these complications and develop strategies to detect them early. Ultimately, these efforts should decrease the morbidity and mortality associated with second cancers and osteoporosis.

References

American Association of Clinical Endocrinologists and American College of Endocrinology. (1996). AACE clinical practice guidelines for the prevention and treatment of postmenopausal osteoporosis. *Endocrine Practice, 2,* 157–171.

American Cancer Society. (2000). *Cancer facts and figures, 2000.* Atlanta: Author.

American Cancer Society. (2001). *Cancer facts and figures, 2001.* Atlanta: Author.

American College of Rheumatology Task Force on Osteoporosis. (1996). Recommendations for the prevention and treatment of glucocorticoid-induced osteoporosis. *Arthritis and Rheumatism, 39,* 1791–1801.

Assikis, V.J., Neven, P., Jordan, V.C., & Vergote, I. (1996). A realistic clinical perspective of tamoxifen and endometrial carcinogenesis [Abstract]. *European Journal of Cancer, 32A,* 1464–1476.

Aventis Pharmaceuticals. (2000). Actonel (risedronate) [Package insert]. Falls Church, VA: Author.

Averette, H., Boike, G.M., & Jarrell, M.A. (1990). Effects of cancer chemotherapy on gonadal function and reproductive capacity. *CA: A Cancer Journal for Clinicians, 40,* 199–209.

Avioli, L.V. (1994). *Clinician's manual on osteoporosis* (2nd ed.). London: Science Press.

Bauer, D.C., Black, D., Ensrud, K., Thompson, D., Hochberg, M., Nevitt, M., Musliner, T., & Freedholm, D. (2000). Upper gastrointestinal tract safety profile of alendronate: The fracture intervention trial. *Archives of Internal Medicine, 160,* 517–525.

Berwick, M. (1999). Skin cancers. In A.I. Neugut, A.T. Meadows, & E. Robinson (Eds.), *Multiple primary cancers* (pp. 445–467). Philadelphia: Lippincott Williams & Wilkins.

Bishop, D.T., & Kolodner, R.D. (1999). DNA repair disorders and multiple primary cancers. In A.I. Neugut, A.T. Meadows, & E. Robinson (Eds.), *Multiple primary cancers* (pp. 197–212). Philadelphia: Lippincott Williams & Wilkins.

Black, D.M., Cummings, S.R., Karpf, D.B., Cauley, J.A., Thompson, D.E., Nevitt, M.C., Bauer, D.C., Genant, H.K., Haskell, W.L., Marcus, R., Ott, S.M., Torner, J.C., Quandt, S.A., Reiss, T.J., & Ensrud, K.E., for the Fracture Intervention Trial Research Group. (1996). Randomized trial of the effect of alendronate on risk of fracture in women with existing vertebral fractures. *Lancet, 348*, 1535–1541.

Blank, R.D., & Bockman, R.S. (1999). A review of clinical trials of therapies for osteoporosis using fracture as an end point. *Journal of Clinical Densitometry, 2*, 435–452.

Bone, H.G., Greenspan, S.L., McKeever, C., Bell, N., Davidson, M., Downs, R.W., Emkey, R., Meunier, P.J., Miller, S.S., Mulloy, A.L., Recker, R.R., Weiss, S.R., Heyden, N., Musliner, T., Suryawanshi, S., Yates, A.J., & Lombardi, A., for the Alendronate/Estrogen Study Group. (2000). Alendronate and estrogen effects in postmenopausal women with low bone mineral density. *Journal of Clinical Endocrinology and Metabolism, 85*, 720–726.

Breast Cancer Linkage Consortium. (1999). Cancer risks in BRCA2 mutation carriers. *Journal of the National Cancer Institute, 91*, 1310–1316.

Carbone, L.D., Kaeley, G., McKown, K.M., Cremer, M., Palmieri, G., & Kaplan, S. (1999). Effects of long-term administration of methotrexate on bone mineral density in rheumatoid arthritis. *Calcified Tissue International, 64*, 100–101.

Cauley, J.A., Seeley, D.G., Enstraud, K., Ettinger, B., Black, D., & Cummings, S.R. (1995). Estrogen replacement therapy and fractures in older women. *Annals of Internal Medicine, 122*, 9–16.

Chesnut, III, C.H., Silverman, S., Andriano, K., Genant, H., Gimona, A., Harris, S., Kiel, D., LeBoff, M., Maricic, M., Miller, P., Moniz, C., Peacock, M., Richardson, P., Watts, N., & Baylink, D., for the PROOF Study Group. (2000). A randomized trial of nasal spray salmon calcitonin in postmenopausal women with established osteoporosis: The prevent recurrence of osteoporotic fractures study. *American Journal of Medicine, 109*, 267–276.

Consensus Development Conference. (1993). Diagnosis, prophylaxis, and treatment of osteoporosis. *American Journal of Medicine, 94*, 646–650.

Cooper, C., Atkinson, E.J., O'Fallon, W.M., & Melton, J.L. (1992). Incidence of clinically diagnosed vertebral fractures: A population-based study in Rochester, Minnesota, 1985–1989. *Journal of Bone and Mineral Research, 7*, 221–227.

Cooper, C., Campion, G., & Melton, L.J. (1992). Hip fractures in the elderly: A worldwide projection. *Osteoporosis International, 2*, 285–289.

Cummings, S.R., Black, D.M., Nevitt, M.C., Browner, W., Cauley, J., Ensrud, K., Genant, H.K., Palermo, L., Scott, J., & Vogt, T.M. (1993). Bone density at various sites for prediction of hip fractures. *Lancet, 34*, 72–75.

Cummings, S.R., Black, D.M., Thompson, D.E., Applegate, W.B., Barrett-Connor, E., Musliner, T.A., Palermo, L., Prineas, R., Rubin, S.M., Scott, J.C., Vogt, T., Wallace, R., Yates, A.J., & LaCroix, A.Z. (1998). Effect of alendronate on risk of fracture in women with low bone density but without vertebral fractures. *JAMA, 280*, 2077–2082.

Cummings, S.R., Eckert, S., Krueger, K.A., Grady, D., Powles, T.J., Cauley, J.A., Norton, L., Nickelsen, T., Bjarnason, N.H., Morrow, M., Lippman, M.E., Black, D., Glusman, J.E., Costa, A., & Jordan, V.C. (1999). The effect of raloxifene on risk of breast cancer in postmenopausal women. *JAMA, 281,* 2189–2197.

Daly, M.B., & Costalas, J. (1999). Breast cancer. In A.I. Neugut, A.T. Meadows, & E. Robinson (Eds.), *Multiple primary cancers* (pp. 303–317). Philadelphia: Lippincott Williams & Wilkins.

Delmas, P.D., Bjarnason, N.H., Mitlak, B.H., Ravoux, A.C., Shah, A.S., Huster, W.J., Draper, M., & Christiansen, C. (1997). Effects of raloxifene on bone mineral density, serum cholesterol concentrations, and uterine endometrium in postmenopausal women. *New England Journal of Medicine, 337,* 1641–1647.

Dempster, D.W., & Lindsay, R. (1993). Pathogenesis of osteoporosis. *Lancet, 341,* 797–801.

Department of Health and Human Services. (1998). *Medicare coverage of and payment for bone mass measurements.* Washington, DC: U.S. Government Printing Office.

Eisen, A., Rebbeck, T.R., Wood, W.C.Y., & Weber, B.L. (2000). Prophylactic surgery in women with a hereditary predisposition to breast and ovarian cancer. *Journal of Clinical Oncology, 18,* 1980–1995.

Eli Lilly & Co. (1997). Evista [Package insert]. Indianapolis, IN: Author.

Eng, C., & Maher, E.R. (1999). Dominant genes and phakomatoses associated with multiple primary cancers. In A.I. Neugut, A.T. Meadows, & E. Robinson (Eds.), *Multiple primary cancers* (pp. 165–195). Philadelphia: Lippincott Williams & Wilkins.

Ettinger, B., Black, D.M., Mitlak, B.H., Knickerbocker, R.K., Nickelsen, T., Genant, H.K., Christiansen, C., Delmas, P.D., Zanchetta, J.R., Stakkestad, J., Gluer, C.C., Krueger, K., Cohen, F.J., Eckert, S., Ensrud, K.E., Avioli, L.V., Lips, P., & Cummings, S.R. (1999). Reduction of vertebral fracture risk in postmenopausal women with osteoporosis treated with raloxifene. *JAMA, 1282,* 637–645.

Felix, C.A. (1999). Chemotherapy-related second cancers. In A.I. Neugut, A.T. Meadows, & E. Robinson (Eds.), *Multiple primary cancers* (pp. 137–164). Philadelphia: Lippincott Williams & Wilkins.

Friedlander, G.E., Tross, R.B., Doganis, A.C., Kirkwood, J.M., & Baron, R. (1984). Effects of chemotherapeutic agents on bone: Short-term methotrexate and doxorubicin (Adriamycin) treatment in a rat model. *Journal of Bone and Joint Surgery, 66,* 602–607.

Ganz, P.A. (2000). Long-term complications after primary therapy of breast cancer. In American Society of Clinical Oncology (Ed.), *ASCO spring educational book* (Vol. 19) (pp. 393–399). Alexandria, VA: American Society of Clinical Oncology.

Gennari, C., Agnusdei, D., & Camporeale, A. (1991). Use of calcitonin in the treatment of bone pain associated with osteoporosis. *Calcified Tissue International, 49*(Suppl. 2), S9–S13.

Gold, D.T. (1996). The clinical impact of vertebral fractures: Quality of life in women with osteoporosis. *Bone, 18*(Suppl. 3), 185S–189S.

Goodwin, P.J., Ennis, M., Pritchard, K.I., Trudeau, M., & Hood, N. (1999). Risk of menopause during the first year after breast cancer diagnosis. *Journal of Clinical Oncology, 17,* 2365–2370.

Greenspan, S.L., Bell, N., Bone, H., Downs, R., McKeever, C., Mulloy, A., Weiss, S., Heyden, N., Lombardi, A., & Suryawanshi, S. (1999). Differential effects of alendronate and estrogen on the rate of bone loss after discontinuation of treatment. *Journal of Bone and Mineral Research, 14*(Suppl. 1), S158.

Guise, T.A., & Mundy, G.R. (1998). Cancer and bone. *Endocrine Reviews, 19,* 18–54.

Hammond, C.B. (1994). Women's concerns with hormone replacement therapy—Compliance issues. *Fertility and Sterility, 62*(6 Suppl. 2), 157S–160S.

Hancock, S.L., & Tucker, M.A. (1998). Second cancers: Can we affect risk? *American Society of Clinical Oncology spring educational book* (Vol. 18) (pp. 74–79). Alexandria, VA: Author.

Harris, S.T., Watts, N.B., Genant, H.K., McKeever, C.D., Hangartner, T., Keller, M., Chestnut, C.H., Brown, J., Eriksen, E.F., Hoseyni, M.S., Axelrod, D.W., & Miller, P.D. (1999). Effects of risedronate treatment on vertebral and nonvertebral fractures in women with postmenopausal osteoporosis. *JAMA, 282,* 1344–1352.

Headley, J.A., Theriault, R.L., LeBlanc, A.D., Vassilopoulou-Sellin, R., & Hortobagyi, G.N. (1998). Pilot study of bone mineral density in breast cancer patients treated with adjuvant chemotherapy. *Cancer Investigation, 16,* 6–11.

Hemminki, K., & Vaittinen, P. (1999). Familial risks in second primary breast cancer based on a family cancer database. *European Journal of Cancer, 35,* 455–458.

Hodgson, S.F., Watts, N.B., Bilezikian, J.P., Clarke, B.L., Gray, T.K., Harris, D.W., Johnson, C.C., Kleerekoper, M., Lindsay, R., Luckey, M.M., McClung, M.R., Mankin, H.R., Petak, S.M., & Recker, R.R. (2001). Medical guidelines for clinical practice for the prevention and management of postmenopausal osteoporosis. *Endocrinologist Practice, 7,* 293–312.

Hunt, A. (1996). The relationship between height change and bone mineral density. *Orthopaedic Nursing, 15*(3), 57–64.

Inskip, P.D. (1999). Second cancers following radiotherapy. In A.I. Neugut, A.T. Meadows, & E. Robinson (Eds.), *Multiple primary cancers* (pp. 91–135). Philadelphia: Lippincott Williams & Wilkins.

Johnston, C.C., Slemenda, C.W., & Melton, L.J. (1996). Bone density measurement and the management of osteoporosis. In M.J. Favus (Ed.), *Primer on the metabolic bone diseases and disorders of mineral metabolism* (3rd ed.) (pp. 142–151). Philadelphia: Lippincott-Raven.

Kalef, J.A., Pavlidis, N., Klouvas, G., Karantanas, A., Hatzikonstantinou, I., & Glaros, D. (1996). Elemental composition of bone minerals in women with breast cancer treated with adjuvant tamoxifen. *Breast Cancer Research and Treatment, 37,* 161–168.

Kanis, J.A. (1994). *Osteoporosis.* Cambridge, MA: Blackwell Science.

Kanis, J.A. (1999). A high incidence of vertebral fracture in women with breast cancer. *British Journal of Cancer, 79,* 1179–1181.

Kayuama, H., Wada, T., & Nishizawa, L. (1977). Cyclophosphamide-induced ovarian failure and its therapeutic significance in patients with breast cancer. *Cancer, 39,* 1403–1409.

Klotzbuecher, C.M., Ross, R.D., Landsman, P.B., Abbott T.A., & Berger, M. (2000). Patients with prior fractures have an increased risk of future fractures: A summary of the literature and statistical synthesis. *Journal of Bone and Mineral Research, 15,* 721–727.

Lane, J.M., Riley, E.H., & Wirganowicz, P.Z. (1996). Osteoporosis: Diagnosis and treatment. *Journal of Bone and Joint Surgery, 78,* 618–632.

Liberman, U.A., Wiess, S.R., Broll, J., Minne, H.W., Quan, J., Bell, N.H., Rodriguez, J.P., Downs, R.W., Dequecker, J., Favus, M., Seeman, E., Recker, R.R., Capizzi, T., Santora,

A.C., Lombardi, A., Shah, R.V., Hirsch, L.J., & Karpf, D.B., for the Alendronate Phase III Osteoporosis Treatment Study Group. (1995). Effect of oral alendronate on bone mineral density and the incidence of fractures in postmenopausal osteoporosis. *New England Journal of Medicine, 333*, 1437–1443.

Lindsay, R. (1996). Prevention of osteoporosis. In M.J. Favus (Ed.), *Primer on the metabolic bone diseases and disorders of mineral metabolism* (3rd ed.) (pp. 256–261). Philadelphia: Lippincott-Raven.

Lindsay, R., & Meunier, P.J. (1998). Osteoporosis: Review of the evidence for prevention, diagnosis and treatment and cost-effectiveness analysis. *Osteoporosis International, 8*(Suppl. 4), S1–S88.

Love, R.R. (1994). Multisystem biological and symptomatic toxicity of tamoxifen in post-menopausal women. In V.C. Jordan (Ed.), *Long-term tamoxifen treatment for breast cancer* (pp. 57–81). Madison, WI: University of Wisconsin Press.

Lufkin, E.G., Wahner, H.W., O'Fallon, W.M., Hodgson, S.F., Kotowicz, M.A., Lane, A.W., Judd, H.L., Caplan, R.H., & Riggs, B.L. (1992). Treatment of postmenopausal osteoporosis with transdermal estrogen. *Annals of Internal Medicine, 117*, 1–9.

Lyles, K.W., Gold, D.T., Shipp, K.M., Peiper, C.F., Martinez, S., & Mulhausen, P.L. (1993). Association of osteoporotic vertebral compression fractures with impaired functional status. *American Journal of Medicine, 94*, 595–601.

Magaziner, J., Simonsick, E.M., Kashner, T.M., Hebel, J.R., & Kenzora, J.E. (1990). Predictors of functional recovery one year following hospital discharge for hip fracture: A prospective study. *Journal of Gerontology: Medical Sciences, 45*(3), 101–107.

Mahon, S.M., Williams, M.T., & Spies, M.A. (2000). Screening for second cancers and osteoporosis in long-term survivors. *Cancer Practice, 8*, 282–290.

May, K.P., Mercill, D., McDermott, M.T., & West, S.G. (1996). The effect of methotrexate on mouse bone cells in culture. *Arthritis and Rheumatism, 39*, 489–494.

McClung, M.R., Geusens, P., Miller, P.D., Zippel, H., Bensen, W.G., Roux, C., Adami, S., Fogelman, I., Diamond, T., Eastell, R., Meunier, P.J., & Reginster, J., for the Hip Intervention Program Study Group. (2001). Effect of risedronate on the risk of hip fracture in elderly women. *New England Journal of Medicine, 344*, 333–340.

Melton, L.J. (1993). Hip fractures: A worldwide problem today and tomorrow. *Bone, 14*(Suppl. 1), S1–S8.

Melton, L.J. (1999). Cost-effective treatment strategies for osteoporosis. *Osteoporosis International, 9*(Suppl. 2), S111–S116.

Melton, L.J., Atkinson, E.J., Cooper, C., O'Fallon, W.M., & Riggs, B.L. (1999). Vertebral fractures predict subsequent fractures. *Osteoporosis International, 10*, 214–221.

Merck & Co., Inc. (1997). Fosamax (alendronate) [Package insert]. Whitehouse Station, NJ: Author.

Merck & Co., Inc. (2000, October 23). *FDA approves once-weekly tablets of Fosamax® or treatment and prevention of postmenopausal osteoporosis* [Press release]. Retrieved June 21, 2001 from the World Wide Web: http://www.prnewswire.com/cgi-bin/stories.pl?ACCT=104&STORY=/www/story/10-23-2000/0001346221&EDATE=

Meunier, P.J. (1998). Calcium and vitamin D are effective in preventing fractures in elderly people by reversing senile secondary hyperparathyroidism. *Osteoporosis International, 8*(Suppl. 2), S1–S2.

Miller, P.D., Bonnick, S.L., & Rosen, C.J. (1996). Consensus of an international panel on the clinical utility of bone-mass measurements in the detection of low bone mass in the adult population. *Calcified Tissue International, 58*, 207–214.

Morris, C.R., Perkins C.I., Wright, W.E., Snipes, K.P., & Young, J.L. (1996). Impact of inclusion of subsequent primary cancers on estimates of risks of developing cancer. *Journal of the National Cancer Institute, 88*, 456–458.

Mundy, G.R. (1996). In M.J. Favus (Ed.), *Primer on the metabolic bone diseases and disorders of mineral metabolism* (3rd ed.) (pp. 16–24). Philadelphia: Lippincott-Raven.

National Dairy Council. (2001). *Calcium counseling resource.* Retrieved July 26, 2001 from the World Wide Web: http://www.nationaldairycouncil.org/dairycs/dcindex.html

National Institutes of Health Consensus Conference. (1994). Optimal calcium intake: NIH Consensus Development Panel of Optimal Calcium Intake. *JAMA, 272*, 1942–1948.

Neugut, A.I., & Gold, D. (1999). Gastrointestinal cancers. In A.I. Neugut, A.T. Meadows, & E. Robinson (Eds.), *Multiple primary cancers* (pp. 347–363). Philadelphia: Lippincott Williams & Wilkins.

Neugut, A.I., Meadows, A.T., & Robinson, E. (1999). Introduction. In A.I. Neugut, A.T. Meadows, & E. Robinson (Eds.), *Multiple primary cancers* (pp. 3–11). Philadelphia: Lippincott Williams & Wilkins.

Nevitt, M.C. (1994). Epidemiology of osteoporosis. *Rheumatic Disease Clinics of North America, 20*, 535–559.

Nevitt, M.C., Thompson, D.E., Black, D.M., Rubin, S.R., Ensrud, K., Yates, A.J., & Cummings, S.R., for the Fracture Intervention Trial Research Group. (2000). Effect of alendronate on limited-activity days and bed-disability days caused by back pain in postmenopausal women with existing vertebral fractures. *Archives of Internal Medicine, 160*, 77–85.

Novartis Pharmaceuticals Corp. (1995). Miacalcin (calcitonin) [Package insert]. Basel, Switzerland: Author.

Obedian, E., Fischer, D.B., & Haffty, B.G. (2000). Second malignancies after treatment of early-stage breast cancer: Lumpectomy and radiation vs. mastectomy. *Journal of Clinical Oncology, 18*, 2406–2412.

Paget, S.A., Gall, E.P., Hochbert, M.C., Jaffee, R., Lindsey, S.M., Mahowald, M.L., Robbins, L., & Simon, L. (1998). *Prevention and treatment of glucocorticoid-induced osteoporosis* [Monograph]. Atlanta: American College of Rheumatology.

Parikh, B., & Advani, S. (1996). Pattern of second primary neoplasms following breast cancer. *Journal of Surgical Oncology, 63*, 179–182.

Perry, H.M., Horowitz, M., Morley, J.E., Fleming, S., Jensen, J., Caccione, P., Miller, D.K., Kaiser, F.E., & Sundarum, M. (1996). Aging and bone metabolism in African American and Caucasian women. *Journal of Clinical Endocrinology and Metabolism, 81*, 1108–1117.

Ravn, P., Bidstrup, M., Wasnich, R.D., Davis, J.W., McClung, M.R., Balske, A., Coupland, C., Sahota, O., Kaur, A., Daley, M., & Cizza, G. (1999). Alendronate and estrogen-progestin in the long-term prevention of bone loss: Four-year results from the Early Postmenopausal Intervention Cohort study. *Annals of Internal Medicine, 131*, 935–942.

Ravnikar, V.A. (1987). Compliance with hormone therapy. *American Journal of Obstetrics and Gynecology, 156*, 1332–1334.

Ray, N.F., Chan, J.K., Thamer, M., & Melton, L.J. (1997). Medical expenditures for the treatment of osteoporotic fractures in the United States in 1995: Report from the National Osteoporosis Foundation. *Journal of Bone and Mineral Research, 12,* 24–35.

Reginster, J.Y., Minne, H.W., Sorensen, O.H., Hooper, M., Roux, C., Brandi, M.L., Lund, B., Ethgen, D., Pack, S., Roumagnac, I., & Eastell, R. (2000). Randomized trial of the effects of risedronate on vertebral fractures in women with established post-menopausal osteoporosis. *Osteoporosis International, 11,* 83–91.

Reid, D., Torgerson, D., Thomas, R., & Campbell, M. (1996). Randomized trial of perimenopausal screening for osteoporosis risk: Effect on HRT uptake and quality of life. *Journal of Bone and Mineral Research, 11*(Suppl. 1), S109.

Ribot, C., Tremollieres, F., & Pouilles, J.M. (1995). Can we detect women with low bone mass using clinical risk factors? *American Journal of Medicine, 98*(Suppl. 2A), 52S–55S.

Riis, B.J. (1995). The role of bone loss. *American Journal of Medicine, 98*(Suppl. 2A), 29S–32S.

Robinson, E. (1999). Clinical characteristics and approach to management. In A.I. Neugut, A.T. Meadows, & E. Robinson (Eds.), *Multiple primary cancers* (pp. 55–66). Philadelphia. Lippincott Williams & Wilkins.

Rodriguez, C., & Ash, C.R. (1996). Cancer therapy: Associated late effects. *Cancer Nursing, 19,* 455–468.

Ross, P.D. (1991). Pre-existing fractures and bone mass predict vertebral fracture incidence in women. *Annals of Internal Medicine, 114,* 919–923.

Ross, P.D. (1996). Osteoporosis: Frequency, consequences, and risk factors. *Archives of Internal Medicine, 156,* 1399–1411.

Roy, J.A., Sawka, C.A., & Pritchard, K.I. (1996). Hormone replacement therapy in women with breast cancer: Do the risks outweigh the benefits? *Journal of Clinical Oncology, 14,* 997–1006.

Rubin, S.M., & Cummings, S.R. (1992). Results of bone densitometry affect women's decisions about taking measures to prevent fractures. *Annals of Internal Medicine, 116,* 990–995.

Schneider, K.A. (1995). *Counseling about cancer: Strategies for genetic counselors.* Wallingford, PA: National Society for Genetic Counselors.

Schottenfeld, D. (1996). Multiple primary cancers. In D. Schottenfeld & J.F. Fraumeni (Eds.), *Cancer epidemiology and prevention* (2nd ed.) (pp. 1370–1387). New York: Oxford University Press.

Silverman, S.L., Chesnut, C., Andriano, K., Genant, H., Gimona, A., Maricic, M., Stock, J., & Gaylink, D., for the PROOF Study Group. (1998). Salmon calcitonin nasal spray (NS-CT) reduces risk of vertebral fracture(s) (VF) in established osteoporosis and has continuous efficacy with prolonged treatment: Accrued 5-year worldwide data of the PROOF study. *Bone, 23*(Suppl. 5), S174.

Smith, T.J., & Hillner, B.E. (2000). Tamoxifen should be cost-effective in reducing breast cancer risk in high-risk women. *Journal of Clinical Oncology, 18,* 284.

Travis, L.B., Curtis, R.E., Boice, J.D., Platz, C.E., Hankey, B.F., & Fraumeni, J.F. (1996). Second malignant neoplasms among long-term survivors of ovarian cancer. *Cancer Research, 56,* 1564–1570.

Van Staa, T.P., Leufkens, H.G.M., Abenhaim, L., Zhang, B., & Cooper, C. (2000). Use of oral corticosteroids and risk of fractures. *Journal of Bone and Mineral Research, 15,* 993–999.

Vassilopoulou-Sellin, R., & Theriault, R.L. (1994). Randomized prospective trial of estrogen-replacement therapy in women with a history of breast cancer. *Journal of the National Cancer Institute Monographs, 16,* 153–159.

Velie, E.M., & Schatzkin, A. (1999). Common environmental risk factors. In A.I. Neugut, A.T. Meadows, & E. Robinson (Eds.), *Multiple primary cancers* (pp. 213–223). Philadelphia: Lippincott Williams & Wilkins.

Wasnich, R. (1993). Bone mass measurement: Prediction of risk. *American Journal of Medicine, 95*(Suppl. 5A), 6S–10S.

Willett, W.C. (1999). Goals for nutrition in the year 2000. *CA: A Cancer Journal for Clinicians, 49,* 331–352.

World Health Organization. (1994). *Assessment of fracture risk and its application to screening for postmenopausal osteoporosis. Report of a WHO Study Group.* Washington, DC: Author.

Wright, C.D., Garrahan, N.J., Stanton, M., Gazet, J.C., Mansell, R.E., & Compston, J.E. (1994). Effect of long-term tamoxifen therapy on cancellous bone remodeling and structure in women with breast cancer. *Journal of Bone and Mineral Research, 9,* 153–159.

Writing Group for the PEPI Trial. (1996). Effects of hormone therapy on bone mineral density: Results from the Postmenopausal Estrogen/Progestin Interventions (PEPI) trial. *JAMA, 276,* 1389–1396.

Zimmerman, R., & Westhoff, C.L. (1999). Gynecologic cancers. In A.I. Neugut, A.T. Meadows, & E. Robinson (Eds.), *Multiple primary cancers* (pp. 397–416). Philadelphia: Lippincott Williams & Wilkins.

CHAPTER 18

Genetic Counseling and Screening

Karen E. Greco, RN, MN, ANP

Introduction

J.D. Watson and F.H.C. Crick first described the complex molecular structure of genes, deoxyribonucleic acid (DNA), in 1953. Watson and Crick shared the Nobel Prize in Physiology or Medicine with M. Wilkins in 1962 for their work in determining the structure of the DNA molecule. An enormous amount of information is present in the 46 chromosomes of a human cell, which are estimated to contain six billion base pairs of DNA. Current technology has allowed people to begin to understand information about their genetic blueprint and identify changes in DNA, which may have implications for risks for certain cancers. As is often the case, scientific discovery and medical technology related to genetic information are advancing faster than is society's ability to deal with the resulting psychosocial, ethical, and medical issues. The discovery of genetic mutations associated with increased cancer risk and the development of cancer predisposition testing is having a tremendous impact on oncology. Patients are concerned about their potential genetic risk for cancer and the risk of those they love. Nurses have a responsibility to help patients and their families to understand genetic information and the implications and uncertainties that come with that information. Nurses must comprehend the issues associated with genetic information related to cancer so that they can answer these questions. This chapter will provide an overview of issues related to genetic information for the purpose of increasing awareness of issues that need to be considered when counseling patients about genetic testing and test results. This information should be helpful to all oncology nurses, whether they are answering basic questions about genetic counseling or providing genetic counseling and predisposition genetic testing services.

Nursing Implications for Genetic Counseling and Screening

Nurses have been involved in genetic counseling and education since the 1960s, when nurses provided services to children with genetic disorders and their families. Forbes (1996) stated that genetic counseling involves the presentation of statistical probabilities while at the same time dealing with the family's knowledge, feelings, and problems related to this information. As part of a multidisciplinary team, nurses fulfill this role by being involved in case finding, detailed history taking, obtaining medical records, pedigree construction, clarification of genetic information, assisting the family to deal with the emotional impact of genetic information, and referral to appropriate resources. Although cancer genetic counseling only began a few years ago, in many respects, the oncology nurse's role in cancer genetic counseling remains largely unchanged. According to Forsman (1994), the only change is the information available and the population to which the information may be applied.

The identification of genetic mutations associated with increased risk for certain cancers and the subsequent development of cancer predisposition testing has created a tremendous need for healthcare professionals who can explain and interpret genetic information through genetic counseling and education. Patients and their families are asking questions about their own cancer risk, whether this genetic information may explain the cancer in their family, the availability of predisposition genetic testing, and how to obtain genetic information they can understand. Oncology nurses, already educated in cancer care and seen as health educators and patient advocates, are on the forefront in providing genetic counseling and education to help to address these questions.

The Oncology Nurse's Role

Cancer genetics is rapidly moving into all areas of cancer practice, and nurses must be able to meet the challenges and take advantage of new opportunities. The Oncology Nursing Society (ONS) recognized this fact and published a position titled "The Role of the Oncology Nurse in Cancer Genetic Counseling" (ONS, 1998). Three levels of oncology nursing practice are addressed in this position: the general oncology nurse, the advanced practice oncology nurse, and the advanced practice oncology nurse with specialty training in cancer genetics. According to this position statement, oncology nurses possess the skills and are well suited to assume expanded roles in genetic counseling. Nurses providing cancer genetic counseling, however, must be advanced practice nurses (APNs) in oncology with specialized education in genetics. Another resource for oncology nurses regarding the genetics nursing role is the *Statement on the Scope and Standards of Genetics Clinical Nursing Practice*, which was published by the American Nurses Association and the International Society of Nurses in Genetics (1998). This statement describes standards of genetics nursing care at both the basic and advanced levels.

Genetic counseling represents only a small component of the cancer genetics continuum of care. A high percentage of patients seen in cancer genetics programs already have been diagnosed with cancer and currently are being seen by oncology healthcare providers who may have instigated the referral. After a patient is seen in a cancer genetics program, often the oncology healthcare providers take the responsibility for ongoing management and surveillance. This may be the area in which oncology nurses have the most to offer patients. Many patients seen in cancer genetics programs only need cancer risk assessment services and do not meet the criteria for cancer predisposition testing. These patients often have a family history of cancer combined with nongenetic risk factors and need education regarding cancer risk reduction and surveillance.

General Oncology Nurses

All oncology nurses, regardless of their practice setting, are likely to encounter questions from patients and family members about genetic services. Part of the nurse's responsibility is to provide at least basic patient education, followed with appropriate referral. Knowledge about available cancer genetics resources is essential. *Genetics in Clinical Practice: New Directions for Nursing and Health Care* (Lea, Jenkins, & Francomano, 1998) provides a good general overview of genetics information and how it applies to nursing. Because it is impossible to be an expert in all areas, knowing where to find appropriate resources is invaluable (Rieger, 1997). Figure 18-1 lists Web addresses for resources, including how to obtain genetic testing pamphlets, a database of cancer genetics information providers, genetics support groups, and a searchable database of genetics nursing literature.

Through nursing assessment, which includes obtaining a personal and family medical history, oncology nurses are in a position to identify red flags that indicate whether an individual may need to be referred for cancer genetic services. In addition, nurses can assess cancer risk factors and identify appropriate community support groups. Oncology nurses also are in an ideal position to educate patients about health maintenance, cancer risk reduction, and cancer surveillance.

Advanced Practice Oncology Nurse
Clinical Practice

Oncology APNs are likely to care for patients and families who may need genetic services. While obtaining a personal and family medical history during the assessment process, they can identify key indicators for referral to cancer genetic counseling or predisposition genetic testing. In addition, they can start the process of documenting cancer diagnoses in a family medical record, educate patients about basic genetic concepts, initiate pedigree construction, and order appropriate cancer surveillance tests. Pedigrees are a diagrammatic way of representing a family history. Gould, Lynch, Smith, and McCarthy (1997) provided detailed instructions for constructing a pedigree. APNs can provide follow-up care to patients with a known genetic mutation that predisposes them to cancer and must be familiar with current cancer surveillance guidelines for people who carry a genetic predisposition for cancer. Knowledge about the risks and benefits of prophylactic surgery, relevant chemoprevention interventions, and other risk-reduction options is critical when providing care to this population.

Figure 18-1. Web Sites[a] Related to Cancer and Genetics

Genetics Alliance Support Groups www.geneticalliance.org/	Nationwide list of genetics support groups
American Society of Clinical Oncology (ASCO) www.asco.org	Under shopping cart button on this Web site, a copy of ASCO's cancer genetics curriculum slides and speaker's notes can be ordered for a fee.
CancerNet[TM] http://cancernet.nci.nih.gov/prevention/genetics.shtml	Can download pamphlets and articles related to genetics
Gene Clinics www.geneclinics.org	Gives an overview of the diagnosis, management, and genetic counseling of individuals and families with specific inherited disorders.
Genetics Education Center www.kumc.edu/gec	A variety of resources for educators at all undergraduate levels who are interested in teaching basic genetics
Genetics Professionals Directory http://cancernet.nci.nih.gov/genesrch.shtml	National Cancer Institute database of cancer genetics service providers nationwide
National Institute of Health's online glossary of genetic terms www.nhgri.nih.gov/DIR/VIP/Glossary/pub_glossary.cgi	Glossary of genetic terms
FORCE (Facing Our Risk of Cancer Empowered) www.facingourrisk.org	This Web site is available for women at high risk for breast or ovarian cancer. An opportunity exists to network with other women at risk for these cancers. This site has a wealth of information that is valuable to nurses, including numerous articles and resources.
Human Genome Project www.nhgri.nih.gov	
International Society of Nurses in Genetics http://nursing.creighton.edu/isong	This Web site contains information about educational opportunities and has links to other genetics-related Web sites.
National Cancer Institute www.nci.nih.gov	Click on "Cancer Information" on the home page, and genetics information is located under "CancerNet."
Oncology Nursing Society www.ons.org	Features a Genetic Resource Area; ONS members have the opportunity to join the Cancer Genetics Special Interest Group.
Women's Cancer Network www.wcn.org/risk	A lay Web site that includes a cancer-risk assessment questionnaire that provides women with information about their risk for breast, ovarian, or colon cancer and also has risk-reduction information

[a] These Web sites were active at the time of this publication.

Research

A critical need exists for APNs to be involved in cancer genetics research. Donaldson (1999) identified six areas of research that are important to genetics nursing practice: (a) health promotion, (b) health and risk assessment, including privacy and confidentiality, (c) health outcomes, (d) health counseling, including ethical issues, (e) family-person coping and experience, and (f) disease prevention/management. Research in cancer genetics often involves complex issues and requires a multidisciplinary approach.

APNs can contribute to the knowledge base of cancer genetics nursing practice in several ways. One option is to work with a team of experienced researchers and oncology nurses involved in a large clinical trial, such as the descriptive study of reactions to disclosure of BRCA1 test results (Lynch et al., 1997). Another option is to carry out a small clinical study in a community setting that replicates the design of a larger clinical trial in a research setting. A third option is to connect with an experienced nurse researcher who is affiliated with a local university and knows how to conduct research but needs a partner with clinical experience in cancer genetics.

Advanced Practice Oncology Nurses With a Subspecialty in Genetics

This group of highly specialized nurses represents the minority of oncology nurses. These nurses often are found in cancer genetics programs where they provide cancer genetic counseling services, order cancer predisposition genetic testing (if within the nurse practice act), provide informed consent, and interpret cancer predisposition genetic test results. APNs who want to order predisposition genetic tests, such as BRCA analysis, are advised to contact the State Board of Nursing in their state to find out if it is within their scope of practice. One of the most important services these nurses offer is developing individualized cancer-surveillance and risk-management plans for patients who have received cancer genetic counseling services, regardless of whether the person receives predisposition genetic testing for cancer. APNs in genetics also are in an ideal position to develop and coordinate cancer genetics programs and services. Figure 18-2 includes a summary of the levels of oncology genetics in nursing practice.

Genetic Cancer Risk Assessment

Cancer risk assessment is a term that usually refers to the evaluation of an individual's cancer risk based on information related to heredity, lifestyle, dietary, hormonal, environmental, and other factors that have been associated with an increased risk for certain cancers. This information then is collated, and some determination is made regarding an individual's cancer risk compared to a standard, such as cancer incidence in the general population. Communicating risk information to patients in a way that facilitates patient understanding and addressing the psychological issues related to the communication of cancer risk information are essential components of cancer risk assessment (Mahon, 1998).

Figure 18-2. Levels of Cancer Genetics Nursing Practice

General Oncology Nurse
• Identify red flags that indicate genetic services may be indicated.
• Provide information about cancer genetics programs and resources.
• Begin collecting a patient and family medical history, which may include beginning pedigree construction.
• Assess cancer risk factors including, but not limited to, heredity, lifestyle, diet, hormone replacement therapy, environment, and occupation.
• Provide basic information about health maintenance, cancer risk reduction, and cancer surveillance.
• Participate as a research nurse in clinical cancer genetics research studies.

Advanced Practice Oncology Nurse (in addition to the above)
• Collect detailed information about the patient's personal and family medical history and construct a pedigree.
• Provide basic patient information concerning what is involved in cancer predisposition genetic counseling and testing.
• Start the process of documenting cancer diagnoses in the family with medical records.
• Order and interpret appropriate cancer surveillance tests.
• Provide follow-up care to patients with a known genetic mutation predisposing them to cancer.
• Provide patient education concerning cancer surveillance guidelines, risks and benefits of prophylactic surgery, relevant chemoprevention interventions, and other risk-reduction options.

Advanced Practice Oncology Nurse With a Subspecialty in Genetics (in addition to the above)
• Provide cancer genetic counseling and cancer-risk assessment services.
• Construct a detailed pedigree, including at least three generations.
• Assess the pedigree and evaluate the likelihood that the cancers in the patient's family may be the result of a hereditary cancer syndrome.
• Provide informed consent for cancer predisposition genetic tests.
• Order cancer predisposition genetic tests, and interpret cancer predisposition genetic test results (if within the state nurse practice act).
• Develop cancer surveillance and risk-management plans for patients who have received cancer genetic counseling services.
• Initiate, coordinate, or participate in clinical cancer genetics research studies.

Approximately 5%–10% of cancers are thought to be related to hereditary factors (Lea et al., 1998). Genetic cancer risk assessment usually refers to the component of assessment that evaluates the probability that the cancer in a person's family is related to an inherited genetic alteration associated with an increased risk for cancer. This involves obtaining a detailed patient and family history of cancer and other medical conditions. A detailed pedigree then is constructed, involving at least three generations. MacDonald (1997) provided a detailed description of how to take a family history. Obtaining information on at least three generations is critical for an accurate evaluation of family history. Each generation is represented on a different level of the diagram, which facilitates identification of patterns of cancer that are passed down through several generations (see Figure 18-3). Cancer diagnoses in the patient, first-degree relatives, and second-degree relatives are documented by obtaining pathology reports whenever possible to increase the accuracy of the family history. A

Figure 18-3. Pedigree Example

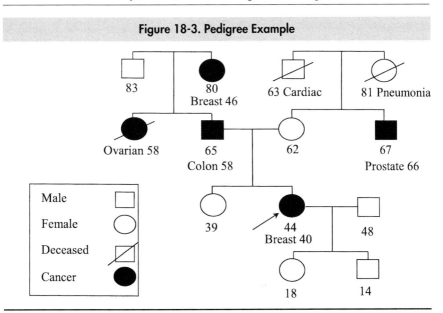

determination then is made concerning how likely it is that a particular family history of cancer is related to a genetic alteration known to be associated with increased cancer risk.

For example, Figure 18-3 is a diagram of a pedigree for a 44-year-old woman who was diagnosed with breast cancer at age 40. The arrow points to the patient whose family history the pedigree represents. This person is referred to as the proband or consultand. First-degree relatives are siblings, parents, and children, and second-degree relatives are grandparents, grandchildren, aunts and uncles, and nieces and nephews.

Hereditary cancer syndromes, such as breast-ovarian cancer syndrome, usually follow an autosomal dominant pattern. This means that if a person carries a genetic alteration that predisposes him or her to cancer, a 50% chance exists of this same genetic alteration being passed on to his or her children. The majority of hereditary breast cancer (approximately 84%) is thought to be related to alterations in two genes, BRCA1 and BRCA2 (Frank, 1998). When these genes are functioning properly, they act as tumor-suppressor genes. A copy that has been damaged is not able to suppress cellular changes that lead to cancer. Most cancer-predisposing genes are autosomal dominant, which means that a person only needs to carry one altered copy of the gene to be at risk for the cancers associated with that particular genetic change (Lea et al., 1998). If a child inherits two normal copies of these genes, then his or her cancer risk will be similar to that of the general population. If one altered copy and one normal copy of either BRCA1 or BRCA2 is inherited, a woman will have a risk of breast cancer about five to six times that of the general population (56%–87% compared to 12%). These genes also are associated with increased risk for other cancers. BRCA1 is associated with a 28%–44% risk of ovarian cancer (compared to 1%–2% in the general population) and an increased risk for colon and prostate cancers. BRCA2 is associated with approximately a 27% risk for ovarian cancer and increased risk for male breast, prostate, and pancreatic cancer (Frank). The proband in Figure 18-3 has one sister who is 39 years old and has never been diagnosed with cancer. Her father was diagnosed with colon cancer at age 58 and is still living; her paternal aunt died of ovarian cancer at age 58; and her paternal grandmother was diagnosed with breast cancer at age 46. Cancer appears in every generation on the paternal side of the family. This is a key indicator that the cancer in her family might be related to a genetic alteration.

Another key indicator is the age at cancer diagnosis. Both the proband and her paternal grandmother were diagnosed with breast cancer in their 40s. Breast, ovarian, and colon cancers all have been associated with mutations in BRCA1. The pedigree for this proband suggests these indicators of hereditary predisposition: cancer in every generation on the paternal side, cancer being diagnosed at earlier ages than the usual onset, and clusters of cancers known to be associated with a hereditary cancer syndrome. This does not mean that the proband carries a cancer predisposing mutation; however, it does mean that further assessment is indicated. Expanding the pedigree to include children of her brother, aunt and uncle, and siblings of her grandparents may give more information about the pattern of cancer in the family.

Confirming the cancers on the pedigree, especially on the paternal side, with pathology reports or death certificates, also is important for accuracy of the genetic assessment. If the ovarian cancer turns out to be uterine cancer, this means that Lynch II, a hereditary colon cancer syndrome, also needs to be considered, which will change the genetic assessment. It is important for the cancer risk assessment to include lifestyle, dietary, hormonal, and environmental factors.

Sometimes it is possible to estimate the probability that a particular cancer-predisposing mutation may be present, given a particular family history pattern based on published research studies. For example, several studies offer genetic risk assessment models that estimate the probability that a person carries an alteration in the BRCA1 or BRCA2 gene (Frank, 1998; Shattuck-Eidens et al., 1995; Strewing et al., 1997). The American Society of Clinical Oncology (ASCO) (1996) recommended that cancer predisposition genetic testing be offered only when the patient has a strong family history of cancer or very early age at onset of disease (with a 10% or greater probability of having a mutation); the test can be interpreted adequately; and the results will influence the medical management of the patient or a family member. The proband in Figure 18-3 would be appropriate for referral to a cancer genetics program for possible genetic testing based on these guidelines. Figure 18-1 includes resources for locating cancer genetic counseling providers in the United States.

When to Refer for Cancer Genetics Services

When is it appropriate to refer a patient to a cancer genetics program? Although no clear answers exist, a few guidelines will be offered. Remember that most cancers are not related to hereditary factors. Certain features of a family history should raise suspicion. Referral indicators include cancer in two or more close relatives on the same side of the family, bilateral cancer in paired organs (e.g., ovaries, breasts), multiple primary cancers in the same person, earlier than usual onset of disease, and specific patterns of cancers known to comprise a cancer syndrome (i.e., breast and ovarian cancers in the same family or individual) (Gould et al., 1997). If a blood relative has been tested and found to carry a mutation known to be associated with increased cancer risk, the patient may benefit from being tested for the same mutation. Men diagnosed with breast cancer are at increased risk for carrying a BRCA2 mutation (Friedman et al., 1997). Ethnic backgrounds also need to be considered when deciding if testing may be appropriate. More than 2% of Ashkenazi Jews are estimated to carry BRCA1 and BRCA2 mutations associated with increased risk for breast, ovarian, and prostate cancers (Strewing et al., 1997).

Counseling Issues Related to Genetic Information

Cancer genetic counseling includes education about the basic principles of cancer genetics; information about relevant cancer syndromes; and assessment, interpretation, and communication of cancer risk information to patients in terminology that they can understand. Counseling sessions also address the risks and benefits of cancer predisposition testing, cancer surveillance and risk-reduction options, and the emotional, family, and psychosocial issues related to genetic information.

Genetic counseling is the process of providing genetic information and the implications of that information to a patient or family in a supportive environment. Traditionally, genetic counseling is nondirective, with sensitivity to the patient's or family's emotional and psychosocial needs, culture, and healthcare beliefs. The focus is on helping patients or family members to understand their own potential genetic risk, presenting current available options, and discussing the complex issues related to genetic information. The patient or family members then use this information in the decision-making process.

Uncertainty of Genetic Information

Patients often seek genetic services thinking they can find concrete answers as to why cancer exists in their family. Genetic testing may be perceived as a diagnostic test that will give clear answers about whether a person will develop cancer. Healthcare providers may want to use genetic information to make decisions about treatment of cancer or precancerous conditions without fully understanding the uncertain nature of genetic information. Probabilities and uncertainties surround genetic information. A positive cancer predisposition test does not mean a person necessarily will get cancer, and a negative cancer predisposition test does not mean a person is free from cancer risk.

Expectations of Patients, Family Members, Support People, and Referral Sources

People seek genetic counseling or predisposition genetic testing services for a number of reasons. Healthcare professionals must understand the patient's motivation and expectations. During the intake process, many questions need to be asked in determining if the program services are likely to meet the patient's needs. Are the patient's expectations realistic? How high does the patient think his or her cancer risk is? How well does the patient understand the issues surrounding genetic information? How does the patient expect to use the information? Through the assessment process, the oncology nurse can evaluate what the patient needs and if genetic services can address those needs.

Several studies have looked at why women might want predisposition genetic testing for breast or ovarian cancer. One study interviewed 105 women with a family history of breast cancer in at least one first-degree relative. The most common reasons for wanting BRCA1 predisposition genetic testing were to learn about one's children's risk, to increase use of cancer screening tests, and to take better care of oneself (Lerman, Seay, Balshem, & Audrain, 1995). A similar study involved 121 first-degree relatives of patients diagnosed with ovarian cancer. The most commonly cited reasons for seeking BRCA1 predisposition genetic testing were to learn about one's children's cancer risks, to increase use of screening tests, to be reassured, to take better care of oneself, and to make childbearing decisions (Lerman, Daly, Masny, & Balshem, 1994). In a series of women's focus groups, the major advantages to BRCA1 predisposition testing that were cited included reducing uncertainty and assisting with decisions about medical treatment, surveillance, and lifestyle changes (Tessare, Borstelmann, Regan, Rimer, & Winer, 1997).

Patients Without Cancer

Patients without cancer often have questions about their personal cancer risk, cancer surveillance plan, or risk-reduction strategies. They are much more likely to be concerned about potential insurance or workplace discrimination if they are found to have a genetic predisposition to cancer. People without cancer who have a family history of cancer may have exaggerated perceptions of their personal cancer risk that can generate unnecessary anxiety (Lerman, Lustbader, et al., 1995). Many patients in this situation will turn out not to be in the high-risk category, and a cancer risk assessment with appropriate health education will help to alleviate anxiety.

Patients With Cancer

People who have been diagnosed with cancer often have different needs when seeking genetic services than people who have not been diagnosed with cancer. The motivation for pursuing cancer predisposition genetic testing may be concern about potential risk for other cancers or the potential cancer risk of a child or other close relative. The possibility of insurance and workplace discrimination based on genetic information is less of an issue for a person with a cancer diagnosis. The individual is already at risk for workplace or insurance discrimination based on their cancer diagnosis. It is not uncommon for a patient to say, "I've already been discriminated against because of my breast cancer."

People recently diagnosed with cancer who are referred for genetic counseling and predisposition genetic testing usually are coping with multiple issues surrounding the cancer diagnosis. They may not want to or be able to deal with the additional psychosocial and family issues that genetic counseling and predisposition genetic testing may bring up.

Family Members and Support People

Genetic information is unique in that implications exist for family members as well as for patients. Because patients receiving genetic counseling often bring other family members to the counseling session, questions usually arise from those family members about their own cancer risk and healthcare issues. Addressing these questions can be challenging. Nurses should help family members to understand what the implications of the genetic information might mean for their own cancer risk and, if appropriate, assist them with obtaining genetic services.

Sometimes, however, the focus of the genetic counseling session can be diverted by questions family members may ask about their own health that are better addressed outside of the genetic counseling session. Examples include, "What kind of cancer screening tests should I have?" "How high is my risk for cancer?" "Should I take hormone replacement therapy with all the cancer in my family?" "Should I have my ovaries removed to decrease my risk for ovarian cancer?" In this situation, the family member has not given written permission to receive services, no provider-patient relationship exists, and no chart is available to document what information was exchanged with the family member during the genetic counseling session. Although the family member is not the patient, the healthcare provider still could be held accountable for advice given during the genetic counseling session. The best approach is to offer to schedule a separate clinic appointment to address family members' healthcare concerns or refer them to appropriate healthcare resources.

Referral Sources

When the referring person is not the patient, which often is the case, the goals and expectations of the referring person and the patient may not coincide. The healthcare provider may want the patient to have cancer risk assessment and predisposition genetic testing so that the patient can use the genetic information to help to make decisions about cancer treatment or prophylactic surgery. The patient, however, may not be ready to deal with the psychological and family issues related to predisposition genetic testing or to make a decision about prophylactic surgery. In addition, the time frame for making a treatment decision usually is much shorter than the time frame needed to undergo genetic counseling and predisposition genetic testing, and the genetic information gained may not necessarily be helpful in making treatment decisions.

Psychosocial Issues and Implications

The communication of genetic information often carries with it an emotional impact that needs to be recognized and addressed. Emotional responses to cancer risk can include anger, fear of developing cancer, fear of disfigurement, fear of dying, grief, guilt, loss of control, negative body image, or a sense or isolation (Schneider, 1994). Patients found to carry a mutation may experience anxiety, depression, anger, feelings of vulnerability, or guilt about possibly having passed the mutation to children. Patients found not to carry a mutation may experience guilt, known as survivor's guilt, especially if close family members are found to carry the mutation. They also may experience regrets if they made major life decisions, such as prophylactic surgery, prior to testing (Geller et al., 1997).

Genetic counseling involves not only communicating genetic information but also addressing the emotional and psychological issues associated with that information. Patients receiving cancer genetic services often have lost loved ones to cancer or have had cancer themselves. Many families have survived multiple losses or have had other family members diagnosed with cancer, and each of these experiences has left an emotional scar. A patient describes her own feelings: "My fear of breast cancer history began 19 years ago when my mother died at age 58, just five months after she was diagnosed with metastatic breast cancer. The agony of watching her die left an emotional imprint on me that can never be erased. In my mind, breast cancer became a disease that could never be survived" (Prouser, 2000).

The psychosocial and medical dimensions of cancer counseling are closely intertwined. How people perceive their cancer risk often depends more on their emotional responses and experiences than the actual numerical risk (Schneider, 1994). Psychological issues may include fear of cancer or medical procedures, past negative experiences with cancer, unresolved loss and sorrow, feelings of guilt about passing on a mutation to children, anxiety about learning test results, and concern about the effect of results on other family members (Botkin et al., 1996). For these reasons, patients should know how to access additional support services such as a psychologist, social worker, nurse counselor, or support group.

Psychological Responses to Predisposition Genetic Testing

Studies looking at psychological outcomes related to BRCA1 testing in women found that noncarriers had lower depressive symptoms and functional impairment compared to carriers and nontested individuals. Mutation carriers, however, did not show increases in depression and functional impairment (Lerman et al., 1996). In a similar study, women carrying a BRCA1 mutation were found to have higher levels of psychological distress than noncarriers. The highest levels of test-related distresses were observed among mutation carriers with no history of cancer or cancer-related surgery (Croyle, Smith, Botkin, Baty, & Nash, 1997). In a study of patients with colorectal cancer undergoing genetic testing for hereditary colon cancer, higher depression scores were associated with being female and having less formal education and fewer sources of social contacts. Increased anxiety was associated with younger age, less formal education, non-White race, and fewer social contacts (Vernon et al., 1997).

The decision to undergo predisposition genetic testing and then waiting for results can be very difficult for patients. For some people, an additional counseling appointment or a referral to a psychologist or social worker can be helpful during this time. From the moment blood is drawn until the results are received may take up to a month. This waiting time can be difficult and can result in increased anxiety, isolation, and depression. Healthcare professionals should maintain telephone contact during this time and offer psychological support. A peer counselor also may be helpful. Peer counselors are trained volunteers who have been through a similar experience and are willing to share how they felt. One individual explained, "I waited about a month to get my blood drawn. I needed some time to process what all of this might mean for my future. I even considered what I saw as a real dilemma. What if I should test negative? I should be happy, but I wondered how would I live, knowing that I was still in that pool of the 1 out of 8 women who will develop breast cancer for nongenetic reasons. And I was so convinced that I would develop it some day that I considered that testing positive might be a relief" (Prouser, 1997).

As nurses learn more about psychological responses to genetic counseling and cancer predisposition genetic testing, they will be better able to structure genetic services to address the needs of patients. Schneider (1994) gave an excellent overview of the psychosocial issues of cancer risk and psychosocial assessment and referral.

Assessing When to Refer for Psychological Counseling

Psychological assessment especially is important when predisposition genetic testing is involved. Receiving test results can be an intensely emotional experience, with the potential for severe depression in some people. Explaining the emotional risks during a genetic counseling session is one thing, but predicting patients' ability to emotionally handle receiving their test results is another story. Ideally, a psychologist or social worker would see every patient, but in clinical practice, this is rarely possible.

Issues for nurses to consider when assessing how individuals might respond to receiving test results include the following.
- Does the patient seem excessively anxious, depressed, or under extreme stress?
- What are the patient's cognitive abilities?
- What coping strategies does the patient use when dealing with difficult situations? Is there a history of ineffective coping?
- How does the patient make difficult decisions, and who does he or she look to for guidance?
- What are the patient's motivations for or against testing?
- Who does the patient look to for emotional and social support?
- Does the patient have a history of unresolved bereavement?
- What is the extent and effectiveness of the patient's support system?
- What are the family dynamics? Is there marital or family discord?
- Has the patient or family experienced multiple crises in a short time span?
- Is the patient interested in a referral to a psychologist or social worker or is psychiatric care indicated?
- Has the patient successfully used these services in the past?

Because of the multiple psychological issues involved in predisposition genetic testing, having a psychologist or social worker available for people who need this additional support is essential. Figure 18-4 gives an overview of when to consider referral for psychological counseling. Experience in working with patients with cancer and an understanding of the psychological and family issues they face are

Figure 18-4. When to Consider Referral for Psychological Counseling

- Symptoms of excessive anxiety, depression, or extreme stress
- Past history or current indications of ineffective coping
- Ineffective social support system
- Indications of distress in making decisions related to genetic information
- History of psychiatric problems
- Unresolved bereavement
- Marital or family discord
- Experiencing multiple crises in a short time span
- Expresses an interest in receiving psychological counseling services

essential for the psychologist or social worker practicing in cancer genetics. Healthcare professionals also need to understand that patients undergoing predisposition genetic testing who have been affected by cancer have different needs than people who have not been affected by cancer.

Who Might Benefit From Cancer Predisposition Testing?

Deciding who may be an appropriate candidate for cancer predisposition testing requires clinical judgment because of the complexity of the issues involved. ASCO (1996) recommended that cancer predisposition genetic testing be offered only when (a) the patient has a strong family history of cancer or very early age of onset of disease (with a 10% or greater probability of having a mutation), (b) the test can be interpreted adequately, and (c) the results will influence the medical management of the patient or family member. The recommendations also list hereditary breast/ovarian cancer syndrome and hereditary nonpolyposis colorectal cancer as two cancer syndromes with a high probability of a mutation detection in a family member, and they give examples of patients who meet their predisposition genetic testing criteria (ASCO). These two hereditary cancer syndromes are the ones oncology nurses are most likely to encounter in clinical practice, and nurses are encouraged to be familiar with these guidelines and any subsequent updates.

Some cancer genetics programs have developed clinical guidelines to assist in the decision-making process. Commercial laboratories offering these tests often have guidelines stating who might benefit from a particular cancer predisposition genetic test. For example, if a blood relative has been tested and found to carry a mutation known to be associated with increased cancer risk, the patient may benefit from being tested for the same mutation. Men diagnosed with breast cancer are at increased risk for carrying a BRCA2 mutation (Friedman et al., 1997). Ethnic background also needs to be considered when deciding if testing may be appropriate.

Eligibility criteria will vary, depending on the mutation, and a complete overview is not included in this chapter. When assessing whether a patient is appropriate for cancer predisposition testing, it often is helpful to discuss the issue in a cancer genetics interdisciplinary team conference or to consult with a medical geneticist. The GeneClinics Web site (www.geneclinics.org) is an excellent resource for information about both hereditary breast and ovarian cancer and familial adenomatous polyposis. Whether patients might benefit from predisposition genetic testing will depend upon their degree of genetic risk, whether testing is likely to address their needs, and the availability of an appropriate cancer predisposition test. Because of the high cost of testing, reimbursement factors also may be an issue. The final decision, however, will depend on whether the patient still is interested in pursuing cancer predisposition testing, after learning the potential risks and benefits.

When deciding whether to pursue cancer predisposition genetic testing, each patient and family member must weigh the options, risks, and benefits in light of their unique situation. The decision is a very personal one, and the issues will be different for each patient. Just because people have a personal or family history that puts them at increased risk for carrying a genetic mutation does not mean they will wish to know their genetic status. For other people, the uncertainty may be causing them great anxiety or interfering with their ability to make informed choices about their health. The physical risks of having a blood sample drawn are minimal; the real risks are associated with the psychological and psychosocial impact of knowing one's genetic status.

Testing of Minors

In general, cancer predisposition testing in minors is discouraged unless there is a clear medical benefit to the child. For example, if someone in the family has tested positive for the adenomatous polyposis coli gene associated with familial adenomatous polyposis, children as young as age 10 could be tested because that is the age recommended to begin annual colon surveillance (Petersen & Brensinger, 1996). If the child has been affected by a cancer diagnosis, such as being diagnosed with osteosarcoma at a young age, and a genetic disorder such as Li-Fraumeni syndrome is suspected, some question still exists about whether the benefits of genetic testing for the p53 gene outweigh the risks. Because no early detection tests are given for the pediatric-onset cancers associated with Li-Fraumeni syndrome, the medical benefits of genetic testing are not clear (Patenaude, 1996). The GeneClinics Web site (www.geneclinics.org) contains information about whether genetic testing of minors is recommended for specific hereditary disorders or syndromes.

Children will not necessarily benefit from test results, and the results may trigger stigmatization by parents, siblings, or others. Children may be given information when they are too young to understand its significance (Dickens, Pei, & Taylor, 1996). Genetic testing of unaffected minors for adult-onset disorders is controversial. Knowing a child's genetic status for adult-onset cancers will not affect the course of the disease or its treatment. When children reach maturity, they can weigh the risks, benefits, and options and make their own decisions about whether to pursue predisposition genetic testing (Gould et al., 1997). Even if a child does not undergo genetic testing, if relatives of that child have tested positive for a mutation associated with a hereditary cancer syndrome, this information has implications for the child's own risk. Decisions still need to be made concerning whether or when to tell the child he or she is at risk for the same hereditary disorder.

In deciding whether to test children or adolescents for a particular hereditary cancer syndrome, many psychological issues need to be considered. If parents choose not to have the child undergo genetic testing, the child may find out the genetic information at a later date and have more difficulty integrating it into his or her self-concept. If parents have the child undergo genetic testing and do not reveal the results, a climate of secrecy may develop within the family. If parents have the child undergo genetic testing and tell the child the results, they may be robbing the child of the autonomy of making his or her own decision about this knowledge later in life. The child also may not be able to understand the difference between being a carrier and being diagnosed with cancer (Fanos, 1997). Even when there is a clear medical benefit to knowing the child's or adolescent's genetic status, the psychosocial consequences of testing of minors need to be considered and genetic counseling provided to the child or adolescent and his or her family.

Understanding the Meaning of Test Results

Clinicians are accustomed to common laboratory tests, such as blood glucose and cholesterol, for which the results are specific numbers representing some type of measurement that can be interpreted relatively easily. Predisposition genetic tests, however, often are a complex maze of probabilities and uncertainties that must be interpreted in a way that patients can understand. Results of predisposition genetic tests generally fall into three categories: positive, negative, or a mutation of uncertain clinical significance.

Positive Test Result

A patient can have a positive test result, which occurs when a known mutation is associated with an increased risk for a particular cancer or syndrome of cancers. The patient is at increased risk for the cancers known to be associated with that mutation. If one or more family members diagnosed with cancer have been tested and found to carry the same mutation, the mutation is probably the reason for the increased number of cancers found in the family. It is possible, however, to have both sporadic and hereditary cancers in the same family. In some families, more than one mutation associated with increased cancer risk has been found, although it is uncommon.

Receiving a positive test result can have a tremendous emotional impact on some patients. Individuals who previously were undiagnosed with cancer may feel as if they have been told they have cancer. Patients may feel isolated from friends who may not understand the feelings associated with learning their genetic status and therefore are unable to offer the necessary support. Patients may have concerns about who should be told in the family, how they will react, and the confidentiality of the information disclosed. Parents may feel guilty for knowing their risk of passing a mutation to a child. Some patients may experience relief knowing their genetic status; it enables them to make healthcare decisions based on this information or at least have a better understanding of why cancer cases exist in their family. A feeling of empowerment can occur because uncertainty is removed and patients are able to move forward in their decision-making process. See Figure 18-5 for a summary of the benefits, risks, and limitations of a positive genetic test result.

Negative Test Result

A negative test can occur in two situations. The first is when a known mutation exists in a family and a family member has been tested specifically for that same mutation. The second situation is when no known mutation exists in the family and the patient is tested for one or more mutations associated with increased cancer risk.

Negative Test Result—Known Mutation in the Family

This occurs when a known mutation exists that is associated with an increased cancer risk that has been found in one or more blood relatives and the patient tests negative for the same mutation. A negative test result does not mean the patient will not get cancer. The patient has the same cancer risk as the general population and is not at increased risk for the cancers associated with the mutation. The patient's cancer risk still may be increased because of nongenetic risk factors related to lifestyle, diet, environment, or carcinogen exposure. In addition, the negative test result only applies to the mutation or mutations tested. The targeted mutation is presumed to have caused cancer in the family; however, a higher risk still could exist from some other mutation associated with increased cancer risk, although this risk is very low (Gould et al., 1997).

Negative Test Result—No Known Mutation in the Family

This occurs when no mutation is found and no blood relative of the patient previously has tested positive for a mutation known to be associated with an increased cancer risk. In this situation, the patient is likely to be the first person in the family to undergo predisposition genetic testing.

In a patient without a cancer diagnosis, three possible interpretations exist for a negative test result. The first possibility is that the cancer in the family is caused by a known mutation for which the patient was tested, and the patient did not inherit it. A second possibility is that the cancer in the family is caused by a different mutation for which the patient was not tested. A third possibility is that the cancer in the family is caused by environmental or other nonhereditary risk factors. Because it is not possible to know which outcome is true for the patient, nurses first should test a blood relative who has been diagnosed with cancer for a mutation known to be associated with that type of cancer. The rationale is that if a mutation exists in the family, it most likely will be found in a family member already diagnosed with cancer. If a mutation is found in an affected family member, then the unaffected family members can be tested for that specific mutation.

A negative test in a patient who previously was diagnosed with a cancer associated with the mutation or mutations for which he or she was tested most likely means the patient's cancer was sporadic or nonhereditary. It still is possible that the

Figure 18-5. Benefits, Risks, and Limitations Associated With Test Results

Benefits Associated With a Positive Test Result
- Removal of uncertainty or reduced anxiety
- Knowing genetic status can facilitate making medical decisions about surveillance, chemoprevention, or prophylactic surgery
- Potential for earlier diagnosis with increased surveillance
- Interventions such as prophylactic surgery, lifestyle changes, or chemoprevention may lower cancer risk.
- Increased motivation to engage in positive health behaviors
- Potential increased support from family and friends
- If the patient chooses to tell other family members that a mutation is present, they may benefit by being able to make more informed healthcare decisions for themselves.

Risks and Limitations Associated With a Positive Test Result
- Feelings such as anger, depression, fear, or hopelessness
- Knowing the risk of passing the mutation on to one's children, which may cause psychological distress
- Potential genetic discrimination by insurance companies or in the workplace
- Family relationships may be strained/under stress.
- Decisions about cancer surveillance, chemoprevention, or prophylactic surgery may cause psychological distress.
- Potential increased healthcare costs from cancer surveillance tests or risk-reduction interventions such as prophylactic surgery

Benefits Associated With a Negative Test Result
- Known mutation in the family
  - Relief in knowing cancer risk related to the mutation is not increased
  - Reduced anxiety, increased happiness
  - Knowing that the mutation will not be passed on to one's children
  - Knowing that additional cancer surveillance or prophylactic surgery may be unnecessary
  - Potential decrease in cancer surveillance
- No mutation in the family
  - Potential relief from learning that mutations known to increase cancer risk for which the patient was tested are not present
  - Potential that the cancer in the family is because of a mutation for which the patient was tested and they did not inherit it

Risks and Limitations Associated With a Negative Test Result
- Known mutation in the family
  - Potential misinterpretation of test result by patient to mean that he or she has no cancer risk
  - Potential decreased adherence to surveillance and risk-reduction behaviors
  - Potential feelings of guilt, especially when loved ones may have been found to have a positive test result ("survivor's guilt")
  - Family members may feel anger or jealousy.
  - Patient may feel excluded by some family members who have bonded based on their shared genetic status.
- No mutation in the family
  - Knowing that the negative test result could mean either the person does not carry the mutation causing the cancer in their family (true-negative test result) or that the cancer in his or her family is because of a mutation for which the patient was not tested may cause feelings of uncertainty.
  - Determining a cancer surveillance plan may be challenging because the level of cancer risk is uncertain.
  - Anxiety about cancer risk may not decrease.

(Continued on next page)

Figure 18-5. Benefits, Risks, and Limitations Associated With Test Results (Continued)

Benefits Associated With a Mutation of Unknown Clinical Significance
- Potential relief from learning that mutations known to be deleterious are not present
- Potential that the mutation is not associated with an increased cancer risk

Risks and Limitations Associated With a Mutation of Unknown Clinical Significance
- Level of cancer risk is uncertain.
- Difficulty in making healthcare decisions regarding cancer surveillance and risk-reduction measures
- Risk of passing a mutation with unknown cancer risk on to one's children
- Potential continued anxiety about one's cancer risk or increased anxiety because of uncertainty
- Whether the cancer in the family is because of the mutation is unknown.

---

patient carries some other mutation associated with increased cancer risk for which he or she was not tested, although this risk is low.

A negative test result can be a relief and result in reduced anxiety about cancer risk. Some patients may experience survivor's guilt if they have not inherited a mutation when loved ones are found to carry the mutation.

In a patient without a cancer diagnosis and without a blood relative known to carry a mutation, a negative test result is difficult to interpret. The patient can be told that known mutations associated with increased cancer risk included in the test are not present. A summary of the benefits, risks, and limitations of a negative genetic test result can be found in Figure 18-5.

Mutation of Uncertain Clinical Significance, Inconclusive Test Result

A test result can be of uncertain clinical significance when a mutation in the DNA is found; however, the risk of cancer associated with that mutation is unknown. This can occur when a new mutation is found or if the mutation is uncommon and not enough information is available to determine if it is deleterious (associated with an increased cancer risk) or harmless. Genes such as BRCA1 and BRCA2 are very large, and hundreds of possible mutations can occur. Not all mutations are deleterious. A mutation can be present and not interfere with cellular function and therefore not increase cancer risk. This is one reason why interpreting predisposition genetic test results is complicated. Until a number of families with the same mutation have been studied, it is not possible to know if an increased cancer risk may be associated with that mutation. This creates a difficult situation for some patients because of the uncertainty it presents.

For patients with a mutation of uncertain clinical significance, it may be helpful to test more family members to find out if the mutation is found only in the affected people, but even this will not give concrete answers. One option is to encourage the patient to become part of a confidential registry for people who carry genetic mutations in the hope that more information about the particular mutation will be known as more people are tested. The patient needs to be informed that, as more information about specific mutations becomes available, it may be possible to determine if the particular mutation found in that patient is deleterious or a polymorphism. In this situation, nurses should suggest that the patient schedule a follow-up visit in a year to discuss any additional information available at that time.

When patients receive a test result with a mutation of uncertain clinical significance, they may experience disappointment, anxiety, anger, or depression because the test result did not give them the information they expected. They also may feel confused and uncertain about how to make healthcare decisions regarding cancer surveillance. It may be reassuring, however, for them to know that, even though the significance of the mutation found is not known, the known mutations associated with cancer risk included in the test are not present. See Figure 18-5 for a summary of the benefits, risks, and limitations of a mutation of uncertain clinical significance.

Oncology Nurse's Role in Interpreting Test Results

To be able to effectively disclose predisposition test results to patients, APNs first must have the clinical background and knowledge to help patients to understand the complexities of genetic information. Equally important is the nurse's sensitivity to the emotional impact of genetic information and ability to support patients and families through this process.

Oncology nurses need to help patients to understand that a positive predisposition genetic test result does not necessarily mean that one will get cancer and a negative test result does not mean that one is free from cancer risk. There is no way to predict when or if an unaffected patient will be diagnosed with cancer or when or if an affected patient will be diagnosed with a different cancer. Predisposition genetic testing sometimes can help nurses to determine how high the probability is that patients may be diagnosed with a certain cancer or cancers in the future. Even correctly estimating the risk for certain cancers is complicated, however, because the cancer risk estimates associated with certain mutations are changing as more information becomes available.

Increased surveillance may lead to earlier detection, or prophylactic surgery may reduce the risk for certain cancers. Insufficient data, however, currently are available to evaluate the effectiveness of these measures, and additional expenses may be associated with these interventions. The Cancer Genetics Studies Consortium, a group sponsored by the National Human Genome Research Institute, has published consensus statements addressing follow-up guidelines for people who carry a BRCA1 or BRCA2 alteration and also for people diagnosed with non-polyposis colon cancer (Burke, Daly, et al., 1997; Burke, Petersen, et al., 1997).

Understanding how to interpret genetic predisposition test results for cancer is more complicated than most laboratory blood tests that both patients and oncology nurses encounter. Patients often expect concrete answers from predisposition testing and do not understand the complexity of interpreting test results. It can be very disappointing for a patient to undergo testing, with the associated psychological distress and expense, only to have the end result be uncertain. Prior to initiating the testing process, patients must understand both the issues associated with predisposition genetic testing and all the potential test

result outcomes. Genetic counseling and testing occur at one point in time; however, the impact of receiving predisposition genetic test results can last a lifetime. Patients with positive test results may go on to have prophylactic surgery and receive long-term clinical services for cancer surveillance. Nurses have a pivotal role in caring for these patients, and their need for emotional support and health education is ongoing. Very little is known about the follow-up needs of patients after they have been through predisposition genetic testing. Nurses need to participate in and initiate nursing research studies to learn more about the long-term needs of these patients.

Counseling Session Content

Genetic counseling involves a communication process by which individuals and families come to learn and understand relevant aspects of genetics. It also involves providing support during the process of integrating personal and family genetic information into their daily lives and making informed healthcare decisions based on genetic information (Lea et al., 1998). Many patients who seek genetic counseling want information about their own or a family member's cancer risk because of a personal or family history of cancer and are not necessarily interested in cancer predisposition testing. Some patients call or are referred for cancer predisposition testing but, after the genetic counseling session, are no longer interested because they are not good candidates for such testing, because the test will not provide the expected concrete answers, because insurance discrimination is a possibility, or because of other issues such as psychosocial and family concerns.

The content of the initial genetic counseling session will vary somewhat, depending on the needs of the patient scheduling the appointment, the outcome of the cancer risk assessment, and whether the patient decides to pursue predisposition genetic testing. When cancer predisposition testing is involved, more than one genetic counseling session is needed.

When patients are first referred to a clinic for genetic services, sending them an initial information packet prior to the genetic counseling appointment often is helpful. Information about the genetic services provided through the program and basic handouts on predisposition genetic testing and cancer risk factors can be included. For example, for questions related to breast-ovarian cancer syndrome and genetic testing for BRCA analysis, the following information could be included: a cover letter describing how to schedule an appointment and what to expect, a brochure about genetic services provided through the healthcare facility (if available), and a copy of the National Cancer Institute brochure *Genetic Testing for Breast Cancer Risk: It's Your Choice* (available online at http://cancernet.nci .nih.gov/peb/genetic_testing/ or by calling the Cancer Information Service at 800-4-CANCER). After reading the information, individuals can call to schedule an appointment if they are interested in pursuing genetic testing.

Structure of Genetic Counseling Sessions

One model that frequently is used for structuring genetic counseling for cancer predisposition genetic testing involves three sessions. The purpose of the first session is to provide a comprehensive cancer risk assessment and cover all of the information patients need to know before they have blood drawn. The purpose of the second session is to verify that patients understand the risks and benefits of the cancer predisposition genetic test being ordered, to obtain written informed consent if they still are interested in predisposition genetic testing, and to have blood drawn and sent to the lab. The third genetic counseling session occurs after the test results have been received for the purpose of disclosure of test results (see Figure 18-6). Because of the complexity of explaining test results and the psychological issues associated with receiving results, it is best to give cancer predisposition genetic test results in person whenever possible.

Methods for Counseling Session Education Delivery

Healthcare professionals must communicate genetic information to patients, evaluate their understanding of the information, and assess their emotional reaction to it. Because of the quantity of information presented, patients very easily can become overwhelmed. Resources are available to assist with the education process (see Figure 18-1).

During the genetic counseling session, use of visual aides such as flip charts or pictures is recommended. To reinforce the learning experience, patients should receive handouts that they can take with them so they can read the materials at a later date and refer back to them as a resource. Videos are available that cover basic information about cancer predisposition testing. If a patient is interested in pursuing testing, he or she can watch a video before the genetic counseling session to help to confirm that decision. Patient-education videos give some background about the issues involved and can facilitate the education process.

Peer counselors also can be a valuable resource by sharing their related personal experiences. Former patients interested in becoming peer counselors should wait at least a year after their own predisposition genetic testing experience before volunteering. Before they contact patients, peer counselors need training that covers confidentiality issues and nondirective communication techniques (e.g., avoiding interpretation, encouraging patients to speak freely).

Some programs offer small group classes lasting an hour or two in which an oncology nurse or a genetic counselor provides basic information about topics such as the genetics of cancer, hereditary and other risk factors, risk reduction, and surveillance options. For many people, this type of setting allows them to obtain information and ask questions in a nonthreatening environment before deciding if they want to schedule an appointment.

Ethical Issues

Potential Workplace and Insurance Discrimination

Many patients are very concerned about releasing information to their insurance companies, fearing that their health insurance will be cancelled or their rates

Figure 18-6. Structure of Genetic Counseling Session Content

Session one (pretest counseling session)
- Determine why the patient is seeking genetic counseling and if it will meet his or her needs. (This also can be performed during the intake telephone call.)
- Take medical and family history (begin documentation process).
- Begin pedigree construction and analysis
- Assess hereditary, clinical, and lifestyle risk factors.
- Explain cancer risk assessment and communicate risk information.
- Perform psychosocial assessment.
- Provide basic explanation of the genetics of cancer (include information on the genetic nature of cancer as a disease, autosomal dominance, and the difference between germline and sporadic mutations).
- Discuss options and limitations for medical surveillance and cancer risk reduction (cancer screening tests, prophylactic surgery, chemoprevention trials, lifestyle and dietary measures).
- Provide information on the specific predisposition genetic test being performed (if the patient wants testing and is an appropriate candidate).
- Discuss fees involved for genetic counseling and predisposition genetic testing and the risks and benefits of applying for insurance coverage for these services.
- Discuss risks and benefits of cancer predisposition genetic testing. (See section on risks and benefits of predisposition genetic testing.)
- Discuss the meaning of potential predisposition genetic test results and the technical accuracy of the test.
- Discuss options without predisposition genetic testing (cancer surveillance, risk-reduction measures, DNA banking, and possible participation in a research study, if available).
- Explain confidentiality of genetic information.

Session two (informed consent and blood draw)
- Answer any questions the patient may have.
- Determine if the patient understands potential risks and benefits of the cancer predisposition test being ordered.
- Offer psychological support and referral to a psychologist, if indicated.
- Discuss who will provide medical follow-up to the patient after test results have been received and whether he or she plans to disclose test results to the care provider.
- Discuss whether the patient intends to discuss test results with family members or friends and the potential impact of this information.
- Discuss option of bringing a companion to the results disclosure visit.
- Discuss format of the results disclosure visit.
- Obtain written informed consent for the predisposition genetic test being ordered.
- Have blood drawn and sent to the laboratory.

Session three (results disclosure visit)
- Disclose results of the cancer predisposition genetic test.
- Allow the patient to process the information and assess his or her response.
- Answer any questions the patient may have.
- Discuss what the test results may mean to the patient and family in relation to cancer risk, psychological issues, and family concerns.
- Discuss medical follow-up, cancer surveillance, and cancer risk-reduction options.
- Discuss any follow-up telephone calls or letters the patient may receive after the session.
- Discuss available resources for additional information, psychological support or counseling, and follow-up.

will increase if they are found to be genetically predisposed to a certain type of cancer. Patients even may fear that an insurance company will discriminate against relatives if they are found to carry a mutation associated with a high cancer risk. Many insurance companies now cover predisposition genetic testing for hereditary breast and ovarian cancer, and some patients are choosing to bill their insurance company for payment of genetic services. Patients seeking predisposition genetic testing need to be informed of potential insurance discrimination issues, what protections exist, and the limitations of those protections.

State and federal laws regulate genetic information and are intended to help to protect the confidentiality of genetic information and prevent insurance discrimination. The most significant federal legislation to date pertaining to genetic information is the Health Insurance Portability and Accountability Act of 1996. A key provision of this legislation is that genetic information may not be treated as a preexisting condition in the absence of a diagnosis of the condition related to such information. Another key provision is that genetic information cannot be used to deny, cancel, or refuse to renew coverage. This provision applies to an individual's eligibility for insurance under a group health plan offered by an employer. In addition, the employer may not require an individual to pay a larger premium than that for another similarly situated individual within the group based on health status of the individual or his or her dependent (Berner, 1996). This legislation only applies to health insurance, not disability or life insurance. Also, individuals who are self-employed or who work for companies with very few employees may not be covered. Several federal bills currently are proposed that would offer additional protections against potential insurance and workplace discrimination, protecting the confidentiality of genetic information.

State legislation regarding these issues varies greatly and is changing rapidly as new legislation is introduced. Understanding the benefits and limitations of these laws and staying abreast of legislative changes can be complicated. An overview of the information on the status of state legislation can be found at the National Human Genome Research Institute Web site (www.nhgri.gov) under "Policy and Public Affairs."

Informed Consent

Informed consent involves more than having a patient sign a consent form. It involves the interaction of healthcare providers and patients in making healthcare decisions. A written consent form is documentation that a patient has been adequately informed and has consented to a medical intervention. Informed consent is defined as the willing acceptance of a medical intervention by patients after adequate disclosure by the healthcare provider of the nature of the intervention, its risks and benefits, and alternatives with their risks and benefits (Jonsen, Seigler, & Winslade, 1992).

Informed consent can be conceptualized as either an event model or a process model. Using the event model, the patient is presented with several options from which to choose; the medical professional usually indicates what he or she thinks is in the patient's best interest; and the patient has the opportunity to agree or disagree. In the event model, the focus of informed consent is on obtaining a written consent form. This model is limited in that it takes place at a single point in time, and this does not reflect how patients make complicated decisions. The process model of informed consent assumes a relationship between the healthcare provider and the patient in which decision making is a multistep process that is shared over time. The decision needs to be consistent with the patient's values and needs, with the patient having an opportunity to confirm and rethink his or her final choice (Geller et al., 1997).

The process model of informed consent has been developed into a model of informed decision making that has been used in studies looking at how well physicians inform patients about routine medical decisions. This process model includes greater involvement of patients in clinical decision making, not merely signing a form. Informed participation of patients in medical decisions is encouraged by providing relevant information about the clinical situation (i.e., predisposition genetic testing), alternatives, risks, and benefits; assessing the patient's understanding of the information; and giving the patient a clear opportunity to voice a preference. Informed participation is the product of a thoughtful dialogue between the healthcare provider and the patient that leads to a decision. This model can be applied to clinical situations involving medical decision making, regardless of whether a written consent form is required (Braddock, Fihn, Levinson, Jonsen, & Pearlman, 1997).

Nurses often are faced with situations in cancer genetics where they are involved in helping patients to make healthcare decisions. The informed consent process is not limited to situations such as predisposition genetic testing and prophylactic surgery, which require written consent forms. Patients' decisions also may involve whether to seek genetic services, making healthcare decisions involving cancer surveillance or hormone replacement therapy, or deciding whether to reveal their genetic status to loved ones or healthcare providers. Oncology nurses can apply the process model of informed decision making in all of these situations. Figure 18-7 outlines the elements of informed decision making.

Informed Consent for Predisposition Genetic Testing

The informed consent process for predisposition genetic testing needs to include both an educational component and a decision-making component. Integral to informed, shared decision making between patients and healthcare providers is

---

Figure 18-7. Elements of Informed Decision Making

1. Discussion of the clinical issue and nature of the decision to be made
2. Discussion of the alternatives
3. Discussion of the pros (benefits) and cons (risks) of the alternatives
4. Discussion of the uncertainties associated with the decision
5. Assessment of patient's understanding
6. Asking the patient to express a preference

Note. From "How Doctors and Patients Discuss Routine Clinical Decisions," by C.H. Braddock, S. Finn, W. Levinson, A. Jonsen, and R.A. Pearlman, 1997, *Journal of General Internal Medicine, 12,* p. 340. Copyright 1997 by Blackwell Science, Inc. Reprinted with permission.

the entire education and counseling process that occurs when patients face a complicated decision, such as whether to pursue predisposition genetic testing. One study found that when women were given information about the limitations and uncertainties of BRCA1 testing, not just its availability, their interest in testing decreased (Geller et al., 1995).

Informed consent for predisposition genetic testing must include the following (ASCO, 1996; Geller et al., 1997).
- Purpose of the specific predisposition genetic test being ordered
- Risks and benefits of the test being ordered
- Amount of blood to be drawn and the associated risks
- Alternatives to predisposition genetic testing
- Cost of testing, when results will be available, and how results will be communicated
- Range of results that might be obtained and what each potential test result might mean
- Name of a contact person who can answer questions
- Psychosocial implications
- Potential insurance risk or employment discrimination
- The understanding that genetic information will be kept confidential, and additional testing will not be performed without informed consent
- Options for obtaining medical follow-up

The goal is to provide enough information to enable patients to come to a decision about predisposition genetic testing based on adequate knowledge of the risks associated with accepting, rejecting, or postponing the testing. This information also should address the risks and benefits of genetic information as it applies to family members as well as the individual being tested (Dickens et al., 1996; Geller et al., 1997). Informed consent should be obtained by the licensed professional ordering the predisposition genetic test and not by support personnel.

The most common method for presenting information about a medical intervention is a one-on-one discussion. Patients' understanding appears to be directly correlated with the amount of time spent with them in the teaching process. Group discussions are another way to present information that offers the advantage of peer interaction. The limitations include embarrassment when speaking in groups and the fear that disclosure may compromise confidentiality and individual needs may not be met (Geller et al., 1997). Other formats that can aid in presenting information include pamphlets, videotapes, and interactive computer programs.

A useful system for documenting the informed consent process in the medical record is the "PARQ," or the Procedure, Alternatives, Risks, and Questions, method.

Procedure: Document that the *procedure* for the predisposition genetic testing process was explained to the patient.

Alternatives: Document that the *alternatives* to predisposition genetic testing were discussed, and briefly note the alternatives.

Risks: Document that the potential *risks* associated with the specific predisposition genetic test were discussed. The patient should have a handout or copy of a signed consent form outlining the potential risks.

Questions: Document that the patient was asked if he or she wanted any more information about the procedure, alternatives, or risks and the patient's response.

A notation needs to be made for each of the four categories. The PARQ method of documenting informed consent is required in some states, such as Oregon (Oregon Medical Association, 1996).

In summary, the informed decision-making model is a useful tool for oncology nurses when decision making regarding predisposition genetic testing is involved. Discussion of predisposition genetic testing issues, alternatives, risks, benefits, and uncertainties are part of the education provided during genetic counseling. Patient education and assessment of patients' understanding of the information presented are both part of the nursing process. Beginning patient education prior to the initial genetic counseling session and allowing patients time to reflect on the information provided at the first genetic counseling visit before their blood is drawn at the second visit affords them the time to rethink and confirm the final decision.

Informed Consent and Release of Information to a Third Party

When insurance coverage for genetic services is involved, informed consent issues arise related to preauthorization. Most insurance companies require preauthorization for genetic counseling and testing before services are provided. This usually involves sending a letter to the insurance company documenting why the services are needed and including medical information specific to an individual's personal and family cancer history. If no patient contact has occurred and a release-of-information form is not on file, this form will need to be sent to the patient to be signed to give informed consent before the letter containing medical information is sent to the insurance company.

Verifying eligibility for predisposition genetic testing also can present challenges to maintaining the confidentiality of family members. One of the eligibility criteria that a number of insurance companies use is that the patient must have a blood relative who carries a mutation known to increase cancer risk. The challenge is how to show that an individual is eligible under these criteria without violating the confidentiality of any family members. With one insurance company, this issue was resolved when the insurance company agreed to accept a letter from the cancer genetics program that contained general wording, such as "this patient has a first-degree relative known to carry a BRCA1 mutation." The insurance company agreed to trust that the cancer genetics program or healthcare provider would verify that a known mutation existed in the family without disclosing any specific information to the insurance company.

Given the sensitivity of genetic information, patients need to know that their genetic information will be confidential in the sense that it will not be released to any third party without their specific written informed consent. Confidentiality and patients' privacy may be violated from the unintentional leakage of genetic information contained in medical records without a patient's consent. Examples might include information in a dictated pathology report for prophylactic surgery stating the reason for the surgery was because of a positive genetic test or a referral letter to a cancer genetics program stating the referral is because the patient is at high risk for carrying a genetic mutation because of a known genetic mutation in the family.

When healthcare providers refer patients to a cancer genetics program for predisposition genetic testing, the patients must sign a written consent form before cancer genetic counseling and predisposition testing information can be released to their healthcare provider. When healthcare providers do not have access to genetic information about patients or their family members, providers are denied information necessary for patient assessment (Dickens et al., 1996). Patients with a positive predisposition genetic test may receive inadequate cancer surveillance, and patients with a negative predisposition genetic test may receive unnecessary cancer surveillance.

Another issue arises when patients tell their healthcare provider that they were found to carry a genetic mutation that predisposes them to some cancers, but they do not want this information put into their medical records. Patients may, however, want the healthcare provider to increase the frequency of physical examinations or order certain cancer screening tests based on this information. An example would be a patient who carries a BRCA1 mutation with no family history of ovarian cancer who does not want this information documented in the medical record but asks the provider to order screening tests for ovarian cancer based on the genetic information. A couple of questions arise from this situation. Will the provider be acting out of accordance with medical standards of practice by ordering ovarian cancer screening tests in the absence of a documented medical need? Also, how can the genetic information truly be private when surveillance behavior has changed based on this information? Prior to testing, it is best to discuss with the patient the importance of sharing their predisposition genetic test results with his or her healthcare provider.

Informed Consent and Secondary Medical Records

The genetic counseling process often involves obtaining patients' medical records from one or more sources, as well as the medical records on one or more family members. The presence of these records in a patient's medical chart creates an additional responsibility in relation to maintaining confidentiality of information. When a patient's medical record contains secondary records (i.e., medical records on a family member or patient records from another institution), these records should not be released to a third party, even with written informed consent from the patient. The third party needs to go to the original source to obtain those records.

Specific Consent Versus General Consent to Release Information

Because of the sensitivity of genetic information and potential insurance and work discrimination issues, specific informed consent is especially important. The standard of practice for people undergoing predisposition genetic testing for cancer is written informed consent. In addition, specific written informed consent is necessary before any genetic information is released to a third party. A general release of information may not be adequate. Standard hospital or outpatient forms often contain a general release-of-information clause, which allows the release of most medical information to the referring primary-care provider or to the insurance company for billing purposes. A general release is not advisable for release of genetic information, such as predisposition genetic test results. This higher standard for a specific written consent release is similar to that required in some states for such sensitive medical information as HIV/AIDS, mental illness, and substance abuse.

State and Federal Laws Relating to Informed Consent

Some states have laws requiring informed consent, including specific forms to be signed, before genetic information is released to a third party, such as a healthcare provider, another cancer genetics program, or an insurance company. Because these laws are rapidly changing, oncology nurses must keep current on the laws affecting genetic information in the states where they practice. Laws such as this protect individuals from being singled out for discrimination because of a specific genetic trait that may or may not affect their future employment or use of health insurance benefits.

Documentation

Documentation in the medical record and maintaining the confidentiality of patient information has long been part of basic nursing practice. More recently, however, the computerization of medical records has increased concerns about patient privacy (Waldo, 1999). Recent federal legislation has been enacted to help to address this concern. The "Standards for Privacy of Individually Identifiable Health Information," which were published by the Department of Health and Human Services (DHHS) in 2000, include detailed guidelines on what constitutes personally identifiable health information, under what conditions the information can be released and to whom, and when informed consent of the individual is needed to protect the privacy of the individual. Copies of these standards can be obtained via the World Wide Web at www.hhs.gov/ocr/regtext.html. Although these standards also apply to genetic information, this important legislation applies to any personal information in a medical record that contains identifying information about the individual. It is important for nurses to not only pay careful attention to accurate documentation of patient information but also ensure that proper safeguards are in place to protect the confidentiality of that information.

Documentation of Information Related to Genetic Counseling and Education

Documentation of genetic counseling sessions and predisposition genetic testing in general follows the same format used when documenting other medical information in a medical chart. The specific format may vary, depending on standard forms used in a particular institution or clinic and any policies concerning documentation and informed consent that may be in place. Because of state and federal regulations and the higher level of confidentiality applied to genetic information than to general patient information, some institutional forms or policies related to documentation may need to be modified. For example, special consent forms that are specific to genetic information may need to be developed and approved.

When cancer predisposition genetic testing is involved, the most important component of the medical chart is documentation reflecting that all of the issues related to informed consent have been documented in writing, indicating they were clearly covered by the healthcare provider. This includes documentation of the specific content covered in the genetic counseling session, whether the patient verbalized understanding of the information discussed, that the patient was asked if he or she wanted additional information, and appropriate signed consent forms.

Forms Usually Found in a Cancer Genetics Medical Record

Forms usually found in a medical record for patients seeking predisposition cancer genetic testing include the following: intake form, progress notes, cancer risk assessment, pedigree, patient and family medical records, patient letters, consent forms, and results of laboratory and diagnostic tests (including predisposition genetic tests). Education records also may be found, which are one method of documenting patient education.

Intake form. An intake form contains basic information about the patient and why he or she is requesting or being referred for genetic counseling. Intake forms might be used if the patient has been referred for genetic counseling a facility at which he or she has not received previous healthcare services.

Progress notes. Progress notes are standard in all medical records. Because genetic counseling services often are multidisciplinary, a progress record that can be used by all team members may be the most useful.

Cancer risk assessment from a genetic perspective. This may consist of a single assessment by the APN or multiple assessments, depending on who sees the patient. Components include a medical and family history; genetic, lifestyle, dietary, hormonal, and environmental cancer risk factors; and psychosocial assessment. An assessment of the patient's risk for the cancer or cancers of concern and the probability that the cancer in the family is the result of an inherited genetic mutation also is included. If a physical exam is conducted, those findings also are included.

Pedigree. As discussed earlier, a pedigree is a diagram of the family history using standard symbols to represent family members, their relationships, who has been affected by cancer or other illnesses, and whether the person is living or deceased. Pedigrees may be hand drawn on a pedigree form or created on a computer using a pedigree software program. A dated copy of the pedigree should be included in the medical record.

Patient and family medical records. Documentation of the patient's reported personal and family history of cancer is important when interpreting the pedigree and assessing cancer risk. For this reason, the chart may contain a number of pathology reports and medical records obtained from other sources pertaining to the patient or family members. These reports also may contain genetic information, especially if a known mutation exists in the family (see Figure 18-8).

Patient letters. Often, a detailed visit summary letter is sent out to a patient after the initial genetic counseling session. This letter frequently includes a review of who was present during the session, the patient's purpose for seeking genetic counseling, what information was exchanged, a summary of the cancer risk assessment, and what was decided as a result of the genetic counseling session. Genetic counselors often send out patient summary letters.

Consent forms. Consent forms most likely to be present include those authorizing predisposition genetic testing and those involving release of information to a third party. With predisposition genetic testing, multiple consent forms may be involved. If an outside laboratory is used, an additional consent form may be required (separate from that of the healthcare institution providing the genetic services).

Laboratory results and diagnostic tests. These may include standard blood work, results of cancer screening tests, or results of cancer predisposition genetic testing. Depending on the format of the clinic and what services are offered, some or all of these may be present.

Education records. Some method of documenting that patient education was provided and that the patient understands the information presented is essential to meet standards of quality-assurance criteria. Standard forms or flow sheets can be used for information that routinely is included in patient education. A more detailed outline of information covered under each patient-education category can be part of a separate document included in the standards of practice. Because each patient will have different educational needs, exceptions to the standard of practice would be addressed in the progress notes. The flow sheet must include each information category covered (e.g., overview of the genetics of breast cancer, risks and benefits of predisposition genetic testing, confidentiality, breast self-examination), the method(s) used for information delivery (e.g., verbal teaching, video, pamphlet), and the method for evaluating if the patient understood (see Figure 18-9).

Protection of Medical Records

Because of the highly sensitive nature of genetic information and the potential for insurance and workplace discrimination, many states have enacted laws requiring specific written authorization from the patient before genetic information can be disclosed (Scanlon, 1998). With the implementation of the DHHS privacy standards previously discussed, which protect all individually identifiable information, genetic information and other information now considered sensitive may no longer need to be singled out, as all medical record information will be held to a higher confidentiality standard. Although the routine use of computers, phones, and fax machines by healthcare professionals has greatly simplified recording and transferring of patient information, it has become all too easy for anyone who walks by a fax machine or logs on to a computer to have access to this information (Reed, 2000). A research study looked at how physicians store cancer predisposition genetic test results and found considerable variability (Wasserman, Jones, Trombold, & Sadler, 2000). Although some physicians

Figure 18-8. Sample Family History of Cancer Form

FAMILY HISTORY OF CANCER					
Who	First Name	Site(s)	Age at Diagnosis	Living? Yes / No	Comments
SELF					
Children					
Mother					
Father					
Brothers					
Sisters					
Maternal (your mother's)					
Grandmother					
Grandfather					
Uncles (your mother's brothers)					
Aunts (your mother's sisters)					
Paternal (your father's)					
Grandmother					
Grandfather					
Uncles (your father's brothers)					
Aunts (your father's sisters)					

(Continued on next page)

758

Figure 18-8. Sample Family History of Cancer Form *(Continued)*

If any cousins have had cancer, please complete this page.

First Name of Aunt or Uncle who is the parent of this cousin	First Name of Cousin	Site(s)	Age at Diagnosis	Still Living? Y/N	Comments
Maternal Cousins					
Paternal Cousins					

put genetic test results in with other laboratory tests in the patients; medical record, other physicians either maintained a separate medical record or did not record genetic test results in the medical record because of confidentiality concerns.

The storage and protection of medical records containing genetic information presents numerous challenges to the oncology nurse. For guidance in addressing how to safeguard medical records, medical records department personnel can be very helpful. Legal services at an institution, if available, can be of assistance in interpreting federal and state legislation related to the privacy and confidentiality of medical record information. The reader is referred to the American Nurses Association publications "Position Paper on Computer-Based Patient Record Standards" and "Privacy and Confidentiality," which are available online at www.nursingworld.org.

Figure 18-9. Patient Teaching Record

PATIENT TEACHING RECORD

Directions: Document date and time teaching is provided. List content of teaching provided in Teaching Content column. Document (1) learner(s), (2) assessment of readiness/barriers, (3) teaching method used, and (4) evaluation using the following codes:

Learner
P: Patient
S: Spouse
SP: Partner
CG: Caregiver
PM: Parent-Mother
PF: Parent-Father
F: Family member
Fri: Friend
*: See Progress Notes

Assessment: Readiness
R: Ready to learn N: Not ready to learn
Assessment: Permanent Barriers to Learning (check one time)
V: Vision impaired - ☐ Uncorrected
☐ Glasses ☐ Contacts
H: Hearing impaired - ☐ Uncorrected
Hearing aid ☐ Right ☐ Left
I: ☐ Interpreter
Variable Barriers to Learning
A: Attention span < 5 min
D: Denies relevance of information
O: Other (speech, etc.)
U: Unable to read
*: See Progress Notes

Teaching Method
D: Demonstration
E: Explanation
H: Printed handout
A/V: Audiovisual
R: Reinforcement
*: See Progress Notes

Evaluation
V: Verbalizes/indicates understanding
D: Demonstrates skill
DP: Demonstrates skill with physical assistance
DV: Demonstrates skill with verbal assistance
N: Needs reinforcement
I: Inability to learn
U: Unsuccessful
*: See Progress Notes

Genetic Testing: Breast Cancer											
Date											
Time											
TEACHING CONTENT	Initials										
Program Overview Genetics of Breast Cancer Overview	learner										
	assess										
	method										
	evaluation										
Risks, Benefits, & Limitations of Genetic Testing,	learner										
	assess										
	method										
	evaluation										
Cost of Testing	learner										
	assess										
	method										
	evaluation										
Confidentiality of Test Results	learner										
	assess										
	method										
	evaluation										
Review Insurance Issues	learner										
	assess										
	method										
	evaluation										
DNA Banking	learner										
	assess										
	method										
	evaluation										
Cancer Risks & Screening Guidelines	learner										
	assess										
	method										
	evaluation										

Copy sent to: _____ _____ _____ _____ _____ _____

Addressing Follow-Up Needs

People undergoing predisposition genetic testing have many issues to consider after test results have been received. Predisposition genetic testing usually is a one-time event; the implications, however, can last a lifetime. For people who test positive, their lives will be altered immediately in some ways. Because of the confidential nature of genetic predisposition testing, bringing people together so they can support one another is not always easy. Outside of large metropolitan areas, not enough people with similar needs may be available to form a support group. The availability of Internet support groups is an option for some, and they can be best used as part of professional healthcare support services. People without a previous cancer diagnosis who test positive may be in need of some type of follow-up psychological support. These patients will not have been involved in support services offered by comprehensive cancer programs and therefore will require referral. Even when these services are available to them, the services may not meet their needs. A patient who tells her own story best illustrates this:

> "Although I've never been told I have cancer, when I was told that I had inherited this gene, I felt as though I'd been told that I did. Living with my family history, it's always been a question of when, not if, I would get breast cancer. And having this gene just made it more of a reality. I felt as though it's been lying dormant, and that it would wake up any day now. Besides one friend, none of my other friends were there for me. I think for most people, there are only two groups of people—those with breast cancer and those without it. To my friends, because I didn't have a diagnosis of breast cancer, I was definitely in the healthy people group. To me, however, I was one degree away from those with breast cancer. And there is a huge gap between those two groups. And no matter how much I assertively talked about this issue, only one friend realized after several months how difficult this was for me" (Prouser, 1997).

Psychological distress can impede patients' ability to receive and process information. For cancer risk counseling to be effective, emotional issues need to be identified and addressed (Peters, 1994). The psychosocial assessment is an ongoing process that takes place as a part of each patient contact and involves verbal, nonverbal, and written cues. Clinical judgment on the part of oncology nurses is involved in deciding how to interpret the gathered information and making appropriate referrals for psychosocial services.

Surveillance and Management of High-Risk Patients

Oncology nurses are in an ideal position to help patients who carry a genetic predisposition to cancer understand the cancer surveillance and risk management options available to them. Their options differ from the general population in that a much more individualized approach is needed for each patient when developing a cancer surveillance and risk-reduction plan. Many factors need to be taken into account. For example, a 35-year-old patient who carries a genetic predisposition to breast and ovarian cancer may not want to consider prophylactic mastectomies, regardless of evidence that shows a significant reduction in breast cancer risk (Hartmann et al., 1999). Although taking tamoxifen for five years reduced the risk of both invasive and noninvasive breast cancer by approximately 50% in women at increased risk for the disease, no data are available on the effect of tamoxifen in women with a genetic predisposition to cancer (Fisher et al., 1998). Basic patient education also should be included, such as instructing women in breast self-examination.

Long-term use of oral contraceptives has been associated with a 50% decreased risk in ovarian cancer in women with either BRCA1 or BRCA2 mutations, so women carrying these mutations may benefit from being informed about this option (Narod et al., 1998). Two articles have been published that address cancer surveillance and risk-reduction options for people who carry a genetic predisposition to cancer (Burke, Daly, et al., 1997; Burke, Petersen, et al., 1997). Mammography is more likely to be started at an earlier age, and clinical breast examinations may need to be more frequent. In addition, a CA 125 tumor marker blood test and vaginal ultrasound are recommended for ovarian cancer screening in the absence of oophorectomy. Although an extreme choice to make, oophorectomy can lower ovarian cancer risk as well as reduce breast cancer risk by approximately 50% in patients known to carry BRCA1 mutations, regardless of whether women are taking hormone replacement therapy (Rebbeck et al., 1999). If a patient undergoes prophylactic bilateral oophorectomy, she will need to be counseled concerning management of early menopause and the need for vitamin D and calcium to reduce the risk for osteoporosis and bone density testing for monitoring. Figure 18-10 provides a summary of what should be included in a cancer surveillance and risk-reduction plan.

As healthcare providers, nurses still have much to learn about the follow-up needs of patients who have been through predisposition genetic testing. The focus has been primarily on surveillance needs and the risks and benefits of prophylactic surgery (Burke, Daly, et al., 1997; Burke, Petersen, et al., 1997; Hartmann et al., 1999; Rebbeck et al., 1999). The psychological impact of receiving predisposition genetic test results can last a lifetime, and little attention has been given to living with the uncertainties associated with genetic risk (Welch & Burke, 1998).

Nurses have a pivotal role in caring for these patients, and their needs for emotional support and health education is ongoing. Patients who test positive for

---

Figure 18-10. Components of a Cancer Surveillance and Risk-Reduction Plan

The following information needs to be included for all common cancers, in addition to any unusual cancers for which the patient may be at increased risk.
• Recommended frequency of suggested cancer screening tests
• Frequency of examinations by a healthcare provider
• Potential risks and benefits of chemoprevention and prophylactic surgery options
• Information about lifestyle, dietary, and environmental factors known to increase cancer risk
• Any follow-up recommendations for additional clinic visits or referrals to outside programs or healthcare providers

---

a genetic mutation may face prophylactic surgery, chemoprevention, and long-term clinical services for cancer surveillance in addition to ongoing health education and psychological support. Nurses need to participate in and carry out nursing research studies to learn more about the long-term healthcare needs of people at genetic risk for cancer. To be effective caregivers, nurses need to know what it is like to live with the uncertainty associated with a genetic risk for cancer. How can nurses best support these patients as they make decisions based on genetic information? What interventions are most helpful in addressing the emotional issues these patients and their families must deal with? The nursing plan of care for psychosocial needs is based on this knowledge.

Conclusion

Nurses must remember that genetic information has implications for the entire family, not just the patient. The predictive nature of genetic information may alter an individual's concept of his or her health, even when no symptoms are present. Genetic information is permanent; current technology cannot alter it. Health decisions are based on this information, and family relationships can be affected. Genetic testing does not provide definite answers and, in some cases, even may increase uncertainty.

Although a predisposition to cancer is not a diagnosis, it may be viewed as one by an insurance company or an employer. This can cause a person to feel "diseased" or "marked" in some way. Feelings of isolation may result when patients are in this unique category of carrying a mutation but not being diagnosed with a disease.

Informed consent and confidentiality issues related to predisposition genetic testing are held to a very high standard of care that oncology nurses must meet. APNs who provide genetic counseling and education are guided by the ethical principles of nursing and have the knowledge, skills, and caring to address the complex issues involved in providing genetic counseling, predisposition genetic testing, and education regarding genetic information.

References

American Nurses Association and International Society of Nurses in Genetics. (1998). *Statement on the scope and standards of genetics clinical nursing practice.* Washington, DC: Author.

American Society of Clinical Oncology. (1996). Genetic testing for cancer susceptibility. *Journal of Clinical Oncology, 14,* 1730–1736.

Berner, S. (1996). Federal protection of genetic information: Congress delivers. *Journal of Women's Health, 5,* 409–410.

Botkin, J., Croyle, R., Smith, K., Baty, B., Lerman, C., Goldgar, D., Ward, J., Flick, B., & Nash, J. (1996). A model protocol for evaluation: The behavioral and psychosocial effects of BRCA1 testing. *Journal of the National Cancer Institute, 88,* 872–882.

Braddock, C.H., Fihn, S.D., Levinson, W., Jonsen, A.R., & Pearlman, R.A. (1997). How doctors and patients discuss routine clinical decisions. Informed decision-making in the outpatient setting. *Journal of General Internal Medicine, 12,* 339–345.

Burke, W., Daly, M., Garber, J., Botkin, J., Kahn, M., Lynch, P., McTiernan, A., Offit, K., Perlman, J., Petersen, G., Thompson, E., & Varricchio, C. (1997). Recommendations for follow-up care of individuals with an inherited predisposition to cancer: BRCA1 and BRCA2. *JAMA, 227*, 997–1003.

Burke, W., Petersen, G., Lynch, P., Botkin, J., Daly, M., Garber, J., Kahn, M.J., McTiernan, A., Offit, K., Thomson, E., & Varricchio, C. (1997). Recommendations for follow-up care of individuals with an inherited predisposition to cancer. I. Hereditary nonpolyposis colon cancer. Cancer Genetics Studies Consortium. *JAMA, 277*, 915–919.

Croyle, R., Smith, K., Botkin, J., Baty, B., & Nash, J. (1997). Psychological responses to BRCA1 mutation testing: Preliminary findings. *Health Psychology, 16*, 63–72.

Dickens, B., Pei, N., & Taylor, K. (1996). Legal and ethical issues in genetic testing and counseling for susceptibility to breast, ovarian, and colon cancer. *Canadian Medical Association Journal, 154*, 813–818.

Donaldson, S.K. (1999). Genetic research and knowledge in the discipline of nursing. *Biological Research for Nursing, 1*, 90–99.

Fanos, J. (1997). Developmental tasks of childhood and adolescence: Implications for genetic testing. *American Journal of Medical Genetics, 71*, 22–28.

Fisher, B., Costantino, J.P., Wickerham, D.L., Redmond, C.K., Kavanah, M., Cronin, W.M., Vogel, V., Robidoux, A., Dimitrov, N., Atkins, J., Daly, M., Wieand, S., Tan-Chiu, E., Ford, L., & Wolmark, N. (1998). Tamoxifen for prevention of breast cancer: Report of the National Surgical Adjuvant Breast and Bowel Project P-1 Study. *Journal of the National Cancer Institute, 90*, 1371–1388.

Forbes, N. (1996). The nurse and genetic counseling. *Nursing Clinics of North America, 1*, 679–688.

Forsman, I. (1994). Evolution of the nursing role in genetics. *Journal of Obstetrics, Gynecology, and Neonatal Nursing, 23*, 481–486.

Frank, T. (1998). Hereditary risk of breast and ovarian carcinoma: The role of the oncologist. *The Oncologist, 3*, 403–412.

Friedman, L., Gayther, S., Kurosaki, T., Gordon, D., Noble, B., Casey, G., Ponder, B., & Anton-Culver, H. (1997). Mutation analysis of BRCA1 and BRCA2 in a male breast cancer population. *American Journal of Human Genetics, 60*, 313–319.

Geller, G., Botkin, J., Green, M., Press, N., Biesecker, B., Wilfond, B., Grana, G., Daly, M., Schneider, K., & Kahn, M. (1997). Genetic testing for susceptibility to adult-onset cancer: The process and content of informed consent. *JAMA, 227*, 1467–1474.

Geller, G., Bernhardt, B., Helzlsouer, K., Holtzman, N., Stefanek, M., & Wilcox, P. (1995). Informed consent and BRCA1 testing, *Nature Genetics, 11*, 364.

Gould, R., Lynch, H., Smith, R., & McCarthy, J. (1997). *Cancer and genetics: Answering patients' questions.* New York: American Cancer Society.

Hartmann, L.C., Schaid, D.J., Woods, J.E., Crotty, T.P., Myers, J.L., Arnold, P.G., Petty, P.M., Sellers, T.A., Johnson, J.L., McDonnell, S.K., Frost, M.H., & Jenkins, R.B. (1999). Efficacy of bilateral prophylactic mastectomy in women with a family history of breast cancer. *New England Journal of Medicine, 340*, 77–84.

Jonsen, A., Seigler, M., & Winslade, W. (1992). *Clinical ethics.* New York: McGraw-Hill.

Lea, D., Jenkins, J., & Francomano, C. (1998). *Genetics in clinical practice: New directions for nursing and health care.* Boston: Jones and Bartlett.

Lerman, C., Daly, M., Masny, A., & Balshem, A. (1994). Attitudes about genetic testing for breast-ovarian cancer susceptibility. *Journal of Clinical Oncology, 12*, 843–850.

Lerman, C., Lustbader, E., Rimer, B., Daly, M., Miller, S., Sands, C., & Balshem, A. (1995). Effects of individualized breast cancer risk counseling: A randomized trial. *Journal of the National Cancer Institute, 87*, 286–292.

Lerman, C., Narod, S., Schulman, K., Hughes, C., Hornez-Caminero, G., Bonney, G., Hold, K., Trock, B., Main, D., Lynch, J., Fulmore, C., Snyder, C., Semon, J., Conway, T., Tonin, P., Lenoir, G., & Lynch, H. (1996). BRCA1 testing in families with hereditary breast-ovarian cancer. *JAMA, 275*, 1885–1892.

Lerman, C., Seay, J., Balshem, A., & Audrain, J. (1995). Interest in genetic testing among first-degree relatives of breast cancer patients. *American Journal of Medical Genetics, 57*, 385–392.

Lynch, H., Lemon, S., Durham, C., Tinley, S., Connolly, C., Lynch, J., Surdam, J., Orinion, E., Slominski-Caster, S., Watson, P., Lerman, C., Tonin, P., Lenoir, G., Serova, O., & Narod, S. (1997). A descriptive study of BRCA1 testing and reactions to disclosure of test results. *Cancer, 79*, 2219–2228.

MacDonald, D.J. (1997). The oncology nurse's role in cancer risk assessment and counseling. *Seminars in Oncology Nursing, 13*, 123–128.

Mahon, S. (1998). Cancer risk assessment: Conceptual considerations for clinical practice. *Oncology Nursing Forum, 24*, 1535–1547.

Narod, S.A., Risch, H., Moslehi, R., Dorum, A., Neuhausen, S., Olsson, H., Provencher, D., Radice, P., Evans, G., Bishop, S., Brunet, J.S., & Ponder, B.A. (1998). Oral contraceptives and the risk of hereditary ovarian cancer. *New England Journal of Medicine, 339*, 424–428.

Oncology Nursing Society. (1998). The role of the oncology nurse in cancer genetic counseling. *Oncology Nursing Forum, 25*, 463.

Oregon Medical Association. (1996). *Oregon legal handbook.* Portland, OR: Author.

Patenaude, A.J. (1996). The genetic testing of children for cancer susceptibility: Ethical, legal, and social issues. *Behavioral Sciences and the Law, 14*, 393–410.

Peters, J. (1994). Breast cancer risk counseling. *Genetic Resource, 8*(1), 20–25.

Petersen, G., & Brensinger, J. (1996). Genetic testing and counseling in familial adenomatous polyposis. *Oncology, 10*(1), 89–94.

Prouser, N. (1997, November). *My story. Breast cancer and genetics.* Symposium conducted by Legacy Cancer Services, Portland, OR.

Prouser, N. (2000). Case report: Genetic susceptibility testing for breast and ovarian cancer: A patient's perspective. *Journal of Genetic Counseling, 9*(2), 153–159.

Rebbeck, T.R., Levin, A.M., Eisen, A., Snyder, C., Watson, P., Cannon-Albright, L., Isaacs, C., Olopade, O., Garber, J.E., Godwin, A.K., Daly, M.B., Narod, S.A., Neuhausen, S.L., Lynch, H.T., & Weber, B.L. (1999). Breast cancer risk after bilateral prophylactic oophorectomy in BRCA1 mutation carriers. *Journal of the National Cancer Institute, 91*, 1475–1479.

Reed, S. (2000). Keeping secrets secret. Legislation to secure patient privacy and confidentiality is still needed. *American Journal of Nursing, 100*(8), 73–74.

Rieger, P.T. (1997). The impact of cancer genetics on oncology nursing practice. *Nursing Interventions in Oncology, 9*, 15–19.

Scanlon, C. (1998). The legal implications of genetic testing. *RN, 61*(3), 61–65.

Schneider, K. (1994). *Counseling about cancer: Strategies for genetic counselors.* Dennisport, MA: Graphic Illusions.

Shattuck-Eidens, D., McClure, M., Simard, J., Labrie, F., Narod, S., Couch, F., Hoskins, K., Weber, B., Castilla, L., & Erdos, M. (1995). A collaborative survey of 80 mutations in the BRCA1 breast and ovarian cancer susceptibility gene. Implications for presymptomatic testing and screening. *JAMA, 273,* 535–541.

Strewing, J., Hartge, P., Wacholder, S., Baker, S., Berlin, M., McAdams, M., Timmerman, M., Brody, L., & Tucker, M. (1997). The risk of cancer associated with specific mutations of BRCA1 and BRCA2 among Ashkenazi Jews. *New England Journal of Medicine, 336,* 1401–1408.

Tessare, I., Borstelmann, N., Regan, K., Rimer, B., & Winer, E. (1997). Genetic testing for susceptibility to breast cancer: Findings from women's focus groups. *Journal of Women's Health, 6,* 317–327.

Vernon, S., Perz, C., Gritz, E., Peterson, S., Amos, C., Baile, W., & Lynch, P. (1997). Correlates of psychologic distress in colorectal cancer patients undergoing genetic testing for hereditary colon cancer. *Health Psychology, 16,* 73–86.

Waldo, B.H. (1999) Managing data security: Developing a plan to protect patient data. *Nursing Economics, 17*(1), 49–52.

Wasserman, L.M., Jones, O.W., Trombold, J.S., & Sadler, G.R. (2000). Attitudes of physicians regarding receiving and storing patients' genetic testing results for cancer susceptibility. *Journal of Community Health, 25,* 305–313.

Welch, H.G., & Burke, W. (1998). Uncertainties in genetic testing for chronic disease. *JAMA, 280,* 1525–1527.

SECTION IV

Cancer Control

OVERVIEW

Section IV

Carol Stoner, MS, RN, and Suzanne M. Mahon, RN, DNSc,
AOCN®, APNG(c)

This section of the textbook is a compilation of a broad range of programs in which nurses have implemented the principles of primary, secondary, and tertiary cancer prevention. Many approaches to cancer control are represented in this section, including mass screening programs, individualized cancer risk assessment and screening programs, cancer genetics counseling programs, government-sponsored programs, and programs that are offered at public events. In each, a great need exists for nursing professionals to coordinate, implement, and help to provide cancer-control and education services. As editors of this section, it was truly amazing to see the scope and creativity of programs. We want to thank each contributor who took the time to share a personal story about a cancer-control program. We hope this section challenges every nurse, no matter what his or her practice setting, to think about the many ways to include and promote cancer prevention and early detection.

Although the programs presented differ in several ways, common themes exist with every program. Nurses need to consider some of these common themes as they begin to develop programs for cancer control. These themes include consideration of the target population, resources of the institution or sponsor, opportunities for and value of collaboration, and resources for and approaches to public education, funding, marketing, and program evaluation.

One of the most frequently overlooked components of successful program development is a detailed and accurate needs assessment prior to the implementation of the program. Ultimately, the success of a particular cancer-screening program can be traced to the amount of effort taken at the beginning to understand the unique needs of the community and population being served (Fitch et al., 1997). A needs assessment can be conducted using focus groups and individual interviews with members of the population to be served. Concerns can be assessed, validated, and discussed to help to discern the best methods to meet the identified need(s).

Every institution needs to select a cancer-control program that not only meets the needs of the population being screened but also fits well with resources available to the institution (or sponsor). Assessing the goals and mission of the institution (or sponsor) is imperative to determine if appropriate support (e.g., clinical services, clerical assistance, billing acumen, marketing expertise, adequate monetary funds, collaborative support opportunities) is available to develop an effective program. Sometimes, piloting a program prior to its mass introduction will help to identify program or institutional deficiencies. If adequate support does not exist at first for a large-scale program, effective smaller programs can be developed incrementally. For example, an institution initially may offer breast self-examination education in conjunction with a mammography program. If this is successful, offering clinical breast examinations and education and counseling about genetic testing may be the next components added. Additionally, adequate physical facilities must be available for performing the cancer-control services and providing patient education (Miller, 1996).

Collaboration is a critical component found in each program description. Objectives for collaboration include assistance with program development or implementation, professional development, or some combination thereof. Some efforts are more traditional in nature (e.g., between institutions, agencies, professional organizations), while others are quite creative (e.g., with organizers of an outdoor bike race). Regardless, each vignette provides evidence that the ability to partner (formally or informally) with those in a position to lend support, knowledge, or even a target audience (e.g., those attending a university football game) can have a positive impact on a program.

All of the programs in this section also include an emphasis on public education, especially as it relates to program-specific health and wellness issues. Procuring or perhaps developing proper patient-education materials is an important task that begins as any cancer-control program is being planned and can be an ongoing challenge. A description of different strategies for providing education on cancer prevention and early detection is provided in Table 1.

A plan for funding the start-up and ongoing costs is critical to the success of any program. Although cancer-control services typically generate meager revenue and often are not reimbursable according to many insurance plans, they often are a source of goodwill on the part of the institution toward the community. If an institution is unable to completely fund a program, other sources of funding (e.g., grants, corporate co-sponsorships, endowments) may be an option. The programs in this section have been funded by a variety of means. Budget items that should be considered in the development of a program include personnel costs and benefits, space rental, office equipment, educational materials, supplies and medical equipment, and marketing.

Regardless of the type of cancer-control program being implemented, a clear program for promoting and marketing the program needs to be identified at the beginning. Consultation with the institution's marketing department can provide much insight on the best ways to promote these programs, considering the target population and the particular geographic area to be served. Continued assessment of how clients become aware of the program and whether the target audience

Table 1. Strategies for Patient Education on Primary and Secondary Cancer Prevention

Educational Material	Strengths	Limitations
Brochures specifically developed for the cancer screening program	• Promote program with phone numbers, logo, addresses etc. • Learn self-examination techniques or information exactly as taught by health professionals in the program. • Can be tailored to meet the specific needs of the program	• Expensive • Require expertise to develop • May require frequent and costly revisions
Brochures from organizations such as NCI, ACS, or the Komen Foundation	• Relatively low cost • Often low-literacy materials available	• Availability may vary • Will not directly promote the program • May present information with different language or technique than taught by health professionals in the program
Brochures from pharmaceutical companies	• Often free • Often have very attractive layout and graphics	• Availability may vary. • Will not directly promote the program • May present information with different language or technique than taught by health professionals in the program • May promote the company's products
Posters	• Often free or low cost • Provide decoration and education in waiting areas or examination rooms	• Can only provide a minimal amount of information • Can become outdated
Free-standing displays/bulletin boards	• Easy way to provide visual information and simple text on a wide variety of topics • Bulletin boards can be changed frequently to promote a topic.	• Free-standing displays can be expensive. • Need room to display
Flip charts	• Can be used free-standing, but best used as an adjunct to patient education • Can be made at institution to meet the specific needs of a program • Do not require much room to use • Can be an effective source of visual education • Relatively low-cost if made at institution	• To be most effective, need to be used with a health professional providing education • Can be expensive if purchased from commercial agencies

(Continued on next page)

Table 1. Strategies for Patient Education on Primary and Secondary Cancer Prevention (Continued)

Educational Material	Strengths	Limitations
VCR/videos	• May be useful for low-literacy clients • Can often find materials that are sensitive to ethnicity issues • Provide a standard message in a short period of time	• Must have the room and equipment to show the tapes • Some tapes may be expensive to purchase.
Computer-assisted education	• Can provide detailed information with appealing graphics • Allows learner to select material and learn at their own pace	• Requires expensive equipment • Must have space for the equipment • Few programs are currently available and many are expensive. • Patients may be intimidated by computers.
Samples (sunscreen, smoking cessation kits)	• Giving the client a sample, may encourage the patient to try the agent. • Usually can be obtained at no costs from pharmaceutical companies	• May require book-keeping of how samples were dispensed (i.e. smoking cessation aids) • Availability may vary
Anatomical models	• Provide visual information to reinforce technically difficult concepts • Can be used to simulate clinical problems, such as a breast lump	• May not be helpful to the patient without an explanation from the healthcare professional • Model may not simulate clinical problem exactly (i.e., breast model may not feel like a woman's breasts) • Can be expensive

Note. From "The Role of the Nurse in Developing Cancer Screening Programs," by S.M. Mahon, 2000, *Oncology Nursing Forum, 27*(Suppl.), pp. 19–27. Copyright 2000 by the Oncology Nursing Press, Inc. Adapted with permission.

actually is using the services will either help-identify successful, cost-effective marketing strategies or necessitate a change in approach.

An important outcome of any cancer-detection program is the assurance that people with abnormal screening results receive appropriate follow-up. Rimer (1996) noted that the ideal strategy to ensure follow-up varies according to the population and the cancer for which screening is being conducted. Before the implementation of any screening program, whether it is for mass screening or a comprehensive program, a strategy for follow-up must be determined. Before instituting any follow-up policy, having a legal analysis of the policy is helpful to be sure it is complete.

Program evaluation is another ongoing challenge in cancer-control programs. Many of the programs presented in this section operate within the context of a larger organizational structure. The strategies used to evaluate such a program optimally are established at the outset and must be indelibly linked to the goals of the program. Without clear program goals to guide the evaluation process, a program's success cannot be evaluated or, worse yet, may be evaluated in a manner that is potentially damaging. For example, there is little chance for program success if the clinician's goal is to provide a service to the community, but administration requires the program to be financially self-supporting. The clinician may have evidence of terrific attendance and participant feedback, but if the program is operating at a net loss, the chances for that program to survive are threatened. Similarly, in this era of institutional consolidations, shifting priorities, and ever-changing insurance reimbursement patterns, program objectives should be revisited periodically to ensure appropriate evaluation methods are being used that will help to support program survival. In addition to determining short and long-term success of a program, evaluation efforts also can provide data for epidemiological research and documentation to funding sources.

Cancer prevention and early detection will continue to grow as a priority for oncology professionals and the institutions where they work. Nurses will continue to play a critical role in the development, management, and success of cancer-control programs. As the examples of cancer control in this section illustrate, oncology nurses are well positioned to accept new and challenging roles in the area of cancer control.

References

Fitch, M.I., Greenberg, M., Levstein, L., Muir, M., Plante, S., & King, E. (1997). Health promotion and early detection of cancer in older adults: Needs assessment for program development. *Cancer Nursing, 20*, 381–388.

Miller, A.B. (1996). Fundamental issues in screening for cancer. In D. Schottenfeld & J.F. Fraumeni (Eds.), *Cancer epidemiology and prevention* (2nd ed.) (pp. 1433–1452). New York: Oxford University Press.

Rimer, B.K. (1996). Adherence to cancer screening. In D.S. Reintgen & R.A. Clark (Eds.), *Cancer screening* (pp. 261–276). St. Louis, MO: Mosby.

CHAPTER 19

The Role of the Nurse in Cancer Control

Claudette G. Varricchio, DSN, RN, FAAN

Introduction

"Cancer control" is not a clearly defined and understood concept. It has many definitions, and the definition is evolving as the science continues to evolve. The earliest use of the phrase seems to have been in 1913 as a part of the name of a newly formed organization, the American Society for the Control of Cancer (Hiatt & Rimer, 1999). This organization became the American Cancer Society in 1945 (New York City Cancer Committee, 1944). The concept entered the healthcare lexicon defining the function of the newly formed National Cancer Institute (NCI) in 1937. The legislative language instructed NCI to "cooperate with state health agencies in the prevention, control, and eradication of cancer." They interpreted cancer control to be the "useful application of their results" (Hiatt & Rimer). This was the application of findings, not cancer control research as we know it. "Cancer control" still was not officially defined.

The enactment of The National Cancer Act of 1971 reaffirmed cancer control within the mission of NCI and authorized a line item in the budget to support cancer control. As a result of this mandate, a working group was formed to define cancer control. They stated that "cancer research seeks to find the means for combating cancer, whereas cancer control is concerned with identifying, community testing, evaluating, and promoting the application of means that are found" (Cancer Control, 1975, p. 2).

The Division of Cancer Prevention and Control, in 1983, stimulated the promulgation of the definition put forth by Greenwald and Cullen (1985). They defined cancer control as "the reduction of cancer incidence, morbidity, and mortality through an orderly sequence from research on interventions and their impact in defined populations to the broad, systematic application of the research results" (p. 543). They proposed a framework of five stages for the logical progression of research: phase I, hypothesis generation; phase II, method development; phase III, controlled intervention trials; phase IV, studies in defined populations; and phase V, demonstration projects.

The most recent definition guiding NCI's cancer-control program was developed and adopted in 1997 "Cancer control research is the conduct of basic and applied research in the behavioral, social, and population sciences that, independently, or in combination with biomedical approaches, reduces cancer risk, incidence, morbidity, and mortality and improves quality of life (Abrams, 1997)."

Sometimes the concept of cancer prevention, or chemoprevention, is incorporated under the umbrella construct of cancer control. Chemoprevention is defined as "the use of pharmacological or natural agents to inhibit the development of invasive cancer. . . . This new science of chemoprevention has been established as an important approach to control malignancy. . . . Chemoprevention is now recognized as both a clinical and basic science" ("Prevention of Cancer," 1999, p. 4743).

These definitions do not give clear guidance to nurses who wish to engage in cancer control research. The role of nursing research as an adjunct to cancer control efforts may be clarified if one keeps in mind that the goals of cancer control are to reduce cancer risk, incidence, morbidity, and mortality and to improve the quality of life through application of research findings (Hiatt & Rimer, 1999).

Examples of national cancer prevention and control trials are the Five a Day Program testing dietary modification to prevent cancer; the breast and prostate cancer prevention trials; the Prostate, Lung, Cervical and Ovarian cancer screening trial; and many specific symptom management, supportive care, and quality-of-life assessment trials sponsored by the cooperative cancer treatment groups.

The Role of Nursing in Cancer Control

Much of nursing research that can be considered cancer control relates to the reduction of cancer-related morbidity. This often is the testing of interventions to manage the symptoms, physiologic and psychologic, that are associated with the diagnosis of cancer done in small local intervention or descriptive studies.

Nurse researchers have explored the impact of being at risk for cancer, the distress of a cancer diagnosis, decision making about cancer treatment or prevention options, and compliance with surveillance recommendations and treatment, as well specific symptom management through drugs or cognitive behavioral interventions. Nurses have been leaders in the field of quality-of-life research and in the management of palliative and end-of-life care. The focus of nurse researchers in cancer control has included family members, caregivers, and systems as well as the person with cancer.

Nurse researchers have begun to conduct multicenter randomized clinical trials over the past few years. This is an area of emerging interest in nursing research. Some adventurous nurse researchers have begun to work with the cooperative cancer treatment groups to develop and implement cancer control protocols using the group resources and infrastructure.

The majority of nurses who are engaged in cancer-control research are able to do so through participation as clinical research associates and data managers for the cooperative clinical trials groups, cancer centers, and community clinical oncology programs. In these roles, nurses recruit subjects, explain the trials, obtain informed consent, and often deliver the interventions. They oversee the data collection and reporting or submission of the data to a central statistical office for analysis.

Much cancer-control research, by its nature, is interdisciplinary. Nurses often are members of these interdisciplinary research teams, but they seldom have been the principal investigators of these teams. Because of this, there has been little nursing input into the design, development, and implementation of the large control clinical trials.

What the Role of Nurses in Cancer Control Research Could Be

Nurses could participate in leadership positions in cancer-control efforts. Much of cancer control is directed at people who have not been diagnosed with cancer. This population is one that may be accessible in other, nononcology, parts of the healthcare system. This is where the potential participants in prevention and screening trials will be found. Nurse-managed clinics could be a vital source of subjects for cancer-control research. Collaborations between nurse clinicians and nurse researchers could be rich and rewarding.

One of the talents of nurses is their ability to communicate well with people in various stressful situations. This makes them ideal partners in cancer-control research where assessment of cancer risk is needed. Nurses can assess comorbidities, especially in the elderly, and recommend screening or surveillance programs or lifestyle changes that are based on research data.

These skills and access lead naturally to recommendations for the establishment of nurse-managed clinics for assessment of disease risk, not only cancer risk. Nurse-directed symptom management clinics are another venue for the conduct and application of cancer-control research. These clinics could include prevention and surveillance activities, as well, and should not be limited to a cancer focus.

Nurses should emphasize the discipline's emphasis on care of the whole person, physical, psychologic, and social. The strength and attractiveness of "one-stop shopping" for risk assessment, screening, symptom management, and rehabilitation interventions should be promoted by nurses. This care delivery system can provide a rich resource for cancer control and other nursing research as well as a place for demonstration projects and research utilization research.

References

Abrams D.B. (1997). *A new agenda for cancer control research: Report of the Cancer Control Review Group.* Bethesda, MD: National Cancer Institute. Retrieved July 5, 2001 from the World Wide Web: http://deainfo.nci.nih.gov/ADVISORY/bsa/bsa_program/bsacacntrlmin.htm

Cancer Control. (1975). *Working Group 8 Report.* Bethesda, MD: National Cancer Institute.

Greenwald, P., & Cullen, J.W. (1985). The new emphasis in cancer control. *Journal of the National Cancer Institute, 74*, 543–551.

Hiatt, R.A., & Rimer, B.K. (1999). A new strategy for cancer control research. *Cancer Epidemiology, Biomarkers and Prevention, 8*, 957–964.

New York City Cancer Committee. (1944). *History of the American Society for the Control of Cancer.* New York: Author.

Prevention of cancer in the next millennium: Report of the chemoprevention working group to the American Association for Cancer Research. (1999). *Cancer Prevention, 59*, 4743–4758.

CHAPTER 20

Local Programs

GatorSHADE™ Sun Protection Program at the University of Florida College of Nursing

Carol Reed Ash, EdD, RN, FAAN, and Jill W. Varnes, EdD, CHES

GatorSHADE™ is a sun-protection program that focuses on increasing awareness of the risks of overexposure to the sun and teaching children and adults the appropriate skills to prevent skin cancer. The program is a joint project of the Colleges of Nursing and Health and Human Performance at the University of Florida in Gainesville. This multifaceted program is designed to provide specific activities based upon the targeted population.

The first GatorSHADE event was a 1994 community awareness campaign that focused on children and adults attending an afternoon football game at the University of Florida. An estimated 85,000 people received the sun-protection message that afternoon. Pocket-sized cards describing sun protection and samples of SPF 30 sunscreen were distributed to all adults. Specially designed hats providing adequate sun protection to the ears and back of the neck were given to the children. Inside the stadium, the electronic message board and the public address system repeated the GatorSHADE message.

Prior to the game, student volunteers circulated in the parking areas to survey the attendees in regard to their planned sun-protective behaviors at the game. This survey was designed to provide some baseline information about the knowledge and behavior of the target group. At the next home game, students again surveyed the crowd to see if the GatorSHADE message was received and retained. Data analysis of the 900 respondents showed a statistically significant increase in awareness related to the need for sunscreen and protective clothing.

The initial GatorSHADE event was accomplished with the support of various colleges in the university and community agencies. Twenty-five thousand dollars was solicited to fund the design and production of the GatorSHADE logo, the 5,000 hats and 45,000 sun-protection cards that were distributed, and the T-shirts for the student volunteers. The 80,000 sunscreen samples were donated. The success of the program was the result of the training, time, and energy of the volunteer students from the Colleges of Nursing and Health and Human Performance. The program also succeeded because of the commitment to the idea and the cooperation of the University Athletic Association in coordinating the event with faculty members.

Since 1994, additional community-focused efforts have been held with other sporting events: summer camps, which included a more intensive educational effort, and school-based programs for fourth graders and special needs children. Nursing students completing community health experiences also emphasized the messages of the sun-protection program when working with various age groups throughout the community.

The program has continued to evolve as the needs of and strategies for delivery of the message varied with the target population. The rationale for the multiple target audiences was based upon a need to educate both the adults and the children simultaneously. Children are more likely to retain a behavior that is supported and encouraged by adults, specifically their parents or primary caregiver.

At this time, the primary focus of the intervention is the school-based educational program. A GatorSHADE sun-protection program has been developed for both fourth grade and special-education students. The program includes a 16-minute "SunScoop" videotape and a curriculum to be used by the teachers. Included in the curriculum book are a teaching plan, word game, crossword puzzle, and board game to reinforce the messages of the videotape. A take-home packet for parents includes the "SunScoop" videotape, a newsletter, and an exercise for the child and parent to do together.

All participating teachers receive a one- to two-hour in-service to review the materials and go over the evaluation process. This in-service allows the teachers to ask specific questions and to clarify their own questions about skin cancer or how to better protect their skin from sun damage. One of the strengths of the program is the take-home component. This curriculum is designed to ensure interaction between the parents and their children related to sun-protective behavior and the need to make this a lifelong habit.

Regardless of the target population, an evaluation component is built in. From the pre- and post-tests of the community awareness campaign to the observations of compliance in the camps, self-reports from the children, and the knowledge tests of the educational program, evidence of increased awareness and knowledge and changes in sun-protective behaviors have been seen. The strongest evidence of the program's impact is its durability.

Since 1994, the GatorSHADE logo and name have become synonymous with sun protection. The initial effort was designed to be a one-time major event. However, increased consumer awareness of the dangers of overexposure to the sun and increased risk of skin cancer, especially in states such as Florida, made the idea seem too good to let go.

Challenges to the program have been multifaceted. Once the initial event concluded, money was not available to continue. Time to work on the program also was a factor. The first GatorSHADE event involved considerable time and effort. Finding the time and money to expand the program consumed many volunteer hours, and obtaining funding to develop the program has required persistence in convincing funding agencies that the program has merit.

Expanding the educational intervention to fourth-grade and special-education students required additional resources, which were provided by the participating colleges and the university's Division of Sponsored Research. Funding from these sources allowed for the production of the GatorSHADE video, workbook, redesigned hats, and follow-up evaluation with the children and families.

The program and all facets of its development, expansion, and evaluation remain the responsibility of Drs. Ash and Varnes. Summary evaluation data are managed within the Colleges of Nursing and Health and Human Performance with the assistance of honors students and graduate research assistants. The program will continue to be offered and tested in a variety of settings and to various age groups as funding becomes available.

The GatorSHADE program has affected the lives of more than 100,000 people. Although long-term follow-up will not be feasible, continued attention to the importance of protecting the skin from overexposure to the sun is vital to decreasing the number of skin cancer cases in the United States.

The Breast and Cervical Cancer Early Detection Program

Sandy Balentine, RN, BBA, OCN®

The National Breast and Cervical Cancer Early Detection Program (NBCCEDP) is a federally funded program that is administered by the Centers for Disease Control and Prevention (CDC). It provides breast and cervical cancer screening and diagnostic services to medically underserved women. The program also provides routine clinical breast examinations, Pap smears, and mammograms. Other covered services include fine needle aspiration, breast ultrasound, and colposcopy, when appropriate. Programs are contracted with private providers, health departments, community health centers, radiology facilities, hospitals, and community groups to provide easy access for women. Arrangements are made with facilities so that women who are diagnosed with cancer can receive appropriate treatment. The CDC has developed standardized data items in collaboration with the states to monitor activities.

The health department in each state designs a program that will work in that state. In Ohio, 12 regions were formed based on the area Agency on Aging county divisions. By responding to a request for proposals, a facility in each region received funding from the Ohio Department of Health to develop, implement, and maintain a comprehensive breast and cervical cancer program in the region.

Beginning in 1994, Good Samaritan Hospital was awarded approximately $300,000 per year to fund the screening and diagnostic services for the priority women (identified in the grant as medically underserved) and provide education and promote outreach to potentially eligible women throughout a nine-county area in southwest Ohio. The continuation grant is applied for annually. Three staff members were hired. A grant/case manager, who is a nurse with oncology experience, manages the day-to-day operations of the grant, provides case management, and supervises staff. The health educator/outreach worker is a social worker with previous experience in social service agencies in the nine counties and provides some case management and health education. The data specialist has experience in collecting, entering, and receiving data collected from the screenings.

Initially, staff members began the process of making the community aware that the funds were available. During this time, they also contracted with providers to perform the services. Start-up was slow. Developing relationships with the minority organizations and building trust took time. The first year showed only small numbers of women in the project, but with enthusiasm and perseverance, the numbers grew.

Eligibility parameters are set at the state level. These require compliance in three areas: women must be older than 40 years of age, be uninsured or underinsured, and meet income requirements of 200% of the federal poverty level or less. There is an emphasis on minority women, such as African Americans, Native Americans, and Hispanics. Women are screened over the phone if they appear to be eligible for grant coverage. Additional information then is collected on their medical and family history.

Reimbursement for services is based on the Medicare part B reimbursement schedule. A specific list of CPT (Current Procedure Terminology) codes for covered services is available to potential providers for their consideration. Contracts must be signed with the funded agency to allow reimbursement. Healthcare workers at the hospital approached numerous levels of providers to meet the facility's care needs and to ensure adequate and accessible services in all nine counties. Private providers and local health departments were contacted; however, most did not or were not willing to provide these services in the facility's areas. The hospital was able to contract with two neighborhood health centers in parts of the urban area in the state's largest county. These health centers provide clinics that are close to areas where much of the target population resides. Physicians who serve a large number of minorities and lower income women also were approached. This was necessary to ensure coverage by gynecologic providers to enable women needing colposcopy and treatment services to have access. Good Samaritan Hospital contracted with at least one mammography provider in each county. Additionally, contracts were established with mobile mammography vans to provide screening services in areas where mammography screening is not easily accessible or available. Mobile mammography services also are used in areas to attract women who will not come in to other facilities. The goal was to ensure that at least one provider was available in each county.

Information was sent to every media source (e.g., television stations, local newspapers, neighborhood newspapers, radio stations). Representatives from the program always were available for interviews. Additional opportunities to advertise the program existed in social service agencies and local coalitions with an interest in women's health. Any opportunity to discuss the program was taken. Each time a grant award was received, a media release was sent to all newspapers. Another effective strategy was to routinely send out media stories that were written in such a manner that the media could insert the article into the paper with little editing or rewriting. This generated a lot of coverage in the neighborhood newspapers. In particular, the project team sent out educational articles that included information about screening services during Breast Cancer Awareness Month, Women's Health Month, Minority Health Month, and any other event that presented itself. Services also were promoted during any educational or community event related to women's health. Flyers were developed to discuss the eligibility requirements for the coverage and what services could be covered. Flyers have been a big source of referrals. These are left in housing projects, beauty salons, laundromats, and department stores and on the sides of soda machines. Brochures also were developed for use in physician offices and clinics. A supply is sent twice a year to numerous social service agencies and facilities.

Eligible women are scheduled for services with a provider who is most convenient for them. Patients are sent reminders about services that are covered, consent forms, and educational materials about breast and cervical health. This is another opportunity to educate women about their health.

Results of screenings are returned to the local project staff. The CDC designed a data system called CAST for this program. Initially, local data were entered in the region and downloaded for state collation. During recent years, it became more appropriate to have all data for the state collected and entered at one location. Data continue to be managed in this way. Data are collected on the demographics for clients and include zip code, age, race, and ethnicity. Results of clinical examinations, radiology studies, and cervical studies are entered onto a data collection form that is printed in duplicate. The local provider maintains one copy, and one copy goes to the local data person, with the original being sent to the state office for data entry. Follow-up time frames also are entered to allow patients to be notified for further studies.

Patients returning for an annual screening are reminded approximately one month prior to their due date with a mailed postcard. They are instructed to call in to verify eligibility and to schedule their appointment. Patients requiring more frequent follow-up are scheduled for services when needs are identified.

The biggest challenge facing the program is in finding ways to make eligible women aware of the grant. At present, a means to enroll large numbers of women in one way or at one location has not been discovered. Women are found one at a time through a flyer, a referral from a physician or friend, or a notice about a mobile health fair.

In the first five years of the program's existence, more than 40 women were diagnosed with breast cancer, and two women were diagnosed with cervical cancer. More than 2,500 women have received services through the project in the nine-county area. All asymptomatic women are reconfirmed for eligibility and reminded to come back for annual examinations. The state provides annual reports to reflect data based on state figures and by the individual regions.

Parameters have been set that include a focus on minority women. All data that are collected are reviewed and considered with the knowledge of the area's population base. These are higher-risk women, with some having a history of poor compliance with follow-up. Although the hospital seeks asymptomatic women, the facility also finds that many women attracted to the program have discovered lumps or other problems. Case management ensures that women who are not completing follow-up or need assistance with follow-up get the needed services. If a woman needs special attention to encourage her to receive follow-up or in finding financial resources, the case manager will provide as much assistance and as many resources as possible.

Data reviewed include

- Demographics—by county, age, and race
- Percent of abnormal clinical breast examinations, pelvic/Pap examinations and mammograms
- Length of time from screening to diagnosis
- Percent of patients diagnosed with cancer who receive treatment
- Percent of patients who return for their annual examination

Education is a key component of the project as well. Screening and education work hand in hand. Education begins with the individual through written materials sent to each eligible patient. Education is provided to groups through presentations and talks. Education also is provided to individuals one on one at health fairs and in medical offices. Women receive information on appropriate techniques for breast self-examination and the importance of clinical breast examinations and mammography. Education also includes a discussion of risk factors for breast and cervical cancer and early detection methods. Physician educational materials have been developed. During the course of this project, an educational program has been developed and taken to locations in eight counties to be presented to healthcare professionals. In 2000, a video/manual continuing-education activity was distributed to all clinical providers in the NBCCEDP.

Another important aspect of this project is maintaining a connection with community agencies and groups. This helps to keep them aware of the project as a resource for women they encounter through their agencies. Types of organizations include the American Cancer Society, task forces, health departments, social service agencies, hospitals, and the Area Agency on Aging. A local coalition helps to provide oversight for the project. This coalition consists of professionals and volunteers who are interested in women's health issues. Information on program progress goes back to the coalition as well as questions and concerns about things that are encountered. The coalition provides resources, ideas for ways to promote the program, and connections with other people/organizations to help to further the program.

Results from this project are numerous. Through the program, healthcare professionals have been able to diagnose women with breast and cervical cancer at an earlier stage because they present for services that they might not otherwise have been able to afford. The program has provided education about good breast and cervical health. The program also strives to develop patterns of behavior in women to encourage them to continue screenings even after they are no longer involved in the grant. Providers are encouraged to monitor their patients for screening time frames and provide them with information about follow-up. The Breast and Cervical Cancer Project is viewed in the community as a resource for information and funding sources related to breast and cervical health.

This program requires a lot of work and energy to make it successful, but the rewards are tremendous. The program touches the lives of a large number of women who become exposed to health information as well as services as a result of the program. The program has resulted in early detection of disease in asymptomatic women, which ultimately improves prognosis and long-term quality of life.

The Regional Hereditary Cancer Evaluation Program

Sandy Balentine, RN, BBA, OCN®, and Faith Callif-Daley, MS

Increased understanding of cancer as a genetic disease has resulted in the need for genetic counseling for families who are concerned about cancer. All cancer is genetic because all cancer cells have genetic alterations that guide their aberrant behavior. This understanding is fueling the development of gene-based cancer treatments. At the same time, some families have a hereditary predisposition to developing cancer. These families are distinguished by unusually early onset of disease, multiple affected family members, bilateral disease in paired organs, and multiple primary cancers. Several genes have been discovered that, when inherited, lead to increased susceptibility to cancer. Families with hereditary cancer are important to recognize because they have much higher chances for cancer than the population at large and, consequently, should be followed more closely for development of malignancies.

The Regional Hereditary Cancer Evaluation Program was a collaborative effort between Samaritan North Cancer Care Center and the Department of Medical Genetics and Birth Defects at Children's Medical Center in Dayton, OH. Services provided include the evaluation of family history, evaluation of cancer risk based on family history, genetic counseling for hereditary cancers, coordination of genetic testing for appropriate families, and education of the medical and lay community about genetic issues in malignancy. Approximately 500 families have been seen through the program. Eighty percent of the cases involved a pediatric cancer and were seen at Children's Medical Center, and the other 20% concerned a cancer in adulthood and were seen at the Samaritan North Cancer Care Center. Personnel involved in the program include a medical geneticist, genetic counselors, an oncology nurse coordinator for the adult program, medical oncologists, pastoral counselor, social worker, psychologist, and nutritionist.

Several methods are used to identify patients for cancer genetics services. In the pediatric setting, the genetic counselor generates a pedigree on all newly diagnosed pediatric patients with cancer at the Children's Medical Center. This takes place in the inpatient or outpatient setting, depending on the child's treatment plan. The genetic counselor also participates in the Long-Term Follow-Up Clinic at the Children's Medical Center, a clinic for childhood cancer survivors, by evaluating the family history and genetic impact of prior cancer treatment. In the majority of families who have a case of pediatric cancer, there is little hereditary cancer risk, but evaluating the family history helps to identify families where there is an increased susceptibility to cancer based on an associated genetic disease, birth defect, or chromosomal or hereditary syndrome.

For adults, referrals to the program come mainly from local physicians or the patients themselves. Most patients have been concerned about hereditary breast/ovarian cancer, but some families have been evaluated for hereditary predisposition to colorectal, thyroid, or other cancers. Recently, the program has begun to evaluate the family histories of the patients in a large gynecology group. Each patient fills out a brief family history questionnaire that is reviewed by the genetic counselor. Someone then will contact those patients with any history of cancer by letter. If, based on their family history, a hereditary cancer syndrome is unlikely, they are informed that genetic counseling is not indicated but are given an option for the service if they are concerned. Patients with a family history associated with a higher personal risk of cancer or probable hereditary cancer syndrome are given a brochure for the program and are informed that genetic counseling could be a helpful service for them.

Regardless of type of cancer or source of referral, the cornerstone of genetic counseling is the pedigree. Families are encouraged to obtain as much information as possible about their family histories and to verify the diagnoses with medical documentation if possible. Because family histories can change with additional information or the new diagnosis of cancer in family members, families are encouraged to contact the genetic counselor with additional changes.

Based on the family history, a risk assessment for the patient and close family members is provided. Using available risk assessment tools and current knowledge of hereditary cancers, the genetic counselor indicates the likelihood that the cancers in the family are hereditary and the related risks for malignancy in at-risk relatives.

All families are given guidelines for cancer surveillance based on their ages and hereditary factors. When appropriate, families are given preliminary information about surgical interventions and chemoprevention opportunities and are referred back to their physician or to appropriate specialists for further discussion.

DNA testing, when available on a research or clinical basis, is offered to families with suspected hereditary cancer syndromes. Informed consent for DNA testing is obtained after a discussion of the advantages, disadvantages, and limitations of testing, turnaround time for results, and the cost of testing. Families are prepared that results of DNA testing could be positive (mutation found), negative (no mutation present), or of uncertain clinical significance (a difference is present but its cancer-causing potential is unknown) and are asked to consider the potential impact of each of these results. Results are disclosed in person, and the family receives a written copy of the results for their records.

Families are asked to consider the financial, psychological, and ethical impact of genetic testing. Specialists are available, as needed, at both hospitals for psychological support, nutritional and social work services, and pastoral care.

Challenges to the program include the financial burden of testing, insurance concerns, the uncertain clinical utility of predictive DNA testing, and the need for continuing education regarding the ever-changing field of cancer genetics. Genetic testing for cancer predisposition costs between $300 and $3,000, depending on the gene or genetic test in question. Tests are less expensive if they involve smaller genes or if mutations are clustered in only certain areas of the gene. For remaining tests, the first person tested, an individual with cancer, pays a more expensive fee to scan the entire gene for the gene mutation lurking in the family. After the familial mutation is established, testing of additional family members is less expensive because it only involves evaluating one genetic change. Research-related testing is available in some cases for no fee; however, in most cases, the turnaround time for research testing is prolonged.

More and more insurers are covering genetic testing for cancer predisposition; however, insurance coverage usually is evaluated on a case-by-case basis, in many cases requiring letters of medical necessity. Many families express concern about insurance reprisals (including increased fees or loss of coverage) related to genetic testing and, on this basis, decide to forgo testing or to pay for the testing themselves. Some statewide and national legal protections are available against insurance discrimination for members of group health plans, but those with other insurance plans remain concerned.

A person who learns that he or she has a gene mutation associated with increased cancer vulnerability can screen for cancer more often, opt for prophylactic surgery, or take chemopreventive medication to help to prevent cancer or find it at its earliest stage. For some types of hereditary cancer, such as multiple endocrine neoplasia and familial adenomatous polyposis, the clinical management guidelines, which include prophylactic surgery, are well established. For other hereditary cancers, including hereditary breast and ovarian cancers, the optimal management strategies currently are unknown and are based on expert opinion.

There is a continuing need for the staff and referring healthcare providers to learn about the latest developments in cancer genetics. Staff members attend conferences, review the medical literature, and participate in cancer genetic programs to develop and maintain skills in the cancer genetics area. Members of the staff have been trained using the American Society of Clinical Oncology's cancer genetics curriculum, and a cancer genetics conference has been arranged for area medical professionals based on that training.

The adult cancer genetics program is promoted through oncology seminars, tumor boards, cancer support groups, and conferences. Initially, direct mailings, including program brochures and guidelines for referral, were sent to physicians in the region. Local TV talk shows, advertisements, and a feature article in local newspapers also have served as promotional tools.

Colon Cancer Screening Program

Deb Bisel, RN, MSN, OCN®

Overview of Program

A free colon cancer screening program is offered through the Spectrum Health Cancer Program in Grand Rapids, MI. The colon cancer screening program offers free fecal occult blood test (FOBT) kits and laboratory interpretation to the community. Spectrum Health is a community hospital on two campuses with approximately 1,000 beds and a 13-county service area. The funding for the colon cancer screening program comes from the Butterworth/Blodgett Foundation. This foundation is sponsored by Spectrum Health and is named for the two hospitals that merged to create Spectrum Health. A generous benefactor donated monies for cancer-related programs that target the local community. The program uses a portion of these funds to purchase hemoccult kits, mailing lists, and the postcards that are sent to the target audience.

The colon cancer screening program was developed when the cancer program was looking for something that would provide early detection of cancer yet not duplicate what already was available in the community. An advisory committee was formed in 1996 to discuss the logistics of providing colon cancer screening to an underserved population in the community. The committee members included three physicians, four RNs, and a representative each from the laboratory and communications department. The medical director of the cancer program, a colorectal cancer surgeon, and a gastroenterologist comprise the physician members. The nurses include the cancer program director, enterostomal therapist, coordinator of the hereditary colorectal cancer clinic, and the coordinator for the cancer program.

The committee decided that offering FOBTs would reach the widest audience, meet one of the American Cancer Society's recommendations for colon cancer screening in a healthy population, be cost effective, and heighten the awareness of the community to colon cancer prevention and early-detection activities. The success of the first event prompted the committee to continue the program yearly and offer it to the entire community rather than only the underserved populations.

The specifics of the program are detailed below and include how healthcare professionals reach the target audience, coordinate the call-in process, set up the lab process, communicate results, and conduct follow-up. Challenges facing the program and data reports also are presented.

Reaching the Target Audience

When the program started in 1996, its goal was to reach the underserved population to encourage them to participate in colon cancer screening. The committee generated several ideas to accomplish this goal. One idea was placing an ad in the local paper inviting the readership to call and receive a FOBT. But members wondered if this would reach the underserved population, many of whom may not subscribe to the local paper. Program members wanted something that would put a piece of paper in each person's hand. They hoped that the majority of recipients would read the information and respond to the invitation to receive a free colon cancer screening kit.

The communications department explained that mailing lists could be purchased based on zip code, age of the occupants living at a particular address, gender, or any other number of demographic characteristics. The committee reacted very favorably to this information and considered mailing a postcard to each household that had an occupant 40 years of age or older. The Grand Rapids area has a population of 200,000 residents, however, and mailing a postcard to this volume of people would be very expensive in terms of postage as well as manpower.

The outcome of this discussion led the committee to decide that it would target specific zip codes where the majority of underserved people reside. The first year, the group identified four zip codes they wished to reach. Criteria established for purchase of the mailing list included the four zip codes with occupants 40 years of age or older. This resulted in a list of approximately 25,000 residents.

The success of the first attempt at reaching the target audience prompted the committee to offer the program every year, targeting a different group of zip codes. A review of the statistics from the state of Michigan revealed that our county diagnosed colon cancers at a more advanced stage than almost every other county in the state. This led us to the conclusion that targeting underserved populations was great, but every resident in the greater Grand Rapids area should be reached. As a result, the colon cancer-screening program has evolved to include the entire community.

Each year, three to four zip codes are identified to participate in the screening. The goal is to reach 20,000 households each year. These households receive a postcard inviting them to call and receive the free kit. The kit we use is the Hemoccult Sensa three-day specimen test. The postcard describes the availability of the kit, its ease of use, and that early detection saves lives (see Table 20-1). It also discusses the number of people diagnosed with colon cancer and the number that die per year in the United States. The postcard identifies who should take the test based on age, personal and family history of cancer, and personal history of bowel-related disorders. Finally, three dates and time frames are listed to call and order the kit, which is mailed within two weeks.

Table 20-1. Results of Kit Mailings

Screening	Kits Mailed	Kits Returned	Negative Results	Positive Results	% Positive
Total for 1999	1,141	327 (29%)	320	7	2%
Total for 1998	685	382 (56%)	370	12	3%
Total for 1997	860	311 (36%)	305	6	2%

Call-In Process

During the call-in days, a phone tree is set up, and the two clerical staff or the nurse coordinator answer the calls. A database is designed and placed on a "shared" drive so that all of the members can enter information from the callers directly into the system, simultaneously. The different departments of the hospital are networked onto a single server within the computer system. For example, the nursing department is on a "nursing server," which provides one drive that can be shared by anyone in nursing. The cancer program has placed files in a database program on this shared drive, including a file for the colon screenings. The people answering phone calls have the file open at the same time and are able to enter information simultaneously.

After obtaining the basic demographic information, a risk assessment for colon cancer, including information about family history, is obtained. The kits are not limited to the person whose name is on the postcard. Any person in the household who meets the criteria can receive a kit. Therefore, callers ask if there is anyone else in the house that would also like a kit.

Laboratory Process

Each participant is assigned a number, which is written in red ink on the return envelope enclosed in the kit. When the laboratory receives the test from the participant, this red number alerts them that this test is part of the colon screening. Sheets are provided to the laboratory, which list the kit numbers in numerical order, the participant's name and address, blank columns for the date received, and three blank "result" columns. Laboratory personnel verify the kit number with the person's name and record the date and results in the columns provided.

Results

The nurse coordinator is responsible for picking up the result sheets from the laboratory weekly. Results of the test are sent to the participant. Results also are sent to the physician identified by the participant. The physician receives a letter that includes the patient's name, date of birth, an explanation that his or her patient chose to participate in the colon screening, and the test results. The physician also is invited to call the nurse coordinator with any questions regarding the colon-screening program.

The participants receive the results in the form of a letter that directs them to either continue FOBTs yearly if there is a negative result or to contact their physician for further testing if positive. The letter also explains the limitations of FOBT, iterating that a negative result does not mean the absence of disease nor a positive result the presence of disease. All participants who return the kit also receive literature detailing the risks, signs and symptoms of colon cancer, and dietary modifications to reduce the risk. The American Cancer Society's guidelines for colon cancer screening are included in the brochure distributed to the participants.

Follow-Up

Those participants with a positive test result receive a phone call from the nurse coordinating the screening about two weeks after receiving the letter. This phone call is designed to encourage, the participant to contact or verify that he or she has contacted his or her physician. If the participant does not have a regular physician, a list of physicians is provided. Physicians are surveyed approximately six months after the screening to determine what follow-up was performed for those individuals who tested positive.

Challenges

The challenges of this program are in receiving the phone calls, sending the results to the physician, and receiving a response from the physician regarding follow-up tests and results for positive participants. During the three-day call-in period, three people answer the phone. Five people would be more efficient. If all three lines are busy, the participant is placed in the phone mail system. The message explains that because of the overwhelming response to the offer, the lines are busy. The message then directs the caller to please leave his or her name, address, phone number, birth date, history of risk factors or family history of cancer, and physician name. This system eliminates the need for making multiple return phone calls.

Another challenge is in sending the results to the physician. Currently, the physician addresses need to be entered manually because not all people know that address at the time they call.

The biggest challenge is finding a way to get the physician's office to complete the questionnaire regarding follow-up of the positive tests. By making the questionnaire a simple checklist, 75% of the physicians typically respond.

Program Data

The following tables outline the numbers of participants in the program over the last three years and the follow-up of the positive tests. The return rate is approximately 39%, with about 2% testing positive (see Table 20-1). Nationally, the average positive test rate is 10%. Workers with the program are unable to explain why their results are so much lower than the national rate. The other interesting note is that no colon cancers were found through this program. However, approximately 24% of the participants with positive results were diagnosed with polyps (see Table 20-2).

Table 20-2. Patient Participation in the Colon Cancer Screening Program

Follow-Up	# Positives	FOBT Repeated	Colonoscopy	Results
1999	7	2	4	2 – Polyps 2 – Hemorrhoids 3 – Unknown
1998	12	3	5	3 – Polyps 2 – Diverticulosis 2 – Hemorrhoids 1 – Crohn's 4 – Unknown
1997	6	2	5	1 – Polyps 2 – Diverticulosis 2 – Hemorrhoids 1 – Normal

Although most colon polyps are benign, adenomatous polyps (or adenomas) are considered to be a precursor to colon cancer. Generally speaking, the larger the adenomatous polyp, the more likely it will be cancerous.

Outreach Versus Income Generator

The free FOBT program also is offered at health fairs and other community events, such as the community-wide prostate screening. Other healthcare professionals also have requested the kits for special projects they are doing. For example, the health department conducts a senior health program, and the hospital provides the kits as a service to this population.

There is no monetary gain to the cancer program for offering this service; however, the project probably is effective as a marketing tool. This aspect never has been measured.

Conclusion

The mission of the cancer program is to encourage prevention and early detection activities among our residents. The purpose of this program is to increase colon cancer awareness in the community. The colon cancer screening project has provided a heightened awareness in the community to pursue cancer-prevention and early-detection activities.

Professional Education for Prevention and Early Detection

Catherine C. Burke, MS, RN, CS, ANP, Jane Williams, MSN, RN, CS, FNP, and Marcia L. Patterson, MSN, RN, CS, ANP, GNP

Professional Education for Prevention and Early Detection (PEPED) at the University of Texas M.D. Anderson Cancer Center was developed in 1975 as a training program for RNs in cancer prevention and screening. It was the first cancer-prevention program in the United States to offer classroom instruction in combination with a clinical rotation. The program is based upon the philosophy that mastery of clinical skills requires a structured curriculum and an opportunity to practice the skills in a supervised environment. PEPED remains one of the few programs that offer participants a clinical experience.

PEPED's primary goals are to promote the practice of cancer prevention and detection among nurses and other healthcare providers and to encourage these providers to become involved in community cancer prevention and detection activities. All faculty members are master's prepared nurse practitioners who are experienced in oncology and nursing education. Additional healthcare professionals, including physicians, complement the PEPED faculty by providing lectures or clinical supervision in their areas of expertise.

PEPED attracts a diverse group of primary healthcare providers. Most participants work in a community public health setting or in an outpatient clinic. The majority (approximately 55%) are RNs prepared at the baccalaureate, diploma, or associate-degree level. Additional participants include nurse practitioners (25%), physicians (20%), and physician assistants (< 1%). PEPED is an approved provider of continuing education in nursing by the Texas Nurses Association and may offer continuing medical education through the institution's office, when appropriate.

The program is divided into modules of site-specific or related cancers. The most popular modules are described in Table 20-3. The aim of each module is to offer participants the basic knowledge and skills needed to provide effective can-

Table 20-3. Professional Education for Prevention and Early Detection Modules

Module/Schedule	Course Content
Breast module • Basic course targeting RNs. May be appropriate for advanced practice nurses who are new to the specialty. • Four days • Combines classroom education with supervised "hands-on" clinical practice	Classroom • Participants learn how to assess breast cancer risk, perform a thorough breast examination, and provide patient education. • Additional lectures—recognizing signs and symptoms of benign and malignant disease, breast cancer genetics, pros and cons of hormone replacement therapy, chemoprevention, nutrition, cancer prevention, cultural issues in cancer screening, and the evaluation of undiagnosed breast problems. Clinical • All participants perform physical examinations, risk assessments, and patient education in a screening clinic. • Additional observational opportunities include high-risk counseling, breast surgery, inpatient/outpatient management of individuals with a breast cancer diagnosis, workup of undiagnosed breast problems, and diagnostic procedures.
Female screening module • Basic course targeting RNs. May be appropriate for advanced practice nurses who are new to the specialty. • Four days • Combines classroom education with supervised "hands-on" clinical practice	Classroom • Participants learn how to assess risk and identify signs and symptoms of gynecologic and colorectal cancers, perform a pelvic examination, obtain a Pap smear, and provide patient education. • Additional lectures—human papillomavirus and cultural issues in cancer screening Clinical • All participants perform physical examinations, risk assessments, and patient education in a screening clinic. • Additional observational opportunities include high-risk counseling, gynecologic surgery, and inpatient/outpatient management of individuals with a gynecologic cancer diagnosis.

(Continued on next page)

Table 20-3. Professional Education for Prevention and Early Detection Modules (Continued)

Module/Schedule	Course Content
Breast and female screening module • Four days • Combination of the two most popular PEPED programs	Classroom • Participants learn how to assess risk and identify signs and symptoms of breast, colorectal, and gynecologic cancers, perform a breast and pelvic examination, obtain a Pap smear, and provide patient education. Clinical • All participants perform physical examinations, risk assessments, and patient education in a screening clinic. • Additional observational opportunities (as listed above)
Colposcopy module • Advanced course, targeting experienced advanced practice nurses and primary-care providers • Three days • Combines classroom education with supervised "hands-on" clinical practice	Classroom • Participants learn how to evaluate and manage the patient with an abnormal Pap smear. • Lectures include colposcopy technique, recognition of normal and abnormal colposcopic findings, managing the pregnant and DES-exposed patient, HPV, vulvar/vaginal dysplasia, and treatment of preinvasive disease Clinical • Participants spend one day in a dysplasia clinic performing colposcopy, cervical biopsies, and endocervical curettage.
Skin module • Basic course targeting registered nurses and primary-care providers • One day, classroom only	Classroom • Participants learn in classrooms how to assess skin cancer risk, perform a total skin examination, recognize melanoma and nonmelanoma skin cancers, and educate the public about skin cancer prevention.

cer prevention and detection services. Core concepts throughout the modules include risk assessment, risk reduction counseling, high-risk counseling, cancer screening examinations, signs and symptoms of cancer, diagnostic tools, follow-up and referral, treatment options, and teaching self-examination methods.

Two modules combine classroom instruction with clinical experiences. The didactic portion of each module is taught in PEPED's classroom. In addition to the lectures, participants receive a complete course syllabus and reference list. The clinical portions of each module primarily are taught in M.D. Anderson's outpatient clinics. Other clinics in the city and surrounding counties are used as appropriate. The clinical faculty to participant ratio is maintained at 1:2, which allows each participant ample opportunity to perform physical examinations, risk assessments, and patient education. Inexperienced participants may require additional practice with a preceptor in his or her facility to gain expertise. Clinical observational opportunities are also available, and these experiences are tailored to each participant's interests and needs.

The colposcopy module is the only program that specifically targets advanced practice nurses, physician assistants, and physicians. It is also the only program that requires nonphysicians to have a designated preceptor as a condition of acceptance. Following the classroom component, participants spend one day performing colposcopic examinations under supervision. However, because both physician and nurse practitioner organizations recommend that novice colposcopists perform approximately 100 examinations under supervision to document proficiency, participants must arrange the majority of the clinical experience for themselves.

The skin workshop does not routinely offer a clinical component. By eliminating the clinical and reducing the workshop cost, PEPED has been able to educate more nurses and primary-care providers about skin cancer prevention and early detection. A clinical experience still is available to those who are interested.

In addition to the on-site programs, PEPED conducts site-specific or generalized cancer prevention and early detection workshops in locations throughout the United States. Each program is customized to meet the needs of the individual site. Programs have included courses in cancer: breast, breast and cervical, male genitourinary, colorectal, and skin. The breast and cervical workshop is PEPED's most frequently requested program, and it usually is offered to primary-care nurses working in rural or underserved communities.

The workshops are typically two days, with participants receiving one day of classroom instruction and one day of supervised clinical practice. PEPED provides all of the learning materials and audiovisual support, and the hosting agency arranges the facilities for both classroom education and clinical experience. The hosting agency also is encouraged to provide the newly trained participants with preceptors and clinical opportunities to develop clinical competency after completion of the workshop.

Two outcomes studies of onsite modules support the effectiveness of PEPED modules on the screening practices of participants. Ford et al. (1997) found that one year after taking the breast module, 41 nurses showed statistically significant increases in general and clinical knowledge, screening skills, incorporation of screening and risk counseling into practice, and involvement in community outreach activities. The total number of people screened, referred, and ultimately diagnosed with breast cancer also was increased; however, this finding was not statistically significant and was attributed to poor compliance with patient log keeping. McCormick, Masse, Cummings, and Burke (1999) evaluated the effectiveness of the original skin cancer module, a five-day program of classroom and clinical education. Thirty-seven nurses who participated in the module were assessed immediately after the program and at three months post-participation. Participant scores were compared to a comparison group of 87 nurses who did not take the module. The findings indicated that nurses who participated in the module gained significant knowledge in general skin cancer and prevention, were better able to perform skin screening, and were more confident in their ability to screen and educate their patients.

Currently, PEPED is evaluating the effectiveness of the off-site breast and cervical workshop. The program includes a basic course evaluation, pre- and post-testing of clinical knowledge and skills, clinical logs that reflect practice patterns before and after training, and an assessment of knowledge and skills following one year of training. The ultimate goal of professional education is to improve the availability of screening and prevention resources for all individuals. The outcome evaluation of this workshop may demonstrate that an abbreviated program also is effective in improving cancer prevention knowledge and clinical skills among participants.

References

Ford, M., Martin, R.D., White-Hilton, L., Ewert-Flannagan, T., Corrigan, G.K., Johnson, G., Hernandez, M.A., Sbach, A., & Lippman, S.M. (1997). Outcomes study of a course in breast cancer screening. *Journal of Cancer Education, 12,* 179–185.

McCormick, L.K., Masse, L.C., Cummings, S.C., & Burke, C. (1999). Evaluation of a skin cancer prevention module for nurses: Change in knowledge, self-efficacy, and attitudes. *American Journal of Health Promotion, 13,* 282–289.

Skin Cancer Awareness at the Races

Marianne E. Casale, MSN, RN, AOCN®, CS

The Philadelphia Area Chapter of the Oncology Nursing Society (PACONS) has sponsored a community-based skin cancer awareness program at the First Union U.S. Pro Championship Bicycle Race the past two years. Children and adolescents were the target populations because they have the potential for high lifetime exposure to the sun. Each year, more than 1,000 spectators stopped to obtain information on being sun smart. The planning team consisted of five oncology nurses, a public health clinical nurse specialist, a medical oncologist, a pharmaceutical representative, and an operational specialist from Threshold Sports. Schering Corporation provided sunscreen samples, and community corporations and pharmaceutical companies provided funding for other resources.

The PACONS educational exhibit at the bicycle race allows the group to inform spectators about sun-sensible behavior. The event is held every June in Philadelphia, PA, with more than 500,000 people attending to watch world-renowned cyclists compete. The increasing popularity of outdoor activities and cycling provide a creative way to introduce PACONS to the community. The recent success of riders like Tour de France Champions Greg LeMond and Lance Armstrong has rekindled a national interest in cycling, resulting in more people spending longer periods of time in the sun.

Planning this event involves several activities: selecting the planning group, establishing goals, developing program objectives, identifying resources, and planning for evaluation. The goal of this program was to make people aware that skin health depends on the habits they develop at a young age. PACONS wanted to educate participants that using prevention strategies would not interfere with outdoor sporting activities, such as cycling.

This primary prevention program was designed to focus on the health of the population and prevent illness. Primary prevention plays a pivotal role in skin cancer. An outdoor lifestyle is associated with an increased risk for skin cancer. Prevention of skin cancer relies on the assumption that reducing sun exposure will decrease the risk of getting the disease. Individuals should stay out of the sun, wear protective clothing, and use sunscreen. Sunscreens should be used to protect against sun exposure, not prolong the amount of time spent in the sun.

Once the objectives have been established, the planning group identifies resources (e.g., personnel, money, educational materials) needed to implement the program. Material resources to give away included T-shirts, sunglasses, cycling water bottles, and a bicycle. Letters requesting support were mailed six months prior to the educational program. PACONS had a 40% response to the request for funding during the first year, but this dropped to 26% the second year.

Implementing this program involved acceptance of the plan, which occurred at several levels. The first level was receiving acceptance from PACONS, First Union Bank, and U.S. Pro Championship promoters. The president-elect of PACONS coordinated the entire effort. Periodic consultation was held every month with members of the planning committee. Other implementation activities included purchasing sunglasses, T-shirts, and bicycles and ordering educational materials from the National Cancer Institute and the American Academy of Dermatology.

The PACONS exhibit was located near the start/finish line, which allowed several spectators to stop and obtain information. They were educated about the ways in which they could reduce the possibility of sun damage. At the end of the mini session, participants who could describe three ways to be sun smart were eligible to win a bicycle. All participants received sunscreen samples, flower seed packets, and educational materials; children also received sunglasses.

The program was evaluated for a couple of reasons: justifying program continuation or expansion and determining the impact of the program. The number of people who stopped to obtain educational information about skin cancer and ask questions related to detection and treatment of other cancers demonstrated that sporting events provide an excellent opportunity to help communities learn about cancer prevention activities. Eighty percent of participants were able to identify three ways to be sun smart. PACONS plays an important role in raising public awareness about the risks of unprotected sun exposure. This educational program will continue at the next year's U.S. Pro Championship Bike Race and hopefully will expand to other outdoor sporting events in Philadelphia.

Comprehensive Breast Center

Dianne D. Chapman, RN, MS

The Comprehensive Breast Center (CBC) operates within the Rush Cancer Institute of Rush-Presbyterian-St. Luke's Medical Center. The Medical Center is a university-based institution located west of the Chicago downtown area. CBC is a specialized center for women at high risk for developing breast cancer and for those requiring consultation for benign and malignant breast disorders. Although the great majority of patients are women, men also are seen. Services include consultation, review of mammograms, cytology/pathology review, diagnostic surgical intervention (fine needle aspiration, core biopsy, ultrasound-guided biopsy, stereotactic biopsy, excisional biopsy, mastectomy, standard axillary dissection, and sentinel node biopsy), screening/diagnostic mammography, ultrasound, and magnetic resounace imaging of the breast.

CBC was conceived and designed by a group of physicians, specializing in the treatment of breast cancer, who believed that women should be presented with options that reflect the most current treatment information available. In the 1980s, as research protocols began indicating that lumpectomy-axillary dissection-radiation therapy was a viable option for many women instead of mastectomy, many patients and families were confused and unsure about which was the best choice. Patients scheduling multiple appointments with different disciplines were having difficulty sorting the information, especially if the opinions conflicted. Additionally, the time lag involved in scheduling these appointments often heightened patient anxiety and possibly resulted in treatment delay. A multidisciplinary clinic was chosen as the best way to convey the information in an understandable manner while fostering a "patient-friendly" atmosphere.

Because breast specialists provide the type of care to properly assess and manage people with complex breast disorders, the founding physicians decided to model CBC into a diagnostic center, opening March 1985. The primary mission was to offer specialized care to women with perceived breast disorders: a lump, mass, or thickening; nipple discharge; an abnormal mammogram; or breast cancer. The management of patients at high risk because of prior breast biopsies or family history also was designated a priority.

Marketing a new program has been carried out in many ways: mass mailings, newspaper ads, radio and television ads, and, more recently, the Internet. Initially, information about CBC was circulated within the institution. Members of the group were guests on radio talk shows, answering questions about breast cancer and discussing lumpectomy versus mastectomy. Other members provided educational presentations to local support groups and cancer societies. Surgical and medical residents also rotated, through CBC and began to refer patients after becoming attending physicians. Some members have appeared on television responding to news items about the treatment of breast cancer. In recent years, the medical center has established a hot line to direct patients to an appropriate physician/clinic. The most successful method of referral for CBC has been word of mouth. Approximately 40% of new patients are self-referred.

CBC enjoyed a steady rise in patient volume from 1985–1992, followed by a decline. The total patient census (new and follow-up patients) has decreased from a high of approximately 1,700 patients in 1992 to 1,100 from 1995–1999. These figures reflect the increase in managed care and preferred provider insurers that limit access to health care. Some patients seeking a second opinion will elect to pay out of pocket for the consultation, despite the fact that they cannot be treated at Rush Cancer Institute.

CBC became part of the Rush Cancer Institute in January 2000. Prior to that date, CBC was an independent corporation that functioned as an affiliate of the Rush Cancer Institute. The medical center provided a clinic facility and workspace for the two full-time employees. The remainder of the expenses (e.g., salaries, computers, office supplies) was the responsibility of CBC. Maintaining an adequate cash flow began to be a problem in the 1990s largely because of insurance restrictions, which affected patient accessibility and reimbursement. The primary restriction CBC experienced resulted from not being included in the institution-negotiated insurance contracts. Consequently, some patients could not come to CBC to see a participating physician, but insurance would reimburse for a visit to see the same doctor in his or her private office, further decreasing CBC patient visits. The business manager negotiated some of CBC's insurance contracts, which lowered current consultation fees because the insurance companies do not recognize the cost effectiveness of a comprehensive consultation. Insurance companies will allow three separate visits to specialists but will not allow the same three physicians to see a patient in concert within CBC. All of these events made it increasingly difficult to maintain independence and continue to meet the operational expenses (salaries for employees and office expenses).

Breast centers are not inherently profitable and often need support from the medical institution. Funding administrators must recognize the additional services generated outside of the breast center, including surgery, diagnostic testing, medical oncology, and radiation oncology. Patients who have had a positive experience at an institution often will request referrals for themselves or family members for other problems. Additionally, an institution that supports a breast cancer center sends a message to the community that women's health is an important issue best served in a comprehensive setting. Unfortunately, that information is difficult to track and document.

CBC is staffed by two full-time employees, a business manager and an advanced practice nurse. The business manager helps with triaging and scheduling patients, coordinates any further diagnostic workup, and handles the billing and reception duties (two afternoons a week). The nurse coordinator triages patient calls, participates in patient/family education and psychosocial support, and handles administrative responsibilities (clinic management, research, community service, and liaison activities between the various services and departments). The nurse holds classes in breast self-examination for employees every three months. The nurse coordinator also participates in formal education programs within the university and for professional organizations that address benign breast disorders, early detection strategies, cancer risk assessment, and genetic testing. The nurse in the CBC also provides counseling and genetic testing for BRCA1 and BRCA2.

CBC also has three to four surgeons, two medical oncologists, and one to two radiation oncologists in the clinic each day. The physicians dedicate a specific afternoon to be present to enhance continuity of care for returning patients. The decision not to have reconstruction surgeons present at CBC was predicated by the number of early-stage breast cancers and the philosophy that breast preservation is offered whenever possible. However, the reconstructive surgeons will see the patients needing mastectomy as expeditiously as possible.

Newly diagnosed patients (post-biopsy, no axillary dissection) see a surgeon, a medical oncologist, and a radiation oncologist. Residents and clinical psychologists from the Department of Psychosocial Oncology are present during clinic hours to provide psychological support to patients with a new diagnosis. Patients are asked to bring all diagnostic information, which may include mammograms, scans, and pathology slides, for review. Each physician examines the patient after reviewing the information. The physicians then consult with one another and come to a consensus regarding the option(s) to be presented to the patient/family. One or more physicians then discuss the recommended option(s) with the patient/family and answer questions. Patients seeking care for a nonmalignant problem usually will see a surgeon, but some patients see both a medical oncologist and a surgeon.

The most frustrating challenge is one that affects all of the comprehensive centers—adequate reimbursement for multidisciplinary services. Insurance company codes do not recognize the advantage of a multidisciplinary consultation. Despite the fact that the fee for a new diagnosis consultation at CBC is less than the fees for three separate appointments, insurance companies will not reimburse accordingly. The situation probably will not change because the tendency with coverage is to restrict rather than expand care options.

The evaluation and treatment of benign and malignant breast disorders is a complex issue, often requiring the expertise of one or more specialists. Women are educated consumers who seek programs that offer specialized care in a "patient-friendly" setting. A dedicated center offering expert opinion regarding surgery, medical oncology, and radiation oncology is best designed to meet these needs.

Establishment of a Breast Cancer High-Risk Registry at Community-Based Institutions

Agnes Masny, RN, MPH, MSN, CRNP

The Fox Chase Cancer Center (FCCC) in Philadelphia, PA, a National Cancer Institute-designated Comprehensive Cancer Center, has conducted cancer risk assessment and research since 1991 through a program called the Family Risk Assessment Program (FRAP), which provides education and counseling to women at risk for breast and ovarian cancer based on their family history. In 1994, the Department of Defense funded a project to establish a Breast Cancer High-Risk Registry (BCHRR) program among the FCCC network hospitals. The Fox Chase Network, a subsidiary corporation of FCCC, is an affiliation of 16 community-based hospital systems, with a total of 19 hospitals established to expand the quality of cancer care at community-based hospitals (see Table 20-4). The purpose of BCHRR was to establish a breast cancer high-risk registry that included both genetic and environmental risk information from a racially and ethnically diverse set of patients with familial breast cancer and from women at

Table 20-4. Network Participation in the Breast Cancer High-Risk Registry Program

	Contact Med. Director	Nurse Trained	Nurse Assigned	Education Resources	Education Initiated	Accrual Begun
New Jersey						
Community/Kimball	X	X	X	X	X	X
Hunterdon	X	X	X	X	X	X
Riverview	X	X	X	X	X	X
South Jersey	X	X	–	–	–	–
St. Francis	X	X	X	X	X	X
Virtua-Memorial	X	X	X	X	X	X
Pennsylvania						
Bon Secours	–	–	–	–	–	–
Conemaugh	–	–	–	–	–	–
Delaware County	X	X	X	X	X	X
Montgomery*	X	X	X	X	X	X
North Penn	–	-	-	–	–	–
Paoli	X	X	X	X	X	X
Pinnacle	X	X	X	X	X	X
Reading	X	X	X	X	–	–
St. Luke's*	X	X	X	X	X	X
St. Mary's	–	X	–	–	–	–

*Inactive

increased risk because of a positive family history. The project, modeled after FCCC's FRAP, was designed to evaluate the feasibility of creating an infrastructure within a network of community-based hospitals for breast cancer risk assessment and research. Moreover, preparing community providers to identify and counsel women at high risk for breast cancer was proposed to serve as a model for transferring genetic information into the public health realm. The services provided corresponded to specific aims of this project. These services included the following.

- Establish a protocol for identifying and recruiting women with one or more first-degree relatives with breast cancer into a regional FCCC network-wide registry of high-risk individuals.
- Establish a computerized database system of comprehensive risk factors, including family history, personal medical history, lifestyle and environmental factors, health practices and beliefs, and psychological variables that will serve as a resource for a spectrum of research activities.
- Develop protocols for the selection of individuals and families for closer genetic investigation and genetic counseling.
- Expand the FCCC/Network Breast Cancer Tissue Registry to include specimens of benign breast lesions as well as serum and DNA from women in the high-risk registry.
- Develop educational tools for primary-care physicians at the community level to prepare them to take a leading role in the identification of women with a family history of breast cancer, in the interpretation of genetic test data, and in its relevance and application to clinical medicine.

- Develop workshops for training nurses at the community level to provide breast cancer risk information, risk assessment, tailored preventive recommendations, and psychosocial support to high-risk women and their families.
- Develop and test behavioral interventions that are sensitive to cultural, ethnic, and racial differences, which will promote positive outcomes to breast cancer risk information, including the results of genetic testing.
- Form a Breast Cancer Risk Advisory Panel to provide guidance and counsel regarding the social, legal, and ethical aspects of genetic testing for breast cancer.

The Department of Defense (Grant DAMD17-94-J-4425) provided funding for four years (1994–1998). The Fox Chase Network Program has provided ongoing support for the project by contributing salary for FCCC "traveling" staff, a part-time genetic counselor, and nurse project manager.

Each hospital has involved the medical director of the respective cancer center for planning and administration, a physician to serve as part of the cancer genetic risk assessment team, and an oncology nurse to coordinate the risk education and counseling. At two hospitals, a social worker was part of the genetics team and one site assigned a part-time secretary to handle telephone intake and correspondence.

Implementation of the
Breast Cancer High-Risk Registry Program

Program implementation began with collaborative meetings with the medical director of each Network Oncology Program. This approach first assessed interest in participation in the program as well as training, education, and administrative needs. These initial meetings laid out the program requirements and time frame for implementation. Those institutions (N = 13) interested in participation were guided through a process that included the development of an administrative and implementation plan; training and preparation of nursing staff to coordinate and conduct the program; training in all protocols and procedures; and ongoing mentoring and monitoring in cancer risk assessment and counseling. Each hospital identified a nurse coordinator and physician team leader. Each nurse coordinator was trained in the cancer risk assessment and counseling process. Educational resources designed to provide genetic cancer risk information regarding breast cancer were supplied to each institution. Use of these resources was accompanied by a training, supervision, and feedback process. All institutions also were supplied with a procedures manual and training for data entry and collection of biologic specimens.

Protocols developed for recruitment included community outreach and education or physician referral. Community outreach included education programs regarding breast cancer risk offered to the community at large. Education regarding risk included personal, biologic, and genetic risk for developing breast cancer as well as information about participation in BCHRR. Physician referral was targeted to patients with breast cancer who were concerned with cancer risk for their family or with a known family history of cancer. These women were referred to the program coordinator for attendance in the education program. BCHRR was described during the education session. Women who were interested in participation in the BCHRR were required to complete a set of questionnaires prior to their individualized risk-assessment session. These questionnaires included the following categories of data.

Demographic data—Date of birth, race, ethnicity, religion, sex, marital status, education, and income.

Family history—Cancer diagnoses, age at onset, cancer deaths, age at death, and place of treatment or death was recorded for all first- and second-degree relatives of network participants. Using our current format, these data readily can be translated into a family pedigree for counseling and teaching purposes. Our success in confirming diagnoses with medical records or death certificates in FRAP supports the reliability of self-report of family history observed by other investigators.

Medical history—Relevant medical conditions (e.g., colonic polyps, benign breast disease), medication use, and weight history were recorded. For females, a thorough review of reproductive events, including menstrual history, pregnancy history, lactation experience, history of spontaneous and induced abortions, and exogenous hormone use, including fertility drugs, was collected.

Epidemiologic risk factors—Radiation and occupational exposures, smoking history, dietary history, alcohol use, and exercise history.

Clinical history (for affected individuals)—Tumor stage, grade, histologic type, prognostic factors (e.g., hormone receptor status for breast cancer), treatment (type of surgery, radiation, and systemic therapy), and disease outcome, as measured by disease-free and overall survival.

Health attitudes and behavior survey—A series of measures was used to assess self-perceived risk for cancer, previous screening behaviors, and attitudes toward genetic testing for individuals and their families.

Annual follow-up—A computer-generated annual follow-up questionnaire provides an update on new cancer diagnoses among participants and their relatives, interval surveillance results, changes in risk status, and disease course in affected individuals.

The program was implemented in 10 of the 13 Fox Chase network institutions that expressed interest. Administrative planning with FCCC medical directors and staff physicians was conducted in 13 network facilities. Nursing staff was trained in those facilities; of these, 11 had a nursing program coordinator assigned. Education and program resources were provided to those 11 hospitals with a nurse coordinator. Ten sites conducted the breast cancer risk education through community education and conducted cancer risk assessment and counseling. Two of the hospitals left the Fox Chase network during the course of the project. Eight network hospitals maintain the program and continue to recruit women for ongoing cancer genetic research studies.

Training Community Nurses

Essential to the success of the project was the development of programs to train nurses at each network hospital for their expanded role in cancer risk identification and counseling. Design of the education materials for nurses began with focus groups to assess training needs. Based on these interviews, a formal three-day training and one-day practicum were developed. The major components of the training included (a) background on breast cancer and cancer genetics, (b) obtaining a medical and family history of cancer, (c) assessment of cancer risk, (d) communication of cancer risk information, (e) tailoring recommendations and support to promote adherence to screening and cancer-control practices, (f) legal, social, and ethical implications of genetic information, and (g) referral for further medical and genetic investigation. Videotaped and case demonstrations of counseling sessions were developed to provide nurses with opportunities for observation and role modeling.

An ongoing mentoring process was developed to assist the network nurses in skill development. This process has included observation and supervision by FCCC staff of the breast cancer risk education session and the individual cancer risk counseling session. All network nurses had the opportunity to observe in FCCC's FRAP. This included an opportunity to attend FCCC's pedigree review committee, a multidisciplinary team review of pedigree and family history, and to observe individual pedigree evaluation sessions. For the initial individual counseling session at the network hospital, the nursing coordinator first observed FCCC staff conducting an individual risk-assessment session. Afterward, FCCC staff supervised the nurse coordinator while she conducted cancer risk counseling sessions. Monthly updates were sent to the nurses regarding advances in genetics and information related to the counseling and testing process. A quarterly in-service training also was conducted. These trainings consisted of updates regarding individual network hospital progress in their FRAPs, review of administrative concerns or issues, and an educational in-service. Additional monitoring of the program was provided by telephone conferencing or site visit.

Recruitment and accrual of women to the BCHRR program occurred in two ways: physician referral of patients with breast cancer and community-education programs on breast cancer risk. In the former, the medical oncologist alerted patients with breast cancer about the program. The patients, in turn, contacted their relatives. To date, a total of 82 education sessions have taken place with 602 women from 10 network hospitals. Sixty-two percent (n = 399) of those attending the education sessions expressed interest in the risk registry and took program questionnaires. Two hundred and forty-eight individuals from 196 families returned the questionnaires and participated in the BCHRR program. The Pedigree Review Committee at FCCC reviewed the family history of these women and gave them a diagnosis for both the maternal and paternal side of the family by cancer type and pattern. The patterns included sporadic or negative (36%), familial (33%), or putative hereditary (31%). Although 95% of maternal patterns included breast or ovarian cancer, only 19% (n = 49) of the paternal case patterns included breast or ovarian cancer. Other varieties of cancer types on the paternal side included prostate, colon, thyroid, kidney, esophageal, and hematopoietic, with the majority, 62%, having a sporadic or negative pattern. Of the families in the program, 54 of them have participated in genetic research studies.

Discussion

The work of FCCC's BCHRR demonstrated that it was feasible to establish cancer risk assessment at community-based hospitals. More than 70% of the institutions participating in the Fox Chase Cancer network implemented BCHRR. The program established a framework for ongoing recruitment whereby research in epidemiology, genetics, and educational and psychological intervention can continue.

Strong physician interest in cancer risk assessment was key to the program implementation. The physicians taking the lead at their respective institutions represented medical, surgical, and radiation oncology as well as family practice. Their active involvement facilitated administrative support for the project, assisted the nurse coordinators in shaping their role, identified marketing and referral strategies, and helped to create contacts with other community physicians.

This project demonstrated that with training and opportunities for practice, oncology nurses were essential to establishing and coordinating the cancer genetic risk assessment and counseling process. The oncology nurses who attended the training showed significant improvement in knowledge in the areas of cancer genetics, genetic testing, and risk models associated with the cancer risk assessment process. After the training course, the network nurses identified an ongoing need for continuing education and access to current genetic information. The nurses cited a lack of confidence in their skills because they often did not have other nurse mentors in their settings with experience in cancer genetics. In contrast, nurses at FCCC had greater access to members of the genetics team to assist in their professional development in cancer genetics through observation, supervision and feedback, case conferencing, and educational opportunities. This project tried to address these continuing-education needs via supervision, mentoring, and in-service training. Additionally, FCCC has developed "Advanced Skills Training for Nurses in Cancer Genetic Risk Counseling" (NCI-R25 CA66061). This training was developed to evaluate a replicable skills-based educational program for nurses who already have acquired a basic understanding of cancer genetics, enhance the practice of skills in identifying and counseling patients at increased risk for cancer, and strengthen their counseling skills in preparing patients for receipt of genetic test information.

The formation of a Breast Cancer Risk Advisory Panel was another facilitating factor for BCHRR. The panel brought together experts in the field of genetics, ethics, and health care and lay consumers. Working groups were established to address the development of counseling protocols, training strategies for healthcare professionals, and ethical issues. Consumers and community-based healthcare professionals broadened the understanding of managed care's influence on the current healthcare environment and the impact of genetic research.

The original program time line estimated that all interested network institutions would have implemented the program within the first two years of the project. On average, three hospitals per year operationalized the program with implementation of new sites that continued into the fourth year of the project. The operational plan required intensive support prior to implementation as well as having trained staff to conduct risk assessment and recruitment. In several settings, appointed and trained staff had job changes; this caused significant delays in program implementation and ongoing recruitment. Furthermore, programmatic materials such as brochures, letters, and informed consents had to be adapted to the specific hospital's conditions. Each hospital had to meet requirements of their respective institutional review boards (IRB), with some settings having a two to three month process before IRB approval. Some of the major IRB issues were confidentiality of genetic information and the concern that research results potentially would not benefit the patient.

Mergers and realignment of healthcare systems affected the implementation process. Two hospitals left the Fox Chase network to affiliate with other hospital or university-based systems. One hospital merged with two other institutions, and program accrual was delayed for more than a year. Economic concerns also were barriers for several network institutions. The current healthcare environment influenced several administrators to weigh the economic advantages and disadvantages of this research project. Unlike other research protocols, there was no financial incentive for accrual. Institutions that perceived a marketing advantage to the genetic research studies were more willing to participate, with the expectation that this project would prepare them to implement cancer genetic services when they become commercially available.

It has been established that 5%–10% of breast cancers are attributed to hereditary cancer syndromes, 70% are attributed as sporadic, and the remaining 20% fall into a familial category (Hoskins et al., 1995). Because hereditary cancer is expected to account for 5%–10% of breast cancers, the proportion of putative hereditary and familial patterns found in participants suggest that the BCHRR program appropriately recruited individuals who carry a higher degree of risk for breast cancer than the general population.

This project determined that the majority of participants had a breast cancer pattern in the maternal line. Ninety-five percent of maternal cases had a breast or breast/ovarian cancer pattern, compared to 19% of the paternal patterns. One explanation is that a misperception persists about the transmission of breast cancer solely through the maternal line. Another explanation is that risk perception of developing breast cancer may be lower when breast cancer occurs on the paternal side. More often these cancers involve second- and third-degree relatives (e.g., grandmother, aunts, cousins). Perceived susceptibility to breast cancer may be higher when a first-degree relative, especially a mother, has had cancer. This suggests that future work in community health education should continue to address modes of transmission for predisposition to breast cancer.

Although the framework of the BCHRR program remains in place to continue recruitment, the program did not achieve its projected accrual of 1,200 participants. However, the number of women receiving education about breast cancer risk was high (n = 602). Although no data were available from this registry study, there were anecdotal reports of women choosing to participate in the first Breast Cancer Prevention Trial after education about breast cancer risk. This suggests that a framework for education about cancer risk can serve as a link to other cancer prevention studies and programs.

Several factors that had an impact on program implementation and accrual to the BCHRR included administrative planning, staff training, and IRB approval. The length of time to train staff and to obtain IRB approval from the respective institutions often slowed the implementation process and, therefore, accrual. Public attitude toward genetic research also affected accrual. Potential participants reported that media attention to genetic issues raised their concerns. Issues related to participation in genetic research included stigmatization, employment and insurance discrimination, misinterpretation of test results, use of genetic information beyond the scope of the research, and lack of legislation to prevent genetic discrimination. Fear of medical insurance discrimination was cited as the major barrier to participation. Clinical trials research indicates that primary reasons for research participation are a perceived benefit to health outcomes, control over the medical course of the disease, and a desire to help future generations (Daugherty et al., 1998; Kennedy et al., 1998). A proportion of the women indicated concern that participation in genetic research would not benefit them. Even with assurances of the privacy measures employed in the study, a subset of women were concerned that genetic information would become known and potentially be harmful to them. Finally, lack of information about genetic research, the needed involvement of family members, and the impact of genetic information on the family have been noted to decrease interest in genetic testing (Holtzman, Bernhardt, Doksum, Helzlsouer, & Geller, 1996).

A subset of women who were interested in the program and who took the program questionnaires never returned them. A sample of these women reported barriers to program participation that included lack of time to complete the family history questionnaire and need to involve other family members. The education, counseling, and informed consent process for those women who consented to participate was lengthy. Under ideal circumstances, the recruitment phase entailed a minimum of three hours of the participant's time. This includes questionnaire completion, group education, and individual risk counseling, with each component taking at least one hour. Needs assessment strategies prior to recruitment and an informed consent process that thoughtfully and directly addresses the participant's perception of genetic research and the time involved in participation are essential to future programmatic design.

Conclusions

This project has demonstrated that it was feasible to create an infrastructure within the community setting to identify patients with breast cancer and women at risk in view of their family history of breast cancer. The program has established a framework for recruitment into this registry and ongoing genetic research whereby we will learn more about the carcinogenic process of breast cancer. Participation in genetic research or a registry has unique informed consent issues not present in prior research studies. Genetic research with both individual and family implications requires academic centers and government agencies to consider a programmatic design that has a broader accrual scope. The need for education and counseling prior to genetic research testing with individuals and extended family members, although labor intensive, is imperative to the informed consent process.

With appropriate training, educational resources, and supervisory support, the transfer of genetic knowledge into community-based practice can be accomplished. To ensure that healthcare professionals are prepared to meet future patient demands for genetic information, professional societies and health education researchers need to make continuing education in genetics a priority.

The FCCC network BCHRR program has provided the opportunity to further epidemiologic and molecular research related to breast cancer risk and to develop and evaluate educational and psychological strategies to optimize breast cancer risk counseling in the community setting. The registry program also has established collaborations with other prevention studies at community-based hospitals, including the first Breast Cancer Prevention Trial and the Study of Tamoxifen and Raloxifene (STAR). These efforts are contributing to further clinical research to help identify the most suitable medical management, surveillance, and chemopreventive therapies for high-risk populations.

References

Daugherty, C.K., Ratain, M.J., Minami, H., Banik, D.M., Vogelzang, N.J., Stadler, W.M., & Siegler, M. (1998). Study of cohort-specific consent and patient control in phase I cancer trials. *Journal of Clinical Oncology, 16,* 2305–2312.

Holtzman, N.A., Bernhardt, B.A., Doksum, T., Helzlsouer, K.A., & Geller, G. (1996). Education about BRCA1 testing decreases women's interest in being tested. *American Journal of Human Genetics, 59*(Suppl. 1), A56.

Hoskins, K.F., Stopfer, J.E., Calzone, K.A., Merajver, S.D., Rebbeck, T.R., Garber, J.E., & Weber, B.L. (1995). Assessment and counseling for women with a family history of breast cancer—A guide for clinicians. *JAMA, 273,* 577–585.

Kennedy, E.D., Blair, J.E., Ready, R., Wolff, B.G., Steinhart, A.H., Carryer, P.W., & McLeod, R.S. (1998). Patients' perceptions of their participation in a clinical trial for postoperative Crohn's disease. *Cancer Journal of Gastroenterology, 12,* 287–291.

Evolution of a Community-Based Family Risk Assessment Program: An Oncology Nursing Perspective

Carol Cherry, RNC, BSN, OCN®

This vignette describes how one institution has implemented the Family Risk Assessment Program at the Fox Chase Cancer Center.

Paoli Memorial Hospital is a 208-bed nonprofit acute-care community hospital located in Paoli, PA, near historic Valley Forge National Park in suburban Philadelphia. The outpatient cancer center is accredited by the American College of Surgeons as a Community Hospital Comprehensive Cancer Program. Paoli Cancer Center is a member of the Fox Chase Network, a select group of community hospitals in Pennsylvania and New Jersey linked with Fox Chase Cancer Center, a National Cancer Institute (NCI)-designated Comprehensive Cancer Center in northeast Philadelphia. This affiliation enables community cancer centers to develop or enhance community-based oncology programs.

The Family Risk Assessment Program (FRAP) offers education and counseling for women with a family history of breast and ovarian cancer. Education, cancer risk counseling, screening recommendations, Mammacare instruction, and the option for genetic testing are provided. FRAP at Paoli was established in 1996 based on the model developed at Fox Chase Cancer Center. Since its inception, 327 women have attended education sessions on the risk factors, screening methods, and genetics of breast/ovarian cancer. These women were predominantly Caucasian and middle class. A small proportion (21%) chose individual cancer risk counseling, and a third of that group opted to participate in genetic testing research protocols. A nurse coordinator oversees all aspects of the program and serves as health educator and cancer risk counselor. An administrative assistant provides part-time support. Three oncologists assist, on an alternating basis, with the education and counseling of women who receive genetic test results. A social worker is available during counseling and for special concerns, as needed. A multidisciplinary steering committee meets quarterly for clinical updates, including ethical issues. The hospital's public relations director coordinates marketing efforts. A "traveling" genetic counselor from FRAP at Fox Chase Cancer Center is present for disclosure of genetic test results. A unique and successful close collaboration exists between the staff in both programs, particularly in mentoring the nurse coordinator. The Department of Defense and the Oncology Nursing Society provided a grant to train the nurse coordinator and establish the program at Fox Chase Cancer Center. Designated cancer program funds donated to the Cancer Center at Paoli Memorial Hospital were used to support marketing and staff time. The services were offered free of charge to the participants.

While working as a radiation oncology nurse at Paoli Cancer Center, an opportunity to attend a training course in Familial Cancer Risk Counseling for Nurses at Fox Chase Cancer Center became available to me. A Department of Defense grant had funded the establishment of a breast cancer high-risk registry among the Fox Chase Network hospitals (smaller community hospitals whose affiliation allows the resources of the NCI-designated comprehensive cancer center to extend to their respective regions). A necessary first step in developing the high-risk registry was to train personnel, with the emphasis being on oncology nurses, to serve as program coordinators and cancer risk counselors.

The intensive three-day training course provided a glimpse of how malignancies develop, offering some hope for a cure. The course also posed a complex challenge—how to take the model of a comprehensive risk assessment program at a major research center and translate it into a workable process in a busy community setting. The reception of the local population and the limited existing personnel were concerns.

Integral to the establishment of FRAP was the formation of an action plan. The hospital vice president of oncology programs was the key administrator who facilitated this process. Several key oncologists and representatives from the public relations, marketing, and community education departments attended the action plan meeting. This group became the core of a multidisciplinary steering committee that later was organized to guide program expansion and discuss ethical issues. The action plan focused on several key components, including more in-depth training for the nurse coordinator and identification of marketing strategies.

A personal commitment of study time to pursue expertise in a complex field like cancer genetics is crucial for a cancer risk counselor. An oncology nursing background along with experience in the clinical aspects of breast and ovarian cancer, as well as family dynamics, provides a foundation on which to build. The challenge to comprehend the intricacies of DNA and gene testing and interpret these issues to the public is a daunting, ongoing process. A series of visits to FRAP at Fox Chase Cancer Center to observe the components of education, individual cancer risk counseling, and the high-risk clinic was useful in the orientation process. The support of a nurse mentor was crucial in adapting the program to the community setting. Quarterly network nurses' meetings held at Fox Chase always were enlightening and provided an inspiring opportunity to share experiences and receive clinical updates. Newly published literature on genetics was forwarded on a regular basis and then disseminated to local FRAP oncologists.

Having colleagues attend trial presentations during lunch breaks is a helpful way to practice delivery of educational session material and develop a comfort level with communicating genetic information and responding to questions. Making the first public presentation to a "friendly" (e.g., breast cancer support group, group familiar to the practitioner) and interested audience is helpful. Having Fox Chase FRAP health educator as a supportive resource also proved beneficial.

A number of marketing strategies were identified to promote the program. Oncologists notified patients who had a family history of breast/ovarian cancer of the new service and invited them to attend free education sessions. The Cancer Center medical director introduced the program to the entire hospital medical staff by letter. Announcements were placed in the bimonthly community education mailer, the weekly employees' newsletter, and news releases to a number of local papers. A brochure was developed and disseminated to the offices of key oncologists, breast surgeons, and gynecologists. After the program was fully under way, a story was pitched to the media, and a full-length feature ran in a local newspaper.

Marketing efforts were successful, and education sessions were offered four times a year as free community meetings. Women older than 20 years of age with a first-degree relative with breast or ovarian cancer were eligible to attend. One-on-one sessions also were available to meet scheduling needs. The hour-long meeting provided an overview of the anatomy and function of the breast or ovary, risk factors, and early-detection practices. The genetics portion presented an overview of the BRCA1 and BRCA2 genes, sporadic, familial and hereditary patterns of cancer, and the benefits, limitations, and risks associated with genetic testing. Attendees were informed of the options for individualized risk assessment counseling and participation in genetic testing protocols. Those interested in pursuing these options were provided with a detailed health history questionnaire and psychological survey tools at the end of the session, to be completed and returned by mail. To date, 327 women have attended education sessions, and roughly half of them picked up the questionnaires.

Of the women who expressed interest in individual risk counseling, approximately 40% of them actually followed through. The questionnaire data entry, generation of pedigrees, and assessment of familial cancer patterns takes place at Fox Chase Cancer Center and is forwarded back to Paoli for review by the nurse and a FRAP oncologist. An individual cancer risk counseling session then is scheduled. In this 1½–2-hour session, the pedigree is expanded, the medical history is recorded, and an interpretation of risk is performed based on the family history that is provided. A letter outlining screening recommendations is reviewed; however, if the woman elects to participate in genetic testing, those recommendations are updated based on the test results. The options for pursuing gene testing are discussed and, if elected, a meeting for informed consent and blood draw is scheduled. Blood is mailed overnight to Fox Chase for genetic analysis.

Test results are provided in a two-step process, the first being predisclosure counseling with a nurse counselor, physician, and optional social worker who are available to review potential results and their implications for the patient and family. A physical examination is performed at this time, if warranted. A second blood sample to validate results also is drawn. When results become available, a disclosure counseling session is planned with the patient, nurse counselor, physician, social worker, and genetic counselor from Fox Chase. A full discussion of prevention options and screening recommendations is reviewed. Patients are encouraged to discuss screening with their personal physicians. At this writing, 25 participants have donated blood for genetic research protocols.

One of the fundamental benefits of this program is the provision of state-of-the-art cancer genetics education to at-risk women, offered as a free community service. Providing the information necessary to reduce cancer risk and make informed decisions about genetic testing is a major strength of the program. For the small number of women who proceed to genetic testing, the opportunity to access the research protocols and expertise of a regional comprehensive cancer center in their local community is a significant benefit.

A major challenge to providing ongoing risk assessment services in a local hospital setting is the fostering of clinical genetics expertise within the busy established practices of community oncology professionals. Physicians at the facility have donated time to pioneer a new program, but as demands increase, discussion has begun regarding fees for service. As the service has gained more visibility in the community, a major corporate donor has emerged to fund the administrative costs. Applying for additional grant funding also has been contemplated.

Receiving strong support is extremely important when developing competence in an evolving specialty while simultaneously juggling the numerous demands of current practice. The uniqueness of this collaborative program provides a practical model for using the inherent resources of both local and comprehensive oncology programs to disseminate cancer genetic risk assessment and prevention information to the community. From a nursing perspective, this opportunity has been an incredible professional challenge and growth experience. Nursing collegiality between the local hospital and comprehensive cancer center nurses has been particularly rewarding. Numerous staff members at both institutions have provided vision and encouragement in the journey.

Development of a Comprehensive Cancer Program

Margaret M. Doyle, RN, BSN, OCN®

The Institution

In 1991, recognizing the impact that cancer has on the health of the community, Hunterdon Medical Center (HMC) designated the development of a comprehensive cancer program as a major initiative. In 1993, Hunterdon Medical Center affiliated with Fox Chase Cancer Center (FCCC) in Philadelphia, PA, and became a member of the Fox Chase Network. This affiliation provided the program an opportunity to offer patients in the community and surrounding area a complete range of cancer services as well as the expertise available at FCCC. In 1999, with the completion of a new facility and the addition of radiation oncology services, the Hunterdon Regional Cancer Program (HRCP) was renamed the Hunterdon Regional Cancer Center (HRCC). Now, patients and families at this 176-bed general acute care, not-for-profit teaching hospital can find a full range of oncology services under one roof—from the prevention, screening, and early detection of cancer to clinical research trials, medical and radiation oncology, as well as social and dietary support services.

Prior to 1993, the public health nurse from the Hunterdon County Department of Health coordinated all educational and screening activities. With the approval of HRCP's participation in the Breast and Prostate Cancer Prevention Trials, a part-time oncology nurse was hired into the role of prevention research nurse (PRN). Included in the responsibilities of this role was the recruitment and education of individuals for participation in these studies. Going out into the community to promote the availability of cancer prevention studies became an opportunity for the public to become aware about cancer screening and early detection. The PRN became a referral resource within the community for upcoming screening events and hospital services. This was the beginning of the HRCP staff attending outside community events on a regular basis to promote cancer program services.

The following year, a new non-nursing role was created—the community liaison. This full-time position was established to coordinate all community screening and educational programs. This individual gradually took over attending community health fairs and coordinated oncology nurse speakers from the HRCP staff, as needed. The PRN and community liaison became the education, early detection, and screening resources within the community. The community liaison collaborated with the local chapters of the American Cancer Society, Department of Public Health, and the County Office on Aging to coordinate annual screening programs. A core of HMC volunteers who worked on specific screenings became familiar with the routines of registration and screening-day participant flow.

The community laiaison role has since been absorbed by the PRN (now full-time) and two outreach staff members (non-nurses). The PRN and the outreach staff members are the main resources within the community regarding prevention and early detection. This would be an insurmountable task if it were not for the collaboration of the entire staff of HRCC. Each staff member understands and is aware of the efforts to be made in the community. Each provides a potential resource for referral to a program. Volunteers provide manpower support in mailing out information and staffing the screening programs. Collaboration with Fox Chase Cancer Center and other agencies (e.g., Department of Public Health of Hunterdon County, the local unit of the American Cancer Society, the state of New Jersey) provides networking opportunities to share ideas and promote the availability of programs and services at HMC. The availability of physicians who voluntarily take the time to provide their expertise to the screening programs and public education also has helped in the success of efforts in the community.

Marketing

Since the creation of the community liaison role, a calendar for public awareness has been created each year, with scheduled education and screening programs. This calendar has become a regular promotional piece. As educational programs, screenings, or the publication of public service announcements are scheduled, the theme of the month is taken into account to enhance the public's awareness of nationally recognized themes (e.g., Skin Cancer Awareness Month, Prostate Cancer Awareness Month). Educational programs are held in conjunction with the screening program. Occasionally, education programs are held at different sites within the community, and those in attendance are given an opportunity to sign up for screening appointments. HMC publishes a monthly calendar in the local papers that promotes educational programs taking place at the hospital. Upcoming screenings and educational sessions are placed in the calendar with a number to call for appointments.

Promotion for all prevention studies and education and screening programs takes place through a variety of media: health fairs, having the PRN go "door-to-door" to physicians' offices, press releases, and calendars in the local newspapers. Quarterly newsletters (for physicians, administrators, and department leaders) allow the promotion of new studies, programs, or staff members. Annual newsletters, published for the general public, allow the promotion of HRCC programs and events. Focusing on a particular topic—women's health, men's health, nutrition and, most recently, prevention—these newsletters provide easy-to-understand information from two reliable resources—FCCC and HRCC.

Screening Programs
Annual Screening

Annual screenings (e.g., skin, prostate, oral) are held at HMC and are coordinated by HRCC in collaboration with the American Cancer Society, Hunterdon Unit, Hunterdon County Department of Public Health, and the Hunterdon County Office on Aging. Each screening program has a volunteer medical advisor who is a member of HMC's staff. The medical advisor helps to determine the times and dates of screenings, occasionally recruits fellow colleagues to assist with the screening process, and acts as an advisor to provide guidance in reviewing screening guidelines and recommended follow-up for suspicious findings. For example, while results of prostate-specific antigen values from the prostate cancer screenings are sent out from the HRCC offices, the medical advisor authors the letters to be sent to participants.

CDC-CEED

Since 1994, breast cancer screening efforts have grown to meet the demands of the community. In 1997, HRCP became the contact agency to coordinate the county's participation in the CDC-CEED (Centers for Disease Control-Cancer Education and Early Detection) Program. Funded by the CDC, this program provides gynecologic and breast cancer screenings to women without adequate insurance coverage who meet eligibility guidelines. An outreach coordinator and outreach worker, whose salaries are funded by the grant, promote the availability of the program within the community. Promotion, also funded by the grant, takes place through a variety of methods including, ads on the back of grocery store receipts, an insert in the local "Value Pac" coupon mailer and flyers that are distributed throughout the community. Area physicians and staff make individual referrals. The outreach coordinator is responsible for overseeing the clinical care that women receive with physicians at HMC. Since the beginning of this project, screening services for high-risk and underinsured people have been expanded to include prostate and colorectal screenings. Funding for these services is supported by the state of New Jersey.

Prevention Studies

Collaborating with medical advisors of the programs has helped in the area of physician recognition and acceptance of new programs. The PRN works closely with the cancer center's principal investigator (PI) of the prevention research studies to promote, recruit, and follow study participants. While the PRN works within the community, the physician acts as a peer resource within the hospital staff. At the time of the first prevention study's approval, with only two oncologists on staff at HMC, the thought of following all prevention research study participants was daunting, especially because they were healthy. The program offered a unique opportunity for research participants to have study-required examinations completed by their own physicians, with the care coordinated by the PRN/PI team.

After the initial education sessions, the participants meet with the PRN to review the consent and discuss follow-up issues. Letters are sent to the primary physicians of potential participants explaining the study and what would be needed of the physicians as their patients participate. After the PI signs the consent and answers final questions, the participant works closely with the PRN and his or her primary physician during study participation. This enhances the patient/PRN relationship (improving compliance), provides the local physician an opportunity to participate in national research studies, and prevents the participant from having to leave a relationship that had been built with a primary physician. The primary physician receives semiannual update letters regarding the study status of his or her patient and is notified of any changes or new information that relates to the study. Although all of this communication with the primary physician may be labor intensive, it helped to create a link between what was a new hospital program and hospital physicians.

Colorectal Awareness

A unique promotional/community education opportunity for collaboration among the HRCC, FCCC, and its network affiliates came in 1997. The "Colorectal Education Initiative" began during National Colon Cancer Prevention Week in September with the mailing of an informational brochure, *Knowledge Is Your Best Defense Against Cancer*, for those 40 years of age and older. The piece had a return card that people could send in requesting information from the HRCC, as well as a free nine-minute video, *What You Should Know About Colorectal Cancer.* This video was produced as a collaborative effort between HRCC and FCCC highlighting HMC, its physicians, and staff.

Family Risk Assessment Program

The affiliation with FCCC has continued to help to promote and advance the services offered through HRCC. A grant funded by the Department of Defense enabled FCCC to bring its high-risk breast and ovarian program to its network hospitals.

The Family Risk Assessment Program (FRAP) at HMC was created in 1996. It is designed to educate individuals and families with a family history of breast and ovarian cancer to help them to understand the hereditary factors that can influence risk for cancer development. FRAP has two medical advisors—a family physician and a medical oncologist. Before the program began, the PRN attended special training at FCCC. This included a week-long seminar at FCCC with classroom and interactive time. A series of short meetings followed to enhance the initial education received at the seminar, as well as expose the PRN to the high-risk program at FCCC. This exposure allowed the PRN to experience participation while learning the role involved in coordinating a program. Once the program began, the PRN had regular opportunities for troubleshooting, sharing of ideas, and enhancement of his or her knowledge base. The PRN promotes the availability of the program and upcoming education sessions, working with the public relations department of the hospital.

One of two medical advisors, along with the PRN, are in attendance during educational sessions and are involved in the consent process and genetic disclosure sessions for those who have genetic testing. The presence of the physician/nurse team provides valuable question-and-answer opportunities for those in attendance and during genetic testing disclosure.

After attending a general education session, participants may opt to have a pedigree (family tree focusing on the presence of disease) created. To create the pedigree, the participant completes a series of questionnaires that are sent to FCCC for pedigree creation and review by the genetics team. The FCCC staff then reviews the pedigree with the PRN. It is the PRN who, while working with the participant, expands and discusses the information that the pedigree provides regarding the risk for the development of disease (e.g., cancer, heart disease, diabetes). Screening guidelines and, if appropriate, the role of genetic testing are reviewed during this meeting. When genetic testing disclosure takes place, the physician, PRN, and a genetic counselor are present. The genetic counselor is involved in the initial review of the pedigree at FCCC, and the PRN updates any information and profiles the family prior to the disclosure meeting. The PRN provides the continuity needed to develop a relationship with the individual/family seeking genetic information.

Initially, FRAP met many challenges. First, it was not a "money maker" for the hospital. It was a labor-intensive program with a small fee for education and pedigree creation services (approximately $25). (Genetic testing, then available only through research studies at FCCC, was free to some individuals.)

Second, physician recognition and acceptance were a challenge initially. At HMC, having a family physician as a medical advisor has proved to be valuable (especially one who interacted with a large portion of the physician population at the hospital and was also an instructor in the family residency program). The medical advisor provides peer guidance to physicians (e.g., current genetic testing recommendations, patient care issues) and refers physicians to the PRN for further information.

Third, community acceptance of the program or, more specifically, community understanding of the program, was extremely challenging. Although it was regarded as a great opportunity to be able to have genetic testing closer to home, communicating who might be eligible for genetic testing and the role of genetic testing proved to be a challenge. Some of the public viewed genetic testing as something simple—a blood test that would indicate whether or not one would develop cancer. It was not always understood that counseling was an integral part of the process.

Educational sessions became important tools in public education by helping to demystify some of the information regarding cancer risk and development. In fact, FRAP education sessions are open to everyone who is interested in breast cancer risk, not just high-risk individuals. Attendance at the first education sessions was very small (perhaps three to five women per session). However, in recent months, with the opening of the Study of Tamoxifen and Raloxifene (for the prevention of breast cancer), FRAP has had an increase in the number of individuals seeking information and taking advantage of pedigree creation to have tools to use when making decisions with physicians regarding breast cancer prevention options. The availability of commercial genetic testing in breast cancer and genetic studies offered by FCCC in areas other than breast cancer (e.g., colon, lung) have made FRAP a more valuable educational resource within the community and to FCCC. With the FRAP available to provide reliable and valuable education regarding risk and cancer development, appropriate individuals can be readily referred to FCCC for other high-risk programs (e.g., FCCC's high-risk prostate or colon programs).

Evaluation

Evaluation mechanisms vary related to the program. Much is accomplished by hand tracking. Each contact is asked how he or she found out about the program. This information is saved, and when beginning to look at a new promotional idea, we look to past response and cost. Annual screening programs are very popular and are filled without allowing repeat participants (individuals must wait at least one year before returning to the program). A database (how, why, which services were used) was created to track those who used HRCC services. FRAP participants receive evaluations at the end of education sessions and in the mail. These are most important when evaluating a program held at one of the hospital's off-site facilities or when press releases are sent.

As this example demonstrates, developing a comprehensive cancer program requires vision, planning, developing collaborative relationships, and tenacious persistence to allow a small program to grow into a viable community resource for cancer prevention and early detection.

Colon Cancer Screening Program: Preventive Healthcare Program Using Nurse Endoscopists

Nancy Eisemon, RN, MPH, CGRN, APN/CNS

Overview

The Colon Cancer Screening Center (CCSC) was developed at a large teaching hospital in Illinois in 1995 and was implemented in November 1997. More than 1,000 patients have been screened as of March 2000. CCSC provides comprehensive colon cancer screening to asymptomatic individuals by a nurse endoscopist. The nurse endoscopist provides hemoccult testing, digital rectal examination, flexible sigmoidoscopy, and preventive health education. The staffing consists of one nurse endoscopist, a customer service representative, and a gastroenterology technician. The customer service representative assists with the pre-evaluation intake form needed for eligibility and with data entry, and also is cross-trained as a gastroenterology technician to assist with the procedure. The gastroenterology technicians are used throughout the screening center of the endoscopy laboratory to assist the nurse endoscopist with biopsies and turn over the room for patients.

The institution identified the need to include a CCSC as part of the comprehensive Gastrointestinal (GI) Oncology Program. Funding for the program came from the GI program. The following goals were identified for the center.
- Provide a unique early cancer detection program in the metropolitan area, which currently is not available to the public.
- Become a leader in early colon cancer detection through screening.
- Provide a referral service to physicians within the institution that provides screening and preventive health education.
- Develop a clinical database to track clinical outcomes and trends in patient compliance.

Description of Program

CCSC provides colon screening by digital rectal examination, hemoccult testing, and flexible sigmoidoscopy to asymptomatic patients who are 50–64 years of

₀e. The program uses one nurse endoscopist who performs the examination and provides patients with cancer preventive health education. Polyps larger than or equal to 7 mm are biopsied. Referrals for colonoscopy are based on the pathology results. Appointments are scheduled in 45-minute intervals, which allows ample time for the nurse endoscopist to prepare the patient for the examination, discuss examination findings, and provide current cancer prevention guidelines. Part of the purpose of CCSC when it was being developed was to decrease embarrassment by providing a comfortable environment, therefore reducing patients' fear and anxiety. Preventive healthcare information on cancer screening guidelines, nutrition, exercise, open chemoprevention trials, and genetic counseling, when appropriate, are discussed with the patient post-examination. Patients are encouraged to share the wellness-related topics with family members.

A primary-care physician directly refers patients to the CCSC, or patients may self-refer, provided that they have a primary-care physician. An eligibility intake form is used to identify average-risk patients. Patients who are at intermediate risk (personal history of colon cancer or adenomatous polyps) or high risk (history of inflammatory disease or a genetic predisposition to colon cancer) are referred back to the primary-care physician for colonoscopy. All Medicare patients are referred back to the primary-care physician. In January 1998, the Health Care Financing Administration expanded Medicare coverage to include colorectal cancer screening. For an average-risk person who is 50 years of age or older, coverage is provided for an annual fecal occult blood test and sigmoidoscopy every four years if performed by a doctor or osteopath. The Medicare restriction of non-physicians performing the examination requires that all patients 64 years of age and older be referred back to the primary-care physician.

The colon screening program generates revenue from referred colonoscopies. Polyps seen during screening flexible sigmoidoscopy are biopsied to determine whether they are hyperplastic polyps (benign) or adenomatous polyps (precancerous). All patients with adenomatous polyps are referred for a colonoscopy. The entire colon is viewed, and all polyps are removed. Patients with adenomatous polyps are classified as intermediate risk and will have follow-up colonoscopy every three to five years, which is determined by the pathological results and the number of polyps seen during the endoscopy.

Program Challenges/Possible Solutions

Several factors have hindered the screening center from attaining its goal of increasing the volume two-fold in one year. Medicare's restrictions definitely had an impact on the volume. A significant number of patients who are 64 years of age and older are referred back to their primary-care physician, therefore decreasing the volume of people at CCSC.

A knowledge deficit appears to exist regarding the appropriate guidelines for colorectal screening by physicians as well as patients. Physicians are either not promoting this type of screening or patients are reluctant to have the procedure. Patients within this institution are having various cancer screening tests performed per the recommended American Cancer Society guidelines, but colon screening is being omitted. High-risk patients and patients with symptoms are inappropriately referred to the screening center. If physicians have to differentiate which patients are appropriate for CCSC and which patients need to be referred to a gastroenterologist, it appears that they find it easier to send all of their patients to a gastroenterologist for further evaluation.

Patients are reluctant to have the examination. More than 23% of patients at CCSC cancel or do not show for the appointment. This patient knowledge deficit creates fears associated with this type of screening examination. Physicians may be suggesting this examination to patients, but the patients are not compliant. Staff members hope that Colon Cancer Awareness Month will change these attitudes and fears.

Advertising strategies for CCSC need to be ongoing. A campaign, which would not only create colorectal cancer screening awareness but also create a new image for the screening, needs to be developed. Emphasis on preventive health teaching in an atmosphere that is nonthreatening should be incorporated in promoting the center. Advertising strategies are needed to change attitudes on screening and correct false impressions and misinformation. The market strategy goal ultimately should be to build familiarity and easy recognition of the center for self-referrals.

Ongoing marketing to physician and patient groups needs to be performed. Brochures and prescription pads with recommended guidelines for colon screening for average-risk individuals are provided to the internal medicine department, family practice physicians, and the OB/GYN department to help to promote screening. Colon Cancer Awareness Month gave the staff an opportunity to provide educational programming for physicians as well as patients. The increased awareness has slightly improved the volume of patients.

Nursing Perspective

Prior to CCSC, only credentialed physicians performed flexible sigmoidoscopy. Many physicians were skeptical of the new role of nurse endoscopist. The institution obtained benchmarked data on nurse endoscopists performing flexible sigmoidoscopy nationally and in the surrounding area. A competency-training program was developed, and qualifications and scope of practice were defined. Various committees in the facility defined and addressed legal issues before training was initiated.

The training program was divided into three phases (see Table 20-5). It took approximately four months for one to feel confident and work independently as a nurse endoscopist. One physician did most of the technical training/mentoring; however, opportunities were available to work with other physicians to observe variations in procedural technique. Even though it was technically possible for an individual to perform the flexible sigmoidoscopy after 25–50 examinations, the comfort level of the patient is compromised with limited examiner experience. Technical skill improves with the number of examinations performed. Performance of a comfortable examination without technical difficulty was achieved after 250 examinations. Background experience as a gastroenterology nurse is extremely helpful. GI nurses who have assisted in thousands of examinations have gained the confidence in identifying pathology.

Table 20-5. Competency Training Program Components

Content of Phase	Learning Objectives
Phase I Cognitive phase providing information needed for competence development and understanding of specific policies/procedures related to the screening center	Describe American Cancer Society guidelines. State indications and contraindications for flexible sigmoidoscopy. Describe patient appropriateness for CCSC. Describe the mission and philosophy of CCSC. Identify normal anatomy of colon and rectum. Discuss techniques used for flexible sigmoidoscopy. Explain care and cleaning of sigmoidoscopes. Describe pre- and post-procedure instructions to patients. Explain referral guidelines for chemoprevention and genetic counseling.
Phase II Development/practice of technical skills needed to perform exam under supervision of gastroenterologist	Demonstrate technical skills to manipulate the sigmoidoscope. Intubate 45–60 cm using various insertion techniques. Identify anatomic or pathologic characteristics. Identify abnormal findings. Demonstrate proficiency in cold biopsy. Demonstrate endoscope withdrawals with good visualization. Document appropriately. Communicate findings to referring physician.
Phase III Independent performance of exam and continued competency and quality monitoring	Maintain quality and competency in performing digital rectal exam and flexible sigmoidoscopy. Participate in quality assurance monitoring of exam by gastroenterologist, 3–5 per quarter.

Note. From Flexible Sigmoidoscopy: A Training Program for the Professional Registered Nurse, by L. Stucky-Marshall, Colon Cancer Screening Center at Northwestern Memorial Hospital, Chicago, IL. Used with permission.

As nurses, we not only focus on the science of medicine, but also on the art of nursing. Patient education and patient satisfaction are of utmost importance. The uniqueness of this center is the length of time for the appointment in which comprehensive cancer prevention education can be provided to the patient and family. It enables the nurse to reassure the patient prior to the procedure and develop a trust that makes the examination easier to perform. Assurance during the examination and the positive progression toward completion of the examination help the patient to relax. Patients do need to have an advocate when the examination is being performed. A job has been performed well when the patient says that "you made an unpleasant experience as pleasant as possible." The role of nurse endoscopist is a very rewarding part of nursing.

The Patient Call Back Tool scores indicate that patients who are screened in CCSC are very satisfied with their care. It is too early to determine if that satisfaction will coincide with compliance for their five-year follow-up examination (see Figure 20-1).

Figure 20-1. Patient Survey

Northwestern Memorial Hospital
Colon Cancer Screening Center Patient Survey
Date: _____

Pre-Examination

1. How did you hear about the Colon Cancer Screening Center?
   ❑ Primary Care Physician   ❑ OB/GYN   ❑ Oncologist   ❑ Corporate Health
   ❑ Northwestern Memorial Hospital publications   ❑ Colon Cancer Screening Center brochure
   ❑ Other (explain) _____

2. Do you know how often you should have your colon screened?   ❑ Yes   ❑ No

   If yes, where did you receive this information?
   ❑ Physician   ❑ Colon Cancer Screening Center brochure   ❑ Newspapers/magazines
   ❑ Television   ❑ Radio   ❑ Staff in the Colon Cancer Screening Center

3. Is this the first time you are having your colon screened by flexible sigmoidoscopy?
   ❑ Yes   ❑ No   Age when screened_____

4. Were the instructions on the enema preparation adequate?
   ❑ Yes   ❑ No
   If no, explain _____

Post-Examination

1. When will you need a screening flexible sigmoidoscopy again?
   ❑ 1 year   ❑ 3 years   ❑ 5 years

2. How often do you need to do the stool test?
   ❑ 1 year   ❑ 3 years   ❑ 5 years

3. Were your questions best answered *before* the examination by
   ❑ a. Written information from the screening center
   ❑ b. Discussion with the nurse endoscopist before the examination
   ❑ c. Discussion with the physician in the office at the time of referral

4. Were your questions *after* the examination answered adequately by the nurse?
   ❑ Yes   ❑ No
   If no, explain _____

5. If you were to choose one thing you liked best about the CCSC, it would be the
   ❑ a. Relaxed atmosphere
   ❑ b. Nurse doing the exam
   ❑ c. Educational information received

6. On a scale of 1–5 (1 = poor—5 = very good) how would you rate your overall satisfaction?
   Score _____

Men Against Cancer Program

Bertie Ford, RN, MS, OCN®, and Jaci Holland, RN, ANP

The Men Against Cancer (MAC) Initiative was started in 1997. The Columbus Chapter of the Black Nurses Association (CCBNA) was provided with $15,000 from the Arthur G. James Cancer Hospital and Solove Research Institute to plan and implement a project that could make a difference in the health of African Americans in central Ohio. CCBNA decided to concentrate its efforts on African American men in the Columbus area.

CCBNA initiated focus groups to find out what men knew or wanted to know about cancer and cancer prevention. The group distributed flyers and invitations to men in fraternities, neighbors, coworkers, and colleagues. The first group of men had a higher-than-average income and education than was expected. When recruiting the second group, the CCBNA members put additional effort in getting less highly educated men. Flyers were passed out at sporting events (e.g., little league baseball games, youth basketball leagues), to hospital housekeeping and maintenance personnel, and to others. This was a very effective method of getting the word out.

The first focus group meeting was held in October 1997; the second was held in January 1998. A monetary incentive and breakfast were provided for the participants, and the meeting was finished by lunchtime. A male facilitator helped ensure personal issues could be discussed freely. With an extensive background in business, labor/human resources, and education, the facilitator did an excellent job of eliciting information. CCBNA members met with approximately 90 men in the two groups. The areas addressed in the focus groups were smoking, nutrition, sources for cancer information and treatment, and general information on lung, prostate, and colon cancer. The men were served a healthy breakfast, and the discussions were initiated with their thoughts about the breakfast food. The men were very interested in screening and early detection, especially with regard to what prostate cancer screening entailed. Some men in the group had previously had the examination, and they were able to share their experiences with others in the group.

In March 1998, an interactive educational session was presented that covered the topics of prostate, testicular, colon, and lung cancers. The topics were chosen because of the incidence of these malignancies in the African American male population. Information about other diseases, such as diabetes and sexually transmitted diseases, also was included. The educational session was based on the Jeopardy® game show format, and the men had an opportunity to win door prizes.

The final effort, with regard to the project, was to expand the target list to 1,000 men. We wanted to assess a larger sample of men in the Columbus area with a survey that ascertained their knowledge, attitude, behaviors, and beliefs. Data were collected in 1999, and a report was generated at the end of that year. CCBNA members used groups such as churches, fraternities, schools, the National Black Leadership Initiative in Cancer, and other civic organizations. Currently, the

CCBNA is in the process of meeting with the executive board of the Arthur G. James Cancer Hospital to plan the next phase with screenings, follow-up, and an educational symposium.

The biggest challenge associated with this program is the time it takes to organize and implement. Thus far, two CCBNA members have performed the majority of the work. Members have collaborated with the Columbus Chapter of the Oncology Nursing Society on the educational component of the project. CCBNA has received $55,000 to fund the project, including the data analyses of the surveys. The main people involved in the project have been registered nurses, a program manager for Community Outreach, and the facilitator of the focus groups, who has expertise in this area.

As African American nurses, CCBNA members believe that they can have an impact on the prevention, detection, and screening behaviors of African American men in the community. We understand the need that the community has in using healthcare professionals who are culturally similar to them. The data collected in the survey provide baseline information for future programming and an opportunity for further analyses. CCBNA aims to provide interventions for the prevention and early detection of cancer in the African American community. They will continue to work for funding to continue the MAC project to decrease barriers to health care and increase early detection of targeted diseases in the community.

Tobacco Free for Good Tobacco Cessation Program

Donna Garrett, RN, MSN, CCRN

The Tobacco Free for Good (TFFG) program is a tobacco cessation program provided, free of charge, to all participants by Spectrum Health and the Kent County Health Department (KCHD). Spectrum Health (formerly Blodgett Memorial Medical Center and Butterworth Hospital) is a tertiary healthcare system in Grand Rapids, MI. Every three years, KCHD conducts a randomized telephone survey with questions regarding the lifestyle habits of the people who live in Kent County. The smoking rate in Kent County is approximately 25%, which is consistent with smoking rates for the state of Michigan (statistics taken from the State Health Department).

Approximately three years ago, a group of individuals within Spectrum Health began to investigate the possibility of offering a free smoking cessation program to the community. Spectrum Health agreed to completely fund a community smoking cessation class as part of their support for the community. In an effort to make the best use of resources within the community, KCHD chose to be a part of this new program. After 18 months of research and planning, the TFFG program was offered to the community, and classes have been offered on a continuous basis.

When the TFFG program was established, only four smoking cessation programs were available in Kent County. The cost to enroll in the programs ranged from $25/participant (a rate based on ability to pay) at KCHD up to $125/participant at other facilities. Attendance at each of the programs averaged 10 or fewer per class, and many of the classes were cancelled because of lack of enrollment. One of the main reasons for offering the class at no charge was to eliminate one of the barriers to attending class. To date, the TFFG program has offered 10 classes and has enrolled approximately 125 participants. Only one class has been cancelled because of low enrollment, and this was a class scheduled during the summer.

At the present time, the program has five instructors, one physician, and five support people from Spectrum Health and KCHD. The instructors either teach as a part of their job or are paid a stipend from Spectrum Health. The support staff has taken on the responsibilities of the program in addition to their regular duties either at Spectrum Health or KCHD. The physician provides his services for the course free of charge. He is a primary supporter of tobacco cessation programs throughout the state.

Description of Program

Enrollment into the TFFG course is handled through the community education department at Spectrum Health. Information is obtained over the phone, as with any other community education offering. The first night of the class is a general overview of the next six sessions. The literature suggested a high dropout rate from the orientation night to the first class session. Our experience has supported this, so the orientation session was designed with that in mind. Individuals are given enough basic information during orientation to assist them with a quit attempt if they choose to try on their own.

The next two sessions begin to prepare the individual for "Quit Night." An individual is assisted in the development of a "Quit Plan," the identification of support people, and identification of those events that will be difficult to get through while quitting. These sessions emphasize three issues that must be dealt with while preparing to quit: (1) nicotine addiction, (2) habits and behaviors associated with smoking, and (3) a psychological dependence on smoking. The third session, "Quit Night," is the part of the course that helps people to quit tobacco use permanently. Often, a ceremony is held to acknowledge that this is a decision that will have an impact on the rest of the participants' lives. Individuals often bring in cherished articles to give away to decrease the temptations to take up smoking again. It is a symbol of their commitment to being tobacco free.

The fourth night is set for 24–36 hours after "Quit Night." The group comes back for support and assistance with particularly difficult situations. At this time, the group has started to form its own support system, and the participants help each other get through this time.

Sessions five and six are follow-up sessions that continue to deal with problems as they arise and emphasize the importance of stress management and a new smoke-free, tobacco-free life.

At the end of the program, participants are asked to take part in the follow-up phone call program, which is optional. Calls are made at 1, 3, 6, 9, and 12 months to determine if the individual is tobacco free and to offer further assistance if a relapse has occurred. The staff person making the calls is not a trained counselor, so an algorithm was established to guide him or her through the questions. Two attempts are made to reach the graduate at the designated time periods. If no response is received after two calling periods, the individual is dropped from the follow-up list. Often, people have moved and no forwarding number is available. If a TFFG graduate has relapsed, he or she is offered an opportunity to come back to the class at no charge, and the phone call follow-up is discontinued.

We found that the highest relapse time was between one and three months. Because of this, we have established a support group that is scheduled to meet monthly for all graduates of the program. This group was started to provide support for individuals on an ongoing basis. At this time, the support group idea has not met with much success.

Results of the program are measured as a "Quit Rate" at the identified call-back times. "Quit Rates" are monitored for up to 12 months. Table 20-6 outlines the "Quit Rates" at the different time periods. The 12-month "Quit Rate" is 27%, which compares to other reported program results.

Table 20-6. Total Number of Follow-Up Calls

Month and Number of Follow-Up Calls	Quit	Relapse	Lost to Phone Follow-Up
1 month, 118	67/57%	29/25%	20/17%
3 months, 112	48/43%	38/34%	28/25%
6 months, 95	32/34%	34/36%	27/28%
9 months, 82	26/32%	32/39%	22/27%
12 months, 67	18/27%	28/42%	19/28%

Many have argued that there should be a fee structure to the TFFG program to increase participants' ownership and desire to succeed once they have enrolled in the program. Although individuals could find a way to purchase their tobacco products, they often had difficulty obtaining the money that was needed for a cessation program. By not charging a fee, the program has opened the opportunity for individuals to participate in a program that, in the past, was cost prohibitive. We also were aware that insurance carriers often do not cover the cost of tobacco replacement products. The combination of cessation that emphasizes behavior modification and stress management and the use of nicotine replacement therapy or bupropion have the highest success rates. A physician presents information in the orientation session, and participants then are referred to their own physician if a prescription is required. All of the instructors can assist the participants in the proper use of the medications.

Smoking cessation is a significant step toward healthier living. The collaboration of Spectrum Health and the KCHD to provide this comprehensive TFFG program demonstrates a serious commitment to cancer prevention.

Enacting Cancer Prevention Clinical Trials in a Community Setting

Cathleen M. Goetsch, MSN, ARNP, AOCN®

Community Clinical Oncology Programs (CCOPs) are grant-supported efforts by the National Cancer Institute (NCI). Their purpose is to provide access to individuals in community settings who might otherwise be limited in their ability to participate in high-quality, large, national cancer clinical trials.

Virginia Mason (VM) Medical Center has been a CCOP site since 1983. Located in Seattle, WA, the main medical center has 336 beds. It is a not-for-profit hospital with more than 400 physicians providing outpatient primary and specialty care in 16 western Washington clinics, in association with a freestanding research center. It is a major referral center for eastern Washington, Montana, and Alaska. Through its CCOP affiliations, it also provides NCI with clinical trial access to five other medical centers: three in western Washington, one in northern Idaho, and one in Alaska. The population base is primarily Caucasian, with strong minority and ethnic communities: 17% Asian American/Pacific Islander, 7% African American, a growing Hispanic representation, and a stable 1% Native American/Eskimo group.

The Cancer Prevention Project has been part of the VM-CCOP structure for approximately seven years. It aims to recruit and maintain participation in NCI-approved clinical trials for primary cancer prevention and prevention of second primary tumors. As a part of these efforts, education about cancer prevention is provided twice a month at community events such as health fairs, community forums, and cancer organization activities. Approximately 15,000 people have been given education materials during the last seven years, and 160 individuals currently are enrolled, with about 25 new entrants added annually. Prevention study participants are offered a "no out of pocket expense" assurance, in which the medical center forgoes charges for study-required examinations, tests, and procedures not covered by insurance.

Because education of the professional community is also a major focus, presentations are made to practicing healthcare providers or student groups about once a month. Venues have included lectures to university students, presentations to professional organizations, participation in resident medical education curriculum, grand rounds, cancer forums, and continuing medical and nursing education program content. More than 1,500 professional attendees participated in these various ways.

As recruitment of participants to the NCI prevention clinical trials began at the institution, it was approached with the same techniques that had proved successful for treatment trials. Early on, it became clear that a different paradigm was required in the prevention setting.

People with cancer seek treatment trials as a means of receiving the most up-to-date care. Drug side effects are a background consideration when saving a life is the potential outcome. Patients with cancer are willing to adhere to awkward, uncomfortable, inconvenient, and costly regimen of treatment and follow-up be-cause they feel the chance of benefit is worthwhile.

Experience with a well population volunteering for prevention studies indi-cated that healthy subjects had a much different motivation and required a differ-ent approach. In these studies where potential benefit was unclear and known side effects existed, altruism most often was the motivator rather than hope of benefit for oneself. Personalizing the concept of study participation was necessary.

Potential participants were intelligent, well read, and inquiring. They had many questions and concerns. They also had lives that did not focus on cancer (unlike patients undergoing treatment). It was imperative that efforts were made to mini-mize the intrusiveness of study participation upon their usual routines.

Designing a position dedicated to meeting the unique needs of this group was a successful strategy. The "Cancer Prevention Nurse" provided community out-reach education that became the basis for recruitment. Flexible follow-up and personalized contact resulted in excellent retention of participants in the face of several adverse situations.

Educating and networking with the primary-care community was recognized as a key element of recruitment. As had been previously reported in several studies, the strongest influence on participants' decisions to join research efforts was their healthcare provider's recommendation to do so. Providing training that was perti-nent to the particular provider and making the study recruitment and follow-up process helpful rather than a hindrance were important aspects. Common to both participant and healthcare provider relationships was consistent, personal contact focusing on their needs rather than the study requirements.

In addition to the cancer prevention nurse/program coordinator, a post-master's prepared nurse practitioner with advanced oncology certification, the personnel involved in the program include the primary investigator, a board-certified on-cologist, three clinical research professionals who provide data management, and off-site nurse support at VM-CCOP affiliated sites.

A computer database system facilitates participant follow-up. Weekly reports are generated noting who is due for what procedures. Mail merge programs are used to assist with patient and provider updating. Personal phone calls are still the gold standard for contacting participants. E-mail and voice mail have helped to streamline and simplify protocol office contacts with providers.

Three nurse practitioners, including the program coordinator, provide follow-up examinations in the outpatient oncology clinic. Alternatively, participants can continue routine care with their usual provider either inside or outside of the VMMC system or VM-CCOP affiliates. In these instances, copies of records are obtained, with the participants' authorization, for study documentation require-ments.

Promotion of the program usually is indirect in association with other educa-tional events in the institution and the community. Letter writing and articles in health publications are aimed separately at lay and professional audiences and have been helpful. Participation in community fund-raising events for cancer pro-grams also is a strategy. National publicity is sometimes provided as new studies begin to spark public awareness and interest.

One measure worthy of mentioning is the usefulness of the program to the parent institution. If it is not valuable to the provider community, it cannot survive. A successful symbiosis is necessary. Existence of the CCOP at the parent institution allows it to meet the American College of Surgeons' requirements for cancer center certification. This is a marketable sign of quality for the medical center.

Because the program is funded by a federal grant, evaluation takes place on an annual basis. Success is measured by meeting present goals for recruitment, retention, protocol adherence, and timeliness and quality of data submission. Although the goals for data quality remain consistently high, the goals for recruitment are raised each year. Outside auditors perform frequent reviews of study documentation to ensure its high caliber. Grant renewal is the reward for meeting these goals. Last year, VM-CCOP's renewal grant was fully funded for another five years, the maximum funding period.

Assessing Hereditary Cancer Risk

Cathleen M. Goetsch, MSN, ARNP, AOCN®

Beginning in the summer of 1996, personal and family cancer risk assessments have been available as a part of a comprehensive cancer care effort. It initially was offered primarily as an adjunct to the care of patients with breast cancer who were seen in the outpatient medical oncology clinic and to women with increased breast cancer risk who were exploring the option of participating in a chemoprevention clinical trial. As the need arose, family members also were served. Primary-care provider awareness of hereditary cancer risk and public knowledge of the availability of testing expanded the patient base to include the "worried well." Initially one new patient/family was seen per month. The current referral rate continues to increase steadily; in the past six months, an average of two new individuals or families have been seen per week.

In addition to in-depth pedigree analysis, personal risk factors, including behavioral and lifestyle risks, are explored. Education regarding recommendations for risk reduction, surveillance, and cancer gene predisposition testing, including pre- and post-test consultation, are offered to individuals and families with indicative histories or expressed interests. Written reports are made to patients and their referring providers. Real-time, two-way, interactive video telemedicine consultation has been used to decrease the challenge of geographic distance that otherwise could limit access to service.

Most patients have had concerns about hereditary breast/ovarian or colon cancer. Li-Fraumeni–type families and individuals with familial melanoma risk also have been served. The scope of practice is restricted to adults and their cancer-related hereditary risk. Non-cancer hereditary syndrome, prenatal counseling, and pediatric syndromes are referred to other community resources.

Primary-care providers, gynecologists, or other healthcare providers may identify initial hereditary cancer risk. For patients with cancer, heredity is considered an aspect of their disease etiology by their surgeon and medical and/or radiation oncologist or oncology nurse. When risk factors are noted or patients express concern about hereditary cancer risk, patients are offered a consultation with the post-master's prepared, advanced oncology certified nurse practitioner who specializes in hereditary cancer risk. After initial consultation, recommendations are made and may include further follow-up, intervention, or testing. This includes availability of cancer prevention clinical trials for patients or their relatives. If indicated, referrals are made to other members of the cancer team. Cases also may be discussed in the weekly interdisciplinary tumor conference.

Providing hereditary cancer risk assessment and management to patients was the impetus for initiating consideration of how such a service might be provided. Beginning with informal referrals by the oncologists—"Why don't you talk to our nurse who specializes in this area?"— word spread to other physicians. As the number of patients needing service increased, a multispecialty team created a referral algorithm.

Because hereditary cancer risk consultation is part of comprehensive cancer care at the institution, each department covers the internal cost of its particular part of the provided service. Services are billed as a part of patients' healthcare evaluation and management. If cancer predisposition gene testing is pursued, insurance coverage issues must be addressed for each individual.

The Community Clinical Oncology Program provides support for screening and recruitment activities to identify people who are eligible for prevention trials (i.e., women at increased risk of developing breast cancer may wish to participate in the Study of Tamoxifen and Raloxifene trial for breast cancer prevention in high-risk, postmenopausal women). The National Cancer Institute has pledged to provide support for the nurse practitioner providing the hereditary cancer risk consultation and to provide the necessary practice requirements (e.g., support personnel, space, supplies) to sustain the service. Marketing to patients and providers outside of the institution awaits the creation of infrastructure to support further increases in patient volume.

Indiana University Nicotine Dependence Program

Deborah M. Hudson, BS, RRT

A dentist (Arden G. Christen, DDS, MA, MSD), who himself is a former smoker, founded the Indiana University Nicotine Dependence Program in 1992. Initially, the program was operated from the Indiana University School of Dentistry in Indianapolis, IN. In 1997, in an effort to reach even more tobacco users, the program moved to a university-affiliated outpatient oncology setting (the Indiana Cancer Pavilion), also in Indianapolis. The move included an expansion of the staff and a name change (addition of "Cancer Center" to the program's name). The founding dentist continues to serve as a co-director to the program; a pulmonologist serves as the other co-director, and a registered respiratory therapist serves as the program coordinator.

The Indiana University Cancer Center Nicotine Dependence Program (IUCCNDP) offers a number of services to a variety of potential patients. The clinical side of the program provides state-of-the-art outpatient tobacco cessation. This intensive, one-on-one program offers a range of treatment options to meet the unique needs of each participant. It has been well documented in the research and clinical literature that nicotine dependence is physical, psychological, and behavioral. To add to the complexity, the intensity of each of these addiction components varies from person to person. Therefore, the staff conducts a very thorough assessment to determine the intensity of each component of nicotine dependence (see Table 20-7).

Table 20-7. Treatment Options for Nicotine Dependence

Interventions	Treatments
Pharmacologic	Nicotine replacement therapy (e.g., transdermal patch, nicotine gum, nicotine inhaler, nicotine nasal spray) Bupropion HCL Combination therapy (e.g., bypropion and patch, nasal spray and patch)
Behavioral	Change daily routines. Identify triggers and plan strategies. Practice relaxation techniques. Exercise regularly.
Psychosocial	Identify potential barriers and a plan to overcome them. Conduct mental rehearsals. Develop coping strategies.

Key components of the assessment include the following
- An extensive assessment questionnaire to obtain a complete smoking and health history
- Biochemical monitoring at each session via a carbon monoxide monitor
- Nicotine dependence diagnostic screens—Fagerstrom (physical dependence), Why Do You Smoke? (psychological dependence)
- Diagnostic consultation—begin educating about nicotine dependence and initial recommendations
- Personalized treatment planning
- Pharmacologic therapy
- Social/family support issues
- Short- and long-term follow-up, including quantifiable measurements
- Relapse prevention
- Relapse management (i.e., if a patient relapses, counselors attempt to help him or her identify why it happened, what to do now that he or she has relapsed, and how to prevent it in the future)

The program staff conducts 3-, 6-, and 12-month follow-ups to verify quit rates and assess patient satisfaction. These are conducted in person if patients still are being counseled, but if they have "graduated," they are completed via phone. If patients do not return calls, a questionnaire is sent via mail. Currently, the database is being renovated to prompt these phone calls. Respiratory therapy students and secretarial staff are responsible for completing these calls in an attempt to ensure that patients will report accurate smoking status without feeling compelled to please the counselor.

The quit rates of patients are used to determine "worth" along with revenue and number of patients seen. The quit rates of patients completing the program rank among the best listed in the literature for formal cessation programs. One-month quit rates are 59%, with the one-year quit rate at 33%. The Agency for Healthcare Policy and Research found a range of 20%–27% for interventions similar to our program structure in their meta-analysis *Clinical Practice Guideline #18, Smoking Cessation.*

IUCCNDP also is committed to educating healthcare professionals about issues related to tobacco control. The staff conducts a day-and-a-half workshop for healthcare professionals to educate them on proper diagnosis, treatment, and management of nicotine dependence. IUCCNDP has provided educational programs locally and to healthcare professionals in Mississippi, Tennessee, and, most recently, Alaska. Every year, a number of medical residents and fellows, respiratory therapy students, and psychology students spend time in the clinic learning how to manage the nicotine-dependent patient.

In addition to clinical services, education, and research, IUCCNDP also provides consultations with managed-care organizations, public health agencies, corporations/businesses, and physician offices and serves as a resource for the state of Indiana on tobacco control.

Although it has met challenges specific to the population of smokers in Indiana, it also has met challenges related to referrals. Patients may self-refer, and the majority of patients at IUCCNDP are self-referrals. Obtaining regular referrals from any specific type of practitioner is a challenge. This does not seem to be because of a lack of physician acceptance but rather the result of a lack of knowledge about the program and nicotine dependence. Pulmonologists, family practice physicians, and dentists refer the most patients to the clinic, with OB/GYNs, pediatricians, oncologists, and surgeons referring the fewest.

The challenge of obtaining referrals from practitioners stems from IUCCNDP's small budget for program promotion. The most effective means for this program's promotion has been "word of mouth." Approximately two years ago, a local healthcare facility obtained funding to subsidize the cost of the program for its employees. With frequent announcements in the organizational newsletter and a significant reduction in the program cost, this became the source of the majority of referrals for the program. Recently, the funding for the project ran out and resulted in a significant increase in the cost to the employees. The clinic has experienced a dramatic decrease in the number of employee enrollments since then. A few television or radio programs have been aired, but they have not produced an abundance of referrals. Newspaper articles have been the most effective means of program promotion, producing a significant number of calls and resulting in patient enrollment.

The other major challenge has been to provide a high-quality, highly effective, clinical program for a cost that patients can afford. Patients are billed directly for services; therefore, IUCCNDP does not have data on insurance reimbursement. Many of our patients report that they have been receiving reimbursement when they obtain a letter of medical necessity from their primary-care physician to accompany the claim. However, most insurance plans in our area require a letter of medical necessity.

During the last eight years, this program has been shaped and molded into a state-of-the-art tobacco cessation program. Following the Agency for Health Care Policy and Research (now the Agency for Healthcare Research and Quality) *Clinical Practice Guideline #18, Smoking Cessation* and the recently updated guideline, *Treating Tobacco Use and Dependence*, and using pharmacotherapy that is approved by the U.S. Food and Drug Administration has led to the success of many of the patients in gaining control over their tobacco addiction. This comprehensive model has been very successful, producing quit rates of 59% at one month and 33% at one year.

University of Colorado Comprehensive Cancer Center Cancer Screening Clinic

Linda U. Krebs, RN, PhD, AOCN®

The Early Years: Initial Program Development

The Cancer Screening Program at the University of Colorado Comprehensive Cancer Center (UCCC) began in 1989 through the vision of a breast cancer nurse specialist in collaboration with another nurse specialist, two oncology clinical nurse specialists (CNSs), and an adult nurse practitioner (ANP). The nurses devised the program, and the physicians of the Cancer Center and the University of Colorado Hospital (UCH) oncology program supported it. The nurses were supported through positions within UCCC, UCH, or the University of Colorado School of Nursing. The clinic was designed to be entirely nurse-run, with medical consultation when needed. The identified clientele were adults who were asymptomatic for cancer. The format included a comprehensive risk assessment and review, a comprehensive physical examination, risk evaluation and counseling, education for self-examinations and risk reduction, and referral to medical healthcare providers, as warranted. The original clinic met one-half day per week and saw between 8 and 12 patients per clinic. Initial barriers to clinic development and implementation included acceptance by the department of nursing and occasional "turf battles" between general internal medicine and the clinic for responsibilities in conducting cancer screenings. Nursing department concerns related to the idea of a somewhat independent nursing practice that would exist outside of the department's direct oversight (the clinic would be a component of UCCC, and only some of the practitioners were employed solely by the hospital) and how direct authority and responsibility for comprehensive nursing practice would be maintained. In general, the physician colleagues were more supportive than the nursing colleagues and have provided medical backup and support throughout. Patients were generated though ads in the paper, flyers, and word of mouth. Patients ranged in age from 10 years to more than 90 years and included almost equal numbers of men and women. The majority of patients were Caucasian with some college education.

The Middle Years: Clinic Revision and Outreach Expansion

In the early 1990s, two clinic staff members wrote a training grant to the Division of Nursing in the Department of Health and Human Services to fund an outreach educational program for rural nurses. This three-year program, which was funded for $496,000, was designed to teach nurses in rural settings how to incorporate cancer screening into daily nursing practice. More than 60 nurses participated in the 20-month curriculum that was conducted in four rural Colorado sites. The nurses participated in five one-and-a-half-day workshops that included both didactic and clinical experiences, culminating in a community clinic that provided a clinical practicum for each student. In between workshops, the participants practiced their screening skills and maintained journals and logs to document skills development. Additionally, students developed educational materials, conducted staff inservices, and identified patient populations for continued screening activities within their communities. As a result of this grant and changes within the institution, several of the original practitioners left the clinic, and an additional CNS from the grant staff joined the screening clinic faculty. The clinic continued on a weekly basis and served as a practicum site/educational experience for undergraduate and graduate nursing students and occasionally as a site for educational experiences for medical students and interns. Patients continued to be generated through intermittent ads placed in local newspapers that announced the availability of low-cost cancer screening at UCCC/UCH. Patients called in for appointments, and usually a long waiting list resulted from each advertisement. The format for the clinic remained unchanged as a nurse-run clinic with medical backup.

For several years, the clinic staff was limited to one or two practitioners who saw patients intermittently. The majority of patients seen were those who previously had been in the clinic and were returning on a yearly basis or who were referred by previous and continuing patients. Clinic services and procedures remained unchanged.

The Current Clinic: Revamping and Expanding

In early 2000, two oncology nurse practitioners (an ANP and a FNP) joined one of the original oncology CNSs (now PhD-prepared) to revamp the clinic and expand services. With support from both UCCC and UCH, the clinic now is available for patient visits four days per week, with evening hours one day per week and early morning hours two days per week. Two practitioners are available to see patients each day. Many challenges have been faced in revitalizing the clinic. Patient accrual has been extremely slow as opposed to previous experience. Ads have been placed in the newspapers and on the radio as part of a major campaign, but they are limited in their information about cancer screening. Thus, the response to these ads has been minimal. Small ads in local papers, including the UCH Senior's newsletter and university publications, have been more successful in drawing patients, many of whom are retired and in their 70s and 80s. Word of mouth continues to provide a number of patients each week. However, if accrual remains low, modifications to the screening clinic schedule, including decreasing the number of days or number of hours per day of clinic operations, may be instituted.

As part of the redevelopment, the role of medical director was instituted, and nurse practitioners developed screening guidelines to ensure congruence among all practitioners about high-risk assessment and routine follow-up procedures. Staff members discussed these guidelines, and members of the appropriate medical staff reviewed them. All clinic materials were reevaluated, and the clinic risk assessment was revised and shortened. The risk assessment is mailed to the patient a minimum of one week prior to the appointment, and the completed form is brought to the appointment. The form is reviewed with the patient prior to the physical examination, and it, along with the findings from the examination, is used to formulate educational interventions and follow-up recommendations. Each patient is provided with a packet of relevant cancer screening education materials and a specific individualized plan for risk reduction, self-examinations, planned follow-up, and appropriate referrals. Referrals may be for follow-up of a suspicious lesion, routine screening such as a mammogram, a chemoprevention or early-detection trial such as a sputum cytology study, or one of the high-risk or hereditary cancer clinics for evaluation and recommendations.

Each practitioner accomplishes patient follow-up. The patients seen are discussed at a weekly conference, and all clinic issues, including program promotion and program-related concerns, are discussed at that time. Reminder systems need to be developed as do a patient database and tracking system. Currently, spreadsheets are used to follow patients through the clinic and for follow-up.

Funding

Funding sources have varied since the clinic's inception. Initially, UCCC, the UCH, and the University of Colorado School of Nursing provided funding. For much of the 1990s, funding was received through federal grant sources and then UCCC and the School of Nursing. Current funding is through the University of Colorado Hospital oncology program, with support from UCCC. Each of the practitioners has additional professional responsibilities. Approximately 40% of each nurse practitioner's time is allocated to screening, and initial support for the PhD-prepared CNS is 50%. Both nurse practitioners independently see patients with cancer and also work in collaboration with the UCCC physicians, primarily in the areas of phase I clinical trials and lung cancer. The CNS has responsibilities at UCCC and the School of Nursing. As the nurse practitioners' responsibilities grow within their own independent and collaborative practices, they may see a decrease in screening clinic responsibilities, particularly if patient participation does not increase. In fall 2000, UCH began to support the CNS 25%. Additional time will be supported through UCCC, as is needed to coordinate and maintain a minimum two-day practice. Currently, the clinic is not income generating, but it is hoped that it will be in the future.

Clinic Evaluation

Since its inception, evaluation procedures have been an essential component of clinic activities. Several small grants were submitted to conduct an evaluation of screening clinic outcomes, and summer students carried out evaluative procedures. Evaluations included satisfaction questions in regard to services provided and follow-up of clinic recommendations. At the time of the initial clinic visit, all patients were invited to participate in short-term follow-up that included a telephone interview about cancer screening practices three to six months after the cancer screening visit occurred. At the time of the visit, the patient was asked about his or her current self-examination and cancer screening practices and information about diet and tobacco use. At the completion of the visit, patients were provided with specific recommendations for risk reduction, self-examination, and referral/follow-up concerning findings. The short-term follow-up call was designed to assess whether patients were following specific recommendations provided by the nurse screeners, why they were or were not following the recommendations, and the outcome of referrals and follow-up visits to other healthcare practitioners. Patients were asked what they remembered of the screening visit; what they were instructed to do in terms of follow-up, self-examination, and diet; and what they had done. The majority of patients stated they had followed-up for suspicious findings, but only about half were practicing routine self-examinations. The most common reason for not doing them was related to continued insecurity with doing the self-examination satisfactorily.

With major changes in clinic structure and the addition of two nurse practitioners, new evaluation measures need to be developed. Current plans include a satisfaction survey, an evaluation of referral patterns (both referrals from the clinic to other services and referrals to the clinic from satisfied customers), and a continuing tally of the numbers of patients seen.

Current Challenges and a Look Toward the Future

Challenges include rebuilding the program with additional practitioners, ongoing discussions of the scope of practice desired, and insurance and payment issues. This clinic has been focused solely on cancer screening, with an emphasis on asymptomatic individuals. However, other models include follow-up of long-term cancer survivors and evaluation of and referral for illnesses other than cancer. In some instances, patients have wanted all care to be managed by the cancer-screening practitioner, which does not fit with the current goals of the program. Insurance issues have been a continual problem, with new guidelines limiting the clinic's ability to charge one low fee to be paid in cash at the time of the appointment and limiting the scope of screening packages that legally can be offered. As with any evolving program, growing pains bring new problems and new solutions that must be discussed and managed if the program is to survive.

Having been a part of the clinic since its inception has allowed me to give a careful evaluation of its evolution. As nursing practice has changed in the last 11 years, so have the focus of cancer care and the role of prevention and early detection. Nurses now have the opportunity to make a positive difference in cancer outcomes through independent and collaborative practices aimed at decreasing cancer risk and facilitating early diagnosis. Nurse-run clinics allow nurses to use all of their skills in promoting health and well-being. This clinic has grown both in size, hours, and scope and is an exciting place to practice quality cancer care and make a difference in patient outcomes.

Tertiary Prevention in Long-Term Survivors of Breast Cancer

Suzanne M. Mahon, RN, DNSc, AOCN®, APNG(c)

As more and more women are successfully treated for breast cancer, there is an ever-growing population of women at risk for developing second malignancies of the breast, colon, ovary, endometrium, and skin, as well as osteoporosis because of estrogen deficiency. These problems can lead to long-term morbidity and mortality in breast cancer survivors. Providing tertiary cancer prevention services is an ever-expanding area of cancer control.

In the fall of 1999, a program was initiated in the outpatient area of the Saint Louis University, Division of Hematology and Oncology, to ensure that women receive education and appropriate screening for second malignancies and osteoporosis. Saint Louis University is located in an urban area of a large Midwestern city. The university serves individuals from a 150-mile radius, many of whom are medically underserved. A large number of phase I, II, and III clinical trials are available to individuals receiving care at the university; many patients seek care here because of these trials.

The development of programs to ensure that long-term survivors of cancer receive screening for second malignancies and osteoporosis has been slow. Findings from a descriptive study of Oncology Nursing Society (ONS) members conducted during 1999 suggested that few research or office protocols exist to ensure that tertiary cancer prevention services are offered to cancer survivors (Mahon, Williams, & Spies, 2000). The program at Saint Louis University was developed to meet this need and has been written as a research protocol to accurately assess the effectiveness of the program. ONS has funded this research.

The program requires the cooperation of physicians, nurses, and staff in the outpatient area. Physicians and their case manager (a registered nurse) who see patients with breast cancer identify women who completed treatment at least two years ago who also have good prognostic factors. These women are scheduled at their next follow-up appointment to not only see the physician, as they routinely do, but also the advanced practice nurse for education and screening recommendations. A one-hour appointment is scheduled for this education. The patients are informed that they will be seeing this nurse and of the purpose of the visit, and they are encouraged to write down any questions they may want to discuss during the appointment. Presently, there is no additional charge to see the advanced practice nurse. It is considered a service provided by the university to the patients in the outpatient area.

On the day of the appointment, the advanced practice nurse completes a risk assessment to better understand the woman's individual risk for second malignancies and osteoporosis. This includes a family history, medication, medical history and, lifestyle history. The information is considered, and risks for second malignancies and osteoporosis are discussed with the woman.

A standardized program of patient education is initiated at this point. The advanced practice nurse has designed a flip chart to ensure that all content is covered in a consistent manner. The flip chart has been produced in Microsoft® PowerPoint® and includes text, pictures, and graphs. Each page is kept in a plastic sheet. This allows pages to be updated, replaced, and added easily. The flip chart is divided into sections: breast cancer, menopause, osteoporosis, gynecologic cancer, colon cancer, and skin cancer. Each section contains information on the incidence of the problem, anatomical illustrations, risk factors, signs and symptoms, methods for primary prevention, methods for secondary prevention, and questions the patient might want to ask for more information.

When appropriate, women are instructed on self-examination of the breast and skin. Women who have had breast surgery are instructed on self-examination of the incision scar and the unaffected breast. This also is usually a good time to check if the woman is having any difficulties with bra or prosthesis fit and to remind the woman about strategies to prevent lymphedema.

The information given during the didactic session and self-examination instruction is supplemented with other patient-education materials the patient can take home, including print pieces and videotapes. This allows patients to learn at their own pace and in their preferred style.

Following the self-examination and other education, there is an opportunity to discuss appropriate screening strategies. If the patient desires, these screening examinations are scheduled at the end of the appointment, or the patient can schedule with their primary-care physician.

A follow-up appointment is made with the advanced practice nurse for the next time the patient is scheduled to see the oncologist. This provides an opportunity to offer additional clarification and review the results of any screening completed. Consideration of the risk assessment and the results of the screening guide future screening recommendations. For example, if a woman is found to have a negative colonoscopy, a follow-up colonoscopy is recommended in five years. If a polyp(s) is detected during colonoscopy, a follow-up colonoscopy is indicated in one year.

To date, 27 women have been evaluated in the program. Many had questions about menopause symptoms and management. This content also is now included in the education. Women repeatedly have commented that they had no idea they were at increased risk for developing colon cancer or osteoporosis. Many are surprised to learn their risk is higher than women in the general population. Few have had prior colorectal cancer screening even if they are older than 50 years of age, when it is routinely recommended in the general population.

Despite the fact that many of the women have been or presently are on tamoxifen, many have experienced bone loss probably related to estrogen deficiency. These women require treatment with an agent such as alendronate. Education about how to appropriately take a bisphosphonate, primary methods of osteoporosis prevention, and follow-up screening are all components discussed in the follow-up appointment. This education is supplemented by videos and written material for patients to use in their home.

Many women also have commented that they appreciate the general information they receive about menopause during the session. This includes information such as what menopause is, risks that increase at menopause, and management of vasomotor symptoms. This need is addressed in both the initial and follow-up appointments. A booklet written by the advanced practice nurse titled *Understanding Menopause and Beyond* is given to women when deemed appropriate. Research suggests that women may find such written materials helpful (Mahon & Williams, 2000).

A key to the success of the program is teaching the staff how to recognize and refer women for the education and screening recommendations. Advanced practice nurses have provided didactic education to the nurses through their journal club, as well as to the residents, fellows, and attending physicians about these risks in survivors. A major responsibility of the advanced practice nurse is to enhance the care the patients receive and conduct continued epidemiologic research on the incidence and effectiveness of screening for second malignancies and osteoporosis. Without the cooperation of all of the members of the multidisciplinary team, it would be impossible to ensure the patients are referred for the screening and education.

As the program continues to grow, care is being taken to ensure that the findings from the screening are considered from an epidemiologic perspective. The exact incidence of second malignancies and osteoporosis in survivors is not known. This program is carefully monitoring the incidence of these complications in cancer survivors, with the goal of ultimately providing more accurate risk assessments and detecting these complications earlier. The impact of the program on quality of life and particularly the adjustment to having a cancer diagnosis also is being considered.

As women are educated and counseled about these risks, it is performed in a nonthreatening manner. Reminding the patients that they should not consider this appointment as "bad news" but as "good news" always opens the session. The physician and others involved in the woman's care believe the prognosis to be good and that the woman could live long enough to develop a second malignancy or osteoporosis. Care is taken to stress that the healthcare providers do not want these complications to go undetected and ultimately compromise quality of life. Services such as tertiary cancer screening are important in the total rehabilitation of the cancer survivor with the goal of ultimately decreasing the morbidity and mortality associated with breast cancer.

References

Mahon, S.M., & Williams, M. (2000). Information needs regarding menopause: Results from a survey of women receiving cancer prevention and detection services. *Cancer Nursing, 23,* 176–185.

Mahon, S.M., Williams, M.T., & Spies, M.A. (2000). Screening for second cancers and osteoporosis in long-term survivors. *Cancer Practice, 8*, 282–290.

Breast Health Outreach

Diane McElwain, RN, OCN®, MEd

The Breast Health Outreach Program began as a project for a newly established cancer center—the York Breast Health Coalition of York County, PA. The organization was formed by several agencies that felt a need to combine resources to plan breast health awareness programs. This group applied for and successfully won three consecutive Avon Breast Health Grants. The awards were as follows: 1994–$15,000, 1995–$29,555, and 1996–$29,310. During the three years with the grant, a program was developed that included flip charts, breast models, packets with breast health information, and videotapes of self-breast examinations and mammograms. Members of the coalition solicited sites for the program to be held (e.g., individuals' homes, church groups, industrial sites, senior centers). In addition to attending the breast health programs, women were able to arrange for a breast examination with a volunteer physician and have an opportunity to schedule a mammogram. During the second year of the grant, two ethnic community health workers were hired to penetrate the African American and Hispanic communities to find women in hard-to-reach areas.

The outcomes of the Breast Health Outreach were multifold. More than 2,800 women were educated in a three-year period in 233 sessions. In addition, women received 370 breast examinations and 161 mammograms. The ethnic range was 45% Caucasian, 21% African American, and 33% Hispanic. More than 45% of the women were older than age 40, a specific requirement of the criteria for the Avon Breast Health Grant. The remaining women were older than 20. Although some teenage ethnic women were educated, the numbers were not recorded because they did not fall within the grant's criteria.

In the follow-up patient survey, 75% of the women found the small group setting very comfortable for sensitive health information. Another 75% said that they would attend another breast health awareness program, suggesting that women prefer to have this type of information repeated more that once. Hiring the two community health workers increased the percentages of ethnic women participating in the program. These workers are necessary to penetrate their ethnic communities and break down barriers such as language and familiarity.

When the grant period ended, the Breast Health Outreach continued under the oncology nurse educator. The York Breast Health Coalition reorganized into a Partner's in Women's Health Coalition and expanded its mission to include information about osteoporosis, heart disease, and breast cancer. The same agency partners exist, but the educational focus has expanded.

The final year of the grant coincided with the Healthy Woman 50+ program from the Pennsylvania Department of Health. This program provided recruitment funds that enabled the hiring of two ethnic community health workers already associated with the Avon Grant. These workers perform one-on-one recruitment and arrange sites for the nurse educator to give breast health programs. These contacts have proven to be very successful in local sites, and the community health workers and nurse have been invited back regularly for Breast Health Outreach.

The Mother's Day Mammogram Program, developed through the Rite Aid Corporation and the Pennsylvania Breast Cancer Coalition, also dovetails with these breast outreach programs. The same nurse educator is the county contact for the toll-free Mother's Day Mammogram phone number. After a short interview with the caller about her need of a Pap smear, the nurse arranges free mammograms and appointments for clinical examinations through the Healthy Woman 50+ program.

The Breast Outreach Program has provided education sessions on breast health for 1,200 women in 39 locations in the fiscal year (7/98 through 6/99). At this point, the program has stopped tracking mammograms and Pap smears because of the variety of settings in which they occur. Referrals can be tracked through the Mother's Day Mammogram Project, numbers seen in the Healthy Woman sites, and free mammogram vouchers through the local American Cancer Society. It has become generally known that the nurse educator can be called at the cancer center to assist women without insurance with annual examinations any time of the year.

In the spirit of the breast health program's success, the nurse educator also started prostate cancer screenings in the community. This has been conducted twice in York with the Black Minister's Association. This program has targeted the African American community and offered prostate-specific antigens (PSAs), rectal examinations, blood pressure checks, and cholesterol and diabetic screenings. The numbers in this effort have been small (56 men in 1998, 12 men in 1999), but the Black Minister's Association has asked that the effort be continued. The cancer center leads the organization of this effort. The oncology nurse educator performs follow-up of the rectal examinations and PSA results. The City Health Department staff follows up on abnormal diabetic, cholesterol, and blood pressure screenings.

The staffing for these programs basically is limited to the oncology nurse educator and two community workers. Help is solicited from the hospital staff for laboratory personnel to perform blood draws and diabetic and cardiac nurse educators. The cost for supplies, mailings, reports, and occasional refreshments is absorbed by the cancer center. The hospital laboratory has a program that covers the cost of the cholesterol screenings and charges the cancer center a fee of $24 per PSA. The total costs for the two prostate screening programs are estimated to be under $500.

Program promotions are a constant challenge. Flyers are distributed throughout the community with the help of various agency partners, the Black Church Network, and local free community newsletters. Sometimes, the program gets effective coverage through a local newspaper article. The program has had excellent physician support for providing clinical examinations when needed. The physician volunteers have included private physicians as well as resident physicians from the York Hospital teaching program.

As always, evaluative efforts are difficult. At this time, the cancer center is interested in distributing information necessary to assist patients in starting an informed conversation with their physician about screening needs. A physician referral system is available for those participants who need this service for follow-up. On the registration forms for the programs, most of the patients served have a physician whom they can contact. Program sites are chosen in areas where we hope to find the medically underserved. So far, since 1993, there have been few problems with clinical follow-up for positive results because the York Hospital is the main provider in the community and has an excellent clinic referral system.

Breast Health Access for Women With Disabilities

Shirley McKenzie, RN, BSN, OCN®

Breast Health Access for Women With Disabilities (BHAWD) is a program that provides breast health education and screening for women age 20 and older who have physical disabilities that prevent them from getting thorough clinical breast examinations (CBEs) and mammograms. BHAWD is an innovative health education and screening model that was initiated to serve women with muscular, skeletal, and neurological disabilities.

BHAWD is a program of rehabilitation services that is located at Alta Bates Medical Center in Berkeley, CA. Services include
- Breast self-examination (BSE) instruction using the MammaCare® method
- CBE using a specially designed examination table that allows many women who use wheelchairs to transfer to the table without assistance
- Mammograms using the Bennett Contour Mammography machine with tilting capability and a pedestal design that accommodates most women in wheelchairs. It is also helpful to women with movement disorders or stamina issues who need to sit for a mammogram.

The program concept originated in December 1994, when a woman with cerebral palsy, who was receiving treatment for breast cancer, asked an oncology nurse what a woman should do if she could not perform BSE. Her question led the oncology nurse to leaders in the disability community in search of resources. When no local programs or resources were identified, each person initially contacted became interested in participating in a committee to develop a solution.

BHAWD was created through the collaboration of Alta Bates Medical Center's Board of Trustees, Comprehensive Breast Center, Foundation, and Rehabilitation Departments. The following community organizations also have been involved: United Cerebral Palsy, Center for Independent Living, and Community Resources for Independent Living. This multidisciplinary committee is composed of a representative from each group that initially researched the issue of lack of access to breast screening for women with disabilities.

Using telephone inquiries and a literature search, committee members discovered that neither major healthcare providers nor social service organizations offered, or knew of, programs with an emphasis on breast health for women in wheelchairs or for those with serious motor, muscular, or neurological conditions. To document the need for this program, a working conference on accessible breast health care was held. Surveys also were conducted in the medical community and among leaders of the disability community. The purpose was to establish a basis for program funding by documenting what previously was learned from these informal conversations. This work led to the successful funding from several organizations and enabled the clinic to be opened.

The BHAWD committee remains the planning and development group for the program. A manager, a scheduler, a nurse practitioner with a rehabilitation specialty, and an oncology nurse with a breast health/breast cancer specialty staff the program. Both nurses are MammaCare specialists.

The clinic opened in April 1997 and is available 20 hours a week, Monday through Friday. Since its opening, BHAWD has provided MammaCare instruction and CBE to more than 500 women with physical disabilities. Many others have been served through outreach efforts, health fairs, and lectures to specific groups such as the deaf community and senior centers. Current outreach targets women whose disabilities occurred later in life through stroke, injury, or chronic illness. Additional outreach efforts focus on educating and increasing awareness among medical professionals and individual organizations that provide cancer screening and early detection.

BHAWD has faced many challenges, with one of the most difficult being educating funding sources regarding the needs of women with disabilities. Until recently, this population was not listed as underserved. Funding organizations did not acknowledge that a significant need for this service existed. Another challenge has been outreach, which is more complex than outreach to other subgroups because women with disabilities do not share a common language or ethnic background.

In addition, outreach needs to target not only a woman with a disability but also her caregiver. Scheduling is complex because it may involve coordinating transportation or an attendant. When an appointment is scheduled, a packet of information is sent to each woman. This includes history and assessment forms that she may need assistance in filling out. Currently, funds are available to assist women in paying for transportation and attendant care if they prefer to bring a trusted person with them. Translation services also are available.

Women seen in the clinic have an initial visit, which includes individualized MammaCare instruction in BSE, and a CBE (see Figure 20-2). The nurse instructs the woman about the nodularity in her breast tissue and assesses her level of ability in performing a BSE. This appointment may last up to two hours but can be divided into two one-hour sessions, depending on the patient's stamina. Yearly follow-up visits are standard for CBE, but a woman may elect to be seen as frequently as quarterly if she cannot do an adequate BSE. There is no charge for these services.

Women who need mammograms are given referrals. If they are uninsured or underinsured, donated funds cover the cost. A research project currently is being conducted to look at the prevalence and type of barriers to breast screening among

Figure 20-2. Breast Self-Exam Instruction Protocol

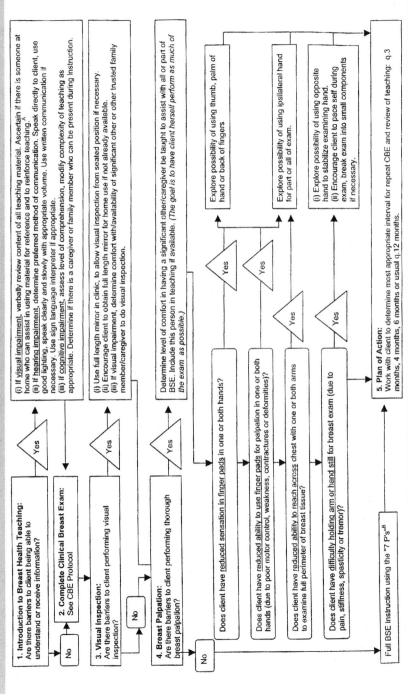

women with disabilities. It also is assessing the outreach, education, and service delivery strategies of BHAWD and what changes are needed. A manual is being developed to outline the BHAWD model and will be available for dissemination at the end of the project.

BHAWD's purpose is to increase breast health awareness among women with disabilities, to provide a clinic where women may come for more frequent CBEs if they are unable to do a BSE, and to increase awareness among healthcare professionals about the needs of this underserved group.

CONVERSATIONS!: The International Ovarian Cancer Connection

Cindy H. Melancon

CONVERSATIONS! is an international newsletter for those fighting ovarian cancer and similarly treated peritoneal and fallopian tube cancers. The purpose of the newsletter is to provide a source of support, hope, and information for women who are diagnosed with these cancers, their loved ones, and the healthcare professionals who care for them. After several years of dedicated work, a cancer control program developed within the unique framework of a simple newsletter. The account of my experience is offered so that other nurses might set out to develop "simple ideas" that have the potential to take on a life of their own.

The newsletter evolved from my personal battle with ovarian cancer. On February 3, 1992, I was diagnosed with stage III-c ovarian cancer. Among all the people I came in contact with during six months of intensive treatment and two major surgeries, I could not find another survivor of ovarian cancer. Needless to say, I felt there was no hope for me. In the summer of 1993, I placed an ad in *Networker*, the quarterly newsletter of the National Coalition for Cancer Survivorship: "Wanted: Contact with someone with a diagnosis of ovarian cancer." Within days of its mailing, 10 women from around the country phoned, and we began a lively exchange of information. One woman would mention a problem and another would offer a solution. Because I was the only one in our group with a computer and word processing skills, I became the hub of our informational wheel.

On Halloween 1993, the first issue was mailed to 10 women. The newsletter had no name, no funding, no special publishing or mailing software, no office, no office equipment, no employees, and no formal mission statement or list of goals. The one thing it did have going for it was a driving need to share and communicate personal feelings and experiences related to ovarian cancer. Each four-page issue was mailed weekly. Within three months, there were about 40 women on the mailing list, all of whom discovered the newsletter through word-of-mouth.

Soon, the concept of the newsletter's mission was clearly articulated: to support those who are fighting ovarian cancer (i.e., the woman who is diagnosed and her family, friends, and healthcare providers). The highest form of emotional support is to give someone hope, and seven areas of hope make up *CONVERSATIONS!*

- Hope for a better today involves sharing tips to cope with side effects of the disease and treatment. To facilitate that sharing, about 400 letters, e-mails, and phone calls are answered each week; tips are compiled into summaries for frequently asked questions; and the Web site (www.Ovarian-news.com) is continually under construction with new features. The questions are answered using scientifically based information and consultations with qualified healthcare providers; other resources are contacted as appropriate. However, the newsletter does not provide medical opinion. The newsletter is liberally sprinkled with humor, reflecting the belief that laughter promotes healing and improves quality of life.

- Hope for a better tomorrow leads to discussions of various treatment options, recently completed clinical research trials, open clinical trials, and experiences of others who have tried treatments that are beyond the standard initial therapy.

- Hope for decreased stress on family and friends demands discovery of useful resources for services (especially free ones), equipment, and other supportive organizations. For those with concerns about cancer prevention in family members, resources for genetic counseling and research about risk-reduction techniques are reported.

- Hope for finding a better treatment involves an ongoing search for books, conferences, and Web sites. Finding and verifying all newsletter content, especially in the area of treatment, is performed by collaborating with an extensive network of specialists and other professionals in various fields.

- Hope for connection and to feel less isolated led to the creation of a pen pal Survivor-to-Fighter matching service, which substantiates that others are dealing with the same things the reader is experiencing. The matching is based upon criteria specified by the requestor (e.g., an unusual treatment, an unusual cell type of ovarian cancer). The requestor is matched with several other subscribers who have given me written permission to share their name with others. Matches can be based upon about 100 different criteria. Frequently, those matched will exchange ideas and become friends. In addition, a listing of support groups is available both on paper and on the Web site.

- Hope for making some sense in the struggle means that the newsletter provides an avenue for contribution of learned lessons, giving each person a voice. Occasionally subscribers are offered the opportunity to participate in an ovarian cancer–focused research study. Opportunities for promoting awareness about ovarian cancer via local, state, and national groups are listed, as well as openings on panels, such as those convened by the National Cancer Institute or the Department of Defense Ovarian Cancer Research Program, which determine the direction for future research in ovarian cancer.

- Hope for survival has produced the newsletter's most unique features. Each month a gold-colored page of Survivor Anniversaries lists the names of those diagnosed in that particular month, arranged by year of diagnosis. This offers tangible proof that it is possible to survive for years after diagnosis, and many subscribers say that they work toward the goal of being featured on this page. Because cancer and its treatment are often impersonal, I have tried to keep the newsletter format and style as personalized as possible. It begins and ends with a vignette and an inspirational thought. The newsletter is formatted in letter style (rather than in columns) to appear more friendly. Drawings are used to illustrate a point, add humor, or soften a stressful concept. Being artistically challenged, my drawings are mostly stick figures or adapted from children's coloring books. The language is clear and informal, and I use simple terms to explain very complex information.

Today, there are more than 3,500 subscribers in 20 countries. The actual number who read the newsletter each month is unknown, as it is frequently copied in large numbers for distribution by physicians, social workers, cancer centers, and support group facilitators. (The newsletter is copyrighted but, in keeping with its mission, permission is given within the header of each issue to make copies for distribution to other cancer fighters.) Over the past nine years, the newsletter has served as a source of support for more than 10,000 subscribers and their families. The newsletter also has made possible access to a large population for survey work. Voluntary donations and the support of my family, including manpower and financial backing, have made this possible. With volunteer help, the financial structure was eventually formalized into a 501-c-3 not-for-profit corporation.

To keep expenses to a minimum, many creative avenues were explored, from doing it all ourselves to having the newsletter printed by a commercial printer and enlisting help from the local Retired Senior Volunteer Program (RSVP) to fold the issues and prepare the mailing. Thankfully, RSVP volunteers are still at it today with 3,500 issues each month. My labor was pro bono until 1999. When I found myself working about 60–80 hours each week, I hired and trained a part-time person. There is a need for another. Because of confidentiality issues and extensive database training requirements, it is difficult to find qualified help. The best candidates for employment have come through friends and church.

In response to increasing postage costs, the newsletter evolved from four pages weekly to four pages every two weeks to a monthly 10-page issue printed with a smaller, clearer font and tighter margins. This shift allows the same information to be sent with one first-class stamp. Rather than using bulk rate for mailing, it was a conscious decision to pay the first-class rate to ensure timely delivery because the newsletter always has time-sensitive information.

Over the years, the newsletter spread from room to room of my house, a little here and a little there. Six months ago, I set up a formal office in one room, but an office outside of the home will be more feasible when additional personnel are trained and affordable office space is found.

Obtaining a large grant would be the answer to funding challenges, but finding and applying for grants is a full-time job in itself. In keeping with the mission of the newsletter, I spend all of my time in providing support for those fighting this disease. In addition, there seem to be very few grants available to fund a newsletter. Another hurdle arises concerning money from pharmaceutical companies. Because the newsletter discusses chemotherapy, accepting funds from drug manufacturers would raise conflict of interest questions in my mind. The last challenge of my venture that I want to mention is related to my initial lack of vision about its future. Because I dealt with an initially very poor prognosis by refusing to look at or plan for the future, and because the newsletter started as a simple exchange of information among friends, I did *not* plan well for its potential for growth. At that critical time in my life, I was unable to dream about anything. Instead, I focused on the day-to-day needs of the newsletter and its subscribers. My clear-cut goal of serving ovarian cancer survivors somehow resulted in a subscriber list that has doubled every 12 months. When evaluating the effectiveness of the newsletter, all that is required is to read the mail or answer the phone. The subscribers are a vocal and responsive group and do not hesitate to provide feedback. Because women find copies in their physicians' waiting rooms, cancer center treatment rooms, or at support group meetings, I know that the newsletter has been found to be medically sound, well balanced between technical and lay language, and worth passing along. Some women report that their oncologists give them copies of the various question-and-answer summaries. However, the best method of evaluating the newsletter's worth is that its readership continues to grow.

Every organization must have a goal for the future. In a newsletter's day-to-day activities, the goals are driven by the needs of the subscribers. Although it is tempting to branch out into other areas, I have chosen to stay focused on providing support for those who are fighting ovarian cancer. My ultimate goal is to play a part in eradicating this disease from the earth for all time. A cure may not come in my lifetime, but it is that hope that sustains me. I want to go out of business because ovarian cancer is preventable and curable!

Buddy Check™ 10: A Breast Cancer Awareness Program

Patti Moser, RN, BSN, OCN®

Buddy Check™ 10 is a breast cancer awareness program offered by Via Christi Cancer Center, a not-for-profit community teaching hospital in Wichita, KS, and KAKE 10 NEWS, a local broadcast news station. The goal of the program is to increase breast cancer awareness by promoting breast self-examination (BSE), clinical breast examination (CBE), and mammograms for all women but especially for those who are at high risk for developing breast cancer. Personnel involved in the program include an oncology certified registered nurse, a hospital marketing department, local broadcast media, a hospital call center, and hospital volunteers. Program funding sources are provided through the oncology service line marketing budget and broadcast media. The program focuses on finding a "buddy" or friend and reminding them to perform monthly BSE and obtain an annual CBE with a mammogram.

Women receive a free packet of information asking them to recognize the importance of breast cancer screening by calling the hospital call center or dropping a postage-paid registration form in the mail. The call center provides a mechanism for participants to register by phone. It is staffed eight hours a day by registered nurses and data entry staff. A voice message can be left to request a Buddy Check 10 packet when the call center is closed. When registering by mail, a buddy is identified, and she is sent a free packet of information as well. Each participant identifies the following baseline information when completing the registration form.

- How to perform BSE
- Level of confidence, from 1–10, in performing accurate BSE
- Frequency of BSE
- Frequency of CBE
- Frequency of mammogram

These baseline data are used to determine increased participant knowledge of how to do a BSE, increased level of confidence in BSE, and increased number of participants following the breast cancer screening guidelines as recommended by the American Cancer Society.

The Buddy Check 10 packet includes a shower card with BSE instructions, information about breast cancer, and reminder stickers to place on a calendar. The calendar stickers are placed on the 10th of each month. On that day, KAKE 10 News evening newscast spotlights a story on breast cancer and reminds each woman to call her buddy to make sure she is performing her monthly BSEs.

Upon registration into the Buddy Check 10 program, each participant receives a quarterly newsletter, *Buddy to Buddy.* The newsletter is produced by the Via Christi Cancer Center and contains up-to-date information about breast cancer (see Appendix 20-1). Some newsletter topics have included current clinical trials, research results, nutrition, BSE in special circumstances, and community resources for free mammograms. Planned future topics include how to determine accurate inernet health information, hormone replacement therapy, and other topics identified by program participants.

The program could not exist without hospital volunteers, who create Buddy Check 10 packets by filling the envelopes with the contents. They also apply mailing labels to the quarterly newsletter.

The program has undergone many changes since its inception two years ago. The program kickoff was February 1998, with a televised broadcast inviting women to sign up for the program. Healthcare professionals from the Via Christi Cancer Center provided staffing for the on-air phone bank, accepting phone registrations and answering questions about breast cancer. At that time, the registration process included a card asking for the participant's name, address, and date of birth. A packet of information was mailed to the participant. The participant then identified their buddy by returning a "Buddy Card" listing her name and address. The buddy then was mailed a packet of information. Of the 4,500 packets distributed within the first year of the program, less than 15% of the "Buddy Cards" were returned. Because of such a low return of these cards for buddy registration, the card was eliminated, and buddy registration was included with participant registration on the new brochure registration forms.

Program data are tracked by the hospital call center. Data collection has changed from tracking the number of packets distributed at each event or activity to a monthly report of the number of packets distributed and the number of participants registered in the database. The data collected were simplified because of the enormous amount of resources used to complete the process required for coding registration cards and packets by event. This process required manual application of a marker code to each registration card, counting registration cards and packets for distribution, and counting the cards and packets after the event for the total distributed.

The stakeholders, including an oncology certified nurse, hospital marketing personnel, a hospital call center registered nurse, and a participant, held a brainstorming session to identify a simplified registration process. The group decided to change the registration card to a brochure with a tear-off postage-paid registration form and a point-of-service display for the brochures. Each lightweight and portable point-of-service display, approximately 12" x 18", described the program and offered mail-in registration brochures in a pocket. Because demographics from the old registration card only identified age and zip code, the brochure registration added the demographics of sex and race. The additional demographic information will help to determine if the program is reaching identified populations.

Finding stories to assist the media for the monthly newscast is challenging. The medical community and professional and community organizations have provided patient stories. The media is informed of upcoming clinical trials, new treatments, and community events addressing breast cancer. Obtaining breast cancer stories using the January 1999 survey (see Appendix 20-2) was unsuccessful.

All registrations are entered into the hospital call center database. This database provides the mailing addresses for the *Buddy to Buddy* newsletter. The first edition of the newsletter was printed in June 1999. Additional newsletters have been mailed in October 1999 and January 2000. Returned mailings helped to identify a limitation with the call center computer software. The database has limited applications for address updates. Updating addresses is a manual process requiring recoding the initial tracking code. This limitation in software is a financial and staffing resource concern. More than 250 newsletters were returned with the January 2000 mailing, an expense of more than $130. Staff resources were used to remove reusable contents of the returned newsletters. The call center is in the process of identifying a software upgrade that will provide a simplified method for address updates.

A January 1999 survey was mailed to 3,578 participants identified in the hospital call center database. The survey objectives were to determine
- Demographics of the participants
- BSE educational needs
- BSE learning modality preference
- Results of BSE
- Changes detected by BSE
- Medical consultation sought upon finding a change during BSE
- Diagnostic intervention(s) recommended
- Program impact on the life of the participant
- Stories to further promote program awareness.

The number of survey returns anticipated was 357, or 10%. The actual number of returned surveys was 480, or 13%. Eighty-three women indicated detecting a change when performing BSE.

The cancer center is interested in determining revenue linked to the Buddy Check 10 program. Currently, the hospital call center database containing participant information does not interface with the hospital's financial reporting system.

The call center manager is in search of a compatible computer software program that will provide a financial reconciliation report to the oncology service line.

In the program's first evaluative efforts, the January 1999 survey results were compiled and analyzed using the Statistics Program for Social Sciences (SPSS®). The survey results provided guidance in the development of the *Buddy to Buddy* newsletter. The baseline data currently being collected on the brochure registration form will be used to measure an increase in breast screening behavior and increased knowledge of how to perform BSE. The evaluation efforts will be completed on an annual basis.

The Buddy Check 10 program is promoted in a variety of ways. Currently, the program is displayed in more than 70 physician offices. Other mechanisms of program promotion include health fairs, the county health department, congregational health ministry, a mobile mammography van, and presentations. A conservative estimate for the number of presentations by cancer center colleagues, community groups, media personnel, and myself is 150 during the past two years. Many calls are generated for information on the program by word-of-mouth from current participants. Several social organizations have selected the program as their community service project. Information packets have been distributed to 6,954 women, and the *Buddy to Buddy* newsletter is mailed to 4,504 participants.

Development of an Oncology Public Education Plan

Patti Moser, RN, BSN, OCN®

The Oncology Prevention and Early Detection Public Education Program provides a mechanism to measure the outcomes of the activities in which the Via Christi Cancer Center (a not-for-profit teaching hospital in Wichita, KS) coordinates or participates. The services offered through the program include presentations, screenings, awareness activities, lifestyle and behavior change counseling, and a supportive environment for patients with cancer and their families. The program has been in existence for one year. Evaluation of the program's first year revealed the following number of activities offered to specific cancer topics/sites: lung (8), prostate (14), breast (45), colon (12), skin (7), and nutrition (1). The number of activities targeting identified populations included women (52), men (29), children (9), Caucasians (62), African Americans (17), and other minorities (2).

Personnel involved in the program include internal and external team members. Internal team members include one oncology certified registered nurse employed by the cancer center, the hospital call center, staffing needs coordinated with other cancer center colleagues (clinical nurse specialist, advanced registered nurse practitioner, and other registered nurses), the oncology service line leadership team, and the hospital marketing department. External team members include local businesses, local broadcast and print media, local physicians, the American Cancer Society, the Leukemia and Lymphoma Society, the Susan G. Komen Foundation, Victory in the Valley, Inc., and Us Too Prostate Cancer Support Group. Funding for the education plan comes from the cancer center's marketing budget, local broadcast and print media, and business partnerships for specific activities.

The cancer outreach coordinator position was developed to coordinate community activities with a focus on prevention and early detection. A variety of awareness and screening programs were in existence before the conception of the outreach coordinator position; however, no measurable method existed to select and prioritize activities in which to participate, no established written goals for the activities or clinical outcomes were established, and there was no well-defined plan to continue the existing programs. Working within the framework of a written plan establishes a path for the public education plan and guides program modification through measurement of goals, outcomes, and year-end evaluation.

Challenges in establishing the public education program included providing a structured educational session to the oncology leadership that explained the mission, objectives, and theory foundation on which the program was designed. The plan is based on the Health Belief Model, which identifies the stages of change. Identifying that the population served could be anywhere in these stages of change assisted the leadership team to recognize a variety of activities that must be offered to meet the needs of the population. Although the cancer outreach coordinator position was a newly created position within the cancer center, it was an adaptation from an old position. This created a challenge for those within the cancer center and the hospital to adopt the revised mission and direction of the program, based on the written plan.

There were additional challenges in establishing the written plan, including creation of a mission statement. Through a series of meetings with stakeholders, the following mission statement was established: "The Via Christi Cancer Outreach Program will promote cancer prevention and early detection in the community and the Via Christi Health Care System." Stakeholders included the cancer outreach coordinator, the hospital call center, the oncology service line leadership team, the medical director of oncology, and the hospital marketing department.

Five high-incidence and high-mortality cancer sites (based on national, state, and local statistics) are targeted for the prevention and early detection program: lung, colon, breast, prostate, and skin. These cancer sites are selected by reviewing statistics from the American Cancer Society, the Kansas Cancer Registry, and the Via Christi Cancer Center Annual Report. National, state, and hospital incidence and mortality numbers provided a benchmark for measuring outcomes in these areas. The criterion for selecting these cancers for the prevention and early detection program was the availability of recognized screening procedures or preventive measures for making a lifestyle change, thereby decreasing cancer risk.

An "Oncology Public Education Program Request" form was developed to help to determine which activities the cancer center would support (see Appendix 20-1). Selected activity parameters include the type of program, intended audience, projected number of participants, how the need was assessed, criteria score, and level of impact. A criterion scoring was established to help in the selection of involvement and to prioritize activities. The "Methods for Selecting Activities" is included in Appendix 20-2. Each activity selected is evaluated relative to the institution's strategic plan.

Impact measurement works closely with criteria scoring. The impact measurement helps to identify whether the selected activity is intended to provide awareness, lifestyle change, or a supportive environment for lifestyle change. The "Evaluation of Program Impact" is included in Appendix 20-3. Previously, the cancer center had been involved in a wide variety of activities with no clear measurement to determine why that activity had been chosen and what the intended impact of the activity had been for the participants.

Evaluation methods are involved with each aspect of the public education plan and are varied dependent upon the delivery of the health promotion activity. Each activity has a designated evaluation or response mechanism. Activities may involve presentations, posters, health fairs, screenings, written articles, or other activities.

Presentation evaluations include teaching objectives with a presenter evaluation. Evaluations of poster activities have included the number of flyers distributed, number of post-presentation phone calls, or the number of promotional materials requested. Health fair evaluations include the number of participants, the targeted audience in attendance, and the number of information handouts taken by participants. Screening evaluation includes the screening event itself, the number of participants, the number of targeted audience members participating, the number of participants who were screened positive, the number of participants responding to follow-up, and the number of participants who were diagnosed with cancer. Written articles may or may not have a response measurement. Responses to an article may include the number of calls or requests for information.

Evaluative efforts are carried out through a variety of mechanisms. Each program occurrence is evaluated, as well as end-of-year program results. Evaluations are tabulated by hand, by computerized retrieval system for phone call response, and by computer programs (Statistical Program for Social Sciences, or SPSS®) after coding evaluation or survey response. Evaluation of each activity involves reviewing the projected versus actual number of participants and degree of outcome achievement.

A year-end 1999 program evaluation revealed that the majority of prevention and early detection efforts had been directed at women, breast cancer, and awareness. Using the 1999 program evaluation results, several improvements have been implemented for the next program year. Requested activities must meet a higher level of criteria scoring, as the scoring was changed to be more restrictive because most of the previous year's activities met the selected criteria (see Table 20-8). Activities are being supported in different ways, such as unmanned versus manned booths, based on the criteria score and the impact level. The greatest number of 1999 programs were directed at the impact level of awareness. Table 20-9 summarizes the number of programs by impact level. For the 2000 plan, increasing the activities that have an impact on levels of lifestyle change and support an environment for a lifestyle change has been targeted.

The cancer center has an excellent process in place for notification of screening results. The first attempt to obtain clinical outcomes from a screening event, a fecal occult blood test, was a survey mailed to 260 participants with a positive screening test. The survey asked for a return mail response identifying if a physician had evaluated the participant, what medical diagnostic testing had been performed, and the definitive diagnosis. This follow-up, which was anonymous, asked

Table 20-8. Oncology Public Education Plan by Criteria Scoring—1999 (See *Evaluating Program Activities,* Appendix 20-2)	
Criteria Scoring	Number of Programs
1	0
2	0
3	0
4	2
5	1
6	4
7	15
8	29
9	22
10	8

Table 20-9. Oncology Public Education Plan by Level of Impact—1999 (See *Evaluating Program Impact,* Appendix 20-3)	
Level of Impact (more than one level may be reflected)	Number of Programs
Level 1 Awareness	70
Level 2 Lifestyle change	62
Level 3 Supportive environment	22
Nonscored	2

for the participants to volunteer their medical diagnosis and occurred six months after the screening event. Although 115 surveys were returned, indicating 86% had contacted their doctor and many had been referred for diagnostic testing, participants did not volunteer the medical diagnosis.

The next phase of development in the follow-up process was to establish a timeline, have a referral system in place, and create a questionnaire allowing capture of the definitive diagnoses. This first attempt with these measures was completed with an employee prostate cancer screening. The follow-up involved a scripted phone call contact or a letter. Precautions were taken to protect confidentiality, addressing the phone calls directly to the participant, not a spouse or other party.

The results of follow-up for the employee prostate cancer screening did not provide the desired information regarding definitive diagnosis. Each participant with a positive screening result received a phone call or letter three months following notification of screening results. The timeframe selected for the follow-up calls/letters did not allow enough time for the participants to receive the diagnosis information from the physician. The timeframe and frequency of calls were limited to eliminate the "harassment" factor. The results indicated that some participants planned to see a physician, had seen a physician, or were not planning to see a physician (see Table 20-10).

Currently, the Via Christi Cancer Center personnel are in the process of developing a written follow-up procedure for all health-screening activities. The rationale for the development of the policy and procedure is based on the Oncology Nursing Society's *Statement on the Scope and Standards of Oncology Nursing Practice*, the American Nurses Association's *Standards of Clinical Nursing Practice*, the Kansas Nurse Practice Act, and textbook listings of "criteria for a screening program."

Promotion of the public education program is self-evolving. All activities are requested through the cancer outreach coordinator position and fall within the

Table 20-10. 1999 Employee Prostate Cancer Screening Outcomes

Patient	Age	Abnormal Prostate-Specific Antigen (PSA)	Abnormal Digital Rectal Examination	Benign Prostatic Hyperplasia (BPH)	Saw Doctor	Further Test	Diagnosis	Made Appointment	Has Doctor
1	51	–	Yes	–	Yes	Biopsy	Pending		
2	62	–	–	Yes	No				
3	66	–	Yes	–	Yes	Biopsy	– Cancer + BPH	No	Yes
4	47	–	Yes	–	Yes	Repeat PSA			
5	57	Yes	–	Yes					
6	56	–	–	BPH					
7	61	Yes	–	BPH					

Physician Recommendations
1—Referred to urologist. Had biopsy. Results pending.
3—Saw an urologist. Had biopsy. Negative results.
4—Primary-care doctor recommended see urologist. PSA redrawn. See primary-care doctor in November.

Other
2—No physician recommendation for follow-up recorded
5—Left message to call. No call received. Certified letter sent and received.
6—Left message to call twice on answering machine. Left message to call with spouse.
7—No home phone. Letters sent in August, November, and December. Certified letter sent and received.

public education program parameters. There are ongoing programs such as a breast cancer awareness program, Buddy Check™ 10, ColoCheck, annual activities with community organizations, and other new programs as health promotion activities develop. The prevention and early-detection activities are used to market the continuum of care offered by the oncology service line.

Vital to the program promotion is communication with community partners, internal departments, the hospital network, oncology service line leadership, and networking within professional groups. The greatest challenge of the program is to meet the current volume of requested activities or programs with limited resources, including financial and personnel.

References

American Cancer Society. (1999). *Cancer facts and figures, 1999*. Atlanta: Author.

Oncology Nursing Society. (1995). *Standards of oncology education: Patient/family and public*. Pittsburgh: Author.

Valanis, B. (1999). *Epidemiology in health care* (3rd ed.). Stamford, CT: Appleton & Lange.

Appendix 20-1. Oncology Public Education Program Request

Oncology Public Education Program Request, Via Christi Cancer Center Cancer Outreach

Name/title _____

Organization _____

Address _____

Phone number _____

Location of program (site, room): _____

Choice of date/time: 1st_____2nd_____

Length of program: ❏ One hour   ❏ One and a half hours   ❏ Two hours
                    ❏ Other _____

Type of program: ❏ Health fair screening   ❏ Article presentation   ❏ Media
                    ❏ Other _____

Cancer topics include: ❏ Colon   ❏ Breast   ❏ Prostate   ❏ Lung   ❏ Skin
                        ❏ Other:

Intended audience: Male: Age____   Female: Age____   Children: Age____

Projected number of participants: ❏ 50 or < 50–100   ❏ 100–150   ❏ 150–200, > 200

Actual number of participants: ❏ 50 or < 50–100   ❏ 100–150   ❏ 150–200, > 200

Other cancer organizations attending: ❏ ACS   ❏ LSA   ❏ GK   ❏ VV
                                        ❏ Other: _____

How need was assessed: _____

Criteria score: 1   2   3   4   5   6   7   8

Required Criteria for Program	**Additional Criteria Total_____** Program meets a minimum five of the six. (7 or >)
• Supports the Cancer Outreach Mission Statement. • Supports or enhances Via Christi Health System initiatives	• Targets the high incidence cancers • Targets populations at high risk • Targets the cancers with the highest mortality rates • Information does not duplicate other event/program offerings. • The projected number of attendees justifies the event/program. • The level of impact justifies the program offering.

Level of impact: Not rated; 1—Awareness; 2—Lifestyle change; 3—Supportive environment

Additional information/comments: _____

Presenter(s) name/title/credentials: _____

Manager approval _____ Date _____

In-house speaker agreement

I agree to provide this program at the date/times indicated. If I am unable to present as agreed, I will be responsible to make every effort to find a qualified substitute presenter. I will provide the following to the Cancer Outreach Coordinator by _____.

Copy of handouts (including bibliography and objectives)

One week after the program offering, _____, I will return the following to the Cancer Outreach coordinator:

Program evaluations and actual number of participants

Signature _____ Date _____

Appendix 20-2. Method for Selecting Activities, January–December 1999

Participation in public education programs will be determined by use of the following criteria. Each criterion is given one point. Program participation will be considered upon achieving a score of six or greater. Other requests will be evaluated on an individual basis.

Program must meet two of the three criteria	Additional criteria total_____ Program meets three to four of the seven
• Supports the Cancer Outreach Mission Statement • Supports or enhances existing Via Christi community affiliations • Enhances existing Via Christi outreach efforts	• Targets the high-incidence cancers • Targets populations at high risk • Targets the cancers with the highest mortality rates • Information does not duplicate other event/program offerings. • Information reinforces or complements other event/program offerings. • The projected number of attendees justifies the event/program (baseline data unavailable). • The level of impact justifies the program offering (baseline data unavailable).

Appendix 20-3. Evaluation of Program Impact

Awareness
• Increases participant's level of awareness or interest in the topic of the program
• Rarely does the participant actually change health behavior or improve health.
• Almost of no value if goal of program is to improve the participant's health.
• Can be used as a direct feeder to the lifestyle change programs.

Lifestyle Change
• Sets lifestyle-related behavior change as the desired outcome
• Improves health status
• Reduces medical problems
• Reduces medical costs
• Is of greater value to the customer than awareness programs

Supportive Environment
• Creates an environment that encourages a healthy lifestyle
• Facilitates maintaining newly acquired healthy lifestyle habits

Health Education Kits: Safe Sun and Don't Get Hooked on Smoking

Patti Moser, RN, BSN, OCN®

Exploration Place, a not-for-profit institution located on the banks of the Arkansas River in Wichita, KS, is a new creative learning and science center funded by county citizens, corporate leaders, and foundations of the community. Exploration Place opened in 2000, and 2,000 adults and children were projected to visit the facility per day.

The Health Discovery Room at Exploration Place offers an opportunity to provide cancer prevention education to children, a patient population rarely addressed by the Via Christi Cancer Center. The target audience for the health education kit is children 10–12 years of age, with a range of children ages 6–14 anticipated to access the kits. A variety of health kits are being developed by representatives from different service lines within Via Christi Regional Medical Center, a not-for-profit community teaching hospital that addresses health concerns of women and children, cardiovascular problems, neurology, nutrition, surgery, and oncology. With the exception of nutrition services, registered nurses represent all service lines for kit development. The cancer outreach coordinator, an oncology certified nurse, represents the oncology service line.

Each health kit developer was given the goals of the kit with instructions to incorporate language arts, math skills, science, health, and critical thinking in an interactive format that is self-directed by the student learner. The goals for each health kit include
- A fun and interactive design for all ages
- A completion time of 10 minutes or less
- A target audience of fourth to sixth graders
- Easy to understand facts
- The concept of "explore it and put it back" not "do it and take it home"
- A thought-provoking question to be placed inside the lid
- Durability and safety—kits cannot contain small pieces that could pose a choking hazard.

The budget for each health kit is $150, provided by Exploration Place.

Including skin cancer and smoking prevention information in the interactive health kit format was not difficult using the Via Christi Cancer Center Oncology Public Education Plan. The Public Education Plan focuses on five cancer sites based on incidence, mortality, disease prevention, screening availability, and scientific research. The five targeted cancers for prevention and early detection include breast, prostate, colon, lung, and skin. Lung and skin cancer development are strongly related to lifestyle choices of smoking and sun exposure. Lung and skin cancer prevention education was selected to increase awareness of behaviors that could reduce the risk of development of these diseases and to reinforce area school programs targeted at smoking prevention, such as Drug Awareness Resistance Education (DARE).

Health Kits

The Safe Sun health kit includes a notebook of activities for the children, which contains the following sections of educational information.

1. Safe Sun Tips using Slip, Slop, Slap, Wrap (American Cancer Society Publication Number 99-300M-No.2012.04-CC)
2. Exposure to sun during certain hours of the day can increase the risk for sunburn.
3. Sunburn can occur on a cloudy day.
4. Wear a sunscreen with a minimum sun protection factor (SPF) of 15.
5. Reapply sunscreen after activity or swimming.
6. Definition of SPF and length of time skin is provided sunburn protection
7. Calculation problem using SPF 15 to determine minutes of sun protection for a stated length of time
8. Basal, squamous, and melanoma skin cancer pictures to examine with a magnifying glass
9. Instructions to complete a Colorforms® picture that would help sunbathers to understand what they can do to protect their skin.

The kit inventory includes the Safe Sun notebook, Colorforms and art board, dry erase board, a magnifying glass made with a plastic lens, and laminated skin cancer pictures. The learning objective of the kit is that each child will create a picture demonstrating behaviors that will protect the skin from the sun.

Don't Get Hooked on Smoking

The activity directed at smoking prevention, Don't Get Hooked on Smoking, includes a notebook containing health information and kit activity instructions. The notebook contains the following sections of educational information and activity directions.

1. Picture of the lung anatomy
2. Directions to examine the enclosed lung model
3. Hold your breath for 40 seconds to demonstrate the amount of life lost with every puff of a cigarette
4. Calculation of the cost of each cigarette in a pack
5. Calculation of the cost of a carton of cigarettes
6. Buy products from the "kids catalog" that are equal to the cost of a carton of cigarettes
7. Read the book *Kids Say Don't Smoke* by Andrew Tobias.
8. Look through magazines and identify what messages the cigarette ads send.
9. Make a poster explaining why people should NOT smoke.

The kit inventory includes the Don't Get Hooked on Smoking notebook, an hourglass shaped like a cigarette, *Kids Say Don't Smoke*, a lung model, markers, drawing pad, magazines, and play money. The learning objective of the kit is that each child will draw an advertisement with an antismoking message.

Each kit developer was challenged to enhance or reinforce other learning activities located within the science center, without duplicating the educational information. The kit is developed with the idea that children can pick up the kit and interact with all or some of the inventory supplies to learn about the subject matter.

It is unknown which component of the kit content each child will find of interest. Trying to include pieces that children could manipulate was difficult, as there were not many hands-on items that met the kit's size constraints.

Computer skills were required to add colorful, eye-catching graphics in the notebook. Identifying health education materials that were targeted at the intended audience and could fit within the confines of the kit space required use of multiple resources. Writing for children was a new experience. Keeping the text age appropriate and health information understandable was a challenge.

Evaluation is to occur by periodic observation of children using the kits to determine if the learning objectives are being met. Children will be observed meeting the Safe Sun health education kit learning objective when they create a Colorforms picture that demonstrates skin protection behaviors. By meeting the learning objective of the Don't Get Hooked on Smoking health education kit, children will learn how to draw a poster with an antismoking message. Other measurable objectives will be the number of visitors to the center, number of children using the kits, and which components of the kit children find of interest and use to meet the learning objective. There is no follow-up mechanism in place for the health information provided by the kits.

While marketing Exploration Place, there is discussion of providing health information presentations in the Health Discovery Room during the school tours and other designated times throughout the calendar year. The information presented by a speaker will further enhance the health message of the kit and other exhibits.

Development of future health kits is projected for the next calendar year. The additional kits will be rotated with existing ones. Children with season passes will have access to new information on a continuous basis. Ideas for new health kits focusing on cancer information include how a normal cell changes to a cancer cell, effects of cancer treatments on cells, and how cancer affects the lives of family members.

Skin Cancer Screening in the Metropolitan Area of Portland, OR

Ann Reiner, RN, MN, OCN®

Four metropolitan-based hospital systems and two professional organizations collaborate to provide a skin cancer screening opportunity for the more than 1.7 million residents of Portland, OR, and Vancouver, WA. The cities are separated by the Columbia River but are joined by two major highways. The systems are Providence Health System, Legacy Health System, Southwest Washington Medical Center (all not-for-profit businesses), and Oregon Health Sciences University, the state's only academic medical center (a public corporation). The professional organizations are the Oregon Chapter of the American Academy of Dermatologists (AAD) and the Pacific Northwest Dermatology Nurses Association.

Once a year for the last four years, on a Saturday morning in May or June, physician and nurse volunteers screen more than 550 adults at four different sites around the metropolitan area. Each hospital system provides a clinic site, most often an ambulatory clinic that is not in operation on weekends. The screening program uses multiple exam rooms—two or three for each physician—reception and waiting areas, telephones, and the staff break room. The clinics only need to provide patient gowns and the use of a VCR and TV monitor. Other sources supply the other supplies (e.g., sunscreen samples, skin cancer literature and videos).

People who wish to be screened call a centralized appointment scheduling service. Arrangements are made with one of the participating Portland-based health systems to use its patient information and resource phone service. The Vancouver site provides its own number and scheduling service. Operators answering calls for Portland-based screening appointments use a scheduling grid made for this event that displays all of the available appointment times per screening site. While speaking with the caller, the operator records the person's first and last name and phone number on the scheduling grid. The grid is a simple online spreadsheet displaying three slots per 15 minutes per each physician at each site. This document, when printed in hard copy, becomes the appointment schedule used on the day of the screening. Each site receives a faxed and final copy of its schedule on Saturday morning, just prior to the opening of the screening clinic.

Operators make every effort to schedule callers on the caller's desired time and location. Portland-based clinics are available in the Northeast, North, and Southwest sections of the city, roughly similar to the city's population densities. Only one location is available in Vancouver; however, a Vancouver-based person could be scheduled at a Portland-based clinic, if so desired. Similar to other border states, citizens of each city frequently cross state lines for work, services, and recreation.

People are asked to arrive 10–15 minutes prior to their scheduled appointment time to fill out the AAD screening forms. Volunteers greet them and give them a form with a clipboard and pen. While waiting, people can watch one of two videos about sun protection. When ready, volunteers escort the person to be screened to an examination room. As with any clinic, an easily understood communication system must be in place to avoid mishaps associated with attending to more than 100 people in four hours.

The person is instructed to undress down to his or her underwear and to put on a patient gown. Physicians perform a visual check and document their findings on the screening form. After the examination, the person meets a nurse who reviews the person's form, looking for any recommendations for follow-up examination or biopsy of a suspicious lesion. If present, that person is directed to a private area where another nurse can discuss and recommend particular clinics or physicians for necessary care. The nurse makes recommendations based on the person's health insurance or screening finding. Those who do not need any further follow-up are directed to another nurse who collects the screening form and distributes skin cancer literature and sunscreen samples. The American Cancer Society and the AAD provide the literature. Sunscreen samples are available from pharmaceutical companies.

The number of physicians, nurses, and volunteers needed on the day of the screening depends on the number of patients that can be accommodated at each clinical site. Generally, if five to six physicians are seeing a total of 240–288 patients, the clinic runs smoothly with three volunteers to greet and register people and distribute screening forms, two to three nurses or volunteers to move people from waiting to examination rooms, and two nurses to conduct exit interviews and make necessary recommendations. If possible, it is helpful to have a nurse familiar with the site who functions only to troubleshoot any problems that might arise.

Supplementary volunteers needed include those on a central planning committee. The committee has representatives from each institutional site and professional organization. The cadre of licensed volunteers for the screening event comes from the recruitment and coordination efforts of this committee's representatives from the professional organizations. The institutional representatives arrange all the details at their respective clinical sites, including site security, refreshments for the volunteers, and the contribution of patient gowns. The committee sees that the work and expenses of the screening event are shared. In addition, one of the institutions accepts the responsibility to collate pertinent information from the screening forms, including patient demographics and results of clinical examinations.

By far, the largest contribution of a particular organization is the charge of coordinating the scheduling. The organization that has a phone call center reviews and implements the particular details and usual procedures of this event. Tasks related to the production and distribution of marketing items, such as flyers and press releases, are divided between organizations. An effort is made to have the story covered by both print and broadcast media. The available appointment slots quickly fill once the story is printed in Portland's only newspaper. Usually a melanoma survivor is profiled in the print story.

The committee also believes this event is for people at high risk for the development of a cancer and includes in that definition those people who are medically underserved. Flyers are sent to nearby senior and retirement centers. People without health insurance or with limited access are targeted through direct mailings to county health clinics, neighborhood associations, community centers, and other agencies that are in communication with this population. Flyers are not distributed within hospital systems so as to discourage the use of the service by those patients and employees who have access to the specialty services of dermatologists.

Despite these efforts, the vast majority of people screened each year have had health insurance (see Table 20-11). In 1999, participants were asked during the registration process to record their responses to two additional questions. Those questions were

- If this screening were not available today, would you be able to receive this service?
- From whom would you receive the screening?

Table 20-11. Data From All Portland-Based Sites

Items	1997	1998	1999	2000
Total number screened	364	490	458	432
% male/female	38/62	37/63	39/61	36/64
Mean age	52	53.7	52.3	54.6
% insured	87.4	88.4	91.0	91.1
% recommended for referral	33	28.8	31.9	39.4
Clinically diagnosed				
Melanoma	17	9	25	18
Squamous cell cancer	3	8	8	13
Basal cell cancer	27	38	38	39

The planning committee was surprised at the results. Again, the vast majority of people screened had health insurance and would rely on their primary-care practitioner to do the screening; however, many were not or would not be satisfied with the results of the practitioner's review. One particular anecdote is notable. The respondent's melanoma was clinically diagnosed at a previous screening, to which she came only after being dissatisfied by her primary-care doctor's assessment of a worrisome mole. She followed the screening dermatologist's advice and continued her workup, resulting in a histologic diagnosis. She was happy to tell us she believes her life was saved because of this screening clinic.

The AAD screening form has multiple copies. One copy is given to the patient, and another is sent to the academy. The Portland-based dermatologist keeps the third copy and agrees to call all the patients identified as needing follow-up evaluation. All participating dermatologists are asked for a commitment to do any of the required follow-up for patients who need it, regardless of their insurance status. A process has been established so that the burden of uncompensated care is not directed at any particular physician group but instead shared throughout a rotation of referrals. The office staff of the dermatologist who calls all the people needing a follow-up appointment records to whom they refer the uninsured patients in a folder, which is considered part of the documents for each subsequent skin cancer screening. In following years, staff then can rotate referrals when necessary.

The central planning committee does another aspect of follow-up. At an agreed date, the members of the committee meet to review the collated data and discuss ways to improve the event. Data are presented by site and by all sites combined.

The committee never has discussed the event's cost-benefit ratio based on potential or actual revenue generated from the screenings. It has discussed increasing the number of screening slots, but some of the sites are at capacity. The committee is pleased with the volunteer commitment. Currently, more than one-third of the metropolitan area's dermatologists participate each year, with many of those returning year to year. There is a strong notion among committee members that the event is the right thing to do for the community. All of the institutions believe in contributing to the health of their community.

Family Cancer Risk Assessment Program

Linda Sveningson, MS, RN, AOCN®, and Carol Grimm, MD, MPH

The Family Cancer Risk Assessment Program, at the Roger Maris Cancer Center in Fargo, ND, began seeing patients for individualized breast cancer risk assessment in January 1999. The Roger Maris Cancer Center is part of the MeritCare Health System, the largest multispeciality medical group in North Dakota, which is comprised of 330 physicians. The healthcare system serves 1.6 million patients per year at 32 clinic locations in a 250-mile wide service area. The program is the only known one of its kind in North Dakota and northwest Minnesota.

The impetus for program development occurred with the advent of commercially available gene testing kits for breast cancer predisposition. This availability raised questions by family members concerned about their history of breast cancer, questioning if they should consider gene testing. The assumption was made that a busy family practice physician or oncologist may not have the time or perhaps the information necessary to counsel these families or individuals. Additionally, it was possible that at-risk patients were not being identified and given options for cancer risk management. Referral centers that are experienced in cancer risk assessment and counseling (a relatively new area of genetic counseling) would require anywhere from a 4–12+ hour drive for individuals residing in North Dakota, a deterrent for many families. Finally, a strong rationale for development of this program was the commitment to provide identification, education, surveillance recommendations, and counseling of high-risk individuals as a standard component of the comprehensive cancer program.

An advisory committee, composed of representatives from medical oncology, administration, education and research, breast clinic, psychology, family practice, ethics committee, and the MeritCare Foundation, formed to discuss program format and funding potential. Others consulted regarding program development included laboratory personnel, a representative from insurance contract management, the attorney for MeritCare Health System, and an MD geneticist from the University of North Dakota. A Service and Technology request for a Breast Cancer Risk Assessment Program was submitted to the MeritCare Health System and the MeritCare Foundation, the philanthropic arm of the health system. Funding was approved for a two-year budget, with 23% of the financial support coming from the MeritCare Health System and 77% from the MeritCare Foundation.

The target population for the first two years of operation has focused on women who have a personal or family history of breast cancer. Based on tumor registry data of individuals diagnosed with breast cancer, it was estimated that 200 women would be referred to the service, with approximately 50 requiring the entire spectrum of program services in the first two years of the program. As the program becomes recognized regionally and statewide, the numbers of individuals requesting program services are anticipated to increase accordingly.

Core staffing for the program consists of a physician medical director, a nurse coordinator, and a secretary. The medical director, in addition to a medical degree, holds a master's degree in public health in the area of clinical prevention. The nurse coordinator is a master's-prepared oncology nurse with 25+ years of oncology expertise. The medical director also works in the breast clinic and provides an invaluable link to referrals to the Family Cancer Risk Assessment Program. In addition to the core staffing, a Cancer Risk Assessment Team, composed of a medical oncologist, gynecologist, medical geneticist, psychologist, and social worker, provide monthly consultative services to the program. The oncologist, geneticist, and psychologist receive a quarterly stipend and CME reimbursement for risk assessment–related educational materials or programs. Additional costs in the first year of program development included consulting fees paid to a program consultant and educational costs allotted for attendance at national workshops and seminars. The goals of the program are designed to address the highly complex issues surrounding risk assessment and genetic testing, such as risk assessment estimates, psychosocial and ethical issues, benefits and risks of genetic testing, and surveillance recommendations based on personal risk. The program consists of four basic components.

- Education for healthcare professionals
- Education for the general public
- Risk assessment and education program for high-risk individuals
- Coordination of services for high-risk individuals who are eligible for and pursue genetic testing

The Cancer Risk Assessment Program is staffed on Tuesdays. Individuals who are referred by their physician or self-referred are invited to participate in Part I of the program, the educational component. Education, provided by the nurse, typically is conducted monthly, with the time of day varying. One-on-one education is provided for those are who are unable to attend the scheduled monthly class. The educational component, which is one-and-a-half hours, provides an overview of breast cancer risk factors, basic principles of cancer development, how cancer is inherited, who might be at risk for inherited breast cancer, and risks and benefits of genetic testing.

Individuals who feel they are at increased risk are encouraged to participate in Parts II and III of the program. Part II involves an individualized intake interview obtaining pertinent medical/family history, construction of the family pedigree, and completion of release of information forms for facilitating family history verification. Typically, Part II takes approximately one-and-a-half to two hours to complete, depending upon the complexity of the family and individual history. If the individual must travel a great distance, the opportunity to complete Parts I and II in one visit is offered.

The Cancer Risk Assessment Program staff members compile the data for each individual, apply various risk assessment models, and submit the case for review by the Cancer Risk Assessment Team. The team meets monthly, reviews the case summaries (family pedigree and medical/family history), and makes assessments regarding level of risk for breast cancer, likelihood of detecting an inherited mutation, appropriateness of genetic testing, and recommendations for surveillance guidelines.

Finally, the medical director of the program meets with the individual/family for Part III of the program and provides a summary of the Cancer Risk Assessment Team's recommendations. Considerable time is spent in providing interpretation of the results and counseling regarding surveillance guidelines. Individuals are advised that the implementation of the surveillance recommendations is their responsibility; however, the program is ready and willing to make referrals upon request. A copy of the assessment, discussion, and surveillance recommendation is given to the individual following the Part III visit. A full consultation also is placed in the individual's medical record. Individuals who choose to pursue genetic counseling and testing consult first with the clinical psychologist to address the complex psychological issues that surround genetic testing. Additional consults may include meetings with a surgeon regarding prophylactic mastectomies, a gynecologist regarding ovarian cancer risk management, or a medical oncologist regarding chemoprevention/research opportunities in cancer prevention. Following the various consults, if the individual chooses to pursue genetic testing, an appointment is set up for the individual to consult with the geneticist for additional counseling, the blood draw for gene testing is coordinated, and the results of the gene testing are reported back.

Individuals participating in the Family Cancer Risk Assessment Program do not pay for services received in Parts I–III of the risk assessment program. The services are provided through the support of the MeritCare Health System and MeritCare Foundation. Consultations with the psychologist, geneticist, surgeon, medical oncologist, and gynecologist are billed to the individual or the individual's healthcare provider. Revenue to the healthcare system, although difficult to track, is anticipated primarily through surveillance procedures and physician consults.

A follow-up phone call, completed by the medical director, is made to each participant one month following completion of Part III. The purpose of the follow-up call is to confirm receipt of the written report, to clarify any questions, to assist with scheduling needs, and to offer continuing support to the individual and her family. Participants also are encouraged and reminded to contact the Cancer Risk Assessment program if any changes in their personal or family medical history occur.

A one-year evaluation of the program revealed that 71 individuals had contacted or been referred to the program, with 23 completing all three parts. Seven participants discussed referrals to the geneticist and two completed gene testing. A program evaluation was mailed to participants completing the entire three-part risk assessment program. Overall, the evaluation indicated high satisfaction with the program services.

The program has been promoted in a variety of ways.
- Program brochures and posters are placed in physician offices.
- Advertisement of the monthly educational session is placed in the local newspaper.
- Television and radio coverage are obtained.
- Presentations are given to physician groups.

The most successful promotion strategy is physician referrals to the program. The Cancer Risk Assessment Program was the featured program in the Fall 2000 Home Run/Walk Race, sponsored by the MeritCare Foundation. Monies from this event went toward continuing support of the program.

Program challenges have been the labor and time intensity required with each participant. We have sought to consolidate the educational component of the program by scheduling monthly group sessions and have been somewhat successful in this regard. However, participant schedules also are very complicated, and situations often require individual scheduling. The program also has seen staff turnover during its first two years of operation. This has required it to fall back in the associated steep learning curve of risk assessment, and this has somewhat slowed our forward progress. The staff is now stable, and the program has become more efficient in its format, so these challenges hopefully are overcome.

The Cancer Risk Assessment Program is entering its third year of operation. Funding has been approved for an additional three years, with continued support from the MeritCare Health Care System and MeritCare Foundation. Plans are under way for the development and implementation of a colon risk assessment program.

The Family Cancer Risk Assessment Program is motivated by the complexity of the issues surrounding risk assessment and the challenge of conveying this information to the program participants in a way that empowers them to design their own plan for risk management. We are extremely grateful for the generous support of the MeritCare Foundation, who sees this service as a unique opportunity to impact the health of people in our community in a positive way.

SECTION V

Issues in Education and Training

Chapter 21.

Preparation of Nurse Generalists for Cancer
Prevention and Detection Practice

Chapter 22.

Advancing the Cancer Control Agenda:
The Role of Advanced Practice Nurses

Chapter 23.

Research Training Opportunities

Chapter 24.

Health-Education Issues for Patients in Cancer
Prevention and Early Detection

Chapter 25.

Information Resources for Patients and Families

OVERVIEW

Section V

Suzanne M. Mahon, RN, DNSc, AOCN®, APNG(c)

Professional and public education about cancer-control issues are critical to the success of any cancer-control program. Before an nurse can implement a cancer-control program, professional education may be necessary to provide the background and clinical skills to develop the program. Once this has been achieved, the nurse must consider appropriate public-education strategies to achieve the desired goal of the cancer-control program. Section V provides insight into how these challenges can be met.

Great strides in providing effective and appropriate cancer-control services have been made during the last decade. This clinical and research knowledge needs to be included in both professional undergraduate and graduate-level course content. It is no longer acceptable to provide a one-hour lecture on cancer control and assume that the student will be adequately prepared to implement these principles into future clinical practice. Programs should have a focus on working with healthy, well individuals, as well as ill individuals. A need exists for practicing clinicians with expertise in cancer control to provide mentorship to students and practicing nurses who want to further develop their cancer-control skills.

A need also exists for intensive continuing education, including both didactic and clinical components, for those nurses in clinical practice who plan to implement a cancer-control program in the clinical setting. Programs such as these are located in various geographic locations and include a variety of teaching strategies. More recently, self-paced, continuing education in both print and electronic format has become available (Jennings-Dozier, 2001).

In Chapter 21, Pearce identifies educational issues at the nurse generalist level. This chapter includes a discussion of undergraduate preparation of nurses in cancer prevention and early detection in selected schools of nursing in Ohio. These examples are used to suggest strategies for teaching cancer prevention and early detection in undergraduate nursing curricula.

Both general and oncology-specific advance practice nurses (APNs) can contribute to improving cancer-control outcomes. In Chapter 22, Cunningham provides a discussion of the role APNs currently play in cancer-control activities and areas for future role development and research. Recommendations for the educational preparation of APNs who practice in cancer control also are included.

Developing a research agenda for nursing in cancer control is important to advance the science of cancer control and train nurse researchers and scholars for the future. In Chapter 23, Wysocki provides an examination of the research training opportunities available for nurses who practice in cancer control. This includes training at the undergraduate level for practicing nurses and APNs.

The direct success of any cancer-control program often can be traced to the public education efforts about wellness. This education is now sometimes referred to as consumer education. The goal of this education is to empower individuals with current and appropriate information in understandable terms so they can make good choices about the prevention and early detection of cancer. Chapter 24 provides a comprehensive review of the considerations that are pertinent to public education. Nurses must carefully consider these theoretical constructs to develop public education programs that are appropriate to the audience they seek to teach. Additional information and resources for public education are provided by Ades in Chapter 25. The reader is encouraged to consult this section for specific resources that may be helpful when developing a cancer-control program. Together, these two chapters provide information on not only what to teach to the patients and families that oncology nurses serve, but how to teach effectively.

Change and new findings continue to emerge in the practice of cancer control. The oncology nurse is challenged to continually learn about these changes and the implications of these changes for clinical practice. This section provides a framework for the integration of professional and public education in cancer control.

Reference

Jennings-Dozier, K.M. (2001). Educational programs in cancer prevention and detection: Determining content and quality. *Oncology Nursing Forum, 27*(Suppl.), 47–54.

CHAPTER 21

Preparation of Nurse Generalists for Cancer Prevention and Detection Practice: Experiences of Associate-Degree Nursing Programs

Jennifer Douglas Pearce, RN, MSN, CNS

Introduction

The shift in the emphasis in health care from an illness to a wellness focus required schools of nursing to make curriculum revisions and find updated clinical experiences to produce graduate practitioners who are prepared to meet the challenges of today's primary healthcare system. According to the World Health Organization (Shoultz & Amundson, 1998), a primary need in health care is to ensure quality education of healthcare professionals for the identification, prevention, and control of prevailing health problems.

The purpose of this chapter is to discuss undergraduate preparation of nurses in cancer prevention and early detection in selected schools of nursing in Ohio and suggest strategies for teaching cancer prevention and early detection in undergraduate nursing curricula.

Considerations in Preparing Nurse Generalists for Cancer Prevention and Detection Practice

Regulations Affecting Nursing Programs and Curriculum Development

Several governing bodies, both legal and professional, affect the way nurse educators develop and evaluate nursing education. The Ohio Board of Nursing (1999) stated that curricula should include courses and content in four major areas, which may be integrated, combined, or presented as separate courses: the nursing process, critical thinking, problem solving, and decision making related to meeting the nursing care and health promotion needs of individuals or groups across the life span. In addition, the content must address the nursing needs of individuals and groups experiencing commonly occurring acute and long-term physical and mental health problems, illness, or adjustments. Nursing curricula should include information regarding health promotion, health maintenance, and restoration of health, as well as methods of dealing with death and dying.

State Boards of Nursing

The board of nursing is an agency organized within the executive branch of the state government that is responsible for administering and enforcing the law regulating the practice of nursing (i.e., Nurse Practice Act) (Ohio Board of Nursing, 1999). Another function of the board is to establish the educational and professional standards for RN licensure. Candidates are required to pass the National Council Licensure Examination (NCLEX-RN) as a prerequisite to licensure as a registered nurse. This system of licensure protects the public and evaluates the graduate's competence to practice nursing safely and effectively. The NCLEX-RN test plan is based on two major components, the phases of the nursing process and patients' needs, with 5%–11% of the questions related to health promotion and maintenance (National Council of State Boards of Nursing, 1997). The test plan explains that nurses will be tested in their knowledge of content on disease prevention, health and wellness, health-promotion programs, health screening, immunizations, lifestyle choices, and techniques of physical assessment.

Pew Health Commission Competencies

According to the Pew Health Commission Competencies for 2005 and the 21 competencies for the 21st century, today's nurses must practice prevention and wellness care (Bellack & O'Neil, 2000). Practitioners also must emphasize primary and secondary preventive strategies in occupational health settings, wellness centers, and self-care programs. In addition, practitioners should provide health-education and health-promotion programs to help individuals, families, and communities to promote and maintain healthy behaviors. Practitioners are encouraged to improve healthcare system operations and accountability by creating partnerships with communities in making healthcare decisions. Practitioners also are urged to continue to learn and help others by anticipating changes in health care and responding by redefining, changing, and maintaining competencies throughout their professional lives.

Oncology Nursing Society Standards on Oncology Nursing Education

In the Oncology Nursing Society's (ONS's) (1995) *Standards on Oncology Nursing Education*, Standard IIIB states that the nurse uses the nursing process systematically to develop an outcome-oriented care plan that is individualized, holistic, culturally sensitive, and cost-effective and incorporates cancer prevention, detection, treatment, rehabilitation, and supportive care. Standards IIID and IIIE state that oncology nurse generalists should assume responsibility for personal professional development in oncology nursing and contribute to the professional growth of others. Standards IIC and IID state that the community should participate in appropriate or recommended cancer-screening activities and identify a course of action for early detection when signs and symptoms of cancer are discovered. The standards emphasize the need for oncology nurses to establish a trusting, collaborative relationship with the community.

American Nurses Association Standards of Clinical Nursing Practice

The purpose of the American Nurses Association's (1998) *Standards of Clinical Nursing Practice* are to promote the educational and professional advancement of nurses so that the public receives high-quality nursing care. The scope of nursing practice includes promoting health and wellness, preventing illness, restoring health, and caring for the dying. Nurses use these guidelines as they engage in individual and community activities to enhance healthy lifestyles, maintain optimal health, and prevent disease. Examples of educational programs that meet these professional standards are stress-management classes; education on healthy nutrition, alcohol use, and smoking cessation; and cancer prevention and early-detection measures.

National League for Nursing

The objective of the National League for Nursing (NLN) is to foster development and improvement of all nursing services and education. This agency provides accreditation for educational programs in nursing. Accreditation from NLN signifies excellence in nursing education. NLN advocates quality nursing education that prepares nurses to meet the needs of diverse populations in an ever-changing healthcare environment. One of the essential elements in the Ohio League for Nursing's *Vision for Nursing in Ohio* (1997) is that nursing educates individuals and communities to care for themselves through informed choices. The document indicates that people often seek solutions to health crises and services to meet basic needs. The profession of nursing accepts the responsibility for this education and care for patients.

Existing Nursing Curriculum and Training in Cancer Prevention and Detection

Nursing has a significant history of incorporating cancer prevention and detection theory and practice into its curriculum and nursing-education activities. However, the quality and amount of time spent on these topics has varied greatly from program to program. Brown, Johnson, and Groenwald (1983) conducted an ONS-sponsored survey of nursing schools to investigate the cancer content taught in the curricula. Nine hundred eighty-two NLN-accredited schools of nursing (diploma, associate-degree, and baccalaureate programs) were surveyed. Each was questioned as to the cancer content in their curriculum, educational resources, preparation of faculty, and areas in need of improvement. Six hundred seventy-two (68%) schools responded. The results showed that only 14.5 hours were spent in classroom presentations. The content included cancer prevention and detection, oncologic emergencies, late effects of treatment, alternative treatments, attitudes toward cancer, home care, social issues, political issues, resources used for assistance (e.g., American Cancer Society [ACS], National Cancer Institute), legal implications, and educational resources for nurses.

Various studies with nursing students identified areas for curriculum revision and examined how experiential learning contributed to the overall application of concepts in cancer detection and prevention.

Post-White, Carter, and Anglim (1993) studied the relationship of the attitudes and behaviors of 220 nursing students and the practice of the recommended guidelines for cancer prevention and early detection following four one-day educational workshops, which included lectures, small-group discussions, and practice of early-detection skills. Of the students from baccalaureate, associate-degree, and practical-nursing programs who participated in the workshops, 179 (81%) responded immediately and 125 (57%) responded at the six-month follow-up. Based on these evaluations, the use of one-day educational workshops increased the nursing students' knowledge of cancer prevention and early-detection recommendations and improved their attitudes regarding the importance and benefits of self-practice, as well as the teaching of patients, family, friends, and peers. Mundt (1996) integrated an ACS patient-education program with didactic and clinical experiences into a basic nursing curriculum. Sixty-five nursing students and their clinical instructors were trained to serve as public-education specialists for the ACS breast health program. Cahill et al. (1998) surveyed 58 accredited associate-degree nursing programs, with 27 (47%) schools responding. The investigators identified the need for these programs to reexamine their curricula in response to specific health needs in the community. They also discussed the integration of community-based clinical experiences within the curricula, focusing on health promotion, disease prevention, and management of both acute and chronic illnesses.

Rushton (1999) described a six-week, three-credit oncology honors elective course, initially taught to undergraduate students at the College of Nursing at Brigham Young University in 1997. Students received three hours of didactic and 15 hours of clinical experience per week. The undergraduate course was developed to teach nursing and non-nursing students basic cancer principles, provide information regarding diagnosis and treatment of disease, and allow students to work with patients with cancer in the nearby area to understand the impact of cancer on patients, families, and the community. A seminar format facilitated active discussion among students, faculty, and guest speakers. For the clinical experience, student teams visited patients with cancer and their families at home and interacted with them during their four visits. Upon completion of the visits, each student wrote a paper discussing the pathophysiology of the patient's disease, a summary of the patient's therapy, and problems requiring solutions. Included was a discussion of any ethical, political, or healthcare issues that arose.

Students reflected on the overall experience as they discussed their perceptions of home visits, cancer knowledge gained as a result, and the community agencies dedicated to holistic cancer care.

Phillips and Belcher (1999) implemented a cancer prevention, screening, and education program into a community-health nursing curriculum, where students assessed hospital employees' cancer risks. Students discovered that hospital employees' lifestyles and work environment exposure placed them at moderate to high risk for certain cancers and that an individualized cancer risk profile could be used in tailoring a cancer-education and screening program for employees. According to Monsen and Anderson (1999), the International Society of Nurses in Genetics is focusing efforts on promoting the integration of genetics information into nursing education.

These examples illustrate how research studies on nursing students and nursing school curricula ultimately influence community health.

Efforts of an Associate-Degree Program

Schools of nursing are taking a proactive stance in the education of students. Schools continue to revisit their curricula, reevaluating the content of courses, selected learning activities, sites for clinical experiences, immediate concerns of students, health needs of society, and use of teaching personnel in economic and efficient ways (Bevis, 1973). For most schools of nursing, a large part of clinical practice has relocated outside the walls of the acute-care setting, and students are more engaged in the care of patients in the community. Schools have entered into partnerships with community agencies, and nursing has assumed the leadership role to coordinate and manage care and to ensure that a multidisciplinary approach to patients' needs is provided.

Background and History of the Raymond Walters College at the University of Cincinnati

Raymond Walters College, an associate-degree program in nursing, has been committed to excellence since its inception in 1967. The two-year program is designed to give students knowledge and technical skills to provide quality nursing care. The curriculum combines nursing courses with general courses in humanities and sciences. In a two-year follow-up survey of the 1997 class, graduates commented on the strengths of their educational experience, including rigor of the program, support from the faculty, gaining the ability to think critically, and receiving comprehensive preparation for boards and general knowledge for nursing (University of Cincinnati, Raymond Walters College, 1997).

To maintain its level of excellence, the nursing curriculum was revised several times in the past 30 years. However, the use of the medical (physiologically based) model has been consistent throughout the nursing program. The most dramatic revision took place during 1994–1996. During the 1994 academic year, the faculty discussed the issues of healthcare reform and its impact on nursing care, the impact of managed care, acute-care agencies as clinical sites, health-promotion issues, and community-health nursing. At least 85% of the faculty was certified in a specialty area, and the literature and faculty networking efforts related to curricular issues supported the belief that the faculty were underpreparing the graduates for the changing healthcare system. At the May 1994 department meeting, the faculty voted to revise the curriculum. Another major decision was made in March 1995, following an associate degree in nursing workshop, at which Tagliareni and Murray (1995) encouraged faculty "not to tinker any longer with curricula, but to create new curricula that look different from the existing ones."

During the next two years, the faculty worked diligently under the leadership of the chairperson and the department's curriculum committee. A facilitator worked with faculty during the discussions on the mission statement, philosophy, theoretical framework, and other elements essential to the curriculum. The faculty adopted the Domains of Nursing (see Figure 21-1) as the organizing framework for the new curriculum. Several recurrent themes were woven into the framework and are reflected in each course (see Figure 21-2). The new philosophy espoused faculty beliefs with regard to nursing practice, the practice of an associate-degree graduate, nursing process, health/wellness, education, and commitment to lifelong learning. During the revision process, questionnaires were sent to community home-health agencies in the Cincinnati area to scan the

Figure 21-1. Domains of Nursing

A. Promotion of well-being
B. Prevention of illness
C. Restoration of health (includes function and rehabilitation)
D. Support through the dying process (includes palliative care)

Figure 21-2. Recurrent Themes in Curriculum

A. Roles of nurse with an associate degree (care provider, care manager, member of the discipline of nursing)
B. Critical thinking
C. Nursing process
D. Communication
E. Caring theory
F. Cultural/spiritual concepts
G. Legal considerations
H. Ethical considerations
I. Teaching and learning
J. Nutrition
K. Promotion of well-being/healthy lifestyle
L. Prevention of illness
M. Restoration of optimal health
N. Health problems
O. Support through the dying process
P. Clinical competence

environment to determine the marketability (i.e., skills, experience, and other requirements) of the associate-degree graduate. Table 21-1 contains a summary of the results of the May 1995 community agencies' survey.

In 1996, the new curriculum was implemented. In the first quarter, students were introduced to the concept of wellness, the domains of nursing (promotion of wellness, prevention of illness, restoration of health, and support through the dying process), and curriculum themes. The operationalization of the theme of health promotion in the curriculum—cancer prevention and early detection—is reflected in Figure 21-3.

Needs Assessment of Cancer Prevention and Detection in Curricula in Other Ohio Schools of Nursing

To determine the degree of emphasis placed on cancer prevention and early detection and health promotion in other nursing schools' curricula, faculty from the Raymond Walters College at the University of Cincinnati conducted an informal survey in Cincinnati, Dayton, and Columbus, OH. Ohio has 61 schools of nursing (30 baccalaureate, 23 associate degree, and 8 diploma), and 13 schools

Table 21-1. Survey Questions and Responses of Community Homecare Agencies in Cincinnati, OH

Questions	n	%
Question #1: Do you hire nurse graduates with an associate degree?		
Yes	22	96
No, but would consider if no BSN was available	1	4
Additional responses		
One year medical-surgical nursing necessary	11	48
Two years of medical-surgical nursing necessary	4	16
Five years medical-surgical/critical care nursing necessary	1	4
Hemodialysis necessary	1	4
Chemotherapy necessary	1	4
Program for new graduates	4	16
Question #2: What areas need strengthening in associate-degree nursing education? Rank the importance of these skills and abilities in home care.		
Physical assessment		
– Most important	20	87
– Very important	1	8
Ability to teach patients and families	21	91
Adaptation of nursing procedure to home setting	19	83
Medication regimen/side effects	18	78
History/interviewing skills	15	65
Legal requirements of safety	13	57
Knowledge of safety factors/risks in the home	12	52

N = 23

Figure 21-3. Cancer Prevention and Early Detection Nursing Curriculum

Promotion of Well-being/Healthy Lifestyle in Nursing: Health and Wellness
(First nursing course)
• Growth and development
• Stress and coping
• Health practices of sexuality (males and females)
• Spirituality

Current health issues
• **Men**
  - Attitudes
  - Prevention
  - Total self-examination
  - Prostate screening

• **Women**
  - Attitudes
  - Prevention
  - Breast self-examination
  - Mammogram
  - Pap smear
  - Osteoporosis

Behaviors that affect adult health
• **Positive**
  - Health examinations
  - Alcohol in moderation
  - Avoidance of sun exposure
  - Minimal stress
  - Smoking cessation
  - Sleep/rest
  - Recreation
  - Awareness and response to warning signs
    of illness
  - Relaxation techniques
  - Imagery
  - Breathing exercises

• **Negative**
  - Substance abuse
  - Sun overexposure
  - High stress
  - Limited/no exercise
  - High-fat, high caloric, or restricted diet
  - Denial/delay of medical intervention

Clinical application
• Four visits to assisted living or independent living areas
• Contact with older adults to complete health interview
• Physical assessment; assessment of health teaching/learning needs
• Implementation of health teaching

Prevention of Illness in Nursing: Acute Illness
(Third nursing course)
• Biohazardous materials
• Chemotherapeutic drug handling, administration, and disposal
• Radiation precautions
• Restoration of health
• Malignant/nonmalignant tumors
• Oncologic emergencies
• Specific tumors

Clinical application
• Care of patients on medical-surgical units with cancer diagnoses
• Care of patients on an oncology unit

(Continued on next page)

Figure 21-3. Cancer Prevention and Early Detection Nursing Curriculum (Continued)

Prevention of Illness in Nursing: Mental Health and Chronic Illness
(Fourth or fifth nursing course)
• Chronic illness trajectory
  - Rehabilitation
• Community resources related to chronic conditions
• Coping tasks of the chronically ill adult
  - Psychosocial assessment
  - Application of cultural/spiritual beliefs
  - Application of nutritional concepts
• HIV/AIDS prevention, education
• Occupational/environmental hazards

Clinical application
• Home visits with case managers to patients with cancer
• Teaching health promotion/early-detection activity to older adults at a senior citizen center

Prevention of Illness in Nursing: Management
(Sixth nursing course)

Clinical application
• Engage in community activities
  - Education/teaching
  - Community services/programs
  - Rehabilitation services
  - Smoking cessation
  - Exercise programs
• Community wellness
  - Assessment of/teaching about environmental pollutants (e.g., Environmental Protection
    Agency, Occupational Safety and Health Administration Standards)

(21%) were surveyed via phone interview or e-mail. The schools were asked the following questions.
• Is cancer content taught in the curriculum?
• Where is cancer content taught in the curriculum?
• How many hours are dedicated to teaching this content, didactic and clinical?
• Are there any discussions on prevention and early detection?
• How is content applied in the clinical setting?
• Are community agencies involved?
• Is there institutional support for this endeavor?
• Are there barriers to this endeavor?

Eight schools responded—one diploma, one associate-degree, and six baccalaureate programs. All schools indicated that some cancer content was taught in their curriculum. Cancer prevention and early detection were taught in a variety of courses (e.g., basic nursing, medical-surgical, community health) and in the discussion of the five types of cancer with high incidence. Two baccalaureate programs offered a cancer nursing elective course. In two other baccalaureate programs in Cincinnati, four to six hours were spent discussing the pathophysiology of cancer and the nursing management and treatment of patients with the most common cancers. Prevention and early-detection measures (e.g., breast self-examination, clinical breast examination, mammography, smoking cessation, prostate-specific antigen) were discussed for specific cancers. The second program indicated that the cancer content in its curriculum was dispersed throughout the program. Students received two hours of didactic content during their sophomore year, eight hours in the junior year, and four hours in the senior year. Curriculum content was driven by the top 10 diseases in morbidity and mortality. Three hours in the junior year were spent on primary and secondary interventions that included epidemiology (host and environmental issues), high-risk populations, screening recommendations, and racial disparities. This school of nursing also offered a three-credit course, Bridging the Gap in Oncology Nursing, in which a maximum of six hours were devoted to prevention, early detection, and screening.

All eight schools used a variety of clinical agencies to provide clinical experiences. However, the oncology clinical hands-on experience was not available to all students. One school included the screening of such high-risk populations as migrant farm workers. Students also conducted community assessments to determine their needs. In four programs, students' clinical experience consisted of caring for patients with cancer. In another program, students were required to attend a local ONS chapter meeting to listen to guest speakers/practitioners discuss oncology-related topics. Four schools in the Cincinnati area also used the community hospice agencies as one of their clinical sites for home visits and inpatient hospice care.

One baccalaureate program in Columbus was in the midst of a curriculum revision, and its content was dispersed throughout its courses. Some clinical content was introduced under the heading of health promotion in the assessment skills component of the foundations course, an integrated course taken during the sophomore year. Specific cancers (e.g., breast, lung, colon) were introduced in the junior-year adult nursing course as medical-surgical conditions with implications for community care (prevention and early detection) and in the older adult course as common conditions. In the senior year, hematologic cancers with multiple complications were covered in the high-acuity course, with James Cancer Hospital as a clinical site. Students in every course have varying degrees of exposure to patient care at this clinical site. Six faculty members who responded either were certified or interested in the specialty of oncology and were recognized as the resource person in the school of nursing.

Implications for Nursing Educators

As illustrated in this brief, informal survey, schools of nursing are providing nurse generalists with some information about cancer and discussion of prevention and early detection and common cancers. However, the hands-on experience that provides reinforcement and application of content to the clinical situation is less than adequate. What can faculty do to provide the necessary combination of theory and practice within the limitation of time and given that other topics are competing for space in the curriculum?

Strategies for Teaching Cancer Content/Prevention and Early Detection in Nursing Curricula

The use of active learning strategies requires students to participate and invest in reading, reflecting, and interacting with faculty and other students (Moffett & Hill, 1997). The faculty member serves as the resource person to provide information, answer questions, facilitate the group process, and guide the discussion (see Tables 21-2 and 21-3).

Table 21-2. Strategies for Student Participation

Teaching Strategy	Activity	Outcome
Debate	Preparation and use of logical arguments for and against use of cancer-preventive measures	Encourages research of a topic, organized thoughts, succinct presentation, improved verbal communication, and critical thinking
Group project	Teaching breast self-examination to classmates, older women at senior citizen centers	Builds skill in critical thinking, teamwork, planning, organization, priority setting, public speaking, needs assessment, and collaboration; builds community relationships
	Discussing health nutrition with high school students, the value of immunization with mothers with young children	
Games	Use of puzzles and games like Jeopardy® and Family Feud®	Promotes group participation and outside preparation, reinforces content from reading, promotes discussion and cooperative group work
	Students develop questions and answers about cancer prevention and early detection, cancer diseases, and treatments	
Case-based teaching, vignettes, and case studies	Review of patient situations with history, signs and symptoms, diagnoses, treatment, and questions	Requires students to problem-solve, respond to specific questions with rationale, discuss actual clinical situations and cluster data, and develop nursing diagnoses; helps students develop an appreciation of patient issues (accessibility of healthcare system; barriers to cancer prevention and early detection; communication; cultural, social; and economic issues)
Narrative-centered teaching	Use of case studies related to cancer prevention and early detection with patient quotes, videotape of personal interviews, and survivor issues	Enhances students' listening skills; enables students to hear and see patient as the expert about his or her life and its meaning; encourages reflection and examination of own values, beliefs, and health behaviors (Swenson & Sims, 2000)

Table 21-3. Strategies for Clinical Application

Clinical Activity	Rationale
Clinical laboratory in which breast self-examination (BSE) and testicular self-examination are taught • Paired student practice with models • Role play of BSE instruction class	Reinforcement of new knowledge Practice of learned skill in structured environment Guided teacher instruction with feedback
Community visits with homecare agencies • Paired student visits for follow-up of patients with cancer and their families, minimum of four visits	Exposure to different types of nursing, collaboration with other health team members; use of communication skills, emphasis on role of provider of care and teacher, opportunity to practice assessment skills, appreciation of patient in home versus acute-care setting, appreciation of coordination of services
Following visits, students wrote a comprehensive paper discussing pathophysiology of disease; summarized patients' therapy; developed solutions to patients' problems; and discussed ethical, political, or healthcare issues experienced by patient, with conclusion supported by two current articles.	Follow-up and evaluation • Application of previously learned knowledge, self-reflection with clarification of issues, use of resources, critical thinking, personal and professional growth, and self-evaluation of learning strengths and needs
A section of the paper also is dedicated to students' personal feelings or experience with a chosen issue; a discussion about students' perception of the home visits and what they learned about cancer from the homecare experience; and their work with a community agency whose mission and purpose is cancer care, support, or education	Comparison of community agencies; appreciation of differences between acute-care setting and community health care
Senior citizen center setting that also provides comprehensive health care for older adults, weekly teaching sessions within their activity schedule, and standard measures of prevention and early detection (smoking cessation classes, breast health and mammography screening, nutritional concepts and meal preparation related to colon cancer, alcohol use, aging and exercise, stress management, well-being and spirituality, overexposure to sun, safe use of medications)	Clinical application of previously learned knowledge, teaching and learning needs, appreciation of and respect for the well and chronically ill older adult, appreciation of measures used to maintain health
Working with community agencies to provide teaching on prevention and early detection • American Cancer Society • American Lung Association • American Red Cross	Community teaching, establishing relationships with community agencies and members of the community

A review of the nursing literature reveals various opinions on teaching cancer content, which often is taught as an elective. Several schools of nursing discuss the need to incorporate primary prevention in their curriculum; however, there is little or no indication that this has been carried out effectively. In the nurse generalist undergraduate curriculum, many competing content areas exist, and too little time is available to address them all. Some of the barriers to teaching cancer prevention and early detection effectively in an undergraduate general school of nursing are listed in Figure 21-4.

Conclusion

Barriers should not be viewed as absolute. A nursing education is grounded in the knowledge of scientific principles, the art of applying these principles during care of the patient, the ability to solve problems by critical thinking, and a commitment to lifelong learning. As long as nursing students integrate these concepts into professional practice, the public will be well served in the areas of cancer prevention, detection, and control.

Figure 21-4. Barriers and Incentives to Teaching Cancer Content/Prevention and Early Detection

Barriers	Incentives
• Too much content in the curriculum	• Identify faculty members interested in the topic/area and encourage them to become involved.
• Reluctance to prioritize content areas	
• Overt or covert sabotage of the process (faculty gatekeepers/blockers of the process)	• Provide administrative support for educating the educator (reimbursement for workshops, joining professional organizations, attendance at ONS Annual Congress, coverage of classroom and clinical experiences to accommodate attendance at ONS Annual Congress).
• Inability to surrender control over strategies and planning	
• Nurse educators' comfort with the biomedical model of traditional nursing, medical-surgical education, pediatrics, psychiatry, and maternity (Covington, 1999)	
• Reluctance to use clinical practitioners to act as preceptors to students in the field	• Recognize certified faculty who are teaching the specialty.
• Reluctance to change the mechanism for student supervision in the field/community (use of pagers and phone versus face-to-face communication)	• Ensure that a clinical coordinator is available to research community agencies, establish contacts for home visits
• Increased travel for faculty and students	• Visit with patients in the community, and maintain relationships with school and community agencies.
• Limited flexibility to attend to other faculty responsibilities	
• Limited administrative support for curriculum changes	

References

American Cancer Society. (2000). *Cancer facts and figures, 1998–1999.* Atlanta: Author.

American Nurses Association. (1998). *Standards of clinical nursing practice* (2nd ed.). Washington, DC: Author.

Bellack, J.P., & O'Neil, E.H. (2000). Recreating nursing practice for a new century: Recommendations and implications of the Pew Health Commission final report. *Nursing and Health Care Perspectives, 21*(1), 14–21.

Bevis, O.E. (1973). *Curriculum building in nursing—A process.* St. Louis, MO. Mosby.

Brown, J.K., Johnson, J.L., & Groenwald, S.L. (1983). Survey of cancer nursing education in U.S. schools of nursing. *Oncology Nursing Forum, 10*(4), 82–83.

Cahill, M., Devlin, M., LeBlanc, P., Lowe, B., Norton, B., Tassin, K., & Vallette, E. (1998). Reexamining the associate degree curriculum: Assessing the need for community concepts. *Nursing and Health Care Perspectives, 19,* 158–165.

Covington, H. (1999). Community involvement: Substance abuse prevention for teens. *Nursing and Health Care Perspectives, 20,* 02–07.

Moffett, B., & Hill, K.B. (1997). The transition to active learning: A lived experience. *Nurse Educator, 22,* 44–47.

Monsen, M.B., & Anderson, G. (1999). Continuing education for nurses that incorporates genetics. *Journal of Continuing Education in Nursing, 30,* 20–24.

Mundt, M.H. (1996). Public education programs in the nursing curriculum. *Nurse Educator, 21,* 31–34.

National Council of State Boards of Nursing. (1997). *NCLEX-RN examination: Test plan for the National Council Licensure Examination for Registered Nurses.* Chicago: Author.

Ohio Board of Nursing. (1999). *Rules promulgated from the law regulating the practice of nursing.* Columbus, OH: Author.

Ohio League for Nursing. (1997). *Vision for nursing in Ohio.* Cleveland, OH: Author.

Oncology Nursing Society. (1995). *Standards of oncology nursing education: Generalist and advanced practice levels.* Pittsburgh: Oncology Nursing Press.

Phillips, J.M., & Belcher, A.E. (1999). Integrating cancer risk assessment into a community health nursing course. *Journal of Cancer Education, 14,* 47–51.

Post-White, J., Carter, M., & Anglim, M.A. (1993). Cancer prevention and early detection: Nursing students' knowledge, attitudes, personal practices, and teaching. *Oncology Nursing Forum, 20,* 743–749.

Rushton, P. (1999). Teaching cancer principles to undergraduate students. *Journal of Nursing Education, 20,* 77–80.

Shoultz, J., & Amundson, M.J. (1998). Nurse educators' knowledge of primary health care. Implications for community-based education, practice, and research. *Nursing Health Care Perspectives, 19*(3), 114–119.

Swenson, M.M., & Sims, S.L. (2000). A narrative-centered curriculum for nurse practitioners. *Journal of Nursing Education, 39,* 109–115.

Tagliareni, E., & Murray, J.P. (1995). Community-focused experiences in the ADN curriculum. *Journal of Nursing Education, 34,* 366–371.

University of Cincinnati, Raymond Walters College. (1997). *Graduate survey.* Cincinnati, OH: Author.

CHAPTER 22

Advancing the Cancer Control Agenda: The Role of Advanced Practice Nurses

Regina S. Cunningham, MA, RN, AOCN®

(Supported by Research Training Grant No. T32NR07035 from the National Institute of Nursing Research and by doctoral scholarships from the ONS Foundation and the American Cancer Society)

Introduction

Since the National Cancer Act was passed more than 30 years ago, cancer prevention and control activities have become an increasingly important component of the National Cancer Program (Loescher & Reid, 2000). Advances in knowledge of molecular mechanisms of cancer, earlier detection of disease through improved technology, and decreased risk factors all have contributed to a slight but sustained decrease in cancer incidence and mortality rates since the early 1990s. If this trend continues over the next decade, by 2015, a 13% and 21% decline in overall cancer incidence and mortality rates, respectively, likely will occur (Byers et al., 1999). Reducing these rates to an even greater extent is possible and should be a goal for all professionals involved in cancer care.

As advocates in the fight against cancer, oncology nurses, particularly those practicing at the advanced level, are uniquely positioned to make meaningful contributions to maintaining the health of individuals, families, and communities by engaging in cancer-prevention activities. The specific competencies associated with the advanced practice role enable these providers to meet the complex challenges that are required to advance the cancer-control agenda. As professionals who are knowledgeable about cancer biology, cancer risk, risk-reduction behaviors, and screening activities, oncology advanced practice nurses (APNs) can work directly in the oncology setting and collaboratively with colleagues in primary care to provide the education and knowledge necessary to allow for the effective incorporation of comprehensive prevention and screening activities into everyday practice. Interactions of this nature are an essential component of an overall strategy to reduce cancer incidence and mortality.

The purpose of this chapter is to discuss the role of APNs in cancer prevention and detection. The focus will be on how both general and oncology-specific APNs can contribute to improving cancer-control outcomes. Several important questions will be explored. How are APNs currently used in the healthcare system? Why are APNs well suited to carry out the prevention and screening activities that are necessary to decrease the incidence and mortality of cancer? What currently is known about the actual cancer prevention and screening practices of APNs? How effective are these activities and what are the education, research, and practice challenges for APNs in the cancer prevention and detection arenas over the next several years?

The chapter is organized into three major sections. The first section defines the roles of APNs and reviews their vast contributions to health outcomes. The second section discusses cancer-control issues and examines the work of APNs within this context. The final section presents recommendations on how APNs can maximize their efforts as a group to advance the cancer-control agenda.

Advanced Practice Nurses

The title *APN* is an umbrella term representing several roles, including certified registered nurse anesthetists (CRNAs), certified nurse midwives (CNMs), clinical nurse specialists (CNSs), and nurse practitioners (NPs). These roles share a common heritage in that they all evolved in response to societal needs. Each of the advanced practice roles has a distinct focus, although skills and knowledge overlap in some areas.

Nurse Anesthetists

CRNAs provide anesthesia and anesthesia-related care. This generally includes preanesthetic preparation and evaluation; anesthesia induction, maintenance, and emergence, including administration of appropriate drugs and local, regional, and general anesthesia, and the establishment of invasive monitoring; care during the postanesthesia period; acute and chronic pain management; and support functions for associated clinical issues, such as respiratory care and emergency resuscitation (American Association of Nurse Anesthetists, 1992).

Nurse anesthesia was the first of the advanced practice specialties to develop after the advent of anesthetic agents in the mid-1800s. Surgeons-in-training provided early anesthesia services. This arrangement was less than optimal, as the focus was on learning the surgical procedure rather than on the safe administration of anesthesia and patient monitoring. Nurses soon were recruited and trained by surgeons to provide anesthesia service and were found to be more effective than their medical predecessors (Diers, 1991).

Certified Nurse Midwives

CNMs are prepared to manage the care of women and newborns. This group of APNs delivers antepartum, intrapartum, and postpartum care as well as neonatal care, family planning, and well-woman gynecology (American College of Nurse Midwives, 1993).

Nurse midwives were the second specialty of nurses to evolve. Their history is somewhat more difficult to trace, as it is commingled with the ancient practices of midwifery. In the United States, nurse midwives gained acceptance during the early 20th century, after studies of maternal and infant mortality rates illustrated the importance of early and continuous prenatal care. In 1925, Mary Breckenridge established the Frontier Nursing Service, an early model of advanced practice. In a rural and economically depressed area of Kentucky, Breckenridge established a network of clinics where midwives, who traveled on horseback, provided healthcare services to Appalachian women and children (Bigbee, 1996).

Clinical Nurse Specialists

The CNS is defined as an expert clinician and patient advocate in a specialty or subspecialty of nursing practice. The CNS may provide direct care, including assessing, diagnosing, planning, and prescribing pharmacologic and nonpharmacologic treatment for health problems, health promotion, and preventive care within the specialized area of practice. In addition to direct practice, subroles of the CNS include that of educator, researcher, and consultant (Hamric & Spross, 1989).

The CNS role evolved during the 1960s, when nursing education reforms furnished funds that enabled schools of nursing to develop graduate education programs. The focus of these efforts was to prepare nurses to work within areas of clinical specialization. New medical discoveries, evolving technologies, and the beginning shift from paternalism to consumerism all fueled the increase in specialty practice that was occurring in health care during this time. Graduates of these new programs were CNSs. These clinicians were prepared to provide social and psychological support to patients, teach patients and families how to manage issues related to illness, act as consultants to other members of the multidisciplinary team, and serve as role models to less-experienced nurses (Bigbee, 1996; Reiter, 1966). The first CNS programs were focused in the area of psychiatric nursing. Over time, continued clinical specialization required diversification of program content to meet emerging needs, such as those in critical care and oncology. In the current system, CNSs represent multiple clinical specialties. Formal educational preparation for these roles occurs uniformly at the graduate level (Galassi, 2000).

Nurse Practitioners

NPs are healthcare providers who use critical judgment in performing expanded health assessments, differential diagnosis, and the prescribing of pharmacologic and nonpharmacologic treatments in the direct management of acute and chronic disease. The practice of NPs promotes wellness and prevents illness and injury. NPs may work autonomously or function within a multidisciplinary team as a resource or consultant. In addition, the role may involve conducting research, providing education, and influencing public policy. NPs may focus on specific areas such as pediatrics, geriatrics, or oncology. They practice in the primary or acute-care setting (American Academy of Nurse Practitioners, 1993; American Nurses Association, 1995; National Alliance of Nurse Practitioners, 1993).

The need for NPs evolved as the trend toward specialization drew increasing numbers of physicians away from primary care, creating a perceived shortage and poor distribution of medical resources. This change spurred the growth and development of the NP movement. Social support for this innovation rested in the potential for NPs to improve access to care, lower costs, and maintain quality (U.S. Congress Office of Technology Assessment, 1986).

Initially, graduate education was not considered essential to NP practice. Early reports described supplemental education or training programs designed to prepare NPs to assume an expanded role in providing primary health care. The Department of Pediatrics at the School of Medicine and the School of Nursing at the University of Colorado jointly developed the first programs. In this setting, nurses received approximately four months of "intensive theory and practice in pediatrics" (Silver, Ford, & Day, 1968, p. 88). Over time, the need for NPs to be prepared at the master's level became more apparent. Since 1992, the American Nurses Credentialing Center has required a master's degree or higher for certification as an adult, pediatric, school, or gerontologic NP. A number of specialty organizations, as well as the American Academy of Nurse Practitioners (1993) and the American Association of Colleges of Nursing (1994), support this position. The majority of NP programs today are at the master's or postmaster's level; by 2007, a master's degree will be required to be eligible for NP certification (American College of Nurse Practitioners, 1998).

Oncology Advanced Practice Nurses

Oncology advanced nursing practice is defined as "expert competency and leadership in the provision of care to individuals with an actual or potential diagnosis of cancer" (Oncology Nursing Society [ONS], 1997b). Minimum preparation for an oncology APN includes a master's degree in nursing, a direct or indirect clinical focus in the care of patients with cancer, and collaborative interactions with colleagues in education, administration, practice, and research (ONS, 1997b).

Trends in Oncology Advanced Practice Nursing

Within oncology nursing, the most common advanced practice roles are that of CNS and NP (Cooley, Spatz, & Yasko, 1996). Fueled by changes in the healthcare environment, shifts in the balance of these groups have occurred during the past decade. CNSs, historically the largest assembly of APNs within oncology, have been decreasing in number while the number of NPs has increased (see Figure 22-1). Many CNSs have returned to school to obtain additional NP training to allow them to practice in either capacity or in a blended role (Bedder, 1998; Much, Cunningham, & Zamek, 1998). The current curriculum guide addressing the specialty of oncology advanced practice nursing was broadened in the late 1990s to support the development of both sets of skills (Galassi, 2000).

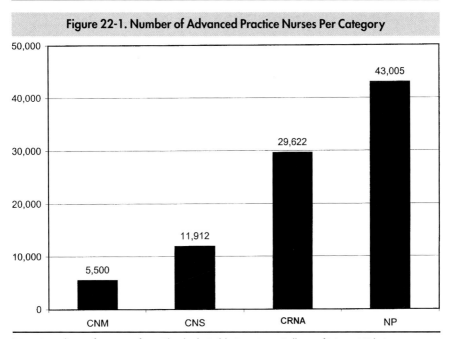

Figure 22-1. Number of Advanced Practice Nurses Per Category

Note. Based on information from Elizabeth Field, American College of Nurse-Midwives, personal communication, May 24, 2000; Steve Horton, American Association of Nurse Anesthetists, personal communication May 24, 2000; Tina Todd, American Nurses Credentialing Center, personal communication, May 24, 2000.

Collaborative approaches using both roles in the oncology-specific environment have been reported. Feuerbach, Miale-Mayer, and Wray (1999) described a professional practice model at a comprehensive cancer center. In this model, CNSs and NPs work collaboratively and share accountability for patient outcomes. The model capitalizes on the strengths of each group theoretically creating synergy, which should result in improved outcomes. Lynch and Lineham (1997) reported improved patient care and enhanced satisfaction outcomes when a similar model was implemented on the oncology service at the Graduate Hospital in Philadelphia.

The increase in the number of oncology NPs has generated keen interest on the work and effectiveness of this group; however, at the present time, very little empirical evidence on the role is available. Kinney, Hawkins, and Hudman (1997) described characteristics and activities of oncology NPs. Their study of 129 oncology-specific NPs indicated that the majority was practicing in university-affiliated, outpatient, and medical-oncology settings in the eastern United States. Most NPs practiced using protocols, many performed procedures, and about half had prescriptive authority. The majority of respondents indicated that they were satisfied with their roles. Interestingly, NPs identified physicians as the group who provided the most support for their role (Kinney et al.).

A pressing need exists for additional descriptive work in this area, as well as studies evaluating the effectiveness of these providers in the oncology-specific context. Several such investigations are in progress, and these data should become available over the next few years.

Oncology Advanced Practice Nursing Role Elements

To identify the elements that compose the role of the oncology APN, a role delineation study was conducted. This investigation involved a sample of 637 master's-prepared nurses in oncology clinical practice and 619 baccalaureate nurses in their first four years of oncology nursing certification. Participants completed a 190-item survey that described activities in five areas reflective of advanced practice, including the role of direct caregiver, researcher, educator, consultant, and administrator/coordinator. The theoretical foundation for the tool was derived from the *Standards of Advanced Practice in Oncology Nursing* (ONS, 1990). Subjects were required to indicate the frequency with which they performed each activity and the importance of the activity to their practice. Results indicated that significant differences existed between the baccalaureate- and master's-prepared groups, with the greatest differences noted in the areas of researcher and consultant. APNs indicated that they performed activities on the direct caregiver and educator subscales more frequently, believing that these behaviors were the most important to their practice. In this sample of APNs, 58% identified their job title as CNS. Only 6% of the sample identified their title as NP; the remainder reported a wide variety of job titles. The results of the study were used to design the blueprint for the Advanced Oncology Nursing Certification (AOCN®) test (McMillan, Heusinkveld, & Spray, 1995).

In light of the changing profile of the oncology APN and the fact that the majority of participants in the initial study were CNSs, concern was expressed that the certification examination might be weighted in favor of CNSs. To address this, a replication role delineation study was undertaken. During the time between the two studies, the number of oncology NPs had increased dramatically (J. Kinzler, personal communication, May 2000); therefore, the second study involved a much more equitable distribution of CNSs and NPs. Respondents again were asked to rate the frequency and importance to practice of 121 activities categorized according to the five role components. The role of direct caregiver again was weighted the most heavily (63%), followed by educator (18%), consultant (10%), administrator/coordinator (5%), and researcher (4%). Fewer than 10% of the items differentiated between CNS and NP respondents. Authors concluded that the blueprint for the AOCN® examination was appropriate for both CNSs and NPs in oncology (McMillan, Heusinkveld, Spray, & Murphy, 1999).

Advanced Practice Nursing Goals and Competencies

As a group of professionals, all APNs share common goals, including improving access to healthcare services, increasing interdisciplinary collaboration, developing an expanded knowledge base for clinical decision making, participating in the development of health and social policy, conducting scholarly investigations, participating in leadership activities, increasing professional autonomy, and providing services in new areas (Barnsteiner, Deatrick, Grey, Hayman, & O'Sullivan, 1993). To achieve these goals, APNs possess a range of competencies that are relevant to the problems and challenges that occur in today's healthcare context. These competencies include providing direct care, coaching, collaboration, ethical decision making, research utilization, and leadership (Spross & Heaney, 2000). Each of the APN goals is congruent with advancing the agenda for cancer control. The defined APN competencies are essential to the group's effectiveness in supporting cancer prevention and detection activities.

Advanced Practice Nursing Effectiveness

Since the inception of advanced practice roles, an evolving body of empirical evidence has documented improvements in health care when APNs manage aspects of care. This body of knowledge provides important background information in that it describes a variety of contexts in which APNs have been able to substantially improve clinical outcomes. Understanding these contributions is essential to realizing the full potential of APNs in the cancer-control arena.

Outcomes Related to Quality

Abundant evidence exists to support APNs' ability to influence the quality of healthcare delivery. Both global and specific health-related outcomes have been positively affected by care delivered or contributed by APNs.

Mortality rates are considered to be an indicator of quality of care. Alice McGaw, an early nurse anesthetist at the Mayo Clinic, reported that she had provided anesthesia care for 14,000 surgical cases without one anesthesia-related death (Thatcher, 1953). Mary Breckenridge's attention to detail in regard to the collection of mortality outcome data was visionary. From the outset, she directed the midwives of the Frontier Nursing Service to keep accurate and detailed records of their activities. When the Metropolitan Life Insurance Company analyzed these data later, they revealed that 8,596 births were attended with a maternal mortality rate of 1.2 per 1,000; this was significantly lower than the national average of 3.4 per 1,000 live births (Varney, 1987). More recently, Levy, Wilkinson, and Marine (1971) and Ellings, Newman, Hulsey, Bivins, and Keenan (1993) reported decreased maternal and infant death rates when APNs managed aspects of care. McCorkle et al. (2000) reported a survival advantage in elderly patients with cancer who received a standardized postoperative intervention provided by APNs in the home setting. Additionally, Hastings et al. (1980) reported a decrease in the rate of suicides in a Florida prison after NPs instituted psychiatric/mental health screening practices.

The quality of APN care frequently has been compared to the quality of the same care provided by physicians. Physician substitution activities are defined as those services historically considered to be within the purview of medicine that can be performed competently by APNs. A substantial body of literature documents the ability of APNs to provide care in certain settings that is equal to or better than that which is provided by physicians. An early report by Sox (1979) reviewed 21 studies and found that primary care rendered by NPs in the office setting was "indistinguishable" from that which was provided by physicians. In 1986, the U.S. Congress Office of Technology Assessment published a policy analysis in response to a request from the Senate Committee on Appropriations. This comprehensive work assessed the contributions of NPs and CNMs in meeting the healthcare needs of the nation and concluded that care provided by these practitioners was of as good or better quality than care provided by physicians. Moreover, Safriet (1992), in a classic analysis, reported that NPs repeatedly have demonstrated superior performance when compared to physicians with respect to access, quality, and cost.

Patient satisfaction outcomes often are used as an indicator of quality of care, and many investigations of APN effectiveness have assessed this variable. Study findings have demonstrated improvements in satisfaction scores after the implementation of APN services. In some cases, patients reported that they were more satisfied with the care provided by APNs than with care rendered by physicians. Reasons for this particular finding were not discussed. Perhaps this level of satisfaction is related to the type or nature of the relationships NPs develop with patients. Several studies alluded to improved communication between patients and providers. Aiken et al. (1993), for example, indicated that patients seen by NPs reported more symptoms than did those who received their care in a physician group. This finding, in part, may be a reflection of the quality of the communication patterns that were established between NPs and patients. Similarly, McCorkle et al. (1989) indicated that patients with lung cancer who received home nursing reported worse health perceptions over time and suggested that this may be because the nurses assisted these patients to acknowledge the reality of their situation. This, again, may be related to the quality of the nurse-patient interaction.

Access-to-Care Outcomes

Historically, because of restrictions on practice, APNs were somewhat limited in the settings in which they could provide care. In many respects, this created an opportunity to operationalize their goal of improving access. Serving populations with limited access to healthcare resources is a resounding theme in the APN literature. Levy et al. (1971) studied midwives who provided perinatal services to women living in a poor, rural, agricultural county. In this setting, midwives had to work with generalist physicians because no obstetricians/gynecologists were available in the area. Spitzer et al. (1974) conceived the idea of using NPs in a thriving family practice to improve access to services. In the Canadian healthcare system, primary care providers were so overburdened that patients had a substantial waiting period before they could receive care. Introducing NPs increased the productivity of the practice and decreased the waiting time for patients. Ross (1981) noted a 27% increase in prenatal visits for Navajo women after a CNM model was implemented. Effectively improving access to care has particular implications in the cancer-control arena. A lack of access to appropriate services has been cited as a common reason for lack of participation in cancer prevention and detection activities (Frank-Stromborg & Cohen, 2000).

Role of Advanced Practice Nurses in Cancer Control

Each of the advanced practice roles has great potential to contribute to advancing the cancer-prevention agenda. Health teaching with a focus on the cause and prevention of disease is an important component of all APN roles. Figure 22-2 illustrates data depicting the number of nurses within each of the advanced practice categories. Figures 22-3 and 22-4 provide a breakdown by specialty within the NP and CNS groups.

Based on their scope of practice and the populations they serve, some groups of APNs have greater potential to have an impact on cancer prevention and detection, and they should be targeted aggressively to actively participate in cancer-control efforts. NPs, because of their expanded perspective and advanced skills, have an extremely important role in cancer-control activities (Frank-Stromborg & Cohen, 2000; Leslie, 1995; Reed & Selleck, 1996; Spencer-Cisek, 1998). NPs often provide primary care, and health-promotion activities are a major component of their practice. According to the American Nurses Credentialing Center (T. Todd, personal communication, May 2000), more than 43,000 NPs currently are practicing in the United States, with the majority of these providers working in adult and family health (see Figure 22-2). Moreover, trends indicate that the number of NPs in the United States is increasing (American Association of Colleges of Nursing, 1997–2000). Coupled with the increased viability of the role in today's healthcare context, this makes NPs a critical group on which to focus cancer-control education and

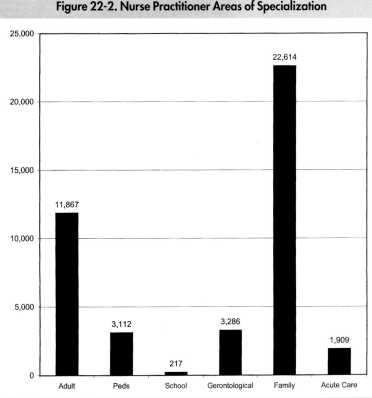

Figure 22-2. Nurse Practitioner Areas of Specialization

Note. Based on information from Tina Todd, American Nurses Credentialing Center, personal communication, May 24, 2000.

Figure 22-3. Clinical Nurse Specialist Areas of Specialization

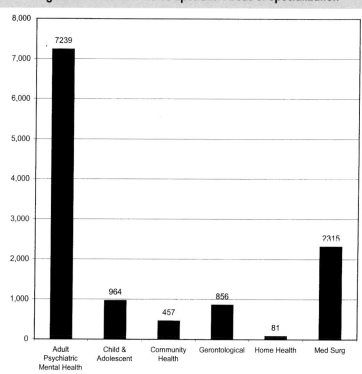

Note. Based on information from Tina Todd, American Nurses Credentialing Center, personal communication, May 24, 2000.

training activities. Ensuring that these practitioners provide their patients with routine prevention education and counseling, as well as systematic opportunities for early detection with appropriate follow-up, could have a substantial impact on cancer incidence and mortality rates.

CNMs also are an important group to target. Although they are smaller in number than NPs, they provide more than five million patient visits annually (Paine et al., 2000). In addition, they have responsibilities similar to those of NPs in terms of managing the health of women. Women represent a potentially vulnerable population, and APNs have a substantial history of working effectively with vulnerable populations. Cancers of the breast and cervix are among those associated with the highest morbidity and mortality rates in the United States (Greenlee, Hill-Harmon, Murray, & Thun, 2001). The 1996 National Institutes of Health consensus statement on cervical cancer identified that substantial subsets of women, specifically ethnic minorities, the elderly, and the uninsured and poor, have not been screened or are not being screened at regular intervals (National Institutes of Health, 1996). CNMs should be actively involved in cancer prevention and detection activities focused on breast and gynecologic malignancies, with particular attention to needy subsets of the population.

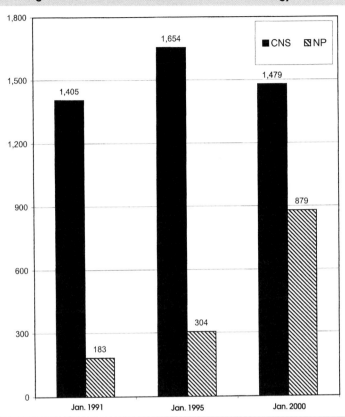

Figure 22-4. Number of Advanced Practice Oncology Nurses

Note. Based on information from Chris Kovac, Oncology Nursing Society, personal communication, June 2, 2000.

The complexity and diversity of CNS activities in the current healthcare system make CNSs another important group on which to focus cancer-control efforts. Although traditionally very different, the practice of CNSs in today's healthcare environment may not be dissimilar to that of NPs. The concept of a "merged" CNS/NP role has been the subject of much discussion and debate over the past decade. Empirical evidence supports similarities in the fundamental knowledge and skills of both groups. Differences primarily are related to time spent in direct versus indirect care activities (Elder & Bullough, 1990; Williams & Valdivieso, 1994). Moreover, several of the studies presented in the previous section clearly demonstrate that CNSs have an established tradition of improving outcomes in a variety of contexts. Many CNSs have roles in which they are assigned accountability for programmatic development. This frequently involves integration of care, coordination of services, public and professional education, quality assurance, and program evaluation, many of which are required to carry out cancer prevention and screening activities effectively.

Despite the fact that they represent a fair percentage of the APN contingency, CRNAs are somewhat more limited in their ability to participate in cancer-control activities because of their circumscribed area of clinical practice. CRNAs, however, should be knowledgeable in regard to cancer-detection activities. In particular, because they frequently are accountable for presurgical histories and physical examinations, they should be well versed in the early warning signs of cancer that might be assessed in this setting.

Current trends in health care have facilitated the development of a myriad of opportunities for APNs in the prevention and detection arenas. The general shift to a wellness orientation has helped to elevate cancer prevention and early detection on the hierarchy of priorities (Hilton, 1999). Moreover, the translation of emerging science in the area of cancer control has created new needs in the clinical setting. The expansion of genetic technology, for example, has created the ability to identify individuals who are at high risk of developing certain types of cancer. This has resulted in the demand for access to genetic testing and information. APNs have responded to these emerging needs through the development of an advanced practice role with a specialty in genetics. Because this role has implications in the cancer-control arena, it will be presented in greater detail later in the chapter. As the delivery of health care continues to evolve and novel needs emerge, new roles and subroles will develop within the APN group.

Cancer Control

Emerging science in the area of cancer control has led to a reconceptualization of cancer prevention. At one time, cancer prevention was thought to encompass all activities that had the potential to limit the progression of the disease at any time during its trajectory. In this model, nursing interventions aimed at cancer control might occur anywhere along the continuum. Newer thinking portends that cancer prevention is achieved when modulation or modification of self-care behaviors or exogenous factors results in decreased cancer risk. Some authors have suggested that prevention interventions relate to particular stages of carcinogenesis. Primary prevention activities, for example, should relate to initiation, secondary prevention to promotion, and tertiary prevention to progression (Byar & Freedman, 1990). The Division of Cancer Prevention and Control of the National Cancer Institute (NCI) currently defines cancer control as the "reduction of cancer incidence, morbidity, and mortality through an orderly sequence from research on interventions and their impact in defined populations to the broad, systematic application of the research results" (Division of Cancer Prevention and Control, 1994, p. 9).

Several approaches to reducing the frequency of cancer exist. Eliminating or modifying well-identified risk factors, such as diet, tobacco, and sun exposure, represent one approach. This can be achieved through education and, in some cases, regulation. A second approach involves host modification. This refers to strategies used to alter the body's internal environment to prevent the initiation or progression of cancer. Approaches to host modification most commonly include immunization and chemoprevention. *Chemoprevention* refers to the use of defined noncytotoxic nutrients or pharmacologic agents to inhibit or reverse the process of carcinogenesis. To date, this approach has been the most tested and promising of the host modification methods (Loescher & Reid, 2000).

Decreasing morbidity and mortality can be achieved through early-detection and screening programs and the application of state-of-the-art cancer treatments. *Early detection of cancer* refers to attempts to diagnose the disease when it is in its earliest stages. Cancer screening involves the use of tests or examinations performed periodically by healthcare professionals to detect disease in an asymptomatic person. Screening is a strategy to detect the disease in its earliest stages, when it will be most amenable to intervention (Frank-Stromborg & Cohen, 2000).

Empirical Evidence Supporting the Role of Advanced Practice Nurses in Cancer Control

Several data sources were used to identify empirical literature reviewing the work of APNs in the area of cancer prevention or detection. An electronic search of the CINAHL® and CANCERLIT® databases was preformed using the key words *cancer prevention, cancer detection, cancer control, cancer screening*, and all titles that would be relevant under the heading Advanced Practice Nurse. Additional references were obtained through a review of the reference lists of selected articles that were retrieved through the electronic search. In addition, a review of published abstracts presented at the ONS Annual Congresses 1997–2000 was conducted to provide evidence on works in progress. The results of this investigation yielded a large number of references focused on the topic.

The literature revealed that APNs are actively involved and use diverse and creative strategies to contribute to cancer-control activities. They are participating in public education, coordinating screening and early-detection programs, and educating colleagues in the area of cancer prevention and control. Many authors supported the role of the APN in carrying out cancer-control activities. Leslie (1995) described how NPs use strategies in their everyday practice to improve breast and cervical cancer prevention. Comprehensive assessment, including family and sexual history, identification of personal risk factors, and appropriate teaching interventions were cited as critical factors in this process. Frank-Stromborg and Cohen (2000) suggested that NPs were well equipped to carry out many of the complex procedures that are components of a comprehensive evaluation. Reed and Selleck (1996) indicated that the activities of NPs and CNMs naturally facilitated cancer prevention and detection. Health promotion, disease prevention and counseling, health maintenance education, screening, and the use of community resources are all activities that are associated with APN practice. Moreover, these activities routinely are taught in APN educational programs and are consistent with functions that APNs view as being within their scope of practice (Reed & Selleck).

Advanced Practice Nursing Cancer-Control Practices

Warren and Pohl (1990) investigated the cancer screening and detection practices of NPs in adult primary-care settings. To assess practice patterns, researchers developed a questionnaire based on the American Cancer Society's (ACS's)

Guidelines for the Cancer-Related Checkup (ACS, 1980) and the cancer detection literature. The instrument was distributed to self-identified NPs practicing in primary-care settings throughout Michigan; the final analysis was conducted using 97 returned questionnaires. Subjects in this sample reported significantly greater frequencies in screening women than in men. Young and early middle-aged adults also were found to have higher rates of screening than older adults. In addition, findings indicated that NPs consider cancer-screening activities to be within their scope of practice, except in areas of male physical examination (e.g., testes, prostate) and invasive procedures such as sigmoidoscopy. When NPs were asked to identify reasons for not implementing screening guidelines, the top four reasons reported were "not feasible because of practice setting," "need to update/do not feel competent," "lack of time," and "cost factors" (Warren & Pohl, p. 150).

Tessaro, Herman, Shaw, and Giese (1996) reported similar findings in a later study. In their investigation, 101 NPs working in 87 health departments indicated that they provided breast and cervical screening services for most women older than 40; however, NPs reported that they were less likely to provide other types of cancer prevention interventions, such as counseling on smoking cessation and dietary risk counseling. The NPs rated their screening skills as excellent. Confidence in educating about cancer risk was rated lower, and NPs indicated that they needed to learn more about the latest recommendations on cancer-prevention practices.

Knowledge and competence also were highly correlated to the frequency of assessment and teaching in work by Maguire-Eisen and Frost (1994). In this study, which was designed to determine how NPs and dermatology and oncology nurses differ in their knowledge of risk factors, preventive measures, and recognition of cutaneous malignant melanoma, dermatology nurses (n = 66) scored higher than NPs (n = 66) or oncology nurses (n = 46) on recognition of all lesions. Knowledge of risk factors did not vary among the groups. Dermatology nurses performed regular skin cancer assessments 58% of the time, whereas NPs reported that they completed this activity only 40% of the time. Interestingly, in this sample, the oncology nurses did not perform routine skin cancer assessments.

The effectiveness of APNs often has been compared to that of physicians. Such a comparison was the subject of work by Mendelblatt et al. (1993), who compared the effectiveness of an NP program that offered low-income elderly African American women breast and cervical screening during routine visits with a control site in which physicians provided care. Postintervention screening rates increased substantially in the NP group. Despite this increase, researchers reported that the rates of screening in this population were below levels targeted by NCI. Authors speculated that these findings might have been attributable to a lack of consensus on screening guidelines, the presence of comorbidities, or the prevalence of hysterectomies in this population (Mendelblatt et al.). Frank-Stromborg and Nord (1979) evaluated patient acceptance of an NP role in a cancer-detection clinic. No significant differences were found in satisfaction with examinations provided by NPs or physicians.

Overview of the Advanced Practice Nursing Role in Prevention and Screening

Screening Initiatives

APNs have demonstrated a strong commitment to cancer control through their consistent and innovative approaches to developing and participating in cancer screening and detection efforts. Multiple examples will be used to provide an overview of these activities.

Colon cancer was expected to account for 21% of all cancer cases in 2001 (Greenlee et al., 2001). Screening tests for colorectal cancer in asymptomatic individuals include digital rectal examination, fecal occult blood testing (Decosse, Tsioulias, & Jacobson, 1994), and sigmoidoscopy (Smith, Mettlin, Davis, & Eyre, 2000). APNs have been actively involved in screening activities for colorectal cancers. Waldman (2000) reported on the development of a colorectal screening clinic in an urban neighborhood that was funded through the Office of Minority Health. APNs coordinated the development and implementation of this program. Successful use of sigmoidoscopy by NPs also has been reported. Rosevelt and Frankl (1984) described the role of NPs in conducting colorectal screening using 60-cm flexible fiberoptic sigmoidoscopy. After receiving training by gastroenterologists, NPs initiated a screening program to evaluate asymptomatic patients older than age 40. Findings were similar to those reported when physicians performed the procedure and substantiated the use of NPs in this capacity. The responses of patients and referring gastroenterologists were positive. Similar results were found in a study in which NPs performed video sigmoidoscopy (Schroy, Wiggins, Winawer, Diaz, & Lightdale, 1988). Froerer (1998) surveyed APNs who were members of the Society of Gastroenterology Nurses and Associates to ascertain whether they believed they should perform endoscopic procedures. More than 70% of the APNs who responded indicated that diagnostic endoscopic procedures were within the scope of their practice. Barriers to performing the procedure, however, included liability, reimbursement, a lack of physician support, and limited training opportunities (Froerer).

APNs have been actively involved in developing screening and early-detection opportunities for many other types of cancer as well. In the majority of these situations, their roles involved that of coordinator or direct caregiver. Coles (1999) reported on the development of an APN-initiated skin cancer screening clinic. In this setting, an oncology CNS convened a multidisciplinary team to coordinate a skin cancer screening initiative. The focus of this effort was to increase awareness by providing education and screening opportunities for local residents. Similarly, Jackson, Moore, and Sobolik (2000) reported on how APNs assumed the leadership role in organizing and implementing free public screenings for prostate, breast, colorectal, and skin cancer. This program was implemented simultaneously at 14 clinics in the metropolitan Atlanta area. APN responsibilities included project organization, strategic selection of sites, staffing, and development and adaptation of screening forms. This work resulted in 1,468 screenings and the identification of 236 suspicious findings.

Waring, Rittenberg, and Bateman (1999) described the role of an oncology CNS in a free breast screening program for uninsured women ages 40–49. In this model, the CNS completed detailed histories and taught participants breast self-examination techniques. When abnormal mammographic findings were identified, the CNS telephoned participants to discuss their results and arrange for follow-up.

The development of a nurse-managed Employee Cancer Screening Clinic to meet the needs of M.D. Anderson Cancer Center's 6,000 employees provides another example of an APN-initiated screening program. In this setting, services provided by nurses included complete histories, physical examinations, nutritional assessments, functional status evaluations, and risk assessments. Issues of education and motivation were addressed, and routine screening opportunities were made available for employees (White, 1989; White & Faulkenberry, 1985).

Improving access to screening is important in reaching many subsets of the general population. An outreach program sponsored by the Markstein Cancer Education and Prevention Center in California and funded by the Susan G. Komen Foundation used a women's health NP to provide educational outreach presentations regarding components of breast cancer screening. Presentations took place at local churches and subsidized housing facilities in an effort to reach low-income women older than age 60—two subgroups that are particularly important to target. The elderly are known to participate less often in screening programs, and lower socioeconomic status is associated with a decreased level of reporting suspicious symptoms (Frank-Stromborg & Cohen, 2000). Participants in this program were given clinical breast examinations, breast self-examination instruction, and mammographies free of charge. Transportation, language translation, and culturally sensitive teaching materials also were provided.

Collaboration and leadership have been identified as key APN competencies (Spross & Heaney, 2000). The two examples that follow demonstrate how APNs have used these skills with organizations and groups to provide screening opportunities.

APNs in the Philadelphia area orchestrated a "Day of Wellness" after completing a community needs assessment. This program provided cancer education and screening for women who belonged to a religious order of sisters in the area. Breast, gynecologic, and colorectal screening by a female gynecologist and an NP also were provided for participants. Successful program evaluations led to additional collaborations and resulted in the development of screening services to meet the healthcare needs for all sisters in the archdiocese of Philadelphia (Boileau, 1998).

An early lung cancer detection initiative at the Cancer Institute of New Jersey provides another example of a unique collaboration. Lung cancer was expected to account for approximately 157,400 deaths in 2001. Estimates suggested that women, in particular, would be affected, with lung cancer being responsible for 25% of all female cancer deaths in 2001. The overall five-year survival rate for the disease is an abysmal 14% (Greenlee et al., 2001). One of the reasons for poor survival is the extent of disease upon clinical presentation; tumors often are not identified until after metastatic infiltration has occurred. In an attempt to rectify this problem, a number of approaches to screening and early detection in this population have been investigated. Evidence thus far has been inconclusive, and no organization currently recommends routine screening (Smith et al., 2000). Recent evidence from the Early Lung Cancer Action Project, however, suggests that low-radiation-dose computed tomography may be useful in detecting early-stage disease, when it would be most amenable to treatment (Henschke et al., 1999). This scan is a component of the early lung cancer detection program at the institute. An APN working in collaboration with a thoracic oncologist coordinates this service. The program represents a joint effort between the institute and a local legislator, who is interested in providing cancer-prevention services in the community. Because the scan is not covered by many health insurance plans, a volume discount was negotiated with the local radiology group for individuals who were eligible to participate. Funding for the program was provided through the local legislator's budget (P. Joyce, personal communication, May 2000).

Cultural and Barrier Issues

One of the points outlined in ONS's *Position Paper on Quality Cancer Care* (ONS, 1997a) was that care should be provided in a cost-effective, ethical, and culturally competent manner. Race and ethnicity are known to affect knowledge and beliefs about cancer (Frank-Stromborg, 1997). The manner in which cultural beliefs and practices influence health behaviors is essential knowledge for developing effective cancer-control activities.

African Americans experience higher cancer incidence and mortality rates than do other Americans (Dignam, 2000; Greenlee et al., 2001). To reduce this disparity, culturally sensitive prevention and early-detection programs must be developed for this population. Robinson, Kimmel, and Yasko (1995) described an excellent example of a comprehensive prevention and screening program targeting African Americans. The African American Cancer Program, developed in 1992 at the University of Pittsburgh Cancer Institute, was designed to enhance cancer awareness and promote prevention, early detection, diagnosis, and treatment in African Americans. Components of this program included the Celebration of Life project, cancer-education programs in the African American community, an anti-smoking campaign in elementary schools in African American neighborhoods, and bimonthly screening opportunities. NPs and physicians conducted screenings at local community centers and included examinations of the head and neck, oral cavity, abdomen, breasts, skin, prostate (digital rectal examination and serum prostate-specific antigen), and cervix (Pap smears). In addition to their role as direct caregivers in this project, APNs were involved in aspects of coordination and administration of the program.

Bartley (1998) reported on the development of a nurse-managed breast cancer screening program within a primary-care clinic serving an inner-city African American population. In this model, an APN was fully integrated into a primary-care clinic. Activities of the APN in this setting included educating physicians and other healthcare providers about screening guidelines, implementing documentation procedures for screening follow-up, placing screening guidelines in examination rooms, and providing culturally appropriate patient-education literature. Program outcomes were measured by tracking patient adherence to initial mammography recommendations and the frequency of return visits for repeat mammography the following year. Of the 323 women who participated in the intervention, 99% received breast self-examination instruction, 94% completed initial mammograms, and 89% of participants older than 50 returned for follow-up (Bartley). Primary-care settings have been identified as an ideal setting for cancer-control activities to take place (Love & Olsen, 1985). This model illustrates how the oncology APN can be used in a general setting to provide services effectively and act as a resource for colleagues working in primary care.

Marinelli, Chin-A-Loy, and Ramsey (1999) reported on an outreach program instituted in Delaware. Distressed by the low response rates of African American men to prostate cancer screening activities, the group formed a special recruitment task force of community volunteers. Participants in this program completed training with specialized instruction on prostate cancer awareness. After implementation, screening rates for African American men rose from 7% to 15%; target goals include increasing participation rates to 25% for this group.

Rural populations represent another "cultural" group. Rural women use mammography at a rate 17% lower than that of women in metropolitan areas. After implementation of the Friend to Friend outreach intervention, coordinated by a public health APN, mammography rates among the sample of rural women tested increased by 29%. In addition, 66% of subjects shared the screening information with nonparticipants (Richards & Kent, 2000). Another study reported on rural Latino women seeking cancer-detection examinations. Surveys of a subset of this sample revealed that Latino women would be more receptive to cervical cancer screening if female NPs conducted examinations. When planning A Day for Latino Women, volunteer family NP (FNP) students from a post-master's FNP course worked with faculty from the Northern Illinois University School of Nursing to provide examinations free of charge (Frank-Stromborg, Wassner, Nelson, Chilton, & Wholeben, 1998). Tailored programs such as these are essential to reach segments of the population that may not otherwise access preventive health services.

Scholarly investigation was one of the goals common to APNs. Several reports indicated that APNs are involved in research activities that examine the influence of cultural beliefs on health-promotion and cancer-prevention practices. The relationship of sociodemographic variables to up-to-date Pap test status in minority urban women was the subject of work by Jennings-Dozier (1999). The probability of a woman being up-to-date with her annual Pap test was found to be associated with age, insurance status, education, marital status, and household size. These findings indicated that screening efforts should target those groups that are less likely to be up-to-date, which include African Americans, Latinos, the elderly, and women who have less than a high-school education, have low socioeconomic status, and are married with large families (Jennings-Dozier).

Advanced Practice Nursing Public-Education Initiatives

Providing the public with information they need to protect and care for themselves is a critical component of the cancer-control process. The public often has misinformation or misperceptions about health issues (Leslie, 1995). Nichols,

Misra, and Alexy (1996) examined the knowledge, attitudes, and behaviors of 172 laypeople to evaluate public knowledge of cancer prevention and detection practices. Findings indicated a substantial lack of understanding of the warning signs of cancer among this group, illustrating the need for public-education programs. APNs, because of their expanded knowledge base and understanding of adult learning principles, are well positioned to provide cancer-prevention education. A number of reports have indicated that APNs spend a significant portion of their time engaged in teaching activities (Hughes, Hodgson, Muller, Robinson, & McCorkle, 2000; White, Given, & Devoss, 1996). Moreover, the original role delineation study, discussed earlier in this chapter, identified that APNs believe that education is one of the most important components of their practice.

APNs have been effective in developing educational programs for the public. A recent report described how APNs coordinated a multidisciplinary team to develop a computerized cancer risk assessment program to be used at senior citizen expos, health fairs, schools, and other sites, as requested. This strategy seemed particularly well conceived because it targeted specific groups. Children, in particular, have been identified as a key group on which to focus cancer-prevention public-education activities (Brethauer & Swenson, 2000).

Children and adolescents were the focus of a public-education program sponsored by the Philadelphia Area Chapter of ONS. This group provided an educational exhibit at the First Union United States Pro Championship Bike Race. The goal of this endeavor was to educate the 500,000 spectators on the risks of skin cancer and teach "sun-sensible" behaviors. Because most lifetime sun exposure occurs early in life, educational strategies were directed to children and adolescents. The success of this effort led the chapter to expand its public-education initiatives to other outdoor sporting events in Philadelphia (Casale, Hostler, & Jackson, 2000).

Jones (2000) described a community-wide approach to reducing the morbidity and mortality of cancer by engaging a group of professionals and the lay community to establish the Committee on Preventable Cancers. Once convened, the group conducted a health needs assessment and developed a plan of action for issues related to breast, skin, and cervical cancer as well as lung and other tobacco-related cancers.

Peer-education methods have been reported to be effective in increasing participation in screening. Weinrich et al. (1998) reported that African American men who received peer-educator interventions, which included a patient testimonial, were more likely to participate in prostate cancer screening activities than were subjects who received standard educational interventions. A similar trial is under way in a different population at the Cancer Institute of New Jersey. In this setting, several members of the APN group are engaged in a breast screening trial. This investigation, which is funded by the Susan G. Komen Foundation, was designed to determine if minority women or those with low socioeconomic status enrolled in a breast cancer screening program are more likely to complete screening and the recommended follow-up if part of the screening involves teaching by a peer who has been treated for breast cancer.

As a part of a breast screening program, either a peer educator or an APN randomly is chosen to teach women. Researchers are testing the hypothesis that peer-taught women will have a higher rate of follow-up mammography and clinical breast examination at one year than the control group. Both APNs and the peer educators have undergone a training session that ensures uniform teaching strategies and information for both groups of subjects in the study. The teaching session includes information on the importance and benefits of mammography, a breast self-examination demonstration, ACS patient-education materials, and information on the role of clinical breast examination. Women in the peer-teaching group also are exposed to a personal vignette from the experience of the peer teacher that stresses the importance of screening (T. Kearney, personal communication, May 2001).

Many of the initiatives discussed in previous sections also included components of public education. Health-promotion teaching, with a focus on healthy lifestyle choices and health-maintenance strategies, has been the focus of many of these activities.

Advanced Practice Nursing Professional-Education Initiatives

The education of colleagues is another strategy that APNs have used to contribute to reductions in cancer incidence and mortality. Education provides knowledge and facilitates the attitude and skill changes that are fundamental to practice changes (Stalker, 1985). APNs frequently are used as a resource in the healthcare community. A recent study evaluated the use of nurse educators to deliver an educational program on colorectal cancer screening to 240 physicians in 120 primary-care practices. Content presented by APNs included a review of colorectal cancer screening guidelines and the standard of care related to research findings (Berry, Kiefer, & Jennings-Dozier, 2000). The effectiveness of this strategy relied heavily upon the expanded clinical knowledge base of APNs as well as their leadership and collaborative skills (A. Berry, personal communication, May 2000).

Emerging Roles for Advanced Practice Nurses in the Cancer-Control Arena

The development of an expanded knowledge base in cancer control has created new needs and subsequent demands on the healthcare system. Guided by its social mandate, nursing has developed strategies to meet the emerging needs effectively. APNs historically have provided leadership in creating opportunities to meet such needs. Two examples of situations where APNs have responded to evolving needs in the healthcare system will be presented to illustrate this point.

Role of Advanced Practice Nurses in Cancer Genetics

Expanding knowledge of genetics and molecular biology has substantially enhanced nurses' understanding of the risk of developing certain types of cancers.

The evolution of genetic technology is beginning to have a profound impact on cancer-prevention strategies. Genetic profiling ultimately will allow customization of health advice, including the application of anticancer interventions. The ability to specifically target appropriate prevention and screening interventions to subgroups of asymptomatic but high-risk individuals will become a reality. Tailored approaches, based on individual need, will minimize the unnecessary anxiety of screening in populations with limited potential to develop the disease. Moreover, this approach will be more acceptable in terms of both associated risks and cost (Engleking, 1994; Peters, 1997).

In addition to the ability to predict and prevent cancers in individuals, genetic and molecular technology is anticipated to enhance clinical diagnostic capability. This may aid in the earlier and more accurate detection of cancers. The diagnosis of cancer is increasingly including specific descriptions of the molecular characteristics of the disease. Moreover, research has suggested that the identification of certain gene mutations may have a useful role as molecular markers in early disease, when treatment is most effective. Clinical practice changes should be anticipated as additional knowledge in the area of molecular pathophysiology in cancer is developed (Peters, 1997).

Oncology APNs already have assumed active roles in managing high-risk populations. Several high-risk evaluation programs have opened in institutions throughout the country. At first, these were located primarily in cancer centers, but, over time, they have become increasingly available in the community setting. These centers provide access to professionals with expertise in the area of cancer genetics who can render comprehensive risk evaluation and counseling, arrange for genetic susceptibility testing, make appropriate follow-up and surveillance recommendations, and provide individual and family education. The coordination of high-risk evaluation programs is an emerging role for APNs. The roles and responsibilities of APNs in these settings often include taking expanded family histories; performing pedigree analysis; obtaining informed consent; providing education and counseling regarding the benefits, limitations, and risks of genetic testing; and coordination and documentation of care. In addition, APNs may function as a resource for professional colleagues in the area of genetics (Dimond, Calzone, Davis, & Jenkins, 1998; Hewitt & Galucci, 1999; J. Much, personal communication, May 2000; Suhayda, 1997).

The psychosocial issues in the "high-risk" population have created new challenges for oncology nurses. Gaining insight into the specialized needs of this group will result from greater experience and research. APNs already have assumed an active role in helping to describe characteristics of the high-risk patient. One study revealed that women who were participating in a comprehensive surveillance program tended to be more anxious than other high-risk women (Gross, McDonough, & Heerdt, 1999). Another investigation explored whether a structured psychosocial intervention improved cancer-risk perception, global depression, cancer worries, and general coping related to genetic cancer-risk assessment. A significant improvement in all psychological measures was noted immediately postintervention; overly high perceptions of cancer risk dramatically declined from baseline to postintervention (Montgomery, Daly, & Masny, 1998).

Complex issues surround the use of genetic information and material. Advances in this area have created numerous ethical and legal dilemmas (Giarelli & Jacobs, 2000), and several authors have identified the need for healthcare professionals, particularly oncology nurses, to be cognizant of the potential problems surrounding genetic issues (Dimond et al., 1998; Engleking, 1994; Giarelli & Jacobs; Peters, 1997). As research evolves, nurses can expect new knowledge to become available on the role that genetics plays in carcinogenesis, cancer initiation, cancer promotion, and disease progression. Nurses must become familiar with new genetic technologies. APNs, because of their skill set and competencies, are uniquely positioned to facilitate the transfer of this information to the practice arena. Moreover, their concern about both ethical and policy issues makes them a good choice to provide leadership on the many complex issues that require attention in this area.

Role of Advanced Practice Nurses in Cancer Prevention Research

Goals of research in the area of cancer control include identifying preventable causes of cancer to reduce cancer incidence by applying preventive strategies to specific populations (Greenwald, Sondik, & Lynch, 1986). NCI has made chemoprevention research a high priority, and more than 400 potential chemopreventive agents are currently under investigation (Swan & Ford, 1997). A myriad of opportunities exist for APNs to actively participate in research activities focused in this area. Cancer-control trials present unique challenges that APNs may be helpful in overcoming. A role for an APN in this capacity may include that of coinvestigator, study coordinator, or project manager. An example will be presented to illustrate how APNs can assume a viable role within the context of cancer-control research.

Study of Tamoxifen and Raloxifene

The Study of Tamoxifen and Raloxifene (STAR) is a chemoprevention trial that was initiated in 1999 at 193 institutions throughout the country. STAR is being conducted by the National Surgical Adjuvant Breast and Bowel Project and is supported by NCI. The study is designed to determine if raloxifene, a selective estrogen-receptor modulator, is either more or less effective than tamoxifen in reducing the incidence of invasive breast cancer in postmenopausal women who are at increased risk for disease. A secondary goal is to determine how well raloxifene compared to tamoxifen reduces the endometrial cancer rate. The study will enroll approximately 22,000 postmenopausal women ages 35 years or older who are at increased risk for breast cancer. Subjects randomly are assigned to receive either 20 mg of tamoxifen plus placebo or 60 mg of raloxifene plus placebo twice daily for five years. While on study, participants will have follow-up examinations that include annual mammograms and gynecologic evaluations.

At several sites, APNs are serving as coinvestigators or study coordinators for the STAR trial. In this capacity, APNs are responsible for a variety of activities, including public and professional education, recruitment of potential subjects, risk analysis, determination of eligibility, obtaining informed consent, and specific follow-up throughout the study period. Follow-up includes completing histories at each visit; providing education and psychological support; monitoring labs, symptoms, and toxicities; assessing adherence; performing clinical breast examinations, pelvic examinations, and Pap smears; ordering mammograms; and making appropriate referrals to meet additional healthcare needs (Aikin, 2000; J. Much, personal communication, May 2001). These activities make an extremely good fit with the competencies of the APN.

Recruitment to cancer-prevention trials presents unique challenges, yet a timely accrual is essential if the questions posed are to be answered. One of the major reasons cited for slow accrual is that these trials involve healthy subjects, and exposure to undo risk is a critical concern. People who are at risk for developing certain types of cancer should be given proper information to make informed decisions about their health. Helping potential subjects to adequately understand the risks and benefits of participation often is laborious and time-consuming. APNs can provide the education and counseling required to obtain fully informed consent. In this capacity, they have great potential to be helpful in expediting recruitment to prevention and control trials.

Cancer-Control Education

Knowledge in the area of cancer control is evolving rapidly. Incorporation of this information into clinical practice is essential if APNs are to effectively contribute to advancing the cancer-control agenda. APNs receive fundamental information on cancer prevention and control during their formal educational preparation. They must take opportunities to build on this knowledge through ongoing participation in continuing-education activities.

Formal Education

Over time, cancer prevention and control content has become increasingly important in nursing curricula. Nursing education at the graduate level has been expanded to include didactic and clinical experiences in primary and secondary cancer prevention (Frank-Stromborg, 1988). Moreover, driven by changes in the practice environment during the past 20 years, graduate programs that prepare APNs have placed an increased importance on the role of the oncology nurse outside of the acute-care setting. Nursing academic programs have broadened their curricula to include cancer-prevention and early-detection concepts and to prepare nurses for active and sometimes nontraditional roles in this area. Longitudinal studies of participants in these programs have demonstrated increased knowledge and incorporation of primary- and secondary-care interventions into their clinical practice. In addition, all cancer-related organizations have stipulated the importance of the nursing role in this context (Frank-Stromborg).

The application of cancer genetics to clinical practice has created substantial educational needs. According to ONS (2000), cancer genetics should be incorporated into all levels of nursing curricula. Olsen (1999) conducted a curricular analysis at the Johns Hopkins University School of Nursing and found that undergraduates receive a total of 19.83 hours of genetics education. In the master's of science curriculum, 79.58 hours are devoted to this topic—12 hours of core content are mandated, and the remainder vary by specialty. Topics covered include normal cell physiology, Mendelian inheritance, gene structure, DNA replication, protein synthesis, mutations, cancer genetics, the public health impact of genetic diseases and associated technology, pharmacogenetics, gene therapy, legal and ethical issues, and high-risk patient identification and referral (Olsen).

Academic faculties have a critical role in ensuring that cancer prevention and control issues are represented adequately in schools of nursing. Recognizing this, ONS has taken an active role in working with nurse educators in regard to their prevention and early-detection knowledge. With funding from NCI, ONS has developed a cancer prevention and detection workshop for nurse educators from historically African American colleges and universities. This workshop seeks to reduce health disparities and cancer mortality among medically underserved African Americans by integrating information about cancer prevention and early detection among African Americans into educational curricula. This two-day workshop will provide nurse educators with training on how to assess cancer risk; develop educational activities related to cancer prevention and early detection among African Americans; plan community-based screening programs; access state-of-the-science cancer information; understand current research efforts relative to this population; communicate with African American cancer survivors; and integrate this information into their nursing curricula. Initiatives of this type make an extremely important contribution to the cancer-control effort.

Continuing Education

In addition to formal education, multiple opportunities exist to provide continuing education on cancer prevention and early detection. One of the most common reasons cited by primary-care NPs for not providing cancer prevention and screening information to patients is that they do not feel competent in these areas (Warren & Pohl, 1990), indicating the need for frequent updates. In a national study to determine how obstetric/gynecologic NPs make practice changes, continuing-education programs were found to be the primary source of information (Flowers, Gay, Buckner, & Lavender, 1989). A recent report indicated that such approaches positively influence cancer-prevention attitudes among nurses. After attending five two-day training sessions during a 20-month period, nurses demonstrated significant differences in attitude scores and confidence ratings, suggesting that they would incorporate cancer prevention and detection skills into their practice. Authors reported that the documentation of such activities following the program was impressive (Howell, Nelson-Marten, Krebs, Kaszyk, & Wold, 1998). Similarly, Post-White, Carter, and Anglim (1993) found that an educational workshop improved knowledge and confidence in regard to cancer prevention and early detection. Participants of this program subsequently taught more patients, family members, friends, and peers about the recommendations they had learned.

A variety of opportunities are available to meet the continuing-education needs of APNs in regard to cancer-control issues. Hospitals, universities, and professional organizations sponsor workshops and conferences devoted to primary and secondary prevention. ONS, for example, hosted a regional cancer prevention workshop developed specifically to teach African American nurses about cancer prevention/early-detection strategies. The purpose of this course was to increase the number of African American nurses who are prepared to participate in cancer-screening activities. Evaluations of the program indicated that the workshop resulted in changes in the practice of participants. Following the course, attendees reported that they provided more education and counseling on primary prevention and early detection to their patients. In addition, they used this knowledge in their own communities (Frank-Stromborg, McCorkle, & Johnson, 1987). ONS continues to offer prevention and early-detection workshops for nurses. ONS convened a group of 250 oncology nurses in 2000 to provide updated information on risk assessment and to develop colon cancer prevention and detection skills (S. Slabe, personal communication, June 2000).

More comprehensive approaches to continuing education on cancer prevention also are available. One of the earliest comprehensive courses developed specifically for nurses was at the University of Texas M.D. Anderson Cancer Center. This course is three weeks long and provides participants with intensive theory and practice in cancer prevention and control. The curriculum covers health education for the public and allied health personnel, techniques for completing medical histories, screening examination techniques for specific organ sites, and documentation and referral information (Goodman, 1982). Although the course is not targeted exclusively for APNs, it provides an excellent opportunity for them to expand their knowledge, skills, and confidence in this area.

Similar programs are available at other cancer centers. In the early 1980s, Memorial Sloan-Kettering Cancer Center in New York designed a program to increase and enhance the ability of NPs in occupational and community settings to address cancer preventive health needs of patients. This program provided content on cancer etiology and prevention, the expanding role of the nurse in preventive health care, and concepts related to preventive health care from the disciplines of sociology, psychology, education, economics, research, and management (Ash, Oberst, Stalker, Park, & Avellanet, 1982).

The effectiveness of comprehensive continuing-education courses has been evaluated. NCI funded the implementation and evaluation of a competency-based course on cancer prevention and early detection that was developed collaboratively by the University of Washington, ACS, and the Fred Hutchinson Regional Cancer Center in Seattle, WA. The goal of the endeavor was to design and evaluate curricular models for NPs and physician assistants that could be replicated for healthcare professional continuing-education programs both nationally and internationally. The curriculum focused on teaching preventive health approaches that could be used specifically to increase cancer prevention and detection practices in primary-care settings. Evaluations of the program were positive; participants scored higher on follow-up examinations, demonstrated stronger beliefs in cancer prevention and the value of patient education related to prevention and detection, and provided significantly more preventive health care to their patients than did matched controls who did not participate in the program (Burdman, Benoliel, Dohner, Schaad, & Strand, 1987).

Many continuing-education offerings are focused in specific areas of cancer control. The role of genetics in cancer prevention, for example, has become an increasingly important topic. Genetics is a complex area, and many nurses practicing today may not have had this content during their formal education. Barse, Grana, and Daly (1998) surveyed oncology nurses to learn about their knowledge and attitudes in regard to familial cancer risk and screening. Almost 700 oncology nurses completed a survey designed to elicit knowledge regarding cancer risk assessment and genetic testing. The majority of respondents indicated that they were interested in receiving further information on this topic.

A number of strategies have been identified to meet the genetics educational needs of practicing oncology nurses. One program at the Fox Chase Cancer Center in Philadelphia provides training workshops for community-based oncology nurses and nurses within the Fox Chase Cancer Network. These workshops are designed to teach nurses how to identify, assess, and communicate familial cancer risk. The course content, which is taught by a multidisciplinary faculty that includes APNs, contains information on basic genetics, patterns of inheritance, molecular genetics of carcinogenesis, and pedigree construction, as well as psychosocial, ethical, and legal implications of genetic risk information. Upon completion of the didactic component of the program, participants are visited in their community hospitals by an APN from the Fox Chase Cancer Center, who provides mentoring as they initiate their roles in familial risk counseling (Suhayda, 1997).

Individual institutions that employ APNs have a responsibility to provide them with ongoing education to ensure their competency. Several institutions have established guidelines or algorithms that govern the practices of APNs in the area of cancer control. These pathways often are based on "best evidence." Institutions may use guidelines that are developed by large organizations such as ACS or NCI, or they may derive their own, based on institutional practices. Memorial Sloan-Kettering Cancer Center (1999), for example, has developed *Screening Protocols for Nurse Practitioners*, which has been reviewed and approved by appropriate bodies internal to the organization. These protocols are designed to serve as a guide for NPs and are to be supplemented with specific patient information. An example of these protocols is provided in Appendix 22-1, which appears at the end of this chapter.

Another source of continuing education for APNs is the literature, which serves as a resource by providing information on practice trends and issues. The oncology-specific literature provides frequent articles focused in the area of cancer prevention and early detection. Table 22-1 provides information on the number of articles concentrating on cancer prevention and detection that have been published in four oncology-specific journals over five recent years. This information was obtained through a review of the tables of contents of the journals listed. Using the same method, five randomly selected APN-specific journals were reviewed to ascertain how frequently articles on cancer prevention or early detection were published. These data, presented in Table 22-2, indicate that the nononcology literature is less likely to be a source of up-to-date information for APNs.

Table 22-1. Quantification of Cancer Prevention, Screening, or Detection Articles From a Sample of Oncology Journals

Oncology Journals	Number of Articles				
	1995	1996	1997	1998	1999
Cancer Practice	3	3	7	9	2
Cancer Nursing	4	5	2	4	3
Clinical Journal of Oncology Nursing[a]	–	–	0	0	0
Oncology Nursing Forum	9	0	4	5	4

[a] Clinical Journal of Oncology Nursing began in 1997.

Table 22-2. Quantification of Cancer Prevention, Screening, or Detection Articles From a Sample of Advanced Practice Journals

Advanced Practice Journals	Number of Articles				
	1995	1996	1997	1998	1999
Clinical Excellence for Nurse Practitioners[a]	–	–	1	1	0
Clinical Nurse Specialist: The Journal for Advanced Nursing Practice	0	1	1	0	0
Journal of the American Academy of Nurse Practitioners	0	4	0	0	0
Journal of Nurse-Midwifery	0	2	0	1	0
Nurse Practitioner Forum	3	0	1	1	0

[a] Clinical Excellence for Nurse Practitioners began in 1997.

Recommendations to Enhance the Role of Advanced Practice Nurses in Cancer Control

APNs are well positioned to contribute substantially to decreasing the incidence and mortality of cancer. Numerous examples of their work in this context have been presented. Although many of these reports clearly demonstrate APNs' ability to perform competently in this area, several identified obstacles prevent them from realizing their full potential. Knowledge deficits, a need for frequent updates, a lack of consensus about screening guidelines, limited training opportunities, and insufficient time all were identified as problems. A variety of strategies should be considered to assist APNs in actualizing their potential to reduce cancer incidence and mortality.

Education

Nursing faculty must ensure that emerging science is incorporated swiftly into APN curricula. Formal educational programs at the graduate level must reflect the state of the science on cancer-control issues. This is particularly challenging because the rate of scientific discovery and the application of technological advances in clinical practice often outpace the formal dissemination of this knowledge. The subsequent application of this information to the clinical setting also is imperative. Offering precepted clinical experiences in a variety of settings will assist new APNs to understand the application of this knowledge and help them to incorporate these skills into the settings where they practice.

In addition to formal educational programs, APNs should have continuing-education opportunities. These should be made available in a variety of locations on a frequent basis. In addition, making available cancer-control programs geared specifically toward an APN audience would be advantageous. In so doing, the special challenges encountered by this group of providers can be addressed. The marketing of these programs to the nononcology APN groups should be used as a strategy to increase participation. Primary-care NPs and FNPs, for example, could participate in joint programs with oncology APNs. Such programs should reflect the collaborations of institutions or organizations. In addition, these forums would provide excellent networking opportunities.

The content and focus of continuing-education programs should reflect research findings. APNs have indicated that additional skills are needed in specific areas. The study by Warren and Pohl (1990) indicated that the level of comfort in performing examinations of the testes and prostate was not adequate. Another report indicated that knowledge about cancer risk and smoking cessation techniques among APNs was limited (Tessaro et al., 1996). Programs in which APNs could acquire these skills should be designed so they can perform them with confidence in the clinical setting. One of the reviews presented identified liability as a concern of APNs in carrying out cancer prevention and detection interventions in their practice. APNs must be educated with regard to the legal risks of conducting cancer-screening examinations and the necessary risk-reduction practices (Frank-Stromborg & Bailey, 1998). This education should be a component of educational programs focused on cancer control.

Programs also need to explore issues of potential bias in providing screening services. More than one of the studies indicated that younger rather than older patients were more likely to receive screening interventions. This is perplexing because increasing age is one of the greatest risk factors for developing cancer (Bright, 1993). Overcoming the barriers of working with the elderly is critical to ensuring adequate cancer control. In a review of barriers to screening, McCool (1994) speculated that existing public attitudes toward the elderly and chronically ill may play a role in providers not promoting screening more aggressively in older women.

Increasing the number of articles focused on cancer control in advanced practice nursing journals represents another educational strategy. The literature serves as a vehicle for the dissemination of timely information. APNs identified that one of the reasons they do not routinely incorporate prevention and detection strategies into their everyday practice is because they feel that they need updated information. As a matter of strategy, oncology APNs should contribute articles focused on specific areas of cancer control to these journals. An update on screening for breast and gynecologic malignancies, for example, probably would be of interest to the readers of the *Journal of Nurse-Midwifery*. Publications such as this would help to heighten awareness of the APN's role in this context as well as to serve as a resource by providing updated information on cancer-control topics. Expanding the number of articles on cancer control in oncology-specific journals also would be an important contribution to the continuing education of APNs.

Practice

The literature presented provides numerous examples of APN practices in the cancer-control arena. All APNs should be knowledgeable about cancer-control topics and incorporate cancer prevention and detection interventions into their everyday practices. This needs to be expanded beyond the oncology-specific setting. The primary-care setting has been suggested as an excellent opportunity for the implementation of a comprehensive program of cancer prevention (Love & Olsen, 1985). A recent editorial challenged oncology nurses to establish stronger alliances with providers in family practice, school health, occupational health, and obstetrics and gynecology so that involvement in cancer prevention and detection can occur more globally (Foley, 2000). Other groups with whom APNs need to consider collaborating include colleagues in nurse-managed clinics and federally qualified health centers. Such programs often provide service for minority populations, who many times are at increased risk and less likely to be able to access preventive health services. Access to services is a vital part of successful screening and detection. APNs have a long history of improving access and working effectively with vulnerable populations.

NCI has designated cancer-prevention research in minorities a priority. Research in this area has indicated that substantial differences exist among cultural groups with regard to prevention and screening practices (Choudhry, Srivastava, & Fitch, 1998; Dibble, Vanoni, & Miaskowski, 1997; Gelfand, Parzuchowski, Rivero-Perry, & Shernoff, 2000; Mack, McGrath, Pendelton, & Zieber, 1993). Kagawa-Singer (1997) outlined the steps that are necessary for oncology nurses to develop effective culturally based early cancer detection and screening programs for ethnic populations. Funders, researchers, practitioners, and patients must work together to develop and deliver available, acceptable, accessible, and appropriate care for multicultural populations. The delivery of culturally competent programs theoretically and clinically can improve the quality of care provided (Frank-Stromborg & Olsen, 1993).

APNs must become more involved in legislative activities as they relate to cancer-control issues. As knowledgeable healthcare providers, APNs have the ability to influence government and form policy. Improved funding and reimbursement for cancer-prevention services is essential to reducing the incidence and morbidity of the disease. Insurance companies often do not provide coverage for preventive patient interventions and counseling. A recent report indicated that patients in health maintenance organizations appear to have higher utilization of cancer screening tests than do patients with fee-for-service insurance (Malin et al., 2000). The uninsured face additional challenges. Poverty is one of the greatest risk factors for developing cancer (Bright, 1993). Overcoming the barriers of working with the socioeconomically disadvantaged is critical to ensuring adequate cancer control. Underwood and Hoskins (1994) challenged the nursing community to advocate for healthcare policies that ensure access to health maintenance services for the socioeconomically disadvantaged. In a poignant article addressing issues of poverty and health, the authors provided a glimpse of the circle of poverty as a mechanism to sensitize providers to the experiences of the poor in acquiring healthcare services. APNs can be instrumental in lobbying for change in this area. A number of initiatives supporting prevention and detection activities already have been submitted.

There is a pressing need to continue to develop the role of the APN with a specialty in genetics. APNs in this specialty undoubtedly will play key roles in the cancer-control arena. Moreover, they will serve a critical function as resources to other healthcare professionals and the public. Many important questions need to be answered in this arena, and APNs who have helped to develop and coordinate high-risk evaluation programs should be involved in these activities.

As an essential component of their practice, APNs act as a resource for others on the healthcare team and in the community with regard to cancer-control activities. APNs are in a position to share advanced knowledge about cancer prevention and early detection with patients, families, and staff. Of equal importance is APNs' commitment to role-model health prevention practices and behaviors. Providing patient and public education is an essential component of their role. This is particularly important in today's healthcare environment, where consumers may have access to so much information that they require assistance in clarifying and tailoring it to their own specific situation.

Finally, APNs must think globally about the issue of cancer control. Hilton (1999), in a recent address, challenged nurses to adopt an international perspective in terms of thinking about screening. Seventy-five percent of the world's population lives in developing countries, and cancer likely will continue to hold its place as one of the leading causes of death worldwide. APNs need to be cognizant of these statistics and work collaboratively with colleagues internationally to share some of the knowledge and resources that are available in the United States to alleviate this burden.

Research

Involvement in research activities that cover all aspects of cancer-control activities should be increased. This should include evaluating cancer-control education strategies and methods as well as designing and testing programs of prevention and screening to evaluate outcomes.

APNs can contribute to advancing the research agenda by serving as co- or principal investigators for studies. Fulfilling the role of study coordinator or project manager, as discussed earlier, represents an alternative strategy. Another approach would include collaborating with researchers to investigate problems that are of joint interest. Partnering with doctorally prepared nurses is an excellent strategy to answer research questions. Benefits to APNs include mentoring from researchers and an opportunity to learn about research design and methods. Benefits to researchers generally include gaining access to the desired patient population and having an advocate at the research site. Poniatowski and Grimm (1999) indicated that the use of doctorally prepared nurses to serve as consultants by providing research expertise to APNs investigating specific problems was a successful strategy.

Conclusion

APNs enrich the healthcare system by adding value to the delivery of health services (Spross & Heaney, 2000). Health teaching focused on the cause and prevention of all cancers is an important role for all APNs. CNMs, NPs, and CNSs, in particular, can have a direct and profound influence on this process. Specifically, these providers are equipped with highly specialized skills that enable them to provide education about risk factors and screening recommendations based on individual characteristics. APNs are involved in a broad array of cancer-control activities. As a group of providers, APNs have a substantial history of improving cost, access, and quality outcomes. Many of their efforts in cancer control have improved access for specific components of the population. The measurement of both quality and cost outcomes needs to be assessed further; however, APNs, by contributing to decreasing cancer incidence and mortality, have the potential to improve quality of life and decrease the economic burden of cancer.

References

Aiken, L.H., Lake, E.T., Semaan, S., Lehman, H.P., O'Hare, P.A., Cole, S., Dunbar, D., & Frank, I. (1993). Nurse practitioner managed care for persons with HIV infection. *Image, 25*, 172–177.

Aikin, J.L. (2000). The Study of Tamoxifen and Raloxifene (STAR): Opportunities and challenges for oncology nursing [Abstract]. *Oncology Nursing Forum, 27*, 324.

American Academy of Nurse Practitioners. (1993). *Standards of practice.* Austin, TX: Author.

American Association of Colleges of Nursing. (1994). *Position statement: Certification and regulation of advanced practice nurses.* Washington, DC: Author.

American Association of Colleges of Nursing. (1997–2000). *Enrollment and graduations in baccalaureate and graduate programs in nursing.* Washington, DC: Author.

American Association of Nurse Anesthetists. (1992). *Guidelines and standards for nurse anesthesia practice.* Park Ridge, IL: Author.

American Cancer Society. (1980). Guidelines for the cancer-related check-up: Recommendations and rationale. New York: Author.

American College of Nurse Midwives. (1993). *Standards for the practice of nurse-midwifery.* Washington, DC: Author.

American College of Nurse Practitioners. (1998). *Letter to health care financing administration.* Retrieved November 20, 2000 from the World Wide Web: http//www.acnp.org

American Nurses Association. (1995). *Nursing facts: Advanced practice nursing—A new age in health care.* Washington, DC: Author.

Ash, C.R., Oberst, M.T., Stalker, M.Z., Park, D., & Avellanet, C. (1982). Cancer prevention: A course for nurse practitioners. New York: Memorial Sloan-Kettering Cancer Center.

Barnsteiner, J., Deatrick, J., Grey, M., Hayman, L., & O'Sullivan, A. (1993). Future of pediatric advanced practice nursing. *Journal of Pediatric Nursing, 19,* 196–197.

Barse, P.M., Grana, G., & Daly, M. (1998). Nurses' survey on knowledge and attitudes about familial cancer risk and screening [Abstract]. *Oncology Nursing Forum, 25,* 334.

Bartley, T.K. (1998). Improved breast cancer screening in African-American women: A nurse managed approach in a primary care community clinic [Abstract]. *Oncology Nursing Forum, 25,* 365.

Bedder, S. (1998). Career planning for advanced practice oncology nurses: Is post-master's nurse practitioner certification right for you? [Abstract]. *Oncology Nursing Forum, 25,* 315.

Berry, A., Kiefer, J., & Jennings-Dozier, K. (2000). The impact of a nurse educator on physician compliance: Implications for colorectal cancer screening outcomes [Abstract]. *Oncology Nursing Forum, 27,* 330.

Bigbee, J.L. (1996). History and evolution of advanced nursing practice. In A.B. Hamric, J.A. Spross, & C.M. Hanson (Eds.), *Advanced practice nursing. An integrative approach* (pp. 3–24). Philadelphia: W.B. Saunders.

Boileau, K. (1998). Developing a screening program for religious women [Abstract]. *Oncology Nursing Forum, 25,* 365.

Brethauer, L.P., & Swenson, C.J. (2000). Development of a cancer risk assessment computer program [Abstract]. *Oncology Nursing Forum, 27,* 314.

Bright, M.A. (1993). Public health initiatives in cancer prevention and control. *Seminars in Oncology Nursing, 9,* 139–146.

Burdman, G.D., Benoliel, J.Q., Dohner, C.W., Schaad, D., & Strand, D. (1987). A focus on cancer: Development of a course on prevention and early detection. *Journal of Continuing Education in Nursing, 18,* 93–96.

Byar, D.P., & Freedman, L.S. (1990). The importance and nature of cancer prevention trials. *Seminars in Oncology, 17,* 413–424.

Byers, T., Mouchawar, J., Marks, J., Cady, B., Lins, N., Swanson, G.M., Bal, D.G., & Eyre, H. (1999). The American Cancer Society challenge goals: How far can rates decline in the U.S. by the year 2015? *Cancer, 86,* 715–727.

Casale, M.E., Hostler, R., & Jackson, G. (2000). PACONS at the races: A community-based skin cancer awareness project [Abstract]. *Oncology Nursing Forum, 27,* 326.

Choudhry, U.K., Srivastava, R., & Fitch, M.I. (1998). Breast cancer detection practices of South Asian women: Knowledge, attitudes, beliefs. *Oncology Nursing Forum, 25,* 1693–1701.

Coles, S.M. (1999). How to plan and host a skin cancer screening clinic [Abstract]. *Oncology Nursing Forum, 25,* 355.

Cooley, M.E., Spatz, D.L., & Yasko, J.M. (1996). Role implementation in cancer nursing. In R. McCorkle, M. Grant, M. Frank-Stromborg, & S.B. Baird (Eds.), *Cancer nursing: A comprehensive textbook* (pp. 25–37). Philadelphia: W.B. Saunders.

DeCosse, J.J., Tsioulias, G.J., & Jacobson, J.S. (1994). Colorectal cancer: Detection, treatment, and rehabilitation. *CA: A Cancer Journal for Clinicians, 44,* 27–42.

Dibble, S.L., Vanoni, J.M., & Miaskowski, C. (1997). Women's attitudes toward breast cancer screening procedures: Differences by ethnicity. *Women's Health Issues, 7,* 47–54.

Diers, D. (1991). Nurse-midwives and nurse-anesthetists: The cutting edge in specialist practice. In L.H. Aiken & C.M. Fagin (Eds.), *Charting nursing's future: Agenda for the 1990s* (pp. 159–180). New York: Lippincott.

Dignam, J.J. (2000). Differences in breast cancer prognosis among African-American and Caucasian women. *CA: A Cancer Journal for Clinicians, 50,* 50–64.

Dimond, E., Calzone, K., Davis, J., & Jenkins, J. (1998). The role of the nurse in cancer genetics. *Cancer Nursing, 21,* 57–75.

Division of Cancer Prevention and Control. (1994). *Annual report.* Bethesda, MD: National Institutes of Health, National Cancer Institute.

Elder, R.G., & Bullough, B. (1990). Nurse practitioners and clinical nurse specialists: Are the roles merging? *Clinical Nurse Specialist, 4,* 78–84.

Ellings, J.M., Newman, R.B., Hulsey, T.C., Bivins, H.A., & Keenan, A. (1993). Reduction in very low birth weight deliveries and perinatal mortality in a specialized, multidisciplinary twin clinic. *Obstetrics and Gynecology, 81,* 387–391.

Engleking, C. (1994). New approaches: Innovations in cancer prevention, diagnosis, treatment, and support. *Oncology Nursing Forum, 21,* 62–71.

Feuerbach, R.D., Miale-Mayer, D., & Wray, C. (1999). Advanced practice nursing: The clinical nurse specialist and nurse practitioner role—A collaborative approach [Abstract]. *Oncology Nursing Forum, 26,* 378.

Flowers, J.S., Gay, J.T., Buckner, E.B., & Lavender, M.G. (1989). How obstetric/gynecologic nurse practitioners make practice changes: A national study. *Journal of the American Academy of Nurse Practitioners, 1,* 132–136.

Foley, G. (2000). Opening the door to new opportunities: Reducing cancer mortality and incidence. *Cancer Practice, 8,* 109.

Frank-Stromborg, M. (1988). Nursing's role in cancer prevention and detection: Vital contributions to attainment of the year 2000 goal. *Cancer, 62,* 1833–1838.

Frank-Stromborg, M. (1997). Cancer screening and early detection. In C. Varricchio (Ed.), *A cancer source book for nurses* (7th ed.) (pp. 43–55). Boston: Jones and Bartlett.

Frank-Stromborg, M., & Bailey, L.J. (1998). Cancer screening and early detection: Managing malpractice risk. *Cancer Practice, 6,* 206–216.

Frank-Stromborg, M., & Cohen, R.F. (2000). Assessment and interventions for cancer detection. In C.H. Yarbro, M.H. Frogge, M. Goodman, & S.L. Groenwald (Eds.), *Cancer nursing principles and practice* (5th ed.) (pp. 150–188). Boston: Jones and Bartlett.

Frank-Stromborg, M., McCorkle, R., & Johnson, J. (1987). A program model for nurses involved with cancer education of black Americans. *Journal of Cancer Education, 2,* 145–151.

Frank-Stromborg, M., & Nord, C. (1979). Nurse practitioner acceptance in a cancer detection clinic. *Nurse Practitioner, 4,* 110–112.

Frank-Stromborg, M., & Olsen, S. (1993). *Cancer prevention in minority populations: Cultural implications for healthcare professionals.* St. Louis, MO: Mosby.

Frank-Stromborg, M., Wassner, L.J., Nelson, M., Chilton, B., & Wholeben, B.E. (1998). A study of rural Latino women seeking cancer-detection examinations. *Journal of Cancer Education, 13,* 231–241.

Froerer, R. (1998). The nurse endoscopist: Fact or fiction? *Gastroenterology Nursing, 21,* 14–20.

Galassi, A. (2000). Role of the oncology advanced practice nurse. In C.H. Yarbro, M.H. Frogge, M. Goodman, & S.L. Groenwald (Eds.), *Cancer nursing: Principles and practice* (5th ed.) (pp. 1712–1727). Boston: Jones and Bartlett.

Gelfand, D.E., Parzuchowski, J., Rivero-Perry, M., & Shernoff, N. (2000). Work-site cancer screening: A Latino case study. *Oncology Nursing Forum, 27,* 659–666.

Giarelli, E., & Jacobs, L.A. (2000). Issues related to the use of genetic material and information. *Oncology Nursing Forum, 27,* 459–467.

Goodman, M. (1982). A cancer screening and detection programme in Texas. *Nursing Times, 78,* 1855–1858.

Greenlee, R.T., Hill-Harmon, M.B., Murray, T., & Thun, M. (2001). Cancer statistics, 2001. *CA: A Cancer Journal for Clinicians, 51,* 15–37.

Greenwald, P., Sondik, E., & Lynch, B.S. (1986). Diet and chemoprevention in NCI's research strategy to achieve national cancer control objectives. *Annual Review of Public Health, 7,* 267–291.

Gross, R.E., McDonough, M., & Heerdt, A.S. (1999). The breast cancer anxiety scale: A pilot project for high risk women [Abstract]. *Oncology Nursing Forum, 26,* 363.

Hamric, A., & Spross, J. (Eds.). (1989). *The clinical nurse specialist in theory and practice.* Philadelphia: W.B. Saunders.

Hastings, G.E., Vick, L., Lee, G., Sasmor, L., Natiello, T.A., & Sanders, J.H. (1980). Nurse practitioners in a jailhouse clinic. *Medical Care, 18,* 731–744.

Henschke, C.I., McCauley, D.I., Yankelevitz, D.F., Naidich, D.P., McGuinness, G., Miettinen, O.S., Libby, D.M., Pasmantier, M.W., Koizumi, J., Altorki, N.K., & Smith, J.P. (1999). Early Lung Cancer Action Project: Overall design and findings from baseline screening. *Lancet, 354,* 99–105.

Hewitt, R., & Galucci, B.B. (1999). Providing comprehensive care to women at high risk for developing breast cancer: The experience of six centers [Abstract]. *Oncology Nursing Forum, 26,* 363.

Hilton, L.W. (1999). The Robert Tiffany Lectureship. Vital signs at the millennium: Becoming more than we are. *Cancer Nursing, 22,* 6–16.

Howell, S.L., Nelson-Marten, P., Krebs, L.U., Kaszyk, L., & Wold, R. (1998). Promoting nurses' positive attitudes toward cancer prevention/screening. *Journal of Cancer Education, 13,* 76–84.

Hughes, L.C., Hodgson, N.A., Muller, P., Robinson, L.A., & McCorkle, R. (2000). Information needs of elderly postsurgical cancer patients during the transition from hospital to home. *Journal of Nursing Scholarship, 32,* 25–30.

Jackson, B., Moore, D., & Sobolik, K. (2000). Development of comprehensive multisite cancer screenings: Advanced practice nursing leadership in action [Abstract]. *Oncology Nursing Forum, 27,* 331.

Jennings-Dozier, K. (1999). Sociodemographic predictors of Pap test up-to-date status among minority Philadelphians [Abstract]. *Oncology Nursing Forum, 26,* 397.

Jones, S.L. (2000). A community-wide approach to reduction of morbidity and mortality due to preventable cancers [Abstract]. *Oncology Nursing Forum, 25,* 333.

Kagawa-Singer, M. (1997). Addressing issues for early detection and screening in ethnic populations. *Oncology Nursing Forum, 24,* 1705–1711.

Kinney, A.Y., Hawkins, R., & Hudman, K.S. (1997). A descriptive study of the role of the oncology nurse practitioner. *Oncology Nursing Forum, 24,* 811–820.

Leslie, N.S. (1995). Role of the nurse practitioner in breast and cervical cancer prevention. *Cancer Nursing, 18*, 251–257.

Levy, B.S., Wilkinson, F.S., & Marine, W.M. (1971). Reducing neonatal mortality rate with nurse-midwives. *American Journal of Obstetrics and Gynecology, 109*, 50–58.

Loescher, L.J., & Reid, M.E. (2000). Dynamics of cancer prevention. In C.H. Yarbro, M.H. Frogge, M. Goodman, & S.L. Groenwald (Eds.), *Cancer nursing: Principles and practice* (5th ed.) (pp. 135–149). Boston: Jones and Bartlett.

Love, R.R., & Olsen, S.J. (1985). An agenda for cancer prevention in nursing practice. *Cancer Nursing, 8*, 329–338.

Lynch, M.P., & Lineham, B. (1997). CNS/NP collaborative practice benefits patients, providers. *Clinical Nurse Specialist/Nurse Practitioner Special Interest Group Newsletter, 4*, 3.

Mack, E., McGrath, T., Pendelton, D., & Zieber, N.A. (1993). Reaching poor populations with cancer prevention and early detection programs. *Cancer Practice, 1*, 35–39.

Maguire-Eisen, M., & Frost, C. (1994). Knowledge of malignant melanoma and how it relates to clinical practice among nurse practitioners and dermatology and oncology nurses. *Cancer Nursing, 17*, 457–463.

Malin, J.L., Kahn, K., Dulai, G., Farmer, M.M., Rideout, J., Simon, L.P., & Ganz, P.A. (2000). Organizational systems used by California capitated medical groups and independent practice associations to increase cancer screenings. *Cancer, 88*, 2824–2831.

Marinelli, C., Chin-A-Loy, S., & Ramsey, M. (1999). A recruitment project: African-Americans and prostate cancer screening [Abstract]. *Oncology Nursing Forum, 26*, 398.

Markstein Cancer Education and Prevention Center. (1999). The Markstein breast cancer early detection and prevention outreach program [Abstract]. *Oncology Nursing Forum, 26*, 365–366.

McCool, W.F. (1994). Barriers to breast cancer screening in older women. *Journal of Nurse-Midwifery, 39*, 283–299.

McCorkle, R., Benoliel, J.Q., Donaldson, G., Georgiadou, F., Moinpour, C., & Goodell, B. (1989). A randomized clinical trial of home nursing care for lung cancer patients. *Cancer, 64*, 1375–1382.

McCorkle, R., Strumpf, N.E., Nuamah, I.F., Adler, D.C., Cooley, M.E., & Lusk, E.J. (2000). A specialized home care intervention improves survival among elderly postsurgical cancer patients. *Journal of the American Geriatrics Society, 48*, 1707–1713.

McMillan, S.C., Heusinkveld, K.B., & Spray, J. (1995). Advanced practice in oncology nursing: A role delineation study. *Oncology Nursing Forum, 22*, 41–50.

McMillan, S.C., Heusinkveld, K.B., Spray, J., & Murphy, C.M. (1999). Revising the blueprint for the AOCN examination using a role delineation study for advanced practice oncology nursing. *Oncology Nursing Forum, 26*, 529–537.

Memorial Sloan-Kettering Cancer Center. (1999). *Screening protocols for nurse practitioners.* New York: Author.

Mendelblatt, J., Traxler, M., Lakin, P., Thomas, L., Chauhan, P., Matseoane, S., & Kanetsky, P. (1993). A nurse practitioner intervention to increase breast and cervical screening for poor, elderly black women. *Journal of General Internal Medicine, 8*, 133–138.

Montgomery, S., Daly, M., & Masny, A. (1998). Psychological outcomes of high-risk women in a cancer genetics education and counseling program [Abstract]. *Oncology Nursing Forum, 25*, 364–365.

Much, J.K., Cunningham, R.S., & Zamek, R. (1998). From novice to expert and back again: Transitioning into the nurse practitioner role [Abstract]. *Oncology Nursing Forum, 25*, 357.

National Alliance of Nurse Practitioners. (1993). *Definition of nurse practitioners.* Washington, DC: Author.

National Institutes of Health. (1996). Cervical cancer: *National Institutes of Health Consensus Development Confrence Statement* April 1–3 1996. Retrieved February 15, 2001, from the World Wide Web: http://adp.ad.nih.gov/consensus/cons/102/102_statement.htm

Nichols, B.S., Misra, R., & Alexy, B. (1996). Cancer detection: How effective is public education? *Cancer Nursing, 19*, 98–103.

Olsen, S.J. (1999). Genetics: A curricular analysis [Abstract]. *Oncology Nursing Forum, 26*, 392.

Oncology Nursing Society. (1990). *Standards of advanced practice in oncology nursing.* Pittsburgh: Author.

Oncology Nursing Society. (1997a). *Position paper on quality cancer care.* Pittsburgh: Author.

Oncology Nursing Society. (1997b). *Statement on the scope and standards of advanced practice in oncology nursing.* Pittsburgh: Author.

Oncology Nursing Society. (2000). *Position on the role of the oncology nurse in cancer genetic counseling.* Pittsburgh: Author.

Paine, L.L., Johnson, T.R., Lang, J.M., Gagnon, D., Declercq, E.R., DeJoseph, J., Scupholme, A., Strobino, D., & Ross, A. (2000). A comparison of visits and practices of nurse-midwives and obstetrician-gynecologists in ambulatory care settings. *Journal of Midwifery & Women's Health, 45*, 37–44.

Peters, J.A. (1997). Applications of genetic technologies to cancer screening, prevention, diagnosis, prognosis, and treatment. *Seminars in Oncology Nursing, 13*, 74–81.

Poniatowski, B., & Grimm, P. (1999, May). *The development of a community cancer center program of nursing research: A research consultant model.* Abstract presented at the Oncology Nursing Society 24th Annual Congress, Atlanta, GA.

Post-White, J., Carter, M., & Anglim, M.A. (1993). Cancer prevention and early detection: Nursing students' knowledge, attitudes, personal practices, and teaching. *Oncology Nursing Forum, 20*, 743–749.

Reed, C.A., & Selleck, C.S. (1996). The role of midlevel providers in cancer screening. *Medical Clinics of North America, 80*, 135–144.

Reiter, F. (1966). The nurse clinician. *American Journal of Nursing, 66*, 274–280.

Richards, L.G., & Kent, B.J. (2000). The use of the friend-to-friend intervention to increase mammography utilization in rural women [Abstract]. *Oncology Nursing Forum, 27*, 331.

Robinson, K.D., Kimmel, E.A., & Yasko, J.M. (1995). Reaching out to the African-American community through innovative strategies. *Oncology Nursing Forum, 22*, 1383–1391.

Rosevelt, J., & Frankl, H. (1984). Colorectal cancer screening by nurse practitioners using 60-cm flexible fiberoptic sigmoidoscope. *Digestive Diseases and Sciences, 29*, 161–163.

Ross, M.G. (1981). Health impact of a nurse midwife program. *Nursing Research, 30*, 353–355.

Safriet, B.J. (1992). Health care dollars and regulatory sense: The role of advanced practice nursing. *Yale Journal on Regulation, 9*, 417–488.

Schroy, P.C., Wiggins, T., Winawer, S.J., Diaz, B., & Lightdale, C.J. (1988). Video endoscopy by nurse practitioners: A model for colorectal cancer screening. *Gastrointestinal Endoscopy, 34*, 390–394.

Silver, H.K., Ford, L.C., & Day, L.R. (1968). The pediatric nurse practitioner program: Expanding the role of the nurse to provide increased health care for children. *JAMA, 204*, 88–92.

Smith, R.A., Mettlin, C.J., Davis, K.J., & Eyre, H. (2000). American Cancer Society guidelines for the early detection of cancer. *CA: A Cancer Journal for Clinicians, 50*, 34–49.

Sox, H.C. (1979). Quality of patient care by nurse practitioners and physician's assistants: A ten-year perspective. *Annals of Internal Medicine, 91*, 459–468.

Spencer-Cisek, P.A. (1998). Overview of cancer prevention, screening, and detection. *Nurse Practitioner Forum, 9*, 134–146.

Spitzer, W.O., Sackett, D.L., Sibley, J.C., Roberts, R., Gent, M., Kergin, D.J., Hackett, B.C., & Olynch, A. (1974). The Burlington randomized trial of the nurse practitioner. *New England Journal of Medicine, 290*, 251–256.

Spross, J.A., & Heaney, C.A. (2000). Shaping advanced nursing practice in the new millennium. *Seminars in Oncology Nursing, 16*, 12–24.

Stalker, M.Z. (1985). Evaluation of a cancer prevention project. *Cancer Nursing, 8*(Suppl. 1), 13–16.

Suhayda, L. (1997). ONS project team member profile: Meet Agnes Masny. *ONS News, 12*(3), 4–5.

Swan, D.K., & Ford, B. (1997). Chemoprevention of cancer: Review of the literature. *Oncology Nursing Forum, 24*, 719–727.

Tessaro, I.A., Herman, C.J., Shaw, J.E., & Giese, E.A. (1996). Cancer prevention knowledge, attitudes, and clinical practice of nurse practitioners in local public health departments in North Carolina. *Cancer Nursing, 19*, 269–274.

Thatcher, V.S. (1953). *A history of anesthesia: With emphasis on the nurse specialist.* Philadelphia: Lippincott.

Underwood, S.M., & Hoskins, D. (1994). Increased nursing involvement in cancer prevention and control among the economically disadvantaged: The nursing challenge. *Seminars in Oncology Nursing, 10*, 89–95.

U.S. Congress Office of Technology Assessment. (1986). *Nurse practitioners, physicians assistants, and certified nurse midwives: A policy analysis.* Washington, DC: U.S. Government Printing Office.

Varney, H. (1987). *Nurse-midwifery* (2nd ed.). Boston: Blackwell Science.

Waldman, A.R. (2000). You want me to do what? Colorectal screening in the community [Abstract]. *Oncology Nursing Forum, 27*, 331.

Waring, A.N., Rittenberg, C.N., & Bateman, M.M. (1999). Measuring the worth of a free breast screening program for younger, uninsured women [Abstract]. *Oncology Nursing Forum, 26*, 382–383.

Warren, B., & Pohl, J.M. (1990). Cancer screening practices of nurse practitioners. *Cancer Nursing, 13*, 143–151.

Weinrich, S.P., Boyd, M.D., Weinrich, M., Greene, F., Reynolds, W.A., & Metlin, C. (1998). Increasing prostate cancer screening in African-American men with peer-educator and client-navigator interventions. *Journal of Cancer Education, 13*, 213–219.

White, L. (1989). Cancer prevention and detection in nursing practice. *Nursing RSA Verpleging RSA, 4,* 27–28.

White, L.N., & Faulkenberry, J.E. (1985). Screening by nurse clinicians in cancer prevention and detection. *Current Problems in Cancer, 4,* 1–42.

White, N.J., Given, B.A., & Devoss, D.N. (1996). The advanced practice nurse: Meeting the information needs of the rural cancer patient. *Journal of Cancer Education, 11,* 203–209.

Williams, C., & Valdivieso, G.C. (1994). Advanced practice models: A comparison of clinical nurse specialist and nurse practitioner activities. *Clinical Nurse Specialist, 8,* 311–318.

Appendix 22-1. Sample Breast Screening Protocol for Nurse Practitioners

Mammogram Requirement
- Women age 40 and older are eligible for a screening mammogram. Mammograms should be performed annually thereafter.
- Younger women will be imaged depending upon their history and physical findings.
- Women who are 10 years younger than a first-degree relative with breast cancer (male relatives included) are eligible for screening and annual mammography. However, if a woman is younger than 25 years old, she should be referred to the 68th or 53rd Street campus for imaging.

Pregnant and Lactating Women
- Pregnant women are not eligible for a screening mammography.
- Women who are unsure of pregnancy must bring documented proof of a negative pregnancy test from their private healthcare provider before being imaged.
- Symptomatic pregnant women should be referred to the physician.
- Asymptomatic lactating women are not eligible for a screening mammography. To be eligible, these women completely have to discontinue breastfeeding or lactation for a minimum of six months before undergoing a screening mammography.
- Symptomatic lactating women, who otherwise would have met the screening requirements, can be imaged before referring to the physician.
- Lactating women, who otherwise would have met the screening criteria, should be referred to the physician.

Women With Mammoplasty
- Women with reduction mammoplasty should be imaged routinely if they meet the screening requirements.
- Women with breast augmentation (implants) are not eligible for screening mammograms at the Breast Education Center at Harlem (BECH). They are to be referred to the 68th or 53rd street campus for imaging. The requisitions must be generated at BECH and the patient referred to the patient navigator.
- Women with augmentation by injection should be imaged routinely at BECH.

Postmastectomy and lumpectomy
- Postmastectomy sites are not imaged.
- Patients who have had lumpectomies are not imaged at BECH; instead, they should follow the protocol for women with implants.

Examination Protocol
- A careful health history should be taken and risk factors identified. The physical examination should be limited to blood pressure, comprehensive breast examination, inspection and palpation of the abdomen, complete pelvic examination, and a rectal examination in women 35 years and older. The standardized physical assessment tool is to be used.

Breast Examination Protocol
- The location, size, shape, consistency, and mobility of a mass, if present, should be documented carefully and a skin marker applied if a mammogram is to be performed.

Education
- Women should be taught breast self-examination using current literature and videotapes.

Management of Clinical Breast Examination Findings
- If during a clinical breast examination a palpable lesion is found and the patient meets mammogram requirements, a mammogram should be requested and the patient referred to the

(Continued on next page)

Appendix 22-1. Sample Breast Screening Protocol for Nurse Practitioners *(Continued)*

physician before the results are available. At the first physician's visit, if a procedure is recommended, the patient is referred to the patient navigator to ensure that follow-up procedures are carried out. The nurse practitioner will continue the screening requirements of the patient on the physician's recommendation.

- If a palpable lesion is detected and the patient does not meet the requirements for a mammogram, she then is referred directly to the physician. The follow-up protocol remains as above.
- Other breast findings, such as atypical nipple discharge, isolated areas of density, asymmetrical breast pattern, axillary masses that are not lymphadenopathies, and skin lesions should be imaged before referring to the physician. However, if mammogram requirements are not met, a direct physician referral is indicated. The nurse practitioner should use clinical judgment in deferring imaging on a patient who may have a skin lesion that is infected or infectious. Occult blood testing should be performed on all atypical nipple discharge.
- All inflammatory processes should be referred to the physician prior to obtaining results from a mammogram.
- Support measures for patients with breast pain without underlying lesions should include, but are not limited to, the use of warm or cold compresses, over-the-counter analgesics, as is necessary, support bras, vitamin E, and the discontinuation of caffeine intake. If no improvement occurs, a record of the pain pattern should be kept and a repeat clinical breast examination performed in three months by the patient's primary care provider. The patient then should resume annual breast cancer screenings.

Management of Clinical Breast Findings Algorithm (CBEF 1 Protocol)

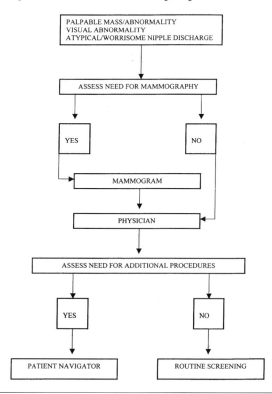

(Continued on next page)

Appendix 22-1. Sample Breast Screening Protocol for Nurse Practitioners *(Continued)*

Management of Mammography Reports
- All mammogram reports must be assigned a BI-RADS score (0–5). Nurse practitioners will analyze all mammogram reports.
- All patients will be given a letter stating the findings of their mammogram.
- Patients with a mammogram report of BI-RADS 0 should have the additional investigation performed within four months. If this is not carried out, the patient should return to the center (BECH) for a repeat mammogram.

Palpable Mass Confirmed by Mammography (BI-RADS 2–5)
- This patient's chart is to be reviewed by the nurse practitioner and the physician. All decisions regarding further management should be the physician's. The nurse practitioner should ensure that the patient is being navigated appropriately. The patient navigator will follow this patient through to resolution to ensure compliance. The nurse practitioner will continue the screening requirements of this patient on the physician's recommendation.

Palpable Lesion Not Confirmed by Mammography (BI-RADS 1 & 2)
- This patient is managed as described above.

Nonpalpable Lesion With Abnormal Mammogram (BI-RADS 0, 3, 4, & 5)
- If radiologists recommend additional investigations, the patient is referred to the patient navigator, who will set up the appropriate appointment. If a physician referral is indicated, the nurse practitioner should make the decision whether the physician's visit should supersede the additional recommended investigation. If the former prevails, then the reports of any other interventions should be available when the patient returns to the physician.
- If the additional investigation is negative (BI-RADS 1 & 2), the patient continues on an annual screening program. If BI-RADS 3, a short-term six-month follow-up is indicated and the patient is given an appropriate appointment.
- If the investigation is abnormal (BI-RADS 4 & 5), the patient is referred to the physician and patient navigator. The patient navigator will track the patient to ensure compliance. Routine follow-up of this patient by the nurse practitioner is conducted on the physician's recommendation.

(Continued on next page)

Appendix 22-1. Sample Breast Screening Protocol for Nurse Practitioners *(Continued)*

Management of Mammography Reports Algorithm

- All mammogram reports should be assigned a BI-RADS score.
- BI-RADS 3 mammogram reports require short-term follow-up.

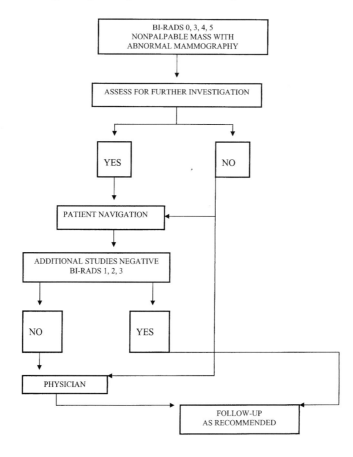

(Continued on next page)

Appendix 22-1. Sample Breast Screening Protocol for Nurse Practitioners *(Continued)*

PATIENT EDUCATION

[ ] BSE   [ ] Video   [ ] Literature   [ ] Supportive Measures

[ ] Lifestyle Modification   [ ] Other

REFERRAL   [ ] STD Screening   [ ] BECH MD   [ ] Other   [ ] Hotline # given

Signature   Date:

DATE	Additional Notes

Results and Recommendation Sheet

1.   **PAP Smear Results**

[ ] 01. Negative for Malignant Cells   [ ] 06. Squamous Cell Cancer

[ ] 02. Infection/Inflammation/Reactive   [ ] 07. Other (specify):
Changes

[ ] 03. Atypical Squamous Cells of   [ ] 09. Not indicated
Undetermined Significance

[ ] 04. Low Grade SIL   [ ] 10. Indicated but not performed
(including HPV changes).

[ ] 05. High Grade SIL   [ ] 11. Pap Smear Specimen Adequacy
                                                           [ ] 1. Satisfactory
                                                           [ ] 2. Satisfactory but limited by

                                                           [ ] 3. Unsatisfactory – Specify

NP's Signature   **Date**

Note. From *Screening Protocols for Nurse Practitioners. Breast Examination Center of Harlem* (pp. 5–10), by W.L. Grant, 1999, New York: Memorial Sloan-Kettering Caner Center. Copyright 1999 by Memorial Sloan-Kettering Cancer Center. Reprinted with permission.

CHAPTER 23

Research Training Opportunities

Annette B. Wysocki, PhD, RN, C

Introduction

Research training opportunities are important for scientists at all stages of their career to develop and maintain a successful program of research. The types of opportunities appropriate for individual investigators will vary, depending on their place on the research trajectory. Opportunities selected will depend on whether investigators are at a very early stage of their research career or are experienced investigators. Regardless of what a nurse's professional position may be, it is wise to stay open to opportunities for learning research. Expanding competency in research is one way to advance a career in nursing.

However, when seeking training in research, one may need to consider what personal factors will affect one's choice of opportunities, such as geographic location, personal finances, young children, or a responsibility to aging parents. In an ideal world, without personal considerations, an investigator would want to find the best possible person to provide the best research training, regardless of location.

The reality for most scientists is that a choice is made after weighing the advantages and disadvantages of each possibility and then selecting the best available opportunity within their personal limitations. A research career that is started as soon as possible allows for more concentrated and protected time because personal responsibilities may be less. This is another reason why individuals who embark on the traditional research path in other disciplines are encouraged to keep moving in the most direct fashion possible from undergraduate to doctoral to postdoctoral training. Although there are other reasons why most basic science disciplines have eliminated awarding master's degrees, investigators who are intent on a research career can complete their training earlier by excluding this step. The result is that they have a longer period of time to be a competitively funded investigator, have an overall impact on a field of research, and be perceived as an expert both within and outside of their area of research expertise.

When contemplating research training opportunities, other aspects should be considered before arriving at a decision: first, spend time assessing training needs and stage of career development, and second, be as careful as possible to choose the best possible mentor. After this process, investigators should start searching for a research training opportunity. When a less-than-ideal choice has been made, the researcher should be aware of the limitations of the decision so he or she can be vigilant in filling any resulting research training gaps.

Assessing Training Needs

Assessing training needs is one factor to consider in selecting a research training opportunity. As individuals move from undergraduate to postdoctoral training, their selection of training opportunities should become more focused and purposeful.

Training Needs During Undergraduate Nursing Education

Nursing students' interest in research may not extend beyond knowing that they are generally curious about the world, like to ask good questions, and would like to understand how the research process works. In this situation, they may want to look around at local universities or research institutions for opportunities. If students have a notion that they would like to work in a bench-based laboratory, then they should look for opportunities in this area. Students should visit laboratories in the molecular/biology, chemistry, physiology, medical, or nursing school. The chairman's office of these various departments is a good place to start. Ask if volunteer work is available in a laboratory. If students are not interested in bench work, then they should look for investigators who conduct research using survey instruments, telephone calls, clinical studies, and interviews. Various departments, such as nursing, sociology, epidemiology, psychology, education, and public policy, conduct these kinds of studies. Students should remember that, depending on where the investigator's project is in the research process, the type of experience gained may vary but always will add new skills to their developing research toolbox. The important overall goal for undergraduates is to gain some general research experience.

During this type of experience, undergraduates probably will be assigned some task on an overall research project. In a bench laboratory, this may include anything from maintaining a cell culture to running gels, measuring protein concentrations, or washing dishes. In general, students will receive an assignment that will give them an overall introduction to a research laboratory and will help them to determine if they want to conduct this kind of research as an independent investigator. If students cannot devote full-time efforts to the laboratory, then, even if their primary task is to wash dishes, they should spend time with graduate and postdoctoral students in the laboratory to learn about their projects. They should ask to look at cells under the microscope, learn how to use a light microscope proficiently, and express an interest in learning some of the assays used in the laboratory. Many times, advanced students will be able to spend time explaining the studies and teaching about cells and tissues.

If undergraduates find that bench science is not their passion, they should look for opportunities with clinical investigators or community-based studies. They can canvass various departments on campus and present themselves as aspiring researchers. In this situation, students may be asked to perform literature searches, retrieve articles from the library, input data into the computer for analysis, assist with copying of instruments, and perform other duties involved in the type of research study being conducted by the principal investigator. If students cannot devote a lot of time to a project, they should be content with learning the research process, seeing it up close, and obtaining hands-on experience. This is an opportunity to ask questions about the research process, learn effective ways to gather data, ask about how to deal with missing data points, begin to know the names of statistical tests, learn how to increase return rates for surveys, or put together a research team. In either a laboratory or nonlaboratory situation, students will gain valuable experience and a research toolbox. Their task after that is to work on the tools to add to the toolbox.

Training Needs During the Novice Years

Once students finish nursing school and begin to practice, they often will start to develop a clear research interest. Research topics often develop out of a clinical experience that fires up the imagination or ignites passion in an area of interest. If practicing nurses suspect that research is in their future, they should look for a position in an academic medical center where they can monitor clinical grand rounds and scientific seminars and presentations. They can contact the dean's office or monitor the university's Web site for a weekly schedule of seminars or presentations. Practicing nurses should attend these sessions and bring a notepad to write down any terms that they are not familiar with or citations of articles that they would like to read at the library. Some speakers are not as skilled and experienced in presenting their research as others, and sometimes students only will understand the first 15 minutes of the presentation. This happens even to established investigators who attend talks outside of their area of research focus, so students should not become discouraged. At the end of the seminar, do not be afraid to speak with the presenter about becoming an investigator in this area or about research opportunities in his or her laboratory or on the research team.

Training Needs During Graduate School

As students move to the graduate level, they will want to start honing some specific skills. By this time, they probably will have had at least one year of clinical experience and perhaps have begun to define the topic of their future research. They also may have eliminated areas that are not of interest. Students' next task is to select a graduate school that is research intensive, has active researchers on faculty who are funded by major research entities (e.g., American Cancer Society [ACS], National Institutes of Health [NIH], American Association of Cancer Research), has faculty members who perform research in their area of interest, has other programs across the campus that can provide a variety of expertise and consultation, and whose faculty members have a good reputation for mentoring. Currently, few nursing programs in the United States have the option to enter a program with a baccalaureate degree and finish with a doctorate; rather, the majority of programs have requirements for a master's degree. Some graduate programs operate jointly with other schools in obtaining students' degrees. Details of these programs can be found elsewhere and are beyond the scope of this chapter. When students choose a university, program of study (major), and degree, they should make the choice that will best prepare them for the kind of research they want to pursue. At the graduate level, they will be adding very substantive tools to their toolbox, and these tools should last a lifetime.

Students may be required to rotate through laboratories or work with members of the faculty who eventually may be on their thesis/dissertation committee. Students should review the literature in their area of interest so they can understand the developments in their field, learn about gaps in the literature, study hot topics, learn research priorities, and anticipate what types of research studies are expected in the future. The literature that students begin to review will help them to identify experts in the field, know their area of research, and learn the necessary terminology. The literature also can point out personal gaps in knowledge or methods that students will need to learn to become top-notch experts in their field. Graduate students should attend seminars presented by experts in their field whenever possible.

Training Needs During the Postdoctoral Period

At the postdoctoral stage, individuals will make a major investment in building a launch pad for their career. This is a critical step toward future research success. The purpose of this period is to spend concentrated time with a senior researcher to remove any glaring deficits in either knowledge or research methods in the individual's area of interest.

To some extent, choosing a postdoctoral experience will be the most important choice students can make in their research career. These are the golden years of most research careers. Individuals will be working long hours with limited compensation, but the chance to concentrate completely on a specific research area is the opportunity of a lifetime.

During postdoctoral study, individuals should engage in other activities to help to free up their minds. Sometimes a trip to an art gallery or an evening at a concert will allow them to meet people from a different background, which will challenge them with other important scientific ideas and discoveries. Some important scientific ideas have occurred not in the lab but on the beach or while driving a car. The sooner individuals reach this stage of their research career and the fewer their personal commitments, the more likely that they will be able to invest time and energy into the experience. At this stage, individuals should make choices that provide the ability to stand head-to-head, toe-to-toe with any expert in the field regardless of their academic stature, affiliation, scientific discipline, or research track record.

Keep in mind that most toolboxes will never be complete, but, at this stage, individuals should make sure that they are rooted firmly in knowledge that will last a lifetime. Individuals should not worry about learning every research method. Methods and approaches to research questions improve or change over time. Knowledge usually is more important than methods, if students have to temper their choice.

The postdoctoral period also is a time when students are likely to meet, develop, and make lifelong colleagues. These are the people with whom students likely will interact as their career develops. At all times, students should try to maintain their own scientific integrity so that they can create opportunities for success. If they meet or hear about individuals who do not aspire to the highest levels of scientific integrity, then students should be prepared to avoid them or to deal with them carefully.

Training Needs for Established Researchers

If individuals are seeking training opportunities as newly independent or established investigators, they will be focusing more on minor knowledge or method deficits. They may have identified an area that will enhance their program of research or broaden the scope of their research efforts. The salient questions to ask here are, Do they need to learn knowledge in a new area? Do they need to learn a new method? Do they need both? In rare instances, established investigators will want to move into a completely new area of study. If this is the case, they should expect to invest more effort to accomplish this transition successfully. In either case, the knowledge or methods that individuals need to learn are likely to be highly focused and very specific. Established investigators should be able to identify individuals who can work or collaborate with them to learn the things they will need to know to remain competitive.

As individuals' research program and experience become more focused, they will be able to identify their training needs. Throughout their research careers, individuals should network with leaders in the field so that they are aware of new trends or methods that can enhance their research program. This vigilance will allow individuals to be aware of the limits of their program of research and know what training opportunities they need to become more successful. Sometimes it is better to locate a training opportunity in a complementary area where the specific topic of that person's research may be different. This strategy can be helpful if the laboratory an individual would like to go to is in direct competition with his or her research agenda. At other times, this strategy can develop into a beneficial collaboration and expand the program of research.

Choosing a Mentor

Choosing a mentor is an important decision at all stages of a research career. Good mentors have the level of scientific expertise that is respected by investigators in the field and can provide entry into an area of lifelong research. They will be able to introduce individuals to leading investigators in the field, provide them with opportunities to meet and talk with postdoctoral colleagues in other laboratories in their department or the laboratories of other colleagues in the field, assist individuals to become recognized leaders in their field, and provide opportunities to publish and present research findings. Identifying a good mentor can take substantial effort. At times, individuals will make what they thought was the best possible choice only to find that the person they are working with is not a good match. As an undergraduate, this may be less important, and students often can limit their experience to a single semester. Individuals should immediately look for another mentor when it becomes obvious that they will not work well together. Never be afraid to walk away from a bad mentor; staying in a bad situation often can cause undue harm to a student's career.

Good mentors are people who have reputations for being passionate about their research, having a sense of justice and fair play, having a record of assisting individuals at all stages of career development if they are willing to invest effort in the project, getting people through the system. They are recognized experts both nationally and internationally and more than likely will develop into a scientific colleague during one's career.

Choosing mentors can sometimes be tricky depending on where the mentor is in his or her stage of career development. Some people will be good mentors no matter where they are in their careers, whereas others will be better mentors once they have achieved tenure or if their laboratory is well funded. Selecting a mentor at the graduate and postdoctoral stage is especially important. When choosing a mentor, visit with them, try to determine their level of egoism versus altruism, ask around the department to determine their reputation, and talk to people in their laboratory or research group. Conduct a literature search to examine their research publications. Is their name always listed first on the publication? Do they move doctoral students through the system in a timely fashion? Do postdoctoral students who work hard in the laboratory get two to six publications out during two to three years? What is the quality of the research? Do others in the field respect them? Are they an opinion leader? Do they present frequently? Do they regularly attend the premier research meetings in their field?

Keep in mind that people may be reluctant to share negative comments, especially in the laboratory. Individuals should try to engage in conversations with people outside of the laboratory environment if they sense a reluctance to speak. Ask questions about how the mentor operates his or her laboratory. Is each person given his or her own project? Do people compete on the same project and whoever gets there first, wins? Try to determine if the mentor operates the laboratory in a constructive or destructive manner. The longer the time spent in the lab, the more important it is to choose wisely.

Independent or established investigators often use a one-year sabbatical or summer for additional training. In these situations, personality may not be the prime issue when choosing a mentor unless the person has an especially bad reputation. For established investigators, the "mentor" may actually be a colleague from their postdoctoral days, and, in this situation, the choice of a mentor or laboratory will be an easy one.

At the graduate level, a mentor should be able to guide students to another good mentor at the postdoctoral level. If the graduate mentor or the chair of the committee cannot carry this through, then it will be more difficult to find a postdoctoral-training opportunity. Sometimes other individuals on a student's committee will be able to assist him or her in identifying a good postdoctoral mentor. If individuals are left to find a mentor on their own after they complete their doctoral training, then they should be prepared to contact individuals via telephone, mail, or e-mail.

Prospective mentors should receive a copy of the individual's curriculum vitae. Students should visit the mentor's laboratory to assess whether it is the right opportunity. Graduate students should start looking for a postdoctoral training experience during the last six months to one year of their doctorate. This will allow the perspective postdoctoral mentor to line up grant funding to sponsor those who do not bring their own funding. Sometimes individuals may only be able to identify a postdoctoral opportunity that is less than ideal, or individuals may identify a better mentor once they arrive at the institution. In this situation, if the current mentor has been good to work with so far, but the project has just started, then the individuals should think carefully about sticking with the opportunity but approach the mentor and telling him or her the future plans. Remember that mentors have invested resources and effort in the trainee, so he or she should remain committed to the lab for the agreed-upon time as long as the mentor has maintained his or her commitment to the trainee with integrity. In some instances, mentors may be able to assist individuals in making the next step. Mentorship is a dynamic interaction. In good situations, the mentor and trainee will develop growing respect for each other over time.

When choosing a postdoctoral mentor, individuals may want to consider one outside of their discipline to expand their horizons. This can often cap off one's research development in a way that adds to the breadth of their knowledge, enabling one to develop knowledge and research capacity at a new level to be even more competitive.

People who have been mentors during the doctoral and postdoctoral years are likely to become the people individual students will list as references. They also may be the same people who will write support letters for one's first grant applications.

One other aspect that deserves attention is the notion of scientific pedigree. The people with whom individuals work during their doctoral and postdoctoral studies will become the generations of their pedigree. Often, these scientific pedigrees are reviewed or touted at scientific venues where someone is being honored with an award or prize. The mentors that students choose will form their pedigree. In his book *The Scientific Attitude*, Grinnell (1992) suggested that if individuals perform their doctoral or postdoctoral work at a university that is counted among the scientific elite, the more likely they will be to join that same group of people, especially if their pedigree can be traced to a member of the National Academy of Sciences or a Nobel prize winner. Although this is not the only criterion on which to judge the best laboratories, it is something individuals should keep in mind if they aspire to be on the cutting edge of science in any discipline.

Some of the skills needed when seeking a mentor will be the same ones needed when identifying the first academic research position. Once individuals have completed their postdoctoral studies, they will look to find the best environment to support their research. They also will be assessing institutions by their reputation or academic atmosphere, the level of productivity of the institutions, the balance or emphasis on research, teaching, and service, and the effects of the location on personal and family life. Lanks (1996) provided information regarding this stage of career development.

Other resources that can be consulted are a collection of personal accounts by prominent women in science (Fort, 1995) and a book on being a mentor (National Academy of Sciences, 1997). In addition, the journal *Science* usually devotes a part of one issue annually to women in science.

In summary, the importance of choosing good mentors, especially at the doctoral and postdoctoral level, cannot be overemphasized. Experiences obtained during doctoral and postdoctoral years will become the fundamental building blocks of a research career launch pad. The better the launch pad, the more likely an individual will be able to propel himself or herself into a successful scientific career. It will take effort, hard work, and planning, but, along the way, individuals will develop good colleagues and friends.

Research Training Opportunities Targeting Cancer Prevention and Detection

The bulk of training opportunities in cancer and other basic and clinical fields are supported by federal sources (e.g., National Cancer Institute [NCI], National Institute of Nursing Research [NINR] of NIH, Agency for Health Care Research and Quality). Sources of nonfederal support may be obtained through ACS or private foundations. Other types of training opportunities are sometimes available at annual research meetings.

A majority of undergraduate, graduate, and postdoctoral training experiences are ones that the mentor can support. In other situations, individuals will have to seek their own source of support to enter the laboratory. At the faculty level, awards are available that also can be used for research training, along with sabbaticals supported by the faculty member's institution.

Extramural

At the federal level, NIH provides sources of extramural and intramural research training. A large number of extramural opportunities can be identified through personal contact, guidance from a mentor, the Internet, attendance at professional meetings, or reviewing journals. Extramural opportunities are available through grants awarded to institutions, National Research Service Awards (NRSAs, T32), or individuals, NRSA predoctoral fellowships (F31), or individual NRSA postdoctoral fellowships (F32).

Almost every institute at NIH awards Institutional Research Training grants (T32) to universities across the country. A list of these grants, their location, and topic can be found by using the CRISP (Computer Retrieval of Information on Scientific Projects) system at https://www-commons.cit.nih.gov/crisp/. These awards are given to a principal investigator at a university for specific types of training opportunities, which are full time and can be at the predoctoral or postdoctoral level. In this situation, applications are made to the institution or principal investigator, who then selects the trainee. The stipend associated with these awards follows guidelines issued by NIH. A recent search of the CRISP system for current awards under the term "cancer" and selecting "Trainee (T)" found 196 hits. Scanning these hits revealed a number of programs targeted at basic, clinical, and epidemiological training. By selecting states or sponsoring institutes, searches can be narrowed to identify specific training opportunities.

Individual NRSAs at the predoctoral (F31) and postdoctoral (F32) levels are awarded to individuals to support research training under the guidance of an identified mentor. For these awards, individuals can tailor the application to match their specific area of research interest and identify a mentor with whom they would like to receive training. Both the individual applying for the training experience and the person who will provide mentorship must complete these applications. Applications for the F31 or F32 can be submitted before the training experience or once it has begun. Individuals who apply for these awards sometimes are viewed more positively later on when looking for a first position or seeking funding because they have learned how to write a grant application. In addition, the awards teach individuals how to handle and manage a small grant by interacting with the institute making the award and the university. This also helps to build a track record of successful funding.

The senior NRSA fellowships (F33) are awarded to scientists who generally have held their doctorate for more than seven years at the time of the award. This award is targeted at assisting scientists at later stages of their career to expand their research capacity, obtain training in a new area, or make major changes in their program of research. The maximum length of this award is two years. Training for this award can be obtained with a mentor at their institution.

Another group of awards where one can obtain training are the so-called "K" awards. Similar to the fellowships, these awards provide research training experiences for those who are not quite ready to submit an investigator-initiated research award and need some additional training to prepare for a competitive application. These awards are especially useful for individuals who cannot leave their current university/geographic setting; they permit these individuals to devote approximately 75% of their time to research. At least three "K" awards are currently available: the Mentored Research Scientist Development Award (K01), the Mentored Patient-Oriented Research Career Development Award (K23), and the Midcareer Investigator Award in Patient-Oriented Research (K24). The K01 is for any area of science, whereas the latter two, K23 and K24, are for patient-oriented research. Details about these awards can be found online at www.nih.gov/ninr/r_restype.html.

Training awards are available through ACS. Information about these opportunities can be found on its Web site at www.cancer.org/research/. ACS offers postdoctoral awards, clinical research awards, and some awards specifically targeted at nursing—Doctoral or Master's Degree Scholarships in Cancer Nursing. Other brief types of training sometimes can be found at annual meetings of various research and professional organizations. These meetings often have preconferences or workshops before or after a meeting for a fee. Depending on the topic and degree of training needed, these types of opportunities often can be a chance for students to see if this is an area in which they would like to invest more effort.

Intramural

At the federal level, other research training experiences can be obtained through the intramural research programs of various NIH institutes. These training opportunities are available for individuals in high school, undergraduate, graduate, or postdoctoral programs and for senior scientists at various stages of their careers. These experiences require that the individual obtain research training at an institute on the campus of NIH in Bethesda, MD, at the National Institute of Aging or the National Institute of Drug Abuse in Baltimore, MD, or the National Institute of Environmental Health Sciences in Research Triangle Park, NC.

For high school, undergraduate, and graduate students, research training opportunities usually are obtained during the summer, and students are paid a modest stipend. Each year, the Office of Education operates a Web site (www.training.nih.gov) that provides information about laboratories that are willing to accept individuals for training opportunities. This Web site also features an online application form. If students are interested in a specific laboratory, they should contact the head of the laboratory, introduce themselves, and express an interest in coming to the laboratory. If possible, they should visit the laboratory before they apply.

At the postdoctoral level, opportunities for research training are available though a variety of programs sponsored by NCI and NINR. Both institutes operate the traditional Intramural Research Training Award (IRTA) program. At the postdoctoral level, this is a full-time training opportunity, and, generally, laboratories will not accept individuals unless they are willing to commit two to three years for training. Thousands of promising young scientists have used this pathway to obtain research training over the last several decades. Individuals who are interested in the IRTA program usually will be asked to submit a curriculum vitae, reference letters, and other materials to support the application. In most cases, the principal investigator of the laboratory will ask individuals to provide a formal presentation and come in for a face-to-face interview.

Currently at NIH, a number of institutes are sponsoring a new group of training opportunities (Wysocki, 1998) using an award mechanism referred to as the K22. Various institutes use different names for the award. NCI named the award the NCI Scholars Award. NINR named the award the NINR Career Transition Award. Regardless of the institute, the overall idea of the award is that it supports postdoctoral training for two to three years at an intramural laboratory and then provides an extramural award to the recipient to help launch his or her research career as a new extramural scientist. Depending on the institute sponsoring the award, the amount of money for each of the intramural and extramural portions of the award varies. Currently, the NINR Career Transition Award provides up to three years of training in an NIH intramural laboratory followed by two years of extramural funding, if progress was satisfactory during the intramural phase. Total direct cost during the extramural phase is $125,000 per year for two years. Of this amount, $50,000 can be used for salary support with 75% effort, and $75,000 can be used for equipment, supplies, and personnel associated with the research project. These awards are given based on a competitive application process, and details about applying for these awards can be found by visiting http://rex.nci.nih.gov/wlcm/

SCHOLARS_MAIN.html for the NCI Scholars Program or www.nih.gov/ninr/r_restype.html for the NINR Career Transition Award.

Other programs operated by NCI include the Cancer Prevention Fellowship Program. This program provides funding for the fellow to obtain a MPH degree within a 12-month period. The program then is linked to a mentored research experience involving a laboratory-based experience, epidemiological laboratory, behavioral science, prevention-related policy research, or research on qualitative and quantitative methodologies. More information about this program can be obtained from the NCI Web site at www.nci.nih.gov/scienceresources/index.html. Another program is the NCI Summer Curriculum in Cancer Prevention. This course typically is about five weeks long, starting in July and concluding in August. The program is broken into two courses: "Principles and Practice of Cancer Prevention and Control" and "Molecular Prevention." The program is open to nurses, physicians, and scientists who are interested in cancer prevention and control. Currently, no fee is charged for the program, but the participant is responsible for room, board, and transportation expenses. Preregistration is required, and information can be found at http://dcp.nci.nih.gov/pob/courses/index.html. NCI's Division of Cancer Epidemiology and Genetics program also sponsors additional training opportunities. A more comprehensive listing of these and other extramural and intramural awards can be found at http://grants.nih.gov/training/extramural.htm, and other types of "K" awards can be found at http://grants.nih.gov/training/careerdevelopmentawards.htm.

Conclusion

When seeking a research training opportunity, individuals should first assess their training needs relative to the stage of their career development. They then should begin to search out available opportunities and mentors, which sometimes can take 6–12 months. Research training opportunities almost always provide investigators with time to expand and enhance their research capacity while allowing them to absorb and immerse themselves in training activities that extend their knowledge so they can emerge ready to meet new research challenges.

References

Fort, D.C. (1995). *A hand up: Women mentoring women in science.* Washington, DC: Association for Women in Science.

Grinnell, F. (1992). *The scientific attitude.* New York: Guilford Press.

Lanks, K.W. (1996). *Academic environment: A handbook for evaluating employment opportunities in science.* Washington, DC: Taylor and Francis.

National Academy of Sciences. (1997). *Adviser, teacher, role model, friend: On being a mentor to students in science and engineering.* Washington, DC: National Academy Press.

Wysocki, A.B. (1998). Launching your research career through postdoctoral training opportunities. *Nursing Research, 47,* 127–128.

CHAPTER 24

Health-Education Issues for Patients in Cancer Prevention and Early Detection

Bessie Woo, RN, MSN, OCN®, Laural A. Aubry, RN, BSN, OCN®, Carol S. Blecher, RN, MS, AOCN®, CNS, C, Janie Eddleman, RN, OCN®, Noella Devolder McCray, RN, MN, and Anne Marie Shaftic, RN, C, BSN, OCN®

Introduction

Patient education, often referred to now as consumer health education, is the number-one way of promoting wellness of the individual and the community at large. Knowledge is power. When people have the knowledge about factors that contribute to wellness, they have the power to change unhealthy habits and adopt practices that improve health. Declines in cancer incidence and mortality rates in the United States, which were first announced in 1996, "can be attributed to a number of factors, including improvements in public and professional education, primary prevention, early detection, and treatment. . . . Tobacco use, lack of exercise, poor diet, and high body mass index may be factors in more than 50% of all cancers in certain age groups" (Seffrin, 2000, pp. 4–5). Nurses and other healthcare professionals can influence each of these factors, whether they work in a hospital or community setting. The efficiency and effectiveness of their efforts can be greatly enhanced if healthcare professionals understand the principles of patient education.

Patient education first was discussed in the literature in the early 1950s (Falvo, 1999). Although healthcare professionals have always provided information to patients on an informal basis, the necessity for offering information in a systematic, measurable manner became increasingly apparent with the advent of managed care. Patient education is both a science and an art. Science is organized knowledge, and patient education uses the knowledge of education models and scientific data on topics such as cancer risk factors, definitions of the target population, studies of effective patient-education programs, and guidelines for selection of patient-education resources. The art of patient education involves applying the knowledge to what is unique about a particular group or individual—not simply finding a practice that applies to all people. Mastery of patient education is an unending process. According to Ames (1997), those who have achieved mastery may have complete command of the skills and even the art of their discipline, but new and increasingly refined aspects of their work continue to appear.

Patient education is like the clothing industry. The demand for clothing has been present since the beginning of civilization, but the styles and fabrics have reflected encounters with new technology, other cultures and climates, as well as the need to make a personal statement. A boutique owner needs to know the clientele's tastes, choose clothing to fit their needs, and present the merchandise in a way that attracts attention to motivate the customers to buy at the boutique. As noted by Lorig (1996), "programs that educate patients do not just happen" (p. 1). A patient educator must be aware of the trends in health care, know the patients' needs, and present health information in a format that is easy to understand and makes the consumer want to take some action. The success of a patient-education project, like the boutique, depends on understanding the needs of those it is intended to serve, offering a product that is perceived as valuable, and developing a trusting relationship.

This chapter will offer nurses ways to tailor the message to the audience to bring about the desired outcomes. It will explore the principles of education that lead to a high standard of care to improve outcomes for individuals and communities. Needs-assessment strategies and development of outcome standards are discussed. Multiple educational challenges, including the special needs of a culturally diverse population, the aging, and those with low literacy skills, are addressed. The development and use of effective educational resources, including the Internet, also are explored. All of these elements continually are evolving in health care. Thoughtful analysis of these challenges, followed by well-designed interventions, can contribute to individual wellness and a healthier society.

Relevance of Patient Education in an Evolving Healthcare System

The focus of the healthcare delivery system is shifting from illness to wellness. Technological advances, changes in diet, and other factors have contributed to increased longevity and an increase in chronic diseases. Increasing healthcare cost-containment efforts has intensified the focus on the measurement of outcomes. Increasing legal and regulatory agency pressures have heightened awareness of the professional's role in providing effective education. "The current healthcare delivery system demands that consumers actively participate in their own care" (Wilson, 2000, p. 114).

Consumers are seeking alternatives and making decisions about their health and wellness, and disease-prevention movements are becoming more prevalent. Individuals are reexamining their diets and lifestyles. Preteens are more aware of the risks of smoking (Nelson et al., 1995). Health-promotion programs are targeting African American men to increase their awareness of their elevated risk for prostate cancer (Eyre & Feldman, 1998). These factors underscore the public's desire and need for effective health education.

Effective education is essential for informed choice and vital to effective health outcomes. According to Wilson (2000), "the objective of patient education is more than disseminating information" (p. 114). Effective education helps individuals to achieve a level of comfort with their self-care needs after receiving acute care and participate in prevention of illness or reduction of complications throughout the continuum of their health care. When individuals and groups understand what is occurring in their health situation, they can partner more effectively with healthcare providers to achieve their health goals. Therefore, effective health education for disease management and prevention is vital throughout the healthcare continuum.

In contacts with individual patients or any target population, nurses need to provide a consistent message. According to the Joint Commission on Accreditation of Healthcare Organizations (JCAHO), patient education should have a multidisciplinary approach that includes physicians, nurses, social workers, physical and occupational therapists, speech therapists, pharmacists, dieticians, exercise specialists, pastoral care, and professionals from any other relevant area. Organizations that are unable to maintain such a comprehensive staff can provide resource listings so patients can gain access to such services. Documentation provides the necessary link between disciplines to support continuity of care.

Fundamentals of Education

Education, by definition, is a two-way process that includes teaching and learning. Although effective teaching depends on the educator's knowledge and skills, effective learning depends on the individual's or group's readiness to learn and the success of addressing learning barriers. Learning barriers may be related to physical disabilities, personality traits, socioeconomic factors, or unique life situations, but the barriers must be recognized (Falvo, 1999).

Although nurses may offer individuals and groups information about their medical condition(s), treatment options, and prevention of diseases or complications, the type and amount of information and the method of communication often varies among practitioners. The variation and degree of effectiveness may be caused by one or more factors, including perceived lack of time, lack of assessment of the need or desire to learn, concern about misinterpretation, concern about creating undue anxiety, professional turf issues over who should communicate particular information, and the individual's expressed desire to be in a more passive role (Falvo, 1999). The challenge is to move beyond the obstacles and improve the health-education process, thus advancing health care.

Effective Education

Although not all nurses may be effective educators, educational skills, like technical skills, can be learned and practiced. Because formal training in the complex process of education often is lacking, many nurses need to acquire knowledge of educational principles and learn specific skills through self-study and peer role models. The nurse who understands the distinctions among providing information, teaching, learning, and education can be a more successful educator.

Information can be provided verbally, through print material, or by video instruction. Providing information alone without any explanations or clarification can contribute to confusion or misunderstanding. **Teaching** involves giving lessons, showing, or demonstrating information. The process of teaching often is one-way and therefore does not ensure that understanding or learning takes place. **Learning** is a process of coming to know, gaining knowledge, or acquiring a skill. **Education** is a process of leading, drawing, bringing, or forming the mind of the learner (Merriam-Webster, 1996). Education requires a two-way communication process of teaching and learning. Learning is the positive outcome of effective education. Individuals who learn about health matters have a logical foundation that encourages the consideration of better lifestyle options (see Table 24-1).

Table 24-1. Differences Between Student and Patient Education and Learning

Student Education (proponents)	Patient Education
Prepare students for adult role position. Bobbitt, 1924; Finney, 1928	Prepare patients to maintain personal health.
Provide students with an orientation to improve the health of society. Kandal, 1941; Kliebard, 1987	Provide an understanding of an individual's influence on the health of society.
Maintain the status quo and reproduce the culture. Broudy, 1982	Maintain the status quo with healthcare provider's dominance over health status.
Provide knowledge that liberates. Anyon, 1980; Friere, 1970	Provide knowledge and understanding that gives patients control over their health status and care.

Note. From "Learning for What Purpose? Questions When Viewing Classroom Learning From a Sociocultural Curriculum Perspective," (p. 33) by S. Chandler in H.H. Marshall (Ed.), *Redefining Student Learning: Roots of Educational Change,* 1992, Norwood, NJ: Ablex Publishing. Copyright 1992 by Ablex Publishing. Adapted with permission.

Principles of Learning

Effective education is more likely when the nurse educator develops a personal knowledge of adult-learning principles and recognizes the components of personal beliefs and other models that describe potential factors in educational outcomes.

Adult Learning

Malcolm Knowles (1970), the father of andragogy, the study of adult learning, identified four characteristics that distinguish the mature adult learner from the child learner. Each characteristic provides direction or goals for educators.

1. Learner's self-concept moves from dependency to self-direction, with responsibility to manage life. The educator who communicates acceptance and support can help the adult learner to express needs and make his or her own choices.
2. Accumulated life experiences are resources for learning. The educator who recognizes positive and negative past experiences effectively can relate each to the new learning situation.
3. Developmental tasks and social roles strongly influence readiness. The educator who recognizes the level of successful mastery of developmental stages and the effect on current roles can relate learning to the individual's ability to succeed. This can be a way of assessing what to teach and who to include in the learning process.
4. Learning is problem-centered and needs immediate application. The educator provides practical answers and helps the learner to apply new knowledge through hands-on practice or verbal role-play.

Learning activities are prioritized by immediacy, perception of need, and promotion of direct problem-solving skills. Characteristics 1 and 4 influence the current need to know. Characteristics 2 and 3 influence the readiness to learn. Through open-ended questioning, the educator can assess the learner's unique learning characteristics. This assessment is key to supporting the individual in knowledge, skill, and behavior mastery.

Health Belief Model

The health belief model also is helpful in understanding motivation to adopt new health behaviors. A group of social psychologists constructed this model in the 1950s (Hochbaum, 1958). It is a tool for understanding the learner's perception of disease or risk. The model originally was developed to help to predict the likelihood of an individual taking recommended preventive action, such as screening tests and check-ups. The model predicts a higher likelihood of using healthcare services if the individual

1. Recognizes the presence of a condition or that high risk exists
2. Recognizes that the condition is harmful and has serious consequences
3. Believes that the suggested health action is of value
4. Believes that the effectiveness of the action is worth the cost of overcoming barriers that may exist.

When nurses understand this reasoning process, they have an increased chance of developing a supportive partnership with the patient. Individuals do not always feel obligated to change health behaviors just because of a healthcare provider's recommendation. Personal belief systems have a major influence. This model also can be applied in community health projects.

The PRECEDE Model

The PRECEDE model, developed by Green et al. (1980), has useful applications for cancer-prevention education programs. The model includes five phases of diagnosis: epidemiological, social, behavioral, educational, and administrative. PRECEDE stands for **p**redisposing, **r**einforcing, and **e**nabling **c**auses in **e**ducational **d**iagnosis and **e**valuation. The model examines what behavior precedes each health benefit and what causes precede each health behavior. The focus is on the final desired outcome. "Why" questions are asked before "how" questions.

One community-health application of this model was the "Food Cent$" project, which was conducted in Australia. The project addressed the risk of nutrition-related diseases when people have little money to buy food. Trained community volunteers were used to help individuals to develop budgeting, shopping, and cooking skills. The study demonstrated that the nutritional quality of the diet could be improved by changing the proportion of money spent on various types of food. Participants were taught to spend more of their food budget on healthy foods and proportionally less on nonhealthy foods (Foley & Pollard, 1998).

Individual Variables

Principles of learning and belief models must be seen in the context of the individual or group demographics. Age, gender, ethnicity, socioeconomic status, educational level, belief systems, and attitudes about cancer are further potential modifiers. Other experiences also may prompt action, such as illness of a family member or friend, media campaigns, or advice from others. For example, the untimely death of a mother because of breast cancer may influence a daughter to take personal action to reduce risk or begin early-detection practices. The nurse must have a complete profile of the individual or group before attempting to gain a commitment to learning healthy behaviors. Individuals often like to tell their unique story. Listening attentively, with thoughtful consideration, gives the nurse an opportunity to identify unique learning needs and readiness to learn and provides a basis for measuring the effectiveness of future interventions.

Information Seeking and Readiness to Learn

Adult learners have positive learning outcomes when they recognize a need to know something and are ready to learn or want to know. Information seeking directs the nurse to develop a partnering or collaborative relationship. During the one-to-one communication process, the educator can assess the level of readiness to learn. Through open-ended questioning, the educator also can identify potential barriers to learning. JCAHO (1997) has incorporated readiness to learn and ability to identify barriers to learning in its standards. Personal feelings, reactions, and responses to an illness, health condition, or general health status strongly influence wellness and prevention activities. Sometimes individuals and groups are unaware of their need to know. They may lack information as basic as the need to use sunscreen to protect themselves against the effects of ultraviolet rays.

Determining Readiness to Learn

Considering the hierarchy of individual needs, the learner and educator realistically can deal with learning needs (Rankin & Stallings, 1996). Needs exist at various levels, and lower-level needs must be met at least partially before a person can meet higher-level needs. Considering the individual's overall needs can help the educator to prioritize educational needs. For example, all nurses know that patients' pain or fear must be dealt with before they can learn about lifestyle adjustments.

Needs Assessment: Who to Target

Lorig (1996) noted that "solid patient education programs are built on carefully executed needs assessments" (p. 1). The goals of a needs-assessment program are to identify and prioritize the needs of the interested parties (Villejo, 1993), such as family members, healthcare providers, and agencies offering services to the target population. Community screenings or surveys also provide an understanding of the needs of the community. The needs of diverse audiences could be the same but may differ. Thus, the goals of an intervention can be nearly uniform, but the interventions may need to be modified to reach each of the various segments of the target audience. A careful needs assessment provides a patient-centered context for the development or selection of patient-education programs and materials. Understanding the needs of the target population leads to developing educational programs that will lead to improved health outcomes.

A Nursing Needs Assessment Model

A nursing practice known as Oncology Transition Services (ONT) was developed in 1989. The primary member of the ONT team was an oncology nurse specialist, who provided individualized assessments for physical, emotional, and educational needs. The specialist also acted as an advocate in assisting in decision making regarding treatments (O'Hare, Yost, & McCorkle, 1993).

Once this model was developed, a study was conducted. This study revealed that patients who had some type of home care had an overall decrease in hospital admissions, including those related to symptom management or a complication of the treatment being administered. This demonstrates the importance of educating the patient or significant other on symptoms of complications related to an illness, which may go unreported. Although this program focuses on the patient with cancer postdiagnosis, a program such as this can be adopted in some fashion for community education. A program related to prevention and early screening especially is valuable to a community with a large elderly population. This model of nursing would allow for the development of a trusting service within a familiar place. Many older adults feel that they no longer need to be screened for cancer because they are elderly and nothing can be done for them.

Perhaps this scenario would help senior citizens to realize they are at a higher risk of developing all types of cancer than the younger population. As nursing students, a group of nurse practitioners started a healthcare clinic in a lower socioeconomic community. In the beginning, they were met with much resistance, but that changed as the community began to trust the nursing staff. After several months, the clinic needed to increase the number of nursing staff to care for the growing number of patients. Because this was a lower socioeconomical area, the number of social workers was increased to assist the patients with their medical needs, such as applying for drug assistance, Medicaid, and food stamp programs. The nurse practitioner students also were involved with a local Catholic school, enabling them to provide education to the older female students about sex education and methods to prevent pregnancy and sexually transmitted diseases. A similarly structured program on prevention and early detection of cancer may be of benefit to all, especially the elderly and lower socioeconomic communities.

Needs assessment is an ongoing process. With each intervention, the needs are reassessed, along with the success or failure of the prior educational efforts. In this way, newly emerging problems may be identified, documented, and resolved at a much quicker pace (O'Hare et al., 1993).

Setting Realistic Goals

As prevention and early detection of cancer methods become more sophisticated and the care of patients becomes more complex, maintaining the standards for education becomes more important. The critical element for effective health outcomes is the achievement of mutually agreed upon health goals, which should be derived from the needs assessment and also be reasonable and measurable. Nurses must understand the values, beliefs, attitudes, life stressors, and previous experiences of the individual or group within the health system. Open communication about what is important for the individual can lead to realistic health goal setting. Recommendations made by nurses may present as an inconvenience or a difficult choice. In making choices that influence health, individuals should consider cost or potential hardships, as well as potential benefits. For instance, a teen who knows about the dangers of smoking may find the future cost of disability or death less costly than ostracism by his or her smoking peers. Yet, when an individual or group chooses not to act on the educator's suggestions, the health educator should try other creative approaches that strengthen communication and eventually lead to behavioral change.

Standards

At intervals throughout the education process, the standards for the education intervention or program need to be reviewed. The standards need to have a purpose, interventions, goals, and a process by which the information will be distributed. Having a method to measure these outcomes provides a tool for judging the success of the intervention.

Jennings, Staggers, and Brosch (1999) identified three categories for patient outcomes. These categories are patient-focused outcomes, which consist of two subsets: disease specific and holistic. The first subset focuses on issues related to a specific disease (i.e., understanding why such a test is performed, the results, and why the results are important in detecting an illness). Holistic indicators go beyond the disease and focus on the patient by offering avenues for prevention. These indicators focus on issues such as quality of life (QOL) and patient satisfaction. In all patient settings, these issues are a major concern, because an illness usually has an impact on both the patient and family. Emotional needs, as well as financial ones, are issues that affect the plan of care that nurses develop for their patients. Patient satisfaction is important to maintain in all types of settings. For example, if a patient has a bad experience in a health clinic, it may deter her from following through with yearly screenings such as mammography.

In educating patients about screening examinations, such as mammography, how to perform a procedure like breast self-examination, or dietary modifications, nurses must consider the individual's financial status. Educating people with limited incomes about the benefits of eating fruits and vegetables to decrease the risk of colon cancer should include suggestions about selecting fruits that are in season at the store or buying from a co-op or farmer's market, where produce is very affordable.

QOL is the best indicator of successful patient education. Improving health habits as a result of what they have learned can lead to a fuller enjoyment of life. Provider-focused outcomes concern methods by which practitioners or family members are able to administer care. Organization-focused outcomes view the institution as a whole. This may relate to rates, such as cost of care or length of stay (Jennings et al., 1999). Although nurses usually are most interested in patient-focused outcomes, an understanding of the different aspects of standard outcomes is helpful.

Fernsler and Cannon (1991) stated that patient education is another compelling rationale for improved patient outcomes. Commonly measured outcomes are patient satisfaction, decreased recovery time following surgery, increased compliance with treatment schedules, and increased ability to handle problems or symptoms related to an illness. Another aspect of weighing outcomes can be the financial status of those involved. As the population lives longer, the elderly may have limited financial resources available to them. The lack of financial resources may cause patients to place other priorities before their healthcare needs, which could affect both the educational process and overall health. Many elderly live on a fixed income and may bypass the need for preventive care, feeling they would not benefit from a screening examination.

Setting Priorities

Once the educational needs are well defined and desired outcomes are formulated, a course of action must be planned. Setting educational priorities can be time efficient when focused on immediate learning needs. Most individuals can learn only one to three new concepts at a time. Therefore, learning needs must be prioritized for health-education goals to be attainable. Overloading learners with information and materials can cause them to feel frustrated, defeated, and dependent. Because time, energy, and resources are at a premium, nurses need to point out what is most important for health promotion. Each encounter with a healthcare provider usually is brief, so having easily accessible teaching materials, which are at an appropriate education level and culturally sensitive, increases the chance of success. Using audiovisuals and interactive methods also increases learning. When the learner is actively engaged in the learning process, retention of information is improved.

With each encounter, learning needs should be reassessed so that the educational goals either can be reprioritized or continued and reinforced. The health educator's goal, therefore, is to provide clear information that leads to understanding and helps learners think for themselves and make informed choices.

Evaluation of Patient-Education Materials

Evaluation of patient-education materials requires the careful balancing of three factors: patients' needs, the purpose of the teaching intervention, and the ease with which the patient can understand the materials. Like a three-legged stool, if one factor is emphasized too much or neglected in relation to the others, the materials will not be solidly grounded. For instance, materials to motivate parents of young children to reduce exposure to sun and advocate the use of sunscreen should have an entirely different approach from materials designed to encourage older adults who already have precancerous lesions to use sun-protective measures. In this scenario, the target populations are members of different age groups and have different lifestyles and interests. In addition, the desired outcomes, although similar, still are different. Therefore, to accomplish their purpose, the materials must be designed for the needs and interests of the target population. The selection and development of materials parallel the patient-education process, and both are most successful if they operate from the patient's perspective (Lumsdon, 1994). This section will discuss needs assessments of target populations and qualities that promote the acceptance and use of patient-education materials. Evaluating the efficacy of patient-education strategies also is discussed.

Why Use Patient-Education Materials?

Although patient education traditionally is conveyed verbally in a medical setting (Foltz & Sullivan, 1998), patients and families find it difficult to remember information unless it is in a written form that they can refer to (Reiley et al., 1996). Written instructions are a cost-effective and time-efficient means of communicating health messages (Wilson, 1996). In the area of cancer prevention, Guidry and Walker (1999) noted that printed materials have become the most common method of educating individuals. The authors stated that printed cancer-education materials are an effective means of delivering cancer-prevention messages.

Other media also may be chosen to reinforce or teach people about the prevention or early detection of cancer. Models, posters, and charts sometimes are needed to demonstrate anatomical relationships or to provide visual clues for patient teaching. At other times, posters may be the media of choice for motivating a target group to some desired action, such as smoking cessation. CD-ROM-based programs are becoming more popular, as are Internet sources of health information. Finally, videotapes are particularly useful to familiarize patients with procedures, equipment, and treatments (Eddleman & Warren, 1994). Studies show that when printed materials were used to reinforce messages on videotapes, subjects were more informed (Guidry & Walker, 1999). Nurses must use their assessment and intervention skills to match the media with the desired message to the target audience.

Assessment of the Target Group

The first step in designing patient-education materials is deciding on the topic (Hussey, 1997). Nurses must identify what the target group needs. Then, they should find out what patients want to learn about the topic. In fact, combining the information the target group wants with what is needed leads to greater acceptance of the program.

Assessment has elements of art and science. The "art" of assessment is in the action that nurses take to understand the target audience's perspective. The "science" of assessment involves data collection and analysis of the audience, an objective determination of what the target audience wants and needs.

After the topic of discussion has been identified and the target audience's needs have been determined, a summary of the findings, which includes a clear description of the target population, is warranted. In addition, learning objectives, goals, and outcomes should be discussed and agreed upon, highlighting educational material(s) to be used in class and distributed as handouts. Whether the patient-education materials are developed within the institution, obtained for free from various agencies, or purchased from commercial sources, the next step is to evaluate the potential materials in relation to the target population, their needs, and the purpose of the materials. The objective is to make the materials effective and easy for patients and families to use.

Criteria for Selecting Patient-Education Materials

When reviewing patient-education materials as a whole, nurses should consider whether the materials show a respect for the audience, promote hope and positive self-esteem, and promote the perception of control over one's own health and well-being.

Content: Focusing content on behaviors that lead to the desired outcome is more important to patients than are the underlying principles (Doak, Doak, & Meade, 1996). This is an important concept. Nurses often feel more comfortable evaluating facts and principles because the medical literature they rely upon also tends to focus on these things. Making facts relevant to patients is a somewhat different process.

1. Provide accurate information. Information should reflect current standards and local practice.
2. Verify that the information is up-to-date. Check the copyright date. When developing materials, include the publication date for ease in reviewing the currency of materials in the future.

Organization: Is the information presented clearly enough for people to "get it?" Organization helps patients to have a clear understanding of the purpose of the materials and anticipate the logic of the argument. It also provides a map to guide them through the information. An organized approach is necessary for all patient-education materials and activities, from verbal interactions to written information, speeches, videotapes, and audiotapes. Overall, organization offers valuable clues to the patient about what the presenter considers important, making those points easy to remember.

1. Have a clear purpose. Informing the patient of the purpose provides a context for the material being presented (Lorig, 1996).
2. Limit educational objectives to one or two (Doak, Doak, & Meade, 1996). The educational objectives should be action oriented. They should state what

the learner would do as a result of using these materials. Besides being measurable and objective, they also should be reasonable.

3. Present the most important information first. Prioritize the information so that the most important information is at the beginning. Assume that the learner only will read the first sentence, the first paragraph, or the first page (Adler, 1991).

4. Limit information to what is needed to meet objectives (Lorig, 1996). A well-organized presentation gives just enough information to meet the objectives. Adding extraneous information, such as underlying principles, adds to the amount of information that patients feel obliged to absorb. "Readers do not need to be presented with an explanation of the underlying principles to understand and carry out the behaviors" (Doak, Doak, & Meade, 1996, p. 1307).

5. Summarize the key points. This acquaints the learner with the important points and helps the patient to understand what needs to be learned or acted upon.

6. Present the context before new information is offered (Lorig, 1996). Research shows that this grammatical device can make a huge difference in comprehension (Doak, Doak, & Meade, 1996). It provides a framework upon which the learner can organize the concept. For instance, "To prevent skin cancers (*the context*), use sunscreen" (*the new information*).

7. Begin with known concepts and logically progress to unknown ones. Similarly, move from general to specific information. These devices are another way of providing a framework or map for learners to make sense of the facts being presented.

8. Repeat important points (Giordano, 1996). Repetition increases the retention of the materials. In addition, repetition indicates that the presenter considers that material important, providing the learner with another clue of what should be retained.

Motivation: Offering clearly stated facts is not enough to change behaviors. Patients are much less interested in facts about cancers than in improving their well-being or solving their problem. Although facts and principles may need to be presented, they will be given more attention and retained better when offered in a problem-solving or behavior context (Doak, Doak, & Meade, 1996).

1. Model desired behaviors (Lorig, 1996). For instance, when explaining breast self-examination, provide an illustration of a woman palpating her breast instead of a diagram of the breast.

2. Present doable behaviors (Doak, Doak, & Root, 1996). The needs assessment will indicate what behaviors are realistic for the target population. For instance, be sure that dietary suggestions respect the targeted cultural group's eating patterns.

3. Ask the readers to do something (Lorig, 1996). Almost any kind of interaction (e.g., checklists, questions to be answered, making a grocery list) improves the retention of information. When materials that required interactions were field tested, they were enjoyed, were learned from, and provided motivation for respondents (Doak, Doak, & Root, 1996). Motivational inter-

actions can be as simple as asking patients to list one or two things they can do to improve their health habits.

Cultural considerations: Cultural issues extend beyond nationality and ethnicity. For example, teens live in a different culture than their parents and grandparents. Because cultural issues are covered more thoroughly elsewhere in this chapter, the topic only is discussed briefly here to ensure that the reader includes the issue in evaluation of materials.

1. Match language, logic, experience, and illustrations to those of a target population (Lorig, 1996). Because people respond favorably to familiar situations, developing culturally relevant approaches to patient education increases acceptance and facilitates learning. Illustrations of people in brochures or characters in videos should look like the target audience. Spokespeople should be members of the target community. When materials are developed for non-English-speaking people, nurses should create them in the ethnic language instead of translating the original English materials literally.
2. Provide positive, realistic, and appropriate cultural images (Doak, Doak, & Root, 1996). Choose images that present the objectives in a favorable context for the targeted population. Materials must convey respect for the culture.

Cost: The cost of materials is a factor that needs to be considered in most patient-education programs. The best materials available may be bypassed because of their impact on the budget. Nurses should look toward creative venues for revenue, such as grants or donations from community groups. If publishing or purchasing a large quantity of materials is unaffordable, a notebook with samples, accompanied by the names and addresses of the source, can be used. Patients and their families may be able to obtain single copies of publications without charge. A library of videotapes may be useful in a clinic setting, where patients tend to wait for appointments, or in a unit's visiting area.

Evaluation Criteria for Written Materials

Although written materials usually are print materials, the following evaluation criteria also can apply to written information presented in videotapes or posters. This list is an attempt to summarize the current literature.

Readability:
1. Match grade level to target population. Detailed information on measuring reading level of materials is provided elsewhere in this chapter.
2. Use one- and two-syllable words. Readability formulas are based on the proportion of short words. Because common words tend to be one or two syllables, they are apt to increase comprehension. On the other hand, readability formulas can be skewed with one- or two-syllable medical terms, such as cervix and prostate. Those medical terms might hinder comprehension, even though they are "short" words.
3. Use short sentences with one idea per sentence. The goal is clear and succinct writing.
4. Use active voice. Active voice almost automatically lowers reading level by several grade levels. Doak, Doak, and Meade (1996) noted that "take your

medicine every day, even when you feel well" is easier to read than "medication should be taken every day, even when one feels well" (p. 1308).

5. Use simple grammatical structures. As a rule, sentences should be limited to 15 words.
6. Use an objective tone, yet keep it personal and informative.
7. Use common words that are explicitly descriptive (Lorig, 1996). Programs on smoking cessation use a common language.
8. Limit use of medical terms. They are like a foreign language to the public. When possible, common terms should be used.
9. Define medical terms. When medical terms are used, they should be defined the first time they appear. They are most effective when placed at the beginning of written material. If the target population has low literacy or learning disabilities, glossaries may hinder comprehension. In addition, poor readers tend to skip difficult words. For those who have difficulty reading, putting the meaning into context or remembering the definition often is difficult. Glossaries only add to the complexity of the material for them.
10. Use a bullet format to stress important points (Giordano, 1996). This format often reduces the number of words and also provides guideposts to enhance comprehension.

Legibility:
1. Choose a style of type that is easy to read and harmonizes with the overall design of materials. Doak, Doak, and Mead (1996) recommended a serif type (e.g., Times Roman), which has strokes at the tips of characters. Hiam (1997) found that Helvetica, which is a sans serif typeface, and Century, a serif typeface, are the most readable.
2. Emphasize text by bolding or underlining rather than using all uppercase letters or italics. When all uppercase letters are used, the text is harder to read. In fact, Hiam (1997) stated that readers read lowercase letters about 13% faster. In addition, readers tend to focus on the capital letters instead of the message. Italics are difficult for people with poor eyesight or reading skills (Hussey, 1997).
3. Use high contrast between color of ink and paper. Dark ink on light-colored paper is most effective.
4. Use at least 10-point type. If a target audience has any visual impairments, use at least 12-point type. Older readers tend to prefer large print.
5. Avoid glossy paper because it may produce a glare, which is distracting and makes for harder reading.

Layout: How a brochure or any other patient-education material looks may determine whether patients read it. Design and layout help to form a first impression.
1. Use adequate spacing and margins. White space aids comprehension.
2. Use topic headings to guide patients through materials. Advanced organizers help readers to gain access to the information. Hussey (1997) recommended using seven or fewer headings for brochures. For patients with low literacy, Hussey recommended reducing the number of headings to three to five. In a study conducted by Thompson and Thiemann (1999), enlarged

content headings increased use of the National Cancer Institute's Physician Data Query database.

3. Develop an uncluttered appearance (Doak, Doak, & Root, 1996). Eliminate distractions. A simple format moves the learner through the material in an orderly manner.

4. Limit fonts and sizes. Changes in fonts and sizes should be used to stress important points or help the reader to navigate through the material. Multiple changes of fonts or sizes are distracting.

5. Left-justified, right-ragged text without hyphenation is easier to read.

Illustrations: Nursing literature has limited information about how to use or evaluate illustrations in patient-education materials. The interpretation of illustrations requires skill that is equivalent to literacy skills (Hussey, 1997). Illustrations increase comprehension and recall of written material (Behan & Reynolds, 1992).

Many of the same concepts applicable to choosing words also apply to the selection of illustrations. Just as common words enhance readability of text, illustrations of familiar objects improve comprehension. Illustrations can be used to attract attention or to guide the reader through the materials. These principles also apply to videotapes, posters, charts, and CD-ROMs.

1. Use illustrations to support or explain the text. Illustrations should relate to the text. They should be placed near the text they are meant to explain or illustrate (Lorig, 1996).

2. Illustrate intended message. Illustrations should meet the intended objectives of the patient-education material. They should support the purpose, not distract from it.

3. Use clearly drawn illustrations (Behan & Reynolds, 1992). Simple drawings free of all nonessential items reinforce the message.

4. Be sensitive to the target audience. Choose illustrations that not only are culturally sensitive but also are familiar to the target audience. Try to view the material through the eyes of the target audience.

5. Provide legible labels (Hussey, 1997). Label the illustration, as needed, to clarify its meaning and relationship to the text. Choose a font size and type that is easy to read.

6. Use diagrams rather than pictures, because they remove superfluous information (Hussey).

7. Know your target audience's preferences. Select colors that attract or transmit the material's message. Remember that colors may have embedded meaning for the target group.

Glossaries: Whereas glossaries seem to be beneficial to readers because they define unfamiliar terms, they have been found to be a barrier for people with reading problems.

Field Testing

Field-testing materials provides invaluable feedback on how a particular target audience views patient-education materials. The careful preparation of a questionnaire focuses the feedback and improves the effectiveness of the evaluation process. Even though all of the guidelines for writing effective patient-education materials may have been followed and a multidisciplinary team may have reviewed the product for accuracy and timeliness of content, field testing by representatives of the targeted population often reveals refinements that can further clarify the intended message. This also applies to the selection of commercially available materials (Lorig, 1996). Doak, Doak, and Meade (1996) also recommended evaluating the materials for attractiveness, comprehension, acceptance, and persuasion.

Although field testing with the target audience is the ideal, occasionally producers of patient-education materials may not have the time or resources for that valuable process. Recognizing this problem, Doak, Doak, and Root (1996) developed and validated a tool, the Suitability Assessment of Materials. It can be used with print material, illustrations, videotapes, and audiotapes. They recommended using the tool to test patient materials or to pinpoint areas for improvement of materials as they are being developed.

Carefully chosen patient-education materials can be effective tools. Understanding the target group's needs and culture to increase the effectiveness of patient-education programs is similar to the boutique owner's creative use of floor space to help shoppers to navigate through the store. Displays and signs help shoppers to quickly find the kind of clothing they want, whereas cluttered shops can confuse the shopper. As new styles emerge, many shoppers need time to adjust to them and consider their suitability. In patient education, the Internet is the newest fashion trend that is expected to be a standard source of health information in the future.

The Internet as a Patient-Education Tool

Information acquired through Internet sources can be used to enhance the nurse/patient relationship. It has become a source where the public can obtain current medical information about cancer detection and prevention (Kotecki & Chamness, 1999) and also has become a very useful resource for nurses. As patients obtain a larger portion of their health information online, nurses have an opportunity to open a channel of communication with patients by discussing Internet resources. In addition to reviewing information obtained by patients, nurses can provide Internet-acquired literature, answer questions, and assist individuals in planning their health goals. This collaborative effort can strengthen the nurse/patient relationship. Improved health outcomes resulting from the communication of accurate prevention and detection information is the nurse's ultimate goal.

Computer technology has rapidly enhanced the communication of health and wellness information. A 1987 National Health Survey evaluating knowledge of cancer-screening procedures gained from electronic media did not list computers as a source for information (Meissner, Potosky, & Convissor, 1992). In the early 1990s, electronic media merely consisted of television and radio. Recently, with increasing computer availability in homes, schools, and libraries, people have greater access to computers as another electronic source for information. From October 1997 through September 1998, approximately 18 million adults within the United States sought health information on the World Wide Web ("Internet

Health Seekers," 1998). The researchers also indicated that the most frequently searched category was related to cancer. As of May 2001, Nielsen Net ratings reported that home Internet access reached 167 million within the United States (Nielsen, 2001). Educational institutions, organizations, and government divisions have developed new Web sites because of an increased demand for information.

Any organization, institution, or individual may design and maintain a Web site. With the emergence of so many Web sites that offer health information, many authors have voiced concern about the accuracy and completeness of the posted information (Berliner, 1998; Fortin, 1998; Kotecki & Chamness, 1999). The Internet is an information source that virtually is unrestricted in content (Clark, 1999). Unscientific information or questionable research data may be published online, which can make potentially harmful information readily accessible. Controversy exists over whether information posted on a Web site should be required to meet certain standards. Although other physician groups advocate quality criteria or guidelines, Rettig (1995) proposed that "caveat lector et viewor—let the reader and viewer beware" should be the mainstay of any information obtained off the Internet. Ultimately, patients will have to determine if the information fits their needs or situation.

To date, no set standards regulate posted information; however, various tools can be used to evaluate Web sites. One such tool, seen in Figure 24-1, can assist the viewer in determining the validity of information and design structure of the site. This site evaluation tool rates a Web site by asking the user questions that require a yes or no response. After answering all of the questions, each response is tallied. Based on the number of yes responses, the Web site is rated as credible, ambivalent, or a red flag site. Nurses and patients who are computer literate will find this tool helpful for Web site evaluation.

Another way individuals may choose to evaluate a Web site is by using principles and codes of conduct, suggested by the Health on the Net Foundation (1997) (see Figure 24-2). The American Medical Association supports these principles, as well (*JAMA* Patient Page, 1998). Additionally, they suggested that dates be posted for updated information, along with the identity of the reviewer. Content of the site, which includes quality, reliability, accuracy, scope, and depth, was cited most frequently in evaluations of Web sites (Kim, Eng, Deering, & Maxfield, 1999). Use of tools, guidelines, and criteria to evaluate the credibility of Web sites will help to minimize misinformation for patients. By becoming knowledgeable about such evaluation tools, nurses can assist patients with their search for reputable Web sites.

The convenience of the Internet as a patient-education tool outweighs the potential for misinformation on the Web. Healthcare experts consider 24-hour availability of information the most important benefit ("Strike It Rich," 1998). Internet access allows patients to browse health-related Web sites when they are ready to learn. Additionally, online information that specifically meets their needs can be printed for future use. Patients no longer are solely dependent on their healthcare professional to provide verbal or written information. Access to the Internet may change the way people learn about healthcare issues and how they use this infor-

Figure 24-1. Health-Related World Wide Web Site Evaluation Tool

Title: _____ URL: http:// _____

Date: _____ Evaluator: _____

Information

Step 1: Check "Y" (Yes) if statement applies "N" (No/Not Sure) if statement does not apply.

Criteria 1: Scope	Y	N
A. Many different aspects of the topic are presented.		
B. Each aspect is presented in depth.		
Tally		

Criteria 2: Accuracy	Y	N
A. The information is consistent with other resources on the topic.		
B. The information presented is properly references.		
C. The information is based on scientific data.		
D. The site includes a disclaimer.		
Tally		

Criteria 3: Authority	Y	N
A. The author(s) organization(s) supplying the information are identified.		
B. The author(s)/organization(s) are recognized in the field.		
C. The credentials of the author(s) are identified.		
D. The author(s) are writing in their discipline.		
Tally		

Criteria 4: Currency	Y	N
A. The information presented is up-to-date.		
B. The information builds on previous knowledge.		
Tally		

Criteria 5: Purpose	Y	N
A. The purpose of the site is identified.		
B. The information is appropriate for the intended purpose.		
C. The intended audience is specified.		
D. The source funding the site is identified.		
Tally		

Step 2: Sum the Y's from each criteria.

C1☐ + C2☐ +C3☐ +C4☐ +C5☐ =☐

Step 3: Rate the site by comprehensiveness of information.

☐ 13-16 = Credible site: Convincing evidence exists
☐ 7-12 = Ambivalent site: inconclusive evidence exists
☐ 0-6 = Red Flag Site: Insufficient evidence exists

Design

Step 4: Check "Y" (Yes) if statement applies "N" (No, Not Sure) if statement does not apply.

Criteria 6: Organization, Structure & Design	Y	N
A. The information presented in the site is well organized.		
B. The terminology used is meaningful to the subject area.		
C. The site contains a table of contents or provides an organizational structure to easily access content.		
D. The site contains specific links to data referenced.		
E. The site contains internal search engines.		
F. The document has a distinguishable header and footer.		
G. The major headings and subheadings are identifiable.		
H. The loading time for the site is reasonable.		

Organization, Structure & Design	Y	N
I. The site's creation date is clearly displayed.		
J. The date of the last revision is clearly displayed.		
K. The reading level and material presented is appropriate for intended audience.		
Tally		

Step 5: Rate the site by "net appeal."

☐ 6-11 = Accomodating site
☐ 0-5 = Hindering site

Step 6: Personal Comments: Now compare this source to other sources you have on this topic.

Note. From "A Valid Tool for Evaluating Health-Related WWW Sites," by J.E. Kotecki and B.E.Chamness, 1999, *Journal of Health Education, 30*(1), p. 57. Copyright 1999 by Association for the Advancement of Health Education. Reprinted with permission.

mation in their daily lives (Berliner, 1998). Web sites that publish guidelines for health screening can have a positive impact on the health of patients and families. For example, many sites list signs and symptoms of colorectal cancer, and others communicate recommendations for breast examination and mammography. Con-

Figure 24-2. Principles to Assess the Quality of Medical Information

- Only medically trained and qualified professionals will give any medical advice that is provided or hosted on this site unless a clear statement is made that a piece of advice offered is from a nonmedically qualified individual/organization.
- The information provided on this site is designed to support, not replace, the relationship that exists between a patient/site visitor and his or her existing physician.
- Confidentiality of data relating to patients' and visitors' identity is respected when they are logged onto a medical Web site.
- Information contained on this site will be supported by clear references to source data and, where possible, have specific HTML links to those data.
- Any claims relating to the benefits/performance of a specific treatment, commercial product or service will be supported by appropriate, balanced evidence in the manner outlined above.
- The designers of this Web site will seek to provide information in the clearest possible manner and provide contact addresses for visitors who seek further information or support. The Webmaster's e-mail address will be displayed clearly throughout the Web site.
- Support for this Web site will be clearly displayed, including the identities of commercial and noncommercial organizations that have contributed funding or services for the site.
- If advertising is a source of funding, it will be clearly stated. A brief description of the advertising policy adopted by the Web site owners will be displayed on the site.

Note. Based on information from Health on the Net Foundation, 1997.

tinued development and use of the World Wide Web as an education source will benefit people who seek readily accessible information related to the prevention and detection of cancer.

With the numerous Web sites available, nurses can offer suggestions to patients on where to find credible information (Cormier, 1997). Self-care is promoted as patients collect information specific to their needs. They then are empowered to make decisions about their health (Fortin, 1998). Suggestions can be individualized to meet specific interests. Table 24-2 lists many Web sites from which individuals can obtain cancer prevention and detection information, including material on disease, diet and nutrition, fitness, and health.

Information from the Internet should not replace verbal communication between nurses and patients. Healthcare professionals should review the information patients present and help them to understand how the data apply to their situation. The nurse's role is to assess if the information is appropriate for the learner's needs. During the educational session, verbal interaction with the patient will promote ongoing evaluation of a patient's understanding. Nurses also can determine whether patients have attained their learning goals. Although electronic media is a useful tool in patient education, verbal interaction with patients is a crucial component leading to the successful understanding and implementation of cancer-prevention and early-detection interventions.

As nurses individualize their patients' educational plans and teaching methods, barriers to computer-related learning must be considered. Children are exposed to computers at an early age through school programs. Developing computer proficiency early in life will help future generations to view and use the Internet as a barrier-free source for health information. Like school-aged children, many working adults use computer equipment and programs on a regular basis. This

Table 24-2. Health-Related Web Sites That Offer Cancer Prevention and Detection Information

Source of Information	Web Address
ACHOO: Internet Health Care Directory	www.achoo.com
American Cancer Society	www.cancer.org
American Medical Association	www.ama-assn.org
Health A to Z	www.healthatoz.com
Health Web	www.healthweb.org
Healthfinder	www.healthfinder.org
Healthtouch	www.healthtouch.com
Susan G. Komen Breast Cancer Foundation	www.komen.org
Mayo Clinic Health Oasis	www.mayo.ivi.com
Medical Matrix	www.medmatrix.org
Medline	www.nlm.nih.gov/databases/freemedl.html
National Alliance of Breast Cancer Organization	www.nabco.org
National Cancer Institute	www.nci.nih.gov
National Library of Medicine	www.nlm.nih.gov
OncoLink	www.oncolink.upenn.edu
Oncology Nursing Society	www.ons.org
Tufts University Nutrition Navigator	www.nagivator.tufts.edu
U.S. Centers for Disease Control and Prevention	www.cdc.gov
U.S. Government	www.healthfinder.gov
Virtual Hospital	www.vh.org
WebMD	www.webmd.com
Wellness Web	www.wellweb.com

experience helps to minimize computer-related barriers in the working adult population. The older population often is intimidated by this relatively new technology. Those who have had little or no exposure to computers are most likely to perceive their lack of computer skills as a barrier to access online information. With more than 50% of cancer cases occurring in people who are older than age 65 (Redman, 1997), a significant effort should be made to have prevention and, especially, early detection information available. The older population, as well as those with no computer skills, can benefit from Internet-acquired prevention and detection information with the help of a person who is computer literate. Local hospital and community libraries usually will provide assistance with computer access. Older adults also may find computer support services through their community's senior center.

An economic barrier, such as the inability to afford personal computer equipment, simply may translate into a convenience issue. Instead of being able to access prevention and detection information at will, people with less money must rely on outside community resources.

As the Internet continues to expand, with more Web sites containing cancer prevention and detection information, it will become difficult to monitor all published data. Therefore, when recommending Web sites to patients, the nurse should suggest those created by "recognized, respected professional societies and organizations" ("Be Leery," 1996). This will improve the patient's chance of obtaining reliable information to determine necessary healthcare interventions and goals.

Patient Education in Special Populations

Teaching Culturally Diverse Patients and Their Families

Nurses should be culturally competent and familiar with cultural concepts. Cultural competence is defined as "being sensitive and responsive to issues related to culture, race, ethnicity, gender, age, socioeconomic status, and sexual orientation" (Brant et al., 1999, p. 3). Nurses need to assess their own beliefs and attitudes; become knowledgeable about other ethnic cultural beliefs and practices; accept and respect patients who have different cultural health beliefs, practices, and values; and negotiate with patients and their family members (Kagawa-Singer, 1997).

Ethnic minority populations are growing at greater rates than the majority White populations (Brant et al., 1999). The population of the United States has become increasingly ethnically diverse during the last decade (Kerner, 1996), and the trend is expected to accelerate. The U.S. Census projects that by 2050, the American population will contain 22.5% Hispanics, 14.4% African Americans, 9.7% Asian Americans, and 0.9% Native Americans (Brant et al.). Nurses will be responsible for recognizing ethnic patients' special needs and developing strategies to meet these needs in patient education (Wilson, 1996).

Educational Barriers in Ethnic Groups

It sometimes is difficult to get ethnic populations to participate in cancer detection and screening programs (Kagawa-Singer, 1997). Recently, researchers found that the lack of a healthcare source because of poverty, different past experiences, limited English proficiency, and cultural differences are the most significant barriers for cancer prevention, early detection, and screening in ethnic populations (Choudhry, Sirvastava, & Fitch, 1998; Kagawa-Singer; Kim, Yu, et al., 1999; Nichols, Misra, & Alexy, 1996; O'Malley, Mandelblatt, Gold, Cagney, & Kerner, 1997). This section discusses these barriers and how to achieve effective patient education in ethnic populations.

Some of the problems associated with reaching out to ethnic groups are related to their lack of a healthcare source because of their low incomes. The lack of economic and social resources is a predictor of invasive cancer and later stage of diagnosis for screenable cancer (Breen & Figueroa, 1996; Kerner, 1996). Many ethnic populations are understudied and underserved (Kerner). For example, a 1997 public health study conducted by UCLA found that nearly 3.9 million Asian and Hispanic immigrants in California were without health insurance. This is significant because the people who have a continual source of health care with regular clinicians who recommend regular tests for early detection and cancer screening often have a higher rate of screening. Therefore, the lack of a health source reduces access to preventive services for many ethnic people (O'Malley et al., 1997).

Elderly people of ethnic populations often are poor and, therefore, have lower rates of participation in cancer-prevention activities. For instance, immigrant women who are age 70 and older are less likely to have mammograms (Choudhry et al., 1998). Many elderly immigrants are not used to detection and screening procedures. Their mothers never performed breast self-examinations or underwent clinical breast examinations or mammograms, and such screening was not readily available in their birthplaces (Choudhry et al.). Therefore, elderly immigrants may not think that these preventive modalities are important. Past experiences, coupled with poverty, need to be addressed in patient-education program planning.

Limited English proficiency affects the ability of many ethnic minorities to read and therefore decreases their knowledge of cancer prevention and early-detection practices. In cervical cancer prevention, studies show that the major reason for many women not having Pap smears was that they did not have disease symptoms (Kim, Yu, et al., 1999). Because English is their second language, some immigrants, even those who had higher education in their birthplace, never have overcome their limited English proficiency. Because of the language barrier, many older ethnic populations live in their own communities for decades and never use the mainstream health system.

Different cultural beliefs and practices in ethnic populations also can create barriers to using preventive modalities. Cultural beliefs and values, in part, give an individual a sense of identity and security (Kagawa-Singer, 1997). Therefore, a new practice that is different from one's culture could be perceived as a threat. Other studies also show that beliefs strongly influence the motivation to comply (Nichols et al., 1996). For example, some cultures believe that blood is a vital force that supports one's health, so blood drawing may be perceived as something that could threaten their health (Woo, 2000). In the mainstream health system, blood drawing is a common practice and screening technique. Some people refuse to seek medical attention because they do not want their blood taken. In some cultures, it is taboo for women to expose their private parts to men, even male healthcare providers (Underwood, Shaikha, & Bakr, 1999). Many women may feel very uncomfortable during breast and pelvic examinations. As a result, they procrastinate or refuse cancer-prevention modalities. When the majority of an ethnic group holds similar beliefs, the entire community may avoid participation in cancer-prevention modalities.

Strategies to Overcome Barriers

How do nurses disseminate cancer-prevention information to ethnic minority groups? Although ethnic minorities are considered by some to be "hard to reach" and "noncompliant" (Chen, Wismer, Lew, & Kang, 1997; Kagawa-Singer, 1997), educators in many communities indicated that ethnic minorities wanted to learn and would attend classes if the education could meet their needs (Kim, Yu, et al., 1999; Woo, 1995). Therefore, conducting needs assessment on a regular basis is essential in successful patient education for cancer prevention and early detection in ethnic populations.

A multidisciplinary approach works well in cancer-prevention programs for ethnic minorities (Breen & Figueroa, 1996). This shows patients and family members that many different people provide care in the mainstream healthcare system, such as nurses, doctors, dieticians, social workers, and therapists. Because many ethnic minorities do not have adequate resources, teaching that includes discussions of possible treatments, costs, and available resources if cancer is detected can reduce patients' fear and worry about cancer. Patients and their family members also should be taught how to use resources appropriately.

Teaching can become more effective if a target population's particular concerns are addressed. For example, most Asian Americans believe that the family as a group is more important than the individual. Applying that cultural belief, smoking cessation programs for Asian Americans should emphasize the effects of smoking on the family. As a result, Asian American smokers are more apt to quit smoking because they value their family members and may not want to see children suffer from the damages caused by passive smoking.

Patient-education materials and activities that do not address cultural needs and bias are not effective teaching tools. A recent study showed that low-income and minority patients usually turn first to family and friends rather than to healthcare providers/educators for nutritional information (Macario, Emmons, Sorensen, Hunt, & Rudd, 1998). When teaching ethnic people about foods that prevent cancer, the suggested foods should be ones that they normally eat. Otherwise, ethnic people will have difficulty in following instructions and will not be able to relate to the role of nutrition in cancer prevention.

In planning education programs, logistics such as duration of class and the convenience of class schedules, locations, transportation, and sufficient funding for free or small-fee classes should be considered. Saturday classes usually have a higher attendance in many cities than do evening classes because people feel safer using public transportation during the daytime. In addition, patients and their family members may be off work, so family members can accompany patients to classes. In many ethnic populations, it is very common for family members to attend classes with patients.

Efforts to use existing community-based information centers should be undertaken. For example, recent reports found that community health centers, churches, hospitals, local schools (Kim, Yu, et al., 1999), and even grocery stores (Sadler, Nguyen, Doan, Au, & Thomas, 1998) are good locations for disseminating information about cancer prevention. These locations tend to be easily accessible by public transportation. Newspapers, radio, brochures, books, and magazines are useful resources for providing ethnic minorities with information on cancer prevention (Kim, Yu, et al.). Televisions and VCRs are popular in many Asian American families; they are useful tools for teaching patients and their families about cancer prevention, early detection, and screening (Kim, Yu, et al). Many ethnic communities have been using the media to discuss smoking cessation, which has raised people's awareness that smoking can cause cancer. Many restaurants and bakeries now post and enforce "no smoking" signs in sitting areas.

Patient-education materials should be improved because cultural content must be an integral part of cancer-education programs for effective practice and care (Boston, 1993; Kagawa-Singer, 1997). Unfortunately, only 4 out of 54 (8.5%) patient-education materials are culturally sensitive (Wilson, 1996). Evaluation of 106 cancer-prevention materials for African Americans found that the majority (56.2%) were culturally insensitive (Guidry & Walker, 1999).

Most patient-education materials, including written and visual, are prepared in English only, with a limited number of materials written in other languages. Monolingual education material can cause a barrier in patient education and break down communication. For instance, in many families, the elderly ethnic populations commonly speak only their native languages and their children who are born in the United States speak only English. As a result, the two groups use a combination of broken English and the ethnic language to communicate. To facilitate learning, patient-education materials should be prepared ideally in both English and in ethnic languages. Many healthcare facilities have a core group of bilingual employees who serve as translators and could make a valuable contribution. Hospitals with a high population of non-English-speaking patients may need to seek out international sources for health-education materials.

Ethnically sensitive materials make culturally diverse patients feel accepted; thus, they are more willing to participate in cancer prevention and early-detection practices. These programs should be planned and implemented by health educators who have studied (or are part of) the ethnic group and are able make the health information relevant and culturally sensitive to overcome language and cultural barriers.

Theoretical information is difficult to absorb and needs reinforcement. Practical information with demonstration and encouragement enhances patient participation in cancer detection and screening (Choudhry et al., 1998). Incorporation of different types of music, art, drama, dance, and exercise into program activities also enhances patient participation (Lorig, 1996). In ethnic groups where patients respect authority, programs in collaboration with a community agency or university can increase patient participation (Chen et al., 1997).

The ability to collaborate with ethnic communities is another very important strategy for effective patient education in cancer prevention and early detection. Gaining trust is crucial in implementing community cancer prevention educational programs. Establishing a good relationship with the community before planning a program and getting the community involved from the beginning is fundamental. Establishing a nurse-managed clinic or other community outreach service helps to build that trust. Working to develop common goals and sharing decision making show respect for the community leaders. Honesty and integrity are the basis of long-term collaborations with communities (Barg & Lowe, 1996; Chen et al., 1997). A strong relationship exists between individual learning and community support. As the ethnic community increases its awareness in cancer prevention, early detection, and screening, community perceptions change. Community education and support can reinforce an individual's knowledge of cancer prevention and facilitate behavior change.

In summary, nurses must be able to identify the barriers that inhibit ethnic patients and their family members from learning about, seeking, and receiving cancer prevention, early-detection, and screening services. A wide variety of strategies could help to overcome a lack of a health source because of poverty, negative past experiences, limited English proficiency, and cultural differences. By using creative and individualized interventions, nurses may find it rewarding to teach and work with ethnic populations.

Educating Patients With Visual Impairment, Hearing Difficulties, or Low Literacy Levels

In the real world of patient education, nurses are presented with numerous barriers to their educational efforts. Many adults and children have visual and auditory difficulties, as well as reading and cognitive disabilities, that challenge nurses' ability to teach. This section will focus on potential visual, auditory, and literacy deficits that have an impact on patient education and the strategies for overcoming these challenges.

Impact of Aging on Vision and Hearing

Normal physiologic aging begins at age 20 and continues through the remainder of the lifespan. The loss of visual and auditory acuity is a normal part of aging. The percentage of individuals in the United States who are older than 65 continually is increasing. Therefore, a significant number of prevention, early-detection, and health-maintenance efforts should be focused on senior citizens. Because of the decreasing visual and auditory acuity in this population, initial evaluations must include assessments of the individual's ability to hear what is being taught and see or read the materials presented.

Visual Impairment

In the United States, approximately 3.5 million Americans are unable to read their mail, drive, sew, or travel independently because of vision loss (Faye, 1998). The three most common causes of this loss in the elderly population are macular degeneration, glaucoma, and cataracts (Weber & Eichenbaum, 1998). As a result, these people may not be able to see gestures, can be incapable of reading well, or may be unable to differentiate facial expressions. Vision loss can result in seeing images in a distorted manner or being incapable of reading signs. In addition, these individuals also may have difficulty identifying colors, especially in the blue/green and yellow/white tones (Faye). In children and teens, visual impairments occur at the rate of 12.2 per 1,000 (National Information Center for Children and Youth with Disabilities [NICHCY], 2000b). The effect on development is dependent on a number of factors, including the severity and type of loss, age of onset, and functional level of the child (NICHCY, 2000b). Some strategies that might improve outcomes in education of people with vision loss are listed in Table 24-3. Resources for those with vision loss are listed in Table 24-4.

Table 24-3. Strategies for Improving Outcomes in Educating Patients With Vision Impairment

Categories	Strategy
Visual aids	Ensure that eyeglasses are worn properly.
	Provide magnifying lenses.
	Provide large-print material.
Light	Position light to come from behind the patient.
	Use nonglare light.
	Allow extra time for eyes to focus during and after presentations.
	Use colored blanks during slide presentations instead of clear ones.
Color	Use black lettering on a white or off-white background.
	Avoid dark colors on dark backgrounds (e.g., black on gray).
	Avoid blues, greens, and violets.

Table 24-4. Resources for Those With Vision Impairment

Name of Resource	Address	Phone/Fax/Internet
American Academy of Ophthalmology	655 Beach St. P.O. Box 7424 San Francisco, CA 94120	415-561-8500 415-561-8533 (fax) www.eyenet.org
American Optometric Association	243 N. Lindbergh Blvd. St. Louis, MO 63141	314-991-4100, ext. 238 314-991-4101 (fax) www.aoanet.org
Lighthouse Inc.	Information and Resource Center 111 East 59th St. New York, NY 10022	800-829-0500, option 2 212-821-9705 (fax) www.lighthouse.org
National Eye Institute	2020 Vision Place Bethesda, MD 20892	301-496-5248 301-402-1065 (fax) http://nei.nih.gov
American Foundation for the Blind	11 Penn Plaza, Suite 300 New York, NY 10001	800-AFB-LIND afbinfo@afb.org (e-mail) www.afb.org
Blind Children's Center	4120 Marathon St. Los Angeles, CA 90029	800-222-3566 info@blindcntr.org (e-mail) www.blindchildrenscenter.org
National Association for Visually Handicapped	22 West 21st St. New York, NY 10010	212-889-3141 staff@navh.org (e-mail) www.navh.org
National Braille Association, Inc.	3 Townline Circle Rochester, NY 14623	716-427-8260 nbaoffice@compuserve.com (e-mail) www.members.aol.com/nbaoffice
National Library Service for the Blind and Physically Handicapped	1291 Taylor St. NW Washington, DC 20542	800-424-8567 nls@loc.gov (e-mail) www.loc.gov/nls

State organizations often provide tactile or Braille patient-education materials for the blind. If computers are being used to educate this population, Braille overlays are available. Braille printers are an effective tool to facilitate information sharing. The National Cancer Institute (1998) has some educational materials available in large-print format for the visually impaired.

Hearing Impairment

The hearing-impaired individual presents the nurse with another set of unique challenges. Hearing impairment in the aging population may be associated with the loss of the ability to discriminate among sounds or the inability to hear clearly. A decrease in the conduction of sound also may be present, along with a loss of auditory capacity in the high frequency ranges. In children, even a mild to moderate hearing loss can affect their speaking ability and understanding, which can impede development (NICHCY, 2000a). Many people are tempted to teach this population by shouting, assuming that a greater volume will overcome the deficits. This usually will not improve communication. In fact, it may further hinder communication because those being addressed may become upset because of the perception that they are being "yelled at."

Some strategies to improve outcomes for the individual with hearing loss are listed in Figure 24-3. Resources for those with hearing impairments are listed in Table 24-5. If the person is deaf, an interpreter will be needed. Family members or significant others may be available to assist in the educational process. In addition, many institutions have lists of people who know American Sign Language and are willing to act as interpreters. Interpreter referral services, which can be accessed on a fee-for-service basis, are available for the deaf through individual states.

Literacy Issues

According to the 1993 National Adult Literacy Survey (National Work Group on Literacy and Health, 1998), 44 million Americans function at the lowest level of literacy. Approximately one-quarter of the population of the United States cannot understand basic written materials, such as the instructions on medication bottles (National Work Group on Literacy and Health). In addition, individuals with low literacy skills have other problems, such as the perception of poor health.

Figure 24-3. Strategies for Educating the Hearing Impaired Individual

- Speak slowly and enunciate clearly.
- Face the learner to facilitate lip reading.
- Address the "good ear."
- Speak in the lower tonal frequencies because high frequencies are where the earliest losses usually occur.
- Ensure that the hearing aid is in place, if the patient uses one.
- Stay within four feet of the hearing-aided ear.
- Decrease extraneous noise.
- Use visual aids to supplement verbal presentations.
- Present the patient with printed materials to take home.
- Write key words/concepts to reinforce verbal communication.
- Do not yell.

Table 24-5. Resources for Those With Hearing Impairment

Name of Resource	Address	Phone/E-mail/Internet
Alexander Graham Bell Association for the Deaf	3417 Volta Place NW Washington, DC 20007	202-337-5220 agbell2@aol.com (e-mail) www.agbell.org
American Society for Deaf Children	P.O. Box 3355 Gettysburg, PA 17323	800-942-2723 asdcl@aol.com (e-mail) www.deafchildren.org
American Speech-Language Hearing Association	10801 Rockville Pike Rockville, MD 20852	800-638-8255 actioncenter@asha.org (e-mail) www.asha.org
Laurent Clere National Deaf Education Center and Clearinghouse	KDES PAS-6, Gallaudet University 800 Florida Ave. NE Washington, DC 20002	202-651-5052 ClearinghouseInfotogo@gallaudet.edu (e-mail) http://clerccenter.gallaudet.edu/infotogo
National Institute on Deafness and Other Communication Disorders Clearinghouse	1 Communication Ave. Bethesda, MD 20892	800-241-1044 nidcdinfo@nidcd.nih.gov (e-mail) www.nih.gov/nidcd
Self-Help for Hard of Hearing People	7910 Woodmont Ave., Suite 1200 Bethesda, MD 20814	301-657-2248 national@shhh.org (e-mail) www.shhh.org

They also consume the greatest volume of healthcare resources (Marwick, 1997; National Work Group on Literacy and Health).

The rationale behind this perception of poor health status has not been fully investigated, but several factors may be involved. These individuals may lack feelings of empowerment and have a general inability to navigate the complexities of the healthcare system. They may not understand prescription information or preprinted instructions and may be unable to perform self-care or health-maintenance activities. The inability to read printed material and the unwillingness to discuss the problem promotes the continuation of the vicious cycle that propagates poor health (Marwick, 1997; National Work Group on Literacy and Health, 1998).

An individual's reading level may be three to five years behind the actual grade level completed (Lee, 1999). Lee indicated that literacy actually is not related to intelligence, as measured by IQ testing, but is correlated to reading ability, comprehension, and the ability to organize information. Individuals who have low literacy levels also tend to think less abstractly than those with better reading ability, which may require nurses to focus on essential skills and decrease the use of abstract terminology (Barnes, 1992).

Empowering people through education can result in the improvement of patient self-care and their ability to navigate the healthcare system (Marwick, 1997). Davison and Degner (1997) explored ways of empowering men who were newly diagnosed with prostate cancer. Patients received an information packet after a discussion of the type of information the men felt that they needed to make treatment decisions. The men also were encouraged to tape their consultation for review at a later date because not all of the information is retained. The results demonstrated that the men who received information about treatment options were more active participants in their treatment decisions and experienced less anxiety.

JCAHO has mandated that patients be provided with education at a literacy level that they can understand. This information must be geared specifically to the individual's educational needs, abilities, and readiness to learn. JCAHO also has specified that patients' understanding of the information must be assessed to ensure that learning has occurred. This becomes a challenge when dealing with low literacy. Today's time constraints force nurses to rely more heavily on printed patient-education materials and videos as a means of supplementing verbal instructions (Revell, 1994). Matching the reading levels of the educational materials to the population is exceedingly difficult because so few printed materials are available for those individuals at the lowest literacy levels. Although approximately one-quarter of the population functions at the lowest literacy level, many others within the United States have difficulty understanding current healthcare literature.

The average reading ability of the U.S. adult population is at the eighth- to ninth-grade level (Meade, Diekmann, & Thornhill, 1992; Revell, 1994; National Work Group on Literacy and Health, 1998). Approximately 50% of the population reads at a ninth-grade level or less; of that group, 18% have reading skills below the fifth-grade level. Yet, American Cancer Society literature is written at a 12th-grade reading level, and information published by the National Cancer Institute is written at a 10th-grade level (Meade et al). This represents a discrepancy of one to four grade levels between the reading comprehension skills of the average adult and current printed healthcare materials. Another report identified that the readability scores of a variety of materials used in a health department, community health center, and home healthcare agency were averaged out to a ninth-grade level, with a range of fifth-grade to postgraduate levels (Wilson, 1995). The readability of materials on the prevention, early detection, and treatment of breast cancer reviewed by Glazer, Kirk, and Bosler (1996) had an average level of 9.15, requiring a reading and comprehension level of at least the ninth grade. The mismatch between these materials and the general population's reading level raises challenges for nurses who educate patients about cancer prevention and early detection. Nurses must be aware of the target population's abilities, and materials need to be reviewed and evaluated to ensure appropriateness for the learner. Table 24-6 lists a comparison of some reading and comprehension tests.

Identifying People With Low Literacy Skills

Individuals with the lowest levels of literacy usually will not tell others that they cannot read. In fact, many individuals who have difficulty reading never share this information with their spouses or children. Parikh, Parker, Nurss, Baker, and Williams (1996) reported that people with low literacy levels have the additional barriers of shame and embarrassment, which block their ability to receive assistance. Patients will attempt to hide their problems at the cost of not seeking health

Table 24-6. Reading Level and Comprehension Tests

Test	Description	Pros	Cons	Source
Wide Range Achievement Test (WRAT)	Subject reads a list of words ranging from simple to complex. Score is based on the number of words pronounced correctly.	• Excellent validity • Excellent reliability	• Not applicable for non-English-speaking people • Does not measure comprehension	Wilson, 1995
CLOZE Technique	Measures comprehension	• Reliable • Valid	• Not applicable for non-English-speaking people • Unusable below a sixth-grade reading level	Wilson, 1995
Rapid Estimate of Adult Literacy in Medicine	Once patients are unable to pronounce several consecutive words, they only say as many of the words as they are able.	• Excellent reliability • Excellent validity • Easily administered • Administered and scored within two to three minutes • Emphasis on medical terminology	• Provides only range estimation of grade level • Not applicable for non-English-speaking people • Does not measure comprehension	Davis et al., 1998
WRAT-3	Essentially the same as WRAT	• Excellent reliability • Excellent validity • Can be administered and scored in three to five minutes • Spanish version available	• Poor readers must struggle until they mispronounce 10 consecutive words. • Does not measure comprehension	Davis et al., 1998
Test of Fundamental Health Literacy in Adults (TOFHLA)	Measures comprehension	• Excellent validity/reliability • Spanish version available (TOFHLA-S) • Measures functional literacy	• Requires 22–30 minutes to administer and evaluate	Parker et al., 1995
SMOG Grading	Measures readability	• Excellent validity • Excellent reliability	• Measures readability	McLaughlin, 1969
Flesh-Kincaid	Microsoft® Word spell check	• Excellent validity/reliability • Usable with various languages		

care or will delay requesting assistance. Low-literacy individuals will find numerous excuses to avoid reading. Some of these include "I forgot my glasses," " I don't want to take the time to read this now; I'll read it later when I get home," "I'll let my family read this to me," or " I'll take this home and let my husband/wife read it first" (Doak, Doak, & Root, 1996; Mayer, 1999; National Work Group on Literacy and Health, 1998; Revell, 1994).

Changes are needed within the healthcare system, through sensitization and education, so that low-literacy individuals can have access to the system without stigmatization (Parikh et al., 1996). Nurses should be able to identify individuals with low literacy skills so that they can be taught effectively.

Assessment for low literacy. Davis, Michiellutta, Ashkov, Williams, and Weiss (1998) noted that adverse effects would be observed if people did not understand the information they were given by the healthcare team. The authors recognized that assessment of literacy levels could provide useful information regarding people's reading ability in the healthcare setting. Doak, Doak, and Root (1996) suggested that literacy testing be performed on each individual to overcome the differences between readability levels and the printed material; this testing would achieve compliance with JCAHO standards. Verifying the understanding of the educational information is important. Davis et al. recommended that people with low literacy skills be identified to provide them with learning experiences that are appropriate to their skill level. To identify these individuals, some type of testing must be performed. Nursing staff within individual practices could perform literacy testing using the Wide Range Achievement Test-3 (WRAT-3) or the Rapid Estimate of Adult Literacy in Medicine. Davis et al. identified two methods for assessing reading skills. One is "aggregate testing," which is the random testing of individuals within the population to provide an average reading level for the population. The other is "individual testing," which can be used alone or in addition to aggregate testing.

Issues identified in conjunction with both types of testing include sensitivity to patient concerns and potential to embarrass people. All test results must be kept confidential because of potential employment problems. A convenient time for both the nurse and patient should be agreed upon. In addition, a private area in which to administer the test and the competency of the individual to accurately administer and score the test must be ensured. Language barriers may limit the use of available testing methods, requiring efforts to secure an interpreter.

In addition to testing for literacy (i.e., actual reading ability), one must ensure comprehension. Wilson (1995) administered the WRAT for reading level, followed by the CLOZE technique for comprehension. A mean of the patients in the study reported completing the 12th grade, with a mean actual reading ability below the eighth-grade level, a variance of four grade levels, and a comprehension level of 58 on CLOZE. In this study, 52% of patients required further directions after reading the printed matter. Thus, nurses cannot merely ask patients what grade level they completed or perform literacy testing. They must ensure comprehension of patient-education materials to improve patient compliance. An easy method of testing understanding is through informal assessment. Patients are asked open-ended questions regarding the material presented to ascertain if they understand what they have read. Patients also may be asked to read a prescription label out loud. Testing must be performed to ensure the ability to read and comprehend printed materials.

Although Brez and Taylor (1997) found that a number of challenges exist in testing people with low literacy skills, particularly regarding disclosure of illiteracy, the hospital was perceived as an area of low threat for people and a place where the secret of illiteracy could be shared safely. Patients may feel more at ease accepting materials at a lower reading level, benefit from them, and not be upset by their simplicity (Mayeaux et al., 1996). The strategies that are used to improve understanding of patients with low literacy abilities also facilitate comprehension in highly literate patients (Doak, Doak, Friedell, & Meade, 1998). Therefore, it is beneficial to have available materials written at a fifth- or sixth-grade reading level and then provide more technical materials if the individual desires.

Strategies for Educating the Low-Literacy Population

Mayeaux et al. (1996) and Doak, Doak, and Root (1996) based the use of adult learning theory in educating patients on research. Patients must find the information to be relevant and recognize the need for this material. Figure 24-4 lists strategies for educating the low-literacy population.

Figure 24-5 identifies salient issues in the development of educational materials. Other suggestions for enhancing patient education include use of audiotapes, videotapes, and interactive multimedia. Whichever method or methods are chosen, nurses must keep in mind that education is a vital part of empowering patients of all literacy levels to become active participants in their health care and health-promotion practices.

Figure 24-4. Strategies for Educating the Low-Literacy Population

- Include adults in planning their educational programs to increase compliance.
- Build upon the previous experiences of the adult learner.
- Ask people what they know and begin the instruction from that point.
- Use examples to demonstrate how the actions taken will be beneficial.
- Use feedback to ascertain understanding.
- Educate family groups and friends simultaneously to increase understanding and facilitate supportive relationships, because people in lower literacy groups frequently turn first to family and friends for health information (Macario et al., 1998).
- Use a combination of methods to provide effective education.
- Use videos and simple printed materials to supplement/complement verbal communication but not to replace it.
- Use written material that is short and simple with colorful illustrations.
- Use vocabulary lists, flash cards, diagrams, and posters to supplement education.

Conclusion

Nurses can have a positive impact on cancer prevention and early detection through increased effectiveness as educators. The multiple challenges and special

Figure 24-5. Salient Issues in the Development of Educational Material

- Plan objectives and be an active writer.
- Use common terminology and short sentences.
- Give examples to explain complex terminology.
- Include questions to ascertain comprehension.
- Increase readability through the use of serif type and 12-point fonts.
- Have adequate white space, otherwise the page appears overwhelming.
- Pictures are important, as many individuals are visual learners.
- Visual clues can enhance learning for every level.
- Do not use all capital lettering, as it is difficult to read.

needs of diverse populations must be met with educational competence. As nurses become more sensitive to patient-education issues, the effectiveness and efficiency of their efforts continually will improve. Nurses then can guide consumers through the explosion of information resources and lead them to informed choices. Effective patient education increases active participation in health care, consumer satisfaction, and health outcomes.

References

Adler, E. (1991). *Print that works: The first step-by-step guide that integrates writing, design, and marketing*. Palo Alto, CA: Bull Publishing Company.

Ames, J.E. (1997). *Mastery: Interviews with 30 remarkable people*. Portland, OR: Rudra Press.

Barg, F., & Lowe, J. (1996). A culturally appropriate cancer education program for African-American adolescents in an urban middle school. *Journal of School Health, 66*, 50–55.

Barnes L.P. (1992). The illiterate client: Strategies in patient teaching. *Maternal Child Nursing, 17*, 127.

Be leery of legal issues when using Internet information. (1996). *Patient Education Management, 3*(11), 122–124.

Behan, B.A., & Reynolds, A. (1992). *Readability of breast self-exam literature*. Retrieved December 29, 1999 from the World Wide Web: www.infotrac.galegroup.com

Berliner, H. (1998). Information management. Key punch. *Health Service Journal, 108*, 24.

Boston, P. (1993). Culture and cancer: The relevance of cultural orientation within cancer education programs. *European Journal of Cancer Care, 2*(2), 72–76.

Brant, J., Ishida, D., Itano, J., Kagawa-Singer, M., Palos, G., Phillips, J., Tejada-Reyes, I., Suhayda, L., Iwamoto, R., & Weekes, D. (1999). *Oncology Nursing Society multicultural outcomes: Guidelines for cultural competence*. Pittsburgh: Oncology Nursing Press, Inc.

Breen, N., & Figueroa, J.B. (1996). Stages of breast and cervical cancer diagnosis in disadvantaged neighborhoods: A prevention policy perspective. *American Journal of Preventive Medicine, 12*, 319–326.

Brez, S.M., & Taylor, M. (1997). Assessing literacy for patient teaching: Perspectives of adults with low literacy skills. *Journal of Advanced Nursing, 25*, 1040–1047.

Chen, A., Wismer, B., Lew, R., & Kang, S. (1997). "Health is strength": A research collaboration involving Korean Americans in Alameda county. *American Journal of Preventive Medicine, 13*(Suppl. 6), 93–100.

Choudhry, U.K., Sirvastava, R., & Fitch, M. (1998). Breast cancer detection practices of South Asian women: Knowledge, attitude, and beliefs. *Oncology Nursing Forum, 25,* 1693–1701.

Clark, P. (1999). How can we coach patients to become critical consumers of information they find on the Internet. *ONS News, 14,* 8.

Cormier, A. (1997). Patients can benefit from information on Internet resources. *Oncology Nursing Forum, 24,* 458.

Davis, T.C., Michiellutta, R., Ashkov, E.N., Williams, M.V., & Weiss, B.D. (1998). Practical assessment of adult literacy in health care. *Health Education and Behavior, 25,* 613–624.

Davison, J., & Degner, L.F. (1997). Empowerment of men newly diagnosed with prostate cancer. *Cancer Nursing, 20,* 187–196.

Doak, C.C., Doak, L.G., Friedell, G.H., & Meade, C.D. (1998). Improving comprehension for cancer patients with low literacy skills: Strategies for clinicians. *CA: A Cancer Journal for Clinicians, 48,* 151–162.

Doak, C.C., Doak, L.G., & Root, J.H. (1996). *Teaching patients with low literacy skills* (2nd ed.). Philadelphia: Lippincott.

Doak, L.G., Doak, C.C., & Meade, C.D. (1996). Strategies to improve cancer education materials. *Oncology Nursing Forum, 23,* 1305–1311.

Eddleman, J., & Warren, C. (1994). Cancer resource center: A setting for patient empowerment. *Cancer Practice, 2,* 371–378.

Eyre, H., & Feldman, G. (1998). Status report on prostate cancer in African Americans: A national blueprint for action. *CA: A Cancer Journal for Clinicians, 48,* 315–319.

Falvo, D.R. (1999). *Effective patient education: A guide to increased compliance.* Gaithersburg, MD: Aspen Publications.

Faye, E.E. (1998). Living with low vision. What you can do to help patients cope. *Postgraduate Medicine, 103,* 167–178.

Fernsler, J., & Cannon, C. (1991). The whys of patient education. *Seminars in Oncology Nursing, 7,* 79–86.

Foley, R.M., & Pollard, C.M. (1998). Food cent$—Implementing and evaluating a nutrition education project focusing on value for money. *Public Health, 22,* 494–501.

Foltz, A., & Sullivan, J. (1998). Get real: Clinical testing of patients' reading abilities. *Cancer Nursing, 21,* 162–166.

Fortin, F. (1998). Internet medicine: From chat room to waiting room. *Professional Medical Assistant, 31*(1), 18–20.

Giordano, B. (1996). Ensuring the readability of patient education materials is one way to demonstrate perioperative nurses' value. *Association of Operating Room Nurses Journal, 63,* 699–700.

Glazer, H.R., Kirk, L.M., & Bosler, F.E. (1996). Patient education pamphlets about prevention, detection, and treatment of breast cancer for low literacy women. *Patient Education and Counseling, 27,* 185–189.

Green, L.W., Kreuter, M.W., Deeds, M.W., & Patridge, K.B. (1980). *Health education planning. A diagnostic approach.* Palo Alto, CA: Mayfield Publishing.

Guidry, J., & Walker, V. (1999). Assessing cultural sensitivity in printed cancer materials. *Cancer Practice, 7,* 291–296.

Health on the Net Foundation. (1997). *Call for standards for Internet health information.* Retrieved December 10, 1999 from the World Wide Web: http://www.ktv-i.com/news/nn04_17_97c.html

Hiam, A. (1997). *Marketing for dummies.* Foster City, CA: IDG Books Worldwide.

Hochbaum, G.T. (1958). *Public participation in medical screening programs.* Washington, DC: Government Printing Office.

Hussey, L.C. (1997). Strategies for effective patient education material design. *Journal of Cardiovascular Nursing, 11,* 37–47.

Internet health seekers reach critical mass. (1998). Retrieved December 10, 1999 from the World Wide Web: http://www.cyberdiologue.com/press/releases/intel_health_day.html

JAMA patient page: Health and the Internet. (1998). *JAMA, 280,* 1380.

Jennings, B., Staggers, N., & Brosch, L. (1999). A classification scheme for outcome indicators. *Image: Journal of Nursing Scholarship, 31,* 381–388.

Joint Commission on Accreditation of Healthcare Organizations. (1997). *Accreditation manual for hospitals.* Oakbrook Terrace, IL: Department of Publications.

Kagawa-Singer, M. (1997). Addressing issues for early detection and screening in ethnic populations. *Oncology Nursing Forum, 24,* 1705–1711.

Kerner, J.F. (1996). Breast cancer prevention and control among the medically underserved. *Breast Cancer Research and Treatment, 40,* 1–9.

Kim, K., Yu, E.S.H., Chen, E.H., Kim, J., Kaufman, M., & Purkiss, J. (1999). Cervical cancer screening knowledge and practices among Korean-American women. *Cancer Nursing, 22,* 297–302.

Kim, P., Eng, T., Deering, M., & Maxfield, A. (1999). Published criteria for evaluating health-related Web sites: Review. *BMJ, 318,* 647–649.

Knowles, M. (1970). *The modern practice of adult education.* New York: Association Press.

Kotecki, J., & Chamness, B. (1999). A valid tool for evaluating health-related WWW sites. *Journal of Health Education, 30,* 56.

Lee, P.P. (1999). Why literacy matters. Links between reading ability and health. *Archives of Ophthalmology, 117,* 100–103.

Lorig, K. (1996). *Patient education: A practical approach.* Thousand Oaks, CA: SAGE Publications.

Lumsdon, K. (1994). Getting real: Study finds success factors in patient education. *Hospitals and Health Networks, 68,* 62.

Macario, E., Emmons, K., Sorensen, G., Hunt, M., & Rudd, R. (1998). Factors influencing nutrition education for patients with low literacy skills. *Journal of the American Dietetic Association, 98,* 559–564.

Marwick, C. (1997). Patients' lack of literacy may contribute to billions of dollars in higher hospital costs. *JAMA, 278,* 971–972.

Mayeaux, E.J., Murphy, P.W., Arnold, C., Davis, T.C., Jackson, R.H., & Sentell, T. (1996). Improving patient education for patients with low literacy skills. *American Family Physician, 53,* 205–211.

Mayer, D.K. (1999). Cancer patient empowerment. *Oncology Nursing Updates, 6*(1), 1–9.

McLaughlin, G.H. (1969). SMOG grading—A new readability formula. *Journal of Reading, 5,* 639–646.

Meade, C.D., Diekmann, J., & Thornhill, D.G. (1992). Readability of American Cancer Society patient education literature. *Oncology Nursing Forum, 19,* 51–55.

Meissner, H., Potosky, A., & Convissor, R. (1992). How sources of health information relate to knowledge and use of cancer screening exams. *Journal of Community Health, 17,* 153–165.

Merriam-Webster's Collegiate Dictionary. (1996). *Education.* Boston: Merriam-Webster Inc.

National Cancer Institute. (1998). *Publications catalogue.* Baltimore: Author.

National Information Center for Children and Youth with Disabilities. (2000a). *General information about deafness and hearing loss.* Washington, DC: Author.

National Information Center for Children and Youth with Disabilities. (2000b). *General information about visual impairments.* Washington, DC: Author.

National Work Group on Literacy and Health. (1998). Communicating with patients who have limited literacy skills. *Journal of Family Practice, 46,* 168–176.

Nelson, D., Giovino, G., Shopland, D., Mowery, P., Mills, S., & Eriksen, M. (1995). Trends in cigarette smoking among U.S. adolescents, 1974–1991. *American Journal of Public Health, 85,* 34–40.

Nichols, B.S., Misra, R., & Alexy, B. (1996). Cancer detection: How effective is public education? *Cancer Nursing, 19,* 98–103.

Nielsen. (2001). *May Internet universe.* Retrieved June 18, 2001 from the World Wide Web: http://www.nielsennetratings.com

O'Hare, P., Yost, L., & McCorkle, R. (1993). Strategies to improve continuity of care and decrease rehospitalization of cancer patients: A review. *Cancer Investigation, 11,* 140–158.

O'Malley, A.S., Mandelblatt, J., Gold, K., Cagney, K.A., & Kerner, J. (1997). Continuity of care and the use of breast and cervical cancer screening services in a multiethnic community. *Archives of Internal Medicine, 157,* 1462–1470.

Parikh, N.S., Parker, R.M., Nurss, J.R., Baker, D.W., & Williams, M.V. (1996). Shame and health literacy: The unspoken connection. *Patient Education and Counseling, 27,* 33–39.

Parker, R.M., Baker, D.W., Williams, M.V., & Nurss, J.R. (1995). The test of functional healthcare literacy in adults: A new instrument for measuring patients' literacy skills. *Journal of General Internal Medicine, 10,* 537–541.

Rankin, S.A., & Stallings, K.D. (1996). *Patient education: Issues, principles, and practice* (3rd ed.). Philadelphia: Lippincott.

Redman, B. (1997). *The practice of patient education* (8th ed.). St. Louis, MO: Mosby.

Reiley, P., Pike, A., Phipps, M., Weiner, M., Miller, N., Stengrevics, S., Clark, L., & Wandel, J. (1996). Learning from patients: A discharge planning improvement project. *Journal on Quality Improvement, 22,* 311–322.

Rettig, J. (1995). *Putting the squeeze on the information fire hose: The need for "neteditors" and "netreviewers."* Retrieved December 10, 1999 from the World Wide Web: http://www.swem.wm.edu/firehose.html

Revell, L. (1994). Understanding, identifying, and teaching the low literacy patient. *Seminars in Perioperative Nursing, 3*(3), 168–171.

Sadler, G.R., Nguyen, F., Doan, Q., Au, H., & Thomas, A.G. (1998). Strategies for reaching Asian Americans with health information. *American Journal of Preventive Medicine, 14,* 224–228.

Seffrin, J.R. (2000). An endgame for cancer. *CA: A Cancer Journal for Clinicians, 50,* 4–5.

Strike it rich: Internet wealth of information. (1998). *Patient Education Management, 5*(6), 73–75, 83.

Thompson, R., & Thiemann, K.B. (1999). Importance of format and design in print patient information. *Cancer Practice, 7,* 22–27.

Underwood, S.M., Shaikha, L., & Bakr, D. (1999). Veiled yet vulnerable: Breast cancer screening and the Muslim way of life. *Cancer Practice, 7*, 285–290.

Villejo, L. (1993). Designing patient education programs for target populations. In B. Giloth (Ed.), *Managing hospital-based patient education* (pp. 357–378). Chicago: American Hospital Publishing Inc.

Weber, C.M., & Eichenbaum, J.W. (1998). Failing vision. A four article symposium. *Postgraduate Medicine, 103*, 113.

Wilson, F.L. (1995). Measuring patients' ability to read and comprehend: A first step in patient education. *Nursing Connections, 8*, 17–25.

Wilson, F.L. (1996). Patient education materials nurses use in community health. *Western Journal of Nursing Research, 18*, 195–206.

Wilson, F.L. (2000). Are patient information materials too difficult to read? *Home Healthcare Nurse, 18*, 107–115.

Woo, B. (1995). The Cantonese women's support group. *Oncology Nursing Forum, 22*, 374.

Woo, B. (2000). Article examines common health beliefs and practices of Chinese Americans. *Oncology Nursing Society Patient Education Special Interest Group Newsletter, 11*, 1.

CHAPTER 25

Information Resources for Patients and Families

Terri B. Ades, MS, APRN-BC, AOCN®

This chapter presents resources about the following topics:
- General cancer information—see page 1002
- Breast cancer—see page 1004
- Gastrointestinal cancer and liver cancer—see page 1006
- Gynecology and women's health—see page 1007
- Kidney cancer—see page 1009
- Lung cancer and tobacco use—see page 1009
- Oral cancer, head and heck cancer—see page 1011
- Prostate cancer—see page 1012
- Skin cancer—see page 1013
- Clinical trials cooperative groups—see page 1014
- Complementary and alternative medicine—see page 1017
- Cancer genetics and hereditary cancers—see page 1017
- Environmental health and consumer safety—see page 1018
- Nutrition—see page 1021
- Groups comprising physicians or cancer centers—see page 1022
- Cancer centers designated by the National Cancer Institute—see page 1024

Every day, thousands of people who are concerned about cancer seek information from call centers and the Internet. Some of these people are concerned about how to prevent cancer, and those with cancer seek information about treatment, what to expect, and how to live with their disease. Many questions pose difficult challenges for the information provider: Do antiperspirants cause breast cancer? I heard that tampons have asbestos in them—is this true? The answers are out there. The resources in this chapter can help you find them.

This chapter presents listings for many organizations that provide information and resources to those concerned about cancer prevention and control. The listings are adapted from information compiled by the American Cancer Society (ACS). ACS updates this information continually and makes the revised listings available to the public in the form of an information database. This information is available by calling ACS's toll-free number, 800-ACS-2345, or by e-mailing ACS through its Web site, www.cancer.org.

General Cancer Information

American Cancer Society
1599 Clifton Road NE
Atlanta, GA 30329
toll-free telephone: 800-227-2345 (seven days a week, 24 hours each day)
www.cancer.org

ACS is a nationwide community-based health organization dedicated to eliminating cancer as a major health problem by preventing cancer, saving lives, and diminishing the suffering caused by cancer. ACS seeks to attain its goals through research, education, advocacy, and service. The society comprises state divisions and more than 3,400 local units. ACS is the largest source of private, nonprofit cancer research funds in the United States. The society's prevention programs focus on tobacco control, sun protection, diet and nutrition, comprehensive school health education, early detection, and treatment. A variety of service and rehabilitation programs are available to patients and their families. Through its advocacy program, ACS educates policy makers about cancer and how it affects the individuals and families they represent.

Cancer Research Institute
681 Fifth Ave.
New York, NY 10022-4209
telephones: 212-688-7515; toll-free, 800-992-2623
fax: 212-832-9376
www.cancerresearch.org
Monday through Friday, 9 am–5 pm ET

The Cancer Research Institute (CRI) supports research aimed at developing new immunologic methods of diagnosing, treating, and preventing cancer. CRI provides
- *The CRI Help Book: What to Do If Cancer Strikes*, a reference guide and resource directory with information about various support services and financial considerations
- *What to Do If Prostate Cancer Strikes* and *Conquering Melanoma*, booklets discussing treatment options for prostate cancer and melanoma
- Answers to questions about cancer immunology
- Assistance in locating clinical trials studying immunotherapy.

Centers for Disease Control and Prevention

1600 Clifton Road NE
Atlanta, GA 30333
telephones: 404-639-3534; toll-free, 800-311-3435
www.cdc.gov
Monday through Friday, 8 am–4:30 pm ET
Spanish-speaking staff; Spanish-language materials available

The Centers for Disease Control and Prevention (CDC) is an agency of the U.S. Department of Health and Human Services. The CDC's mission is to promote health and quality of life by preventing and controlling disease, injury, and disability. The CDC provides information about many chronic health problems, including cancer, and information about related topics such as genetics and exposure to radiation.

The CDC Web site includes an online database of health topics and access to publications, products, and software for healthcare professionals and the public. These items can be ordered or downloaded. The site provides links to all centers and offices of the CDC.

National Cancer Institute

NCI Public Inquiries Office
Building 31, Room 10A31
31 Center Drive, MSC 2580
Bethesda, MD 20892-2580
telephones: 301-435-3848; toll-free, 800-422-6237 (answers as "Cancer Information Service")
TTY: 800-332-8615
fax: 301-402-5874 (To obtain a list of the information available by fax, dial the fax number from a fax machine and use the machine's handset to hear recorded instructions.)
www.nci.nih.gov
Monday through Friday, 9 am–4:30 pm ET
Spanish-speaking staff; Spanish-language materials available

The Cancer Information Service, the telephone service of the National Cancer Institute (NCI), provides accurate, up-to-date information about cancer to patients and their families, healthcare professionals, and the general public. NCI's Web site, called CancerNet, presents materials for healthcare professionals, patients, and the public. Cancerlit, a part of the site, is a bibliographic database. The site provides access to PDQ (Physician's Data Query), a database that allows the user to enter queries about cancer treatment, screening, prevention, supportive care, and clinical trials. See the NCI site at http://cancertrials.nci.nih.gov for information about participating in clinical trials and news about breakthroughs in research. NCI also makes information available via e-mail, through its CancerMail service. To obtain a list of materials available via e-mail, send an e-mail message to cancermail@icicc.nci.nih.gov. Type the word "Help" in the subject line of the message and, in the body, ask for a contents list.

Oncology Nursing Society
501 Holiday Drive
Pittsburgh, PA 15220-2749
telephone: 412-921-7373
fax: 412-921-6565
www.ons.org
Monday through Friday, 8:30 am–5 pm ET

The Oncology Nursing Society (ONS) is a national membership organization devoted to promoting excellence in oncology nursing. Nonmembers can access the ONS Web site to find information about cancer prevention, detection, screening, diagnosis, and treatment; survivorship; and end-of-life issues. Through ONS, oncology nurses can learn about continuing education and certification opportunities.

Breast Cancer

Encore^plus Program of the YWCA
Office of Women's Health Advocacy
1015 18th St. NW, Suite 700
Washington, DC 20036
telephones: 202-467-0801; toll-free, 800-953-7587
fax: 202-467-0802
www.ywca.org/html/B4d1.asp
Monday through Friday, 9 am–5 pm ET

Encore^plus is a national system of health promotion that works through education, clinical service delivery, and advocacy. The community-based program helps medically underserved women who need early-detection education, breast and cervical cancer screening, and support services. To women who are receiving treatment and recovering from breast cancer, Encore^plus offers a unique program that combines peer-group support and exercise.

Susan G. Komen Breast Cancer Foundation
5005 LBJ Freeway, Suite 250
Dallas, TX 75244
telephones: 972-855-1600; toll-free, 800-462-9273
fax: 972-855-1605
toll-free order line: 877-745-7467 (to order materials)
www.breastcancerinfo.com
Monday through Friday, 9 am–4:30 pm CT
Spanish-language materials available

The Susan G. Komen Breast Cancer Foundation is a nonprofit organization dedicated to eradicating breast cancer as a life-threatening disease by advancing research, education, screening, and treatment. The foundation offers the Breast Care Helpline telephone service, through which trained volunteers provide information about breast cancer, breast health, and local support services. The foundation also offers printed materials and referral to local support groups. The Web site includes a news section that features current developments regarding breast cancer, online discussion forums, a calendar of foundation events, and an interactive breast health quiz. The foundation organizes the Race for the Cure and Lee National Denim Day.

National Alliance of Breast Cancer Organizations

9 East 37th St., 10th Floor
New York, NY 10016
telephones: 212-889-0606; toll-free, 888-806-2226 (voice mail with daytime callbacks; 24-hour voice mail)
fax: 212-689-1213
www.nabco.org
Monday through Friday, 9:30 am–5:30 pm ET

The National Alliance of Breast Cancer Organizations (NABCO) provides information and assistance to anyone with questions about breast cancer and acts as a voice for breast cancer survivors and women at risk. NABCO provides printed materials about breast cancer; referral to support groups; and a publication, *The NABCO Breast Cancer Resource List* ($3). The NABCO Web site includes
- Information about breast cancer and breast health
- A calendar of events across the United States that are related to breast cancer
- A text version of *The NABCO Breast Cancer Resource List*
- A list of local breast cancer support groups
- A list of clinical trials related to breast cancer.

National Breast Cancer Coalition

1707 L St. NW, Suite 1060
Washington, DC 20036
telephones: 202-296-7477; toll-free, 800-622-2838
fax: 202-265-6854
www.stopbreastcancer.org
Monday through Friday, 9 am–5:30 pm ET

The National Breast Cancer Coalition (NBCC) is a grassroots membership organization whose mission is to eradicate breast cancer through action and advocacy. Founded in 1991, NBCC comprises more than 300 member organizations.

Y-ME National Breast Cancer Organization

212 W. Van Buren St., Suite 500
Chicago, IL 60607-3908
telephones: 312-986-8338; toll-free, 800-221-2141 (support line, English), 800-986-9505 (support line, Spanish)

fax: 312-294-8597
www.y-me.org
24-hour Y-ME National Breast Cancer Hot Line
Spanish-speaking staff; Spanish-language materials available

Y-ME is a nonprofit organization serving men and women with breast cancer, as well as their families and friends. Y-ME includes chapters throughout the United States. Y-ME materials and services include
- A national hot line staffed by trained peer counselors who are breast cancer survivors (male and female)
- Materials about breast health (including fibrocystic breast changes) and breast cancer
- Monthly educational and support meetings throughout the United States
- Information about comprehensive breast care centers and treatment and research hospitals
- Referral to support groups nationwide
- Wig and prosthesis banks.

The Y-ME Web site includes information about all the services the organization provides, general information about breast cancer and breast health, a way to send questions by e-mail, a list of Y-ME chapters, and a list of publications with an electronic order form for ordering them.

Gastrointestinal Cancer and Liver Cancer

American Gastroenterological Association
7910 Woodmont Ave., Suite 700
Bethesda, MD 20814
telephone: 301-654-2055
fax: 301-654-5920
www.gastro.org
Monday through Friday, 8:30 am–5 pm ET
Spanish-speaking staff; Spanish-language materials available

The American Gastroenterological Association (AGA) is a nonprofit specialty medical society. AGA—along with the American Society for Gastrointestinal Endoscopy and the American Association for the Study of Liver Diseases—is a partner in the American Digestive Health Foundation, which supports research and education regarding digestive diseases.

The AGA publishes wellness brochures, which cover topics such as heartburn, cirrhosis of the liver, pancreatitis, gallstones, colorectal cancer screening, inflammatory bowel disease, irritable bowel syndrome, and hemorrhoids. The association also publishes a bimonthly digestive health and nutrition magazine.

The AGA Web site provides an online resource center that focuses on digestive disorders and a directory of gastroenterologists who are members of the association.

American Liver Foundation
75 Maiden Lane, Suite 603
New York, NY 10038
telephones: 973-256-2550; toll-free, 800-465-4837 or 800-223-0179
fax: 973-256-3214
www.liverfoundation.org
Monday through Thursday, 9 am–7 pm ET; Friday, 9 am–6 pm ET
Spanish-speaking staff; Spanish-language materials available

The American Liver Foundation (ALF) is a nonprofit health agency dedicated to preventing, treating, and curing hepatitis and all liver diseases through research, education, and support. ALF provides information about liver diseases and conditions that can lead to liver disease, and it provides referrals to local chapters and support groups. The foundation offers information about raising funds for liver transplantation. *Note:* ALF has very limited information about primary liver cancer. The foundation does not provide information about cancer that has metastasized to the liver.

Gynecology and Women's Health

American College of Obstetricians & Gynecologists
409 12th St. SW
P.O. Box 96920
Washington, DC 20090-6920
telephones: 202-638-5577, 202-863-2518 (Resource Center)
fax: 202-484-5107
www.acog.org
Monday through Friday, 9 am–9 pm ET
Spanish-speaking staff; Spanish-language materials available

The American College of Obstetricians & Gynecologists (ACOG) is a nonprofit organization that advocates for quality health care for women; promotes patient education and patient understanding of, and involvement in, medical care; increases awareness among its members and the public of the changing issues facing women's health care; and maintains standards of clinical practice and continuing education for its members. Through the ACOG Resource Center, the college provides brochures for patients about gynecologic topics, including cancer. The center also offers a list of members that is categorized by location. The ACOG Web site provides a member physician directory and online gynecologic wellness information.

Gynecologic Cancer Foundation
401 N. Michigan Ave.
Chicago, IL 60611
telephones: 312-644-6610; toll-free 800-444-4441 (referral directory)

fax: 312-527-6640
www.wcn.org/gcf
Monday through Friday, 8:30 am–5 pm CT

The Gynecologic Cancer Foundation (GCF) was established by the Society of Gynecologic Oncologists as a nonprofit charitable organization to support philanthropic programs benefiting women who have gynecologic cancer or who are at risk for developing it. GCF's automated information line allows a caller to request a booklet on maintaining gynecologic health, a list of local gynecologic oncologists, or a directory of all GCF members practicing in the United States. GCF maintains the Woman's Cancer Network, an interactive Web site that includes an interactive gynecologic cancer risk survey and a gynecologic oncologist locator.

National Ovarian Cancer Coalition

500 NE Spanish River Blvd., Suite 14
Boca Raton, FL 33431
telephones: 561-393-0005; toll-free, 888-682-7426 (to order materials)
fax: 561-393-7275
www.ovarian.org
Monday through Friday, 9 am–2 pm ET

National Ovarian Cancer Coalition (NOCC) is a nonprofit organization founded by ovarian cancer survivors. Their mission is to raise awareness about ovarian cancer and to promote education about this disease. NOCC provides general information and materials about ovarian cancer, a list of gynecologic oncologists, and a network of people who have been affected by ovarian cancer. In addition, NOCC publishes a newsletter. The Web site offers a frequently-asked-questions section, a gynecologic oncologist locator, and an NOCC chapter locator.

National Women's Health Information Center

8550 Arlington Blvd., Suite 300
Fairfax, VA 22031
toll-free telephone: 800-994-9662
fax: 703-560-6598
www.4woman.org
Monday through Friday, 9 am–6 pm ET
Spanish-speaking staff; Spanish-language materials available

The National Women's Health Information Center (NWHIC) is a federally funded women's health information and referral service. The center is staffed by information specialists who answer questions, identify appropriate federal and private sector referral organizations, and order selected materials for callers. The NWHIC Web site contains links to an exceptionally wide variety of information about women's health, including dictionaries, glossaries, journals, and links to other organizations. The site also includes links to information about minority health and information written in Spanish as well as English.

Gilda Radner Familial Ovarian Cancer Registry

Roswell Park Cancer Institute
Elm and Carlton Streets
Buffalo, NY 14263-0001
telephones: 716-845-4503; toll-free, 800-682-7426
fax: 716-845-8266
www.ovariancancer.com
Monday through Friday, 9 am–5 pm ET

The Gilda Radner Familial Ovarian Cancer Registry conducts research and provides diagnostic information and literature about ovarian cancer. The registry provides referrals to support groups and offers communication with other patients with ovarian cancer across the United States. The Web site provides general information about ovarian cancer and an online version of the registry newsletter.

Kidney Cancer

National Kidney Foundation

30 E. 33rd St.
New York, NY 10016
telephone: 212-889-2210; toll-free, 800-622-9010
fax: 212-689-9261
www.kidney.org
Monday through Friday, 8:30 am–5:30 pm ET
Spanish-language materials available

The National Kidney Foundation (NKF) is dedicated to the detection, prevention, and treatment of diseases of the kidney and urinary tract. NKF provides information and materials about kidney and urinary tract diseases, kidney cancer, and organ donation. The organization also offers referrals to support groups, a quarterly newsletter, professional education programs, and some financial assistance to kidney dialysis and transplantation patients. The NKF Web site includes information about kidney disease, a list of NKF's affiliate offices, and an online newsletter.

Lung Cancer and Tobacco Use

Alliance for Lung Cancer Advocacy, Support, and Education

1601 Lincoln Ave.
P.O. Box 849
Vancouver, WA 98666
telephone: 360-696-2436; 800-298-2436 (U.S. only)

fax: 360-735-1305
www.alcase.org
Monday through Friday, 8 am–5 pm PT

The Alliance for Lung Cancer Advocacy, Support, and Education (ALCASE) helps people with lung cancer improve their quality of life. All ALCASE services are provided free of charge. ALCASE provides
- Detailed information about lung cancer, including *The Lung Cancer Resource Guide* and *The Lung Cancer Manual*
- Referral to lung cancer support groups
- "Phone buddies," peers who support each other over the telephone
- Information about clinical trials
- A list of positron emission tomography (PET) sites in the United States
- A quarterly newsletter.
The alliance's Web site provides information about all its offerings and links to other sites. Web information is in English and Italian.

American Lung Association
1740 Broadway
New York, NY 10019
telephones: 212-315-8700; toll-free, 800-586-4872 (connects caller to a local office)
fax: 212-265-5642
www.lungusa.org
Monday through Friday, 9 am–5 pm ET
Spanish-speaking staff may be available; Spanish-language materials available

The American Lung Association (ALA) is a nonprofit agency devoted to fighting lung disease. The association provides printed materials about topics related to lung health, including lung cancer, asthma, tobacco control, and environmental health. In addition, ALA sponsors smoking-cessation programs and support groups for patients and their families. The ALA Web site includes
- Detailed information about lung disease
- Information about ALA programs and events
- A list of publications that can be ordered online
- An ALA chapter locator
- Many features in Spanish as well as English.

Nicotine Anonymous—World Services
P.O. Box 126338
Harrisburg, PA 17112-6338
telephone: 415-750-0329 (24-hour voice mail)
fax: 714-969-4493
www.nicotine-anonymous.org
Spanish-language materials available

Nicotine Anonymous is an anonymous support fellowship based on the 12-step concept. Its members are people who want to live free of nicotine addiction. Meetings consist of two or more people. No member of Nicotine Anonymous pays dues or fees. For more information, worldwide meeting schedules, and printed materials, call the organization or visit the Web site. In addition, the site provides answers to frequently asked questions about nicotine addiction and nicotine cessation and information in Portuguese, French, Swedish, and German, as well as in English.

Office on Smoking and Health
National Center for Chronic Disease Prevention and Health Promotion/CDC
4770 Buford Highway NE, Mailstop K-50 (Rhodes Building)
Atlanta, GA 30341-3724
telephone: 770-488-5705; toll-free, 800-232-1311 (to receive recorded or faxed information only)
www.cdc.gov/tobacco
Monday through Friday, 8:30 am–5 pm ET
Spanish-language materials available

The Office on Smoking and Health (OSH), a unit of the Centers for Disease Control and Prevention, maintains a database regarding the prevalence and epidemiology of smoking. Information specialists provide answers to tobacco-related health questions, bibliographic and reference services, and publications and other materials. The OSH Web site offers
• Access to the bibliographic database
• A list of available publications
• Text of selected publications
• News bulletins on tobacco issues.

Oral Cancer, Head and Neck Cancer

American Dental Association
211 E. Chicago Ave.
Chicago, IL 60611
telephones: 312-440-2500, 312-440-2593 (for consumer information)
fax: 312-440-7494
www.ada.org
Monday through Friday, 8:30 am-5 pm CT
Spanish-language materials available

The American Dental Association (ADA) is a professional association of dentists dedicated to serving both the public and the profession of dentistry. The ADA provides
• Printed information about oral health care, dental procedures, and oral cancer

- Information about dentists who are ADA members
- Referrals to state dental associations
- An avenue to voice complaints about ADA dentists.

The ADA Web site contains a section for patients and consumers that provides answers to frequently asked questions; information about dental care and procedures; and information about disease prevention and dental insurance.

Prostate Cancer

American Foundation for Urologic Disease

1126 N. Charles St.
Baltimore, MD 21201-5559
telephones: 410-468-1800; toll-free, 800-242-2383 (for ordering materials only)
fax: 410-468-1808
www.afud.org
Monday through Friday, 8:30 am–5 pm ET
Spanish-language materials available

The American Foundation for Urologic Disease supports national urologic research, education, awareness, and advocacy programs. The foundation provides information and literature about urologic diseases and disorders, a national directory of prostate cancer support and self-help groups, and a prostate cancer resource guide. The Web site includes

- Information about urologic conditions, including prostate cancer, bladder cancer, kidney cancer, benign prostatic hypertropy, prostatitis, urinary incontinence, and erectile dysfunction
- Text of the prostate cancer resource guide
- A urologist locator

CaP Cure (The Association for the Cure of Cancer of the Prostate)

1250 Fourth St., Suite 360
Santa Monica, CA 90401
telephones: 310-458-2873; toll-free, 800-757-2873, 800-777-3035 (for information about clinical trials)
fax: 310-458-8074
www.capcure.org
Monday through Friday, 8:30 am–5:30 pm PT

CaP Cure is a nonprofit public charity dedicated to finding a cure for prostate cancer. CaP Cure provides general information about prostate cancer and nutrition, information about clinical trials, and stories about survivors. *Note:* CaP Cure does not provide medical advice other than clinical trial information. The Web site presents a limited amount of treatment information.

US TOO! International

930 N. York Road, Suite 50
Hinsdale, IL 60512
telephones: 630-323-1002; toll-free, 800-808-7866
fax: 630-323-1003
www.ustoo.org
Monday through Friday, 8:30 am–5 pm CT
Spanish-language materials available

US TOO! is an independent network of support-group chapters for men with prostate cancer and their families. The organization offers a hot line to answer callers' inquiries, and it provides literature and makes referrals to its network of support groups. The Web site provides
• Information about prostate cancer
• A list of local support groups
• A list of clinical trials
• An online form for ordering literature
• Newsletter articles
• Many links to related sites.

Skin Cancer

American Academy of Dermatology

930 N. Meacham Road
Schaumburg, IL 60173
telephones: 847-330-0230; toll-free, 888-462-3376 (24-hour automated information line)
www.aad.org
Monday through Friday, 8:30 am–5 pm CT

The American Academy of Dermatology is a professional organization of practicing dermatologists in the United States and Canada. Through the automated information line, the academy provides information about skin disorders and skin cancer and a dermatologist locator. The Web site includes
• Information about skin disorders and skin cancer
• A list of publications and an online order form
• A dermatologist locator that includes information about individual doctors
• A means of locating skin cancer screening facilities
• A list of organizations that provide related information and support
• A skin cancer risk assessment.

Skin Cancer Foundation

P.O. Box 561
New York, NY 10156
telephones: 212-725-5176; toll-free, 800-754-6490 (for an information packet only)

fax: 212-725-5751
www.skincancer.org
Monday through Friday, 9 am–5 pm ET

The Skin Cancer Foundation is a nonprofit organization that conducts public and medical education programs about skin cancer and provides support for medical training and research regarding skin cancer. Materials available from the foundation include information about various types of skin cancer and skin cancer prevention, books and audiovisual materials, a packet that directs a self-examination of skin, and a quarterly newsletter. For a list of available materials, call or send a self-addressed, stamped envelope. The foundation's Web site includes information about skin cancer, pictures and descriptions of skin cancers, and information about sun safety.

Clinical Trials Cooperative Groups

A clinical trial is a study designed to answer questions by using the scientific method. A clinical trial regarding cancer, for example, could be designed to determine if a particular investigational drug has the ability to prevent cancer under certain conditions. Another trial could be designed to determine if existing drugs, used in combination, are effective in cancer treatment or if specific screening techniques are more effective than others in providing early diagnoses. A clinical trial might monitor the quality of life or the psychological impact of cancer. Trials are sometimes conducted by a cooperative group, a network of researchers, physicians, and healthcare professionals—at public and private institutions—who collaborate to design and manage clinical trials. Advances in cancer treatment have occurred largely because of the knowledge gained in large clinical trials.

More information about clinical trials for specific types of cancer is available by calling the National Cancer Institute at the toll-free number 800-422-6237 or by checking the Internet at http://cancertrials.nci.nih.gov/.

This section presents information about cooperative groups conducting cancer clinical trials.

American College of Surgeons Oncology Group

633 N. Saint Clair St.
Chicago, IL 60611-3211
telephone: 312-202-5400
fax: 312-202-5011
www.acosog.org

Cancer and Leukemia Group B

208 S. LaSalle St., Suite 2000
Chicago, IL 60604-1104
telephone: 773-702-9171
fax: 312-345-0117
www.calgb.org

Children's Oncology Group
440 E. Huntington Drive
P.O. Box 60012
Arcadia, CA 91066-6012
telephone: 800-458-NCCF
fax: 626-445-4334
www.nccf.org/nccf/AboutCCG/Ccg_who.htm

Children's Oncology Group Soft Tissue Sarcoma Committee
Soft Tissue Sarcoma Committee
Operations Office
440 E. Huntington Drive
P.O. Box 60012
Arcadia, CA 91066-6012
telephone: toll-free, 800-458-6223
fax: 626-447-6359
http://rhabdo.org

Eastern Cooperative Oncology Group
ECOG Coordinating Center, Frontier Science
303 Boylston St.
Brookline, MA 02445-7648
telephone: 617-632-3610
fax: 617-632-2990
http://ecog.dfci.harvard.edu

European Organization for Research and Treatment of Cancer
EORTC Central Office
Av. E. Mounier 83, BTE 11
1200 Brussels
Belgium
telephone: 32 2 774 16 41
www.eortc.be

Gynecologic Oncology Group
1234 Market St., Suite 1945
Philadelphia, PA 19107
telephone: 215-854-0770
fax: 215-854-0716
www.gog.org

National Cancer Institute of Canada Clinical Trials Group
Queen's University
82-84 Barrie St.
Kingston, Ontario K7L 3N6

Canada
telephone: 613-533-6430
fax: 613-533-2941
www.ctg.queensu.ca

National Surgical Adjuvant Breast and Bowel Project
East Commons Professional Building
Four Allegheny Center, Fifth Floor
Pittsburgh, PA 15212-5234
telephone: 412-330-4600
fax: 412-330-4660
www.nsabp.pitt.edu

North Central Cancer Treatment Group
NCCTG Operations Office, Plummer Building
200 First St. SW
Rochester, MN 55905
telephone: 507-284-5999
fax: 507-284-1902
http://ncctg.mayo.edu

Quality Assurance Review Center
825 Chalkstone Ave.
Providence, RI 02908
telephone: 401-456-6500
fax: 401-456-6550
www.qarc.org

Radiation Therapy Oncology Group
1101 Market St., 14th Floor
Philadelphia, PA 19107
telephone: 215-574-3150
fax: 215-928-0153
www.rtog.org

Southwest Oncology Group
14980 Omicron Drive
San Antonio, TX 78245-3217
telephone: 210-677-8808
fax: 210-677-0006
http://swog.org

Complementary and Alternative Medicine Resources

National Center for Complementary and Alternative Medicine
P.O. Box 8218
Silver Spring, MD 20907-8218
toll-free telephone: 888-644-6226
fax: 301-495-4957
http://nccam.nih.gov
Monday through Friday, 8:30 am–5 pm ET
Spanish-speaking staff

The National Center for Complementary and Alternative Medicine (NCCAM) conducts and supports research and training and disseminates, to practitioners and the public, information about complementary and alternative medicine. NCCAM provides general information about alternative medicine, fact sheets and information packages, and bibliographies. The NCCAM Web site includes a database of bibliographic references and the text of NCCAM's general information packet. *Note:* NCCAM does not provide medical referrals to individual practitioners of alternative medicine.

Cancer Genetics and Hereditary Cancers

David G. Jagelman Inherited Colorectal Cancer Registry
The Cleveland Clinic Foundation/Medical Genetics/T10
9500 Euclid Ave.
Cleveland, OH 44195
telephones: 216-445-5686; toll-free, 800-998-4785
fax: 216-445-6935
www.clevelandclinic.org/registries
Monday through Friday, 9 am–5 pm ET
Some Spanish-language materials available

The David G. Jagelman registry is the largest registry for inherited forms of colorectal cancer in the United States. The registry includes more than 400 families with familial polyposis, hereditary nonpolyposis, and familial colon cancers. Also included are data about kindred with juvenile polyposis and Puetz-Jeghers syndrome. The main purpose of the registry is to prevent needless deaths from colon cancer. In addition, staff members ensure that each patient diagnosed with one of the tracked diseases is aware of the necessary screenings and follow-up visits to a physician. The staff sends patients and their families annual letters about screenings, informational booklets, and newsletters. Also available are materials about risk assessment, preventive measures, screening, detection, treatment, and research.

Hereditary Cancer Prevention Clinic
Department of Preventive Medicine
Creighton University
2500 California Plaza
Omaha, NE 68178
telephone: 402-280-1796 (answers as: "Department of Preventive Medicine");
    toll-free, 800-648-8133 (for patients)
fax: 402-280-1734
http://medicine.creighton.edu/medschool/PrevMed/HC.html
Monday through Friday, 8 am–5 pm CT

The purpose of the Hereditary Cancer Institute is to evaluate and identify families at high risk for a hereditary cancer. Once a family is identified as having a hereditary cancer syndrome, institute staff members educate the family about the syndrome and make specific recommendations about surveillance or early detection. In addition, the institute provides educational publications for families and physicians.

National Cancer Institute Cancer Genetics Services Directory
International Cancer Information Center
9030 Old Georgetown Road, Attn: CIAT
Bethesda, MD 20892-2650
toll-free telephone: 800-422-6237 (answers as: "Cancer Information Service")
fax: 301-402-6728
http://cnetdb.nci.nih.gov/genesrch.shtml
Monday through Friday, 9 am–4:30 pm ET

In regard to cancer genetics, the National Cancer Institute offers the PDQ Cancer Genetics Services Directory (previously called the Genetic Counselors Directory), a database of individuals who provide services related to cancer risk assessment, genetic counseling, genetic susceptibility testing, and other aspects of cancer genetics. Each person listed must be licensed, certified, or eligible for board certification and must have specific training in cancer genetics. He or she also must be a member of a National Genetics Society or a national oncology society and be willing to accept referrals. The directory, which is available on the Internet only, is searchable by the provider's name, city, state, or country or by specific cancers or genetic conditions. About 200 providers are currently in the directory.

Environmental Health and Consumer Safety

Consumer Product Safety Commission
[The commission does not accept inquiries by mail.]
Washington, DC 20207
toll-free telephone: 800-638-2772 (recorded information available seven days a
    week, 24 hours each day)

toll-free TTY: 800-638-8270
fax: 301-504-0127
www.cpsc.gov
Monday through Friday, 9 am–5 pm ET
Spanish-speaking staff, Spanish-language materials available

The Consumer Product Safety Commission (CPSC) provides information about product hazards, recalls, defects, and injuries sustained in using products. Information is available by telephone calls to commission staff, via recorded telephone messages, in publications, and on the CPSC Web site. The site contains a section for children that discusses safety measures kids should know. In addition, the commission provides an avenue to file complaints against unsafe products. *Note:* The CPSC only provides information about products used in and around the home, excluding automobiles, car seats for children, food, prescriptions, cosmetics, warranties, advertising, repairs, and maintenance.

Environmental Protection Agency
Ariel Rios Building
1200 Pennsylvania Ave. NW
Washington, DC 20460-2403
telephone: 202-260-2090
www.epa.gov
Monday through Friday, 8 am–6 pm ET

The mission of the Environmental Protection Agency (EPA) is to protect human health and safeguard the natural environment. The EPA provides information about many topics, including
- Radon
- Hazardous waste
- Air pollution
- Water pollution
- Environmental tobacco smoke
- Pesticides
- Drinking water
- Programs and activities of the EPA.

The EPA provides a number of toll-free hot lines, including the Indoor Air Quality Information Hot Line (800-438-4318) and the Asbestos Ombudsman Hot Line (800-368-5888). See www.epa.gov/epahome/hotline.htm for a complete list of hot lines. See www.epa.gov/epahome/topics.htm to find lists of publications and other available information.

National Institute for Occupational Safety and Health
4676 Columbia Parkway
Cincinnati, OH 45226-1998
telephones: 513-533-8573; toll-free, 800-356-4674 (automated information available at all hours)

www.cdc.gov/niosh/homepage.html
Monday through Friday, 9 am–4 pm ET

The National Institute for Occupational Safety and Health (NIOSH) conducts research and makes recommendations for the prevention of work-related injuries and illnesses, including cancer. NIOSH also investigates potentially hazardous working conditions as requested by employers or employees. NIOSH information specialists and the NIOSH Web site provide information on many work-safety topics, including
• Lung diseases
• Cancer
• Asbestos and other chemical hazards
• Indoor air quality
• Electric and magnetic fields
• Personal protective equipment.

Occupational Safety and Health Administration

U.S. Department of Labor
200 Constitution Ave. NW
Washington, DC 20210
telephone: 202-693-1999; toll-free, 800-321-6742
www.osha.gov
Monday through Friday, 8 am–5 pm ET

The Occupational Safety and Health Administration (OSHA) is responsible for creating and enforcing workplace safety and health regulations. The OSHA Web site provides
• Lists of known and suspected carcinogens
• Standards and guidelines for occupational exposure to chemicals
• Information about reproductive hazards
• Links to material safety data sheets (MSDSs).

Radiation Exposure Compensation Program

U.S. Department of Justice
P.O. Box 146, Ben Franklin Station
Washington, DC 20044-0146
toll-free telephone: 800-729-7327
www.usdoj.gov/civil/torts/const/reca/index.htm
Monday through Friday, 9 am–5 pm ET

The Radiation Exposure Compensation Act of 1990 authorizes the attorney general of the United States to make lump-sum compensation payments to individuals who have contracted certain illnesses following exposure to radiation during employment in underground uranium mines or following radioactive fallout emitted during the government's atmospheric nuclear tests. The Radiation Exposure Compensation Program provides a way to make a claim for compensation. A copy of the regulations, claim forms, and guidebooks that describe claim-eligibility requirements are available by calling the toll-free number, writing to the program, or using the program's Web site.

Nutrition

American Dietetic Association
216 W. Jackson Blvd., Suite 800
Chicago, IL 60606-6995
telephone: 312-899-0040; toll-free, 800-877-1600, 800-366-1655 (for information and dietitian referral)
fax: 312-899-1979
www.eatright.org
Monday through Friday, 9 am–4 pm CT

The American Dietetic Association (ADA) is the world's largest organization of food and nutrition professionals. The ADA serves the public by promoting nutrition, health, and well-being. The ADA operates a consumer nutrition hot line, which provides referrals to registered dietitians (including professionals specializing in nutrition for patients with cancer) in the caller's locale. The hot line also provides recorded information about food and nutrition. The ADA Web site presents information about diet and nutrition and a registered-dietitian locator service.

Meals on Wheels of America
1414 Prince St., Suite 202
Alexandria, VA 22314
telephone: 703-548-5558
fax : 703-548-8024
www.projectmeal.org
Monday through Friday, 9 am–5 pm ET

Meals on Wheels is an association of about 900 programs that provide home-delivered and congregate meals. The goal of the organization is to improve the quality of life of the needy, particularly the elderly, disabled, and homebound. Some programs provide other health and social services, such as transportation, recreation, nutrition education, information, referrals, and case management.

U.S. Department of Agriculture Food and Nutrition Information Center
National Agricultural Library, Room 304
10301 Baltimore Ave.
Beltsville, MD 20705-2351
telephone: 301-504-5719 (main), 301-504-5414 (for inquiries to dietitians and nutritionists)

fax: 301-504-6409
www.nal.usda.gov/fnic
Monday through Friday, 8 am–4:30 pm ET
Spanish-speaking staff; Spanish-language materials available

The Food and Nutrition Information Center (FNIC) is an information center associated with the National Agricultural Library. FNIC provides dietitians and nutritionists to answer inquiries, and the center provides publications about food and nutrition, resource lists, and bibliographies. The FNIC Web site includes information about
- Dietary supplements (vitamin, mineral, and herbal)
- Food safety
- Dietary guidelines
- The "food pyramid"
- Food composition facts (including facts about fast food)
- A list of available publications.

Groups Comprising Physicians or Cancer Centers

American Board of Medical Specialties
1007 Church St., Suite 404
Evanston, IL 60201-5913
telephone: 847-491-9091; toll-free, 866-275-2267 (Please refer to the Web site when possible.)
fax: 847-328-3596
www.abms.org
Monday through Friday, 8:30 am–5 pm CT

The American Board of Medical Specialties (ABMS) is the umbrella organization for the 24 approved medical specialty boards in the United States. The ABMS maintains a list of all board-certified physicians. Consumer information about a physician's certification status can be obtained through the ABMS Web site. The ABMS also provides a list of board-certified physicians by specialty and geographic area (physicians must subscribe to be included in this list). The list is available through the ABMS Web site or in printed form as *The Official ABMS Directory of Board Certified Medical Specialists*. Specialists also are listed in the yellow pages of local telephone directories, under the heading "American Board of Medical Specialists." *Note:* To better serve the needs of the public and at the request of the ABMS, please refer to the ABMS Web site (rather than calling ABMS) when possible.

American College of Surgeons
633 N. Saint Clair St.
Chicago, IL 60611-3211
telephones: 312-202-5000, 312-202-5085 (Cancer Department)

fax: 312-202-5001
www.facs.org
Monday through Friday, 8 am–5 pm CT

The American College of Surgeons (ACOS) is a scientific and educational association of surgeons that was founded to improve the quality of care for surgical patients by setting high standards for surgical education and practice. ACOS accredits the cancer programs of U.S. healthcare organizations. The list of approved programs is updated at least twice each year. Information about the status of an institution's cancer program and services can be obtained on the ACOS Web site or by calling the American College of Surgeons.

American Medical Association
515 N. State St.
Chicago, IL 60610
telephones: 312-464-5000; toll-free, 800-621-8335 (order placement)
fax: 312-464-5600
www.ama-assn.org
Monday through Friday, 8:30 am–4:30 pm CT

The American Medical Association (AMA) is a membership organization comprising American medical doctors and certain allied health professionals. The AMA Web site includes AMA Health Insight, an online health information source about a broad range of medical topics; AMA Hospital Select, a hospital locator providing information about almost every U.S. hospital; and AMA Physician Select, a physician locator providing information about almost every licensed U.S. physician. *Note:* The AMA does not provide names or information about individual physicians over the telephone. The AMA can refer callers to local medical societies for lists of physicians in the caller's locale who are accepting patients.

American Society of Clinical Oncology
1900 Duke St., Suite 200
Alexandria, VA 22314
telephone: 703-299-0150
fax: 703-299-1044
www.asco.org
Monday through Friday, 8:30 am–5:30 pm ET

The American Society of Clinical Oncology (ASCO) is an international medical society comprising cancer specialists involved in clinical research and patient care. The society publishes the *Journal of Clinical Oncology*. The ASCO Web site includes
- ASCO guides for patients: *Follow-Up Care for Lung Cancer, Advanced Lung Cancer Treatment*, and *Questions and Answers About Pain Control*
- A glossary of cancer terms
- A locator that helps users find ASCO oncologists
- Links to related sites.

American Society of Plastic Surgeons
444 E. Algonquin Road
Arlington Heights, IL 60005
telephones: 847-228-9900; toll-free, 888-475-2784 (24-hour referral service)
fax: 847-228-7099
www.plasticsurgery.org
Monday through Friday, 8:30 am–4:30 pm CT
Spanish-language materials available

The American Society of Plastic Surgeons (ASPS) assists the public in searches for board-certified plastic surgeons. ASPS provides brochures about plastic surgery, including breast reconstruction and choosing a qualified surgeon; referrals to board-certified surgeons in the requestor's area who specialize in specific procedures; and verification of a physician's board certification. The ASPS Web site includes the information services above as well as answers to frequently asked questions.

Association of Community Cancer Centers
11600 Nebel St., Suite 201
Rockville, MD 20852-2557
telephone: 301-984-9496 (answers as: "Triple C")
fax: 301-770-1949
www.accc-cancer.org
Monday through Friday, 9 am–5:30 pm ET

The Association of Community Cancer Centers (ACCC) is a membership organization comprising physicians, cancer centers, and hospitals across the United States. For patients, ACCC provides a free brochure, *Cancer Treatments Your Insurance Should Cover.* The ACCC Web site contains profiles of the cancer programs of more than 500 member institutions. *Note:* ACCC does not provide referrals or profile information by telephone.

Cancer Centers Designated by the National Cancer Institute

The National Cancer Institute (NCI) supports research-oriented institutions across the United States that are characterized by scientific excellence and their ability to integrate and focus a diversity of research approaches on the cancer problem. NCI supports three types of cancer centers; the centers are categorized according to their degree of research specialization.
- Cancer center: The research at cancer centers is very focused (i.e., cancer center researchers conduct basic research or epidemiology research).
- Clinical cancer center: Researchers at clinical cancer centers usually integrate strong basic science with strong clinical science (i.e., the research is patient-oriented).

- Comprehensive cancer center: Researchers at comprehensive cancer centers integrate basic science; clinical science; and expertise in population science and disease prevention and control.

Many of the clinical cancer centers and all of the comprehensive cancer centers conduct outreach, education, and information activities in their communities. The goals of such activities are to enhance disease prevention and improve care and related services.

The contact for general information about NCI designations for cancer centers is Cancer Centers Branch, Office of the Deputy Director for Extramural Science National Cancer Institute
6116 Executive Blvd., Suite 700, MSC 8345
Bethesda, MD 20892-7383 (For Express Mail, use Rockville, MD 20852.)
telephone: 301-496-8345
fax: 301-402-0181
www.nci.nih.gov/cancercenters/default.html

The list that follows shows the centers that were NCI-designated at the time this book was being prepared for publication; each listing cites the appropriate designation. NCI updates the list from time to time. For an up-to-date list, see www.nci.nih.gov/cancercenters/centerslist.html, a page on the NCI Web site.

ALABAMA
UAB Comprehensive Cancer Center
1824 Sixth Ave. S
Birmingham, AL 35294-3300
telephones: 205-975-8222; toll-free, 800-822-0933
www.ccc.uab.edu
NCI designation: Comprehensive Cancer Center

ARIZONA
University of Arizona Comprehensive Cancer Center
1515 N. Campbell Ave.
P.O. Box 285024
Tucson, AZ 85724
telephones: 520-626-6044; toll-free, 800-622-2673
www.azcc.arizona.edu
NCI designation: Comprehensive Cancer Center

CALIFORNIA
The Burnham Institute Cancer Center
10901 N. Torrey Pines Road
La Jolla, CA 92037-0658

telephone: 858-455-6480, ext. 3209
www.burnhaminstitute.org
NCI designation: Cancer Center

Chao Family Comprehensive Cancer Center
University of California, Irvine
Building 23, Route 81
101 The City Drive
Orange, CA 92868
telephone: 714-456-8200
www.ucihs.uci.edu/cancer
NCI designation: Comprehensive Cancer Center

City of Hope National Medical Center
1500 E. Duarte Road
Duarte, CA 91010-3000
telephone: 626-359-8111
www.cityofhope.org
NCI designation: Comprehensive Cancer Center

Jonsson Comprehensive Cancer Center
University of California, Los Angeles
Factor Building, Room 8-684
Los Angeles, CA 90095-1781
telephone: 310-825-5268
www.cancer.mednet.ucla.edu
NCI designation: Comprehensive Cancer Center

Salk Institute Cancer Center
10010 N. Torrey Pines Road
La Jolla, CA 92037-1099
telephone: 858-453-4100
www.salk.edu
NCI designation: Cancer Center

UCSD Cancer Center
9500 Gilman Drive, Mail Code 0658
La Jolla, CA 92093-0658
telephone: 858-534-7600
http://cancer.ucsd.edu
NCI designation: Clinical Cancer Center

University of California, San Francisco Comprehensive Cancer Center
Box 0128
2340 Sutton St.
San Francisco, CA 94143-0128

telephones: toll-free, 800-888-8664 (cancer referral line); 415-476-2201 (general information)
http://cc.ucsf.edu
NCI designation: Comprehensive Cancer Center

USC/Norris Comprehensive Cancer Center
1441 Eastlake Ave.
Los Angeles, CA 90033-0804
telephones: 323-865-3000 (general information); toll-free, 800-872-2273 (patient referral)
http://ccnt.hsc.usc.edu
NCI designation: Comprehensive Cancer Center

COLORADO
University of Colorado Cancer Center
Box E 190
4200 E. Ninth Ave.
Denver, CO 80262
telephones: 303-372-1550 (main); toll-free, 800-621-7621 (cancer referral line)
http://uch.uchsc.edu/uccc
NCI designation: Comprehensive Cancer Center

CONNECTICUT
Yale Cancer Center
Yale University School of Medicine
333 Cedar St.
P.O. Box 208028
New Haven, CT 06520-8028
telephone: 203-785-4095 (administrative office)
www.info.med.yale.edu/ycc
NCI designation: Comprehensive Cancer Center

DISTRICT OF COLUMBIA
Lombardi Cancer Center
Georgetown University Medical Center
3800 Reservoir Road NW
Washington, DC 20007
telephone: 202-784-4000
http://lombardi.georgetown.edu
NCI designation: Comprehensive Cancer Center

FLORIDA

H. Lee Moffitt Cancer Center & Research Institute at the University of South Florida

12902 Magnolia Drive
Tampa, FL 33612-9497
telephone: 813-972-4673
www.moffitt.usf.edu
NCI designation: Clinical Cancer Center

HAWAII

Cancer Research Center of Hawaii

University of Hawaii
1236 Lauhala St.
Honolulu, HI 96813
telephone: 808-586-3010
www.hawaii.edu/crch
NCI designation: Clinical Cancer Center

ILLINOIS

Robert H. Lurie Comprehensive Cancer Center of Northwestern University

710 North Fairbanks Court, Olson Pavilion 8250
Chicago, IL 60611-3013
telephone: 312-908-5250
www.lurie.nwu.edu/
NCI designation: Comprehensive Cancer Center

University of Chicago Cancer Research Center

5841 S. Maryland Ave.
Chicago, IL 60637-1470
telephones: 773-702-8200; toll-free, 888-824-0200 (new patients)
www-uccrc.bsd.uchicago.edu
NCI designation: Comprehensive Cancer Center

INDIANA

Indiana University Cancer Center

Room 455
535 Barnhill Drive
Indianapolis, IN 46202
toll-free telephone: 888-600-4822
http://iucc.iu.edu
NCI designation: Clinical Cancer Center

Purdue University Cancer Center
Hansen Life Sciences Research Building
S. University St.
West Lafayette, IN 47907-1524
telephone: 765-494-9129
www.pharmacy.purdue.edu/~ccenter
NCI designation: Cancer Center

IOWA
Holden Comprehensive Cancer Center at the University of Iowa
5970-Z John Pappajohn Pavilion
200 Hawkins Drive
Iowa City, IA 52242-1009
toll-free telephones: 800-777-8442 (patient referral); 800-237-1225 (general information)
www.cancer.vh.org
NCI designation: Comprehensive Cancer Center

MAINE
The Jackson Laboratory
600 Main St.
Bar Harbor, ME 04609-0800
telephone: 207-288-6000 (main); 207-288-6051 (public information)
www.jax.org
NCI designation: Cancer Center

MARYLAND
Johns Hopkins Oncology Center
600 N. Wolfe St.
Baltimore, MD 21287-8943
telephone: 410-955-8964
www.hopkinscancercenter.org
NCI designation: Comprehensive Cancer Center

MASSACHUSETTS
Dana-Farber Cancer Institute
44 Binney St.
Boston, MA 02115
telephone: 617-632-3000 (main)
www.dana-farber.net
NCI designation: Comprehensive Cancer Center

MIT Center for Cancer Research
77 Massachusetts Ave., Room E17-110
Cambridge, MA 02139-6403
telephone: 617-253-6400
http://web.mit.edu/ccrhq/www
NCI designation: Cancer Center

MICHIGAN
Barbara Ann Karmanos Cancer Institute
Wertz Clinical Cancer Center
4100 John R
Detroit, MI 48201-1379
toll-free telephone: 800-527-6266
www.karmanos.org
NCI designation: Comprehensive Cancer Center

University of Michigan Comprehensive Cancer Center
1500 E. Medical Center Drive
Ann Arbor, MI 48109-0943
toll-free telephone: 800-865-1125
www.cancer.med.umich.edu
NCI designation: Comprehensive Cancer Center

MINNESOTA
Mayo Clinic Cancer Center
200 First St. SW
Rochester, MN 55905
telephone: 507-284-2111 (appointments)
www.mayo.edu/cancercenter
NCI designation: Comprehensive Cancer Center

University of Minnesota Cancer Center
Box 806 Mayo
420 Delaware St. SE
Minneapolis, MN 55455
telephone: 612-624-8484
www.cancer.umn.edu/
NCI designation: Comprehensive Cancer Center

MISSOURI
Siteman Cancer Center
Washinton University School of Medicine
600 S. Euclid Ave., Box 8100
St. Louis, MO 63110-1093
telephone: 314-747-7222

fax: 314-454-5300
NCI designation: Clinical Cancer Center

NEBRASKA
University of Nebraska Medical Center/Eppley Cancer Center
600 S. 42nd St.
Omaha, NE 68198-6805
telephone: 402-559-4238
www.unmc.edu/cancercenter
NCI designation: Clinical Cancer Center

NEW HAMPSHIRE
Norris Cotton Cancer Center
Dartmouth-Hitchcock Medical Center
One Medical Center Drive
Lebanon, NH 03756-0001
telephone: 603-650-6300
www.nccc.Hitchcock.org
NCI designation: Comprehensive Cancer Center

NEW JERSEY
The Cancer Institute of New Jersey
Robert Wood Johnson Medical School
195 Little Albany St.
New Brunswick, NJ 08901
telephone: 732-235-2465 (appointments)
http://130.219.231.104
NCI designation: Clinical Cancer Center

NEW YORK
American Health Foundation
320 E. 43rd St.
New York, NY 10017
telephone: 212-953-1900
www.ahf.org
NCI designation: Cancer Center

Cold Spring Harbor Laboratory
P.O. Box 100
Cold Spring Harbor, NY 11724
telephone: 516-367-8383
www.cshl.org
NCI designation: Cancer Center

Albert Einstein Cancer Research Center
Albert Einstein College of Medicine
1300 Morris Park Ave.
Bronx, NY 10461
telephone: 718-430-2302
www.ca.aecom.yu.edu
NCI designation: Comprehensive Cancer Center

Herbert Irving Comprehensive Cancer Center
Columbia Presbyterian Center, New York-Presbyterian Hospital
PH 18, Room 220
622 W. 168th St.
New York, NY 10032
telephones: 212-305-8610, 212-305-9327 (administration office)
www.ccc.columbia.edu
NCI designation: Comprehensive Cancer Center

Kaplan Comprehensive Cancer Center
New York University Medical Center
550 First Ave.
New York, NY 10016
telephone: 212-263-6485
http://kccc-www.med.nyu.edu
NCI designation: Comprehensive Cancer Center

Memorial Sloan-Kettering Cancer Center
1275 York Ave.
New York, NY 10021
telephone: 212-639-6561
www.mskcc.org
NCI designation: Comprehensive Cancer Center

Roswell Park Cancer Institute
Elm and Carlton Streets
Buffalo, NY 14263-0001
telephone: 800-767-9355
www.roswellpark.org
NCI designation: Comprehensive Cancer Center

NORTH CAROLINA
Comprehensive Cancer Center at Wake Forest University
Medical Center Blvd.
Winston-Salem, NC 27157-1082
telephone: 336-716-4464
www.bgsm.edu/cancer
NCI designation: Comprehensive Cancer Center

Duke Comprehensive Cancer Center

Duke University Medical Center
Box 3843
Durham, NC 27710
telephone: 919-684-3377
http://cancer.duke.edu
NCI designation: Comprehensive Cancer Center

UNC Lineberger Comprehensive Cancer Center

University of North Carolina at Chapel Hill
Campus Box 7295
Chapel Hill, NC 27599-7295
telephone: 919-966-3036
http://cancer.med.unc.edu
NCI designation: Comprehensive Cancer Center

OHIO

Ireland Cancer Center at University Hospitals of Cleveland and Case Western Reserve University

11100 Euclid Ave.
Cleveland, OH 44106-5065
telephones: 216-844-5432; toll-free, 800-641-2422
www.irelandcancercenter.org
NCI designation: Comprehensive Cancer Center

The Ohio State University Comprehensive Cancer Center

The Arthur G. James Cancer Hospital and Richard J. Solove Research Institute
300 W. 10th Ave., Suite 519
Columbus, OH 43210-1240
toll-free telephone: 800-293-5066
www.jamesline.com/output/content/CCCsite/ccc
NCI designation: Comprehensive Cancer Center

OREGON

Oregon Cancer Institute

Oregon Health Sciences University Clinical Cancer Center
3181 S.W. Sam Jackson Park Road
Portland, OR 97201-3098
telephone: 503-494-1617
www.ohsu.edu/occ
NCI designation: Clinical Cancer Center

PENNSYLVANIA

Fox Chase Cancer Center

7701 Burholme Ave.
Philadelphia, PA 19111

telephones: 215-728-2570 (appointments); toll-free, 888-369-2427 (patient services)
www.fccc.edu
NCI designation: Comprehensive Cancer Center

Kimmel Cancer Center

Thomas Jefferson University
Bluemle Life Sciences Building
233 S. 10th St.
Philadelphia, PA 19107-5541
toll-free telephones: 800-533-3669, 800-654-5984 (for the hearing- and speech-
    impaired)
www.kcc.tju.edu
NCI designation: Clinical Cancer Center

University of Pennsylvania Cancer Center

16th Floor, Penn Tower
3400 Spruce St.
Philadelphia, PA 19104-4283
telephones: 215-662-6300 (main number); toll-free, 800-789-2366 (referral and
    appointments)
www.oncolink.upenn.edu
NCI designation: Comprehensive Cancer Center

University of Pittsburgh Cancer Institute

Iroquois Building, Suite 206
3600 Forbes Ave.
Pittsburgh, PA 15213-3410
telephone: 800-237-4724
www.upci.upmc.edu
NCI designation: Comprehensive Cancer Center

Wistar Institute

3601 Spruce St.
Philadelphia, PA 19104-4268
telephone: 215-898-3926
www.wistar.upenn.edu/internet/intro.html
NCI designation: Cancer Center

TENNESSEE
St. Jude Children's Research Hospital

332 N. Lauderdale St.
Memphis, TN 38105-2794
telephone: 901-495-3300 (main)
www.stjude.org
NCI designation: Clinical Cancer Center

Vanderbilt-Ingram Cancer Center

Vanderbilt University
649 The Preston Building
Nashville, TN 37232-6838
telephones: 615-936-1782; toll-free, 800-811-8480
www.vanderbilt.cancer.org
NCI designation: Comprehensive Cancer Center

TEXAS
San Antonio Cancer Institute

8122 Datapoint Drive
San Antonio, TX 78229-3264
telephone: 210-616-5590
www.ccc.saci.org
NCI designation: Comprehensive Cancer Center

University of Texas M.D. Anderson Cancer Center

1515 Holcombe Blvd.
Houston, TX 77030
toll-free telephone: 800-392-1611
www.mdanderson.org
NCI designation: Comprehensive Cancer Center

UTAH
Huntsman Cancer Institute

University of Utah
2000 Circle of Hope
Salt Lake City, UT 84112
toll-free telephone: 877-585-0303
www.hci.utah.edu
NCI designation: Clinical Cancer Center

VERMONT
Vermont Cancer Center

University of Vermont Medical Alumni Building
Burlington, VT 05401
telephone: 802-656-4414
www.vermontcancer.org
NCI designation: Comprehensive Cancer Center

VIRGINIA
The Cancer Center at the University of Virginia

P.O. Box 800334

Charlottesville, VA 22908
telephones: 804-924-9333; toll-free, 800-223-9173
www.med.virginia.edu/medcntr/cancer/home.html
NCI designation: Clinical Cancer Center

Massey Cancer Center

Virginia Commonwealth University
401 College St.
Richmond, VA 23298-0037
telephone: 804-828-0450
www.vcu.edu/mcc
NCI designation: Clinical Cancer Center

WASHINGTON

Fred Hutchinson Cancer Research Center

FM-252, 1100 Fairview Ave. N
Seattle, WA 98109-1024
telephones: 206-667-5000; 206-667-7222 (appointments and referral)
www.fhcrc.org
NCI designation: Comprehensive Cancer Center

WISCONSIN

McArdle Laboratory for Cancer Research

University of Wisconsin
1400 University Ave., Room 1009
Madison, WI 53706-1599
telephone: 608-262-2177 or 7992
http://mcardle.oncology.wisc.edu
NCI designation: Cancer Center

University of Wisconsin Comprehensive Cancer Center

600 Highland Ave., K4/666
Madison, WI 53792-0001
telephones: 608-262-5223; toll-free, 800-622-8922 (cancer information)
www.cancer.wisc.edu
NCI designation: Comprehensive Cancer Center

INDEX

Index

strengths/limitations of, 424*f*
second primary cancers associated with,
687-688
self-examination for, 11, 23-24, 160-
161, 430-431, 843*f*
staging for, 164
and tamoxifen use, 23, 46*t*, 54, 161, 179,
182, 214
Breast Cancer High-Risk Registry
(BCHRR) program, 800–808, 801*t*,
808-811
Breast Cancer Prevention Trial (BCPT),
of NSABP, 50*f*, 179, 182, 263
breast-conserving surgery, vs. mastectomy, 54
Breast Health Access for Women With
Disabilities (BHAWD), 841-844,
843*f*
Breast Health Outreach Program
(Pennsylvania), 839-841
breast premalignancies, 161-163, 162*f*
breast self-examination (BSE), 11, 23-24,
160-161, 430-431, 843*f*
bronchioloalveolar carcinomas, 156
Buddy-Check™ 10 breast cancer
awareness program, 847-850
budget considerations. *See* costs
for intervention planning, 93
bupropion, for nicotine dependence, 297

C

CA 15-3, 164
CA 27.29, 164
CA 125 testing, 147-148, 154, 558
calcitonin, for osteoporosis treatment,
713-714, 714*f*
calcium
in chemoprevention, 260*f*, 261
and colorectal cancer, 457, 477
dietary sources of, 707*t*
and osteoporosis prevention, 706
Canadian Cancer Registry, 47
cancer centers, information resources on,
1000-1014
Cancer Chemotherapy National Service

Center, formation of, 10
Cancer Chromosome Aberration Project
(CCAP), 111
Cancer Control Review Group, of
National Cancer Institute, 80
Cancer Genetics Special Interest Group,
of ONS, 130-131
Cancer Genome Anatomy Project
(CGAP), 111
Cancer Information Service, 10
Cancer Nursing Service, 13
A Cancer Source Book for Nurses (ACS,
1957), 11
cancer surveillance, 66-68, 67*f*-68*f*, 761-
763, 762*f*
cancer survivors
ethical issues concerning, 180-181
osteoporosis in, 696
second primary cancers in, 684-693
surveillance of. *See* tertiary cancer
prevention
cancer treatment trials, 54, 56*t*. *See also*
clinical trials
carcinoembryonic antigen (CEA), 154,
167
carcinogenesis
in breast, 400-402
mutations and, 119-121, 120*f*-121*f*,
123-125, 124*t*-125*t*
process of, 257-259, 258*f*
carcinogens, known/probable, 356*t*-359*t*
carcinomas, definition of, 151
carcinosarcoma, definition of, 156
care, ethic of, 196*t*, 200-201
carrier testing, 127
case-based reasoning, 196*t*, 197
case-control studies, 44*t*-45*t*, 47-48, 48*t*,
50-52, 51*t*
case-fatality rates, 39-40
formula for calculating, 40
case finding screening, 62
case reports, 43, 45*t*
case series, 43, 45*t*
casuistry, 196*t*, 197
cause-specific survival, 70
Celera Genomics Corporation, 110

D